Diagnostic Cytopathology Board Review and Self-Assessment

Walid E. Khalbuss • Qing Kay Li
Editors

Diagnostic Cytopathology Board Review and Self-Assessment

Springer

Editors
Walid E. Khalbuss
Professor of Pathology
GE Clarient Diagnostic Services
Aliso Viejo, CA, USA

Qing Kay Li
Associate Professor of Pathology
The Johns Hopkins University School of Medicine
Baltimore, MD, USA

ISBN 978-1-4939-1476-0 ISBN 978-1-4939-1477-7 (eBook)
DOI 10.1007/978-1-4939-1477-7
Springer New York Heidelberg Dordrecht London

Library of Congress Control Number: 2014948199

Printed on acid-free paper

Springer is part of Springer Science+Business Media (www.springer.com)

I dedicate this book to my beloved family, my teachers, mentors, and trainees

Walid E. Khalbuss

I dedicate this book to my parents, my husband, my son Ray, as well as Liz and Nathaniel

Qing Kay Li

Preface

This book provides a comprehensive review of nongynecological cytology including cytomorphology, pitfalls, and ancillary testing. The material is presented in a high-yield review and board-type questions with detailed discussions. It is an excellent review and self-assessment tool for practicing pathologists, cytologists, as well as cytology trainees (e.g. pathology residents, cytopathology fellows, and cytotechnology students). The book includes 13 chapters covering nongynecological cytology including one chapter dedicated to ancillary testing as related to diagnostic cytology. Most chapters contain introductory high-yield reviews on the subject in a series of tables with key points emphasizing useful criteria and concepts needed to make diagnoses in common and uncommon cases.

The book contains a wealth of full high-quality color photomicrographs with over 886 images, 54 tables, and over 963 MCQs that focus on practical diagnostic knowledge that will be useful to cytology trainees seeking basic information and also those with more experience who would like to fine-tune their skills.

The book is written by nine academic cytopathologists who are involved in practicing cytology and teaching cytopathology to residents, fellows, cytotechnologists, and cytotechnology students.

Aliso Viejo, CA, USA — Walid E. Khalbuss
Baltimore, MD, USA — Qing Kay Li

Acknowledgment

We are indebted to Drs. Cynthia Benedict (Pathology, LLC; Indianapolis, IN) and Ehab A. ElGabry (University of Pittsburgh Medical Center, Dept. of Pathology, Pittsburgh, PA) for their meticulous review of this entire book and for sharing their pearls of wisdom with us.

Contents

1 **Lung Cytopathology (Bronchial and Aspiration Cytology)** ... 1
Qing Kay Li and Walid E. Khalbuss

2 **Serous Fluid Cytopathology** ... 121
Qing Kay Li and Walid E. Khalbuss

3 **Cerebrospinal Fluid (CSF) Cytology** ... 199
Marilyn M. Bui, Ehab A. ElGabry, and Walid E. Khalbuss

4 **Thyroid Fine-Needle Aspiration** ... 241
Reda S. Saad, Jan F. Silverman, and Walid E. Khalbuss

5 **Lymph Node Cytopathology** ... 305
Matthew A. Smith and Walid E. Khalbuss

6 **Salivary Gland Fine-Needle Aspiration** ... 353
Abdelmonem Elhosseiny and Walid E. Khalbuss

7 **Liver Fine-Needle Aspiration** ... 409
Qing Kay Li and Walid E. Khalbuss

8 **Pancreatic Fine-Needle Aspiration** ... 469
Abdelmonem Elhosseiny and Walid E. Khalbuss

9 **Gastrointestinal and Bile Duct Brushing Cytology** ... 521
Qing Kay Li and Walid E. Khalbuss

10 **Renal and Adrenal Fine-Needle Aspiration** ... 573
Qing Kay Li and Walid E. Khalbuss

11 **Urine Cytopathology** ... 617
Ehab A. ElGabry and Walid E. Khalbuss

12 **Soft Tissue and Bone Fine-Needle Aspiration** ... 669
Ehab A. ElGabry and Walid E. Khalbuss

13 **Application of Molecular Diagnostics to Cytopathology** ... 717
Momin T. Siddiqui

Erratum to ... E1

Index ... 735

Contributors

Marilyn M. Bui, MD, PhD Department of Anatomic Pathology (MCC), Moffitt Cancer Center, Tampa, FL, USA

Ehab A. ElGabry, MD University of Pittsburgh Medical Center (UPMC)-Shadyside, Department of Pathology, Pittsburgh, PA, USA

Abdelmonem Elhosseiny, MD Fletcher Allen Health Care, University of Vermont, Department of Pathology, Burlington, VT, USA

Walid E. Khalbuss, MD, PhD, FIAC GE Clarient Diagnostic Services, Pathology Department, Aliso Viejo, California, USA

Qing Kay Li, MD, PhD The Johns Hopkins University School of Medicine, The Johns Hopkins Bayview Medical Center, Baltimore, MD, USA

Reda S. Saad, MD, PhD, FRCPC Department of Pathology, Organization Hotel Dieu Grace Hospital, Windsor, ON, Canada

Momin T. Siddiqui, MD Department of Pathology and Laboratory Medicine, Emory University Hospital, Atlanta, GA, USA

Jan F. Silverman, MD Department of Pathology, Allegheny General Hospital, Pittsburgh, PA, USA

Matthew A. Smith, MD Department of Pathology, University of Pittsburgh Medical Center-Shadyside, Pittsburgh, PA, USA

1 Lung Cytopathology (Bronchial and Aspiration Cytology)

Qing Kay Li and Walid E. Khalbuss

Contents

1.1 **Image-Based Questions 1–82** 4

1.2 **Text-Based Questions 83–142** 86

1.3 **Answers and Discussion of Image-Based Questions 1–82** 92

1.4 **Answers and Discussion of Text-Based Questions 83–151** 108

Reading List 119

Q.K. Li, MD, PhD (✉)
Department of Pathology, The Johns Hopkins University School of Medicine, The Johns Hopkins Bayview Medical Center, 4940 Eastern Avenue, AA Building, Room 154B, Baltimore, MD 21224-2780, USA
e-mail: qli23@jhmi.edu

W.E. Khalbuss, MD, PhD, FIAC
Department of Pathology, GE Clarient Diagnostic Services, 31 Columbia, Aliso Viejo, California, 92656, USA
e-mail: Walid.khalbuss@ge.com

W.E. Khalbuss, Q.K. Li (eds.), *Diagnostic Cytopathology Board Review and Self-Assessment*, DOI 10.1007/978-1-4939-1477-7_1, © Springer Science+Business Media New York 2015

Table 1.1 Benign component in lung cytopathology

	Descriptions	Differentials
Benign bronchial epithelium	Clusters, sheets, or picket fence arrangement of cells with cilia, may have a mild nuclear atypia	Cells are well organized and with cilia. Nuclei show mild variation in size and multinucleation DD: well-differentiated adenocarcinoma
Reactive bronchial cells (Creola body)	Three-dimensional clusters of bronchial epithelial cells with cilia, marked variation of nuclear size, and mild to moderate nuclear atypia	Small nucleoli, no chromatin hyperchromasia, or markedly nuclear atypia DD: adenocarcinoma
Bronchial reserve cells (basal cells)	Tight clusters or sheets of small hyperchromatic cells with mild nuclear crowding	Small "dark" cells with smudgy chromatin, no mitoses or necrosis DD: small cell carcinoma
Squamous cells	Scattered individual cells with small pyknotic nuclei, and dense cytoplasm, indicating cytokeratin formation (orangeophilic color with Papanicolaou stain)	Cells have a oval or spindle shape, low N/C ratio, and benign nuclear features DD: squamous cell carcinoma
Bronchoalveolar macrophages	Loose clusters or individual cells with centrically located small round nuclei, benign nuclear features, and foamy cytoplasm	Cells have cytoplasmic pigments (anthracotic pigments in smokers) or vacuoles DD: well-differentiated adenocarcinoma
Type II pneumocytes	Intermediate-sized cells with large nuclei, coarse chromatin, prominent nucleoli, smooth nuclear membrane, and scant cytoplasm	Single cells and/or cluster of cells with benign nuclear features, may be associated with acute lung injury DD: adenocarcinoma
Goblet cells	Sheets and clusters of cells with abundant mucin-filled cytoplasm and eccentrically located nuclei with "signet ring" appearance	Cells are without nuclear atypia DD: mucinous adenocarcinoma, signet ring-cell carcinoma
Cryptococcosis	Yeast-form budding fungus with variable size, mucin capsule, and refractile center	Narrow-based budding yeast with 4–15 μm in diameter DD: histoplasmosis, blastomycosis
Pneumocystis jiroveci (carinii) pneumonia (PCP)	Extracellular and/or intracytoplasmic amorphous material with Papanicolaou stains	Methenamine silver stain highlights numerous tiny cup-shaped cysts with a black dot in the center of the cyst DD: coccidiomycosis
Candidiasis	Budding yeast with pseudohyphae	Pseudohyphae are 2–10 μm in diameter and branch at a 90° angle DD: aspergillosis
Aspergillosis	Hyphae with septate	Hyphae are 10–30 μm in diameter and branch at a 45° angle DD: candidiasis
Birefringent calcium oxalate crystals	Needle-shaped, polarizable crystals; they may form rosettes or wheat sheaf-like clusters	Associated with *Aspergillus* infection DD: Charcot–Leyden crystals
Charcot–Leyden crystals	Needle-shaped orangeophilic color crystal, by-product of eosinophil degranulation	Associated with allergy DD: calcium oxalate crystals
Ferruginous bodies	Dumbbell-shaped mineral fibers, 5–200 μm in length, golden-yellow to black color with Papanicolaou stain	Associated with Asbestos exposure DD: Charcot–Leyden crystals
Curschmann spiral	Coils and strands of mucus. Purple helices with Papanicolaou stains	Represent mucus and commonly seen in chronic pulmonary disease. Non-specific finding DD: parasite infection
Granulomas (sarcoidosis)	Clusters of epithelioid histiocytes with elongated nuclei, admixed with lymphocytes, scattered multinucleated giant cells, and reactive bronchial cells	Nodular aggregates of histiocytes and lymphocytes in a background of scattered multinucleated giant cells DD: well-differentiated adenocarcinoma

Table 1.2 Neoplastic lesions in lung cytopathology

Conditions	Descriptions	Differentials
Adenocarcinoma	Three-dimensional and acinar/papillae arrangement of columnar cells with high N/C ratio, prominent nucleoli, and "lacy" cytoplasm with vacuolization (cytoplasmic mucin)	Large hyperchromatic nuclei with irregular nuclear membranes, coarse chromatin, prominent nucleoli DD: poorly differentiated non-keratinizing squamous cell carcinoma
Squamous cell carcinoma	Discohesive and scattered individual polymorphic cells with hyperchromatic smudgy chromatin, dense cytoplasm with or without keratinization	Polygonal cells and elongated or tadpole-shaped cells with large hyperchromatic nuclei and dense cytoplasm DD: poorly differentiated adenocarcinoma
Small cell carcinoma	Tight clusters of small hyperchromatic cells (two- to threefold of mature lymphocytes), fine (salt-and-pepper) chromatin, nuclear molding and crowding, nuclear stripes (broken down nuclear material), inconspicuous nuclei, scant cytoplasm	Fine chromatin texture and nuclear crowding and molding, mitosis, necrosis, and apoptotic body DD: lymphoma, basaloid squamous cell carcinoma, and poorly differentiated adenocarcinoma
Undifferentiated large cell carcinoma	Loosely cohesive clusters, syncytial sheets, or scattered polymorphic large cells with coarse chromatin, single or multiple prominent nucleoli, and feathery cytoplasm	Large cells with large prominent nucleoli. Numerous mitoses DD: poorly differentiated adenocarcinoma, sarcoma
Carcinoid	Loosely cohesive clusters and scattered individual cells arrange in rosette-like structures. Tumor cells are relatively uniform in size, with fine ("salt-pepper") chromatin, and moderate cytoplasm	Monomorphic appearance of tumor cells, with fine chromatin, inconspicuous nucleoli. Branching capillaries in the background. No mitosis or necrosis DD: small cell carcinoma, atypical carcinoid
Lymphoma	Discohesive and scattered individual cells with vesicular nuclei, clumped (soccer-ball-like) chromatin, irregular nuclear membrane, and scant cytoplasm. Lymphoglandular body in the background	Monomorphous population of cells, with clumped (soccer-ball-like) chromatin, irregular nuclear membranes, conspicuous nucleoli, and scant cytoplasm DD: small cell carcinoma, carcinoid

1.1 Image-Based Questions 1–82

Fig. 1.1

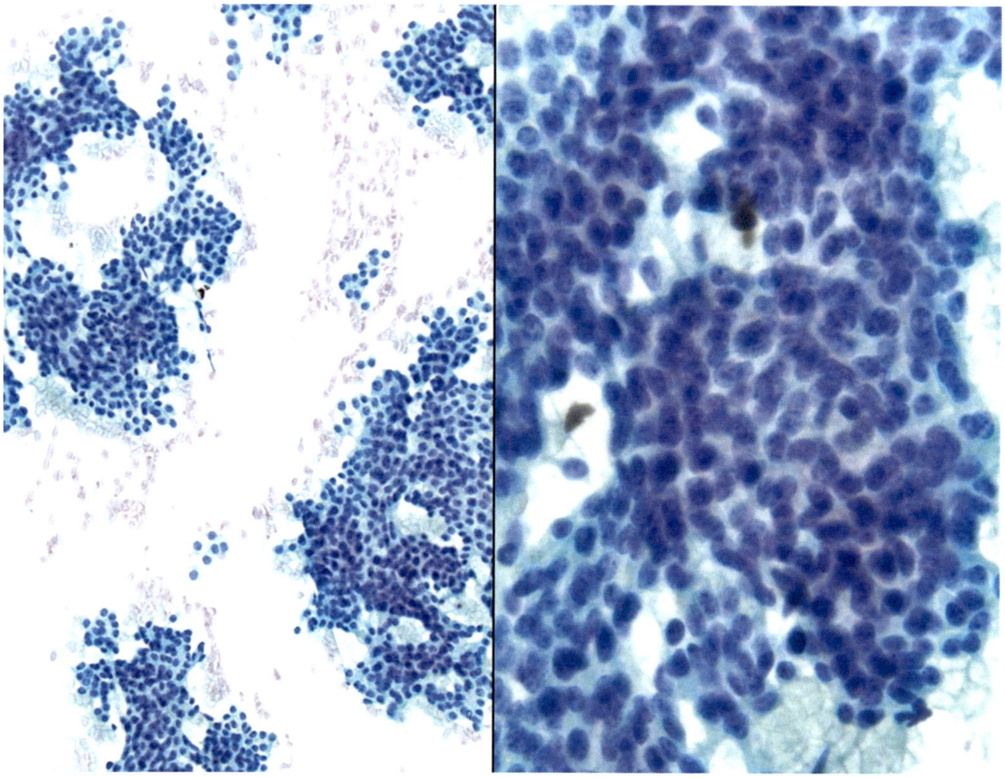

Q-1. What is the diagnosis of this specimen?
(a) Lymphoma
(b) Poorly differentiated adenocarcinoma
(c) Reactive lymphocytes
(d) Carcinoid

Fig. 1.2

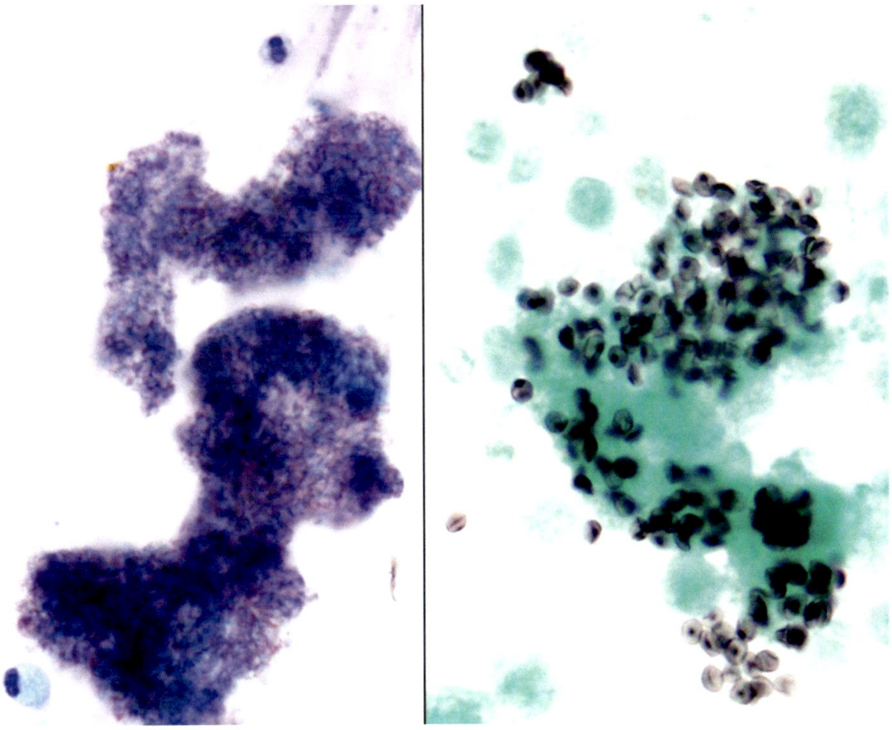

Q-2. A HIV-positive patient presented with cough and fever. Computed tomography (CT) scan revealed bilateral lung infiltrations. A BAL was performed. What is the diagnosis?

(a) *Pneumocystis jiroveci (carinii)* pneumonia (PCP)
(b) Aggregates of red blood cell (RBC) ghost cells
(c) Alveolar proteinosis
(d) Aspergillosis

Fig. 1.3

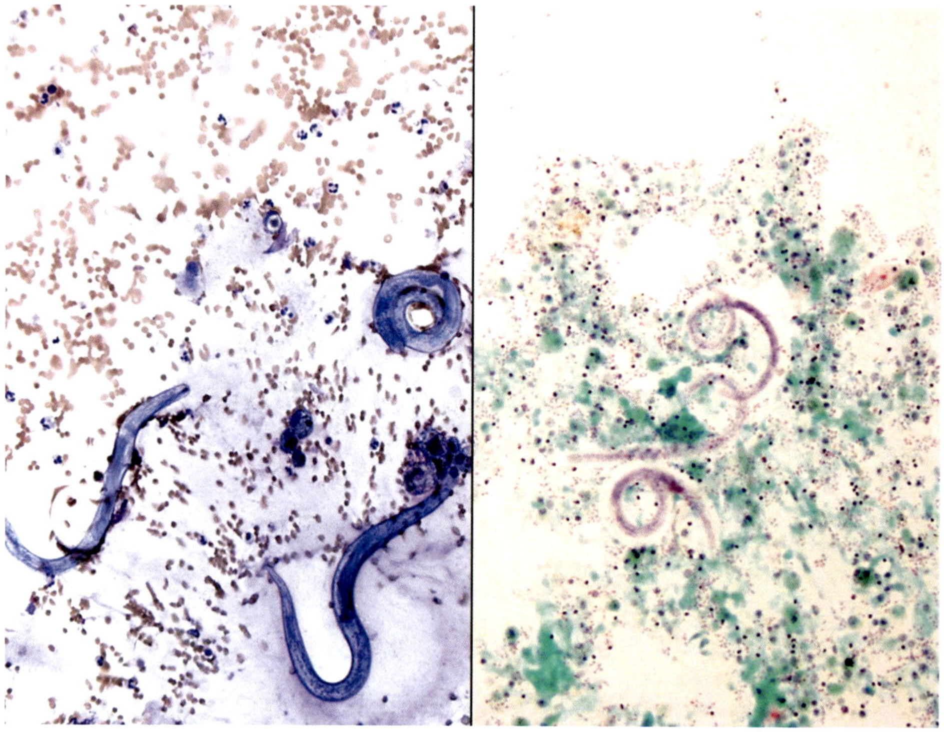

Q-3. A HIV-positive patient presented with hemoptysis and fever. CT scan revealed bilateral lung infiltrations. A BAL was performed. What is the diagnosis?

(a) *Pneumocystis jiroveci (carinii)* pneumonia (PCP)
(b) Strongyloidiasis
(c) Alveolar proteinosis
(d) Aspergillosis

Fig. 1.4

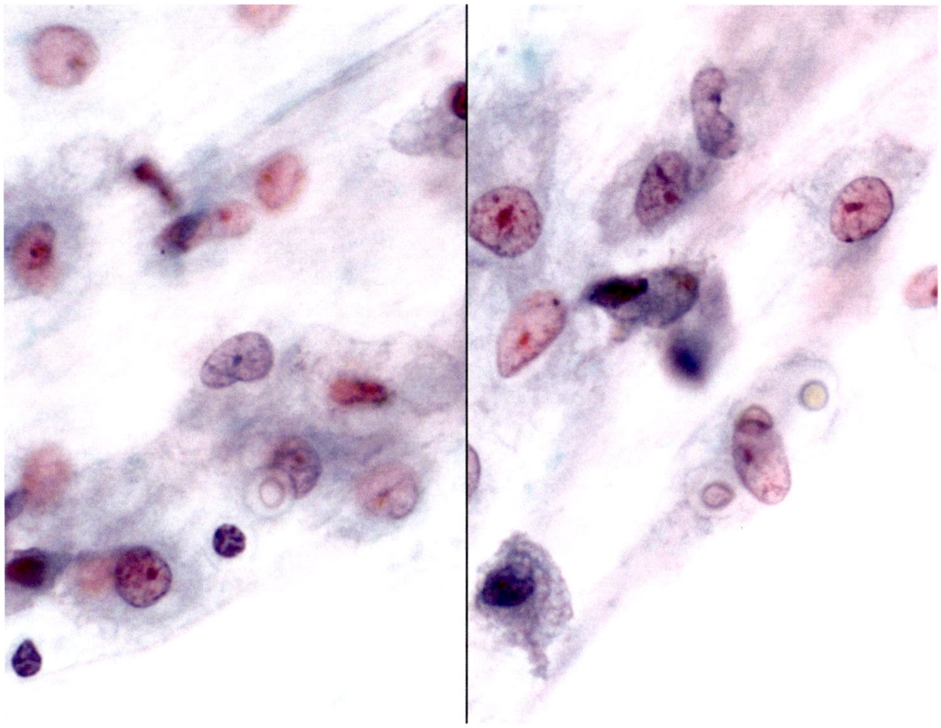

Q-4. A patient presented with productive cough, fever, and weight loss. CT scan revealed bilateral lung infiltrations. A bronchoalveolar lavage (BAL) was performed. What is the diagnosis?
(a) Blastomycosis
(b) Histoplasmosis
(c) Cryptococcosis
(d) Aspergillosis

Fig. 1.5

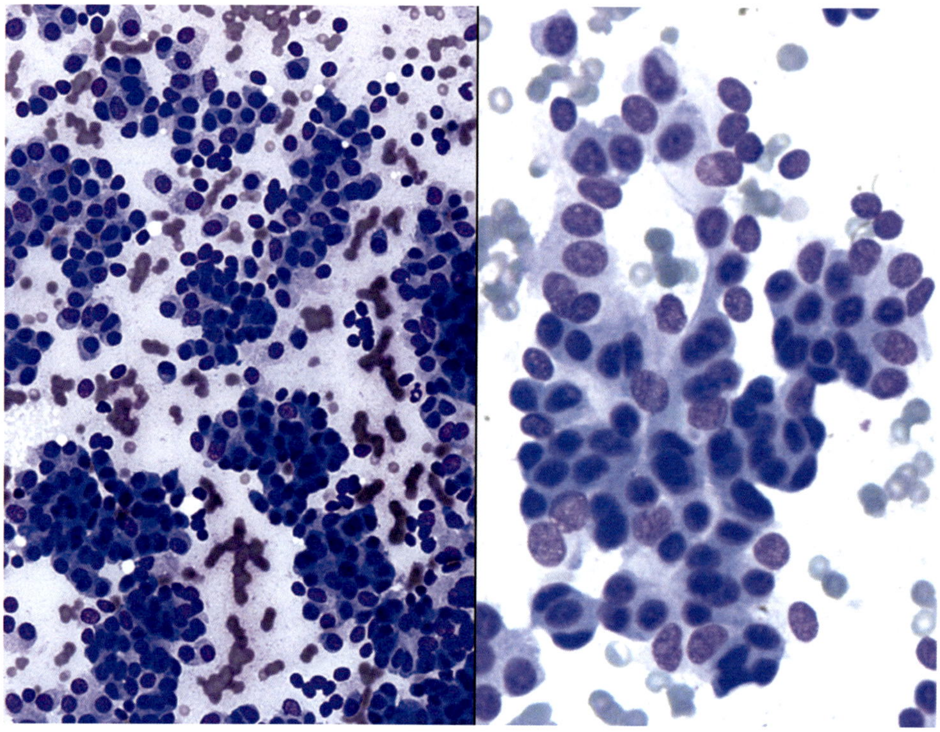

Q-5. What is the diagnosis of this lung fine-needle aspiration (FNA)?
(a) Well-differentiated adenocarcinoma
(b) Carcinoid
(c) Poorly differentiated adenocarcinoma
(d) Reactive bronchial cells.

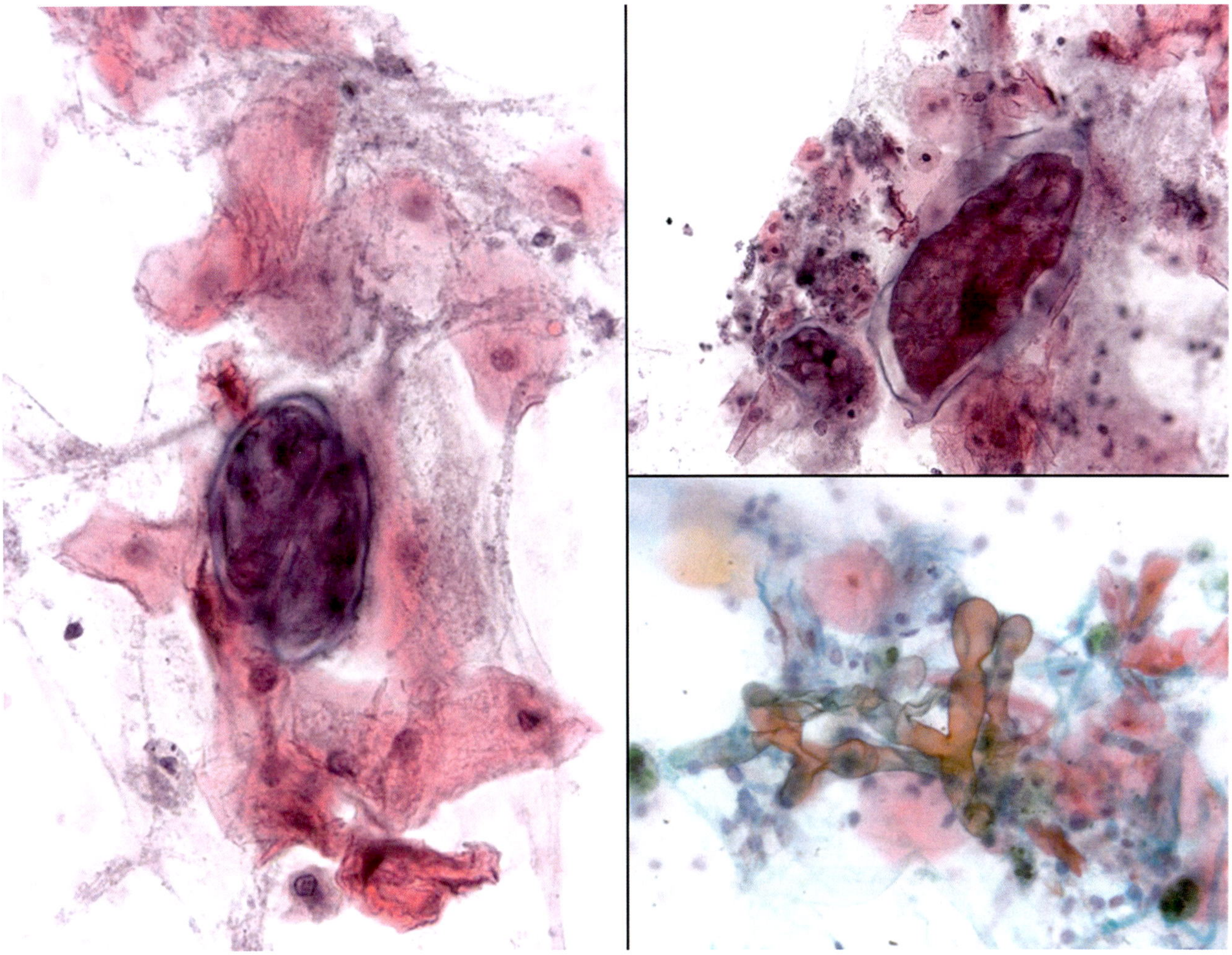

Fig. 1.6

Q-6. This sputum specimen was collected from a lung cancer patient who presented with neutropenia. What is the diagnosis?

(a) Blastomycosis
(b) Mucormycosis (zygomycosis)
(c) Aspergillosis
(d) Paragonimus eggs

Fig. 1.7

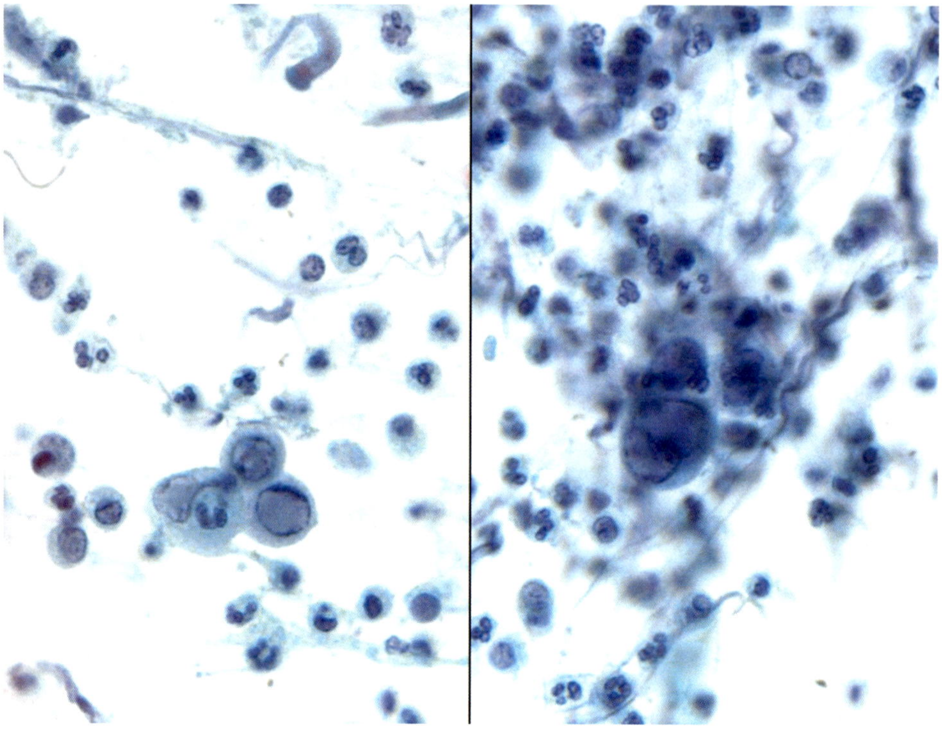

Q-7. This BAL specimen was collected from a patient with the history of colon adenocarcinoma, who presented with respiratory distress. What is the diagnosis?
(a) Markedly reactive bronchial cells and alveolar macrophages
(b) Poorly differentiated adenocarcinoma
(c) Squamous cell metaplasia
(d) *Herpes simplex virus* (HSV) infection

Fig. 1.8

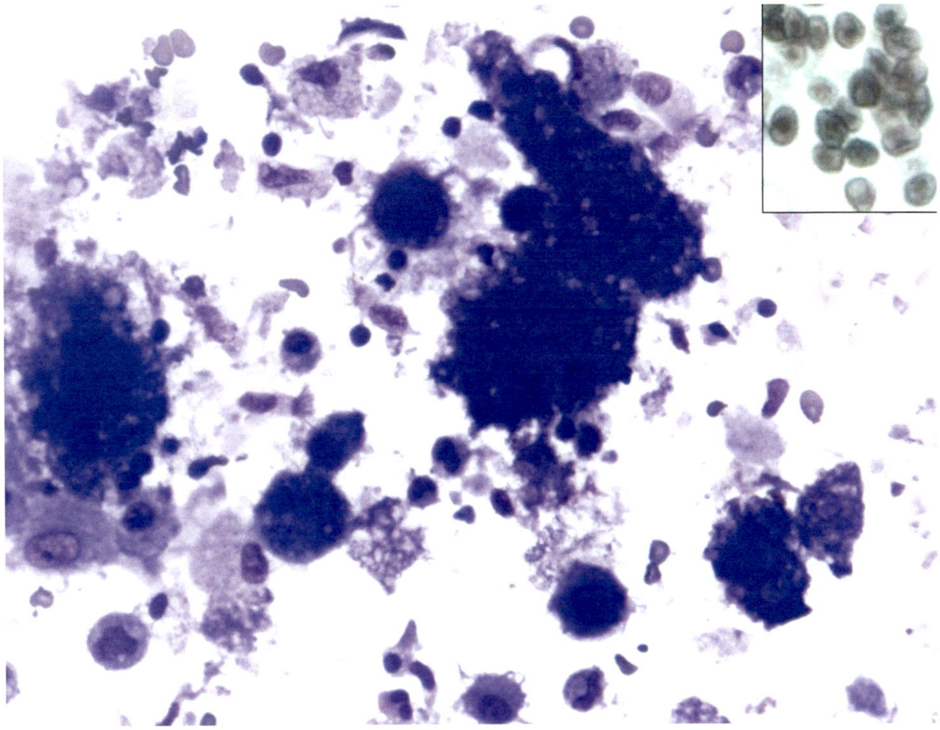

Q-8. A HIV-positive patient was clinically suspicious for *Pneumocystis jiroveci* (*carinii*) pneumonia (PCP) infection of the lung. A BAL was performed. What is the diagnosis?

(a) *Pneumocystis jiroveci* (*carinii*) pneumonia
(b) *Cryptococcus* infection
(c) Alveolar proteinosis
(d) Lysed red blood cells

Fig. 1.9

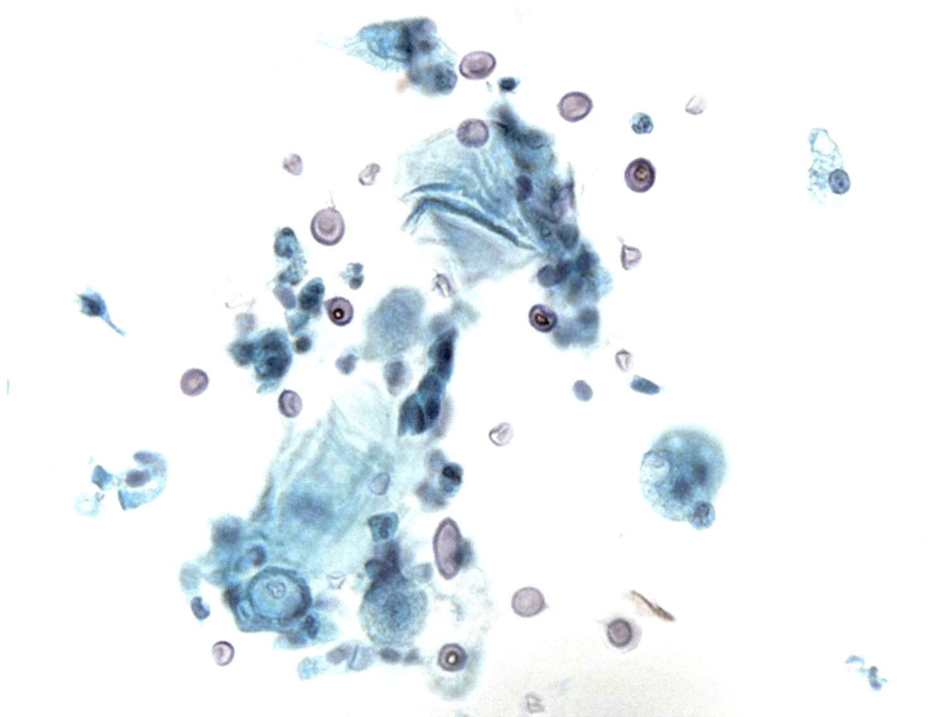

Q-9. A patient presented with multiple lung nodules and hilar lymphadenopathy. A transbronchial lung FNA of the lung nodule was performed. What is the best diagnosis?

(a) Reactive bronchial cells and alveolar macrophages
(b) Poorly differentiated adenocarcinoma
(c) Histoplasmosis
(d) *Pneumocystis jiroveci* (*carinii*) *pneumonia* (PCP)

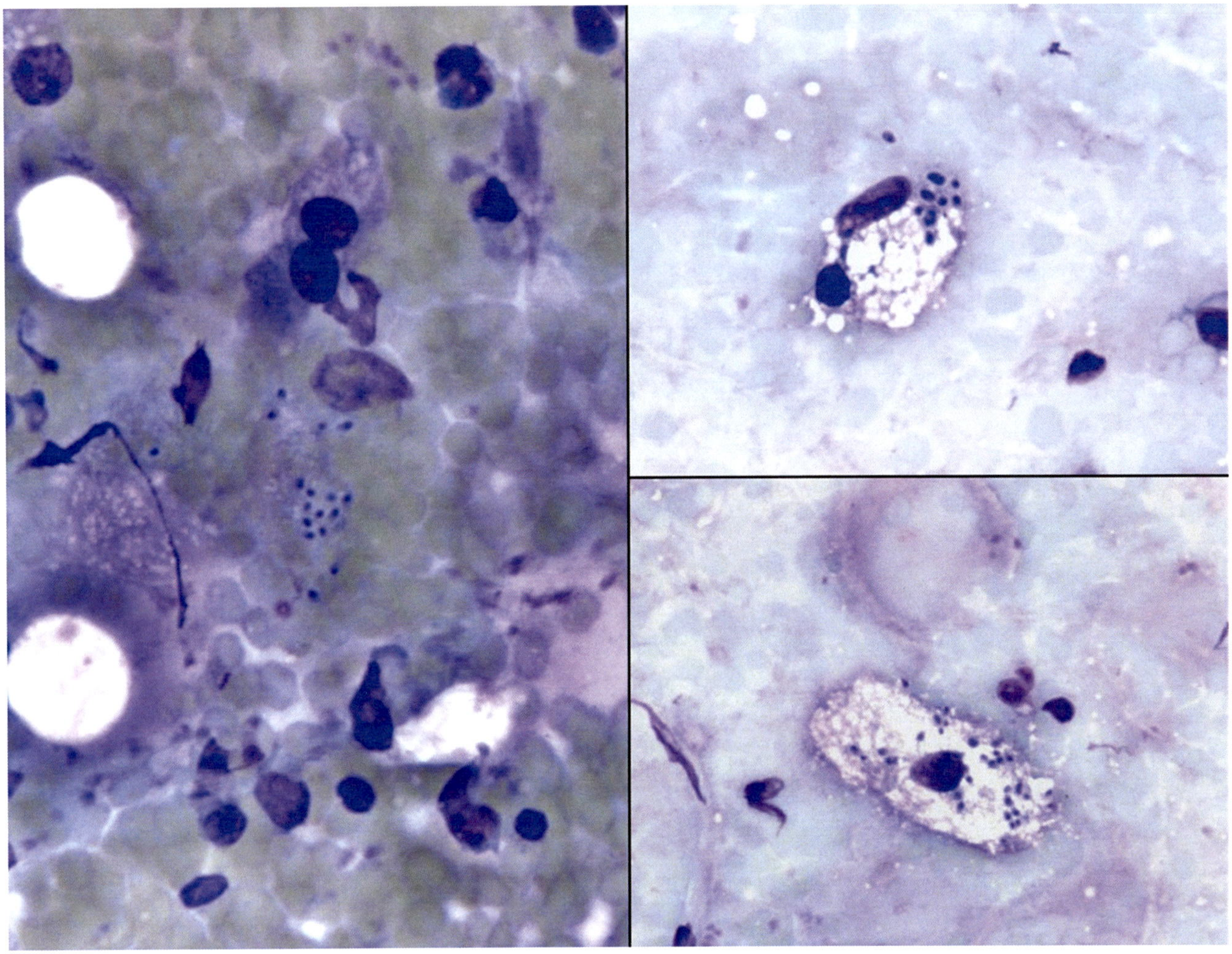

Fig. 1.10

Q-10. A patient presented with lung and liver cystic masses. The CT-guided FNA of the lung lesion was performed. What is the diagnosis?
(a) Echinococcosis (Hydatid disease)
(b) Strongyloidiasis
(c) *Entamoeba histolytica* infection
(d) Paragonimus eggs

Fig. 1.11

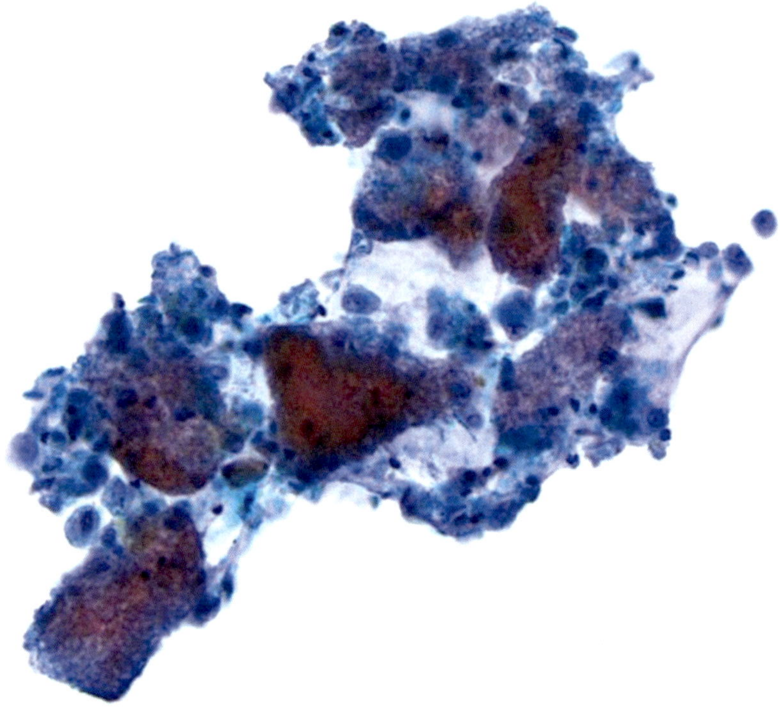

Q-11. A HIV-positive patient presented with cough and hemoptysis. The chest x-ray revealed a cavitary lung lesion. A FNA of the lung lesion was performed. What is the diagnosis?

(a) Blastomycosis
(b) Mucormycosis (zygomycosis)
(c) Aspergillosis
(d) Candidiasis

Fig. 1.12

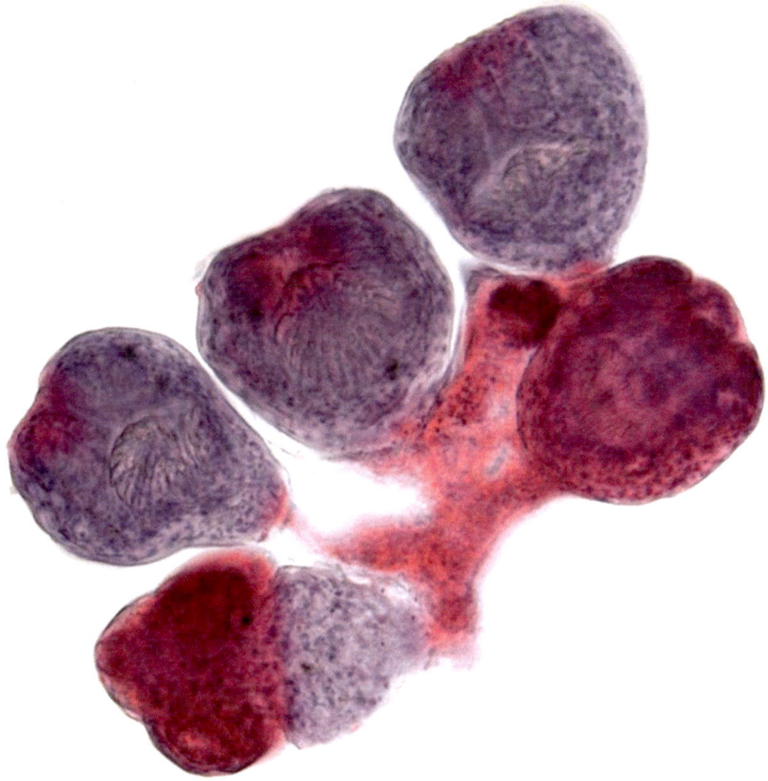

Q-12. An immunocompromised patients presented with cough, fever, pneumonia, and bilateral lung infiltrations. What is the diagnosis of this BAL specimen?
(a) Poorly differentiated adenocarcinoma
(b) *Cytomegalovirus* (CMV) infection
(c) Squamous cell metaplasia
(d) *Herpes simplex virus* (HSV) infection

Fig. 1.13

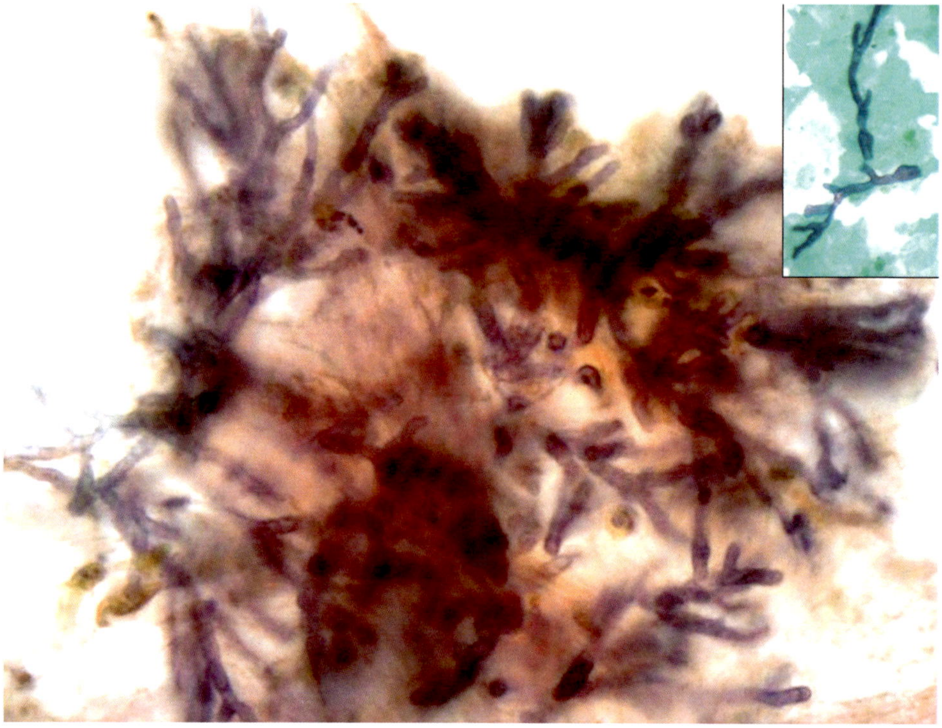

Q-13. A 32-year-old man presented with chronic cough, hemoptysis, and bilateral lung infiltrations. A sputum specimen was collected. What is the diagnosis?
(a) Echinococcosis (Hydatid disease)
(b) Strongyloidiasis
(c) *Entamoeba gingivalis* infection
(d) Paragonimus eggs

Fig. 1.14

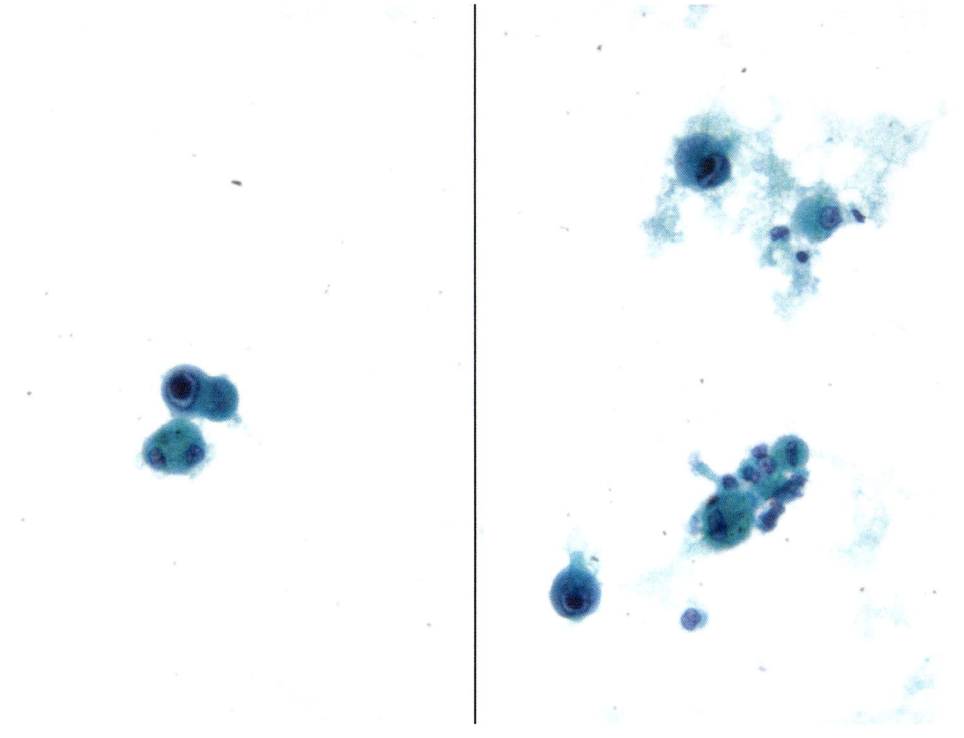

Q-14. A 67-year-old transplant patient presented with chronic cough and multiple lung nodules. A BAL was performed. What is the best diagnosis?
(a) Reactive bronchial cells and alveolar macrophages
(b) Poorly differentiated adenocarcinoma
(c) Histoplasmosis
(d) *Pneumocystis jiroveci* (*carinii*) *pneumonia* (PCP)

Fig. 1.15

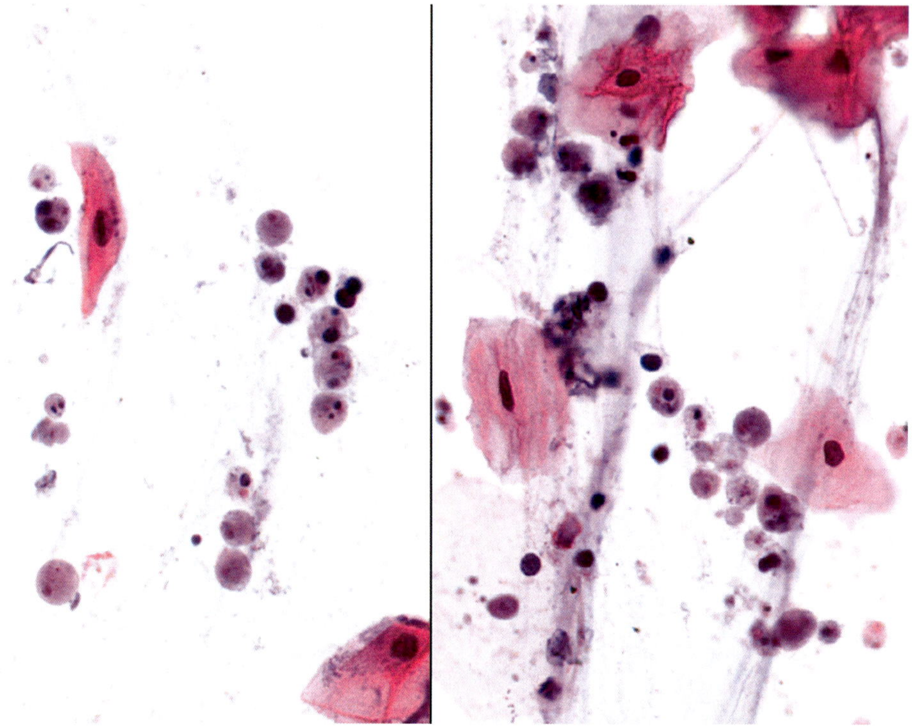

Q-15. A 33-year-old non-smoking man presented with a 3 cm lung nodule. A transbronchial FNA of the lung lesion was performed. What is the diagnosis?

(a) Cryptococcosis
(b) Coccidioidomycosis
(c) Histoplasmosis
(d) *Pneumocystis jiroveci* (*carinii*) *pneumonia* (PCP)

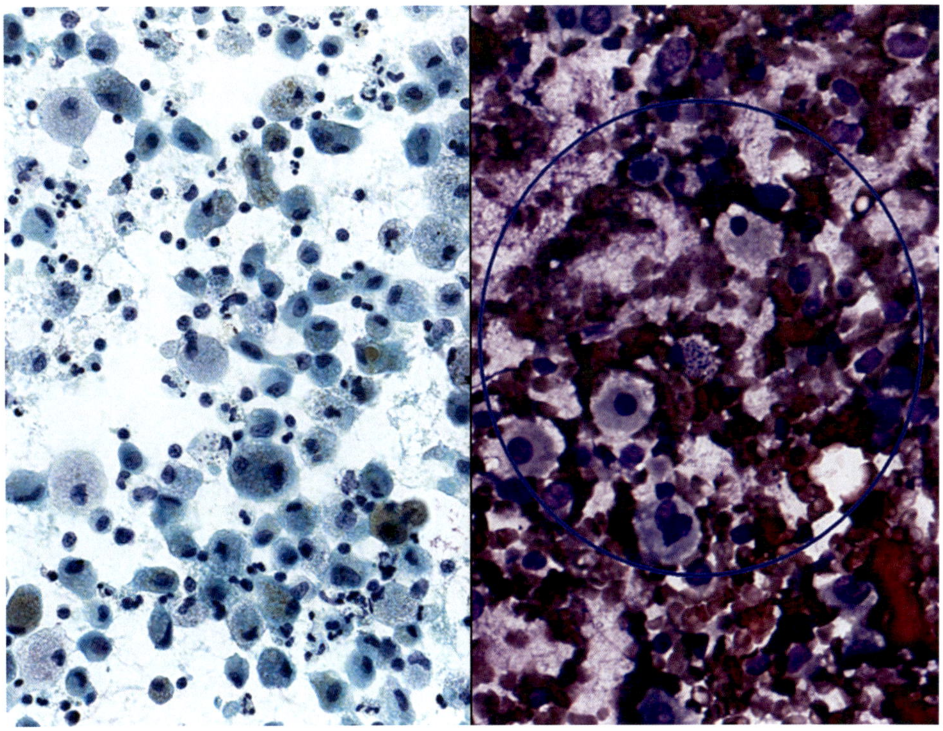

Fig. 1.16

Q-16. A 33-year-old non-smoking man presented with a 3 cm lung nodule. A transbronchial FNA of the lung lesion was performed. What is the diagnosis?

(a) Cryptococcosis
(b) Coccidioidomycosis
(c) Histoplasmosis
(d) *Pneumocystis jiroveci* (*carinii*) *pneumonia* (PCP)

Fig. 1.17

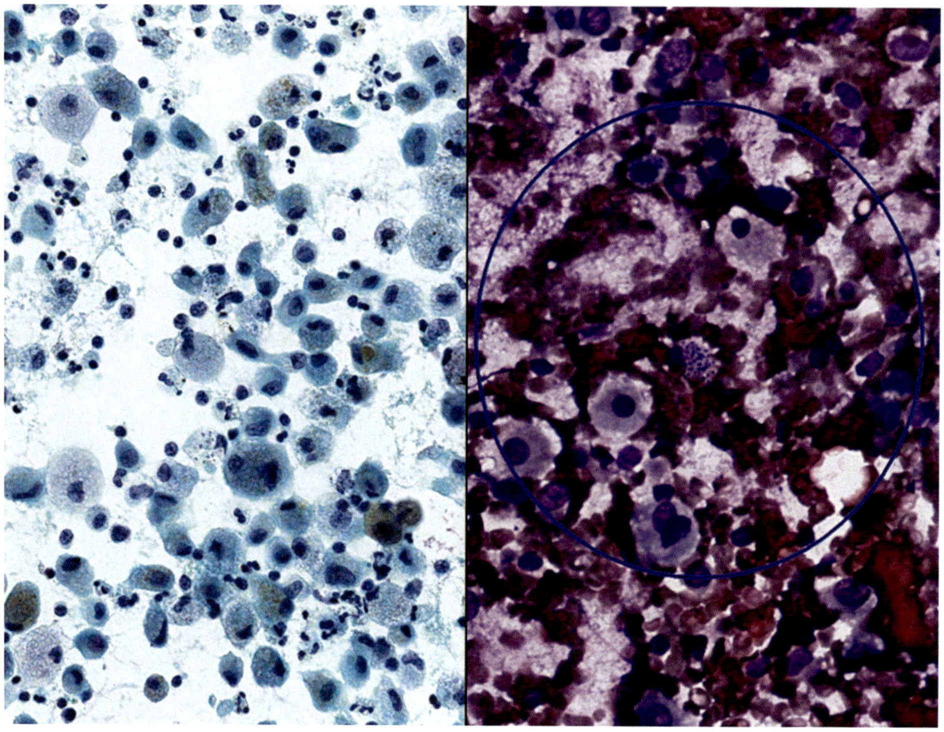

Q-17. A 53-year-old female presented with chronic cough, night sweats, fever, weight loss, and fatigue. CT scan showed bilateral cavitary lung lesions. A transbronchial FNA of the lung lesion was performed. What is the diagnosis on this Diff-Quik smear?

(a) Cryptococcosis
(b) Histoplasmosis
(c) Tuberculosis
(d) *Pneumocystis jiroveci* (*carinii*) *pneumonia* (PCP)

Fig. 1.18

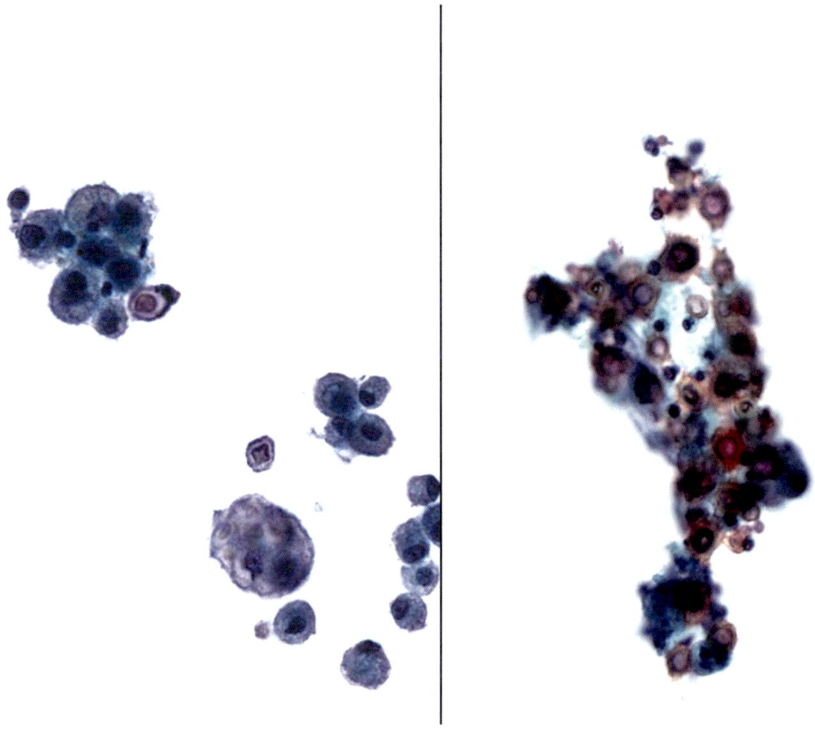

Q-18. This BAL specimen was collected from a transplant patient. What is the diagnosis of the BAL?
(a) *Pneumocystis jiroveci (carinii) pneumonia* (PCP)
(b) Histoplasmosis
(c) Tuberculosis
(d) Toxoplasmosis

Fig. 1.19

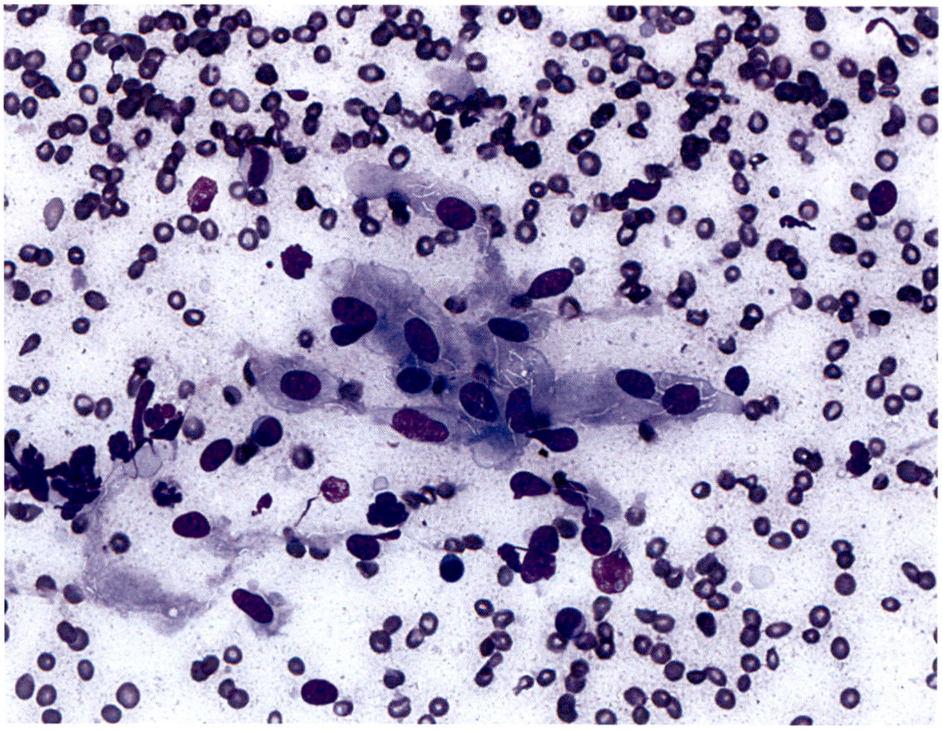

Q-19. An immunocompromised patients presented with cough, fever, pneumonia, and bilateral lung infiltrations. What is the diagnosis of this BAL specimen?

(a) *Pneumocystis jiroveci* (*carinii*) *pneumonia* (PCP)
(b) Cytomegalovirus (CMV) infection
(c) Co-infection with CMV and PCP
(d) *Herpes simplex virus* (HSV) infection

Fig. 1.20

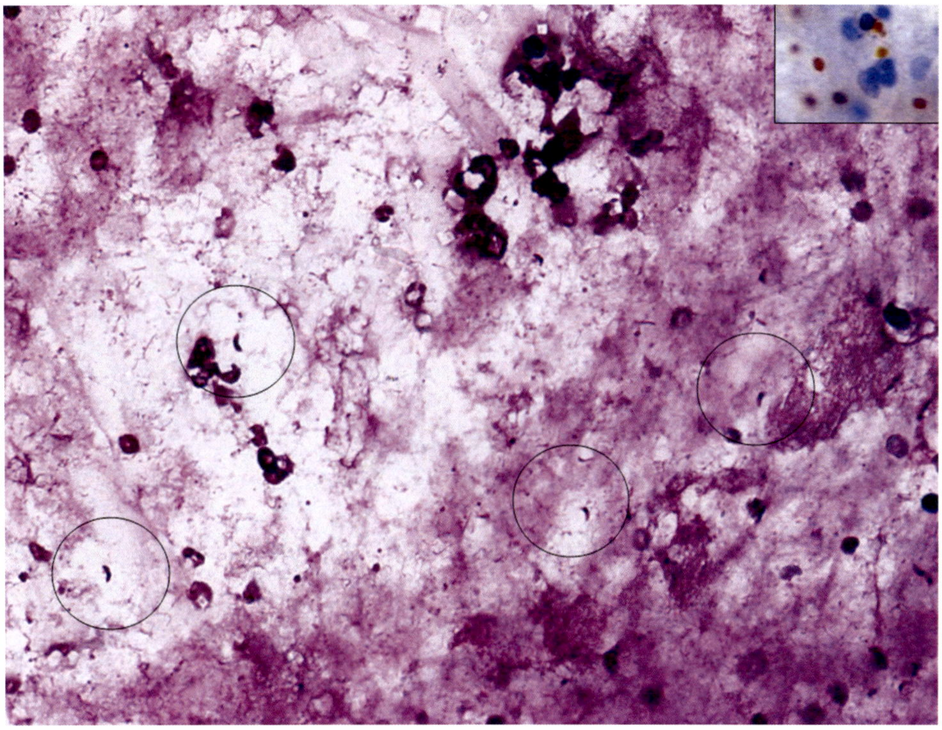

Q-20. The structures seen in photos are most likely found in a patient with:

(a) Asthma
(b) *Pneumocystis jiroveci (carinii) pneumonia* (PCP)
(c) Aspergillosis
(d) Asbestos exposure

Fig. 1.21

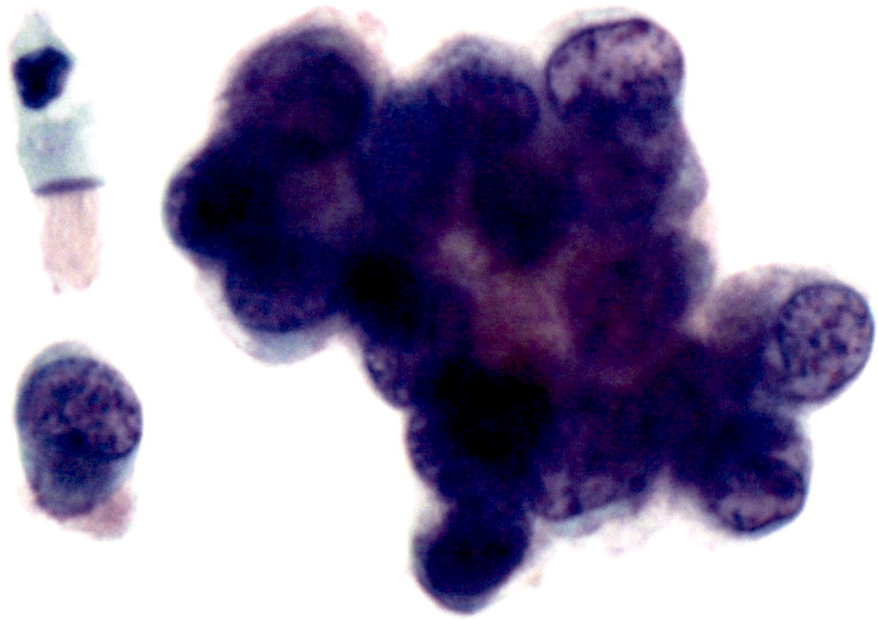

Q-21. What is the diagnosis of this image?
(a) Well-differentiated adenocarcinoma
(b) Reactive bronchial epithelium
(c) Creola body
(d) Bronchoalveolar macrophages

Fig. 1.22

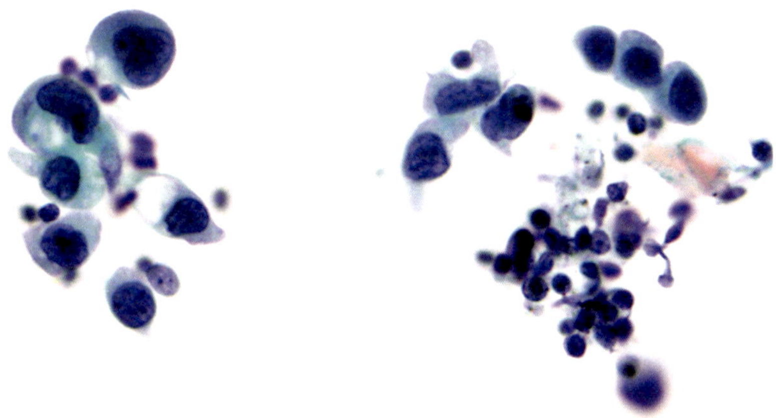

Q-22. What is the diagnosis of this image?
(a) Reactive bronchial epithelium
(b) Creola body
(c) Bronchoalveolar macrophages
(d) Adenocarcinoma with cytoplasmic mucin

Fig. 1.23

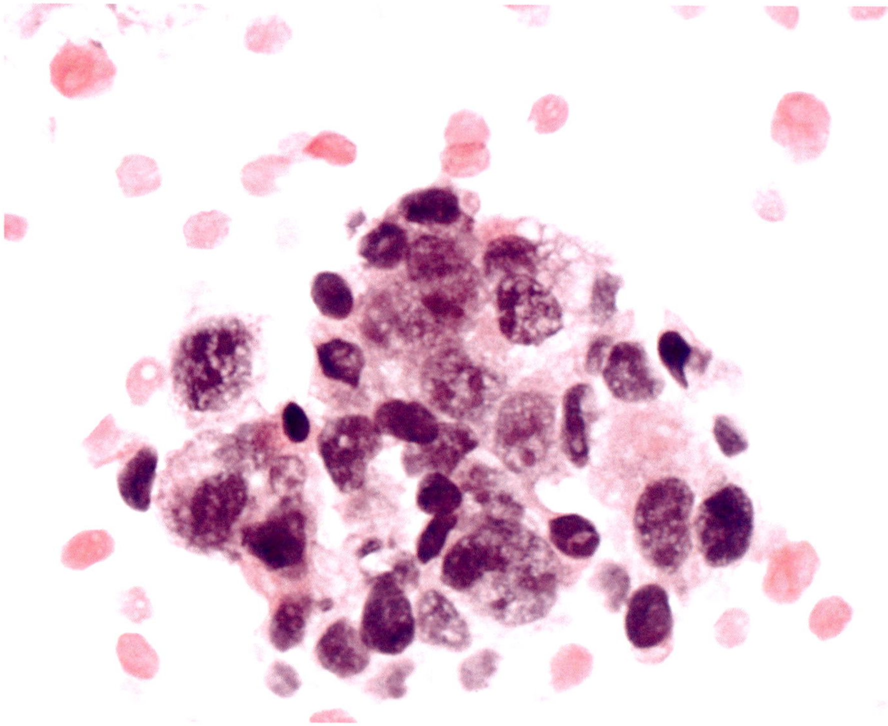

Q-23. What is the diagnosis of this cell block preparation?

(a) Bronchoalveolar macrophages
(b) Goblet cell hyperplasia
(c) Adenocarcinoma
(d) Reactive bronchial epithelium

Fig. 1.24

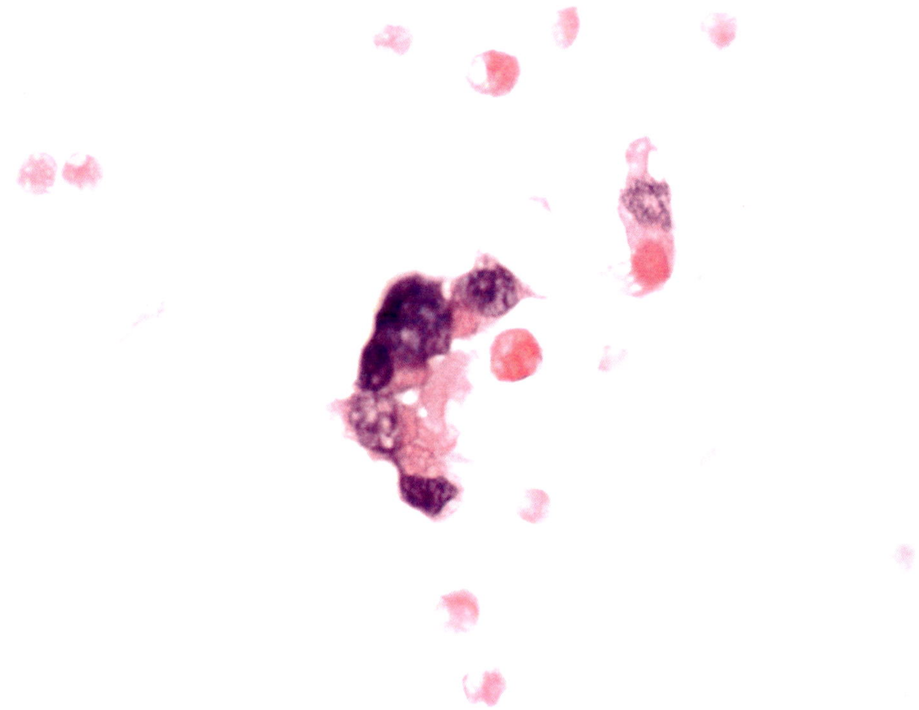

Q-24. A 67-year-old female smoker had bilateral lung infiltration. What is the diagnosis of this cell block preparation?

(a) Bronchoalveolar macrophages
(b) Goblet cell hyperplasia
(c) Adenocarcinoma
(d) Reactive bronchial epithelium

Fig. 1.25

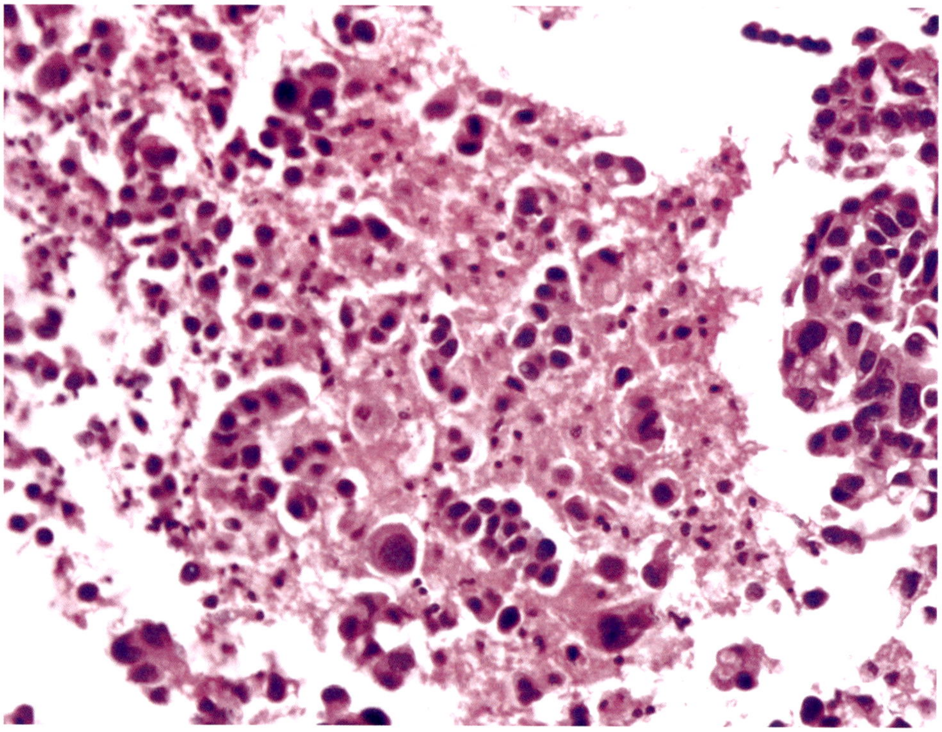

Q-25. This is a transbronchial fine-needle aspiration from a 78-year-old male smoker who has a right upper lobe lung nodule. What is the diagnosis of this cell block preparation?

(a) Squamous cell carcinoma
(b) Bronchoalveolar macrophages hyperplasia
(c) Adenocarcinoma
(d) Reactive bronchial epithelium

Fig. 1.26

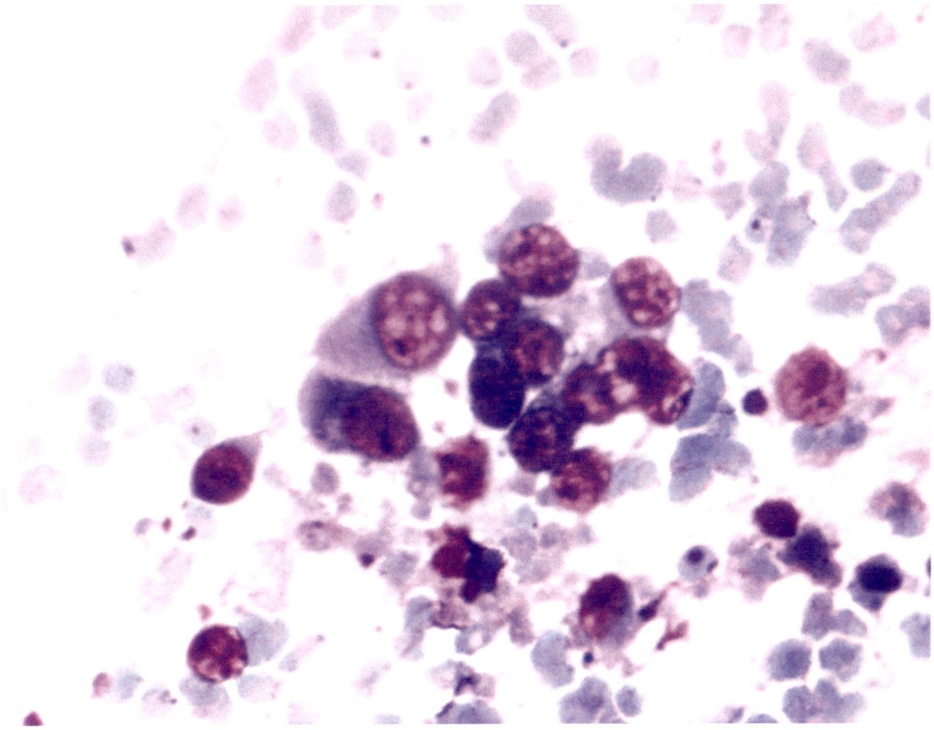

Q-26. This is an on-site evaluation of a transbronchial fine-needle aspiration. What is the diagnosis of this Diff-Quik preparation?

(a) Reactive bronchial epithelium
(b) Squamous cell carcinoma
(c) Bronchoalveolar macrophages hyperplasia
(d) Adenocarcinoma

Fig. 1.27

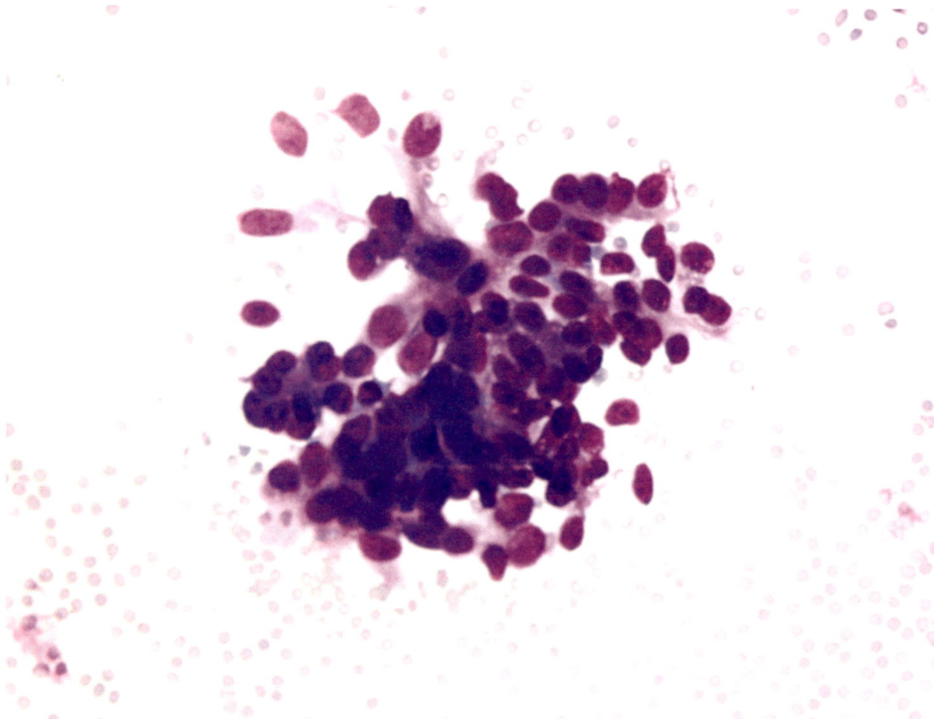

Q-27. This is an on-site evaluation of a transbronchial fine-needle aspiration from a 52-year-old female with clinical history of a breast cancer, who now has developed bilateral lung nodules. What is the diagnosis of this Diff-Quik preparation?

(a) Reactive bronchial epithelium
(b) Squamous cell carcinoma
(c) Metastatic carcinoma of the breast
(d) Adenocarcinoma of the lung

Fig. 1.28

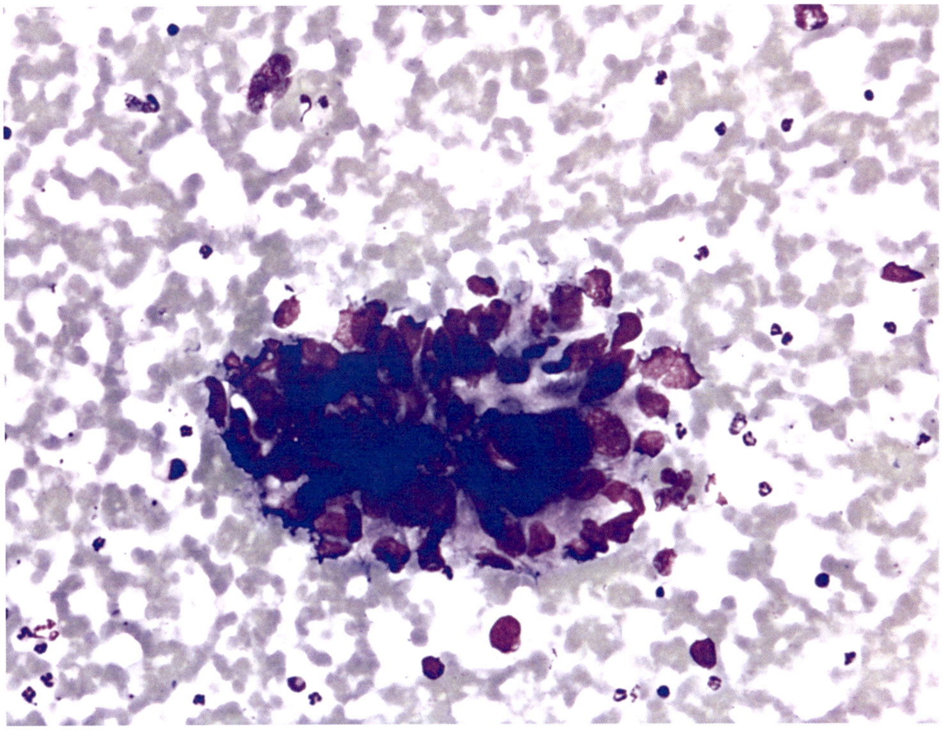

Q-28. This is an on-site evaluation of a transbronchial fine-needle aspiration from a 68-year-old male with clinical history of a colon cancer, now developed bilateral lung nodules. What is the diagnosis of this Diff-Quik preparation?
(a) Reactive bronchial epithelium
(b) Squamous cell carcinoma
(c) Metastatic adenocarcinoma of the colon
(d) Adenocarcinoma of the lung

Fig. 1.29

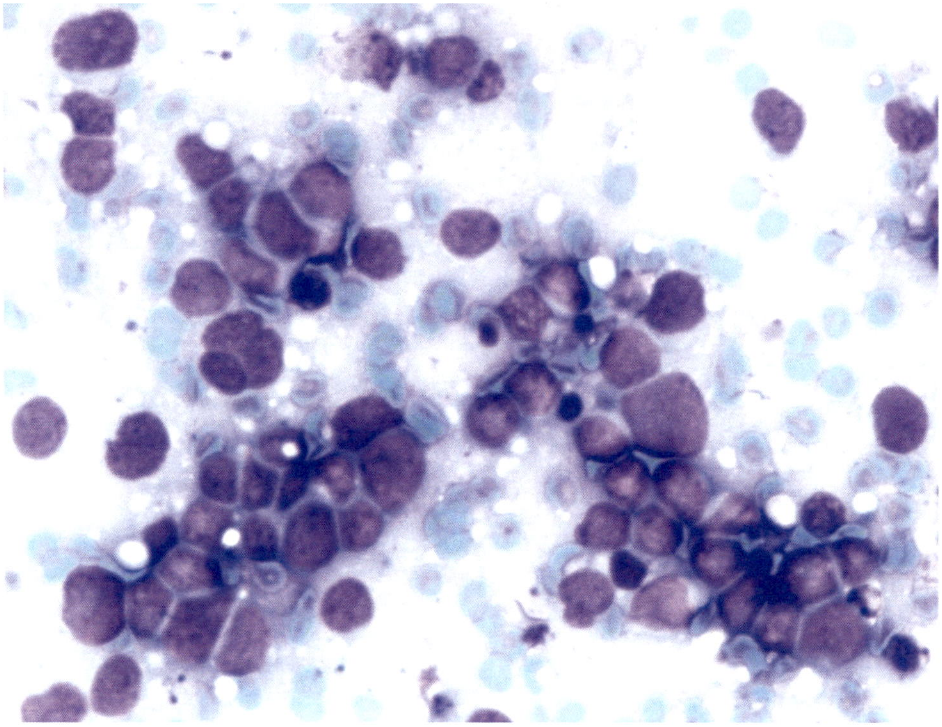

Q-29. This is an on-site evaluation of a transbronchial fine-needle aspiration from a 68-year-old male smoker with a large hilar mass. What is the diagnosis of this Diff-Quik preparation?

(a) Reactive bronchial epithelium
(b) Reactive lymphocytes
(c) Poorly differentiated squamous cell carcinoma
(d) Small cell carcinoma

Fig. 1.30

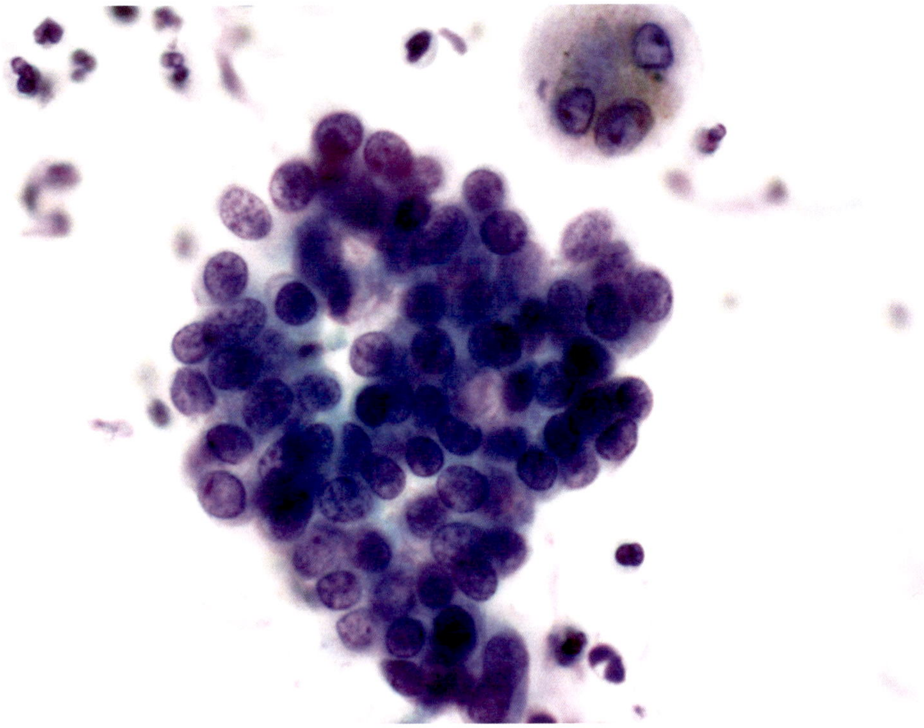

Q-30. This is a transbronchial fine-needle aspiration from a 74-year-old female with clinical history of a breast cancer, now developed bilateral lung nodules. What is the diagnosis of this Papanicolaou preparation?

(a) Reactive bronchial epithelium
(b) Squamous cell carcinoma
(c) Metastatic carcinoma of the breast
(d) Adenocarcinoma of the lung

Fig. 1.31

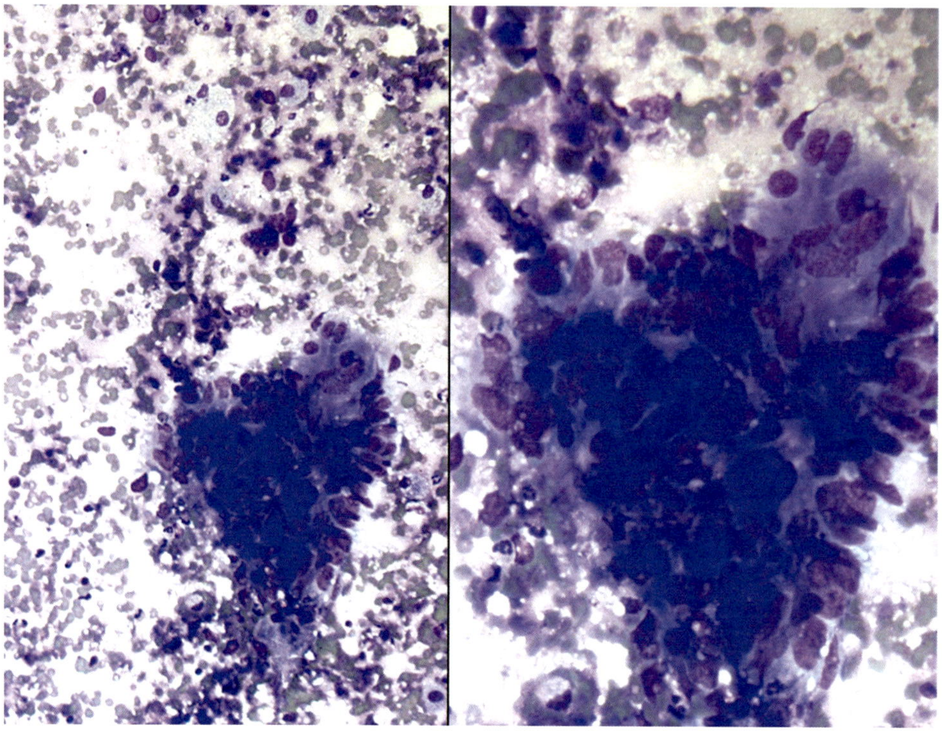

Q-31. This is a transbronchial fine-needle aspiration from a 68-year-old male with clinical history of a colon cancer, who now has developed bilateral lung nodules. What is the diagnosis of this Papanicolaou preparation?
(a) Reactive bronchial epithelium
(b) Squamous cell carcinoma
(c) Metastatic adenocarcinoma of the colon
(d) Adenocarcinoma of the lung

Fig. 1.32

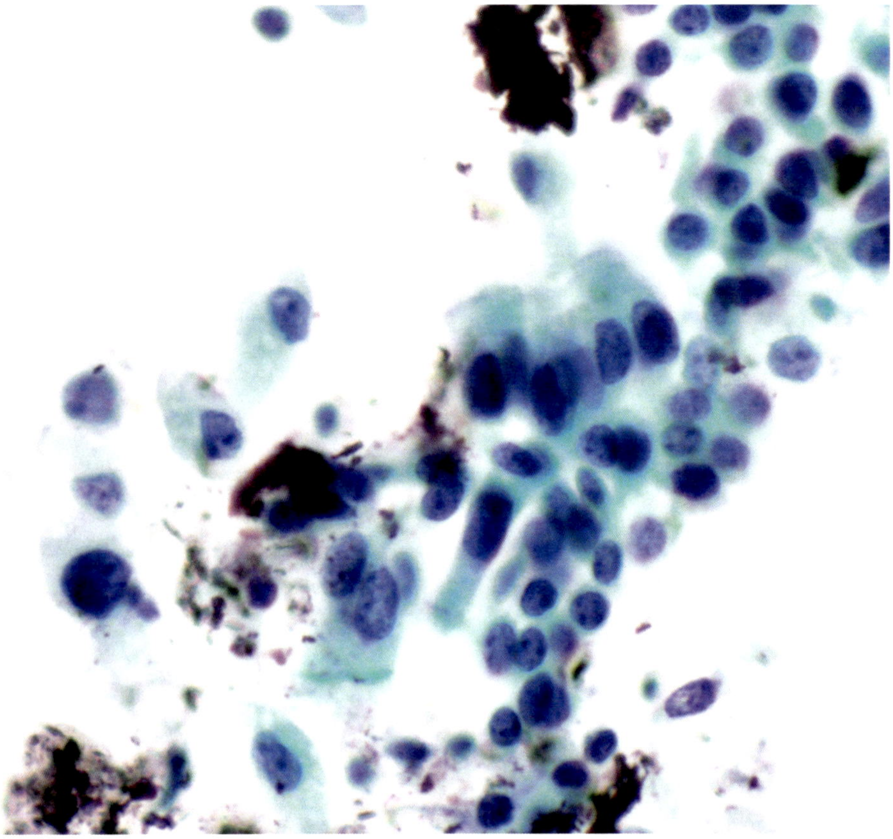

Q-32. This is a transbronchial fine-needle aspiration from a 70-year-old male with clinical history of a colon cancer, who now has developed bilateral lung infiltration. What is the diagnosis of this Papanicolaou preparation?

(a) Reactive bronchial epithelium
(b) Squamous cell carcinoma
(c) Metastatic adenocarcinoma of the colon
(d) Well-differentiated adenocarcinoma of the lung

Fig. 1.33

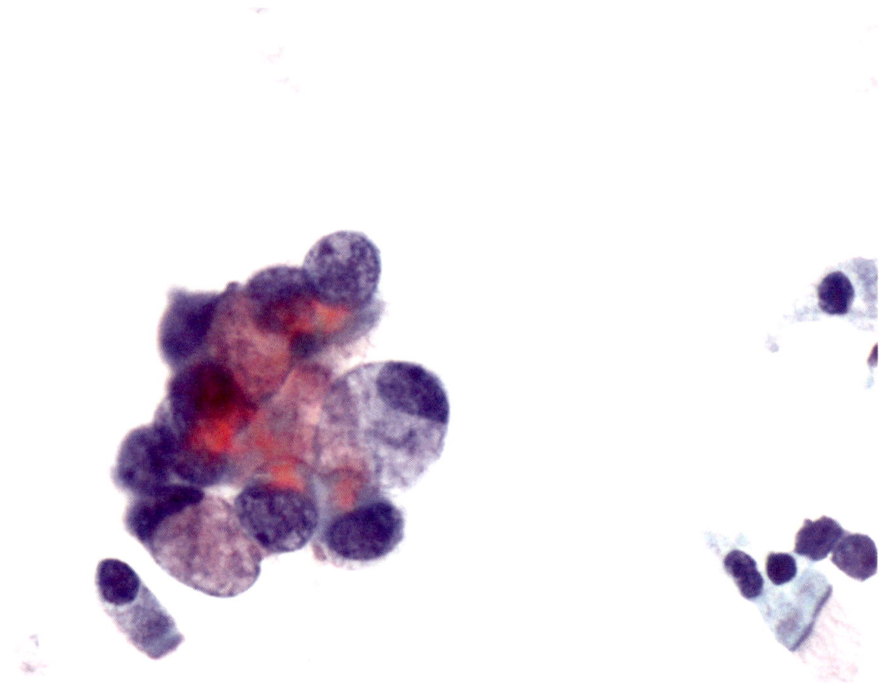

Q-33. This is a transbronchial fine-needle aspiration from a 70-year-old male smoker with bilateral lung infiltration and productive cough. What is the diagnosis of this Papanicolaou preparation?
(a) Reactive bronchial squamous cells
(b) Goblet cell hyperplasia
(c) Squamous cell carcinoma
(d) Adenocarcinoma

Fig. 1.34

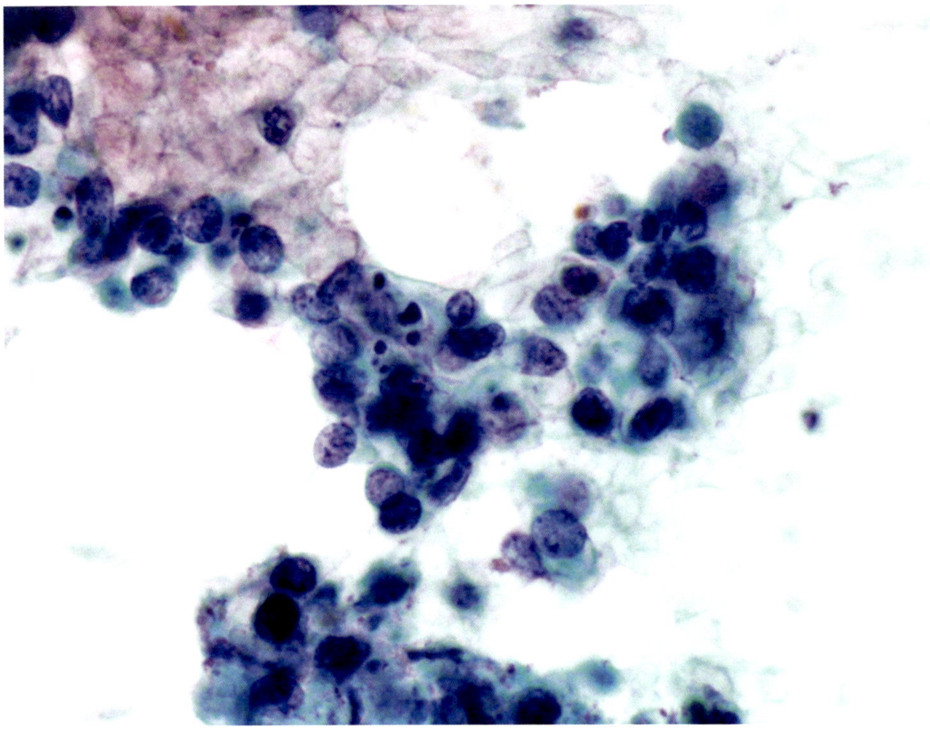

Q-34. This is a transbronchial fine-needle aspiration from a 66-year-old male smoker with left lung mass and brain metastasis. What is the diagnosis of this Papanicolaou preparation?
(a) Reactive bronchial squamous cells
(b) Small cell carcinoma
(c) Squamous cell carcinoma
(d) Adenocarcinoma

Fig. 1.35

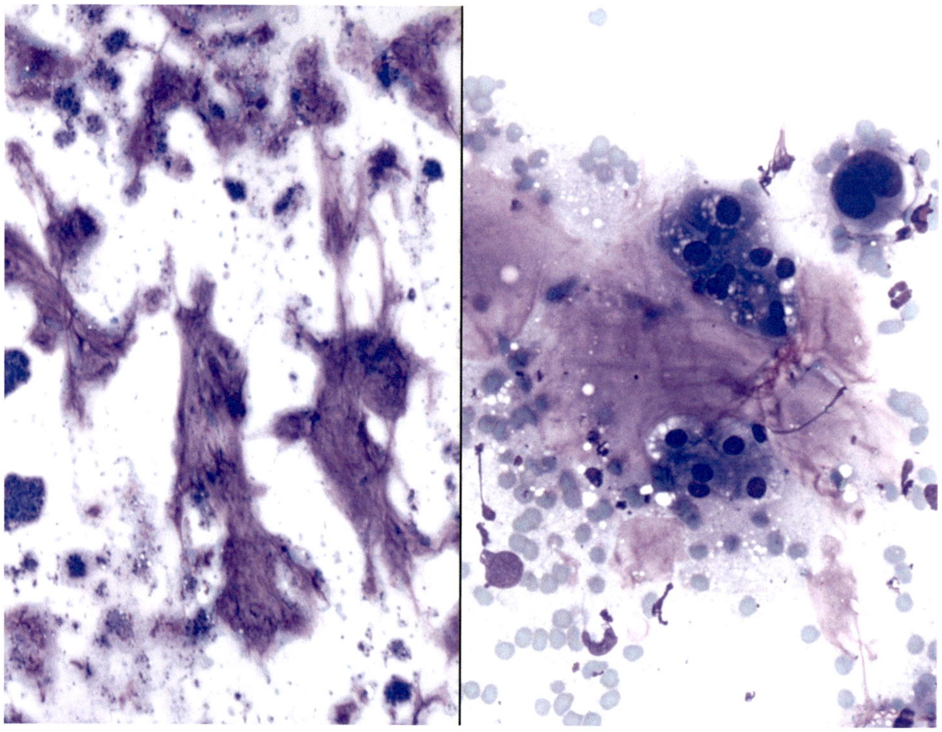

Q-35. This is a sputum specimen from a 58-year-old male smoker with a lung mass. What is the diagnosis of this Papanicolaou preparation?
(a) Reactive bronchial cells
(b) Small cell carcinoma
(c) Goblet cells
(d) Adenocarcinoma with mucinous features

Fig. 1.36

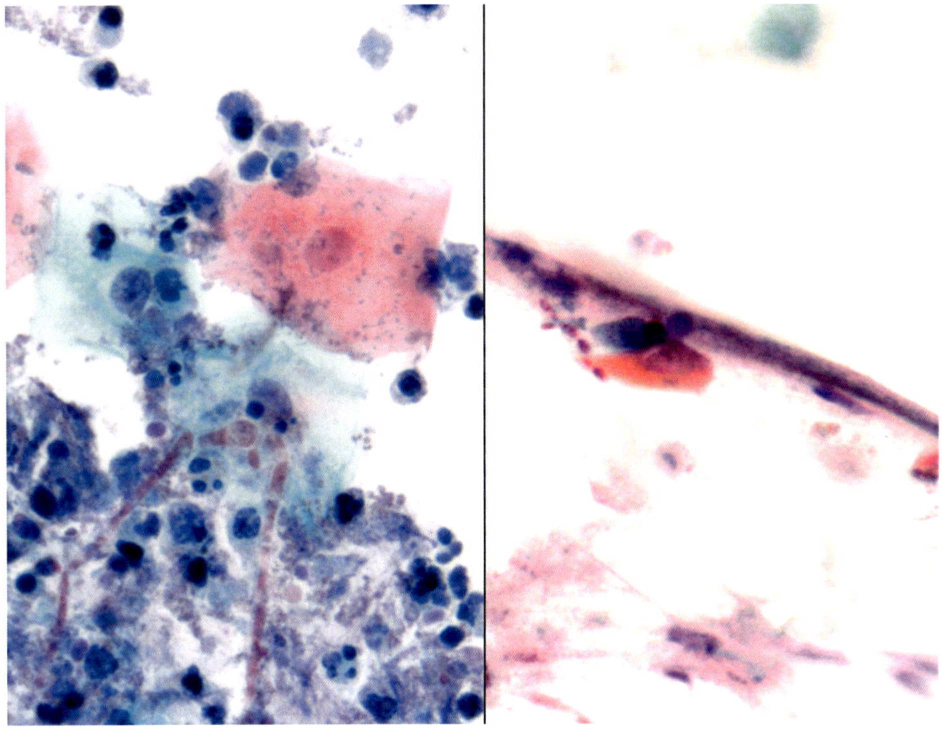

Q-36. This is a BAL specimen from a 55-year-old female smoker with diabetics, who has developed cough and fever. What is the diagnosis of this Papanicolaou preparation?

(a) Reactive bronchial cells and *Candida*
(b) Aspergillosis
(c) Squamous cell carcinoma
(d) Adenocarcinoma

Fig. 1.37

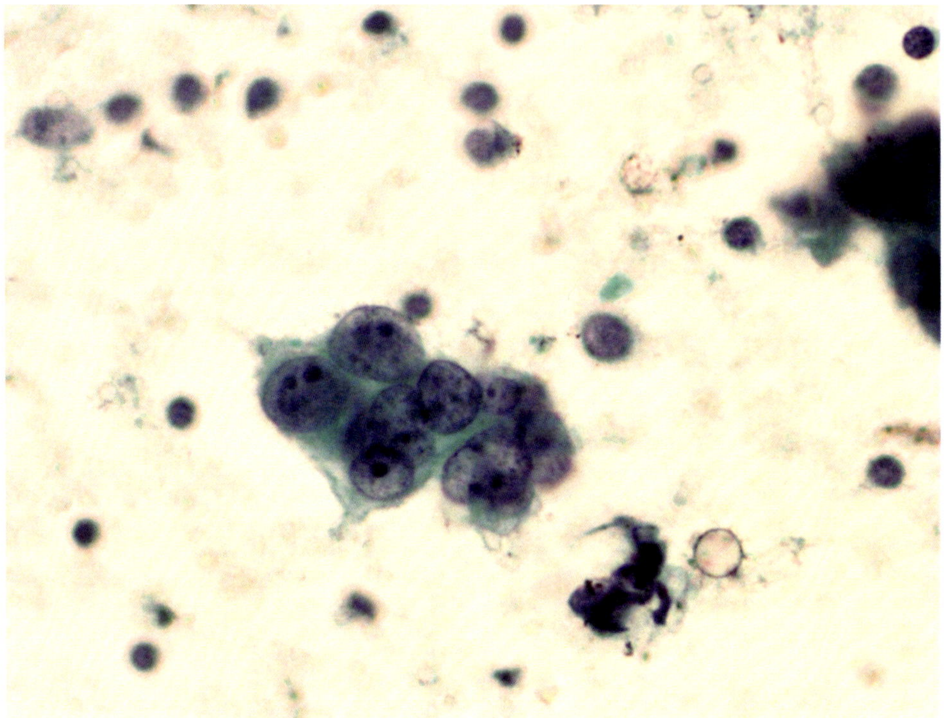

Q-37. This is a BAL specimen from a 71-year-old female smoker with a right lower lobe lung mass. What is the diagnosis of this Papanicolaou preparation?

(a) Reactive bronchial cells
(b) Small cell carcinoma
(c) Squamous cell carcinoma
(d) Adenocarcinoma

Fig. 1.38

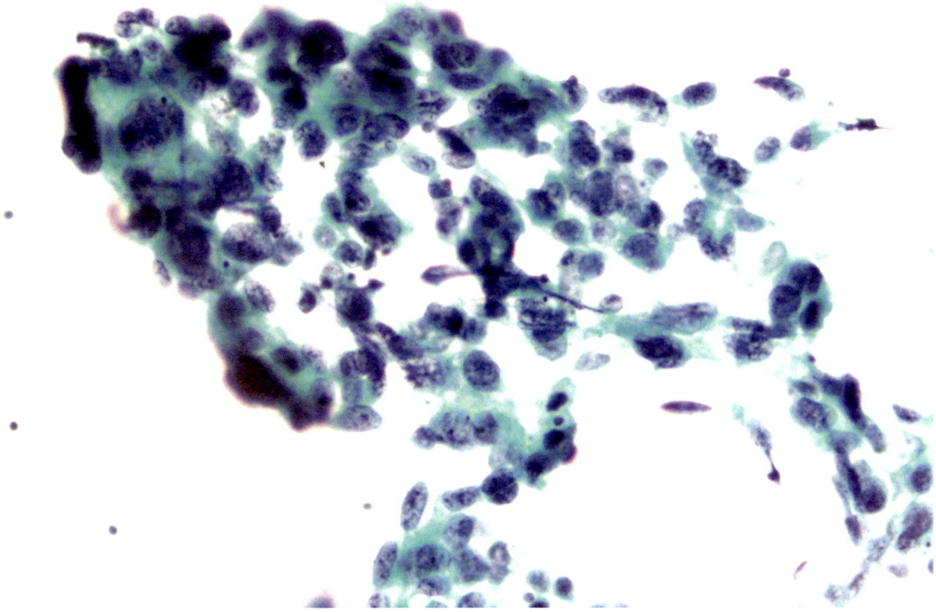

Q-38. This is a transbronchial fine-needle aspiration specimen from a 58-year-old male smoker with a left lower lobe lung mass. What is the diagnosis of this Papanicolaou preparation?

(a) Reactive bronchial cells
(b) Small cell carcinoma
(c) Squamous cell carcinoma
(d) Adenocarcinoma

Fig. 1.39

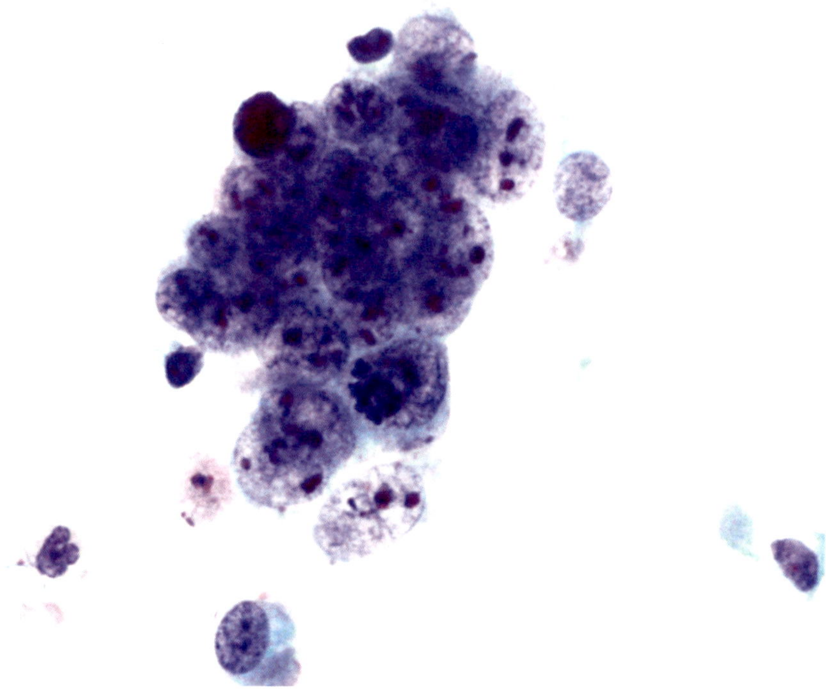

Q-39. This is a transbronchial fine-needle aspiration specimen from a 58-year-old male smoker with a left lower lobe lung mass. What is the diagnosis of this Papanicolaou preparation?
(a) Reactive bronchial cells
(b) Small cell carcinoma
(c) Squamous cell carcinoma
(d) Poorly differentiated adenocarcinoma

Fig. 1.40

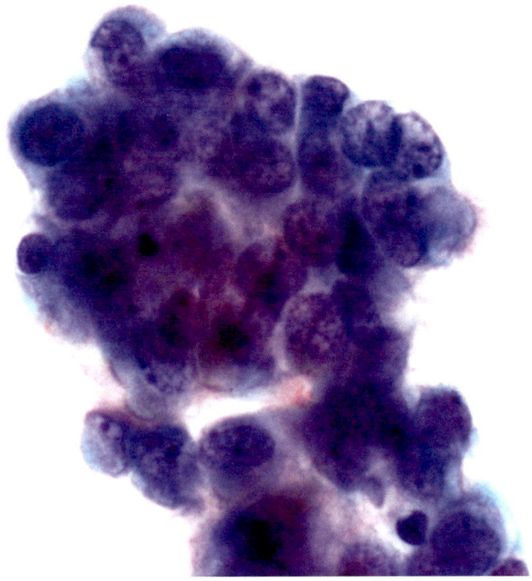

Q-40. This is a transbronchial fine-needle aspiration specimen from a 20-year-old male smoker with a left lower lobe lung lesion. What is the diagnosis of this Papanicolaou preparation?

(a) Reactive bronchial epithelial cells
(b) Small cell carcinoma
(c) Squamous cell carcinoma
(d) Well-differentiated adenocarcinoma

Fig. 1.41

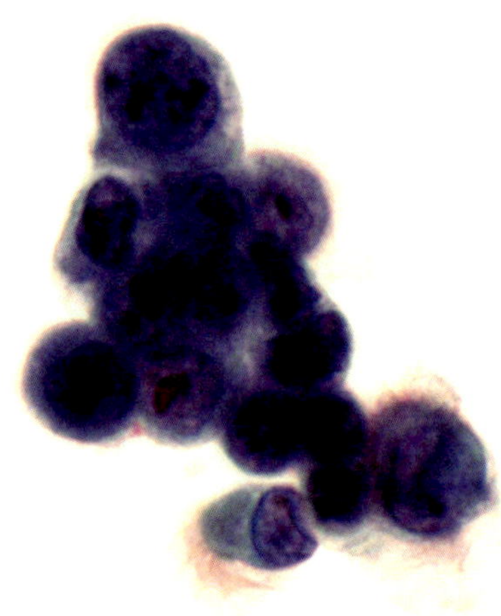

Q-41. This is a BAL specimen from a 60-year-old male smoker with lower lobe lung lesions. What is the diagnosis of this Papanicolaou preparation?
(a) Reactive bronchial epithelial cells
(b) Small cell carcinoma
(c) Squamous cell carcinoma
(d) Well-differentiated adenocarcinoma

Fig. 1.42

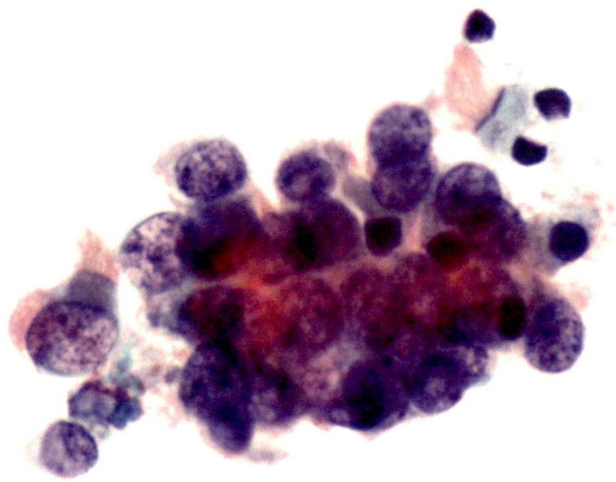

Q-42. This is a transbronchial fine-needle aspiration specimen from a 70-year-old male smoker with bilateral lung lesion. What is the diagnosis of this Papanicolaou preparation?

(a) Well-differentiated adenocarcinoma
(b) Small cell carcinoma
(c) Squamous cell carcinoma
(d) Reactive bronchial epithelial cells

Fig. 1.43

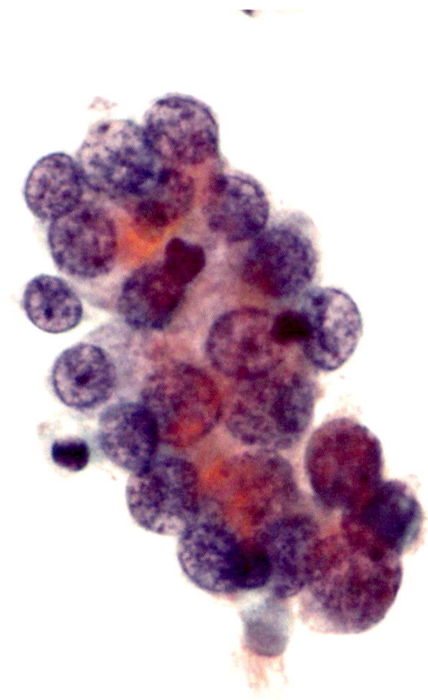

Q-43. This is a transbronchial fine-needle aspiration specimen from an 80-year-old male smoker with a hilar lung lesion. What is the diagnosis of this Papanicolaou preparation?
(a) Small cell carcinoma
(b) Reactive bronchial epithelial cells
(c) Squamous cell carcinoma
(d) Well-differentiated adenocarcinoma

Fig. 1.44

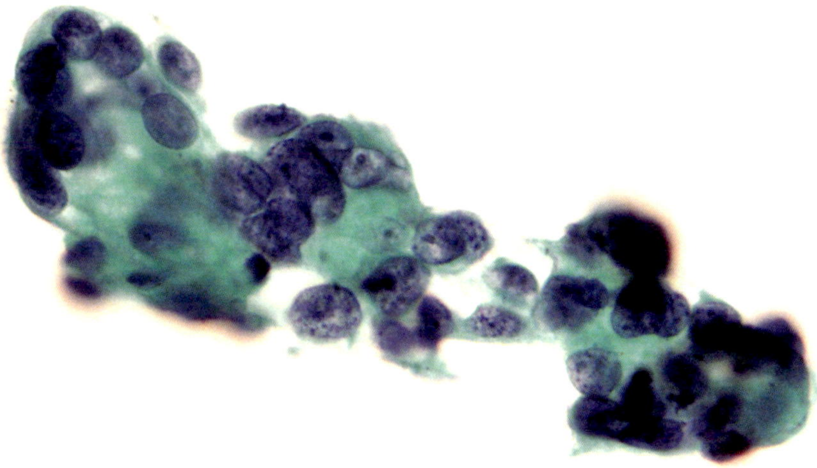

Q-44. This is a transbronchial fine-needle aspiration specimen from a 79-year-old male smoker with a peripheral right lung lesion. What is the diagnosis of this Papanicolaou preparation?

(a) Small cell carcinoma
(b) Reactive bronchial epithelial cells
(c) Squamous cell carcinoma
(d) Adenocarcinoma

Fig. 1.45

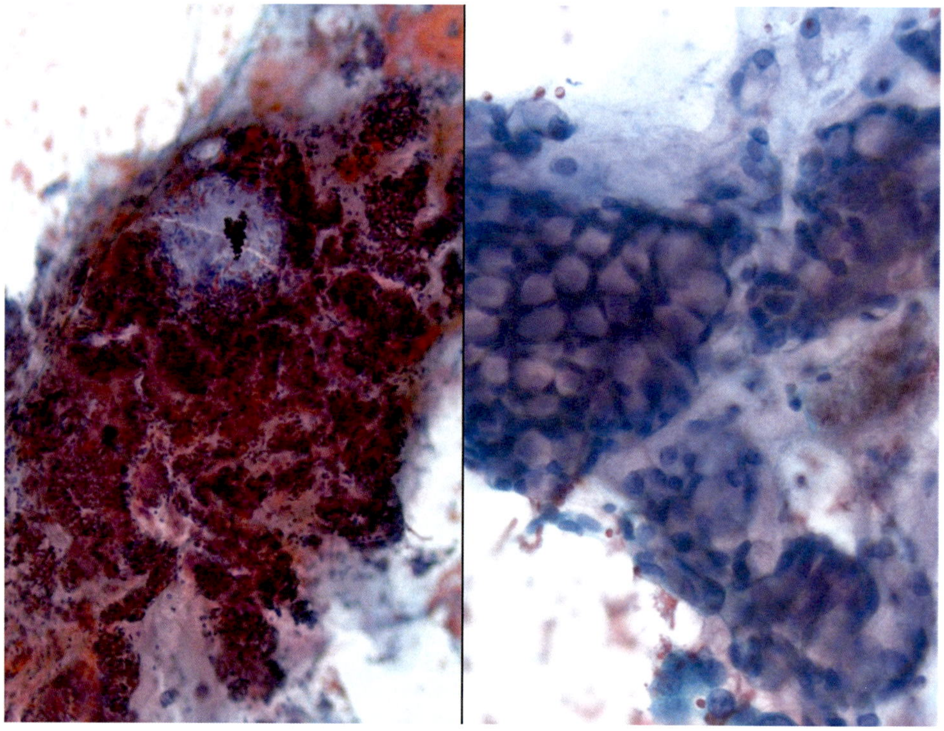

Q-45. What is the diagnosis of this Papanicolaou preparation from the endobronchial ultrasound (EBUS) specimen?

(a) Small cell carcinoma
(b) Reactive bronchial epithelial cells
(c) Goblet cell hyperplasia
(d) Adenocarcinoma

Fig. 1.46

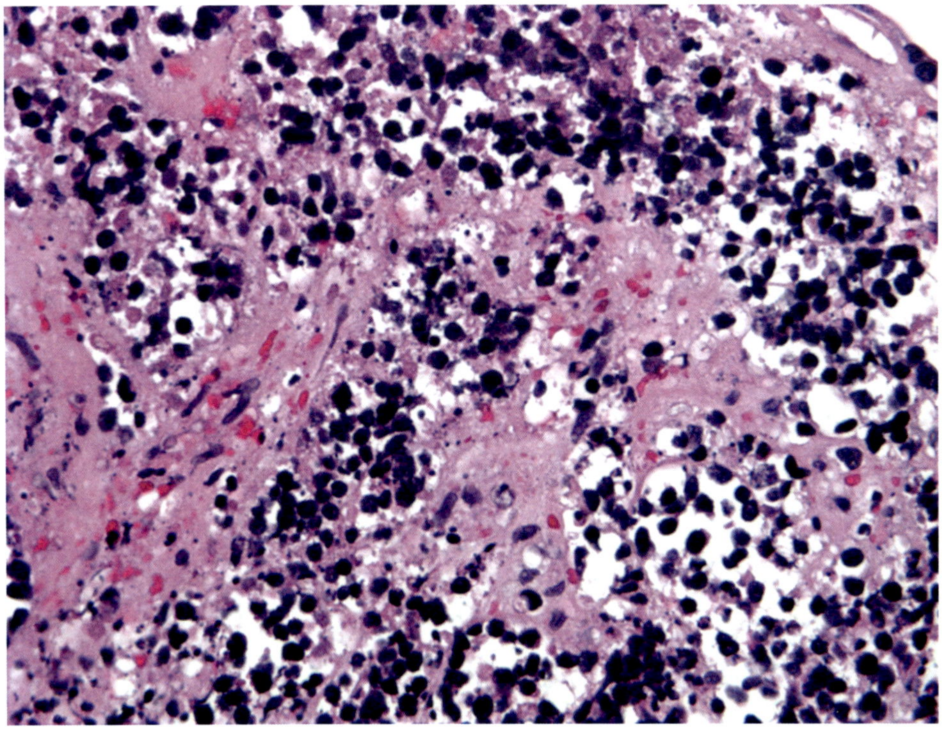

Q-46. This is a transbronchial fine-needle aspiration specimen from a 69-year-old male smoker with a centrally located lung mass. What is the diagnosis of this cell block preparation?

(a) Small cell carcinoma
(b) Reactive bronchial epithelial cells
(c) Reactive lymphocytes
(d) Adenocarcinoma

Fig. 1.47

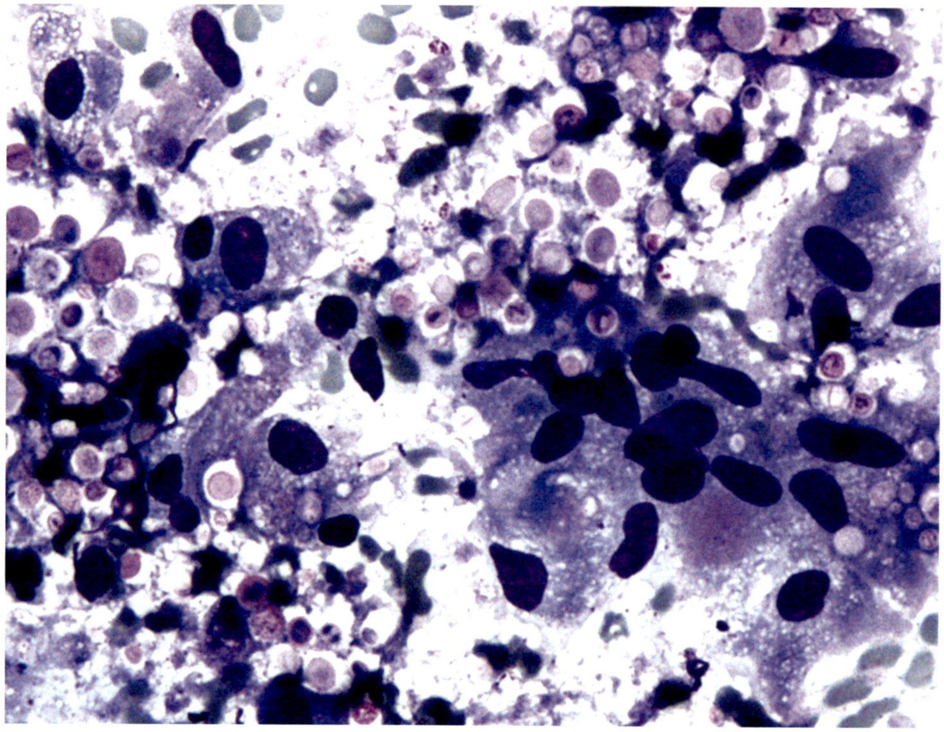

Q-47. This is a BAL specimen from a 32-year-old male smoker with HIV-positive serum test and lung lesions. What is the diagnosis of this Papanicolaou preparation?

(a) Reactive goblet cells
(b) Histoplasmosis
(c) Cryptococcosis
(d) Blastomycosis

Fig. 1.48

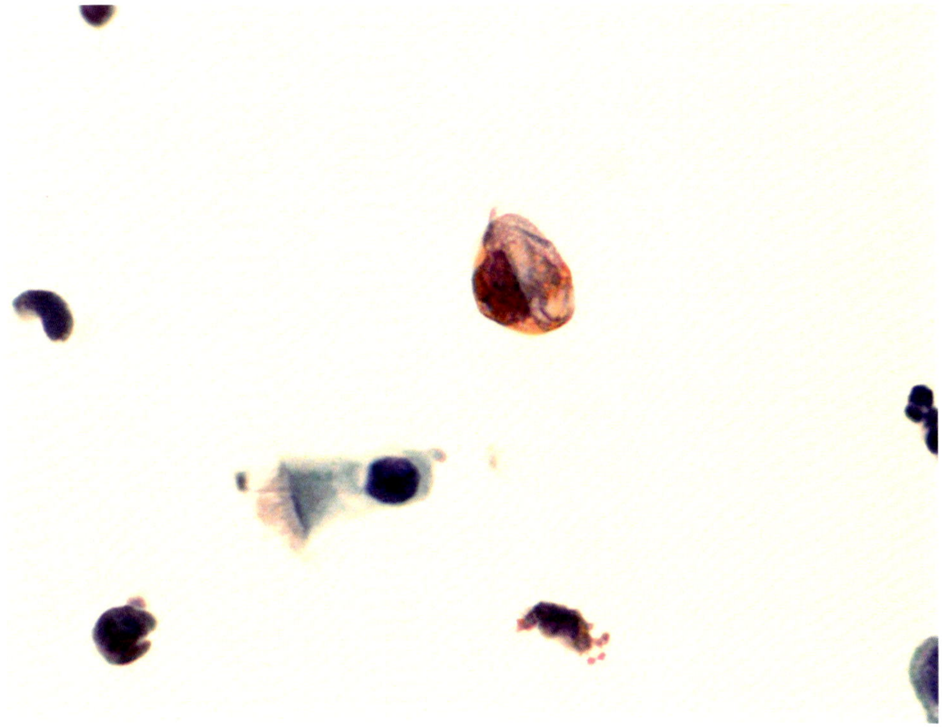

Q-48. This is a BAL specimen from a 25-year-old male without clinical history of malignancy. What is the diagnosis of this large non-ciliated cell?
(a) Signet ring cell carcinoma
(b) Reactive bronchial epithelial cells
(c) Degenerated alveolar macrophages
(d) Adenocarcinoma

Fig. 1.49

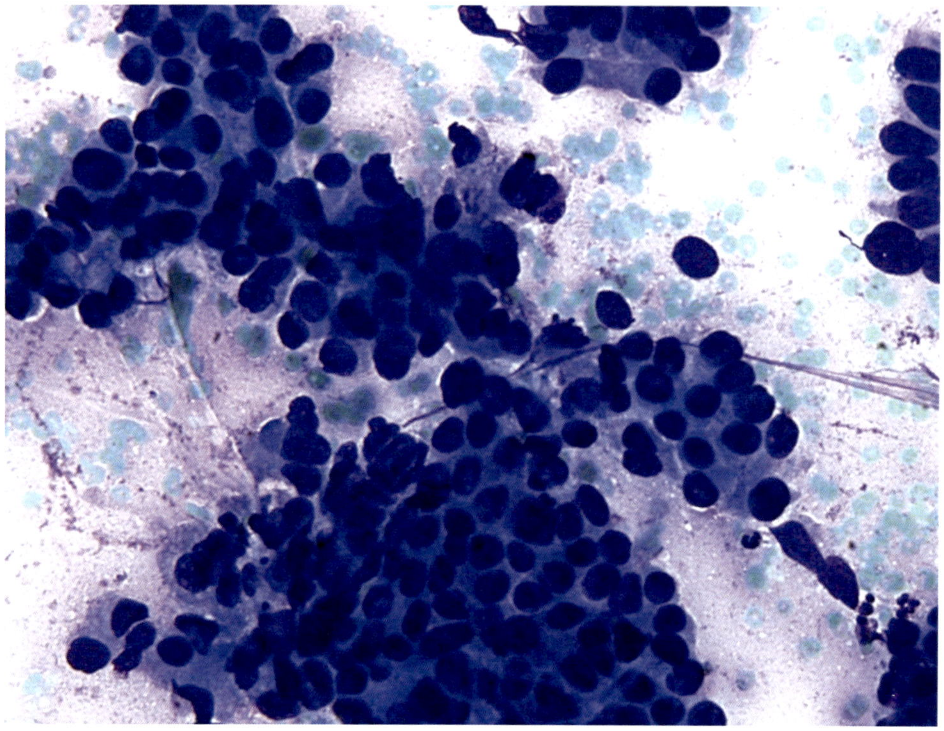

Q-49. This is a transbronchial fine-needle aspiration specimen from an 80-year-old male smoker with a peripheral lung lesion. What is the diagnosis of this Diff-Quik preparation?

(a) Small cell carcinoma
(b) Reactive bronchial epithelial cells
(c) Squamous cell carcinoma
(d) Adenocarcinoma

Fig. 1.50

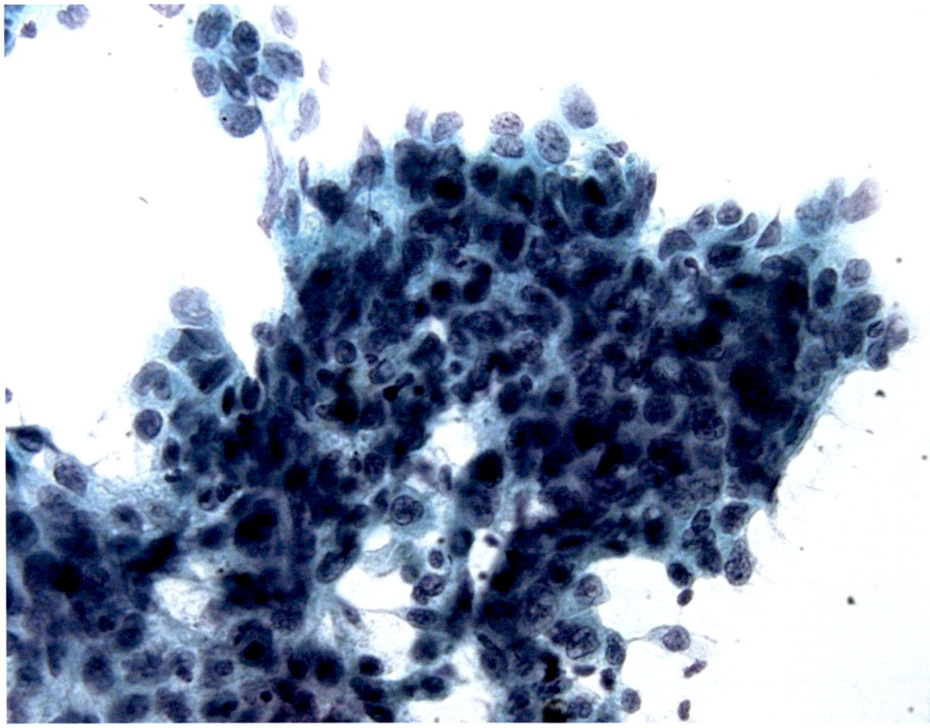

Q-50. This is a transbronchial fine-needle aspiration from an 84-year-old male smoker with a large hilar mass. What is the diagnosis of this Papanicolaou preparation?

(a) Reactive bronchial epithelium
(b) Adenocarcinoma
(c) Squamous cell carcinoma
(d) Small cell carcinoma

Fig. 1.51

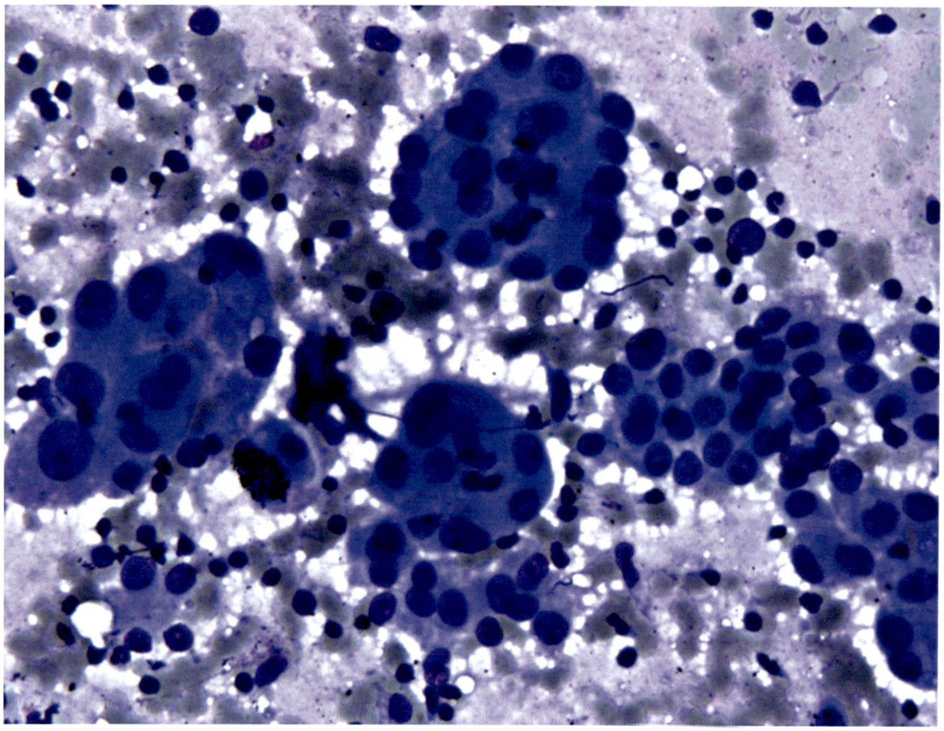

Q-51. What is the diagnosis of this Diff-Quik preparation?
(a) Reactive bronchial epithelium
(b) Adenocarcinoma
(c) Poorly differentiated squamous cell carcinoma
(d) Small cell carcinoma

Fig. 1.52

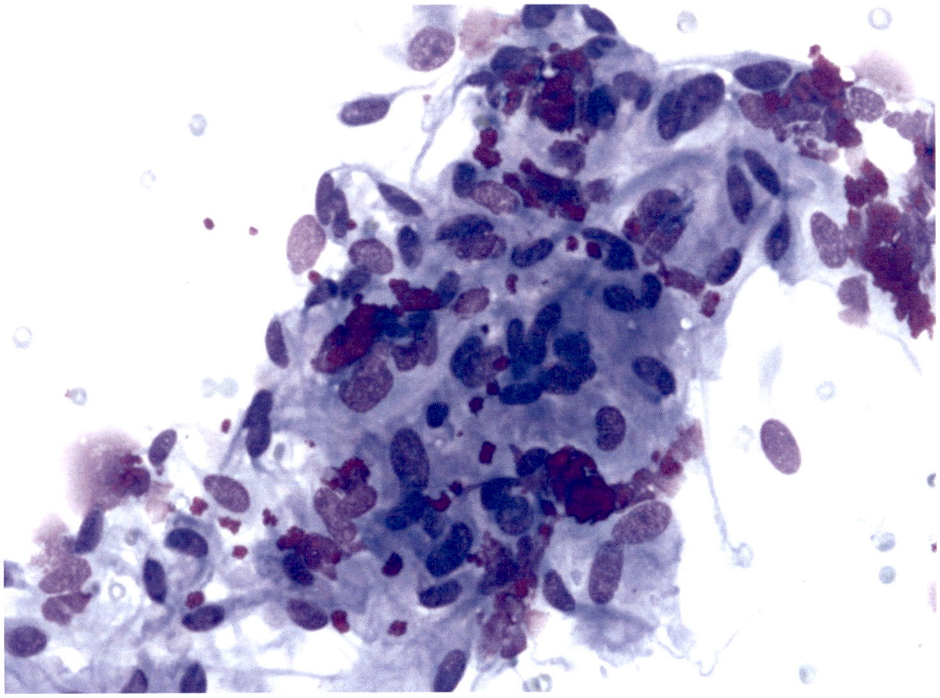

Q-52. This is a transbronchial fine-needle aspiration from a 48-year-old African American female with bilateral lung infiltration. What is the diagnosis of this Diff-Quik preparation?
(a) Reactive lymphocytes
(b) Adenocarcinoma
(c) Poorly differentiated squamous cell carcinoma
(d) Granulomatous inflammation

Fig. 1.53

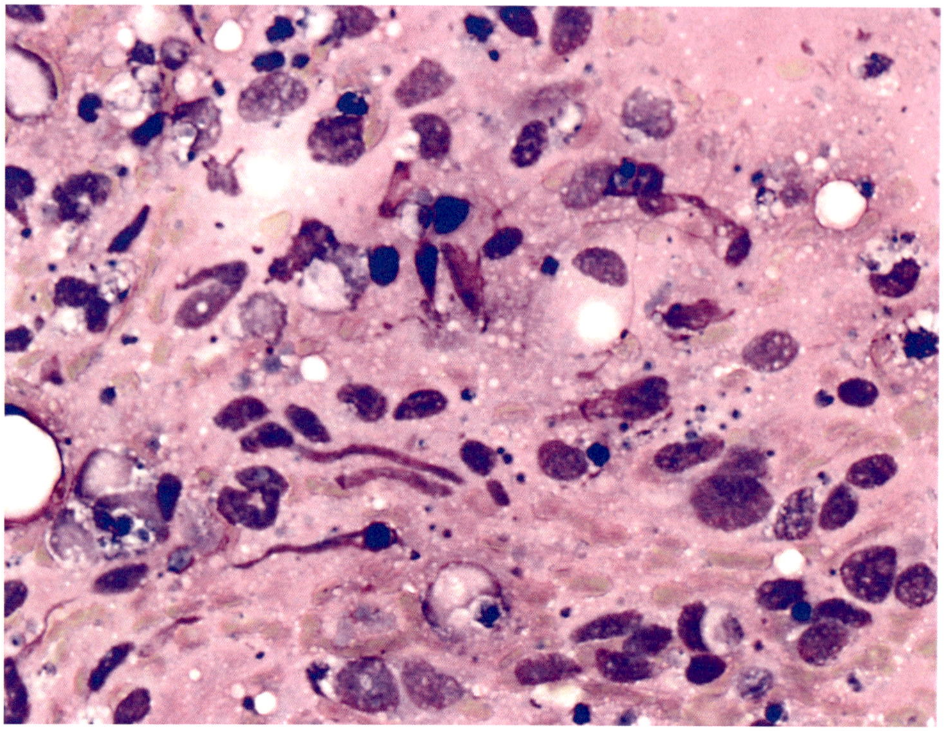

Q-53. This is a transbronchial fine-needle aspiration from a 55-year-old male with a clinical history of synovial sarcoma, who developed bilateral lung infiltrations. What is the diagnosis of this Diff-Quik preparation?

(a) Reactive lymphocytes
(b) Adenocarcinoma
(c) Poorly differentiated squamous cell carcinoma
(d) Metastatic synovial sarcoma

Fig. 1.54

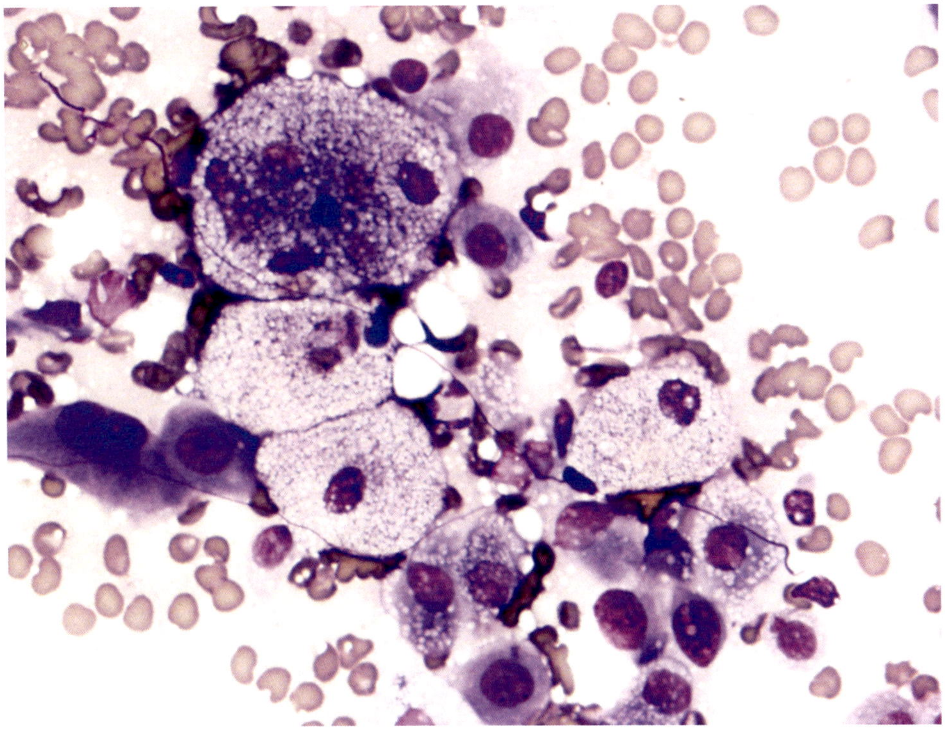

Q-54. What is the diagnosis of this Diff-Quik smear?
(a) Goblet cells
(b) Adenocarcinoma
(c) Metastatic renal cell carcinoma
(d) Bronchioalveolar macrophages

Fig. 1.55

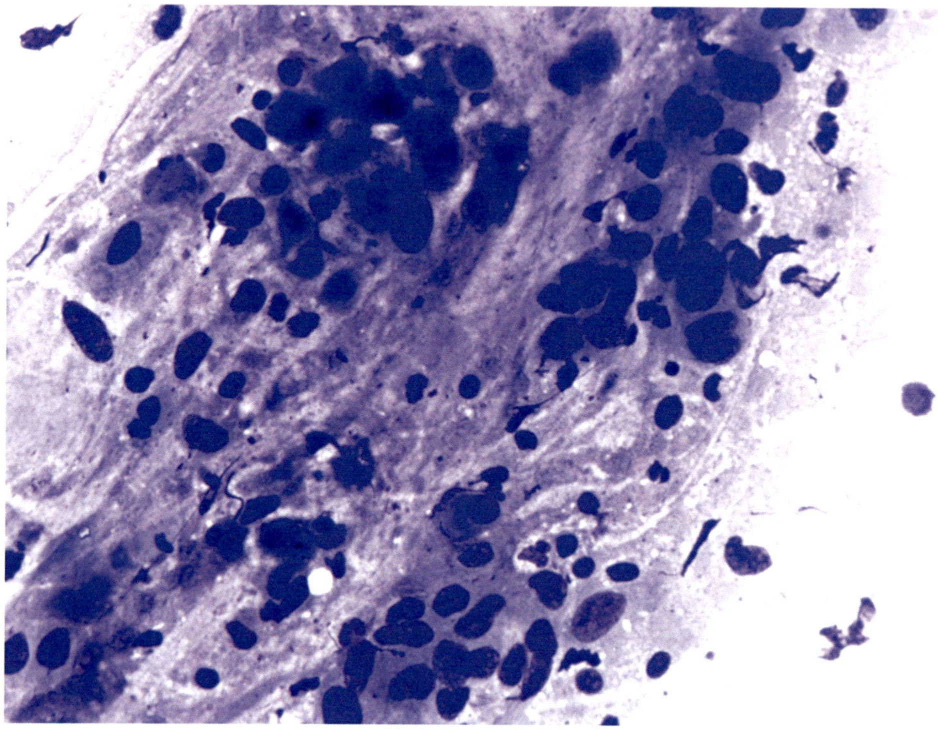

Q-55. This is an on-site evaluation of a transbronchial fine-needle aspiration from a 74-year-old male smoker with a large left upper lung mass. What is the diagnosis of this Diff-Quik preparation?
(a) Reactive bronchial epithelium
(b) Adenocarcinoma
(c) Poorly differentiated squamous cell carcinoma
(d) Small cell carcinoma

Fig. 1.56

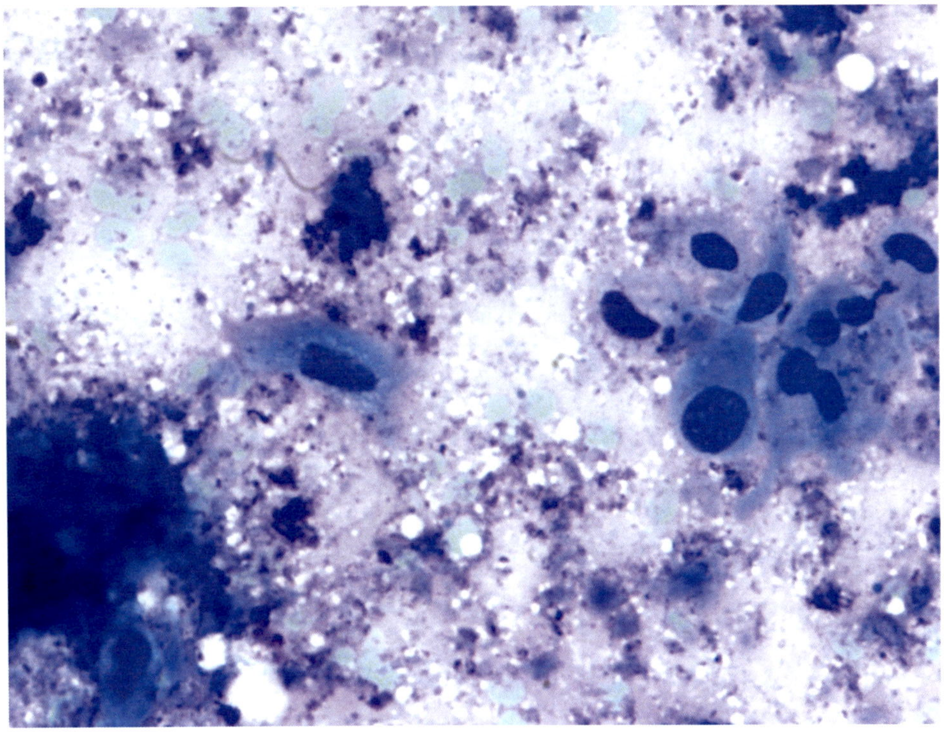

Q-56. What is the diagnosis of this Diff-Quik smear?
(a) Goblet cells
(b) Adenocarcinoma
(c) Squamous cell carcinoma
(d) Bronchioalveolar macrophages

Fig. 1.57

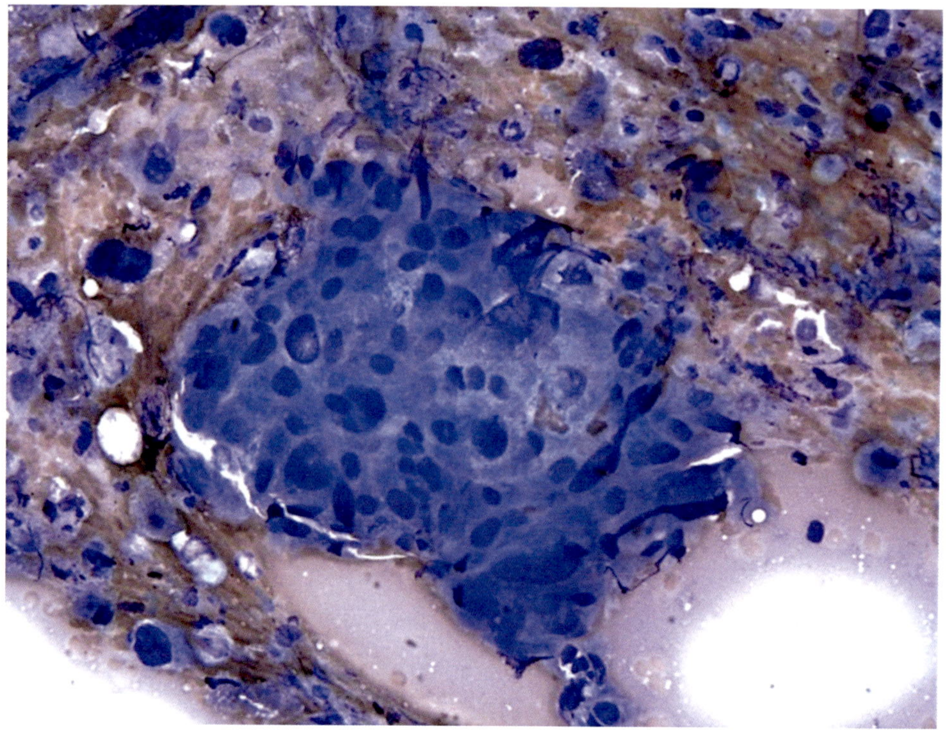

Q-57. What is the diagnosis of this Diff-Quik smear?
(a) Granuloma
(b) Adenocarcinoma
(c) Squamous cell carcinoma
(d) Bronchioalveolar macrophages

Fig. 1.58

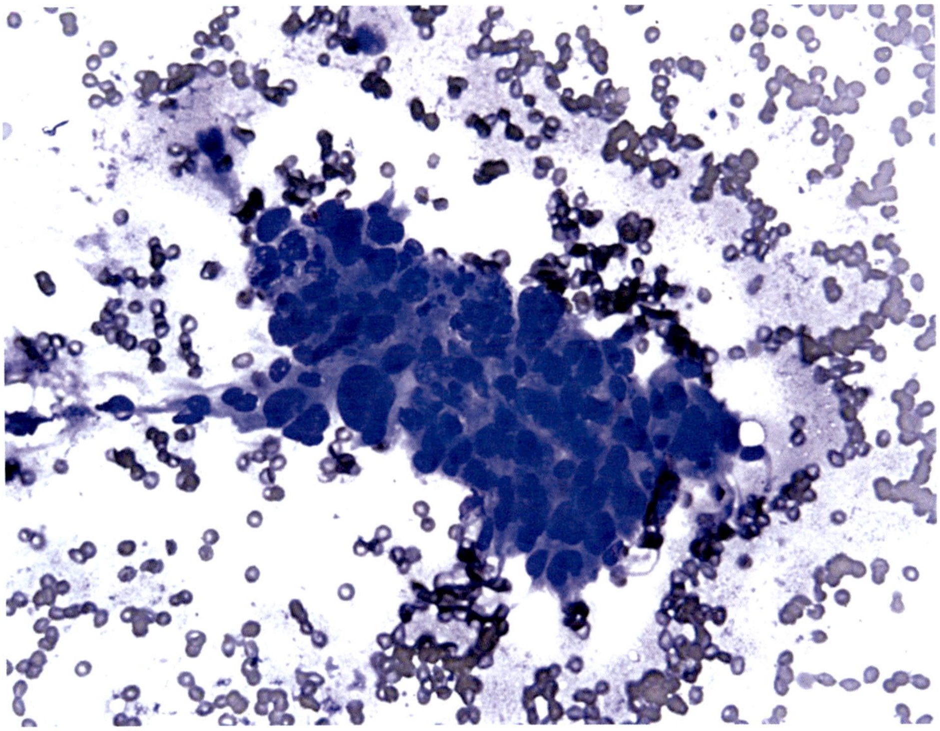

Q-58. What is the diagnosis of this Diff-Quik smear?
(a) Granuloma
(b) Adenocarcinoma
(c) Squamous cell carcinoma
(d) Bronchial reserve cell hyperplasia

Fig. 1.59

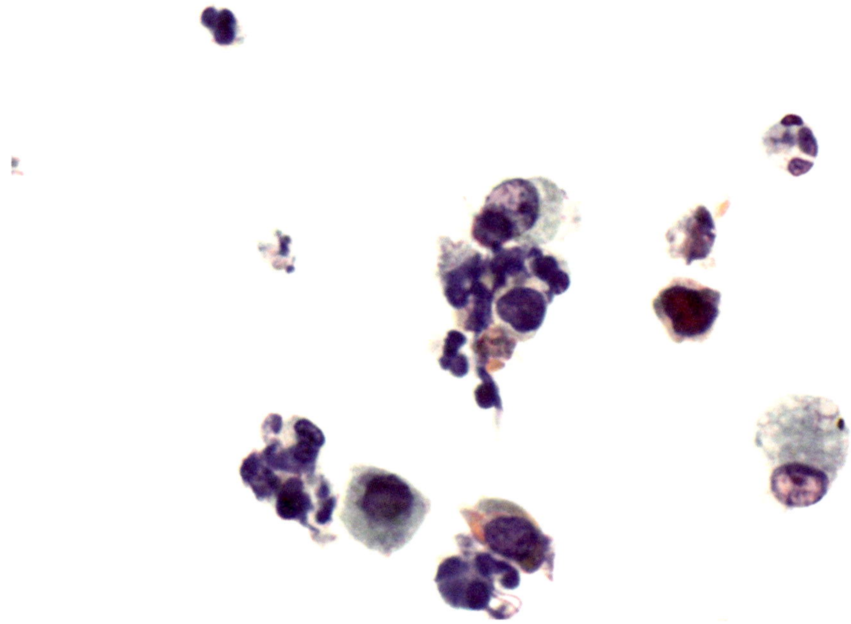

Q-59. This is a bronchoscopic washing from a 25-year-old female with chronic cough. What is the diagnosis?
(a) Granuloma
(b) Adenocarcinoma
(c) Squamous cell carcinoma
(d) Degenerated bronchioalveolar macrophages

Fig. 1.60

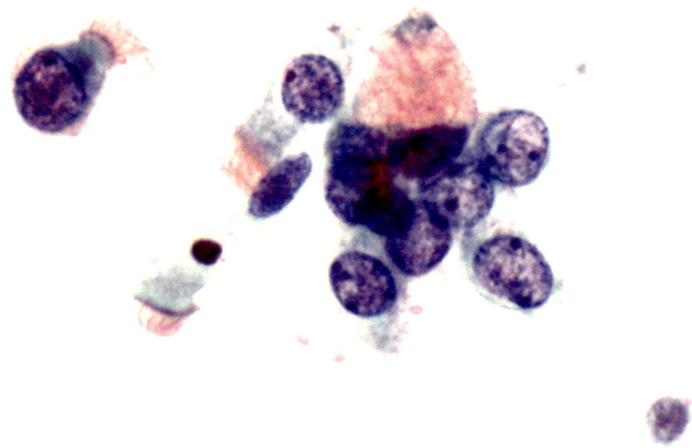

Q-60. This is a bronchoscopic washing from an 18-year-old female with clinical history of cystic fibrosis. What is the diagnosis?
(a) Goblet cell
(b) Adenocarcinoma
(c) Signet ring cell carcinoma
(d) Small cell carcinoma

Fig. 1.61

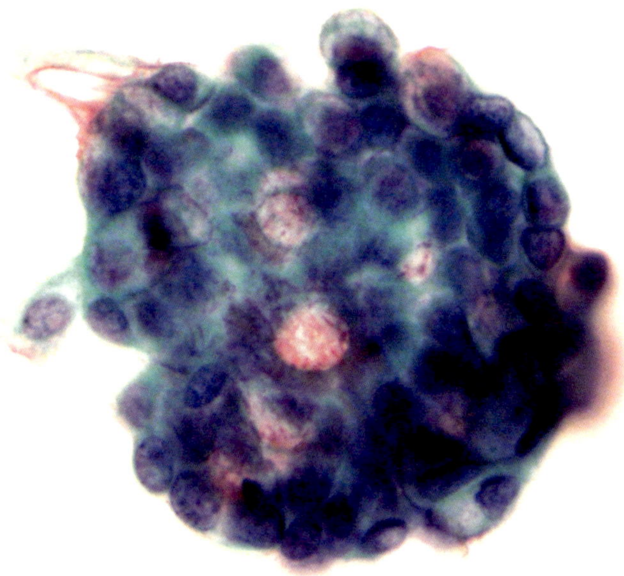

Q-61. This is a transbronchial fine-needle aspiration from a 35-year-old African American female with bilateral lung infiltration. What is the diagnosis of this Papanicolaou preparation?

(a) Small cell carcinoma
(b) Adenocarcinoma
(c) Granuloma
(d) Goblet cell hyperplasia

Fig. 1.62

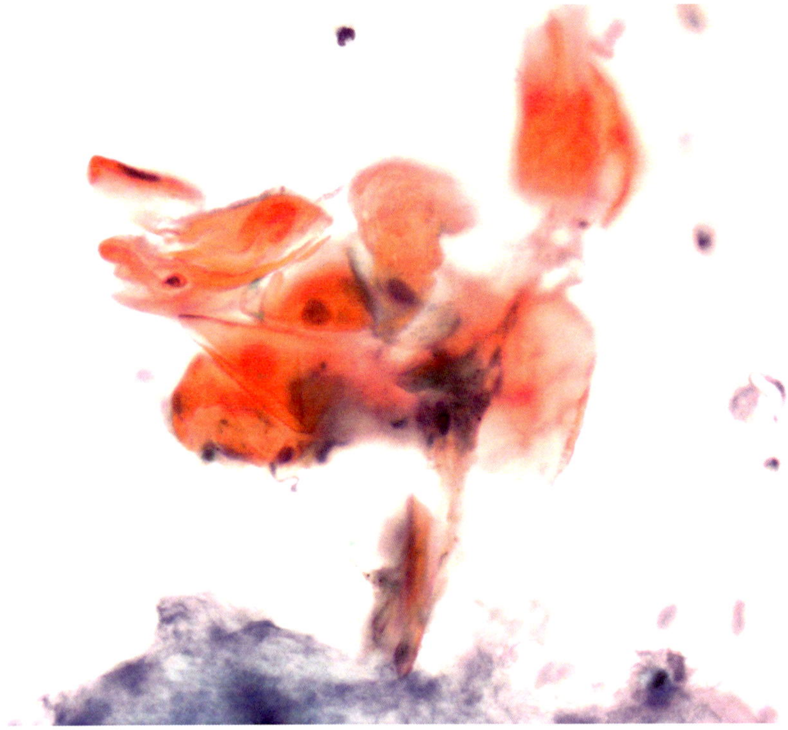

Q-62. This is a sputum specimen from a 59-year-old smoker with lung lesions. What is the diagnosis?
(a) Squamous cells with reactive atypia
(b) Adenocarcinoma
(c) Squamous cell carcinoma
(d) Bronchial goblet cell hyperplasia

Fig. 1.63

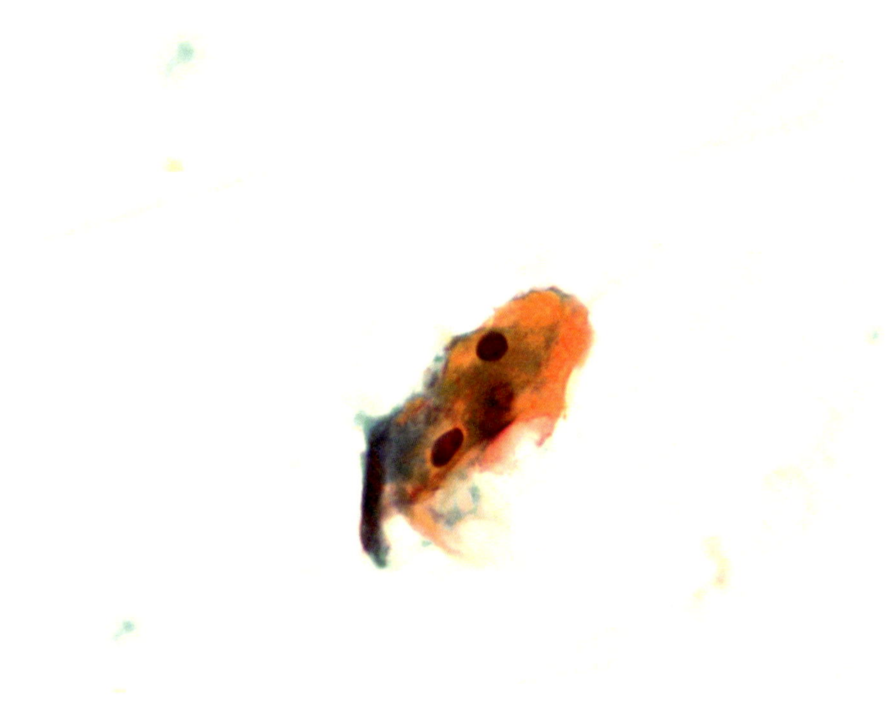

Q-63. This is a transbronchial fine-needle aspiration from a 62-year-old smoker with lung lesions. What is the diagnosis?
(a) Adenocarcinoma
(b) Reactive squamous cells
(c) Squamous cell carcinoma
(d) Bronchial macrophages

Fig. 1.64

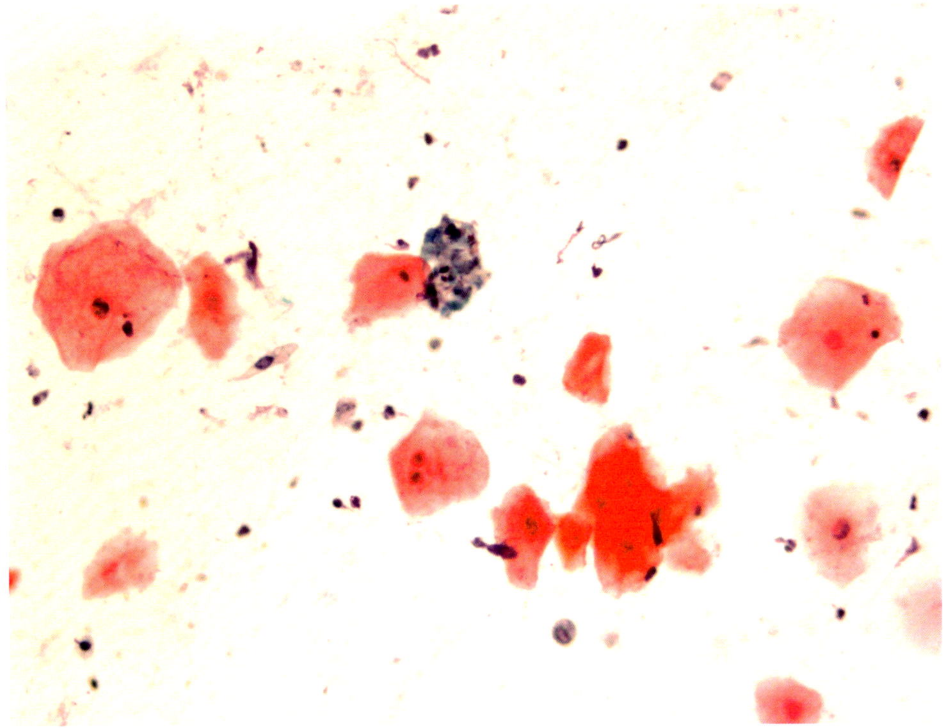

Q-64. This is a sputum specimen from a 79-year-old smoker with lung lesions. What is the diagnosis?
(a) Non-diagnostic specimen
(b) Reactive squamous cells
(c) Squamous cell carcinoma
(d) Bronchial macrophages

Fig. 1.65

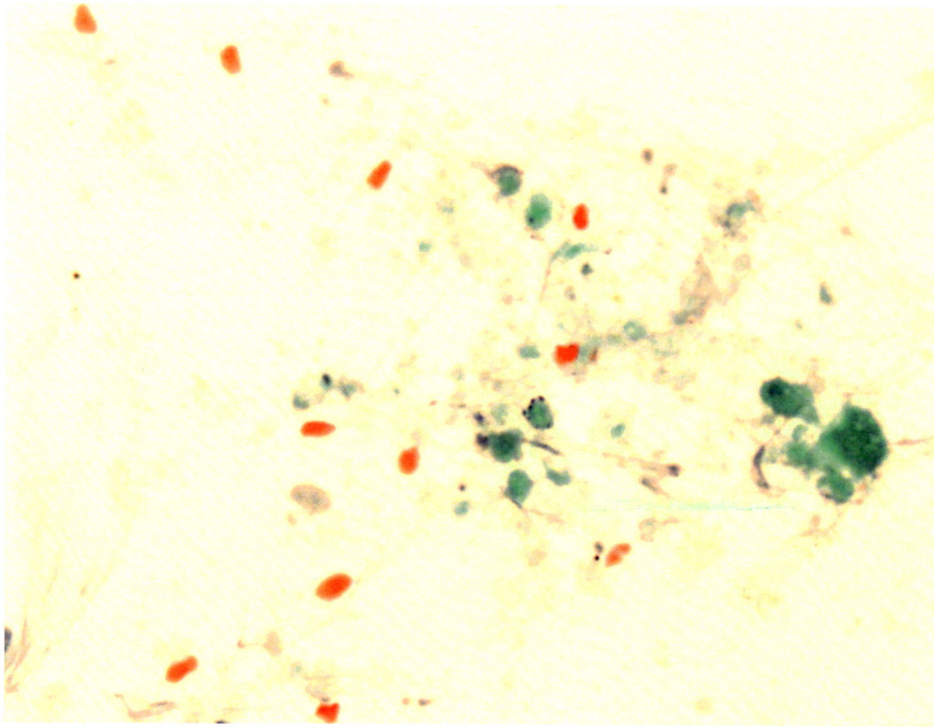

Q-65. This is a transbronchial fine-needle aspiration from a 67-year-old smoker with a large lung mass, a squamous cell carcinoma is clinically suspected. What is the best interpretation of this slide?
(a) Metaplastic squamous cells
(b) Reactive squamous cells
(c) Karetin debris and it is necessary to repeat the biopsy
(d) Squamous cell carcinoma

Fig. 1.66

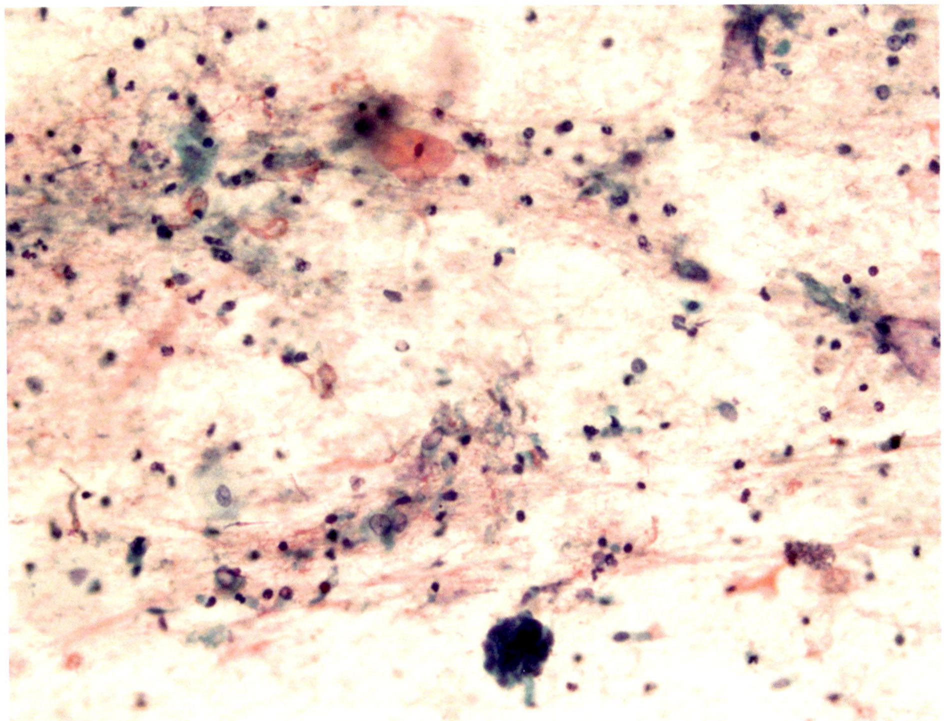

Q-66. This is a BAL specimen from a 45-year-old smoker with lung lesions. What is the diagnosis?
(a) Non-diagnostic specimen
(b) Adenocarcinoma
(c) Squamous cell carcinoma
(d) Reactive bronchial epithelium

Fig. 1.67

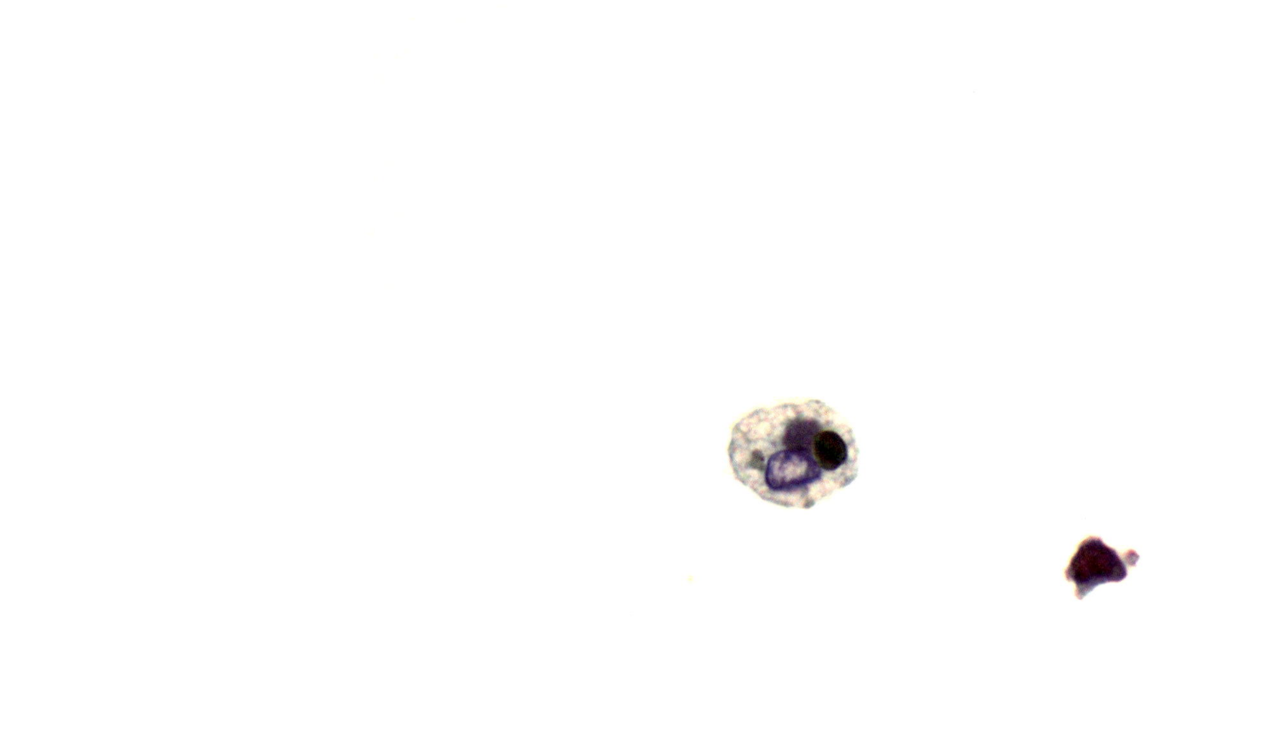

Q-67. This is a BAL specimen from a 45-year-old smoker with lung lesions. What is the diagnosis?
(a) Signet ring cell carcinoma
(b) Adenocarcinoma
(c) Bronchioalveolar macrophages
(d) Reactive bronchial epithelium

Fig. 1.68

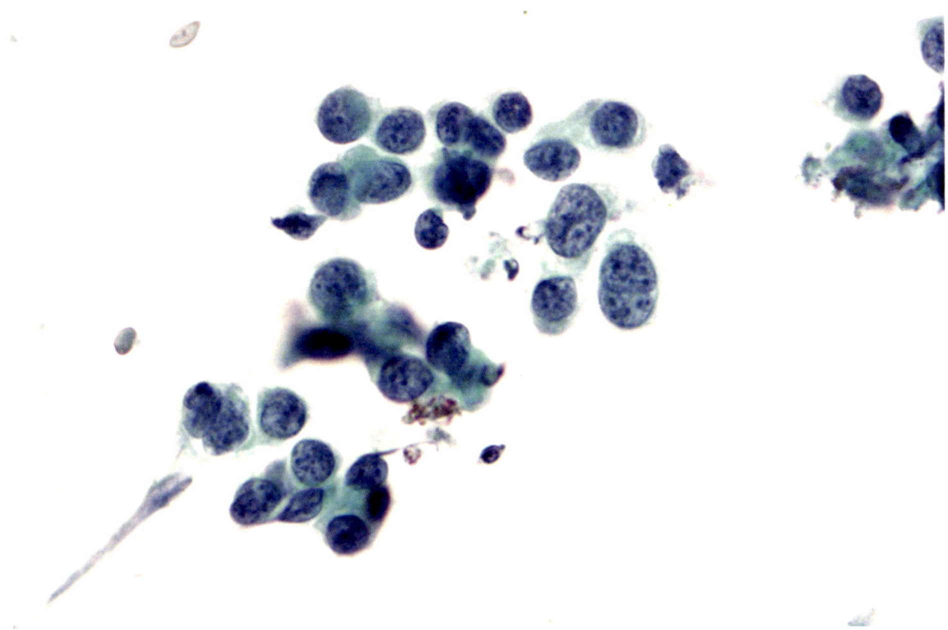

Q-68. This is a BAL specimen from a 73-year-old smoker with lung lesions. What is the diagnosis?
(a) Squamous cell carcinoma
(b) Adenocarcinoma
(c) Bronchioalveolar macrophages
(d) Reactive bronchial epithelium

Fig. 1.69

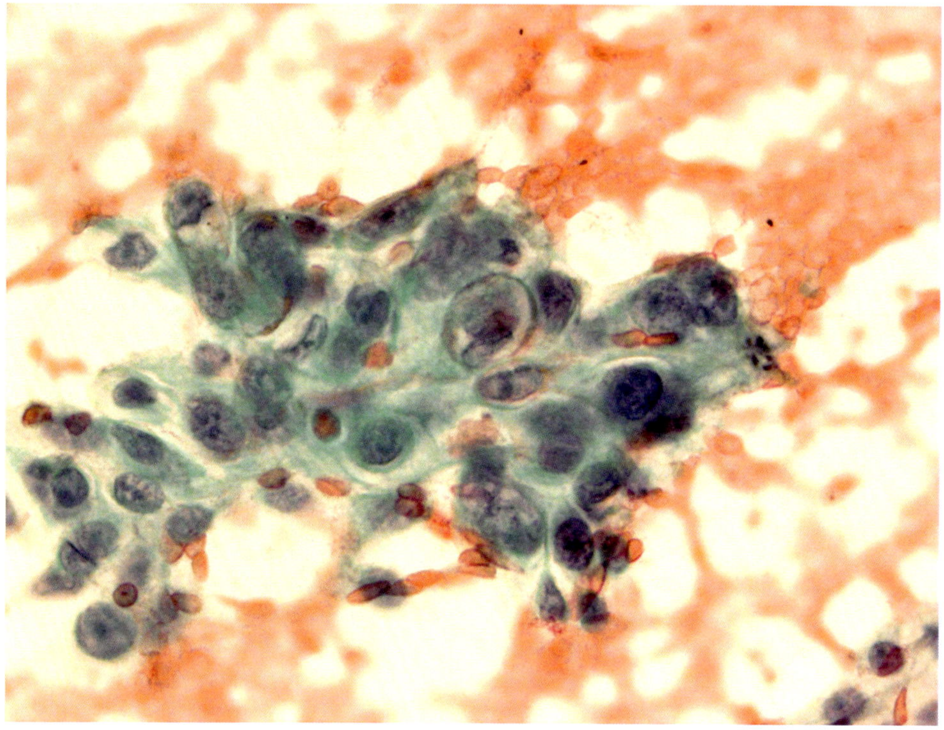

Q-69. This is a transbronchial fine need aspiration specimen from a 70-year-old smoker with a lung lesion. What is the diagnosis?
(a) Poorly differentiated squamous cell carcinoma
(b) Adenocarcinoma
(c) Bronchioalveolar macrophages
(d) Reactive bronchial epithelium

Fig. 1.70

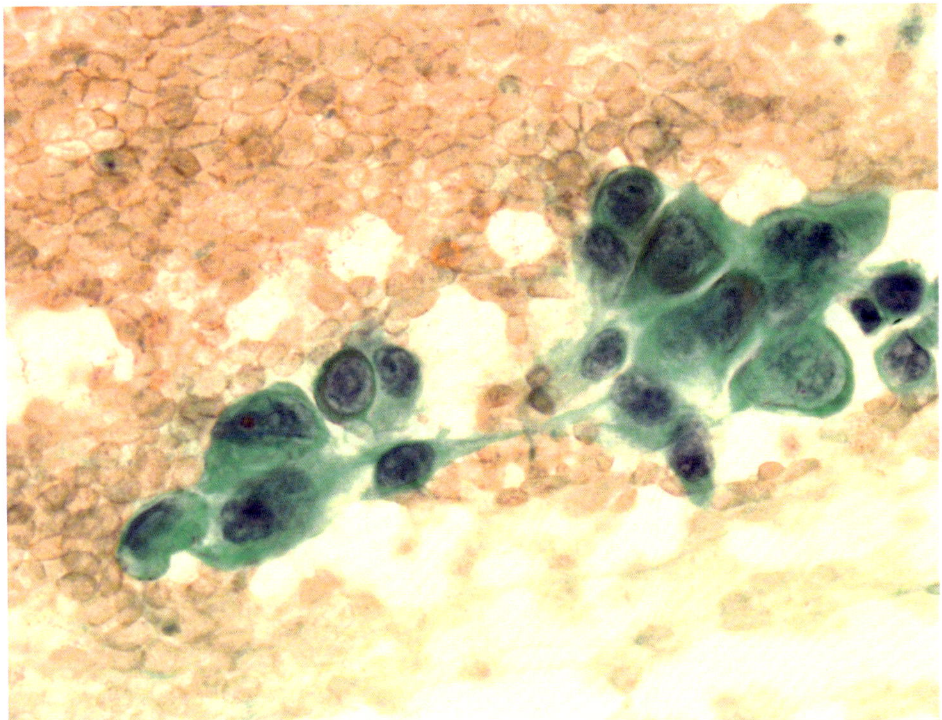

Q-70. What is the diagnosis of this Papanicolaou preparation?
(a) Poorly differentiated squamous cell carcinoma
(b) Adenocarcinoma
(c) Bronchioalveolar macrophages
(d) Reactive bronchial epithelium

Fig. 1.71

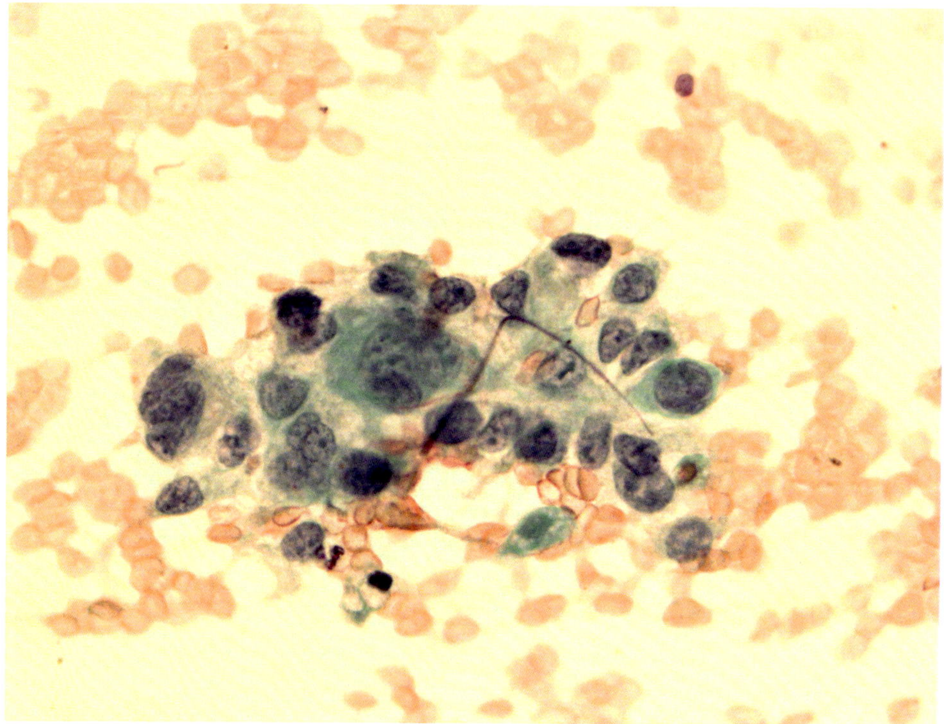

Q-71. What is the diagnosis of this Papanicolaou preparation?
(a) Poorly differentiated squamous cell carcinoma
(b) Adenocarcinoma
(c) Bronchioalveolar macrophages
(d) Reactive bronchial epithelium

Fig. 1.72

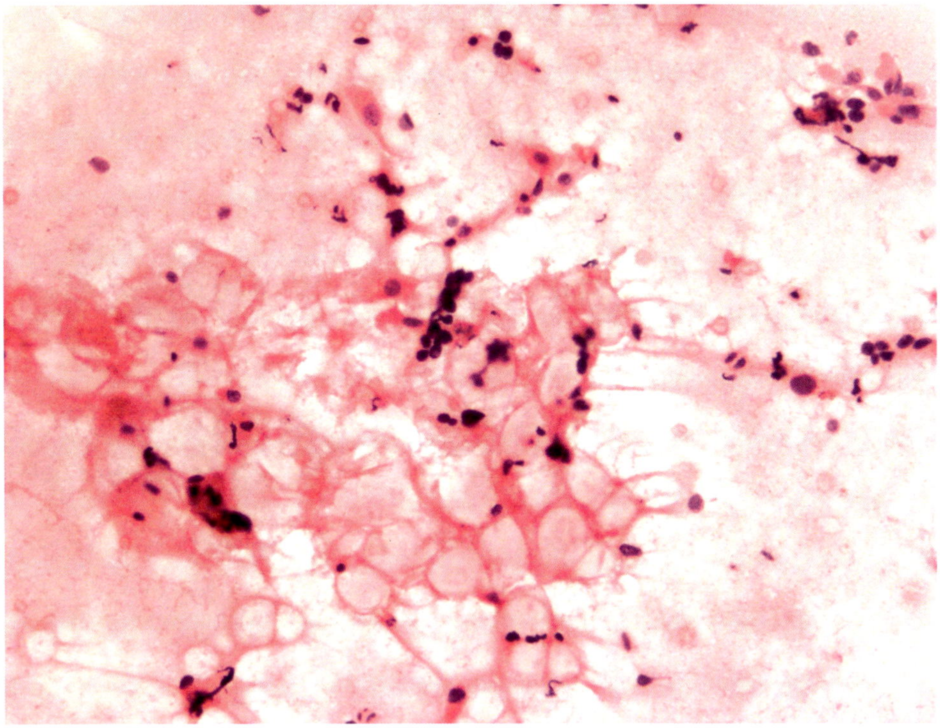

Q-72. What is the diagnosis of this BAL specimen?
(a) Vegetable cells
(b) Goblet cells
(c) Reactive bronchial cells and mucin vacuole
(d) Adenocarcinoma

Fig. 1.73

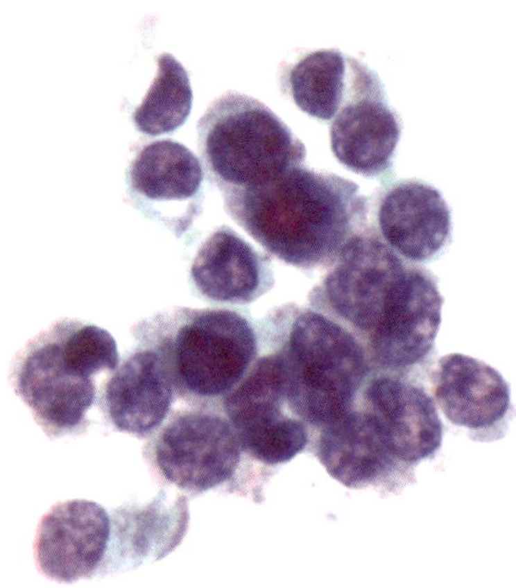

Q-73. What is the diagnosis of this BAL specimen?

(a) Small cell carcinoma
(b) Goblet cells
(c) Reactive bronchial epithelial cells
(d) Adenocarcinoma

Fig. 1.74

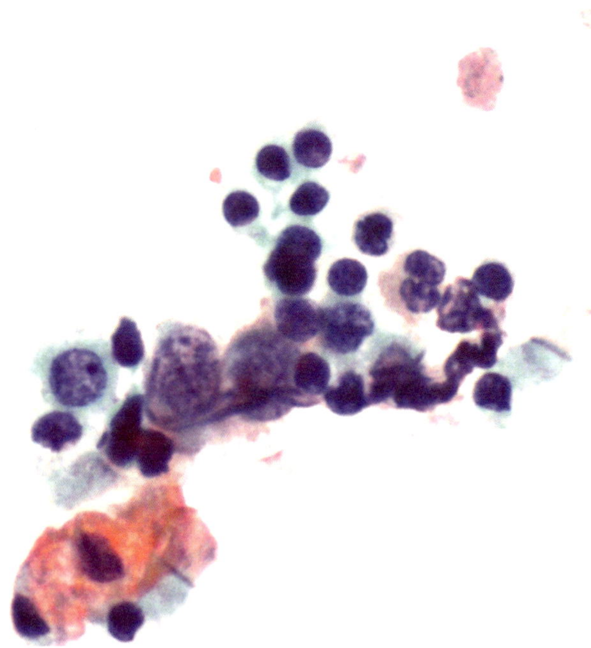

Q-74. What are these small hyperchromatic cells in this BAL specimen?
(a) Vegetable cells
(b) Lymphocytes
(c) Small cell carcinoma
(d) Bronchial reserve cells

Fig. 1.75

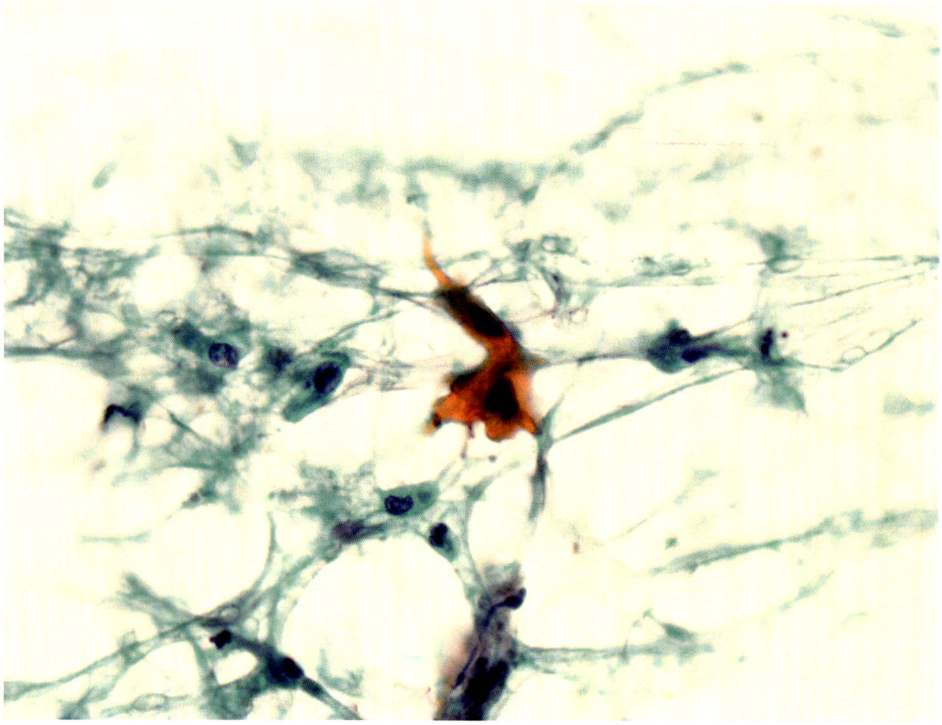

Q-75. What is the diagnosis of this sputum specimen?

(a) Reactive squamous cells
(b) Squamous cell carcinoma
(c) Reactive bronchial cells
(d) Adenocarcinoma

Fig. 1.76

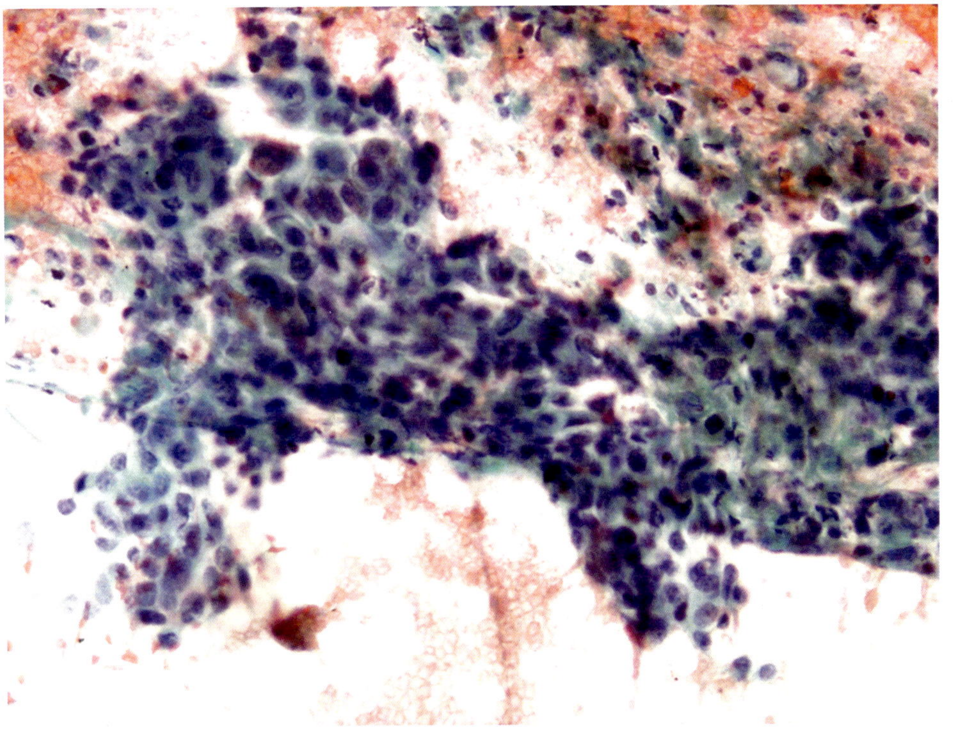

Q-76. This is a transbronchial fine need aspiration specimen from a 60-year-old smoker with a lung lesion. What is the diagnosis?
(a) Squamous cell carcinoma
(b) Adenocarcinoma
(c) Bronchioalveolar macrophages
(d) Reactive bronchial epithelium

Fig. 1.77

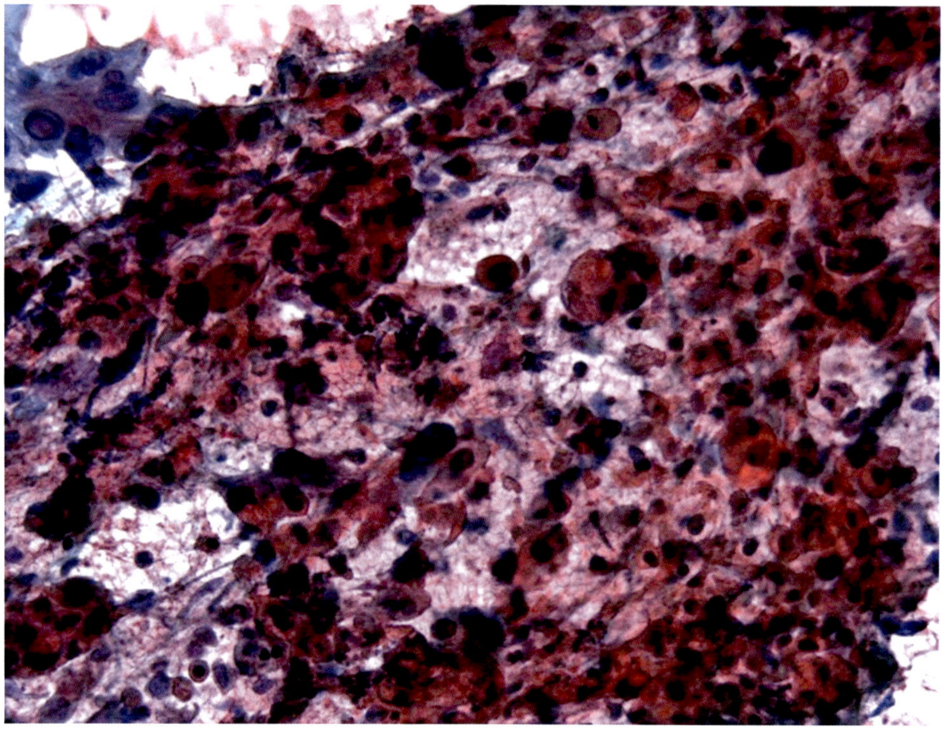

Q-77. This is a transbronchial fine need aspiration specimen from a 48-year-old smoker with a lung lesion. What is the diagnosis?
(a) Squamous cell carcinoma
(b) Adenocarcinoma
(c) Bronchioalveolar macrophages
(d) Reactive squamous cells

Fig. 1.78

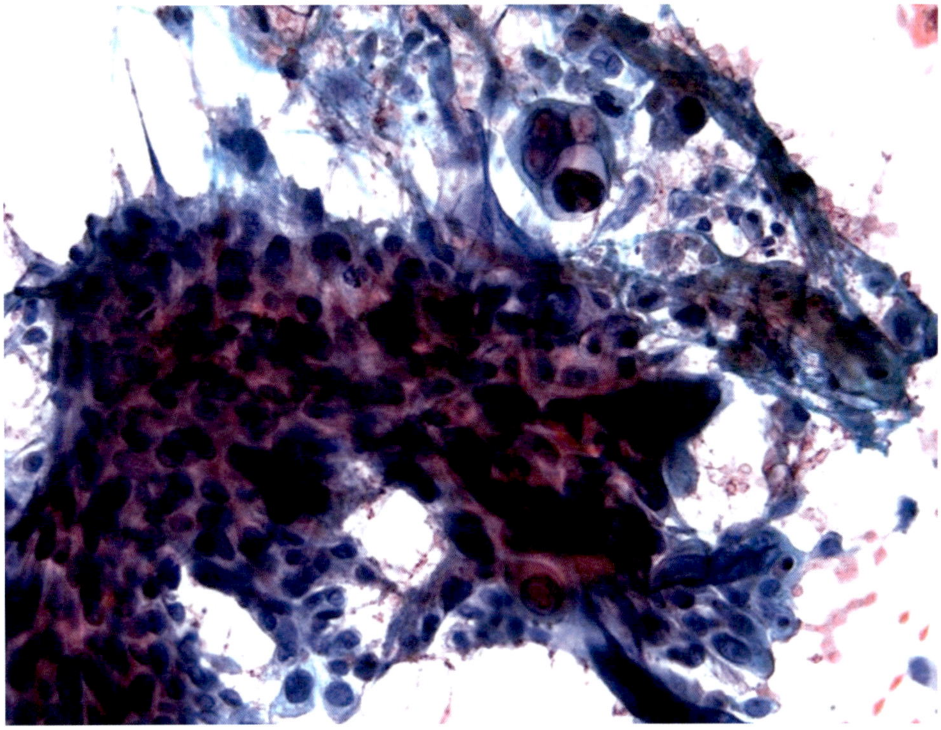

Q-78. This is a transbronchial fine need aspiration specimen from a 71-year-old smoker with a lung lesion. What is the diagnosis?
(a) Reactive squamous cells
(b) Adenocarcinoma
(c) Bronchioalveolar macrophages
(d) Squamous cell carcinoma

Fig. 1.79

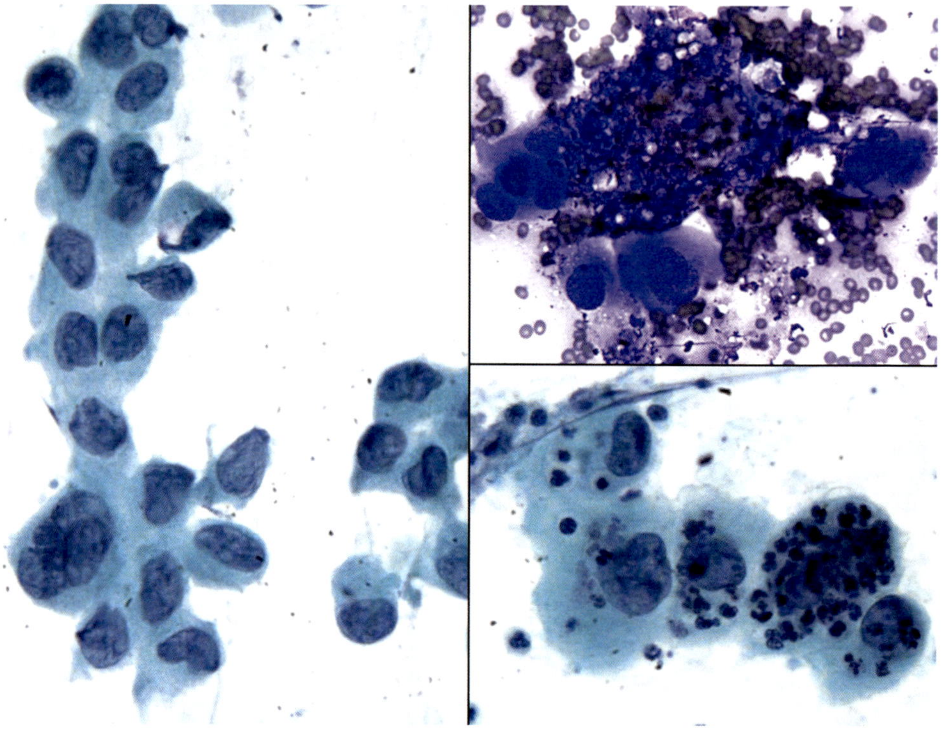

Q-79. This is a transbronchial fine need aspiration specimen from a 71-year-old smoker with a lung lesion. What is the diagnosis?
(a) Reactive squamous cells
(b) Adenocarcinoma
(c) Bronchioalveolar macrophages
(d) Poorly differentiated squamous cell carcinoma

Fig. 1.80

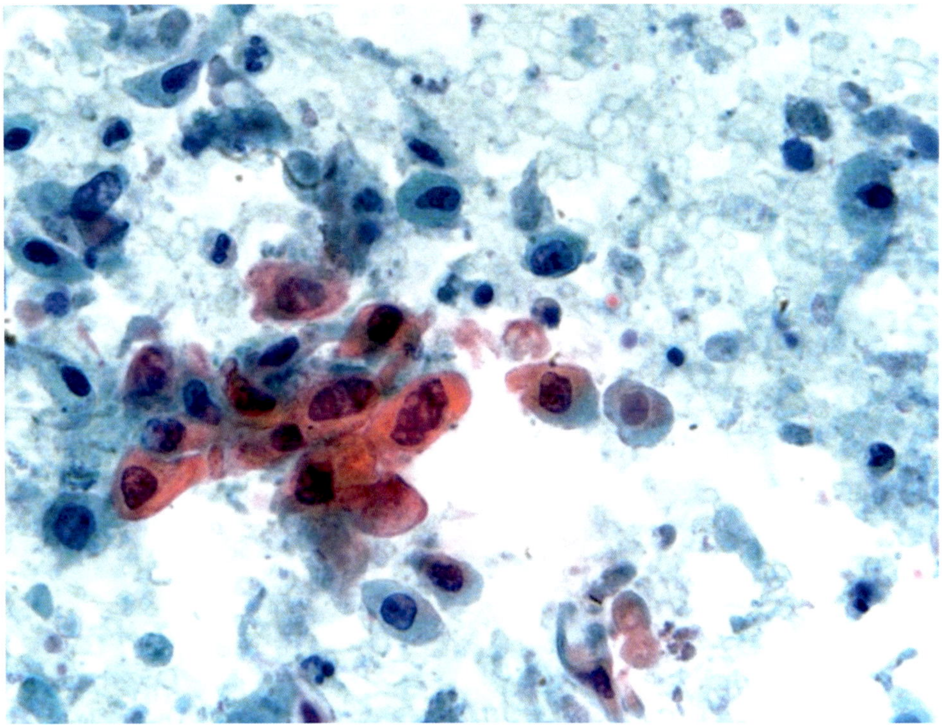

Q-80. What is the diagnosis of this specimen?
(a) Reactive squamous cells
(b) Adenocarcinoma
(c) Bronchioalveolar macrophages
(d) Squamous cell carcinoma

Fig. 1.81

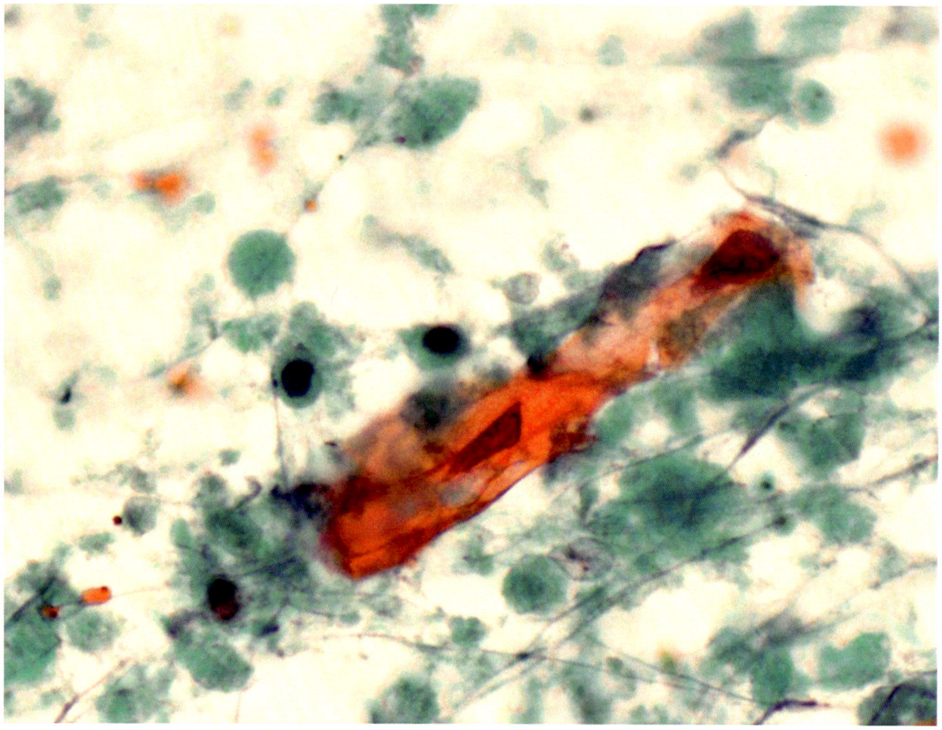

Q-81. What is the diagnosis of this sputum specimen?
(a) Reactive squamous cells
(b) Squamous cell carcinoma
(c) Reactive bronchial epithelial cells
(d) Adenocarcinoma

Fig. 1.82

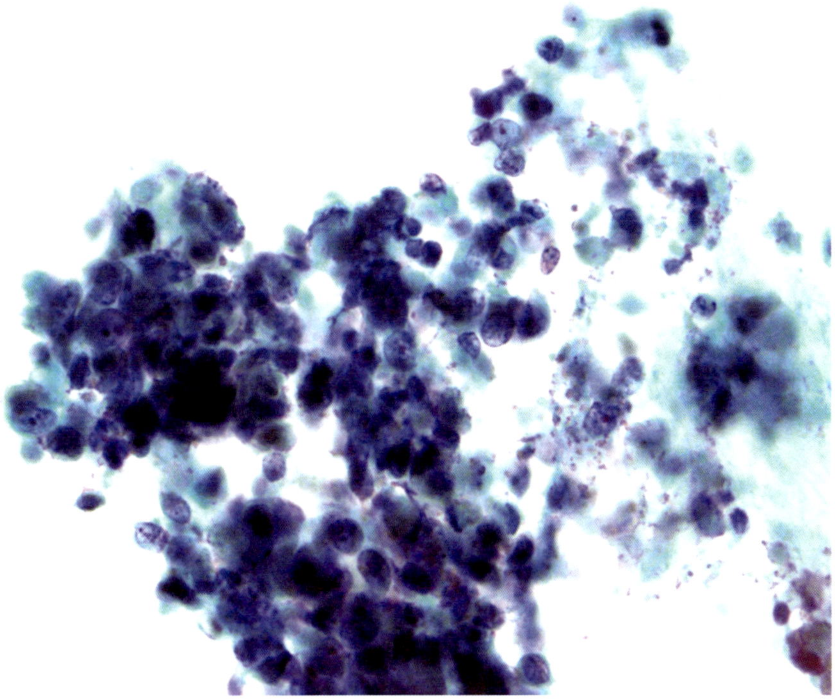

Q-82. What is the diagnosis of this specimen?
(a) Reserve cells
(b) Poorly differentiated adenocarcinoma
(c) Reactive lymphocytes
(d) Small cell carcinoma

1.2 Text-Based Questions 83–142

Q-83. For a sputum sample, including both spontaneous and induced specimens, the presence of which of the following cells and/or material is considered to be an adequate specimen?
(a) Abundant squamous cells and inflammatory cells
(b) Alveolar macrophages or Curschmann spirals
(c) Inflammatory cells and bacterial colonies
(d) Abundant squamous cells and neutrophils

Q-84. Which pair of technique and adequacy criteria is correct?
(a) Bronchoscopic brushing and washing—well preserved, properly fixed, and stained respiratory epithelium
(b) Bronchoscopic fine-needle aspiration (FNA)—representative cells/material of the lesion
(c) Bronchoalveolar lavage (BAL)—abundant alveolar macrophages
(d) All of the above

Q-85. Which type of fine-needle aspirate (FNA) is more often used for staging of lung cancers?
(a) CT-guided transthoracic
(b) Ultrasound-guided transcutaneous
(c) Endoscopic transesophageal FNA with or without ultrasound guidance
(d) Endoscopic transbronchial FNA with or without ultrasound guidance

Q-86. Which of following lung cancer patients is more likely to harbor the *ALK* gene rearrangement?
(a) A 55-year-old female never smoker
(b) A 70-year-old male heavy smoker
(c) A 30-year-old male HIV-positive patient
(d) A 60-year-old male lung transplant recipient

Q-87. Which one of the following is the most useful feature for separating reactive bronchial epithelium (reactive atypia) from a well-differentiated lung adenocarcinoma?
(a) Two- or three-dimensional clusters of bronchial epithelium with nuclear variations
(b) Multinucleated bronchial epithelium
(c) Normal N/C ratio
(d) Clusters of ciliated bronchial epithelium (Creola bodies)

Q-88. The presence of cartilage on a transbronchial fine-needle aspiration biopsy is diagnostic of lung hamartoma, true or false?
(a) True
(b) False

Q-89. Radiation- and chemotherapy-induced bronchial epithelium changes include all of the following, EXCEPT:
(a) Cytomegaly with proportionate nuclear enlargement
(b) Multinucleation and a vesicular chromatin pattern
(c) Prominent nucleoli
(d) Hyperchromatic nucleoli and clumped chromatin

Q-90. Currently EGFR and KRAS mutations are routinely tested in non-small cell lung cancer patients. In addition to adequate tumor cells in the specimen, the following specimens can be used for mutational tests, EXCEPT:
(a) A small transbronchial FNA biopsy specimen of a large lung mass
(b) A biopsy specimen of a lymph node with metastatic lung adenocarcinoma
(c) A surgical resection specimen of lung adenocarcinoma
(d) A biopsy specimen of a bone lesion with metastatic lung adenocarcinoma

Q-91. In sputum and bronchial washing specimens, the finding of which type of cells are considered to be an adequate specimen?
(a) Abundant neutrophils and scattered lymphocytes
(b) Squamous cells and inflammatory cells
(c) Scattered ciliated bronchial epithelial cells and inflammatory cells
(d) Abundant alveolar macrophages

Q-92. A transthoracic CT-guided fine-needle aspiration is performed on a 65-year-old male who has a large right lower lobe lung mass. Sheets of relatively uniform epithelioid cells with well defined cell borders and intercellular "windows" are identified on aspiration smears. What is the most likely diagnosis?
(a) Benign mesothelial cells
(b) Well-differentiated adenocarcinoma of the lung
(c) Benign bronchial epithelium
(d) Mesothelioma

Q-93. All of the following features can be seen in a squamous cell carcinoma, EXCEPT:
(a) Smudgy chromatin
(b) Dense cytoplasm
(c) Prominent nucleoli
(d) Shared cell borders

Q-94. A 40-year-old male smoker presents with a 2 cm lung mass. During the on-site evaluation, the smear of a transbronchial fine-needle aspiration reveals "necrotic debris." What is the best next step?
(a) Tell the pulmonologist to stop the procedure because no cancer is identified.

(b) Send the specimen for microbiology culture.
(c) Send the specimen for microbiology culture and biopsy the peripheral area of the lesion.
(d) Tell the pulmonologist that the lesion is an "infection."

Q-95. Reactive and reparative changes of bronchial epithelium include all of the following features, EXCEPT:
(a) Prominent nucleoli
(b) Multinucleation
(c) Variation of nuclei
(d) Irregular nuclear membrane and hyperchromasia

Q-96. Which of the following lung tumors is more likely to shed diagnostic cells in sputum?
(a) A 3 cm adenocarcinoma involving the pleural surface
(b) A 3 cm squamous cell carcinoma involving the main bronchi
(c) A 3 cm adenocarcinoma involving the right lower lobe
(d) A 3 cm squamous cell carcinoma involving the left upper lobe

Q-97. All the following tumors have been reported to contain "pseudointranuclear inclusions," EXCEPT:
(a) Lung adenocarcinomas with lepidic growth pattern (bronchoalveolar carcinoma)
(b) Melanomas
(c) Hepatocellular carcinomas
(d) Renal cell carcinomas

Q-98. Cytological features of so-called neuroendocrine tumors may include all of these features, EXCEPT:
(a) Fine (salt-and-pepper) chromatin pattern
(b) Nucleoli
(c) Scant to moderate cytoplasm
(d) Nuclear grooves

Q-99. A 60-year-old male patient presents with mediastinal lymphadenopathy. Endoscopic transbronchial fine-needle aspiration (FNA) of a station 7 lymph node was performed. Which of the following features is considered an "abnormal" lymph node?
(a) Polymorphous population of lymphocytes
(b) Monomorphous population of lymphocytes
(c) Tingible body macrophages
(d) Lymphoglandular bodies

Q-100. Which of the following tumors is most likely to be mistaken for "reactive atypia" on transbronchial fine-needle aspirations?
(a) Adenocarcinoma with lepidic growth pattern (bronchoalveolar carcinoma)
(b) Mucinous adenocarcinoma
(c) Basaloid squamous cell carcinoma
(d) Small cell carcinoma

Q-101. In the sputum, the finding of birefringent calcium oxalate crystals is suggestive of which of the following diagnoses?
(a) Papillary adenocarcinoma
(b) Adenocarcinoma with lepidic growth pattern (bronchoalveolar carcinoma)
(c) *Pneumocystis jiroveci (carinii)* pneumonia (PCP)
(d) Aspergillosis

Q-102. A mediastinal mass was biopsied. The main differentiation diagnosis of the mass is lymphoma verse thymoma. Of the following tests/markers, the single most important diagnostic test/marker is:
(a) Immunostains of T and B cells
(b) Flow cytometry for lymphoma markers
(c) Immunostains of CD45 and CD5
(d) Immunostains of cytokeratin

Q-103. Which one of the following bronchoscopic specimens has the lowest sensitivity in the diagnosis of malignancy?
(a) Bronchoscopic brushing
(b) Bronchoscopic washing
(c) Bronchoalveolar lavage
(d) Transbronchial fine-needle aspiration

Q-104. The contraindications of percutaneous ultrasound-guided fine-needle aspiration for lung lesions are all the following, EXCEPT:
(a) Uncontrollable cough
(b) Severe pulmonary hypertension
(c) Suspected echinococcal cyst
(d) Bilateral lung infiltrations

Q-105. Which of the following findings is not the cytological feature of bronchial reserve cell hyperplasia?
(a) Mitosis and necrosis
(b) Tightly packed small-sized cells
(c) Dark chromatin and scant cytoplasm
(d) Nuclear molding

Q-106. Which of the features is NOT seen in benign degenerated squamous cells?
(a) Smudgy nuclei
(b) Nuclei with marked variation in size and shape
(c) Pyknotic nuclei
(d) Cytokeratin formation

Q-107. Most squamous cell carcinomas can be distinguished from adenocarcinomas of the lung based on the presence of the following features, EXCEPT:
(a) Keratinization
(b) Mucin production (cytoplasmic mucin)
(c) Pseudoacinar arrangement of tumor cells
(d) Prominent nucleoli

Q-108. Cytological preparations from a mucinous adenocarcinoma showed uniform cells with pale nuclei, vesicular chromatin, inconspicuous nucleoli, and foamy cytoplasm, which of the following findings is the most useful feature and can help you to make the diagnosis of adenocarcinoma?
(a) Nuclear pseudoinclusion
(b) Multinucleated giant cells
(c) Three-dimensional cluster of cells
(d) Clusters of bronchial epithelial cells without cilia

Q-109. In a well-differentiated adenocarcinoma, tumor cells can be arranged in a variety of architectural patterns, such as two- and three-dimensional clusters, flat sheets, acinar and papillary arrangements.
(a) True
(b) False

Q-110. A bronchoalveolar lavage was performed on a 65-year-old male smoker who presented with an opaque right upper lobe infiltration. On the cytological preparations, large sheets and tight clusters of "signet ring-like" cells are identified. What is the differential diagnosis?
(a) Adenocarcinoma of the lung
(b) Goblet cell hyperplasia
(c) A metastatic adenocarcinoma from stomach
(d) All of the above

Q-111. The pulmonary primary epithelioid hemangioendothelioma (EHE) and epithelioid angiosarcoma (EAS) are positive for vascular markers CD31 and CD34, but negative for cytokeratin, true or false?
(a) True
(b) False

Q-112. A transbronchial fine-needle aspiration smear reveal sheets and two-dimensional clusters of spindle cells, the differential diagnosis of the lesion include all of the following, EXCEPT:
(a) Spindle cell carcinoma
(b) Leiomyosarcoma
(c) Spindle cell carcinoid
(d) Poorly differentiated adenocarcinoma

Q-113. The presence of numerous small- to medium-sized lymphocytes in a BAL specimen from the patient with autoimmune disease is a suspicious feature of a mucosa-associated lymphoid tissue (MALT) lymphoma. What is the best next step of actions?
(a) Perform immunostain of B-cell markers
(b) Perform flow cytometry
(c) Perform immunostain of T-cell markers
(d) Perform immunostain of cytokeratin

Q-114. A transbronchial fine needle biopsy reveals scattered small but well formed non-necrotizing granulomas with little surrounding inflammation. Special stains for microorganisms are all negative. The diagnosis of sarcoidosis is made. Sarcoidosis is generally a self-limiting process, and most of the patients do not progress to pulmonary fibrosis, true or false?
(a) True
(b) False

Q-115. A CT scan from an asymptomatic 50-year-old smoker revealed bilateral ground glass opaque lesions. A BAL specimen from the patient showed numerous alveolar macrophages and eosinophilic acellular material, the most likely diagnosis is:
(a) *Pneumocystis jiroveci (carinii)* pneumonia (PCP)
(b) Alveolar proteinosis
(c) Amyloid
(d) Aspergillosis

Q-116. Which panel of immune markers is most useful for the differential diagnosis of mesothelioma and lung adenocarcinoma?
(a) Calretinin, CK7, TTF, BerEP4, and CEA
(b) Desmin, D2-40, WT1, CK7, TTF, BerEP4, and CEA
(c) Calretinin, p53, WT1, TTF, BerEP4, CEA, and CD15
(d) P63, p53, WT1, TTF, BerEP4, CEA, and CD15

Q-117. A 50-year-old female developed a chronic cough, chest x-ray showed bilateral small opaque infiltrates. The on-site evaluation of the transbronchial fine-needle aspiration of the lesion revealed scattered clusters of epithelioid histiocytes. What is the next step of action?
(a) Microbiology culture and core biopsy of the lesion
(b) Microbiology culture only
(c) Core biopsy the lesion
(d) Do nothing

Q-118. A HIV-positive patient was clinically suspicious for *Pneumocystis jiroveci (carinii)* pneumonia (PCP) of the lung. A BAL was performed. What is the best next step of actions?
(a) Make cell block and perform silver stain
(b) Make cell block and perform PAS stain
(c) Make cell block and perform serial H&E stains
(d) Make cell block only

Q-119. On a FNA specimen, which one of the following features is commonly seen in a metastatic breast carcinoma to the lung?
(a) Monotonous appearance of tumor cells
(b) Tight three-dimensional clusters and/or acini arrangements of tumor cells
(c) Frequently intracytoplasmic lumen
(d) All of the above

Q-120. A primary lung adenocarcinoma intestinal subtype can be reliably differentiated from a metastatic colonic adenocarcinoma to the lung with immunostaining of CK20 and CDX2, because the primary lung adenocarcinoma intestinal subtype is negative for both CK20 and CDX2, true or false?
(a) True
(b) False

Q-121. A transbronchial fine-needle aspiration of a lung mass from a patient with multiple lung nodules was performed and found to be an adenocarcinoma. Tumor cells revealed a distinctively tall columnar "picket fence" appearance, hyperchromatic nuclei, and "dirty" necrosis. Which one is the most likely primary site of the tumor?
(a) Breast
(b) Liver
(c) Colon
(d) Uterus

Q-122. Which option is the best one for the diagnosis of a metastatic melanoma involving a hilar lymph node of the lung?
(a) Using unstained slides to perform IHC markers S100, HMB45, and Melanin A
(b) Using unstained slides to perform IHC markers S100, HMB45, and Melanin A with red chromogenics rather than the one with brown chromogenics
(c) Using unstained slides to perform IHC marker Melanin A only
(d) Using unstained slides to perform IHC marker S100 only

Q-123. All of following cytological features can be seen in a small cell carcinoma of the lung, EXCEPT:
(a) The size of tumor cells are two- to threefold of mature lymphocytes
(b) Paranuclear blue bodies in the cytoplasm
(c) Nuclear crowding and molding
(d) Prominent nucleoli

Q-124. Which of the following is NOT associated with a small cell carcinoma?
(a) Lambert–Eaton syndrome
(b) Cushing's syndrome
(c) Hyponatremia
(d) Pancoast tumor

Q-125. Which of the following statements is CORRECT?
(a) Atypical carcinoid can be easily separated from typical carcinoid
(b) Atypical carcinoid shares many cytological features with typical carcinoid
(c) Necrosis can be easily identified in an atypical carcinoid
(d) Increased mitotic figures is the only cytological criterion for diagnosing of atypical carcinoids

Q-126. Which of the following features can be used to separate typical carcinoids from atypical carcinoids and small cell carcinomas?
(a) The prominent nucleoli
(b) Fine (salt-and-pepper) chromatin pattern
(c) The lower mitotic rate and the absence of necrosis
(d) Organoid and/or pseudorosette arrangement of tumor cells

Q-127. Which of the following cytological features is the most helpful one in the differential diagnosis of large cell neuroendocrine tumor?
(a) Fine (salt-and-pepper) chromatin pattern
(b) Organoid and/or pseudorosettes arrangement of tumor cells
(c) The mitotic rate and the focal necrosis
(d) Carcinoid tumor-like nuclei with markedly atypia and enlargement

Q-128. Which of the following statements of pulmonary hamartoma is CORRECT?
(a) Involving the *HMGI*(Y) gene on chromosome 6p21
(b) The presence of cartilage on the smear is diagnostic
(c) It often involves several members from the same family
(d) It is a infiltrating tumor

Q-129. In lung transplant patients, bronchoalveolar lavage (BAL) is routinely performed to monitor a patient's condition. Which statement is INCORRECT?
(a) Neutrophils are normally seen within the first 3 months after transplantation.
(b) Increased number of macrophages can be seen for years after transplantation.
(c) The most common fungal infection is Candida.
(d) Neutrophils can be seen in 1 year after transplantation.

Q-130. Anaplastic lymphoma kinase (*ALK*) gene rearrangement has been detected in a subset tumor of lung adenocarcinomas. *ALK* gene rearrangement has also been detected in which of the following tumors?
(a) Leiomyosarcoma
(b) Inflammatory myofibroblastic tumor (IMT)
(c) Rhabdomyosarcoma
(d) Desmoplastic small blue cell tumors

Q-131. In lung adenocarcinomas, both *EGFR* and *KRAS* mutations can occur in the same tumor, true or false?
(a) True
(b) False

Q-132. Which of the following statements is NOT correct?
(a) Mutation and overexpression of the *EGFR* gene lead to cancer cell overgrowth, but not tumor progression.
(b) Mutations of the *EGFR* gene lead to cancer cell overgrowth and tumor progression.
(c) Mutations of the *EGFR* gene stimulate tyrosine kinase activity.
(d) Erlotinib and gefitinib are tyrosine kinase inhibitors (TKIs) that target the *EGFR* signaling pathway.

Q-133. Which of the following statements is NOT correct?
(a) The KRAS protein stimulates downstream activity of EGFR tyrosine kinase.
(b) *KRAS* mutations lead to a constitutive activation of RAS signaling pathway.
(c) EGFR tyrosine kinase inhibitors (TKIs) cannot block the activity of mutated KRAS proteins.
(d) *KRAS* mutations are more likely to be found in non-smokers.

Q-134. Rearrangements of the gene encoding anaplastic lymphoma kinase (*ALK* gene rearrangements) have been found in a subset of lung adenocarcinomas. Which of the following statements is CORRECT?
(a) The most common *ALK* rearrangement in non-small cell lung carcinoma is *EML4-ALK* fusion.
(b) *EML4-ALK* rearrangements are found in tumor with *KRAS* mutations.
(c) *EML4-ALK* rearrangements are found in tumor with *EGFR* mutations.
(d) *EML4-ALK* rearrangements are more common found in adenocarcinomas of heavy smokers.

Q-135. In a transthoracic fine-needle aspiration (FNA) of a lung lesion, what is the most important cytological feature to separate reactive methothelial cells from a well-differentiated adenocarcinoma?
(a) Sheets of intermediate-sized epithelioid cells
(b) Prominent nucleoli
(c) Intercellular "windows"
(d) Three-dimensional clusters of hyperchromatic cells

Q-136. Which one of the following cytological findings is the most useful feature in the separation of reactive squamous cell atypia from squamous cell carcinoma?
(a) Prominent nucleoli
(b) Significant variation of nuclear size and shape
(c) Dispersed individual cells
(d) Necrotic debris

Q-137. In a percutaneous fine-needle aspiration (FNA) of the lung lesion, the presence of mesothelial cells, muscle cells, and adipose tissue is a common finding, true or false?
(a) True
(b) False

Q-138. Numerous benign appearing liver cells were found on a transthoracic fine-needle aspiration (FNA) specimen from a patient with a right lower lobe lung mass. No other type of cells was identified. The differential diagnosis of this FNA includes all of the followings, EXCEPT:
(a) Benign liver cells
(b) Small cell carcinoma
(c) Adenocarcinoma
(d) Hepatocellular carcinoma

Q-139. Which of the following crystals/structures is commonly seen in a BAL specimen from an asthma patient?
(a) Ferruginous bodies
(b) Psammoma bodies
(c) Charcot–Leyden crystals
(d) Corpora amylacea

Q-140. Which of the following statements regarding *EGFR* mutations is CORRECT?
(a) *EGFR* mutations are often found in adenocarcinoma with micropapillary and/or the lepidic growth pattern.

(b) *EGFR* mutations are not found in Asian patients.
(c) Tumors with *EGFR* mutation have a poor response to EGFR tyrosine kinase inhibitor therapy.
(d) *EGFR* mutation can be detected in a tumor with *KRAS* mutations.

Q-141. *KRAS* mutations are found in non-small cell lung carcinomas. Which of the following statements is NOT correct?
(a) *KRAS* mutations are less commonly seen among Asian descents.
(b) *KRAS* mutations are more commonly seen among non-smokers.
(c) Patients with *KRAS* mutations seem to have a poorer prognosis.
(d) Patients with *KRAS* mutations seem to be resistant to EGFR tyrosine kinase inhibitor therapy.

Q-142. According to the laboratory regulation policy of the Health Care Financing Administration (HCFA), the following items must be included on the requisition form for a BAL specimen, EXCEPT:
(a) Date and time of the sample collected
(b) Date of the sample received in the laboratory
(c) Time of the sample received in the laboratory
(d) The color and volume of the specimen

1.3 Answers and Discussion of Image-Based Questions 1–82

A-1. **(d) Carcinoid**
In carcinoids, tumor cells are arranged in acini and pseudorosette structures, and dispersed individual cells with monomorphic appearance. Tumor cells reveal vesicular nuclei, fine (salt-and-pepper) chromatin, and inconspicuous or small nucleoli. No obvious mitotic activity or tumor necrosis. Although mitotic account plays an important role in the classification, it is not always seen on cytological smears. Therefore, careful evaluation of cytomorphology on slides and immunostain of Ki67 on cell block section may be necessary for an accurate classification. In lymphomas, tumor cells are discohesive and have coarse chromatin, prominent nucleoli and irregular nuclear membranes, and lymphoglandular bodies.

A-2. **(a) *Pneumocystis jiroveci* (formerly called *carinii*) pneumonia (PCP)**
The cytological features of PCP on the BAL specimen include predominantly foamy macrophages, amorphous material, and rare inflammatory cells. In foamy macrophages and amorphous material, numerous casts (rounded masses of organisms), staining purple color with Diff-Quik and blue color with Papanicolaou stain, are identified. The spherical or cup-shaped organisms are 4–8 μm in diameter and slightly smaller than RBC. On careful view, ill-defined central or eccentric dots are present and best seen with silver stains such as the Gomori methenamine silver stain, which are revealed black in color. PCP infection usually involves immunocompromised patients. Alveolar proteinosis reveals coarsely granular eosinophilic to cyanophilic debris; they are positive for periodic acid–Schiff stain and negative for sliver stain.

A-3. **(b) Strongyloidiasis**
The infection involves in immunocompromised patients such as HIV infection, transplantation, and chemotherapy; and caused by the nematode *Strongyloides strecoralis*, which is usually identified in the form of long round worms that are 200–400 μm in length. Infection of the lung is due to the hematogenous migration of the infective larva from the GI tract or skin. The organism can be found in sputum and/or BAL specimens. The strongyloidiasis is differentiated from other hookworms by its short buccal cavity and notched tail.

A-4. **(c) Cryptococcosis**
Cryptococcosis is caused by infection of *Cryptococcus neoformans*, the inhabitants in the soil with bird droppings. The infection occurs in both immunocompromised and immunocompetent patients worldwide and may involve many body sites; however, lung involvement is more common. In a BAL specimen, the fungus reveals as yeast forms with narrow and pinched buddings, refractile centers, and mucoid capsules (clear zone around the stained organisms). The capsule is positive with periodic acid–Schiff, alcian blue, and mucicarmine stains. In histoplasmosis, numerous small budding yeasts are seen in the cytoplasm of histiocytes. The infection is most commonly seen in the Ohio and Mississippi river valleys. In blastomycosis, specimen reveals large broad-based budding yeasts and thick cell walls. The yeast is bigger than Cryptococcus.

A-5. **(b) Carcinoid**
Typical carcinoid tumors are usually centrally located and may appear as an exophytic endobronchial lesion. In the peripheral location, they may have a spindle cell morphology. The cytopathological features include loosely cohesive clusters with rosette formation or single plasmacytoid cells with uniform nuclei containing "salt-and-pepper" stippled chromatin. In some cases, atypical carcinoid tumors show more mitoses, a higher proliferation index, and associated necrosis than in typical carcinoids, but do not reach the level of pleomorphism seen with small cell carcinoma. The cytological features include findings similar to carcinoid, but with more mitoses than carcinoid and some necrosis. In general, the cells tend to have more cytoplasm and less nuclear atypia than small cell carcinoma. In lymphomas, tumor cells are discohesive and have coarse chromatin, prominent nucleoli and irregular nuclear membranes, and lymphoglandular bodies.

A-6. **(b) *Mucormycosis* (*zygomycosis*)**
Pulmonary mucormycosis (zygomycosis) rarely occurs in immunocompetent hosts. The risk factors include diabetes mellitus, neutropenia, sustained immunosuppressive and chronic prednisone therapies, iron chelation therapy, broad-spectrum antibiotic use, severe malnutrition, and primary breakdown in the integrity of the cutaneous barrier such as trauma, surgical wounds, needle sticks, or burns. This invasive fungal infection is caused by mycelia-forming fungi of the *Mucorales* (e.g., *Rhizopus*, *Mucor* spp.) and

Entomophthorales (e.g., *Conidiobolus* and *Basidiobolus* spp.). In the sputum specimen, it reveals terminal chlamydoconidia and hyphae. Terminal chlamydoconidia are thick-walled spherical structures (Pap stain, intermediate magnification on the left, and high magnification on the right upper images), whereas, hyphae are characterized by irregularly shaped, broad ribbon-like, non-septated hyphae with right-angle branching (Pap stain, high magnification on the right lower image). In aspergillosis, hyphae form fungi are seen, characterized by the presence of true septate and relatively straight branching. The calcium oxalate crystal is also associated with aspergillosis. In blastomycosis, it reveals large round yeast (5–15 μm), characterized by double-contoured thick cell walls and broad-based budding. In parasite infections, the size of Paragonimus eggs is much larger than that of fungi, and reveals a thick, double contour shell with an operculated end.

A-7. (**d**) **Herpes simplex virus** (**HSV**) **infection**
HSV infection commonly occurs in neonates and immunocompromised patients. Clinical manifestations of HSV infection of the lung include necrotizing and/or diffuse interstitial pneumonia. On BAL specimen, it reveals a cellular specimen containing large atypical cells (metaplastic squamous cells) with intranuclear inclusions (cytopathic virus effects). Two forms of characteristic inclusions may be seen, including Cowdry type A inclusions (distinct eosinophilic intranuclear inclusions surrounded by a clear halo due to margination of chromatin material) and Cowdry type B inclusions (eosinophilic ground glass "smudge nuclei" with margination of the chromatin material) (shown in the image). These inclusions can be found within metaplastic squamous cells when the inflammation is centered around airways or in multinucleated giant cells within necroinflammatory debris in the interstitial form of disease. Virus-infected cells may also display prominent nuclear molding. The background of the slide may reveal acute inflammatory cells and necrotic debris. In other conditions, cells may reveal multinucleation and prominent nucleoli; however, no characteristic virus cytopathic inclusion is present. In difficult case such as scant specimen with rare atypical cells, immunostain of HSV may help to confirm the diagnosis of HSV infection.

A-8. (**a**) ***Pneumocystis jiroveci*** (***carinii***) **pneumonia**
Pneumocystis jiroveci (carinii) pneumonia (PCP) infection usually involves immunocompromised patients, such as HIV infection, organ transplantation, chemotherapy, and cancer patients. The infection typically involves the distal airspaces and is associated with a foamy or frothy exudate. The cytological findings of PCP on the BAL specimen include numerous alveolar macrophages and amorphous/foamy material. Cup-shaped microorganisms (cysts) can be seen in the cytoplasm of alveolar macrophages and in the extracellular amorphous/foamy material by both Diff-Quik and Papanicolaou stains, but organisms are stained poorly or not at all with Papanicolaou method. In silver stains, such as Grocott's methenamine silver (GMS) stain, the cell wall of the organisms stains with black color. The cysts tend to aggregate together, and should not be confused with *Histoplasma* or *Cryptococcus* which typically do not aggregate. Alveolar proteinosis reveals amorphous material without the finding of cup-shaped cysts. The cell block preparation and silver stain may help to identify the cup-shaped microorganisms and confirm the diagnosis of PCP. Other useful ancillary tests include immunocytochemistry using a specific *Pneumocystis* immunostain and polymerase chain reaction (PCR).

A-9. (**c**) **Histoplasmosis**
Histoplasmosis is caused by the inhalation of infective spores (microconidia), dimorphic fungus *Histoplasma capsulatum*, which primarily affect alveolar macrophages. Pulmonary histoplasmosis can present clinically with pneumonia, lung nodule, cavitary lung disease, mediastinal or hilar lymphadenopathy. It is not uncommon for localized infections to mimic cancer. On the cytological preparation, slides reveal numerous intracellular yeasts measuring 3–5 μm, with narrow-based budding, within alveolar macrophages. When cells are disrupted, they may also be seen in the extracellular location. Special stains (GMS and PAS stains) are positive for intra- and extracellular yeasts. In PCP, cytological preparations reveal numerous cup-shaped microorganisms (cysts) in the cytoplasm of alveolar macrophages and in the extracellular amorphous/foamy material. In reactive bronchial epithelium and adenocarcinoma, atypical bronchial cells with enlarged nuclei and prominent nucleoli are usually seen. In difficult cases, fungal culture and antigen detection (enzyme immunoassay using urine, blood, or bronchoalveolar lavage fluid) may confirm the diagnosis.

A-10. (**a**) **Echinococcosis** (**Hydatid disease**)
Echinococcosis (Hydatid disease) is the most common cestode (tapeworm species) infection to the lung and is caused by the larvae of *Echinococcus granulosus*. The infection has a worldwide distribution

including South America, the Mediterranean and Middle East countries, Russia, and China. Dogs are the definitive host for *E. granulosus* and harbor the adult worms in their gut. The eggs shed in dog feces and contaminate food sources. After ingestion of contaminated food, the eggs travel to the liver or lungs and slowly develop into hydatid cysts over a period of several months or years. Although most cysts form in the liver, 20–30 % form in the lung. Occasionally, lung cysts form after transdiaphragmatic spread of parasites following the rupture of liver cysts. Patients may be asymptomatic for many years. FNA of the lesion usually contains hydatid sand with hooklets and detached (free) refractile hooklets (resembling shark's teeth) and the thick granular material. Cell blocks may contain portions of a cyst wall that consists of three layers: (1) host layer with giant cells, fibroblasts, and eosinophils; (2) middle acellular laminated membrane; and (3) inner germinal layer. A primary hydatid cyst of the chest may mimic a neoplasm. However, it is controversial whether suspected hydatid cysts should be aspirated as fluid leakage could result in anaphylaxis or disseminated disease. In strongyloidiasis, it reveals *Strongyloides strecoralis*, a long roundworm measuring 200–400 μm in length.

A-11. (**c**) **Aspergillosis**

Aspergillosis is caused by the inhalation of airborne conidial forms (fruiting body) of fungus *Aspergillus*. Infections mainly affect individuals with underlying lung disease such as cystic fibrosis and/or immunocompromised patients such as transplant and AIDS patients. There are four types of lung disease caused by *Aspergillus*: (1) allergic bronchopulmonary aspergillosis, (2) aspergilloma (fungus ball or mycetoma), (3) chronic necrotizing pneumonia, and (4) invasive pulmonary aspergillosis, which may cause lung infarction and dissemination to other organs. On cytological preparations, usually only the hyphal form is seen, characterized by septated hyphae with relatively straight walls and 45° (dichotomous) branching. Conidial forms (fruiting bodies) may be seen when the organism is exposed to air (e.g., abscess cavity or involvement of large airways). Calcium oxalate crystals, which are strongly birefringent under polarized light, may be seen and are highly suggestive of aspergillosis. In mucormycosis (zygomycosis), it reveals terminal chlamydoconidia and hyphae. Terminal chlamydoconidia are thick-walled spherical structures (Pap stain, intermediate magnification on the left, and high magnification on the right upper images), whereas, hyphae are characterized by irregularly shaped, broad ribbon-like, non-septated hyphae with right-angle branching. In blastomycosis, it reveals large round yeast (5–15 μm), characterized by double-contoured thick cell walls and broad-based budding. In candidiasis, it reveals pseudohyphae (elongated yeast joined together) and budding yeasts. Several clinical tests may be used to confirm the diagnosis of aspergillosis, such as immunocytochemistry using an immunostain specific to the *Aspergillus* genus (but not species-specific), aspergillosis antibody test, and fungal culture.

A-12. (**b**) **Cytomegalovirus (CMV) infection**

CMV is one of the most common causes of opportunistic infections involving the respiratory tract. In the respiratory tract, CMV mainly targets pulmonary macrophages, endothelial cells, and fibroblasts, but virtually any cell can be infected by the virus. CMV pneumonia is frequently seen in recipients of organ transplants, patients with HIV/AIDS, or elderly patients. The diagnostic features of CMV infection include cytomegaly, large amphophilic intranuclear inclusions with perinuclear halos and chromatin margination ("owl eye" inclusion), and small basophilic cytoplasmic inclusions. The number of cells showing cytopathic changes varies with the severity of infection or as a result of patients receiving prophylactic antiviral therapy. In HSV infection, it reveals intranuclear inclusions, including Cowdry type A inclusions (distinct eosinophilic intranuclear inclusions surrounded by a clear halo due to margination of chromatin material) and Cowdry type B inclusions (eosinophilic ground glass "smudge nuclei" with margination of the chromatin material). In adenocarcinomas, tumor cells form tight three-dimensional clusters with hyperchromatic nuclei, prominent nucleoli, irregular nuclear membrane, and high nucleus:cytoplasm (N:C) ratio. In squamous cell metaplasia, cell reveals normal in size with dark nuclei and dense cytoplasm (cytokeratin formation); no intranuclear inclusion is seen. Most cases of the CMV infection do not need ancillary studies to confirm the diagnosis. In difficult cases, immunocytochemistry or in situ hybridization for CMV, molecular testing (PCR), and viral culture may be performed to confirm the diagnosis.

A-13. (**c**) ***Entamoeba gingivalis*** **infection**

E. gingivalis is a parasitic protozoan of the oral cavity. In patients with poor oral hygiene, aspiration can result in a lung infection. The morphological appearances of *E. gingivalis* and *E. histolytica* (causing amebic enteritis and liver abscess) are quite similar, although the trophozoites of *E. gingivalis* tend to be comparably larger (10–35 vs. 15–20 μm) and, unlike with *E. histolytica*, there is no associated cyst stage. *E. gingivalis* is also the only species of amebae that can phagocytose white and red blood cells as well as ingest bacteria. Amebae have a histiocyte-like morphology and typically contain ingested RBCs in their cytoplasm. Trophozoites are, however, slightly larger than macrophages and have smaller nuclei with coarser chromatin than histiocytes. In the Echinococcosis (Hydatid disease), it reveals hydatid sand with hooklets and detached (free) refractile hooklets (resembling shark's teeth) and the thick granular material. In Paragonimus eggs, the size of Paragonimus eggs is much larger than that of *E. gingivalis*, and it has a thick, double contour shell with an operculated end.

A-14. (**c**) **Histoplasmosis**

Histoplasmosis is caused by the inhalation of infective spores (microconidia), dimorphic fungus *Histoplasma capsulatum*, which primarily affect alveolar macrophages. Pulmonary histoplasmosis can present clinically with pneumonia, lung nodule, cavitary lung disease, mediastinal or hilar lymphadenopathy. It is not uncommon for localized infections to mimic cancer. On the cytological preparation, slides reveal numerous intracellular yeasts measuring 3–5 μm, with narrow-based budding, within alveolar macrophages. When cells are disrupted, they may also be seen in the extracellular location. Special stains (GMS and PAS stains) are positive for intra- and extracellular yeasts. In PCP, cytological preparations reveal numerous cup-shaped microorganisms (cysts) in the cytoplasm of alveolar macrophages and in the extracellular amorphous/foamy material. In reactive bronchial epithelium and adenocarcinoma, atypical bronchial cells with enlarged nuclei and prominent nucleoli are usually seen. In difficult cases, fungal culture and antigen detection (enzyme immunoassay using urine, blood, or bronchoalveolar lavage fluid) may confirm the diagnosis.

A-15. (**b**) **Coccidioidomycosis**

Coccidioidomycosis is caused by the inhalation of arthroconidia of *Coccidioides immitis* or *Coccidioides posadasii*. The infection is endemic in Arizona, California, Nevada, New Mexico, Texas, Utah, and northern Mexico. Most people are asymptomatic following initial respiratory exposure to arthroconidia. Those who become ill typically develop respiratory symptoms, such as cough, fever, and pneumonia. *C. immitis* infection typically causes a necrotizing granulomatous inflammation, pulmonary nodules, cavities, diffuse reticulonodular pneumonia, and rarely pleural disease. Fungemia can also produce multiple septic pulmonary emboli, especially in immunocompromised patients. Cytological preparations reveal thick walled spherules (measuring 10–80 μm) that contain endospores (measuring 2–5 μm). There are generally very few spherules present in most specimens. Sometimes the spherules may be collapsed and appear as empty structures, surrounded by scattered endospores all over the slide. Wet preparation of fresh samples using saline or potassium hydroxide solution can be utilized to demonstrate spherules. Calcofluor staining is positive. In histoplasmosis, it reveals numerous intracellular yeasts measuring 3–5 μm with narrow-based budding in alveolar macrophages. In cryptococcosis, it reveals round- to oval-shaped yeast (measuring 5–20 μm) with narrow-based budding. Yeasts may resemble Pneumocystis cysts, but tend to be more variable and often larger in size. Encapsulated cryptococcal organisms are surrounded by a thick capsule which is positive with mucicarmine, alcian blue, and colloidal iron stains. In PCP, cytological preparations reveal numerous cup-shaped microorganisms (cysts) in the cytoplasm of alveolar macrophages and in the extracellular amorphous/foamy material.

A-16. (**a**) **Cryptococcosis**

Humans are infected by *Cryptococcus neoformans* and *Cryptococcus gattii* due to the inhalation of basidiospores or yeast. The course and clinical presentation of the disease depends on whether yeast are encapsulated (encapsulated yeast may cause a granulomatous reaction) and the patient's immune status. Invasive cryptococcosis has become increasingly common among HIV-positive and transplant patients. Clinical manifestation of the lung infection varies from asymptomatic airway colonization to a slowly progressive lung mass (cryptococcoma), pneumonia, and acute respiratory distress syndrome (ARDS), to pleural effusion. On slides, it reveals round- to oval-shaped yeast (measuring 5–20 μm) with narrow-based budding. Yeasts may resemble Pneumocystis cysts, but tend to be more variable and often larger in size. Encapsulated cryptococcal organisms are surrounded by a thick capsule which is positive with mucicarmine, alcian blue, and colloidal iron stains. In coccidioidomycosis, it reveals thick-walled spherules (measuring 10–80 μm) that contain endospores (measuring 2–5 μm). In histoplasmosis, it reveals numerous intracellular yeasts measuring 3–5 μm, with narrow-based budding, within alveolar macrophages. In PCP, cytological preparations reveal numerous cup-shaped microorganisms (cysts) in the cytoplasm of alveolar macrophages and in the extracellular amorphous/foamy material.

A-17. (**c**) **Tuberculosis**
Pulmonary tuberculosis (TB) is caused by the bacterium *Mycobacterium tuberculosis*. Pulmonary TB may be due to primary or reactivation (chronic) infection. Manifestations of pulmonary TB include bronchopneumonia, caseating pneumonia, nodular disease (tuberculoma), tracheobronchitis, milliary disease, hilar lymphadenopathy, and pleural disease. Individuals at risk for infection are those who are immunosuppressed, the elderly, and infants. The main cytomorphological findings of pulmonary TB arc granulomas that show clusters of epithelioid histiocytes with or without lymphocytes, Langhans and/or foreign body-type multinucleated giant cells, with/without a necrotic background. A negative image of extracellular mycobacteria may be notable with Diff-Quik, Giemsa, or other Romanowsky-type stains. The diagnosis of mycobacterial infection can be made on the basis of the identification of microorganisms with acid-fast (AFB) stains. In cytological preparation, mycobacteria of *M. tuberculosis* may be rare and require careful and lengthy scrutiny of slides. Mycobacteria may be weakly gram-positive and will stain with GMS. Fluorescence microscopy with fluorochrome dyes such as auramine O or auramine–rhodamine are more sensitive and specific than AFB stains. PCR for diagnosis and subclassification can be done on cell block material. Mycobacteria are slow growing and culture can take weeks (6–8 weeks with conventional Lowenstein-Jensen medium and 3 weeks with Middlebrook liquid and solid media). The differential diagnosis includes other AFB-positive microorganisms that cause necrotizing granulomatous inflammation such as *Nocardia*, *Rhodococcus*, and *Legionella micdadei*, and non-infectious causes of granulomatous lung disease such as sarcoidosis.

A-18. (**d**) **Toxoplasmosis**
Toxoplasma pneumonia is being recognized with increased frequency, especially in immunocompromised patients. Particularly, lung involvement occurs with severe disseminated infection (toxoplasmosis). Respiratory specimens like BAL require close inspection for crescent or banana-shaped free (extracellular) trophozoites, as they measure only around 5–7 μm in length. These banana-shaped extracellular trophozoites have prominent central nucleus with Giemsa stain. The parasites are barely visible with the Pap stain. Alveolar macrophages may be seen containing several parasites. The trophozoites need to be distinguished from similar-sized *Histoplasma* (which exhibit narrow-neck budding) and *Leishmania* (which also contain a kinetoplast). In addition to the Giemsa stain, an immunohistochemical stain for Toxoplasma is also available for the confirmation of the diagnosis. In PCP, cytological preparations reveal numerous cup-shaped microorganisms (cysts) in the cytoplasm of alveolar macrophages and in the extracellular amorphous/foamy material.

A-19. (**c**) **Co-infection with CMV and PCP**
CMV is one of the most common causes of opportunistic infections involving the respiratory tract. As CMV is frequently found in immunocompromised patients, it may be seen together with other opportunistic pathogens infections such as fungi including *P. jirovecii*. Co-infection with CMV and *P. jirovecii* is shown in this BAL specimen. The slides reveal characteristic "owl eye" nuclear inclusions in cells. Multinucleation is rare in CMV infection, but can occur. Pneumocystis infection resulted in the cast of frothy material, containing cup-shaped organisms with a central dot in Pap stain. In HSV infection, it reveals intranuclear inclusions, including Cowdry type A inclusions (distinct eosinophilic intranuclear inclusions surrounded by a clear halo due to margination of chromatin material) and Cowdry type B inclusions (eosinophilic ground glass "smudge nuclei" with margination of the chromatin material).

A-20. (**a**) **Asthma**
The structures in photos are Curschmann spirals and Charcot–Leyden crystals. Curschmann spirals are coiled strands of mucus, and associated with chronic pulmonary disease. Although non-specific findings, they are commonly seen in asthma patients. Charcot–Leyden crystals are needle-shaped orangeophilic color crystal and by-products of eosinophil degranulation. They can be found in asthma patients. In aspergillosis, birefringent calcium oxalate crystals (needle-shaped, polarizable crystals) are common findings, and they may form rosettes or wheat sheaf-like clusters. In PCP, cytological preparations reveal numerous cup-shaped microorganisms

(cysts) in the cytoplasm of alveolar macrophages and in the extracellular amorphous/foamy material. In asbestos exposure, ferruginous bodies are usually seen; they are dumbbell-shaped mineral fibers, 5–200 μm in length, golden-yellow to black color with Papanicolaou stain.

A-21. (a) **Well-differentiated adenocarcinoma**
The Papanicolaou stain shows three-dimensional clusters or acinar/papillae arrangement of columnar cells with hyperchromatic nuclei and coarse chromatin, irregular nuclear membranes, "lacy" cytoplasm, and cytoplasmic vacuolization. Tumor cells are large in size and have high N:C ratio, and without cilia. Adjacent to tumor cell clusters, there is a benign reactive bronchial cells with cilia. Creola bodies are three-dimensional clusters of reactive bronchial cells with marked variation of nuclear sizes, and without malignant nuclear features, cells still have cilia. Bronchoalveolar macrophages have abundant cytoplasm and eccentrically located nuclei.

A-22. (d) **Adenocarcinoma with cytoplasmic mucin**
The Papanicolaou stain shows predominantly dispersed individual tumor cells with hyperchromatic nuclei and coarse chromatin, irregular nuclear membranes, "lacy" cytoplasm, and cytoplasmic vacuolization (intracytoplasmic mucin). The differential diagnosis includes primary lung adenocarcinoma verse a metastatic adenocarcinoma with mucin production such as gastric and breast carcinoma. IHC study of TTF1 and Napsin A is necessary to confirm the lung primary. The most important differential diagnosis is bronchoalveolar macrophages. Bronchoalveolar macrophages have abundant vacuolated cytoplasm and eccentrically located nuclei, without nuclear atypia.

A-23. (c) **Adenocarcinoma**
The cell block preparation shows loosely formed two-dimensional clusters of large epithelial cells with hyperchromatic nuclei, coarse chromatin, prominent nucleoli, irregular nuclear membranes, "lacy" cytoplasm, and cytoplasmic vacuolization. In reactive bronchial epithelium, cells reveal marked variation of nuclear sizes, without malignant nuclear features, and cells still have cilia. In goblet cell hyperplasia, it reveals clusters of cells in honeycomb arrangement, with abundant mucin-filled cytoplasm and eccentrically located nuclei; no malignant nuclear features are identified. In reactive bronchial epithelium, cells are arranged in three-dimensional clusters, with marked variation of nuclear sizes, without malignant nuclear features, cells still have cilia.

A-24. (c) **Adenocarcinoma**
In lung adenocarcinomas, particularly in adenocarcinomas with lepidic growth pattern (formerly bronchioalveolar adenocarcinomas), radiographic studies may reveal bilateral infiltrate of the lung. The cell block preparation shows loosely formed clusters and dispersed large epithelial cells with hyperchromatic nuclei, coarse chromatin, prominent nucleoli, irregular nuclear membranes, "lacy" cytoplasm, and cytoplasmic vacuolization. In goblet cell hyperplasia, it reveals clusters of cells in honeycomb arrangement, with abundant mucin-filled cytoplasm and eccentrically located nuclei; no malignant nuclear features are identified. In reactive bronchial epithelium, cells are arranged in three-dimensional clusters, with marked variation of nuclear sizes, without malignant nuclear features, cells still have cilia.

A-25. (c) **Adenocarcinoma**
The cell block preparation shows loosely formed clusters and dispersed large epithelial cells with hyperchromatic nuclei, coarse chromatin, prominent nucleoli, irregular nuclear membranes, and "lacy" cytoplasm. In reactive bronchial epithelium, cells reveal marked variation of nuclear sizes, without malignant nuclear features, and cells still have cilia. Bronchoalveolar macrophages reveal clusters of cells with abundant vacuolated cytoplasm and nuclei without malignant nuclear features. In squamous cell carcinomas, tumor cells are predominately arranged in dispersed individual cells, with large nuclei, hyperchromatic smudgy chromatin, marked variation of nuclear size and shape, and dense cytoplasm (cytokeratin formation). In addition, spindle-shaped cells and bizarre tumor cells are also commonly seen.

A-26. (d) **Adenocarcinoma**
The Diff-Quik stain shows loosely formed clusters with acini arrangement and dispersed large epithelial cells with hyperchromatic nuclei, coarse chromatin, prominent nucleoli, irregular nuclear membranes, and "lacy" cytoplasm. In reactive bronchial epithelium, cells reveal marked variation of nuclear sizes, without malignant nuclear features, and cells still have cilia. Bronchoalveolar macrophages may be arranged in clusters, and cells reveal abundant vacuolated cytoplasm and nuclei without malignant nuclear features. In squamous cell

carcinomas, tumor cells are predominately arranged in dispersed individual cells, with large nuclei, hyperchromatic smudgy chromatin, marked variation of nuclear size and shape, and dense cytoplasm (cytokeratin formation). In addition, spindle-shaped cells and bizarre tumor cells are also commonly seen.

A-27. (**c**) **Metastatic carcinoma of the breast**
The Diff-Quik preparation shows tight three-dimensional clusters of cells with acini arrangements. Cells are intermediate in size and relatively uniform in appearance; they may or may not have pseudointranuclear inclusions (best seen on Papanicolaou stain). Tumor cells reveal hyperchromatic nuclei, coarse chromatin, "lacy" cytoplasm and cytoplasmic vacuolization, and high N/C ratio. In adenocarcinomas of the lung, tumor cells are larger in size, and form clusters and dispersed individual cells with hyperchromatic nuclei, coarse chromatin, prominent nucleoli, irregular nuclear membranes, and "lacy" cytoplasm. IHC stains of breast carcinoma markers (ER, PR, GCDFP, mammaglobin, and GATA3) and lung carcinoma markers (TTF1 and Napsin A) may help with the differential diagnosis.

A-28. (**c**) **Metastatic carcinoma of the colon**
In metastatic colonic adenocarcinoma, tumor cells are large in size and form three-dimensional cluster and acinar arrangements, with elongated nuclei and tumor necrosis. In adenocarcinoma of the lung, tumor cells are arranged in clusters and dispersed individual cells with hyperchromatic nuclei, coarse chromatin, prominent nucleoli, irregular nuclear membranes, and "lacy" cytoplasm. IHC stains of colon carcinoma markers (CK20 and CDX2) and lung carcinoma markers (CK7, TTF1, and Napsin A) may help with the differential diagnosis.

A-29. (**d**) **Small cell carcinoma**
The Diff-Quik preparation shows tight clusters of small hyperchromatic cells (two to three times of the size of mature lymphocytes) with scant cytoplasm, fine chromatin ("salt-and-pepper" appearance), nuclear molding and crowding, inconspicuous nucleoli (best seen on Papanicolaou stain), nuclear stripes (broken down nuclear material), mitosis, necrosis, and apoptotic bodies. In reactive lymphocytes, cells are discohesive and have coarse chromatin. Lymphoglandular bodies are present on the slide.

A-30. (**c**) **Metastatic carcinoma of the breast**
Breast carcinoma is a common tumor which metastases to the lung, due to its anatomic location. Metastatic breast carcinomas have many cytological features that overlap with primary lung adenocarcinomas. In metastatic breast carcinomas, tumor cells are intermediate in size and arranged in tight three-dimensional clusters and/or acini. Tumor cells reveal a monotonous appearance, with hyperchromatic nuclei, prominent nucleoli and frequently with intracytoplasmic lumen. In lung adenocarcinomas, tumor cells may have more pleomorphic appearance and variation in size and shape of nuclei. In difficult cases, immunostains of breast cancer markers (estrogen receptor (ER), progesterone receptor (PR), gross cystic disease fluid protein (GCDFP-15), mammaglobin and GATA-3) and lung markers (TTF1 and napsin A) may help for the differential diagnosis.

A-31. (**c**) **Metastatic carcinoma of the colon**
In metastatic colonic adenocarcinoma, tumor cells are large in size and form three-dimensional clusters and acinar arrangements, with elongated nuclei and tumor necrosis. In adenocarcinoma of the lung, tumor cells are arranged in clusters and dispersed individual cells with hyperchromatic nuclei, coarse chromatin, prominent nucleoli, irregular nuclear membranes, and "lacy" cytoplasm. IHC stains of colon carcinoma markers (CK20 and CDX2) and lung carcinoma markers (CK7, TTF1, and Napsin A) may help with the differential diagnosis.

A-32. (**a**) **Reactive bronchial epithelium**
It can be difficult to distinguish reactive bronchial epithelial cells (reactive atypia) from a well differentiated adenocarcinoma. In reactive atypia, bronchial epithelial cells form sheets and/or loose cluster of cells with mildly to moderately enlarged nuclei, vesicular chromatin, single or multiple small nucleoli, abundant cytoplasm, and normal N:C ratio. The important clue for reactive atypia is the presence of cilia on bronchial epithelial cells. In a well-differentiated adenocarcinoma, tumor cells are arranged in two- or three-dimensional clusters or in disorganized sheets. Tumor cells have round nuclei, vesicular chromatin, small nucleoli and foamy cytoplasm, and high N:C ratio. However, no cilia are identified in tumor cell clusters.

A-33. (**b**) **Goblet cell hyperplasia**
In goblet cell hyperplasia, it reveals clusters and/or honeycomb sheets of cells with abundant mucin-filled cytoplasm and eccentrically located nuclei ("signet ring" appearance); no malignant nuclear features are identified. In reactive bronchial epithelium,

cells are arranged in three-dimensional clusters, with marked variation of nuclear sizes, without malignant nuclear features, cells still have cilia. In adenocarcinomas, tumor cells are arranged in two- or three-dimensional clusters or in disorganized sheets. Tumor cells reveal large round to oval nuclei, coarse chromatin, prominent nucleoli and foamy cytoplasm, and high N:C ratio. However, no cilia are identified in tumor cell clusters.

A-34. (b) **Small cell carcinoma**
The Papanicolaou preparation shows tight clusters of small hyperchromatic cells (two to three times of the size of mature lymphocytes) with scant cytoplasm, fine chromatin ("salt-and-pepper" appearance), nuclear molding and crowding, inconspicuous nucleoli (best seen on Papanicolaou stain), nuclear stripes (broken down nuclear material), mitosis, necrosis, and apoptotic bodies. In reactive squamous, cells are large in size, discohesive, and have pyknotic nuclei with smudgy chromatin. The cytoplasm is dense with cytokeratin. In adenocarcinomas, tumor cells are arranged in two- or three-dimensional clusters or in disorganized sheets. Tumor cells reveal large round to oval nuclei, coarse chromatin, prominent nucleoli and foamy cytoplasm, and high N:C ratio.

A-35. (d) **Adenocarcinoma with mucinous features**
The Papanicolaou stain shows three-dimensional clusters of malignant hyperchromatic cells with extra and intracytoplasmic mucin. The differential diagnosis includes primary lung adenocarcinoma verse a metastatic adenocarcinoma with mucin production, such as adenocarcinoma of stomach, breast, and colon. IHC study (TTF1 and Napsin A) is necessary to confirm the lung primary. In goblet cell hyperplasia, it reveals clusters and/or honeycomb sheets of cells with abundant mucin-filled cytoplasm and eccentrically located nuclei ("signet ring" appearance); no malignant nuclear features are identified. In reactive bronchial epithelium, cells are arranged in three-dimensional clusters, with marked variation of nuclear sizes, without malignant nuclear features, cells still have cilia.

A-36. (a) **Reactive bronchial cells and *Candida***
In candidiasis, budding yeasts with pseudohyphae are identified. Pseudohyphae are 2–10 μm in diameter and branch at a 90° angle. *Candida* is also a common finding of oral contamination in sputum. Aspergillosis is characterized by the presence of mucus plugs containing fungal organisms admixed with birefringent calcium oxalate crystals, inflammatory cells, and eosinophils. *Aspergillus* are characterized by true septate hyphae with 45° angle branching. The uniform thickness (3–6 μm in width) and the septa of hyphae differentiate *Aspergillus* from other fungus such as *Mucor* and *Candida*. Aspergillosis can also cause reactive atypia mimicking of non-small cell lung cancers, particularly a squamous cell carcinoma.

A-37. (d) **Adenocarcinoma**
The Papanicolaou preparation shows three-dimensional clusters of cells with acini arrangement. Tumor cells reveal high N/C ratio, hyperchromatic nuclei, "lacy" cytoplasm, and cytoplasmic vacuolization. Nuclei are large with irregular nuclear membranes, coarse chromatin, and prominent nucleoli. In reactive bronchial epithelium, cells are arranged in three-dimensional clusters, with marked variation of nuclear sizes, without malignant nuclear features, cells still have cilia.

A-38. (d) **Adenocarcinoma**
The Papanicolaou preparation shows clusters of cells with acini arrangement and dispersed individual tumor cells with elongated nuclei. Tumor cells reveal high N/C ratio, hyperchromatic nuclei, "lacy" cytoplasm, and cytoplasmic vacuolization. Nuclei are large with irregular nuclear membranes, coarse chromatin, and prominent nucleoli. In reactive bronchial epithelium, cells are arranged in three-dimensional clusters, with marked variation of nuclear sizes, without malignant nuclear features, cells still have cilia. In squamous cell carcinomas, tumor cells are predominately arranged in dispersed individual cells, with large nuclei, hyperchromatic smudgy chromatin, and marked variation of nuclear size and shape. In addition, spindle-shaped cells and bizarre tumor cells are also commonly seen. Tumor cells of squamous cell carcinomas also reveal dense cytoplasm with cytokeratin formation.

A-39. (d) **Poorly differentiated adenocarcinoma**
The Papanicolaou preparation shows tightly formed three-dimensional clusters of tumor cells with high N/C ratio, "lacy" cytoplasm, and cytoplasmic vacuolization. There is no obvious acini arrangement as seen in a well-differentiated adenocarcinoma. Nuclei of tumor cells are large with irregular nuclear membranes, coarse chromatin, and multiple prominent nucleoli. In reactive bronchial epithelium, cells are arranged in three-dimensional clusters, with marked variation of nuclear sizes, without malignant nuclear features, cells still have cilia.

A-40. (**a**) **Reactive bronchial epithelial cells**
It can be difficult to distinguish reactive bronchial epithelial cells (reactive atypia) from a well-differentiated adenocarcinoma. In reactive atypia, bronchial epithelial cells form sheets and/or cluster of cells with mildly to moderately enlarged nuclei, vesicular chromatin, single or multiple small nucleoli, abundant cytoplasm, and normal N:C ratio. The important clue for reactive atypia is the presence of cilia on bronchial epithelial cells. In a well-differentiated adenocarcinoma, tumor cells are arranged in two- or three-dimensional clusters or in disorganized sheets. Tumor cells have round nuclei, vesicular chromatin, small nucleoli and foamy cytoplasm, and high N:C ratio. However, no cilia are identified in tumor cell clusters.

A-41. (**a**) **Reactive bronchial epithelial cells**
It can be difficult to distinguish reactive bronchial epithelial cells (reactive atypia) from a well-differentiated adenocarcinoma. In reactive atypia, bronchial epithelial cells form sheets and/or cluster of cells with mildly to moderately enlarged nuclei, vesicular chromatin, single or multiple small nucleoli, abundant cytoplasm, and normal N:C ratio. The important clue for reactive atypia is the presence of cilia on bronchial epithelial cells. In a well-differentiated adenocarcinoma, tumor cells are arranged in two- or three-dimensional clusters or in disorganized sheets. Tumor cells have round nuclei, vesicular chromatin, small nucleoli and foamy cytoplasm, and high N:C ratio. However, no cilia are identified in tumor cell clusters.

A-42. (**d**) **Reactive bronchial epithelial cells**
It can be difficult to distinguish reactive bronchial epithelial cells (reactive atypia) from a well-differentiated adenocarcinoma. In reactive atypia, bronchial epithelial cells form sheets and/or cluster of cells with mildly to moderately enlarged nuclei, vesicular chromatin, single or multiple small nucleoli, abundant cytoplasm, and normal N:C ratio. The important clue for reactive atypia is the presence of cilia on bronchial epithelial cells. In a well-differentiated adenocarcinoma, tumor cells are arranged in two- or three-dimensional clusters or in disorganized sheets. Tumor cells have round nuclei, vesicular chromatin, small nucleoli and foamy cytoplasm, and high N:C ratio. However, no cilia are identified in tumor cell clusters.

A-43. (**b**) **Reactive bronchial epithelial cells**
It can be difficult to distinguish reactive bronchial epithelial cells (reactive atypia) from a well-differentiated adenocarcinoma. In reactive atypia, bronchial epithelial cells form sheets and/or cluster of cells with mildly to moderately enlarged nuclei, vesicular chromatin, single or multiple small nucleoli, abundant cytoplasm, and normal N:C ratio. The important clue for reactive atypia is the presence of cilia on bronchial epithelial cells. In a well-differentiated adenocarcinoma, tumor cells are arranged in two- or three-dimensional clusters or in disorganized sheets. Tumor cells have round nuclei, vesicular chromatin, small nucleoli and foamy cytoplasm, and high N:C ratio. However, no cilia are identified in tumor cell clusters.

A-44. (**d**) **Adenocarcinoma**
The Papanicolaou preparation shows clusters of cells with acini arrangement and dispersed individual tumor cells with elongated nuclei. Tumor cells reveal high N/C ratio, hyperchromatic nuclei, "lacy" cytoplasm, and cytoplasmic vacuolization. Nuclei are large with irregular nuclear membranes, coarse chromatin, and prominent nucleoli. In reactive bronchial epithelium, cells are arranged in three-dimensional clusters, with marked variation of nuclear sizes, without malignant nuclear features, cells still have cilia. In squamous cell carcinomas, tumor cells are predominately arranged in dispersed individual cells, with large nuclei, hyperchromatic smudgy chromatin, and marked variation of nuclear size and shape. In addition, spindle-shaped cells and bizarre tumor cells are also commonly seen. Tumor cells of squamous cell carcinomas also reveal dense cytoplasm with cytokeratin formation. In small cell carcinomas, tumor cells are small and with "salt-and-pepper" chromatin, nuclear crowding and molding.

A-45. (**c**) **Goblet cell hyperplasia**
In goblet cell hyperplasia, it reveals clusters and/or honeycomb sheets of cells with abundant mucin-filled cytoplasm and eccentrically located nuclei ("signet ring" appearance); no malignant nuclear features are identified. In reactive bronchial epithelium, cells are arranged in three-dimensional clusters, with marked variation of nuclear sizes, without malignant nuclear features, cells still have cilia. In adenocarcinomas, tumor cells are arranged in two- or three-dimensional clusters or in disorganized sheets. Tumor cells reveal large round to oval nuclei, coarse chromatin, prominent nucleoli and foamy cytoplasm, and high N:C ratio. However, no cilia are identified in tumor cell clusters. In small cell carcinomas, tumor cells are small and with "salt-and-pepper" chromatin, nuclear crowding and molding.

A-46. (a) **Small cell carcinoma**
The cell block preparation shows tight clusters of small hyperchromatic cells with scant cytoplasm, nuclear molding, and crowding. In small cell carcinomas, tumor cells are relatively small in size and approximately two- to threefold of mature lymphocytes. Tumor cells reveal scant cytoplasm and high N:C ratio, large nuclei with fine chromatin (salt-and-pepper) pattern, nuclear crowding and molding, and paranuclear blue bodies in the cytoplasm. Numerous "blue strips" may be seen on smears due to crush artifacts and the breakdown of nuclei DNA material. The nucleoli are inconspicuous in small cell carcinomas. In some cases, tumor cells may reveal rare nucleoli, but they are small in size. In reactive lymphocytes, cells are discohesive and have coarse chromatin. Lymphoglandular bodies are present on the slide. In adenocarcinomas, tumor cells are arranged in two- or three-dimensional clusters or in disorganized sheets. Tumor cells reveal large round to oval nuclei, coarse chromatin, prominent nucleoli, and foamy cytoplasm.

A-47. (c) **Cryptococcosis**
Cryptococcosis is caused by infection of *Cryptococcus neoformans*, the inhabitants in the soil with bird droppings. The infection occurs in both immunocompromised and immunocompetent patients worldwide and may involve many body sites; however, lung involvement is more common. In a BAL specimen, the fungus reveals as yeast forms with narrow and pinched buddings, refractile centers, and mucoid capsules (clear zone around the stained organisms). The capsule is positive with periodic acid–Schiff, alcian blue, and mucicarmine stains. In histoplasmosis, numerous small budding yeasts are seen in the cytoplasm of histiocytes. The infection is most commonly seen in the Ohio and Mississippi river valleys. In blastomycosis, specimen reveals large broad-based budding yeasts (8–20 μm in diameters) with thick cell walls. The yeast is bigger than Cryptococcus.

A-48. (c) **Degenerated alveolar macrophages**
In BAL specimen, alveolar macrophages are arranged in loose clusters or individual cells with benign nuclear features and foamy cytoplasm. Cells may reveal cytoplasmic pigments (anthracotic pigments in smokers) or vacuoles (in the lipid pneumonia). In degenerative changes, cells may reveal hyperchromatic nuclei and slightly irregular nuclear membrane. In adenocarcinomas and signet ring cell carcinomas, tumor cells are arranged in two- or three-dimensional clusters or in disorganized sheets. Tumor cells reveal large round to oval nuclei, coarse chromatin, prominent nucleoli, foamy cytoplasm, and high N:C ratio.

A-49. (d) **Adenocarcinoma**
The Diff-Quik preparation shows clusters of cells with acini arrangement and dispersed individual tumor cells. Tumor cells reveal high N/C ratio, hyperchromatic nuclei, "lacy" cytoplasm, and cytoplasmic vacuolization. Nuclei are large with irregular nuclear membranes, coarse chromatin, and prominent nucleoli. In reactive bronchial epithelium, cells are arranged in three-dimensional clusters, with marked variation of nuclear sizes, without malignant nuclear features, cells still have cilia. In squamous cell carcinomas, tumor cells are predominately arranged in dispersed individual cells, with large nuclei, hyperchromatic smudgy chromatin, and marked variation of nuclear size and shape. In addition, spindle-shaped cells and bizarre tumor cells are also commonly seen. Tumor cells of squamous cell carcinomas also reveal dense cytoplasm with cytokeratin formation. In small cell carcinomas, tumor cells are small and with "salt-and-pepper" chromatin, nuclear crowding and molding.

A-50. (b) **Adenocarcinoma**
The Papanicolaou preparation shows predominantly dispersed individual tumor cells and clusters of cells with acini arrangement. Tumor cells reveal high N/C ratio, hyperchromatic nuclei, "lacy" cytoplasm, and cytoplasmic vacuolization. Nuclei are large with irregular nuclear membranes, coarse chromatin, and prominent nucleoli. In reactive bronchial epithelium, cells are arranged in three-dimensional clusters, with marked variation of nuclear sizes, without malignant nuclear features, cells still have cilia. In squamous cell carcinomas, tumor cells are predominately arranged in dispersed individual cells, with large nuclei, hyperchromatic smudgy chromatin, and marked variation of nuclear size and shape. In addition, spindle-shaped cells and bizarre tumor cells are also commonly seen. Tumor cells of squamous cell carcinomas also reveal dense cytoplasm with cytokeratin formation. In small cell carcinomas, tumor cells are small and with "salt-and-pepper" chromatin, nuclear crowding and molding.

A-51. (b) **Adenocarcinoma**
The Diff-Quik preparation shows predominantly clusters and dispersed individual tumor cells with acini arrangement. Tumor cells reveal high N/C ratio, hyperchromatic nuclei, "lacy" cytoplasm, and

cytoplasmic vacuolization. Nuclei are large with irregular nuclear membranes, coarse chromatin, and prominent nucleoli. In reactive bronchial epithelium, cells are arranged in three-dimensional clusters, with marked variation of nuclear sizes, without malignant nuclear features, cells still have cilia. In squamous cell carcinomas, tumor cells are predominately arranged in dispersed individual cells, with large nuclei, hyperchromatic smudgy chromatin, and marked variation of nuclear size and shape. In addition, spindle-shaped cells and bizarre tumor cells are also commonly seen. In a poorly differentiated squamous cell carcinoma, tumor cells may have prominent nucleoli, mimicking adenocarcinomas, however, tumor cells of squamous cell carcinomas also reveal dense cytoplasm with cytokeratin formation, separating them from adenocarcinomas. In small cell carcinomas, tumor cells are small and with "salt-and-pepper" chromatin, nuclear crowding and molding.

A-52. (**d**) **Granulomatous inflammation**
The Diff-Quik preparation shows clusters of epithelioid histiocytes admixed with inflammatory cells, scattered multinucleated giant cells, and reactive bronchial cells. Granulomatous inflammation may be found in both benign such as sarcoidosis and malignant lesions. Sarcoidosis is an idiopathic disease characterized by non-necrotizing granulomas. It typically involves mediastinal lymph nodes and the lung. However, it can be a systemic process and involve other organs, such as the heart, central nerve system, and skin. The disease usually occurs in middle-aged African-American females. The patient may need steroid therapy. In adenocarcinomas, tumor cells reveal high N/C ratio, hyperchromatic nuclei, "lacy" cytoplasm, and cytoplasmic vacuolization. Nuclei are large with irregular nuclear membranes, coarse chromatin, and prominent nucleoli.

A-53. (**d**) **Metastatic synovial sarcoma**
The Diff-Quik slide shows predominately dispersed individual tumor cells with pleomorphic, spindle- to oval-shaped nuclei, and scant cytoplasm. The nuclei are hyperchromatic with coarse chromatin and small nucleoli. Mitosis is frequent. Tumor cells are positive for AE1/AE3, EMA, CD99, and vimentin. The main differential diagnosis is poorly differentiated carcinoma. In squamous cell carcinomas, tumor cells are predominately arranged in dispersed individual cells, with large nuclei, hyperchromatic smudgy chromatin, marked variation of nuclear size and shape, and cytokeratin. In addition, spindle-shaped cells and bizarre tumor cells are also commonly seen, however, tumor cells of squamous cell carcinomas also reveal dense cytoplasm with cytokeratin formation. In a poorly differentiated adenocarcinoma, it reveals predominantly dispersed individual tumor cells and clusters of cells with acini arrangement. Tumor cells reveal high N/C ratio, hyperchromatic nuclei, "lacy" cytoplasm, and cytoplasmic vacuolization.

A-54. (**d**) **Bronchioalveolar macrophages**
In BAL specimen, alveolar macrophages are arranged in loose clusters or individual cells with benign nuclear features and foamy cytoplasm. Cells may reveal cytoplasmic pigments (anthracotic pigments in smokers) or vacuoles (in the lipid pneumonia). In degenerative changes, cells may reveal hyperchromatic nuclei and slightly irregular nuclear membranes. In adenocarcinomas and signet ring cell carcinomas, tumor cells are arranged in two- or three-dimensional clusters or in disorganized sheets. Tumor cells reveal large round to oval nuclei, coarse chromatin, prominent nucleoli, irregular nuclear membranes, foamy cytoplasm, and high N:C ratio.

A-55. (**c**) **Poorly differentiated squamous cell carcinoma**
In squamous cell carcinomas, tumor cells are predominately arranged in dispersed individual cells, with large nuclei, hyperchromatic smudgy chromatin, marked variation of nuclear size and shape, and cytoplasmic keratin. In addition, spindle-shaped cells and bizarre tumor cells are also commonly seen. In a poorly differentiated squamous cell carcinoma, tumor cells may have prominent nucleoli, mimicking adenocarcinoma; however, tumor cells of squamous cell carcinomas also reveal dense cytoplasm with cytokeratin formation, separating them from adenocarcinomas. In adenocarcinomas, tumor cells are arranged in two- or three-dimensional clusters or in disorganized sheets. Tumor cells reveal large round to oval nuclei, coarse chromatin, prominent nucleoli, foamy cytoplasm, and high N:C ratio. In small cell carcinomas, tumor cells are small and with "salt-and-pepper" chromatin, nuclear crowding and molding.

A-56. (**c**) **Squamous cell carcinoma**
Diff-Quik stain shows polygonal, rounded, elongated, or tadpole-shaped cells with large hyperchromatic nuclei and dense cytoplasm. In squamous cell carcinomas, tumor cells are predominately arranged in dispersed individual cells, with large nuclei, hyperchromatic smudgy chromatin, marked variation

of nuclear size and shape, and cytoplasmic keratin. In addition, spindle-shaped cells and bizarre tumor cells are also commonly seen. In a poorly differentiated squamous cell carcinoma, tumor cells may have prominent nucleoli, mimicking adenocarcinomas, however, tumor cells of squamous cell carcinomas also reveal dense cytoplasm with cytokeratin formation, separating them from adenocarcinomas. In adenocarcinomas, tumor cells are arranged in two- or three-dimensional clusters or in disorganized sheets. Tumor cells reveal large round to oval nuclei, coarse chromatin, prominent nucleoli, foamy cytoplasm, and high N:C ratio. In goblet cells and bronchioalveolar macrophages, cells reveal abundant foamy cytoplasm and cytoplasmic vacuoles, without malignant nuclear features.

A-57. (c) **Squamous cell carcinoma**
Diff-Quik stain shows polygonal, rounded, elongated, or tadpole-shaped cells with large hyperchromatic nuclei and dense cytoplasm. In squamous cell carcinomas, tumor cells are predominately arranged in dispersed individual cells, with large nuclei, hyperchromatic smudgy chromatin, marked variation of nuclear size and shape, and cytoplasmic keratin. In addition, spindle-shaped cells and bizarre tumor cells are also commonly seen. In adenocarcinomas, tumor cells are arranged in two- or three-dimensional clusters or in disorganized sheets. Tumor cells reveal large round to oval nuclei, coarse chromatin, prominent nucleoli, foamy cytoplasm, and high N:C ratio. In granulomas, it reveals clusters of epithelioid histiocytes admixed with inflammatory cells, scattered multinucleated giant cells, and reactive bronchial cells.

A-58. (c) **Squamous cell carcinoma**
Diff-Quik stain shows polygonal, rounded, elongated, or tadpole-shaped cells with large hyperchromatic nuclei and dense cytoplasm. In squamous cell carcinomas, tumor cells are predominately arranged in dispersed individual cells, with large nuclei, hyperchromatic smudgy chromatin, marked variation of nuclear size and shape, and cytoplasmic keratin. In addition, spindle-shaped cells and bizarre tumor cells are also commonly seen. In adenocarcinomas, tumor cells are arranged in two- or three-dimensional clusters or in disorganized sheets. Tumor cells reveal large round to oval nuclei, coarse chromatin, prominent nucleoli, foamy cytoplasm, and high N:C ratio. In granulomas, it reveals clusters of epithelioid histiocytes admixed with inflammatory cells, scattered multinucleated giant cells, and reactive bronchial cells. In bronchial reserve cell hyperplasia, cells are arranged in cohesive sheets or clusters with nuclear overlapping and crowding. The nuclei reveal dark smudgy chromatin, inconspicuous nucleoli, smooth nuclear membrane, and scant cytoplasm. The N:C ratio is in normal range or slightly increased.

A-59. (d) **Degenerated bronchioalveolar macrophages**
The slide reveals dispersed intermediate cells with normal N:C ratio, cytoplasmic vacuoles, breakdown of nuclei membranes, and smudgy chromatin. In BAL specimen, alveolar macrophages are arranged in loose clusters or individual cells with benign nuclear features and foamy cytoplasm. Cells may reveal cytoplasmic pigments (anthracotic pigments in smokers) or vacuoles (in the lipid pneumonia). In degenerative changes, cells may reveal hyperchromatic nuclei and slightly irregular nuclear membranes. In adenocarcinomas and signet ring cell carcinomas, tumor cells are arranged in two- or three-dimensional clusters or in disorganized sheets. Tumor cells reveal large round to oval nuclei, coarse chromatin, prominent nucleoli, irregular nuclear membranes, foamy cytoplasm, and high N:C ratio.

A-60. (a) **Goblet cell**
In a bronchial washing and/or BAL specimen, goblet cells are arranged in clusters and/or honeycomb sheets of cells with abundant mucin-filled cytoplasm and eccentrically located nuclei ("signet ring" appearance); no malignant nuclear features are identified. In adenocarcinomas and signet ring cell carcinomas, tumor cells are arranged in two- or three-dimensional clusters or in disorganized sheets. Tumor cells reveal large round to oval nuclei, coarse chromatin, prominent nucleoli and foamy cytoplasm, and high N:C ratio. No cilia are identified in tumor cell clusters. In small cell carcinomas, tumor cells are small and with "salt-and-pepper" chromatin, nuclear crowding and molding.

A-61. (d) **Goblet cell hyperplasia**
In goblet cell hyperplasia, it reveals clusters of cells and sheets of cells in honeycomb arrangement, with abundant mucin-filled cytoplasm and eccentrically located nuclei ("signet ring" appearance). Cells are without nuclear atypia. In adenocarcinomas and signet ring cell carcinomas, tumor cells are arranged in two- or three-dimensional clusters or in disorganized sheets. Tumor cells reveal large round to oval nuclei, coarse chromatin, prominent nucleoli and foamy cytoplasm, and high N:C ratio. No cilia are identified in tumor cell clusters. In small cell

carcinomas, tumor cells are small and with "salt-and-pepper" chromatin, nuclear crowding and molding. In granulomas, it reveals clusters of epithelioid histiocytes with elongated and curved nuclei admixed with lymphocytes.

A-62. (**a**) **Squamous cells with reactive atypia**
The slide reveals discohesive clusters and scattered individual cells with keratinization, small pyknotic nuclei, and normal N:C ratio. Reactive squamous cells have several cytological features overlapping with well-differentiated squamous cell carcinomas. In reactive squamous cells, cells may be arranged in small two-dimensional clusters and dispersed individual cells. They reveal mildly enlarged nuclei with minimal variation in size and shape, and abundant dense cytoplasm. The N:C ratio of the cell is normal or slightly increased. In squamous cell carcinomas, tumor cells are predominately arranged in clusters and dispersed individual cells, with large nuclei, hyperchromatic smudgy chromatin, marked variation of nuclear size and shape, and dense cytoplasm (cytokeratin formation). In addition, spindle-shaped cells and bizarre tumor cells are also commonly seen. Prominent necrotic debris in the background is also a feature for squamous cell carcinomas.

A-63. (**b**) **Reactive squamous cells**
In reactive squamous cells, cells may be arranged in small two-dimensional clusters and dispersed individual cells. They reveal mildly enlarged nuclei with minimal variation in size and shape, and abundant dense cytoplasm. The N:C ratio of the cell is normal or slightly increased. In squamous cell carcinomas, tumor cells are predominately arranged in clusters and dispersed individual cells, with large nuclei, hyperchromatic smudgy chromatin, marked variation of nuclear size and shape, and dense cytoplasm (cytokeratin formation). In addition, spindle-shaped cells and bizarre tumor cells are also commonly seen. Prominent necrotic debris in the background is also a feature for squamous cell carcinomas.

A-64. (**a**) **Non-diagnostic specimen**
It is a non-diagnostic specimen, due to the lack of bronchoalveolar macrophages. The criteria for an adequate sputum specimen include the presence of alveolar macrophages and/or Curschmann spirals, which indicate a representative collection of the lower respiratory tract material. Other cells and material in specimens such as squamous cells, neutrophils, and chronic inflammatory may represent oral contaminations. Sometimes, ciliated respiratory epithelial cells can be identified in the sputum, but they do not necessarily represent cells that come from the lower respiratory tract, since ciliated respiratory epithelial cells can be found in the lining of sinonasal passage of the upper respiratory tract.

A-65. (**c**) **Karetin debris and it is necessary to repeat the biopsy**
This is a non-diagnostic specimen; it predominantly contains keratin debris and no tumor cells seen. Prominent keratin and necrotic debris in the background of the slide is a feature commonly seen in a squamous cell carcinomas, however, the feature can also be seen in benign lesions. Therefore, a repeat biopsy of the viable tumor is necessary to establish the diagnosis of a squamous cell carcinoma.

A-66. (**d**) **Reactive bronchial epithelium**
The slide reveals three-dimensional clusters and dispersed individual columnar cells. It can be difficult to distinguish reactive bronchial epithelial cells (reactive atypia) from a well-differentiated adenocarcinoma. In reactive atypia, bronchial epithelial cells form sheets and/or cluster of cells with mildly to moderately enlarged nuclei, vesicular chromatin, single or multiple small nucleoli, abundant cytoplasm, and normal N:C ratio. The important clue for reactive atypia is the presence of cilia on bronchial epithelial cells. In a well-differentiated adenocarcinoma, the tumor cells are arranged in two- or three-dimensional clusters or in disorganized sheets. Tumor cells are intermediate in size with round nuclei, vesicular chromatin, small nucleoli and foamy cytoplasm, and high N:C ratio. However, no cilia are identified in tumor cell clusters.

A-67. (**c**) **Bronchioalveolar macrophages**
The slide reveals a large cell with round nuclei, normal N:C ratio, vacuolated cytoplasm, and cytoplasmic red blood cells. In BAL specimens, alveolar macrophages are arranged in loose clusters or individual cells with benign nuclear features and foamy cytoplasm. Cells may reveal cytoplasmic pigments (anthracotic pigments in smokers) or vacuoles (in the lipid pneumonia). In degenerative changes, cells may reveal hyperchromatic nuclei and slightly irregular nuclear membranes. In adenocarcinomas and signet ring cell carcinomas, tumor cells are arranged in two- or three-dimensional clusters or in disorganized sheets. Tumor cells reveal large round to oval nuclei, coarse chromatin, prominent nucleoli, irregular nuclear membranes, foamy cytoplasm, and high N:C ratio.

A-68. (**b**) **Adenocarcinoma**
The Papanicolaou preparation shows two-dimensional clusters and acini of hyperchromatic tumor cells with high N/C ratio, "lacy" cytoplasm, and cytoplasmic vacuolization. Nuclei are large with hyperchromatic coarse chromatin, irregular nuclear membranes, and prominent nucleoli. In squamous cell carcinomas, tumor cells are predominately arranged in clusters and dispersed individual cells, with large nuclei, hyperchromatic smudgy chromatin, marked variation of nuclear size and shape, and dense cytoplasm (cytokeratin formation). In addition, spindle-shaped cells and bizarre tumor cells are also commonly seen.

A-69. (**a**) **Poorly differentiated squamous cell carcinoma**
Papanicolaou stain shows discohesive and scattered individual polygonal tumor cells with large hyperchromatic nuclei and dense cytoplasm. Some of tumor cells show prominent nucleoli. In a poorly differentiated squamous cell carcinoma, tumor cells may be arranged in clusters and round up with prominent nucleoli, less or no cytokeratin formation. These features may be confused with adenocarcinomas. In adenocarcinomas, tumor cells are arranged in tight three-dimensional clusters. Tumor cells of adenocarcinomas have hyperchromatic nuclei, coarse chromatin, prominent nucleoli and vacuolated and feathery cytoplasm (indication of mucin production).

A-70. (**a**) **Poorly differentiated squamous cell carcinoma**
Papanicolaou stain shows discohesive and scattered individual polygonal tumor cells with large hyperchromatic nuclei and dense cytoplasm. Some of tumor cells show prominent nucleoli. In a poorly differentiated squamous cell carcinoma, tumor cells may be arranged in clusters and round up with prominent nucleoli, less or no cytokeratin formation. These features may be confused with adenocarcinomas. In adenocarcinomas, tumor cells are arranged in tight three-dimensional clusters. Tumor cells of adenocarcinomas have hyperchromatic nuclei, coarse chromatin, prominent nucleoli and vacuolated and feathery cytoplasm (indicative of mucin production).

A-71. (**a**) **Poorly differentiated squamous cell carcinoma**
Papanicolaou stain shows discohesive and scattered individual polygonal tumor cells with large hyperchromatic nuclei and dense cytoplasm. Some of tumor cells show prominent nucleoli. In a poorly differentiated squamous cell carcinoma, tumor cells may be arranged in clusters and round up with prominent nucleoli, less or no cytokeratin formation. These features may be confused with adenocarcinomas. In adenocarcinomas, tumor cells are arranged in tight three-dimensional clusters. Tumor cells of adenocarcinomas have hyperchromatic nuclei, coarse chromatin, prominent nucleoli and vacuolated and feathery cytoplasm (indicative of mucin production).

A-72. (**c**) **Reactive bronchial cells and mucin vacuole**
The slide reveals dispersed bronchial epithelial cells admixed with mucin vacuoles. In vegetable cells, it reveals sheets of rectangular shape, uniform cells with cellulose walls. Vegetable cells have large nuclei, resembling tumor cells of squamous cell carcinomas.

A-73. (**c**) **Reactive bronchial epithelial cells**
The diagnosis is reactive bronchial cells. The Papanicolaou preparation shows two- or three-dimensional clusters of columnar cells with cilia, benign nuclear features, and some variation of nuclear size. It can be difficult to distinguish reactive bronchial epithelial cells (reactive atypia) from a well-differentiated adenocarcinoma. In reactive atypia, bronchial epithelial cells form sheets and/or loose cluster of cells with mildly to moderately enlarged nuclei, vesicular chromatin, single or multiple small nucleoli, abundant cytoplasm, and normal N:C ratio. The important clue for reactive atypia is the presence of cilia on bronchial epithelial cells. In a well-differentiated adenocarcinoma, the tumor cells are arranged in two- or three-dimensional clusters or in disorganized sheets. Tumor cells are intermediate in size with round nuclei, vesicular chromatin, small nucleoli and foamy cytoplasm, and high N:C ratio. However, no cilia are identified in tumor cell clusters.

A-74. (**d**) **Bronchial reserve cells**
The slide reveals loose clusters of small "dark" cells with smudged chromatin and scant cytoplasm. In BAL and/or bronchial washing specimens, bronchial reserve cells are arranged in clusters and sheets. They are small in size and have hyperchromatic nuclei with nuclear crowding. Nuclei are "dark" with smudged chromatin, no mitoses or necrosis. The main differential diagnosis of bronchial reserve cells is small cell carcinoma. In small cell carcinomas, tumor cells are relatively small in size and approximately two- to threefold of mature lymphocytes. Tumor cells reveal scant cytoplasm

and high N:C ratio, nuclei with fine chromatin (salt-and-pepper) pattern, nuclear crowding and molding, and paranuclear blue bodies in the cytoplasm. Numerous "blue strips" may be seen on smears due to crush artifacts and the breakdown of nuclear DNA material.

A-75. (**b**) **Squamous cell carcinoma**

Papanicolaou stain shows discohesive and scattered individual polygonal tumor cells with large hyperchromatic nuclei and cytokeratin. In squamous cell carcinomas, tumor cells are predominately arranged in clusters and dispersed individual cells, with large nuclei, hyperchromatic smudgy chromatin, marked variation of nuclear size and shape, and dense cytoplasm (cytokeratin formation). In addition, spindle-shaped cells and bizarre tumor cells are also commonly seen. Prominent necrotic debris in the background is also a feature for squamous cell carcinomas. In reactive squamous cells, cells may be arranged in small two-dimensional clusters and dispersed individual cells. They reveal mildly enlarged nuclei with minimal variation in size and shape, and abundant dense cytoplasm. The N:C ratio of the cell is normal or slightly increased.

A-76. (**a**) **Squamous cell carcinoma**

Papanicolaou stain shows discohesive sheets and scattered individual polygonal tumor cells with large hyperchromatic nuclei and cytokeratin. In squamous cell carcinomas, tumor cells are predominately arranged in clusters and dispersed individual cells, with large nuclei, hyperchromatic smudgy chromatin, marked variation of nuclear size and shape, and dense cytoplasm (cytokeratin formation). In addition, spindle-shaped cells and bizarre tumor cells are also commonly seen. Prominent necrotic debris in the background is also a feature for squamous cell carcinomas. In reactive squamous cells, cells may be arranged in small two-dimensional clusters and dispersed individual cells. They reveal mildly enlarged nuclei with minimal variation in size and shape, and abundant dense cytoplasm. The N:C ratio of the cell is normal or slightly increased. In adenocarcinomas, the tumor cells are arranged in two- or three-dimensional clusters or in disorganized sheets. Tumor cells have high N:C ratio, round nuclei with vesicular chromatin, small nucleoli, and foamy cytoplasm.

A-77. (**a**) **Squamous cell carcinoma**

Papanicolaou stain shows discohesive sheets and scattered individual polygonal tumor cells with large hyperchromatic nuclei and cytokeratin. In squamous cell carcinomas, tumor cells are predominately arranged in clusters and dispersed individual cells, with large nuclei, hyperchromatic smudgy chromatin, marked variation of nuclear size and shape, and dense cytoplasm (cytokeratin formation). In addition, spindle-shaped cells and bizarre tumor cells are also commonly seen. Prominent necrotic debris in the background is also a feature for squamous cell carcinomas. In reactive squamous cells, cells may be arranged in small two-dimensional clusters and dispersed individual cells. They reveal mildly enlarged nuclei with minimal variation in size and shape, and abundant dense cytoplasm. The N:C ratio of the cell is normal or slightly increased. In adenocarcinomas, the tumor cells are arranged in two- or three-dimensional clusters or in disorganized sheets. Tumor cells have high N:C ratio, round nuclei with vesicular chromatin, small nucleoli, and foamy cytoplasm.

A-78. (**d**) **Squamous cell carcinoma**

Papanicolaou stain shows discohesive sheets and scattered individual polygonal tumor cells with large hyperchromatic nuclei and cytokeratin. In squamous cell carcinomas, tumor cells are predominately arranged in clusters and dispersed individual cells, with large nuclei, hyperchromatic smudgy chromatin, marked variation of nuclear size and shape, and dense cytoplasm (cytokeratin formation). In addition, spindle-shaped cells and bizarre tumor cells are also commonly seen. Prominent necrotic debris in the background is also a feature for squamous cells carcinoma. In reactive squamous cells, cells may be arranged in small two-dimensional clusters and dispersed individual cells. They reveal mildly enlarged nuclei with minimal variation in size and shape, and abundant dense cytoplasm. The N:C ratio of the cell is normal or slightly increased. In adenocarcinomas, the tumor cells are arranged in two- or three-dimensional clusters or in disorganized sheets. Tumor cells have high N:C ratio, round nuclei with vesicular chromatin, small nucleoli, and foamy cytoplasm.

A-79. (**d**) **Poorly differentiated squamous cell carcinoma**

Papanicolaou stain shows discohesive and scattered individual polygonal tumor cells with large hyperchromatic nuclei. Some of the tumor cells show prominent nucleoli. In a poorly differentiated squamous cell carcinoma, tumor cells may be arranged in clusters and round up with prominent nucleoli, less or no cytokeratin formation. These features may be confused with adenocarcinomas. In adenocarcinomas, tumor cells are arranged in tight three-dimensional clusters. Tumor cells of adenocarcinoma have hyperchromatic nuclei, coarse chromatin, prominent nucleoli, and vacuolated and feathery cytoplasm (indication of mucin production).

A-80. (**d**) **Squamous cell carcinoma**
Papanicolaou stain shows clusters/sheets and scattered individual polygonal tumor cells with large hyperchromatic nuclei and dense cytoplasm (cytokeratin formation). In squamous cell carcinomas, tumor cells are predominately arranged in clusters and dispersed individual cells, with large nuclei, hyperchromatic smudgy chromatin, marked variation of nuclear size and shape, and dense cytoplasm (cytokeratin formation). In addition, spindle-shaped cells and bizarre tumor cells are also commonly seen. Prominent necrotic debris in the background is also a feature for squamous cell carcinomas. In reactive squamous cells, cells may be arranged in small two-dimensional clusters and dispersed individual cells. They reveal mildly enlarged nuclei with minimal variation in size and shape, and abundant dense cytoplasm. The N:C ratio of the cell is normal or slightly increased. In adenocarcinomas, the tumor cells are arranged in two- or three-dimensional clusters or in disorganized sheets. Tumor cells have high N:C ratio, round nuclei with vesicular chromatin, small nucleoli, and foamy cytoplasm.

A-81. (**b**) **Squamous cell carcinoma**
The sputum specimen shows scattered individual polygonal tumor cells with large hyperchromatic nuclei and dense cytoplasm (cytokeratin formation). In squamous cell carcinomas, tumor cells are predominately arranged in clusters and dispersed individual cells, with large nuclei, hyperchromatic smudgy chromatin, marked variation of nuclear size and shape, and dense cytoplasm (cytokeratin formation). In addition, spindle-shaped cells and bizarre tumor cells are also commonly seen. Prominent necrotic debris in the background is also a feature for squamous cell carcinomas. In reactive squamous cells, cells may be arranged in small two-dimensional clusters and dispersed individual cells. They reveal mildly enlarged nuclei with minimal variation in size and shape, and abundant dense cytoplasm. The N:C ratio of the cell is normal or slightly increased. In adenocarcinomas, the tumor cells are arranged in two- or three-dimensional clusters or in disorganized sheets. Tumor cells have high N:C ratio, round nuclei with vesicular chromatin, small nucleoli, and foamy cytoplasm.

A-82. (**d**) **Small cell carcinoma**
The slide reveals tight clusters of small hyperchromatic cells with nuclear molding and crowding, mitosis, necrosis, and apoptotic body. In small cell carcinomas, tumor cells are relatively small in size and approximately two- to threefold of mature lymphocytes. Tumor cells reveal scant cytoplasm and high N:C ratio, nuclei with fine chromatin (salt-and-pepper) pattern, nuclear crowding and molding, and paranuclear blue bodies in the cytoplasm. Numerous "blue strips" may be seen on smears due to crush artifacts and the breakdown of nuclear DNA material. In BAL and/or bronchial washing specimens, bronchial reserve cells are arranged in clusters and sheets. They are small in size and have hyperchromatic nuclei with nuclear crowding. Nuclei are "dark" with smudged chromatin, no mitoses or necrosis. The main differential diagnosis of bronchial reserve cells is small cell carcinoma. In reactive lymphocytes, cells reveal coarse chromatin, scant cytoplasm, and lymphoglandular bodies, without nuclear crowding and molding.

1.4 Answers and Discussion of Text-Based Questions 83–151

A-83. **(b) Alveolar macrophages or Curschmann spirals**
Sputum specimens, including both spontaneous and induced specimens, are routinely used for the evaluation of respiratory tract lesions. A "good" sputum specimen is considered a specimen containing cellular material from the lower respiratory tract. Although they are easy to obtain, they are often contaminated with oral cells and material. Therefore, the first step in the cytological evaluation of sputum is to determine the adequacy of the specimen. The criteria for an adequate sputum specimen include the presence of alveolar macrophages and/or Curschmann spirals, which indicate a representative collection of the lower respiratory tract material. Other cells and material in sputum specimens such as squamous cells, neutrophils, mucus, bacteria, and Candida are considered oral contents, and they represent an unsatisfactory specimen. Sometimes, ciliated respiratory epithelial cells can be identified in the sputum, but they do not necessarily represent cells that come from the lower respiratory tract, since ciliated respiratory epithelial cells can be found in the lining of sinonasal passage of the upper respiratory tract.

A-84. **(d) All of the above**
For bronchoscopic procedures, including brushings, lavages/washings, and FNA specimens, an adequate specimen is crucial for an accurate diagnosis. Several factors are considered to play important roles in the process for accurate diagnosis, including (1) representative cells and material from the lesion, (2) a proper fixation of the specimen, and (3) crushing and drying artifacts. Furthermore, abundant ciliated bronchial epithelial cells may be present in the bronchoscopic specimen in a lung cancer patient, but the specimen should still be considered an inadequate and/or a non-diagnostic specimen due to lack of diagnostic tumor cells. In the BAL and washing specimens, as in sputum specimens, the finding of abundant alveolar macrophages is considered to be a satisfactory specimen.

A-85. **(d) Endoscopic transbronchial FNA with or without ultrasound guidance**
Endoscopic transbronchial FNA with (EBUS-TBNA) or without ultrasound guidance (TBNA) are commonly used procedures for the diagnosing and staging of lung cancers. Although both of them are useful for sampling mediastinal lymph nodes, EBUS-TBNA has a higher sensitivity and specificity than conventional TBNA in the staging of lung cancer patients. EBUS-TBNA can sample small lung lesions and small lymph nodes with the guidance of a built-in ultrasound probe. Otherwise, those small lesions and/or small mediastinal lymph nodes cannot be sampled by conventional TBNA. Endoscopic transesophageal FNA with (EUS-FNA) or without ultrasound guidance is also used for staging of lung cancer patients, but it can only sample certain locations of mediastinal lymph node. Both CT-guided transthoracic and ultrasound-guided transcutaneous fine needle biopsy (FNA) are more commonly used for diagnosis of lung lesions.

A-86. **(a) A 55-year-old female never smoker**
Recently, it has been reported that genomic abnormalities in the gene of anaplastic lymphomakinase (*ALK*) are detectable in a subset of 4 % (range: 0.9–13 %) of non-small cell lung cancer (NSCLC). In these tumors, a small paracentric inversion within the short arm of chromosome 2 results in an *ALK* gene rearrangement, causing a fusion gene *EML4-ALK* gene, which leads to a consecutive expression of the ALK kinase protein. Tumors containing *ALK* rearrangements are almost exclusive of adenocarcinomas without mutations of epidermal growth factor receptor (*EGFR*) gene or V-Ki-ras2 Kirsten rat sarcoma viral oncogene homolog (*KRAS*) gene, and preferentially involve in female non-smokers. Crizotinib, the ALK inhibitor, has been used as a targeted therapy in patients who have *ALK* gene rearrangement and shown to improve survival rates of patients. *ALK* gene rearrangement can be tested/detected by an FDA-approved ALK-FISH assay.

A-87. **(d) Clusters of ciliated bronchial epithelium (Creola bodies)**
Reactive bronchial epithelium hyperplastic changes (reactive atypia) can be caused by a variety of reasons, such as chemo- and radiation therapy, inflammation, chronic irritation, smoke, and others. Bronchial epithelium hyperplasia results in papillary-like mucosal folds. Bronchial epithelial cells are arranged in two- and three-dimensional clusters. The most characteristic finding is the presence of cells with cilia and/or Creola bodies, which are three-dimensional clusters of ciliated bronchial epithelium with slight variation of nuclei. Cells of Creola bodies have mild to moderate enlarged nuclei, vesicular chromatin, small nucleoli, and smooth nuclear membrane. The important differential diagnosis of

reactive atypia is a well-differentiated adenocarcinoma. In adenocarcinomas, tumor cells form tight three-dimensional clusters with hyperchromatic nuclei, prominent nucleoli, irregular nuclear membrane, and high N:C ratio. The important clue for reactive atypia is the presence of cilia on bronchial epithelial cells.

A-88. **(b) False**
Fragments of cartilage on a transbronchial fine-needle aspiration biopsy are common findings, they are not indicative of a lung hamartoma. During the procedure of transbronchial fine-needle aspiration biopsy, a wire stylet is placed within the lumen of the aspiration needle to prevent and to remove possible intraluminal bronchial epithelium and cartilage, that may obstruct the needle lumen. Then, the stylet is removed, and a VacLok syringe is attached to the instrument in order to aspirate biopsy material under a negative suction pressure. Therefore, the presence of cartilage should not be interpreted as a hamartoma. In hamartomas, in addition to cartilage, other diagnostic features include the presence of ciliated bronchial epithelium, bland spindle cells, adipocytes, and background of myxoid material.

A-89. **(d) Hyperchromatic nucleoli and clumped chromatin**
In reactive/reparative bronchial epithelium, including radiation and chemotherapy-induced changes, epithelial cells form cohesive sheets and/or two-dimensional clusters. These cells can be big (cytomegaly), but the nuclear enlargement is proportional to the cytoplasm with a normal N:C ratio. Multinucleation and prominent nucleoli are common. However, hyperchromatic nuclei, clumped chromatin, and irregular nuclear membrane are not features seen in reactive atypia. The presence of these features indicates malignant lesions. The differential diagnosis of reactive changes includes non-small cell lung carcinomas, particularly a well-differentiated adenocarcinoma. In adenocarcinomas, tumor cells form tight three-dimensional clusters with hyperchromatic nuclei, prominent nucleoli, irregular nuclear membrane, and high N:C ratio. The important clue for adenocarcinoma is the loss of cilia on bronchial epithelial cells.

A-90. **(d) A biopsy specimen of a bone lesion with metastatic lung adenocarcinoma**
Any type of formalin-fixed and paraffin-embedded specimens can be used for molecular and mutational analyses. However, bone biopsy material of a metastatic carcinoma is usually not a good sample for molecular analyses/tests, because the decalcification procedure is usually needed in order to cut blocks for hematoxylin and eosin (H&E) stain. The decalcification may destroy tumor cell DNA, and may potentially affect the sensitivity and accuracy of molecular tests. Therefore, decalcified bone biopsy material is not a good specimen for molecular tests. For all types of specimens, the diagnosis and the presence of adequate tumor cells must be confirmed by a pathologist prior to sending the specimen for any molecular tests.

A-91. **(d) Abundant alveolar macrophages**
The finding of abundant alveolar macrophages is considered an adequate specimen, particularly for a sputum specimen. The criteria for an adequate specimen include the presence of alveolar macrophages and/or Curschmann spirals, which indicate a representative collection of the lower respiratory tract material. Other cells and material in specimens such as squamous cells, neutrophils, and chronic inflammatory may represent oral contaminations. Sometimes, ciliated respiratory epithelial cells can be identified in the sputum, but they do not necessarily represent cells coming from the lower respiratory tract, since ciliated respiratory epithelial cells can be found in the lining of sinonasal passage of the upper respiratory tract. In bronchial washing specimens, scattered inflammatory cells, including neutrophils and lymphocytes, are also identified. An increased number of inflammatory cells is considered abnormal. Abundant neutrophils may be suggestive of an acute pneumonia. Numerous lymphocytes may be indicative of a chronic inflammation or a lymph proliferative disorder.

A-92. **(a) Benign mesothelial cells**
In a transthoracic CT-guided fine-needle aspiration, the presence of benign mesothelial cells is a common finding. They should not be confused with mesothelioma and/or adenocarcinoma. Benign mesothelial cells are arranged in flat sheets. The cells have round and/or oval nuclei, vesicular chromatin, abundant cytoplasm, and "windows" between cells. In case of mesothelioma, tumor cells form three-dimensional clusters with scalloped (knobby) edges. The high power view reveals that tumor cells have centrally placed round nuclei, coarse chromatin, prominent nucleoli, dense cytoplasm with peripheral "halo" and intercellular "windows." In adenocarcinomas, tumor cells are arranged in three-dimensional clusters with smooth edges. Tumor cells have hyperchromatic nuclei, irregular nuclear membranes, prominent nucleoli, scant cytoplasm, and without intercellular

"windows." In difficult cases, immunostains of mesothelial cell marker (calretinin, D2-40, WT1, p53) and adenocarcinoma markers (TTF, Napsin A, BerEP4) could be performed to separate mesothelial cells from adenocarcinoma.

A-93. (**d**) **Shared cell borders**

Tumor cells of squamous cell carcinomas form loose clusters or dispersed individual cells with hyperchromatic nuclei, smudgy chromatin, dense cytoplasm and cytokeratin formation, and a distinct cell border. In a well-differentiated tumor, numerous spindle-shaped malignant cells with prominent cytoplasmic keratin are identified. Cytokeratin stains purple to blue color with Diff-Quik method and orangeophilic with Papanicolaou method. In a poorly differentiated squamous cell carcinoma, tumor cells may be arranged in clusters and round up with prominent nucleoli, and less or no cytokeratin formation. In adenocarcinomas, tumor cells are arranged in tight three-dimensional clusters. Tumor cells of adenocarcinomas have hyperchromatic nuclei, coarse chromatin, prominent nucleoli, and vacuolated and feathery cytoplasm (indication of mucin production). Therefore, shared cell borders are not a feature of squamous cell carcinomas, and it is more often seen in adenocarcinomas.

A-94. (**c**) **Send the specimen for microbiology culture and biopsy the peripheral area of the lesion**.

During the transbronchial biopsy, the identification of necrotic debris warrants a microbiology culture. A variety of benign and malignant lesions can present with necrosis. For example, squamous cell carcinoma is often associated with tumor necrosis. Benign lesions such as granulomas may also present as a mass with or without central necrosis. Therefore, biopsy of peripheral area of the lesion is crucial for the establishment of the diagnosis. The cytological findings should be corrected with radiographic findings. If an image study is suggestive of a malignant lesion, necrotic debris are found on the FNA specimen during the on-site evaluation, several passes from the peripheral area of the lesion are definitely needed to make an accurate diagnosis.

A-95. (**d**) **Irregular nuclear membrane and hyperchromasia**

In reactive and reparative cellular changes, bronchial epithelial cells reveal a mild to moderate atypia. Cytological features include sheets and/or loose clusters of epithelial cells with mildly to moderately enlarged nuclei, vesicular chromatin, single or multiple small nucleoli, and abundant cytoplasm. N:C ratio is normal in reactive cells. The important clue for reactive atypia is the presence of cilia on bronchial epithelial cells. In adenocarcinomas, tumor cells form acini and/or three-dimensional clusters or many discohesive individual tumor cells with large hyperchromatic nuclei, coarse chromatin, irregular nuclear membranes, prominent nucleoli, overlapping nuclei, and high N:C ratio. Therefore, careful evaluation of nuclear features is crucial in the differential diagnosis of reactive atypia from adenocarcinoma.

A-96. (**b**) **A 3 cm squamous cell carcinoma involving the main bronchi**

Squamous cell carcinoma accounts for 30–40 % of non-small cell lung cancers. The majority of these tumors are located at main bronchi/hilar area (central area) of the lung; therefore, tumors are more likely to shed diagnostic cells into the sputum. Patients with a squamous cell carcinoma often present with hemoptysis and obstructive pneumonia. On image studies, a cavitary lesion is often identified. Tumor cells of squamous cell carcinomas form loose clusters or dispersed individual cells with hyperchromatic nuclei, smudgy chromatin, dense cytoplasm and cytokeratin formation, and a distinct cell border. In a well-differentiated tumor, numerous spindle-shaped malignant cells with prominent cytoplasmic keratin are identified. Cytokeratin stains purple to blue color with Diff-Quik method and orangeophilic with Papanicolaou method. In a poorly differentiated squamous cell carcinoma, tumor cells may be arranged in clusters and round up with prominent nucleoli, and less or no cytokeratin formation. These features should not be confused with adenocarcinoma.

A-97. (**d**) **Renal cell carcinoma**

"Pseudointranuclear inclusions" are formed by the protrusion of cytoplasm into the nuclei, and they have been described in a variety of malignant tumors, such as hepatocellular carcinoma, melanoma, a subset of lung adenocarcinomas, papillary thyroid carcinoma, meningioma, and others. Therefore, the finding of "pseudointranuclear inclusion" is nonspecific. However, it is usually not seen in renal cell carcinomas. The cytological features of renal cell carcinomas (clear cell renal cell carcinomas) include cohesive clusters of tumor cells with centrally located nuclei, vesicular chromatin, and abundant clear cytoplasm. The presence of nucleoli is variable depending on the Fuhrman grade. The nucleoli is inconspicuous in a low grade tumor, whereas the nucleoli is prominent in a high grade tumor.

A-98. (**d**) **Nuclear grooves**
Neuroendocrine tumors (NET) are a spectrum of neoplasms. The World Health Organization (WHO) classifies NET into three main categories: (1) well-differentiated neuroendocrine tumors with benign behavior; (2) well-differentiated (low grade) neuroendocrine carcinomas with low-grade malignant behavior; and (3) poorly differentiated (high grade) neuroendocrine carcinomas with aggressive clinical course, such as the large cell neuroendocrine and small cell carcinomas. All NET have common phenotypic characteristics, despite differing embryological origin. The cytological features of tumor cells are characterized by fine granular chromatin (salt-and-pepper chromatin) pattern, inconspicuous nucleoli, and scant cytoplasm. Mitosis may be rare or abundant depending on the differentiation of the tumor. Nuclear crowding and molding are often seen in small cell carcinomas; however, nuclear groove is not a feature of neuroendocrine tumors. In addition, cellular proliferative rate (Ki67 labeling) has been considered as a useful marker for the classification of NET.

A-99. (**b**) **Monomorphous population of lymphocytes**
Reactive lymphoid hyperplasia contains a heterogeneous mixture of lymphocytes, including small lymphocytes, centrocytes/centroblasts, immunoblasts, tangible-body macrophages, and other cells. There is a great variation of cellular sizes and appearances, characteristic of polymorphous population of cells. Monomorphous population of lymphocytes is usually seen in lymph proliferative disorders and/or lymphomas, particularly in small lymphocytic lymphomas/chronic lymphcytic leukemia (SLL/CLL). It represents a monoclonal proliferation of lymphoma cells. Other cytological features of SLL/CLL include discohesive tumor cells with hyperchromatic nuclei, clumped (soccer-ball-like) chromatin, irregular nuclear membranes, inconspicuous nucleoli, and scant cytoplasm and rare or absence of tangible body macrophages.

A-100. (**a**) **Adenocarcinoma with lepidic growth pattern (bronchoalveolar carcinoma)**
Adenocarcinoma with lepidic growth pattern (formerly bronchoalveolar carcinoma), particularly the minimal invasive variant, is considered a well-differentiated adenocarcinoma. It can be difficult to distinguish reactive bronchial epithelial cells (reactive atypia) from a well-differentiated adenocarcinoma. In reactive atypia, bronchial epithelial cells form sheets and/or loose cluster of cells with mildly to moderately enlarged nuclei, vesicular chromatin, single or multiple small nucleoli, abundant cytoplasm, and normal N:C ratio. The important clue for reactive atypia is the presence of cilia on bronchial epithelial cells. In a well-differentiated adenocarcinoma, the tumor cells are arranged in two- or three-dimensional clusters or in disorganized sheets. Tumor cells are intermediate in size with round nuclei, vesicular chromatin, small nucleoli and foamy cytoplasm, and high N:C ratio. However, no cilia are identified in tumor cell clusters. In mucinous adenocarcinomas, large tumor cells reveal hyperchromatic nuclei and cytoplasmic mucin. In basaloid squamous cell carcinomas, tumor cells form tight three-dimensional clusters with smudgy and/or coarse chromatin and scant dense cytoplasm. In small cell carcinomas, tumor cell reveals fine (salt-and-pepper) chromatin with nuclear crowding, molding, apoptosis, necrosis, and blue strips of DNA material. The tumor also has a high N:C ratio.

A-101. (**d**) **Aspergillosis**
Aspergillosis is characterized by the presence of mucus plugs containing fungal organisms admixed with birefringent calcium oxalate crystals, inflammatory cells, and eosinophils. Calcium oxalate crystals are needle-shaped, polarizable crystals; they may form rosettes or wheat sheaf-like clusters. Fungus microorganisms are characterized by true septate hyphae with 45° angle branching. The uniform thickness (3–6 μm in width) and the septa of hyphae differentiate *Aspergillus* from other fungus such as *Mucor* and *Candida*. Aspergillosis can also cause reactive atypia mimicking of non-small cell lung cancers, particularly a squamous cell carcinoma. Aspergillosis may be found in cancer patients, too. In *Pneumocystis jiroveci (carinii)* pneumonia (PCP) infection, extracellular and intracytoplasmic amorphous material containing cup-shaped microorganisms are seen.

A-102. (**d**) **Immunostains of cytokeratin**
Thymoma is the most common primary mediastinal neoplasm. Most patients are asymptomatic. When present, symptoms of cough, chest pain, and dyspnea are commonly seen. There are two major subtypes of thymomas (type A and type B) by WHO classification. In type A thymoma, tumor epithelioid cells reveal bland spindle or oval-shaped nuclei and without lymphocytic infiltrates, whereas, in type B thymoma, tumor epithelioid cells reveal polygonal appearance and admixed with different extent of lymphocytic infiltrates. The cytological features of thymoma vary widely, ranging from lymphocyte predominant to a biphasic population

of epithelial cells and lymphocytes, to exclusively epithelial cells. The neoplastic epithelial cells are in spindle and oval shape, or polygonal with abundant cytoplasm and well-defined cell borders. The nuclei are bland with evenly distributed chromatin and small inconspicuous nucleoli. In type B tumors, neoplastic epithelial cells present as clusters or as scattered individual tumor cells in a background of lymphocytes. Therefore, the most important single test/marker for the differential diagnosis of thymoma from lymphoma is cytokeratin stain. Cytokeratin is positive for thymoma and negative for lymphoma. Other lymphoid markers such as CD45, CD5, and T/B cell markers could be positive in thymomas and lymphoma. Finally, it is difficult to distinguish benign from malignant thymomas by cytomorphology alone. The presence of pleomorphism, markedly nuclear atypia and increased mitotic figures may be indicative of a thymic carcinoma.

A-103. (**b**) **Bronchoscopic washing**
Bronchoscopic washing has the lowest diagnostic sensitivity among all procedures. Its sensitivity ranges from 30 to 70 % depending on the location and the size of the lesion. In BAL, the sensitivity is 40–80 %. Bronchial brushing has a higher sensitivity than washing and BAL. Transbronchial fine-needle aspiration has a sensitivity of 60–90 %. Cell block preparations during these procedures can markedly increase the detection sensitivity, since it may provide additional diagnostic cells and/or material.

A-104. (**d**) **Bilateral lung infiltrations**
Bilateral lung infiltrations can be seen in both benign disease and malignant tumors. In benign lesions, such as infections, granulomas, and interstitial lung diseases, the clinical presentation and radiographic findings can present as bilateral lung infiltrations. The malignant tumors, such as adenocarcinomas with lepidic growth pattern (formerly bronchoalveolar adenocarcinoma) and advanced stages of lung cancers, can also present as bilateral lung infiltrations. The condition is not a contraindication for lung fine-needle aspiration. Other conditions, such as uncontrollable cough, severe pulmonary hypertension, and suspected echinococcal cysts are contraindications for fine-needle aspiration of the lung, due to the potential risk of damage to the lung parenchyma and the dissemination of the disease.

A-105. (**a**) **Mitosis and necrosis**
All features can be seen in bronchial reserve cell hyperplasia, except mitosis and necrosis. In reserve cell hyperplasia, cells are arranged in cohesive sheets or clusters with nuclear overlapping and crowding. The nuclei reveal dark smudgy chromatin, inconspicuous nucleoli, smooth nuclear membrane, and scant cytoplasm. The N:C ratio is slightly increased. There is no mitosis or necrosis seen. Bronchial reserve cell hyperplasia is a mimic of small cell carcinomas. In small cell carcinomas, tumor cell reveals fine (salt-and-pepper) chromatin with nuclear crowding, molding, apoptosis, necrosis, and blue strips of DNA material. The tumor also has a high N:C ratio.

A-106. (**b**) **Nuclei with marked variation in size and shape**
Degenerated squamous cells can be seen in a variety of lung diseases and almost any type of injury to the lung, such as infection, pneumonia, chemotherapy, sepsis, and diffuse alveolar damage. The cytological features of degenerated squamous cells reveal single and loosely formed clusters of cells with slightly enlarged pyknotic nuclei, smudgy chromatin, cytoplasmic keratin, and normal N:C ratio. The marked variation of size and shape of the nuclei is the feature of squamous cell carcinomas. In squamous cell carcinomas, numerous spindle-shaped and polygonal malignant cells with hyperchromatic nuclei, smudgy chromatin, cytokeratin, and high N:C ratio are identified.

A-107. (**d**) **Prominent nucleoli**
In squamous cell carcinomas, tumor cells form loosely clusters or dispersed individual cells with hyperchromatic nuclei, smudgy chromatin, dense cytoplasm and cytokeratin formation, and a distinct cell border. In a well-differentiated tumor, numerous polygonal and spindle-shaped malignant cells with hyperchromatic nuclei and high N:C ratio are identified. Cytokeratin stains purple to blue color with Diff-Quik method and orangeophilic with Papanicolaou method. When tumors are poorly differentiated, the distinction between squamous cell carcinomas and adenocarcinomas may become difficult. In a poorly differentiated squamous cell carcinoma, tumor cells may be arranged in clusters and round up with prominent nucleoli, and with less or no cytokeratin formation. These features should not be confused with adenocarcinomas. In adenocarcinomas, tumor cells form acini and/or three-dimensional clusters or many

discohesive individual tumor cells with large hyperchromatic nuclei, coarse chromatin, irregular nuclear membranes, prominent nucleoli, and vacuolated cytoplasm (cytoplasmic mucin production).

A-108. (**d**) **Clusters of bronchial epithelial cells without cilia**

The cytological features of a mucinous adenocarcinoma include relatively uniform tumor cells with pale nuclei, vesicular chromatin, inconspicuous nucleoli, and foamy cytoplasm. Tumor cells are arranged in tight clusters and dispersed individual cells with inconspicuous cytological atypia, and resemble macrophages. Therefore, careful evaluation of nuclear features and the presence or absence of cilia is critical for the diagnosis. Features such as nuclei enlargement with irregular nuclear membrane and absence of cilia in cellular clusters should be considered malignancy.

A-109. (**a**) **True**.

In lung adenocarcinoma, a significant morphological heterogeneity can be seen in tumors. The WHO classification of adenocarcinoma of the lung includes many subtypes, such as acinar, papillary, solid, mucinous, clear, and mixed subtypes. Cytological arrangements of adenocarcinomas may be seen as three-dimensional clusters, acinar and papillary groups, honeycomb-like sheets, and/or dispersed individual tumor cells. In general, tumor cells reveal large round or oval-shaped nuclei, coarse chromatin, irregular nuclear membranes, prominent nucleoli, and cytoplasmic vacuolization. The N:C ratio of tumor cells is high. Increased mitosis and tumor necrosis may also present on the slide.

A-110. (**d**) **All of the above**

The differential diagnosis of so-called "signet ring" cells in cytological specimens is broad, including both benign (goblet cells) and malignant (adenocarcinomas of the lung and stomach) conditions. A careful evaluation of the nuclear features is important for distinguishing between benign and malignant lesions. The nuclear features of carcinomas include large nuclei, hyperchromatic chromatin, irregular nuclear member, and large prominent nucleoli. Although signet ring cell carcinomas are more commonly seen in stomach carcinomas, a subset of lung adenocarcinomas may have signet ring cell features. Therefore, the finding of signet ring morphology in a lung lesion may be mistaken as a metastatic carcinoma of the stomach. Immunostains of TTF and CDX2 may not help in the differential diagnosis of primary from metastatic adenocarcinoma, since the TTF may be negative and CDX2 may be focally positive in a primary lung mucinous adenocarcinoma. Thus, cytological findings should be correlated with clinical and radiographic findings in order to render the correct diagnosis.

A-111. (**b**) **False**

Vascular tumors EHE and EAS can occur as a primary tumor of the lung. EHE is a low-to-intermediate grade tumor, whereas EAS is a high-grade tumor. In EHE, tumor cells are arranged in small clusters and cords and reveal epithelioid appearance with abundant eosinophilic cytoplasm. The nuclei are round in shape with hyerchromatic chromatin, prominent nucleoli, and irregular nuclear membranes. In EAS, tumor cells are arranged in dispersed individual cells with marked nuclear pleomorphism. Increased mitotic activity, focal spindle shaped cells, and tumor necrosis are also present. Both tumors have intracytoplasmic vacuoles, representing small vascular lumina, which may mimic cytoplasmic mucin. Therefore, they may be confused with adenocarcinoma due to the epithelioid appearance and the cytoplasmic vacuoles. The diagnosis of both EHE and EAS often requires the immunostain of vascular markers CD31 and CD34. In addition, about one-third of the vascular tumors are immunoreactive with cytokeratin.

A-112. (**d**) **Poorly differentiated adenocarcinoma**

The differential diagnosis of a spindle cell lesion in FNA cytology is broad, including spindle cell carcinoma, leiomyoma, leiomyosarcoma, melanoma, nerve tumors, fibrous tumors, and others. In a leiomyosarcoma, tumor cells have "cigar-shaped" nuclei and finely granular cytoplasm. Naked nuclei and increased mitosis are also common in the tumor. IHC stains of tumor cells are positive for desmin and myogenin. In spindle cell carcinomas, tumor cells form clusters with epithelioid appearance, such as large hyperchromatic nuclei, coarse chromatin, irregular nuclear membranes, prominent nucleoli, and scant cytoplasm. In spindle cell carcinoids, tumor cells reveal neuroendocrine cell features with uniform oval nuclei, fine chromatin, inconspicuous nucleoli, and abundant cytoplasm. The cytological features of a poorly differentiated adenocarcinoma include predominantly dispersed individual pleomorphic tumor cells and three-dimensional clusters. Tumor cells reveal large round or oval-shaped nuclei with hyperchromatic coarse chromatin, irregular nuclear membranes, prominent nucleoli, and vacuolated cytoplasm. The spindle cell appearance is not the feature of a poorly differentiated adenocarcinoma.

A-113. (**b**) **Perform flow cytometry**
The FNA of a MALT lymphoma reveals a discohesive population of lymphoma cells, resembling small lymphocytes, centrocytes, or monocytes. Lymphoma cells have round or irregular nuclei, coarse granular chromatin, inconspicuous nucleoli, and scant cytoplasm. In the background of the slide, a few or no tingible-body macrophages are identified. There is no specific IHC marker for diagnosing MALT lymphoma. CD20 stain is diffusely positive for tumor cells, and aberrant coexpression of CD43 by neoplastic B cells is found in up to 50 % of cases. Immunophenotyping such as flow cytometry study is necessary in a suspicious patient to establish the diagnosis. The MALT lymphoma can be confused with a reactive lymphoid hyperplasia and/or reactive lymph node. In reactive lymphoid hyperplasia, in addition to small lymphocytes, centrocytes, and tingible-body macrophages, the dendritic lymphocytic aggregate can be identified. The dendritic lymphocytic aggregate is a loose cluster of small lymphocytes and dendritic cells, dendritic cells reveal vesicular (pale) nuclei, fine chromatin, and delicate cytoplasm.

A-114. (**a**) **True**
Sarcoidosis is an idiopathic disease characterized by non-necrotizing granulomas. It typically involves mediastinal lymph nodes and the lung. However, it can be a systemic process and involve other organs, such as the heart, central nerve system, and skin. The disease usually occurs in middle-aged African-American females. The patient may need steroid therapy. Only a small percentage of patients progress to pulmonary fibrosis and require lung transplantation.

A-115. (**b**) **Alveolar proteinosis**
Alveolar proteinosis is an idiopathic disease; however, it can occur in a variety of conditions such as infections, occupational exposures, and malignancies. BAL is often performed for the therapeutic purpose. The patient usually has an excellent prognosis. On BAL slides, numerous alveolar macrophages and eosinophilic granular material are revealed by the Papanicolaou stain. In amyloid, it reveals acellular dense waxy material which has a characteristic birefringent "apple green" appearance by the Congo-red stain under the polarized microscope. PCP infection occurs in immunocompromised patients, and reveals intracytoplasmic cup-shaped microorganisms. In aspergillosis, fungal hyphae are identified.

A-116. (**c**) **Calretinin, p53, WT1, TTF, BerEP4, CEA, and CD15**
The cytomorphological distinction between mesotheliomas and adenocarcinomas can be difficult due to overlapping cytological features. Therefore, immunostains are necessary to establish the diagnosis. A panel of immunomarkers, including both adenocarcinoma markers and mesothelioma markers, is usually performed. Commonly used adenocarcinoma markers include TTF, BerEP4, CEA, B72.3, MOC-31, and CD15 (Leu-M1), whereas commonly used "mesothelioma markers" include calretinin, p53, D2-40, and WT1. Mesothelioma is positive for Calretinin, p53, and WT1, whereas, adenocarcinoma of the lung is positive for TTF, BerEP4, CEA, B72.3, MOC-31, and CD15.

A-117. (**a**) **Microbiology culture and core biopsy of the lesion**
The cytological finding of this on-site evaluation indicates a granulomatous inflammation. The granuloma can be found in both benign and malignant lesions. Therefore, the best action is to send specimens for microbiology culture and to perform a core needle biopsy. The microbiology culture will be helpful for the differential diagnosis of infections. The core biopsy material is important for the microscopic evaluation of the lesion and to perform immunostudies of the lesion if it is needed.

A-118. (**a**) **Make cell block and perform silver stain**
Pneumocystis jiroveci (carinii) pneumonia (PCP) infection usually involves immunocompromised patients, such as HIV infection, organ transplantation, chemotherapy and cancer patients. The cytological findings of PCP infection on the BAL specimen include numerous alveolar macrophages and amorphous material. Cup-shaped microorganisms can be seen in the cytoplasm of the macrophages and in amorphous material by Papanicolaou stain, but organisms are stained poorly or not at all with Papanicolaou method. In silver stains, such as Grocott's methenamine silver (GMS) stain, the cell wall of the organisms stains with black color. The cell block preparation and silver stain may help to identify the cup-shaped microorganisms and confirm the diagnosis.

A-119. (**d**) **All of the above**

Breast carcinoma is a common tumor which metastases to the lung, due to its anatomic location. Metastatic breast carcinomas have many cytological features that overlap with primary lung adenocarcinomas. In metastatic breast carcinomas, tumor cells are arranged in tight three-dimensional clusters and/or acini. Tumor cells reveal a monotonous appearance, with hyperchromatic nuclei, prominent nucleoli, and frequently intracytoplasmic lumen. In lung adenocarcinomas, tumor cells may have more pleomorphic appearance and variation in size and shape of nuclei. In difficult cases, immunostains of breast cancer markers (estrogen receptor (ER), progesterone receptor (PR), gross cystic disease fluid protein (GCDFP-15), mammaglobin and GATA-3), and lung markers (TTF1 and napsin A) may help for the differential diagnosis.

A-120. (**b**) **False**

In a primary lung adenocarcinoma intestinal subtype and/or mucinous subtype, tumors reveal tall glandular or columnar cells with abundant cytoplasmic mucin. In this subtype, tumor cells frequently stain negative for TTF1, but positive for CK20 and CDX2. Therefore, this subtype of primary lung adenocarcinoma cannot be reliably differentiated from a metastatic colonic adenocarcinoma by immunomarkers of CK20 and CDX2. For differential diagnoses, the patient's clinical history (presence or absence of malignant history or colon lesions), radiographic information (single verse multiple lung nodules), and colonoscopic evaluation (presence or absence of colonic lesions) should be considered and correlated with cytological findings.

A-121. (**c**) **Colon**

The metastatic colonic adenocarcinoma has characteristic cytological features. Tumor cells are arranged in three-dimensional clusters and acini structures with distinctive tall columnar and glandular cells, showing a "picket fence" appearance. Tumor cells reveal oval hyperchromatic nuclei, coarse chromatin, prominent nucleoli, irregular nuclear membranes, high N:C ratio, and "dirty" necrosis. In metastatic breast carcinomas, tumor cells are arranged in tight three-dimensional clusters and/or acini with a monotonous appearance. In metastatic hepatocellular carcinomas, tumor cells are predominately arranged in dispersed individual cells with polygonal appearance, large nuclei, prominent nucleoli, and dense granular cytoplasm. In metastatic uterine carcinomas, tumor cells may reveal several different cytomorphologies, ranging from malignant glandular cells to clear cells, depending on the subtype of the primary tumor.

A-122. (**b**) **Using unstained slides to perform IHC markers S100, HMB45, and Melanin A with red chromogenics rather than the one with brown chromogenics.**

Tumor cells of a metastatic melanoma produce dark brown to black color melanin pigment. Macrophages in lymph nodes of the lung contain anthracotic pigment, they can be confused with melanin pigment. Therefore, routine IHC marker using brown color chromogenics will cause false-positive staining. Therefore, using IHC markers with red color chromogenics is more specific for the detection of a metastatic melanoma in the lymph node containing anthracotic pigment. Alternatively, one can use bleached slides to perform routine IHC markers S100, HMB45, and Melanin A. Recently, a nuclear transcript factor SOX10 has been used for the detection of melanomas. It has been reported that SOX10 has a 100 % sensitivity and specificity for the identification of melanomas, particularly in desmorplastic melanoma which is negative for many melanoma markers.

A-123. (**d**) **Prominent nucleoli**

In small cell carcinomas, tumor cells are relatively small in size and approximately two- to threefold of mature lymphocytes. However, in small cell carcinoma large cell variant, the size of tumor cells can be much larger. Tumor cells show scant cytoplasm and high N:C ratio, large nuclei with fine chromatin (salt-and-pepper) pattern, nuclear crowding and molding, and paranuclear blue bodies in the cytoplasm. Numerous "blue strips" are seen on the slides due to crush artifacts and the breakdown of nuclear DNA material. The nucleoli are inconspicuous in small cell carcinomas. In some cases, tumor cells may reveal rare nucleoli, but they are small in size. The prominent nucleolus is not usually seen in a small cell carcinoma, and it can be seen in atypical carcinoid and/or large cell neuroendocrine tumors.

A-124. (**d**) **Pancoast tumor**

An apical squamous cell carcinoma in the superior sulcus is called the "Pancoast tumor" and characterized by rib destruction, neural invasion, and Horner syndrome (enophthalmos, ptosis, miosis, and ipsilateral decreased sweating). Other syndromes, such as Lambert–Eaton syndrome (weakness or loss of movement of muscles, vision changes, and nerve system symptoms), Cushing's syndrome, and hyponatremia are usually associated with a small cell carcinoma.

A-125. (**b**) **Atypical carcinoid shares many cytological features with typical carcinoid**
Atypical carcinoid shares many cytological features with typical carcinoid, including cellular arrangement and tumor cell morphology. In atypical carcinoids, tumor cells are arranged in acini and pseudorosette structures. Tumor cells may have more pleomorphic appearance and are larger in size than that of typical carcinoids. Atypical carcinoids also reveal vesicular nuclei, fine (salt-and-pepper) chromatin, and slightly increased mitotic activity and focal tumor necrosis. The presence of nucleoli can be seen in both atypical and typical carcinoids. In general, the mitotic figures range from 2 to 10 per 10 high power fields in atypical carcinoids. Although mitotic account plays an important role in the classification, it is not always seen on cytological smears. Therefore, careful evaluation of cytomorphology on slides and immunostain of Ki67 on cell block sections may be necessary for an accurate classification. The distinction between atypical and typical carcinoids usually requires a surgical specimen.

A-126. (**c**) **The lower mitotic rate and the absence of necrosis**
All neuroendocrine tumors share many cytological features, such as fine (salt-and-pepper) chromatin and acini and pseudorosette arrangement of tumor cells. The prominent nucleoli can be seen in large cell neuroendocrine tumors and atypical carcinoids, but is inconspicuous in small cell carcinomas, and typical carcinoids can have a small nucleoli. The separation from typical carcinoids from small cell carcinomas is easier than from atypical carcinoids. In small cell carcinomas, tumor cells reveal hyperchromatic nuclei with nuclear crowding and molding, scant cytoplasm, numerous apoptotic bodies and mitoses, and tumor necrosis. Typical carcinoid is separated from atypical carcinoid by several criteria, such as a lower mitotic rate, absence of tumor necrosis, and uniformity of tumor cells. The presence of nucleoli can be seen in both atypical and typical carcinoid. It has been considered that the mitotic rate is less than 2, and 2–10 per 10 high power field in a typical and atypical carcinoid, respectively. Although mitotic account plays an important role in the classification, it is not always seen on cytological smears. Therefore, careful evaluation of cytomorphology on slides and immunostain of Ki67 on cell block sections may be necessary for an accurate classification. The distinction between typical and atypical carcinoids usually requires a surgical specimen.

A-127. (**d**) **Carcinoid tumor-like nuclei with markedly atypia and enlargement**
In large cell neuroendocrine tumors (LCNEC), tumor cells are large in size with more pleomorphic appearance and moderate to abundant cytoplasm. They are arranged in nests, acini, and pseudorosettes. Tumor cells also have carcinoid tumor-like nuclei with markedly atypia and enlargement, vesicular or salt-and-pepper chromatin, and prominent nucleoli. The mitotic rate is very high and typically more than 11 (average of 50–70) per 10 high power fields. A large area of tumor necrosis is also a common finding.

A-128. (**a**) **Involving the *HMGI*(Y) gene on chromosome 6p21**
Pulmonary hamartoma is a benign neoplasm and involves the *HMGI*(Y) gene on chromosome 6p21. The cytological features include benign glandular cells, fibromyxoid material, spindle cells (smooth muscle), cartilage, and adipocytes. There is no evidence of familiarity with this tumor. Clinically, the tumor is a well-circumscribed lesion and usually presents as an incidental finding. Surgical resection of the tumor can cure the disease and the patient has an excellent prognosis.

A-129. (**d**) **Neutrophils can be seen in 1 year after transplantation**.
In the lung transplant patient, BAL procedure is routinely performed to monitor the patient. In such type of specimens, neutrophils are normally seen within the first 3 months after the transplantation. After this period, the finding of neutrophils in the BAL specimen should be carefully evaluated to determine the presence of potential infections. It is also important to look for fungal, viral, and PCP infections, since transplant patients are immunocompromised, whereas an increased number of macrophages in BAL specimens can be seen for years after transplantation.

A-130. (**b**) **Inflammatory myofibroblastic tumor** (**IMT**)
IMT is a myofibroblastic tumor in children and young adults involving lung, liver, as well as retroperitoneal and pelvic soft tissues. It has a low malignant

potential and indolent clinical course. In the past, a variety of names have been used to describe this lesion, including inflammatory pseudotumor, plasma cell granuloma, inflammatory myofibroblastic proliferation, and pseudosarcomatous myofibroblastic proliferation. Currently, it has been recognized by WHO classification as IMT. The tumor consists of bland spindle cell proliferation in a background of plasma cells, lymphocytes, neutrophils, and eosinophils. Positive immunoreactivity with antibodies against ALK protein and molecular study of *ALK* gene arrangement can be detected in approximately 40–50 % of patients, and help in the differential diagnosis.

A-131. (**b**) **False**
EGFR and *KRAS* mutational rates are found in 10–20 % and 15–30 % of lung adenocarcinomas in the United States, respectively. *EGFR* and *KRAS* mutations are mutually exclusive in non-small cell lung carcinomas, and have not been found to occur in the same tumor. In lung adenocarcinomas, patients with *EGFR* mutations are associated with a good response to tyrosine kinase inhibitors therapy, whereas *KRAS* mutations are associated with a resistance to tyrosine kinase inhibitor therapy, and with poor prognosis. Therefore, the tests of *EGFR*, *KRAS*, and other genetic mutations in lung cancer patients are critical for targeted therapies.

A-132. (**a**) **Mutation and overexpression of the *EGFR* gene lead to cancer cell overgrowth, but not tumor progression**.
In non-small cell lung carcinomas, mutation of *EGFR gene* induces intrinsic protein tyrosine kinase activity of EGFR receptor and constitutive activation of EGFR signaling pathway, which leads to cell proliferation and uncontrolled cell division. Therefore, activation mutations and overexpression in the tyrosine kinase domain of the *EGFR* gene involve in tumor overgrowth and progression. Currently, EGFR signaling pathway has been successfully targeted by several tyrosine kinase inhibitors, such as Erlotinib and gefitinib. These tyrosine kinase inhibitors of the EGFR signaling pathway have been used to treat non-small cell lung cancer patients, particularly in lung adenocarcinoma patients. A marked improvement of overall survival rate has been shown in patients with *EGFR* mutations. Finally, *EGFR* mutations are more often found in tumors with micropapillary morphology and the lepidic growth pattern (formerly known as bronchioloalveolar carcinoma).

A-133. (**a**) **The KRAS protein stimulates downstream activity of EGFR tyrosine kinase**
KRAS belongs to the *RAS* family of oncogenes. *KRAS* mutations have been detected in approximately 15–30 % of non-small cell lung carcinomas, especially in lung adenocarcinomas. The mutations cause an impaired GTPase activity and subsequently a constitutive activation of RAS signaling pathway, which is located downstream of EGFR signaling. The constitutive activation of RAS signaling pathway leads to activation of anti-apoptotic pathways and cell proliferation. *KRAS* mutations have been associated with primary resistance to EGFR tyrosine kinase inhibitor therapy in non-small cell carcinomas. It has been found that *KRAS* mutations occur more commonly in adenocarcinomas from elderly patients and heavy smokers. Patients with *KRAS* mutations are unlikely to respond to EGFR tyrosine kinase inhibitor therapy and are associated with a poor prognosis.

A-134. (**a**) **The most common *ALK* rearrangement in non-small cell lung carcinoma is *EML4-ALK* fusion**
The most common *ALK* gene rearrangement in non-small cell lung carcinomas is *EML4-ALK* rearrangement, which involves the 5′ end of the *EML4* gene and the 3′ end of the *ALK* gene on chromosome 2p23. *ALK* gene rearrangements occur in non-small cell carcinoma patients with a younger age, who are never smokers. Females are more likely to have the mutation than males. *EML4-ALK* gene rearrangements have not been found to be associated with *EGFR* and *KRAS* mutations, therefore, patients with *ALK* gene rearrangements do not benefit from EGFR-specific tyrosine kinase inhibitor therapy. Crizotinib (Xalkori®, Pfizer) is the FDA-approved ALK tyrosine kinase inhibitor therapy for patients whose tumors are positive for *ALK* rearrangements.

A-135. (**c**) **Intercellular "windows"**
The cytological features of mesothelial cells reveal sheets and loosely formed clusters of intermediate-sized cells with large centrally located nuclei, vesicular chromatin, small prominent nucleoli, dense cytoplasm, and intercellular "windows." The nuclei of mesothelial cells may reveal mild to moderate variation in size and shape, particularly in reactive mesothelial cells; therefore, they may be confused with a well-differentiated adenocarcinoma. In adenocarcinomas, tumor cells are commonly arranged in tight three-dimensional clusters and acinar structures. Tumor cells are large in size, with high N/C ratio, and

hyperchromatic nuclei. The nuclei contain coarse chromatin, prominent nucleoli, and irregular nuclear membranes. The cytoplasm of tumor cells is "lacy" and with cytoplasmic vacuolization. The finding of intercellular "windows" is a reliable feature for the separation between mesothelial cells and adenocarcinomas.

A-136. (**b**) **Significant variation of nuclear size and shape**
Reactive squamous cells have several cytological features overlapping with squamous cell carcinomas. In reactive squamous cells, cells may be arranged in small two-dimensional clusters and dispersed individual cells. They reveal mildly enlarged nuclei with minimal variation in size and shape, and abundant dense cytoplasm. The N:C ratio of cells is normal or slightly increased. In squamous cell carcinomas, tumor cells are predominately arranged in dispersed individual cells, with large nuclei, hyperchromatic smudgy chromatin, marked variation of nuclear size and shape, and dense cytoplasm (cytokeratin formation). In addition, spindle-shaped cells and bizarre tumor cells are also commonly seen. Prominent necrotic debris in the background is also a feature for squamous cell carcinomas.

A-137. (**a**) **True**
Percutaneous FNA is a transthoracic procedure and usually performed under CT and/or ultrasound guidance. Therefore, it is important to recognize that several types of cells and tissue fragments can be found on the cytological slides, and they should not be misinterpretated as a lesional component. For example, mesothelial cells from pleura, smooth muscle, and adipose tissue from chest walls are quite common findings. The benign appearances of these cells separate them from a potential lesion. The most important differential diagnosis of mesothelial cells is adenocarcinoma. In adenocarcinomas, tumor cells reveal tight three-dimensional clusters and acinar structures, with high N/C ratio, hyperchromatic nuclei, coarse chromatin, prominent nucleoli, and irregular nuclear membranes. No intercellular "windows" characteristic of mesothelial cells is identified in adenocarcinomas.

A-138. (**b**) **Small cell carcinoma**
In this situation, several differential diagnoses should be considered in a transthoracic FNA of a right lower lobe lung mass, including lung adenocarcinoma with hepatocellular features, benign liver cells, and/or a hepatocellular carcinoma. In a lung adenocarcinoma of hepatocellular variant, tumor cells reveal prominent nucleoli and dense granular cytoplasm, mimicking hepatocellular carcinomas, however, tumor cells are arranged in tight three-dimensional clusters, with hyperchromatic nuclei, irregular nuclear membrane, and a high N:C ratio. In hepatocellular carcinoma, numerous dispersed individual tumor cells and naked nuclei are characteristic findings. Benign liver cells are arranged in honeycomb sheets and small clusters; cells reveal centrally located nuclei with small nucleoli and a normal N:C ratio. Small cell carcinomas with nuclear crowding and molding should not be confused with liver cells.

A-139. (**c**) **Charcot–Leyden crystal**
Charcot–Leyden crystal is a needle-shaped, orangeophilic structure derived from degenerated eosinophils. It can be found in a variety of lung diseases associated with increased eosinophils; however, it is more commonly seen in specimens from asthma patients. Ferruginous bodies are dumbbell-shaped, golden yellow to black-colored mineral fibers, and associated with asbestos exposure. Psammoma bodies are structures with concentrically laminated calcification and a circumferential thin layer of epithelial cells; it is commonly seen in both carcinomas and benign conditions. Corpora amylacea are round structures with circumferential and radiating lines; they are a non-specific finding in BAL and sputum specimens.

A-140. (**a**) ***EGFR* mutations are often found in adenocarcinoma with micropapillary and/or the lepidic growth pattern**.
Based on the new adenocarcinoma classification proposed by the International Association for the Study of Lung Cancer, American Thoracic Society, and European Respiratory Society, *EGFR* mutations have been found to be frequently associated with the micropapillary subtype and the lepidic growth pattern (formerly known as bronchioloalveolar carcinoma). Although *EGFR* mutations are only identified in 10–20 % of surgically resected lung adenocarcinomas in the United States and Europe, they are identified in approximately 50 % of Asians. *EGFR* and *KRAS* mutations are mutually exclusive in non-small cell lung carcinomas, and have not been found to occur in the same tumor. In lung adenocarcinomas, patients with *EGFR* mutations are associated with a good response to EGFR tyrosine kinase inhibitors therapy, and a better survival rate than patients without *EGFR* mutations. Therefore, the tests of *EGFR*, *KRAS*, and other genetic mutations in lung cancer patients are critical for targeted therapies

A-141. **(b) *KRAS* mutations are more commonly seen among non-smokers.**

KRAS mutations are found in 15–30 % of adenocarcinomas in the United States and Europe. However, they are less commonly seen in tumors of Asian descents. It has been found that *KRAS* mutations occur more commonly in adenocarcinomas from elderly patients and heavy smokers. Patients with *KRAS* mutations are unlikely to respond to EGFR tyrosine kinase inhibitor therapy; thus, they are associated with a poor prognosis.

A-142. **(d) The color and volume of the specimen**

According to the laboratory regulation policy of the Health Care Financing Administration (HCFA), the time and date of the sample collected, and the time and date of the sample received by the laboratory must be included and/or documented on the requisition form. The color and volume of the specimen is not required to include on the requisition form by the HCFA.

Reading List

Bibbo M, Wood MD, Fitzpatrick BT. Peritoneal washings and ovary. In: Bibbo M, Wilbur D, editors. Comprehensive cytopathology. 3rd ed. Philadelphia: Saunders/Elsevier; 2008.

Cibas ES. Peritoneal washings. In: Cibas ES, Ducatman BS, editors. Cytology: diagnostic principles and clinical correlates. Philadelphia: Saunders/Elsevier; 2009.

DeMay RM. The art and science of cytopathology, exfoliative cytology, vol. 1. 2nd ed. Chicago: ASCP Press; 2012.

Feller-Kopman D, Yung RCW, Burroughs F, Li QK. Cytology of endobronchial ultrasound-guided transbronchial needle aspiration (EBUS-TBNA). A study of 135 cases with histology correlation. Cancer Cytopathol. 2009;117:482–90.

Khalbuss WE, Yang H, Lian Q, Elhosseiny A, Pantanowitz L, Monaco SE. The cytomorphologic spectrum of small-cell carcinoma and large-cell neuroendocrine carcinoma in body cavity effusions: a study of 68 cases. Cytojournal. 2011;8:18.

Khalbuss WE, Monaco SE, Pantanowitz L. Chapter 12. Lung and respiratory cytopathology. In: The ASCP Quick Compendium (QC) of cytopathology. Chicago: ASCP Press; 2013. p. 212–57.

Lindeman NI, Cagle PT, Beasley MB, Chitale DA, Dacic S, Giaccone G, Jenkins RB, Kwiatkowski DJ, Saldivar JS, Squire J, Thunnissen E, Ladanyi M. Molecular testing guideline for selection of lung cancer patients for EGFR and ALK tyrosine kinase inhibitors: guideline from the College of American Pathologists, International Association for the Study of Lung Cancer, and Association for Molecular Pathology. J Mol Diagn. doi:10.1016/j.jmoldx.2013.03.001. pii: S1525-1578(13)00041-X. [Epub ahead of print]. 2013;15:415–53.

Monaco SE, Pantanowitz L, Khalbuss WE. Comparing endobronchial ultrasound-guided fine needle aspiration specimens with and without rapid on-site evaluation. Cytojournal. 2012;9:2.

Munfus-McCray D, Adams C, Harada S, Askin F, Clark DP, Gabrielson E, Li QK. *EGFR* and *KRAS* mutations in metastatic lung adenocarcinomas. Hum Pathol. 2011;42:1447–53.

Munfus-McCray D, Cui M, Zhang Z, Askin F, Gabrielson E, Li QK. Comparison of *EGFR* and *KRAS* mutations in primary and unpaired metastatic lung adenocarcinoma with potential chemotherapy effect. Hum Pathol. 2013;44:1286–92.

Stoll LM, Johnson MW, Burroughs F, Li QK. Cytological diagnosis and differential diagnosis of lung carcinoid tumors: a retrospective study of 63 cases with histological correlation. Cancer Cytopathol. 2010;118:457–67.

Serous Fluid Cytopathology

2

Qing Kay Li and Walid E. Khalbuss

Contents

2.1 **Image-Based Questions 1–50 (50 Images)**........................ 124

2.2 **Text-Based Questions 51–100**.. 174

2.3 **Answers and Discussion of Image-Based Questions 1–50**.. 179

2.4 **Answers and Discussion of Text-Based Questions 51–100**.. 188

Reading List.. 197

Q.K. Li, MD, Ph.D. (✉)
Department of Pathology, The Johns Hopkins University School of Medicine, The Johns Hopkins Bayview Medical Center, 4940 Eastern Avenue, AA Building, Room 154B, Baltimore, MD 21224-2780, USA
e-mail: qli23@jhmi.edu

W.E. Khalbuss, MD, PhD, FIAC.
Department of Pathology, GE Clarient Diagnostic Services, 31 Columbia, Aliso Viejo, California, 92656, USA
e-mail: walid.khalbuss@ge.com

W.E. Khalbuss, Q.K. Li (eds.), *Diagnostic Cytopathology Board Review and Self-Assessment*,
DOI 10.1007/978-1-4939-1477-7_2, © Springer Science+Business Media New York 2015

Table 2.1 Benign components in serous fluid

	Descriptions	Differentials
Mesothelial cells	Sheets and/or dispersed individual cells with round nuclei, small nucleoli, granular chromatin, dense cytoplasm and clear outer rim, and "windows" between cells	Organized cellular arrangements and/or dispersed individual cells. Nuclei may show mild atypia, but with smooth nuclear membrane; no hyperchromasia DD: well-differentiated adenocarcinoma
Reactive mesothelial cells	Small clusters of cells (less than10–20 cells) or dispersed individual cells with enlarged nuclei, coarse chromatin, prominent nucleoli, dense cytoplasm and clear outer rim, and "windows" between cells	A spectrum of changes ranges from normal to markedly atypical cells. Binucleation and multinucleation are common DD: well-differentiated adenocarcinoma
Histiocytes	Loosely formed two-dimensional clusters or dispersed individual cells, with coffee bean-shaped nuclei, fine chromatin, inconspicuous nucleoli, and foamy cytoplasm	Cells have coffee bean-shaped nuclei, cytoplasmic vacuoles and normal N/C ratios DD: well-differentiated adenocarcinoma
Eosinophils	Granulocytes with brick-red cytoplasmic granules after staining with eosin (a red dye) using the Papanicolaou stain method	Cells with eosinophilic intracytoplasmic granules DD: neutrophils
Lupus erythematosus (LE) cells	Neutrophils or macrophages with intracytoplasmic hematoxylin bodies	Cells with eccentric nuclei and large homogeneous intracytoplasmic bodies (hematoxylin bodies) DD: signet ring cells
Hematoxylin body	Homogeneous and glassy intracytoplasmic body (denatured nuclear material), green or blue or purple in color with the Papanicolaou stain, and magenta in color with the Diff-Quik stain	Presence in the cytoplasm of neutrophil or macrophage (LE cells), commonly seen in lupus pleuritis
Psammoma body	Round collections of calcium which is covered with a thin layer of benign mesothelial cells. It stains purple in color with the Papanicolaou method	Calcium in the center of the spheres. It may be found in both benign and malignant conditions DD: collagen ball
Magenta body	Variably sized red-to-purple perinuclear inclusions seen by the Diff-Quik stains	Seen in metastatic breast carcinomas
Collagen ball	Spheres of collagen which is covered with a thin layer of benign mesothelial cells	Nonspecific finding DD: psammoma body. Metastatic mucinous adenocarcinomas, papillary serous carcinomas of the ovary, and mesotheliomas
Charcot–Leyden crystal	Needle-shaped orangeophilic color crystal, a by-product of eosinophil degranulation	Associated with allergy DD: calcium oxalate crystals

Table 2.2 Malignant conditions in serous fluid

Conditions	Descriptions	Differentials
Mesothelioma	Numerous three-dimensional clusters (with more than 20–30 tumor cells). Tumor cells have large nuclei, coarse chromatin, and irregular nuclear membrane	Cellular clusters with scallop border and cytoplasmic vacuoles. Tumor cells may maintain low N/C ratios and "windows" between cells. Cytoplasm is dense with "hyaluronic acid mucin" DD: adenocarcinoma
Adenocarcinoma	Three-dimensional cell clusters with smooth border and/or acinar/papillae arrangements of columnar cells. Tumor cells have high N/C ratios, prominent nucleoli, and "lacy" cytoplasm with vacuolization	Columnar cells have high N/C ratios with irregular nuclear membrane, coarse chromatin, prominent nucleoli, and cytoplasmic vacuole (mucin production). No "window" between cells DD: mesothelioma, poorly differentiated nonkeratinizing squamous cell carcinoma
Squamous cell carcinoma	Discohesive and scattered individual polymorphic cells or loosely formed two-dimensional cell clusters with or without keratinization	Polygonal, rounded, elongated, or tadpole-shaped cells with large pyknotic nuclei, smudgy chromatin and dense cytoplasm. No "window" between cells DD: poorly differentiated adenocarcinoma
Small cell carcinoma	Tight clusters of small hyperchromatic cells (two to three times the size of mature lymphocytes) with nuclear molding and crowding, nuclear stripes (breakdown of nuclear material), inconspicuous nuclei, scant cytoplasm	Fine chromatin (salt-and-pepper appearance), mitoses, necrosis, and apoptotic bodies DD: lymphoma, basaloid squamous cell carcinoma, and poorly differentiated adenocarcinoma
Undifferentiated large cell carcinoma	Loosely cohesive clusters, syncytial sheets or scattered polymorphic large cells with high N/C ratios, single or multiple prominent nucleoli and feathery cytoplasm	Malignant cells are huge with large nucleoli. Numerous mitoses DD: poorly differentiated adenocarcinoma and sarcomas
Melanoma	Scattered individual large cells with prominent nucleoli and cytoplasmic melanin pigments. Binucleation with "mirror" arrangement. Pseudointranuclear inclusions	Discohesive malignant cells with prominent nucleoli DD: poorly differentiated carcinoma, Hodgkin lymphoma
Lymphoma (non-Hodgkin lymphoma)	Dispersed individual atypical lymphoid cells with clumped chromatin and irregular nuclear membrane. Increased mitotic activity. Lymphoglandular bodies in the background of the slide	The size of tumor cells ranges from small to large depending on the type of lymphoma. Monomorphous population of lymphocytes is a characteristic of SLL/CLL DD: reactive lymphocytes, small cell carcinoma, poorly differentiated carcinoma
Non-epithelial cell neoplasma	Individual or clusters of spindle cells, small round cells or pleomorphic tumor cells	DD: muscle, nerve tumors, small round cell tumor, and sarcomas

2.1 Image-Based Questions 1–50 (50 Images)

Fig. 2.1

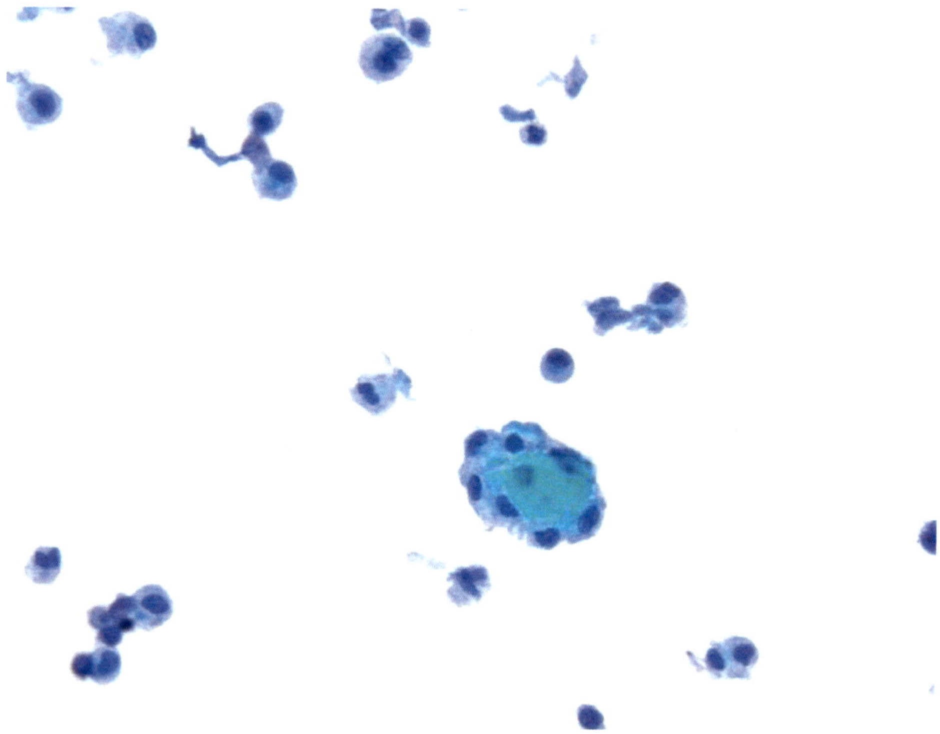

Q-1. What is the diagnosis of this peritoneal washing specimen?
(a) Metastatic adenocarcinoma
(b) Serous carcinoma of ovary
(c) Collagen ball
(d) Mesothelioma

Fig. 2.2

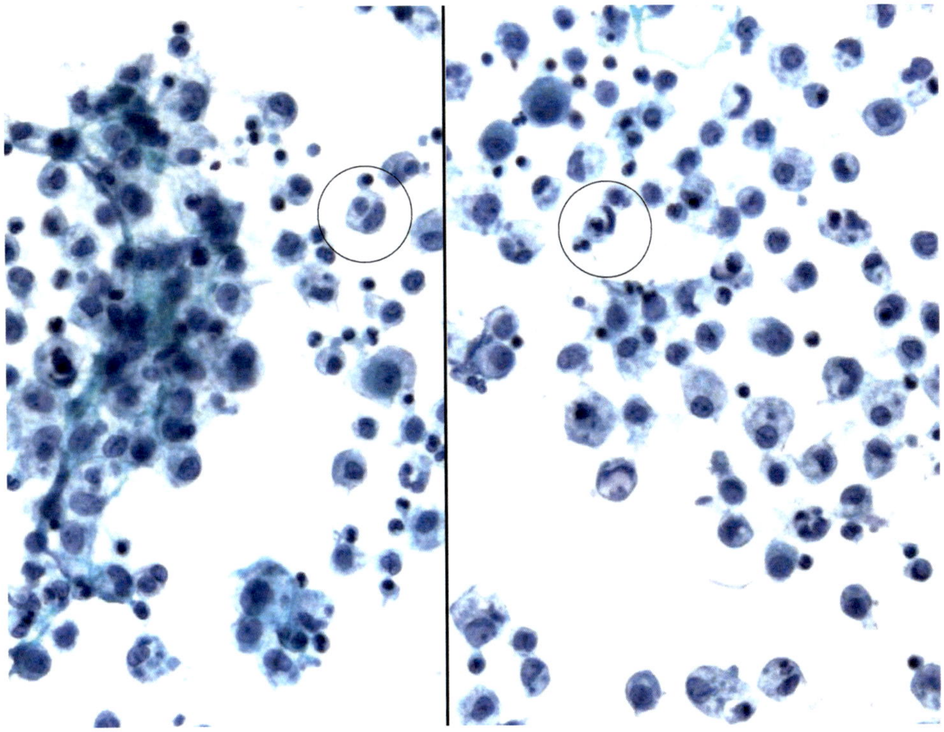

Q-2. What is the diagnosis of cells seen in the pleural effusion from a patient with systemic lupus erythematosus?

(a) Lupus erythematosus (LE) cells
(b) Tart cells
(c) Reactive mesothelial cells
(d) Mucin-producing cells

Fig. 2.3

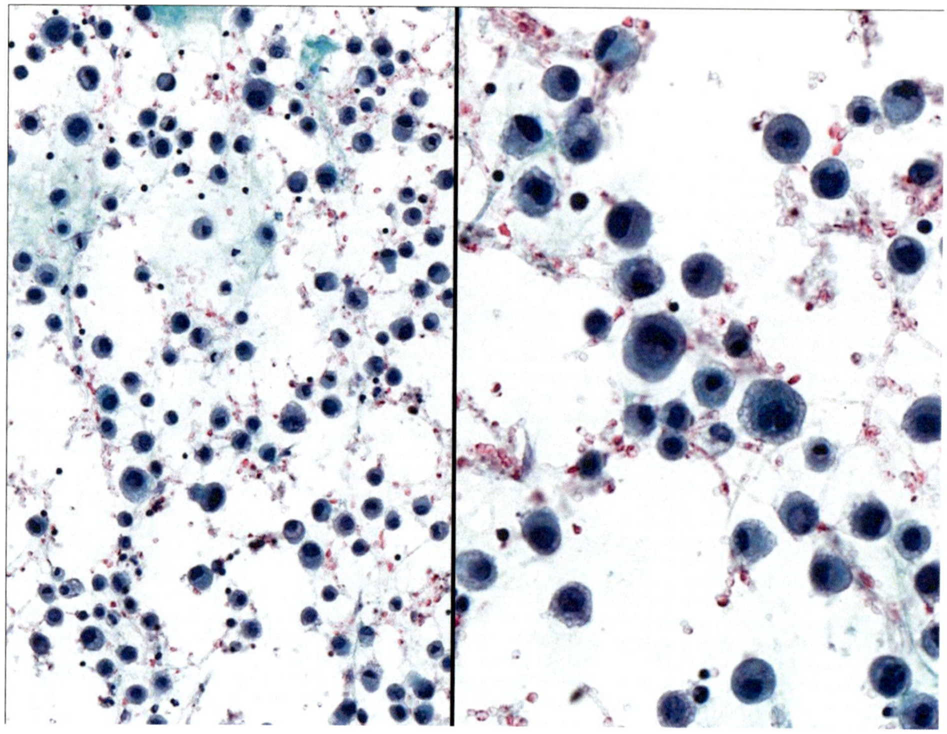

Q-3. What is the diagnosis of cells seen in this pericardial effusion from a 52-year-old female patient with a history of breast carcinoma and melanoma?

(a) Metastatic lung adenocarcinoma
(b) Reactive mesothelial cells
(c) Metastatic melanoma
(d) Metastatic breast lobular carcinoma

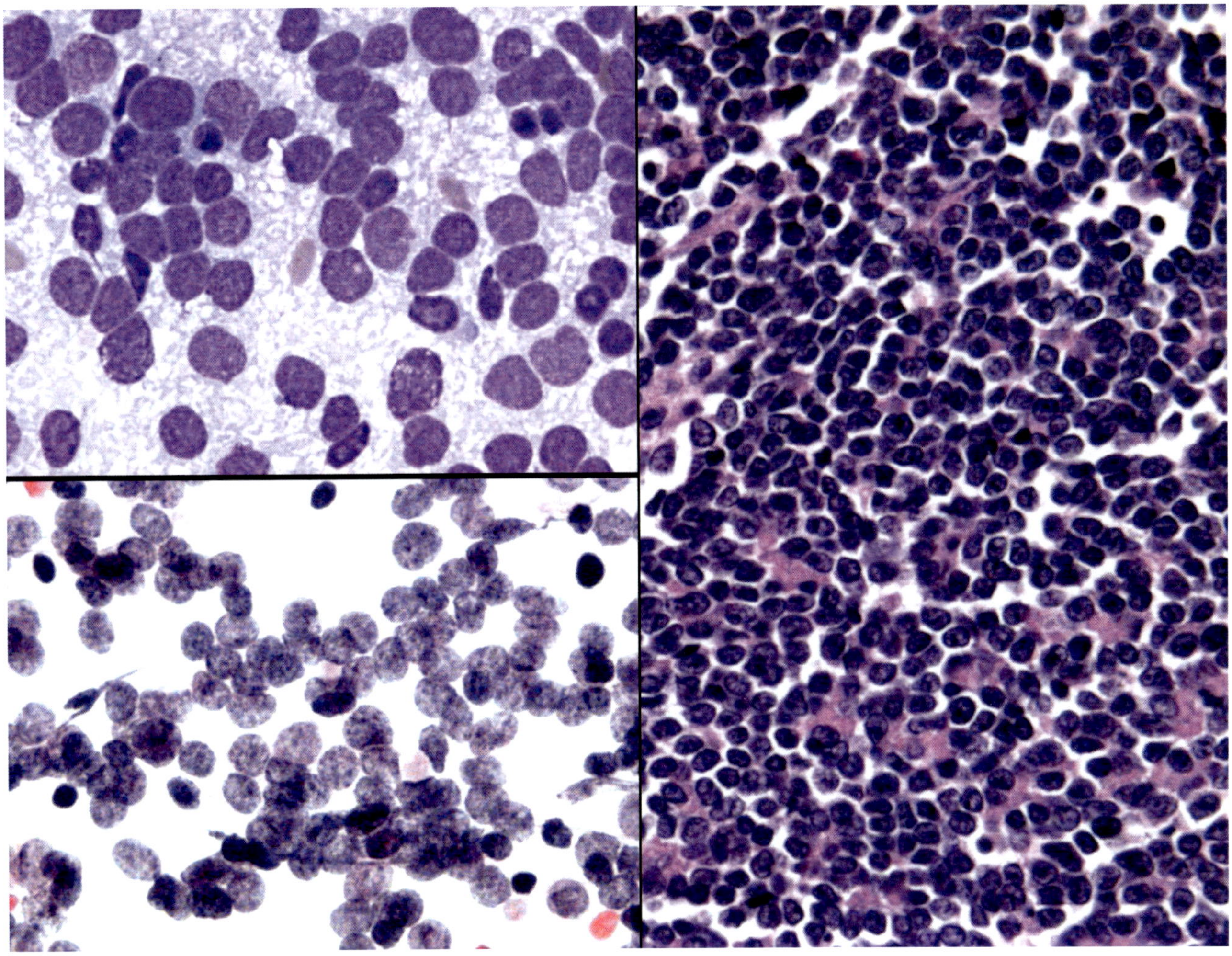

Fig. 2.4

Q-4. What is the diagnosis of cells seen in this ascites from a 24-year-old male with a retroperitoneal mass?
(a) Small cell carcinoma
(b) Lymphoma
(c) Ewing's sarcoma
(d) Metastatic adenocarcinoma

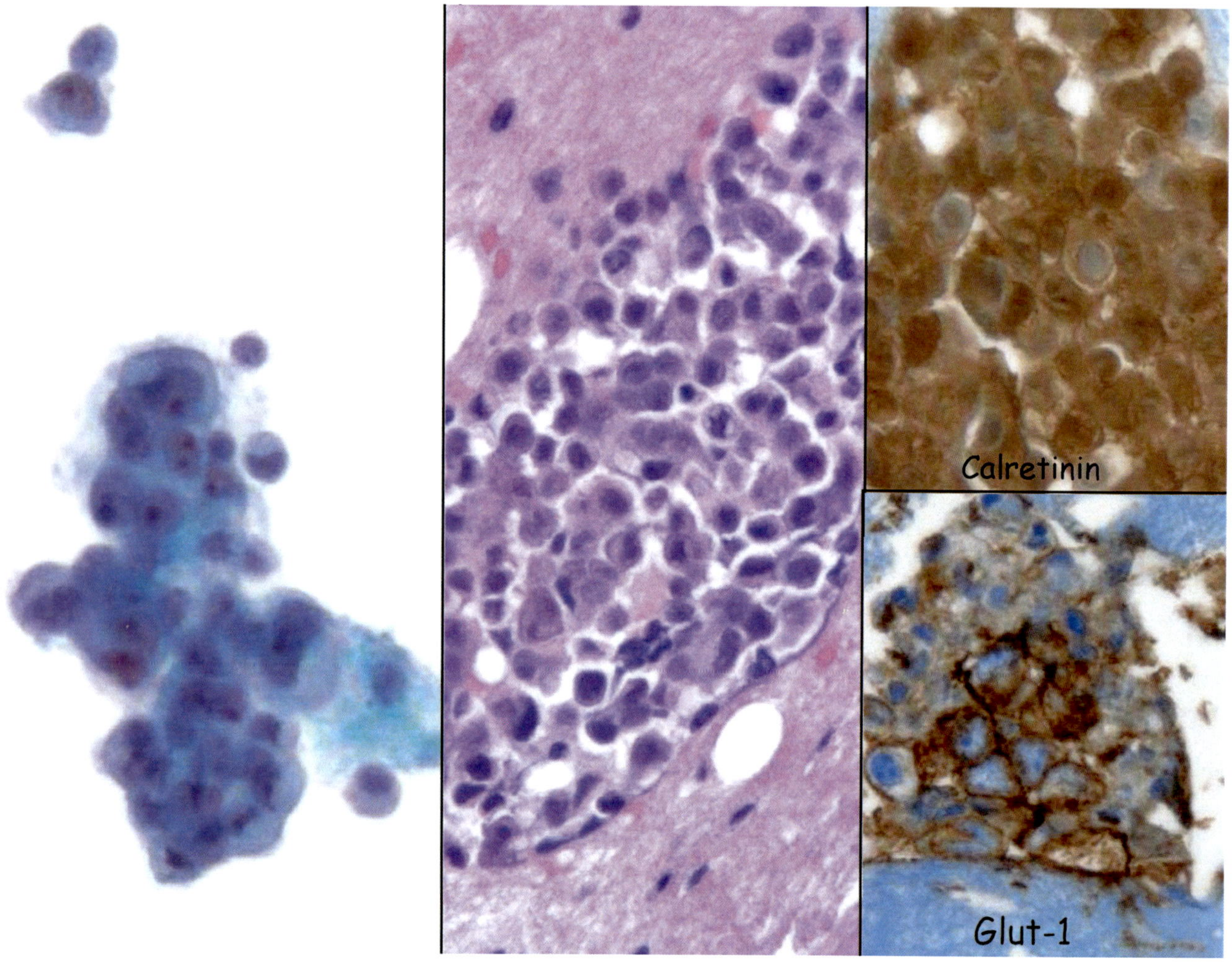

Fig. 2.5

Q-5. What is the diagnosis of cells seen in this pleural effusion from a 78-year-old female patient with pleural thickening?
(a) Metastatic lung adenocarcinoma
(b) Reactive mesothelial cells
(c) Metastatic melanoma
(d) Mesothelioma

Fig. 2.6

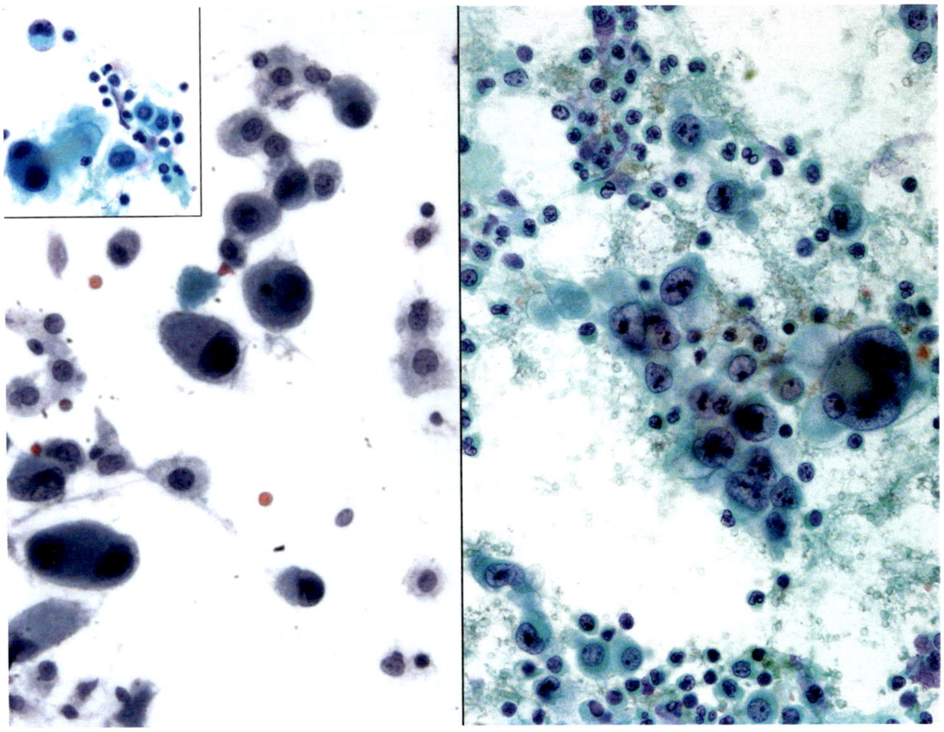

Q-6. What is the diagnosis of cells seen in this ascites from an 8-year-old boy with a retroperitoneal mass?
(a) Metastatic adenocarcinoma
(b) Reactive mesothelial cells
(c) Metastatic melanoma
(d) Metastatic rhabdomyosarcoma

Fig. 2.7

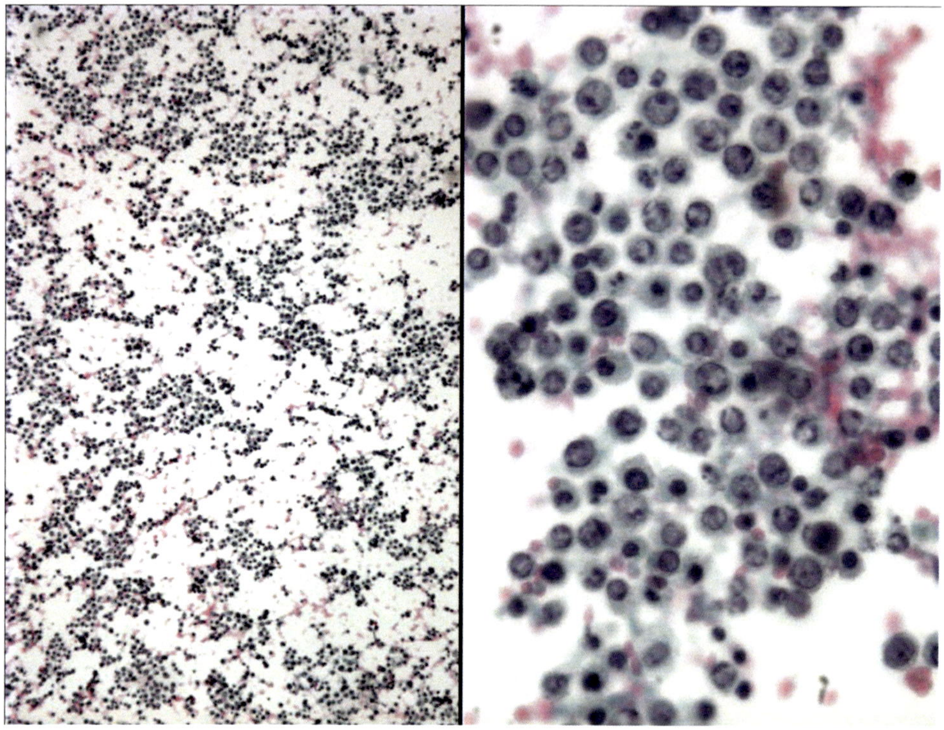

Q-7. An 83-year-old male patient with lymphadenopathy developed pleural effusions. The specimen consists predominately of a monomorphous population of lymphocytes with apoptosis. Which one the following diagnoses is correct?

(a) Metastatic poorly differentiated adenocarcinoma
(b) Small cell carcinoma
(c) Metastatic melanoma
(d) Lymphomatous effusion most consistent with malignant lymphoma

Fig. 2.8

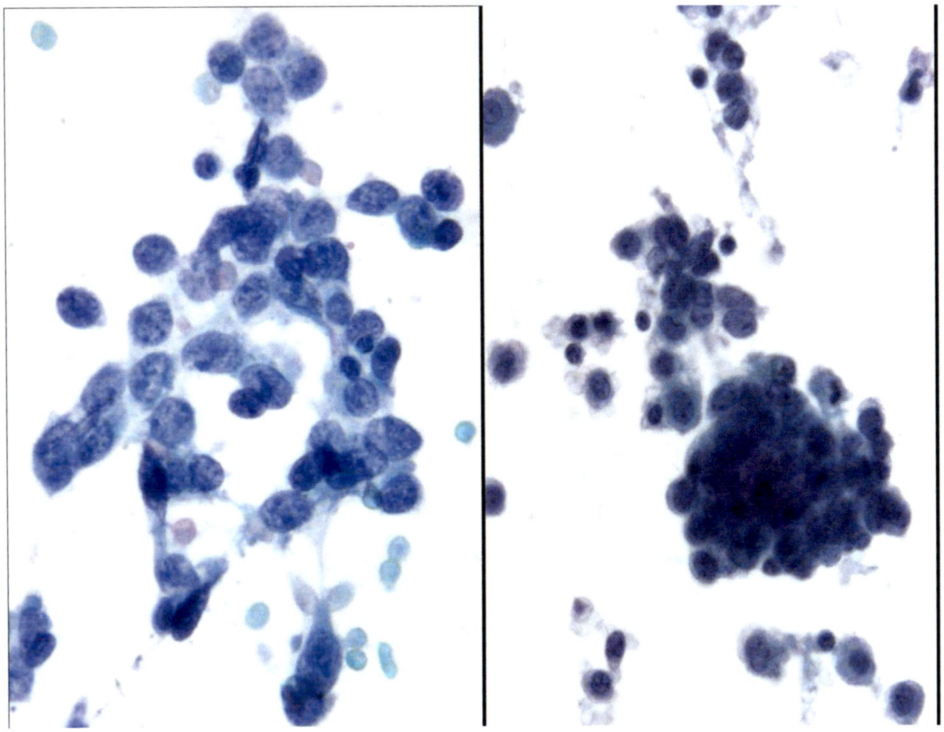

Q-8. A 77-year-old male smoker with a right upper lung mass developed a pleural effusion. Which one of the following diagnoses is correct?

(a) Metastatic poorly differentiated adenocarcinoma
(b) Metastatic small cell lung carcinoma
(c) Metastatic melanoma
(d) Lymphoma

Fig. 2.9

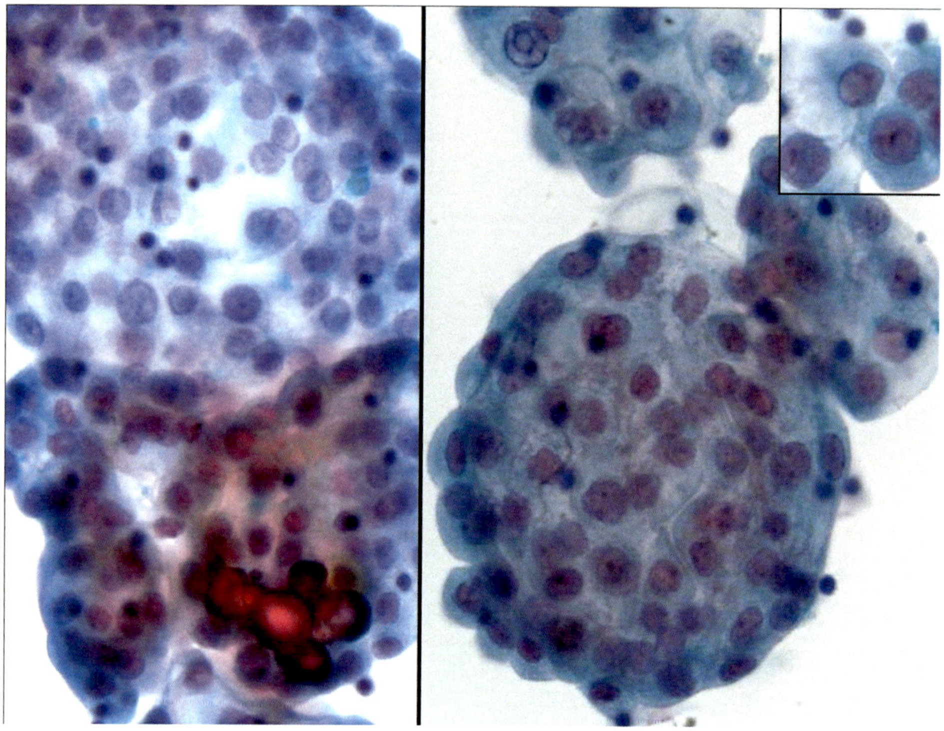

Q-9. In this ascites from a 58-year-old female, the cytological findings are shown in this photo. What is the correct diagnosis?
(a) Metastatic ovarian serous carcinoma
(b) Mesothelial cell hyperplasia
(c) Endosalpingiosis
(d) Metastatic adenocarcinoma

Fig. 2.10

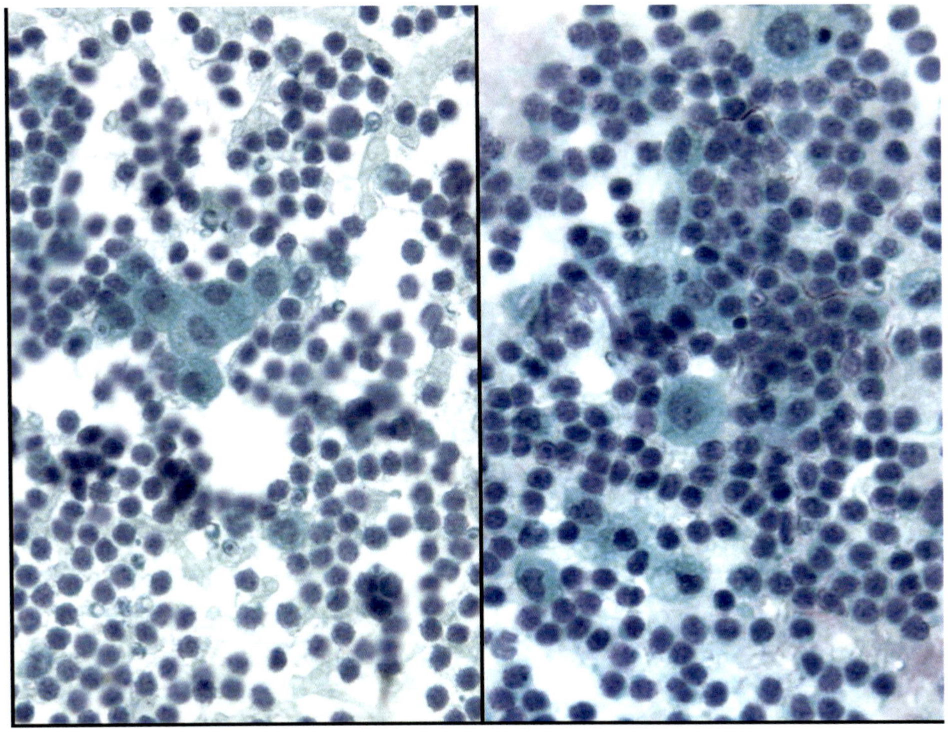

Q-10. A 64-year-old female smoker with a lung mass developed a pleural effusion. On cytospin preparation, the smear consists of predominantly small- to intermediate-sized lymphocytic cells with evenly distributed chromatin. Which one of the following diagnoses is correct?
(a) Metastatic poorly differentiated adenocarcinoma
(b) Metastatic small cell lung carcinoma
(c) Lymphoma
(d) Lymphocytosis (lymphocytic effusion)

Fig. 2.11

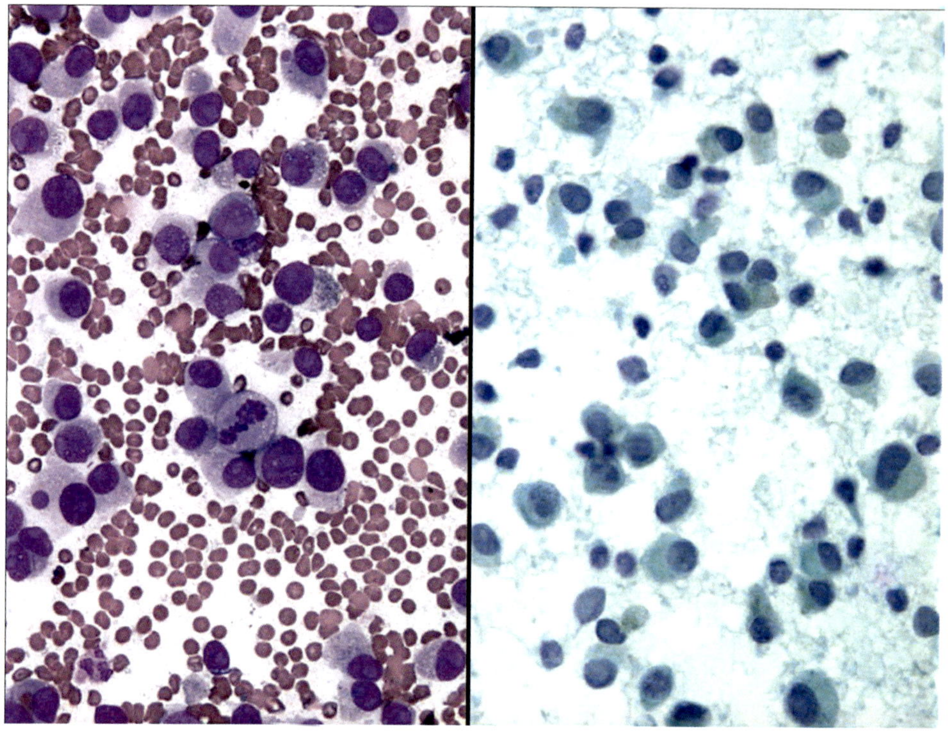

Q-11. A 34-year-old female with a history of melanoma now develops a lung mass and pleural effusion. Which one the following diagnoses is correct?
(a) Metastatic poorly differentiated adenocarcinoma of the lung
(b) Metastatic small cell lung carcinoma
(c) Metastatic melanoma
(d) Lymphoma

Fig. 2.12

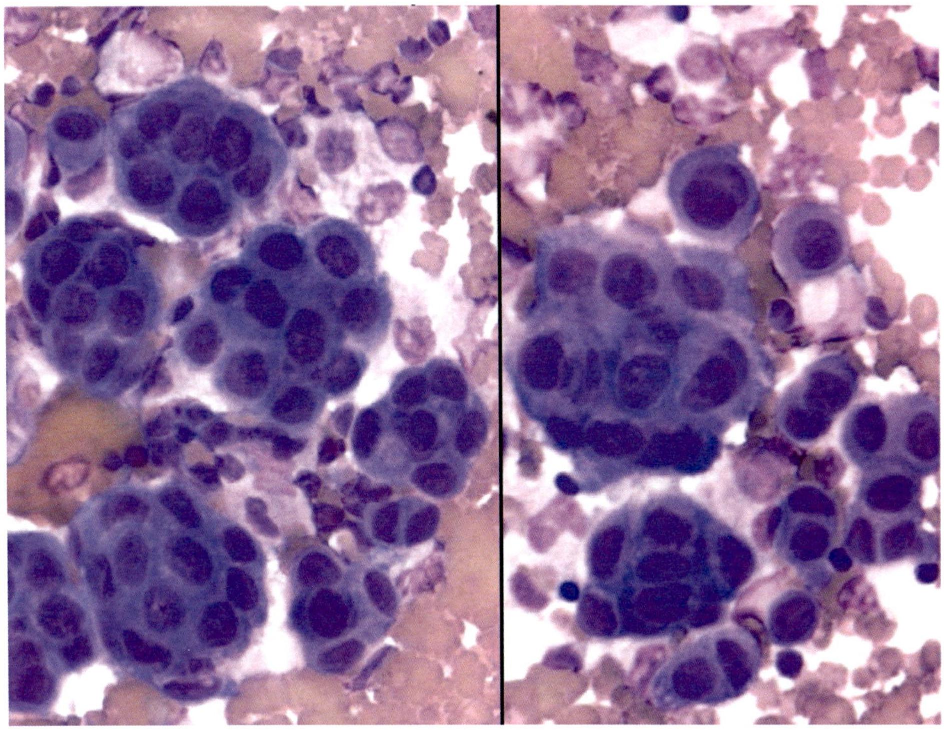

Q-12. What is the diagnosis of cells seen in this pleural effusion?
(a) Metastatic lung adenocarcinoma
(b) Reactive mesothelial cells
(c) Metastatic melanoma
(d) Mesothelioma

Fig. 2.13

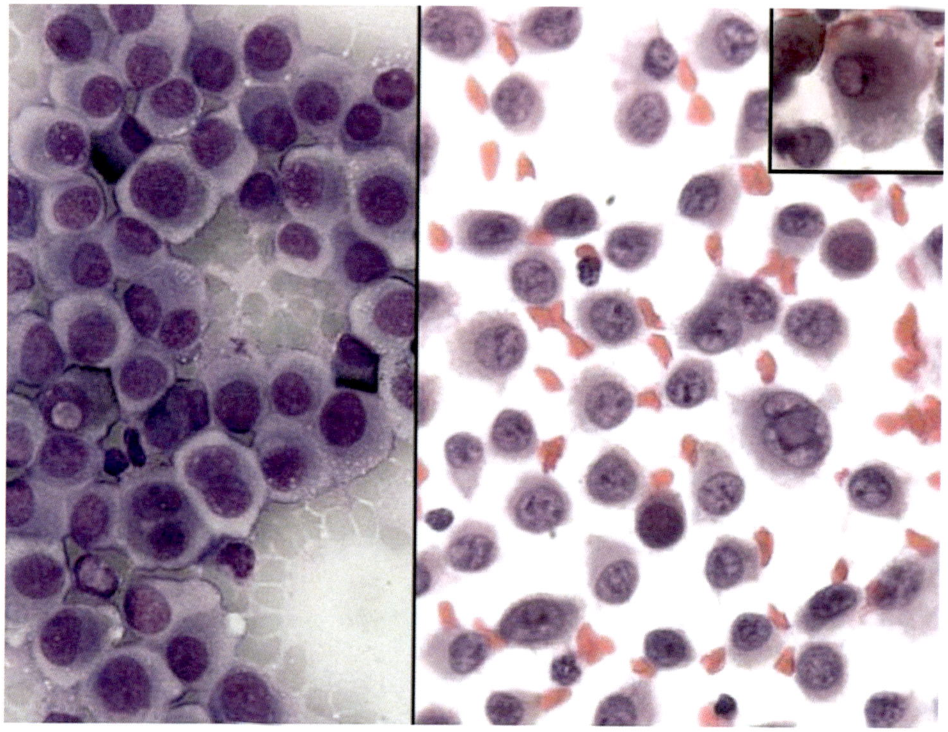

Q-13. A 48-year-old female with a history of melanoma now develops a pleural effusion. Which one of the following diagnoses is correct?
(a) Metastatic renal cell carcinoma
(b) Metastatic small cell lung carcinoma
(c) Metastatic melanoma
(d) Lymphoma

Fig. 2.14

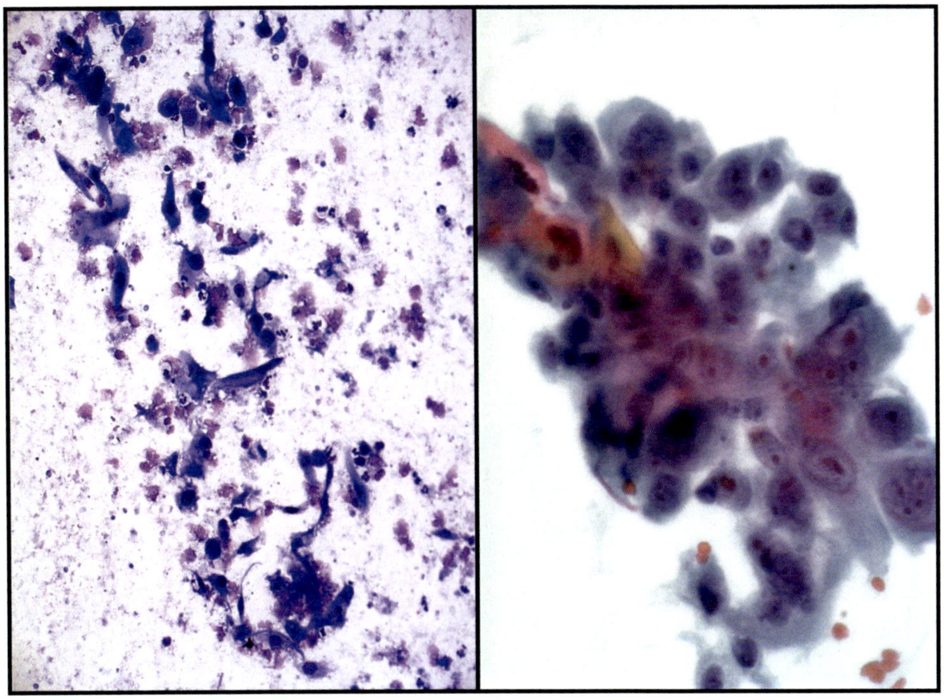

Q-14. A 68-year-old male with a head and neck mass now develops a pleural effusion. Which one of the following diagnoses is correct?
(a) Metastatic squamous cell carcinoma
(b) Metastatic poorly differentiated adenocarcinoma
(c) Metastatic melanoma
(d) Lymphoma

Fig. 2.15

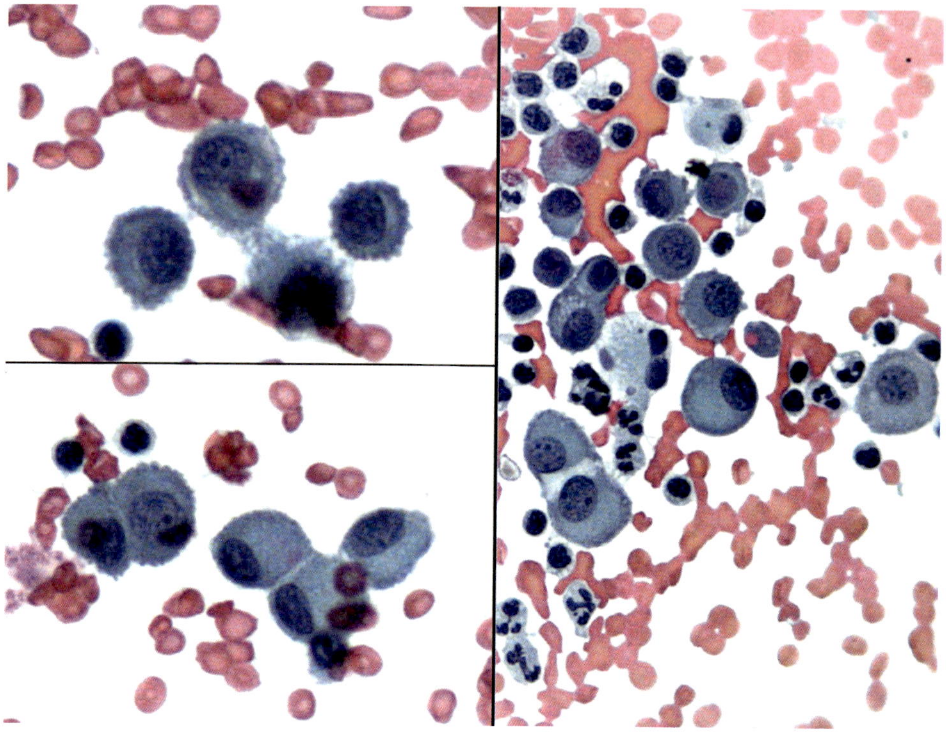

Q-15. A 48-year-old female with a history of melanoma now develops a lung mass and pleural effusion. What is the diagnosis of cells seen in this pleural effusion?

(a) Metastatic lung adenocarcinoma
(b) Reactive mesothelial cells
(c) Metastatic melanoma
(d) Mesothelioma

Fig. 2.16

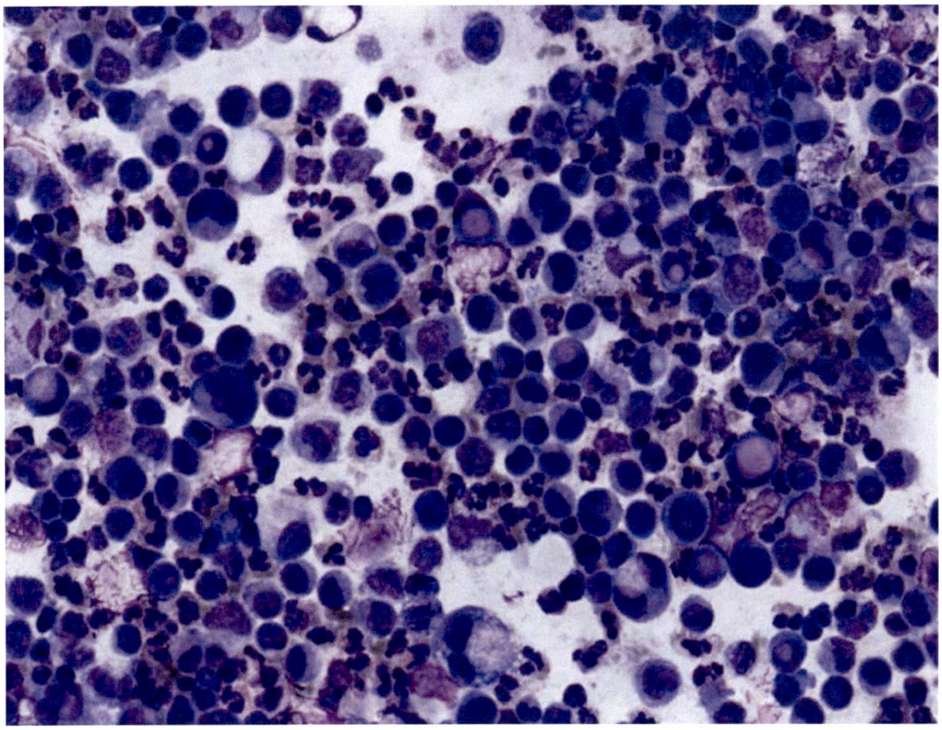

Q-16. A 62-year-old female with a history of "carcinoma" now develops a pleural effusion. What is the diagnosis of cells seen in this pleural effusion?
(a) Metastatic renal cell carcinoma
(b) Reactive mesothelial cells
(c) Metastatic melanoma
(d) Metastatic signet ring cell carcinoma

Fig. 2.17

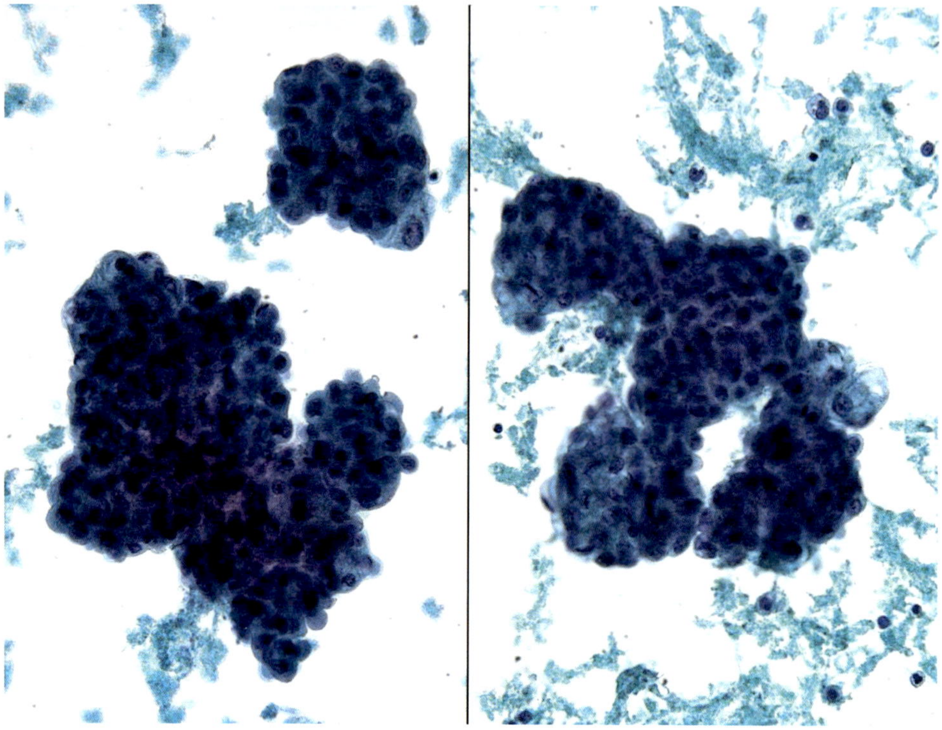

Q-17. A 70-year-old female with a history of right "kidney tumor" develops a right-side pleural effusion. What is the diagnosis of cells seen in this pleural effusion?
(a) Metastatic papillary renal cell carcinoma
(b) Reactive mesothelial cells
(c) Mesothelioma
(d) Metastatic poorly differentiated adenocarcinoma of the lung

Fig. 2.18

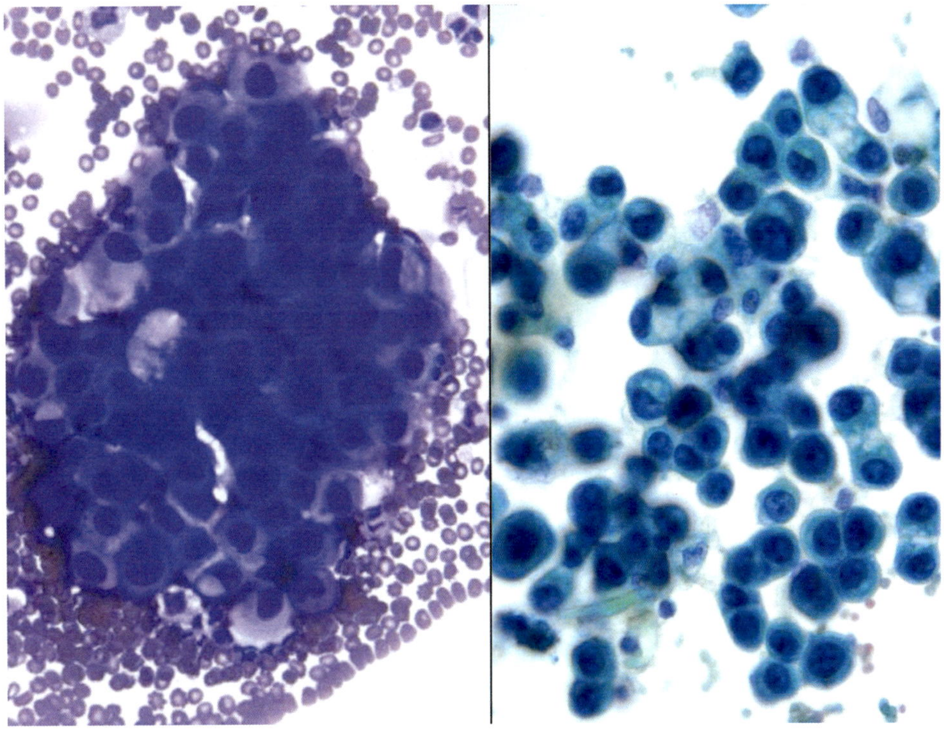

Q-18. A 61-year-old male with a clinical presentation of a lung mass develops a left pleural effusion. What is the diagnosis of cells seen in this pleural effusion?

(a) Metastatic adenocarcinoma of the lung
(b) Reactive mesothelial cells
(c) Mesothelioma
(d) Metastatic poorly differentiated small cell carcinoma

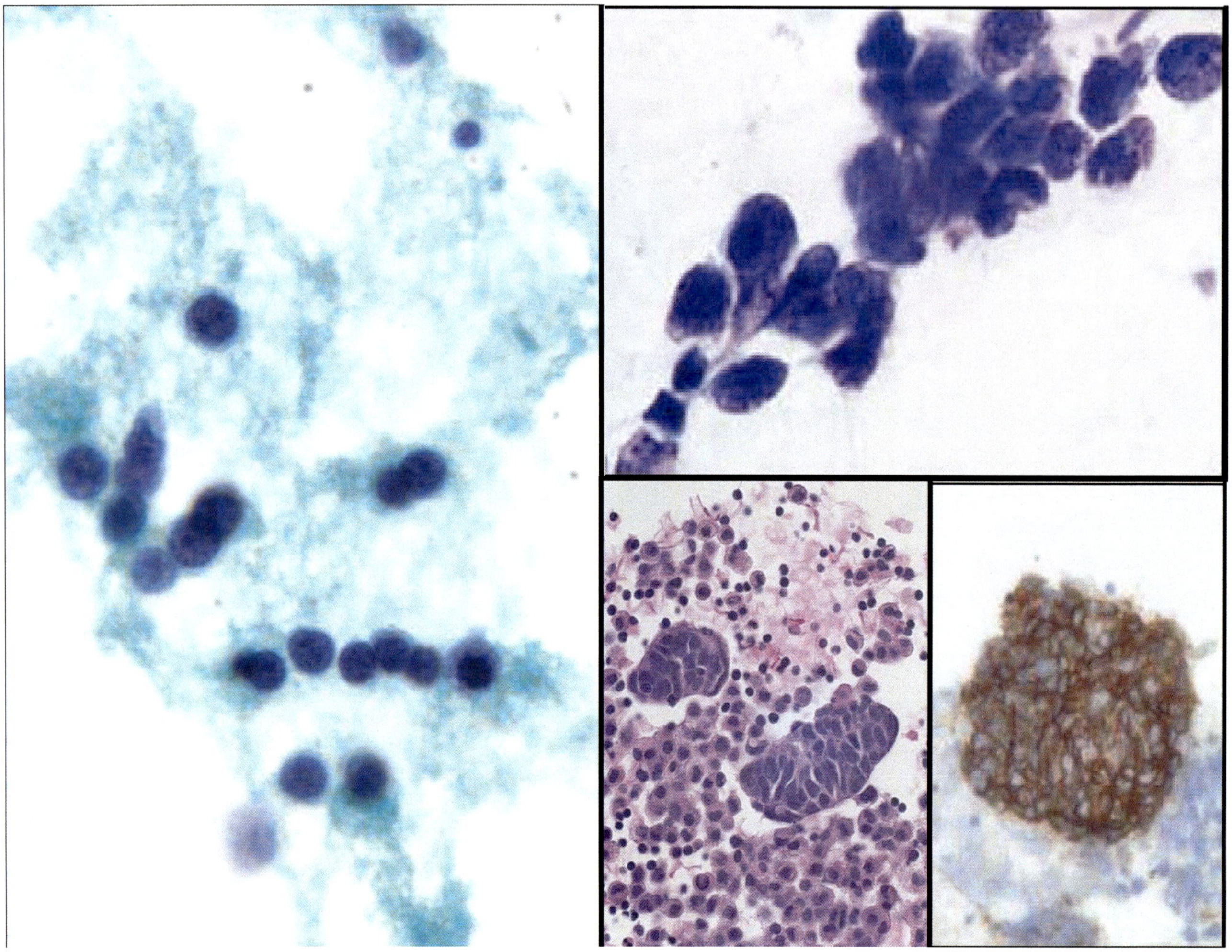

Fig. 2.19

Q-19. Which one of the following immunomarkers has a better sensitivity for this metastatic carcinoma of the lung?
(a) TTF1 (thyroid transcription factor 1)
(b) Synaptophysin
(c) Chromogranin A
(d) CD56

Fig. 2.20

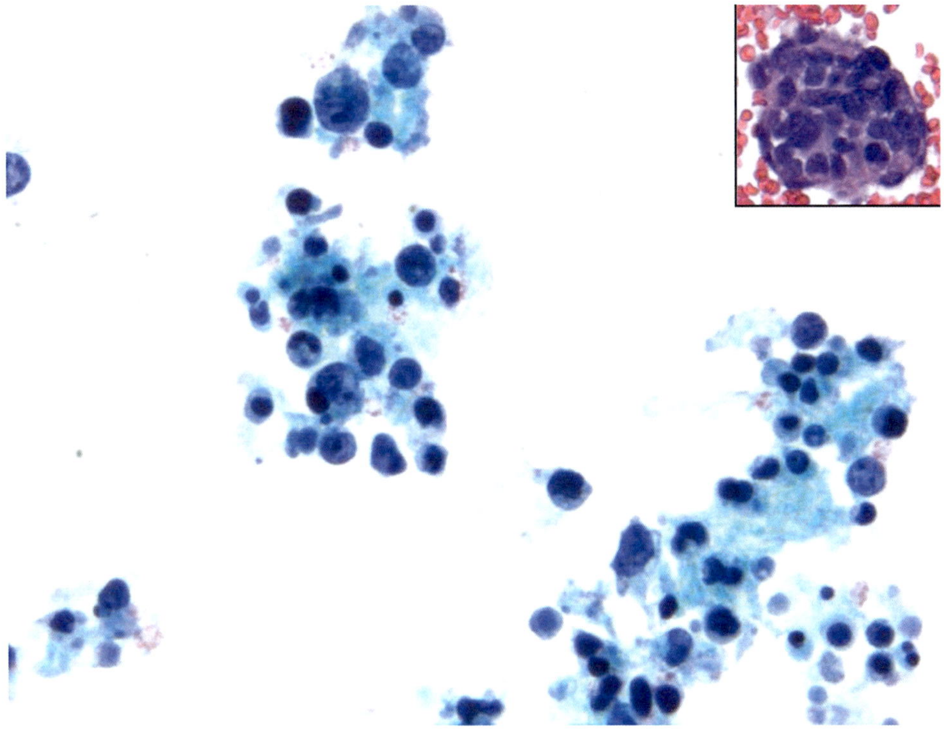

Q-20. A 2-year-old female with an abdominal mass developed ascites. On surgical resection specimen, Homer–Wright rosettes are identified. The ascites cytospin was shown here. Which panel of following immunomarkers can help you confirm the diagnosis?

(a) Cytokeratin and TTF1
(b) Neuron-specific enolase (NSE), synaptophysin, S100, and glial fibrillary acidic protein (GFAP)
(c) Chromogranin A, synaptophysin, and CD56
(d) CD20, CD3, and CD56

Fig. 2.21

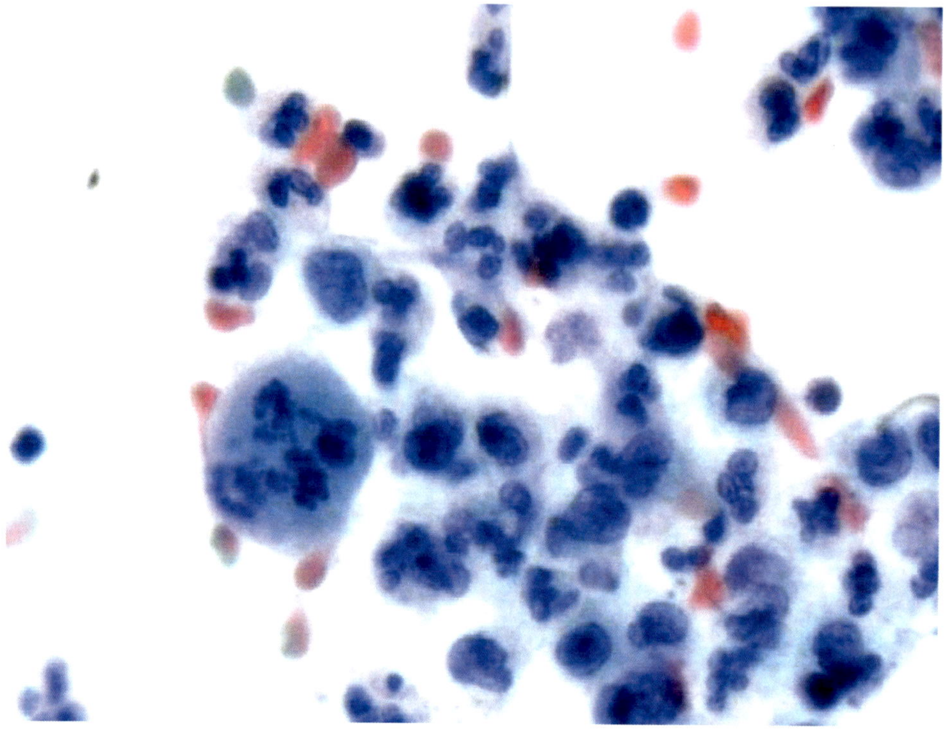

Q-21. A 70-year-old male with a liver mass and lung masses develops a left pleural effusion. What is the diagnosis of cells seen in this pleural effusion?

(a) Metastatic poorly differentiated adenocarcinoma of the lung
(b) Reactive mesothelial cells
(c) Metastatic hepatocellular carcinoma
(d) Metastatic poorly differentiated squamous cell carcinoma

Fig. 2.22

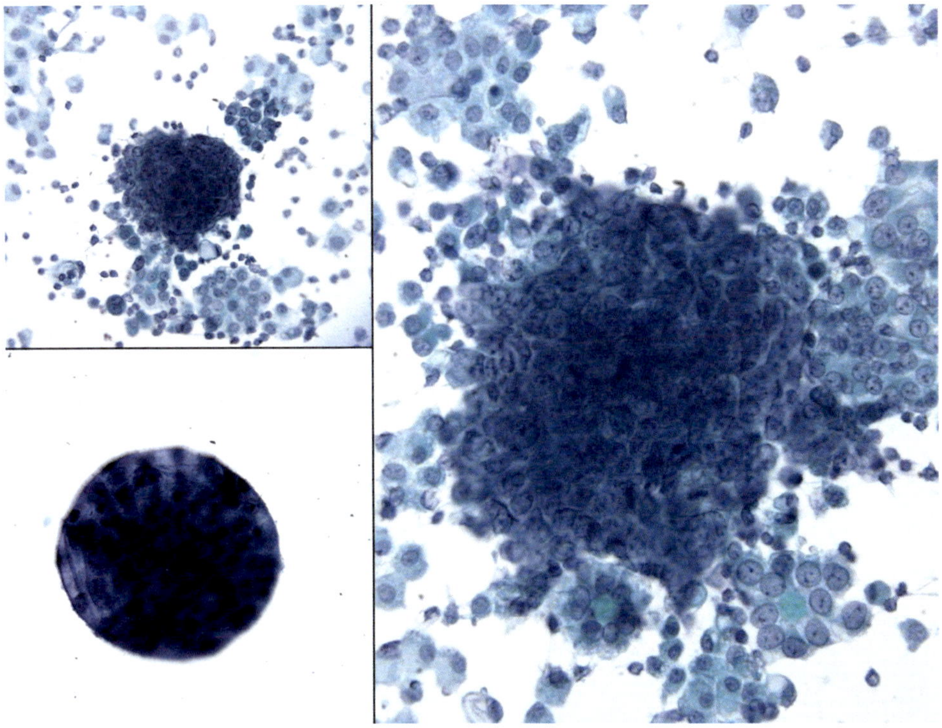

Q-22. A 72-year-old female with a history of colon cancer now develops a lung mass and pleural effusion. What is the diagnosis of cells seen in this pleural effusion?
(a) Metastatic carcinoma of the breast
(b) Reactive mesothelial cells
(c) Metastatic colonic adenocarcinoma
(d) Mesothelioma

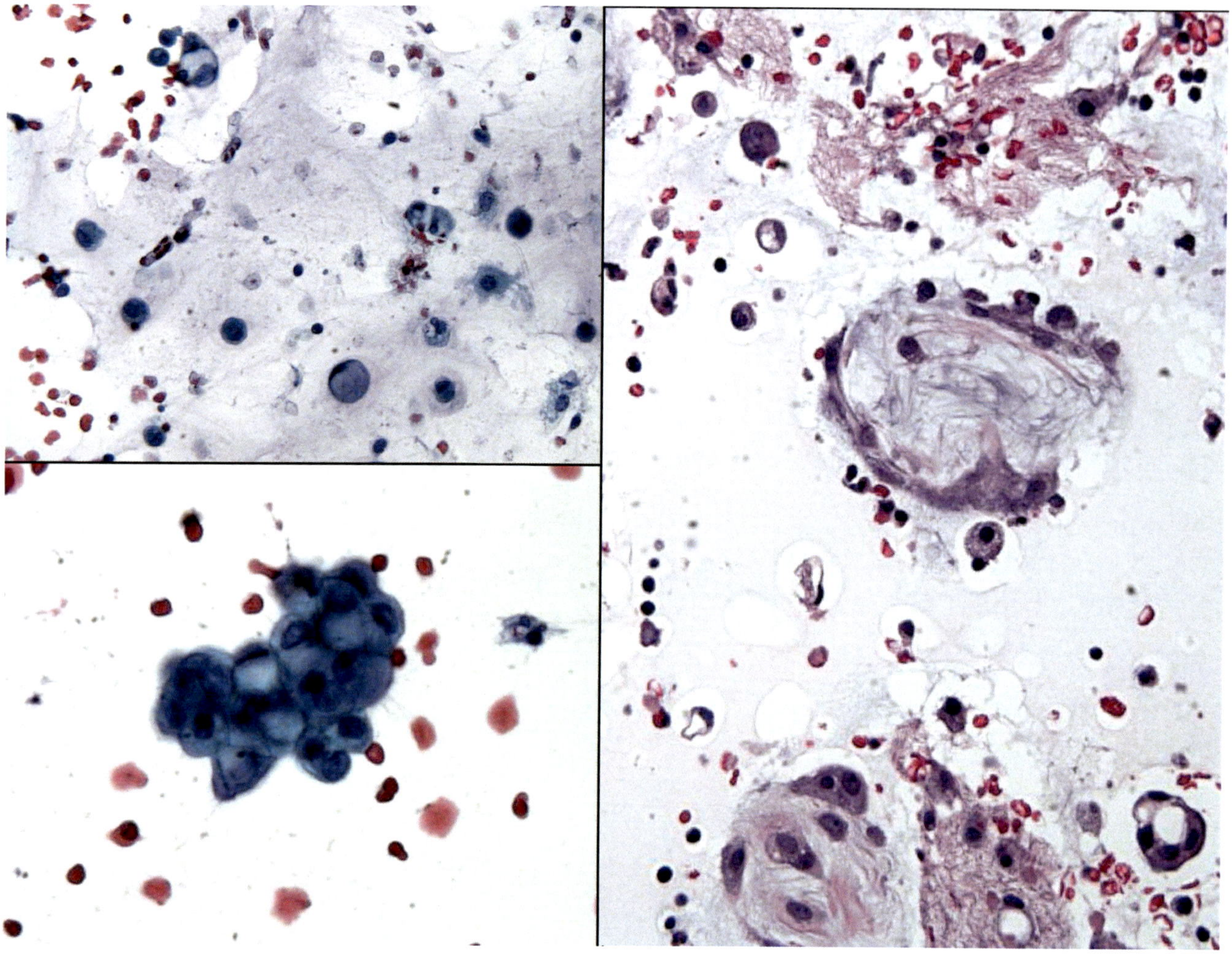

Fig. 2.23

Q-23. A 69-year-old male smoker presents with a right lung mass and pleural effusion. What is the diagnosis of cells seen in this pleural effusion?
(a) Metastatic papillary adenocarcinoma of the lung
(b) Reactive mesothelial cells
(c) Metastatic colonic adenocarcinoma
(d) Metastatic mucinous adenocarcinoma of the lung

Fig. 2.24

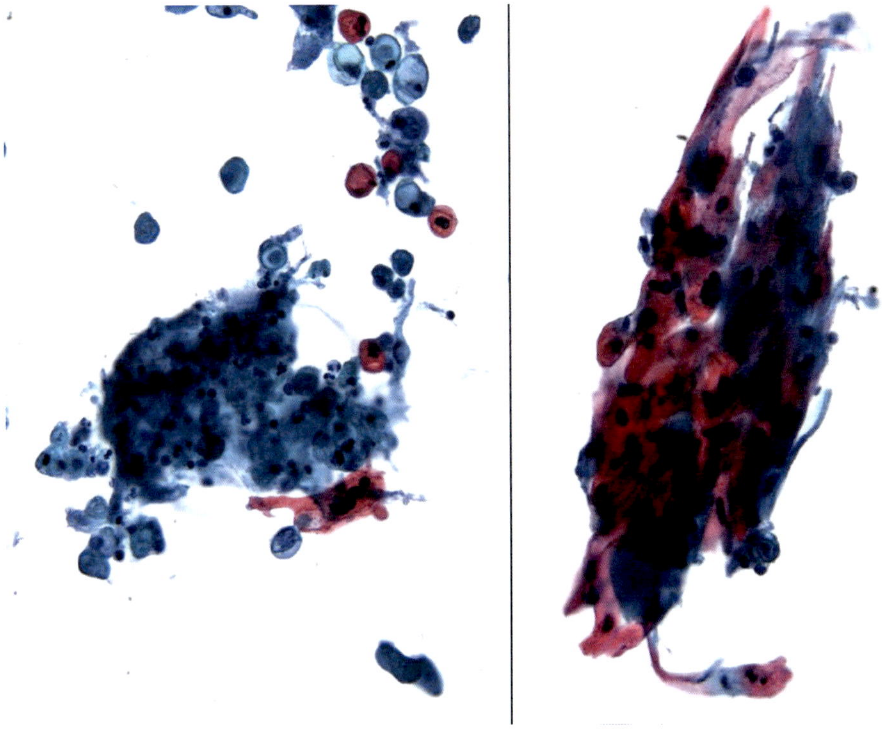

Q-24. What is the diagnosis of cells seen in this pleural effusion?

(a) Metastatic adenocarcinoma
(b) Reactive mesothelial cells
(c) Mesothelioma
(d) Metastatic squamous cell carcinoma

Fig. 2.25

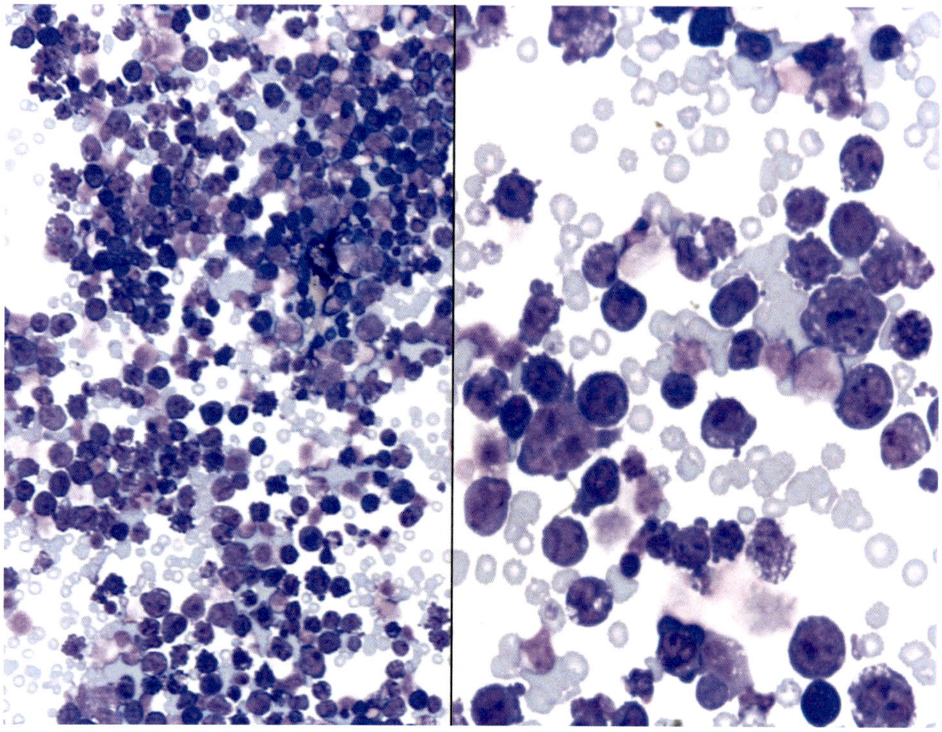

Q-25. An HIV-positive patient develops bilateral pleural effusions. What is the diagnosis of cells seen in this pleural effusion?

(a) Metastatic adenocarcinoma
(b) Primary effusion lymphoma
(c) Reactive mesothelial cells
(d) Metastatic squamous cell carcinoma

Fig. 2.26

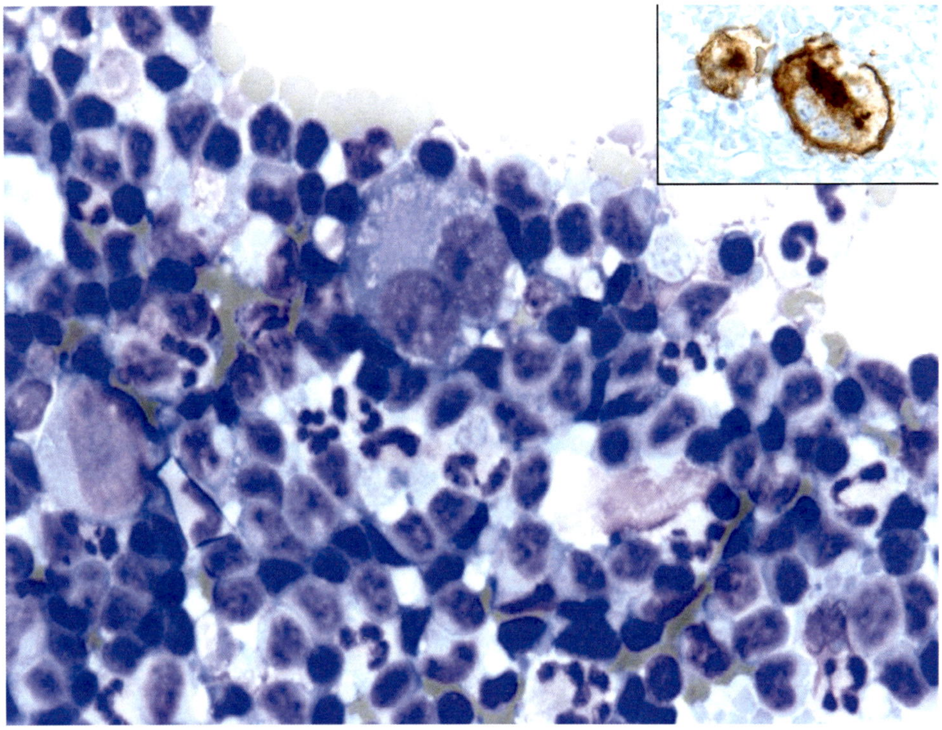

Q-26. A 79-year-old patient with neck lymphadenopathy and mediastinal mass develops bilateral pleural effusions. What is the diagnosis of cells seen in this pleural effusion?

(a) Metastatic adenocarcinoma
(b) SLL/CLL
(c) Reactive mesothelial cells
(d) Hodgkin lymphoma

Fig. 2.27

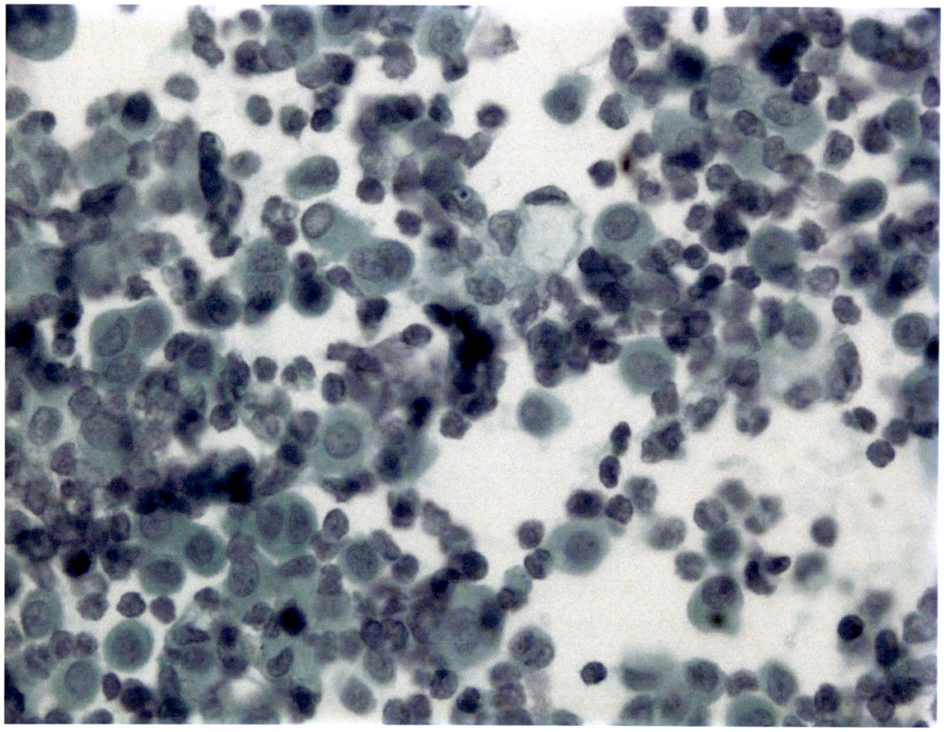

Q-27. A 47-year-old male with history of hepatitis C and numerous liver nodules develops pleural effusion and ascites. What is the diagnosis of cells seen in this pleural effusion?
(a) Metastatic signet ring cell carcinoma
(b) SLL/CLL
(c) Reactive mesothelial cells
(d) Hodgkin lymphoma

Fig. 2.28

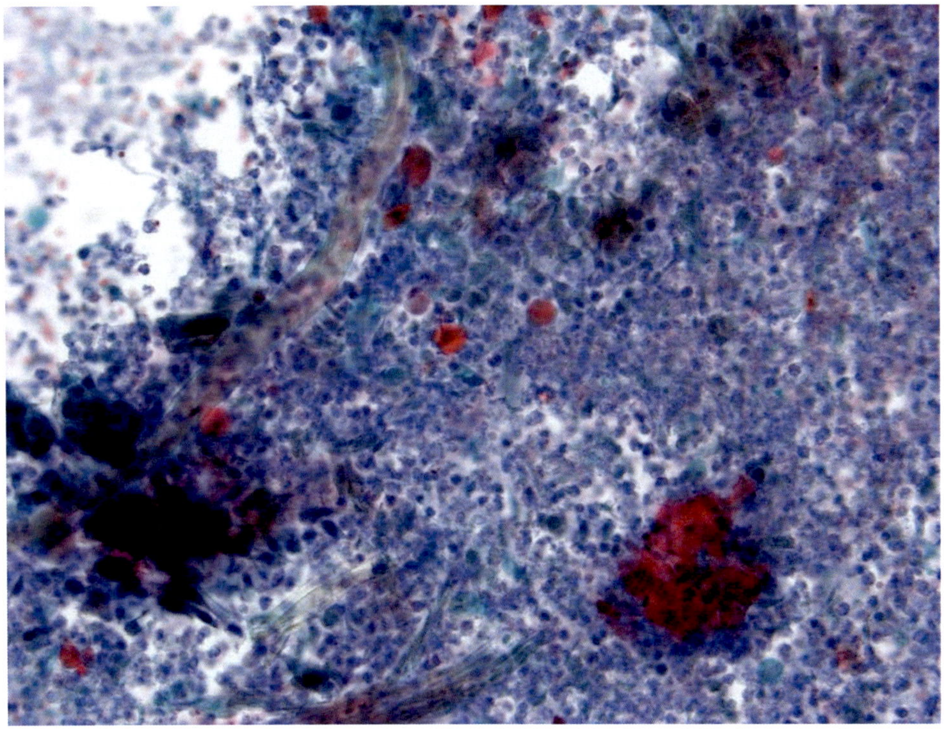

Q-28. A 58-year-old male smoker with history of "lung cancer" develops a pleural effusion. What is the diagnosis of cells seen in this pleural effusion?

(a) Metastatic adenocarcinoma
(b) Metastatic squamous cell carcinoma
(c) Reactive mesothelial cells
(d) Metastatic melanoma

Fig. 2.29

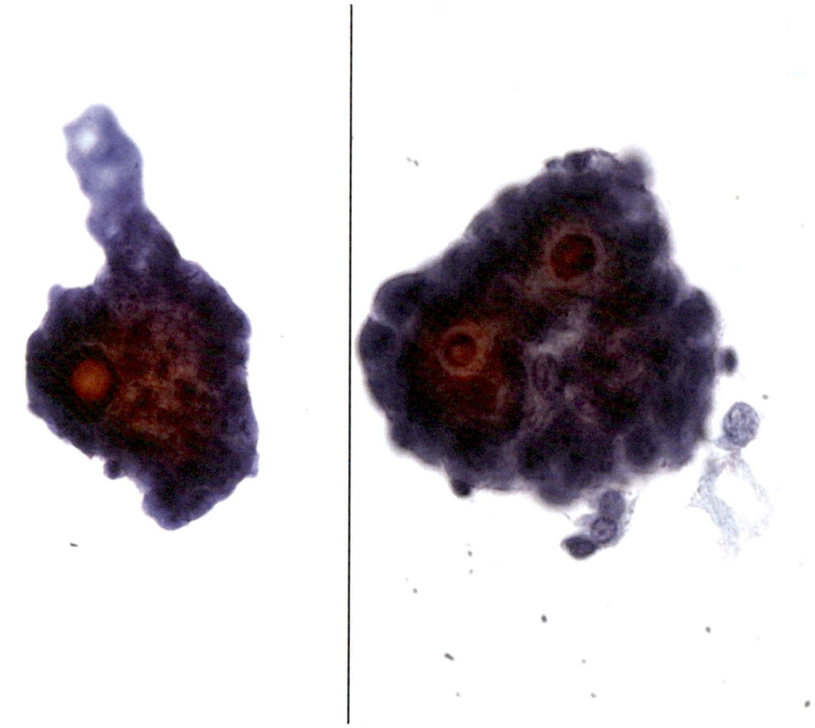

Q-29. Surgical peritoneal washing was performed for staging purpose. What is the diagnosis of this cytological specimen?

(a) Metastatic adenocarcinoma of the colon
(b) Metastatic squamous cell carcinoma
(c) Reactive mesothelial cells
(d) Metastatic serous carcinoma

Fig. 2.30

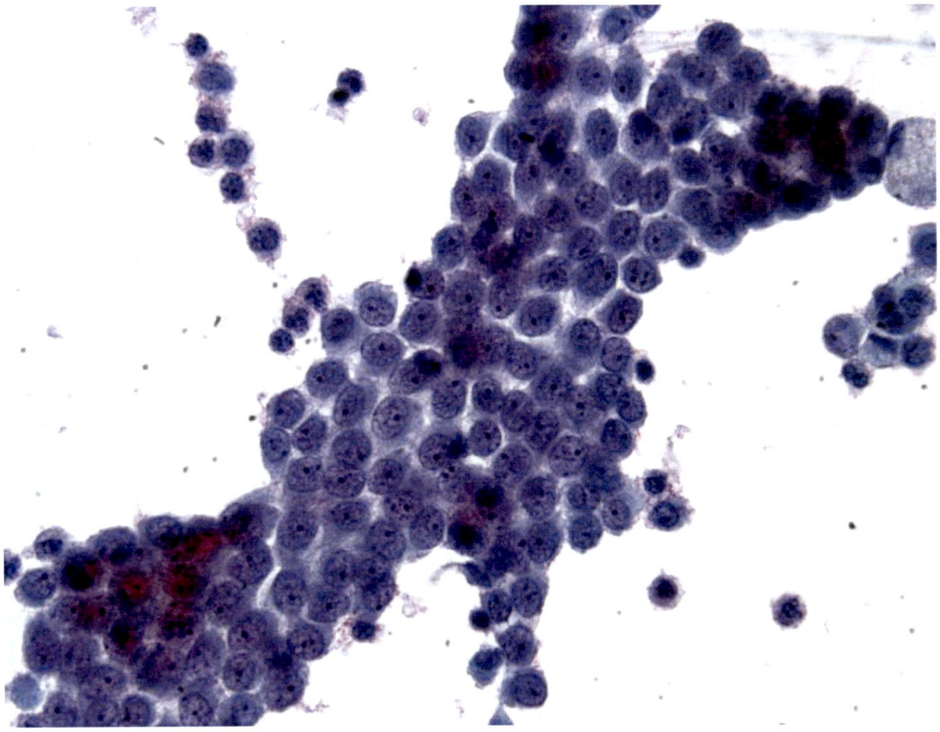

Q-30. A 58-year-old female with history of breast cancer and radiation and chemotherapy develops a pleural effusion. What is the diagnosis of cells seen in this pleural effusion?
(a) Metastatic adenocarcinoma
(b) Metastatic squamous cell carcinoma
(c) Reactive mesothelial cells
(d) Metastatic melanoma

Fig. 2.31

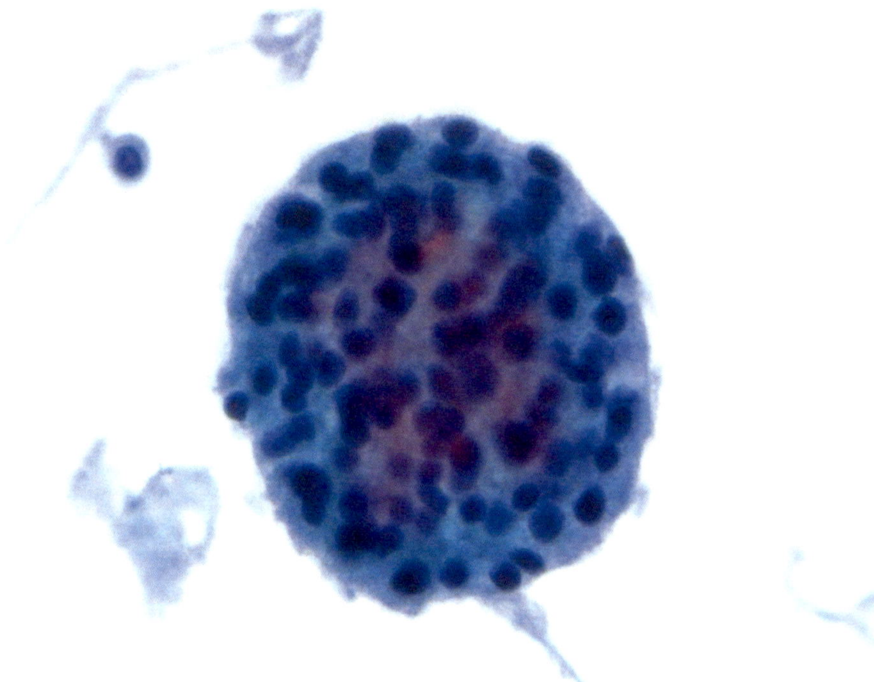

Q-31. The diagnosis of a malignant pleural effusion was made in this specimen. Which panel of immuno-markers can help you confirm the diagnosis?

(a) Cytokeratin and CK7
(b) Calretinin, TTF, and BerEP4
(c) Chromogranin A, synaptophysin, and CD56
(d) CD20, CD3, and CD56

Fig. 2.32

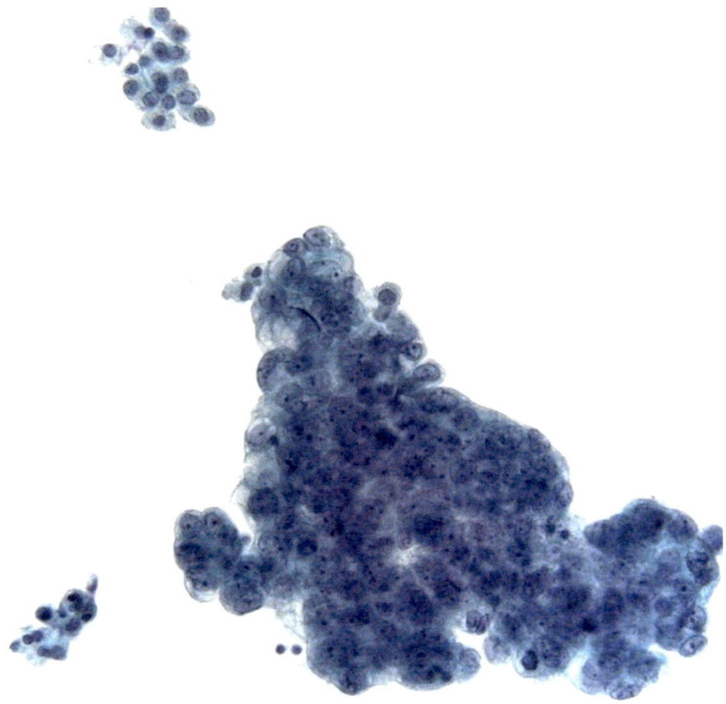

Q-32. The diagnosis of a malignant pleural effusion was made on this specimen. What is the diagnosis of cells seen in this pleural effusion?

(a) Metastatic mucinous adenocarcinoma
(b) Metastatic squamous cell carcinoma
(c) Reactive mesothelial cells
(d) Metastatic small cell carcinoma

Fig. 2.33

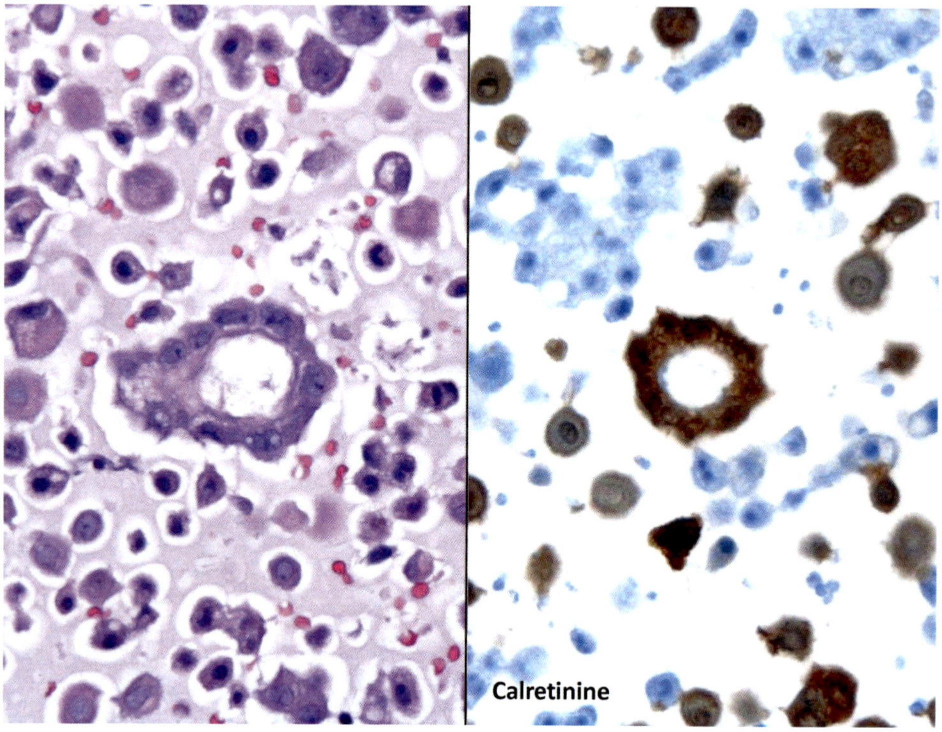

Q-33. Surgical peritoneal washing was performed. What is the diagnosis of this cytological specimen (cell block preparation)?
(a) Metastatic adenocarcinoma of the colon
(b) Mesothelioma
(c) Reactive mesothelial cells
(d) Metastatic serous carcinoma of the ovary

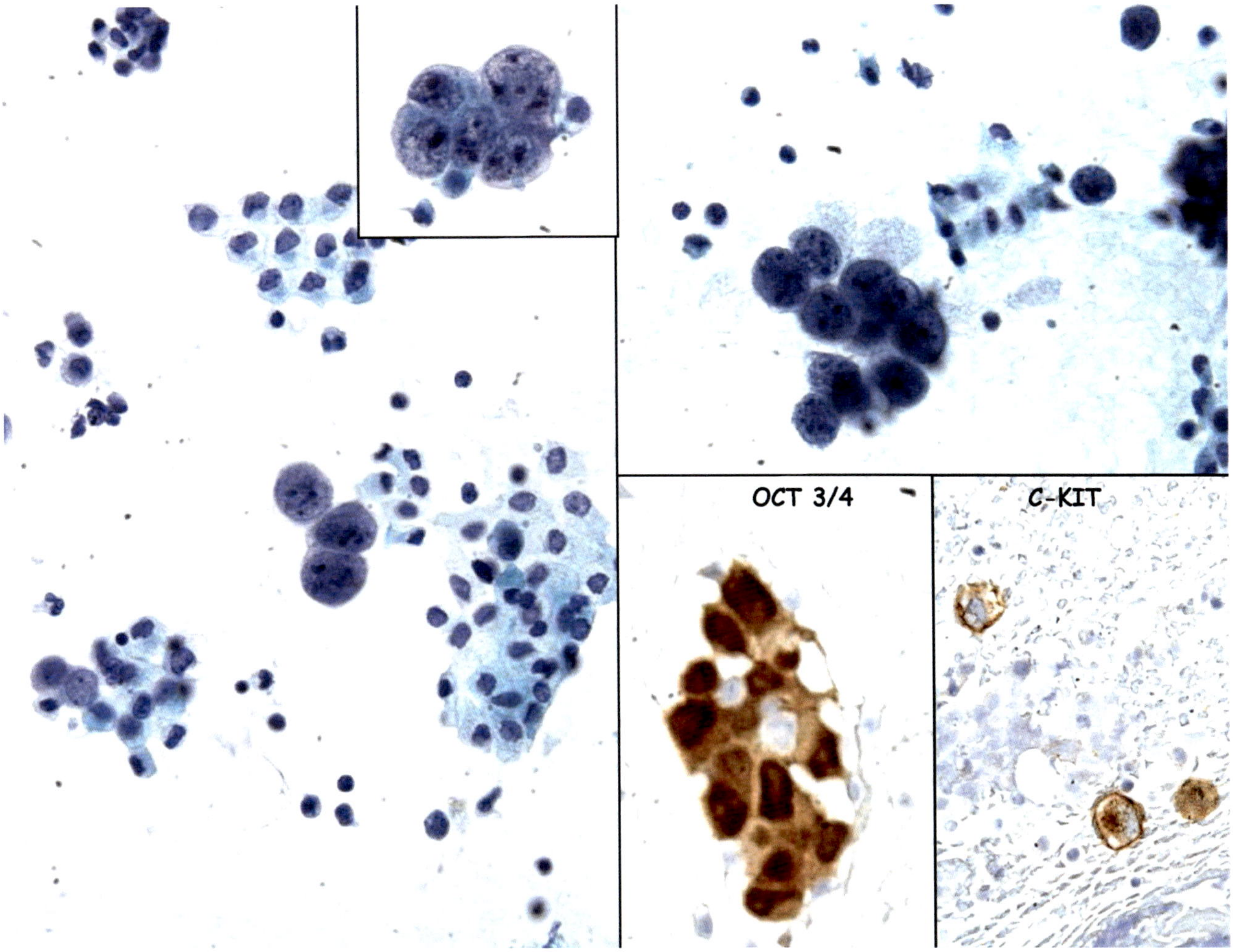

Fig. 2.34

Q-34. A 22-year-old female with an ovarian mass. During her surgery, pelvic washing was performed. What is the diagnosis of this cytological specimen?
(a) Metastatic adenocarcinoma of the colon
(b) Metastatic dysgerminoma
(c) Reactive mesothelial cells
(d) Metastatic serous carcinoma of the ovary

Fig. 2.35

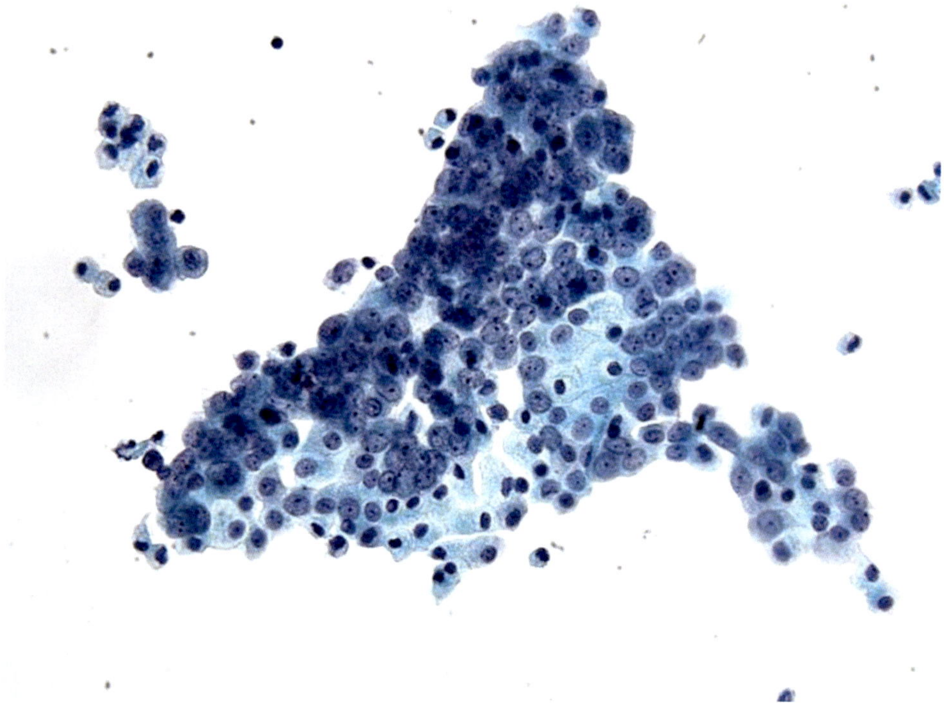

Q-35. Surgical peritoneal washing was performed. What is the diagnosis of this cytological specimen?
(a) Metastatic adenocarcinoma of the colon
(b) Mesothelioma
(c) Reactive mesothelial cells
(d) Metastatic serous carcinoma of the ovary

Fig. 2.36

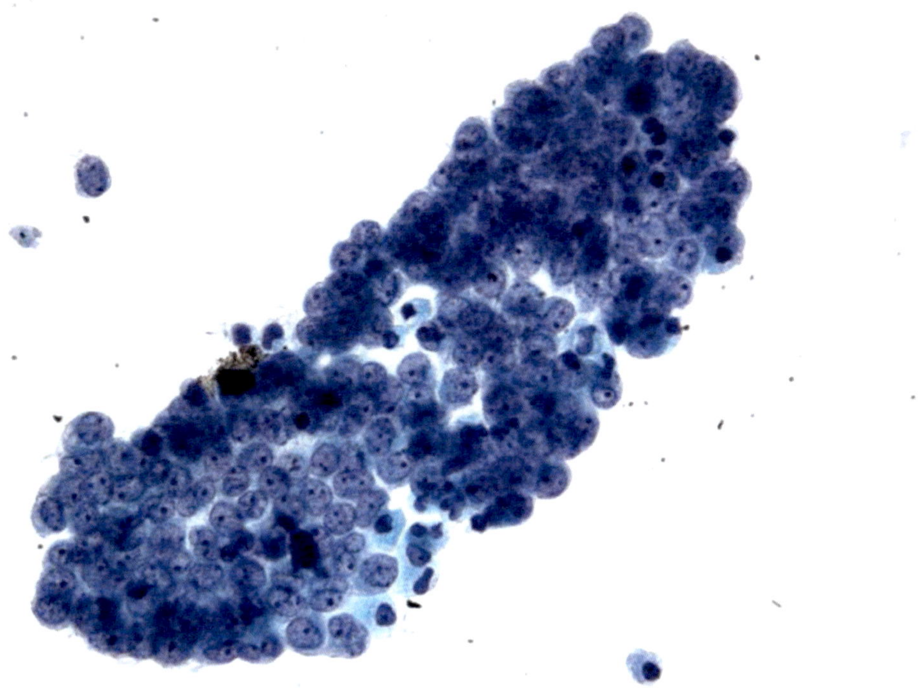

Q-36. Surgical peritoneal washing was performed. What is the diagnosis of this cytological specimen?
(a) Metastatic adenocarcinoma of the colon
(b) Mesothelioma
(c) Reactive mesothelial cells
(d) Metastatic serous carcinoma of the ovary

Fig. 2.37

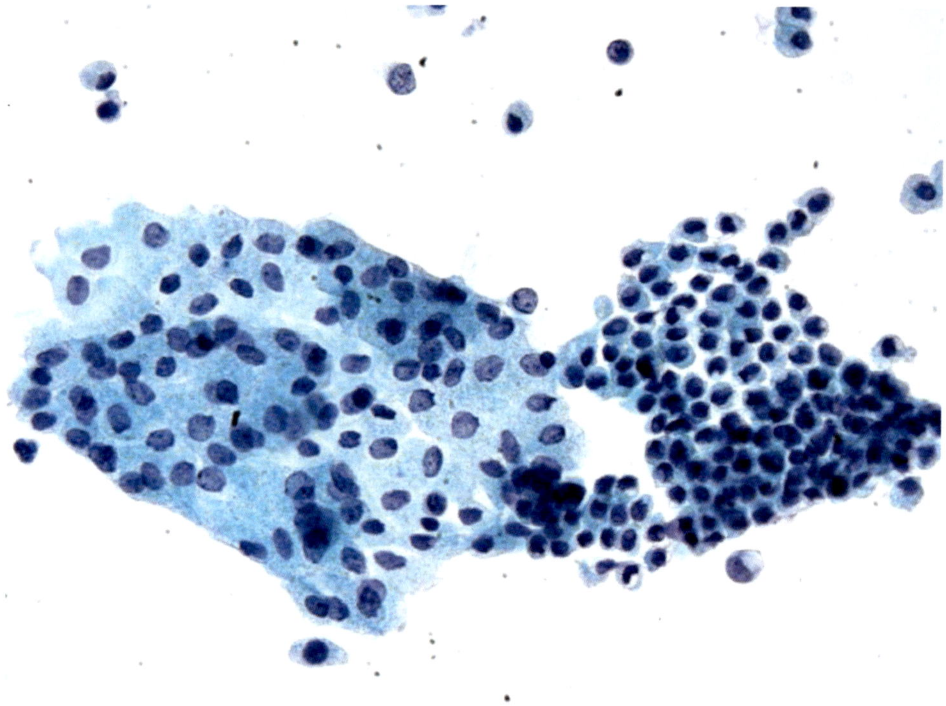

Q-37. Surgical peritoneal washing was performed. What is the diagnosis of this cytological specimen?
(a) Metastatic adenocarcinoma of the colon
(b) Reactive mesothelial cells
(c) Mesothelioma
(d) Metastatic serous carcinoma of the ovary

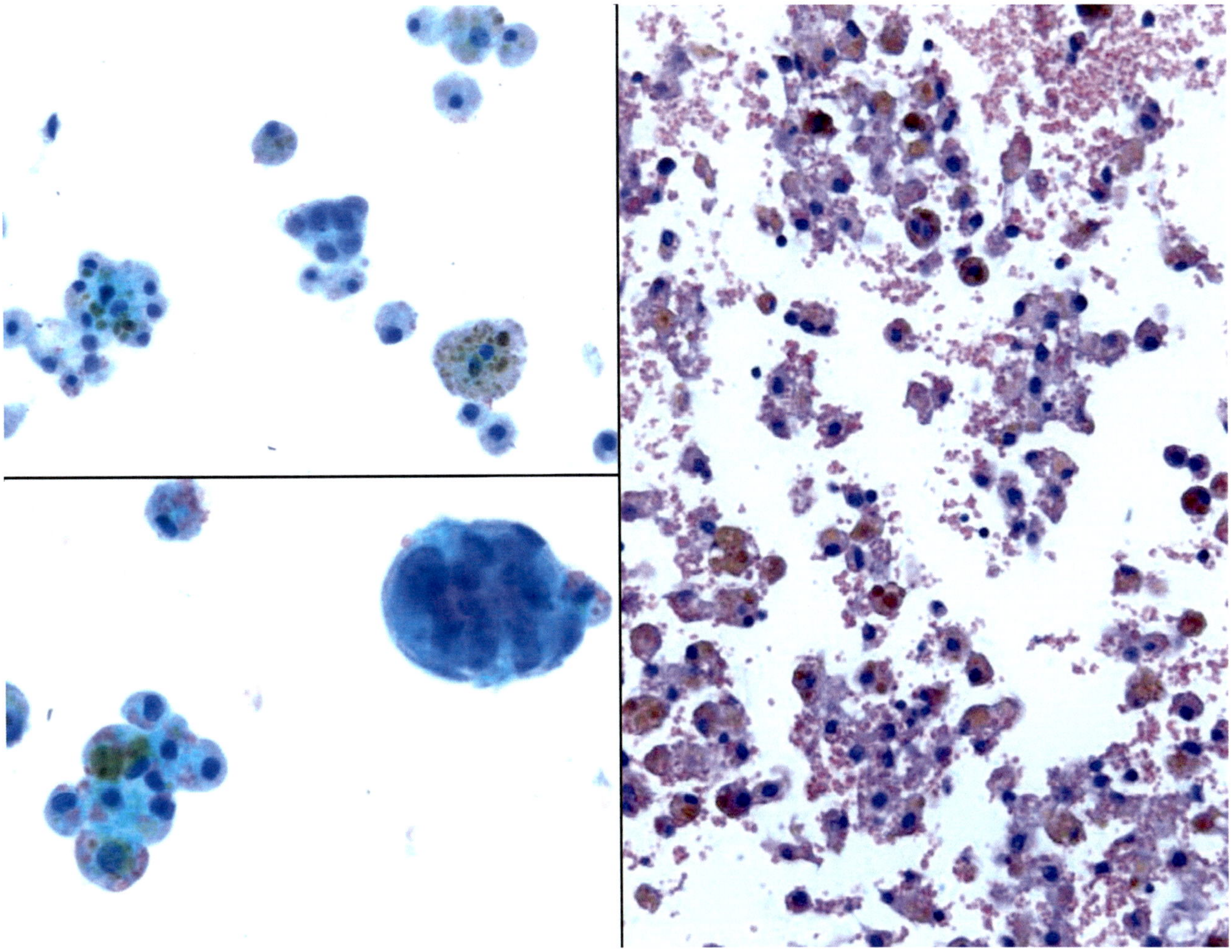

Fig. 2.38

Q-38. A 35-year-old with an ovarian mass had a surgical resection of the lesion. Pelvic washing was performed during the procedure. The resected lesion reveals a hemorrhagic cyst. What is the diagnosis of this pelvic washing specimen?

(a) Metastatic adenocarcinoma of the colon
(b) Reactive mesothelial cells
(c) Endometriosis
(d) Metastatic serous carcinoma of the ovary

Fig. 2.39

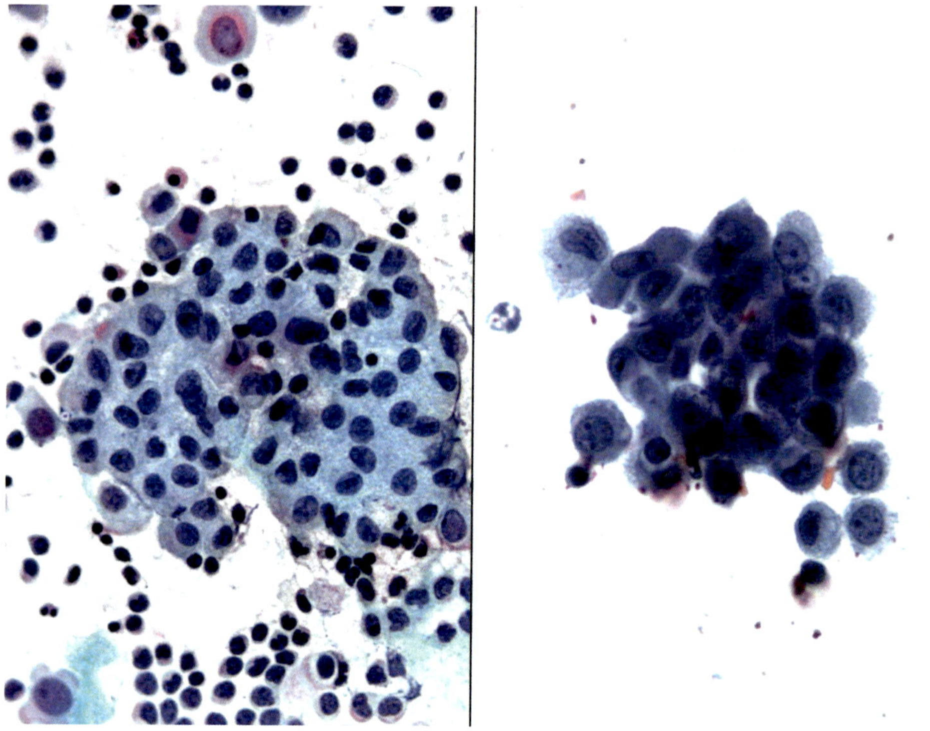

Q-39. Surgical peritoneal washing was performed. What is the diagnosis of this cytological specimen?
(a) Metastatic adenocarcinoma
(b) Reactive mesothelial cells
(c) Mesothelioma
(d) Metastatic serous carcinoma of the ovary

Fig. 2.40

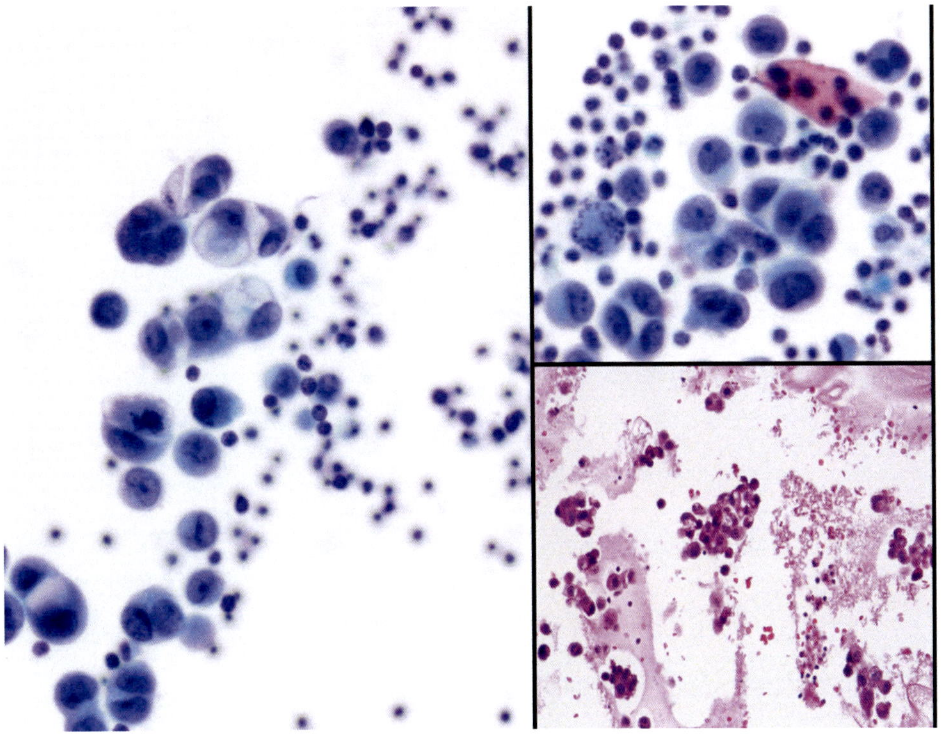

Q-40. An 87-year-old female nonsmoker with a lung mass develops a pleural effusion. What is the diagnosis of this cytological specimen?
(a) Metastatic adenocarcinoma of the lung
(b) Reactive mesothelial cells
(c) Metastatic melanoma
(d) Metastatic squamous cell carcinoma

Fig. 2.41

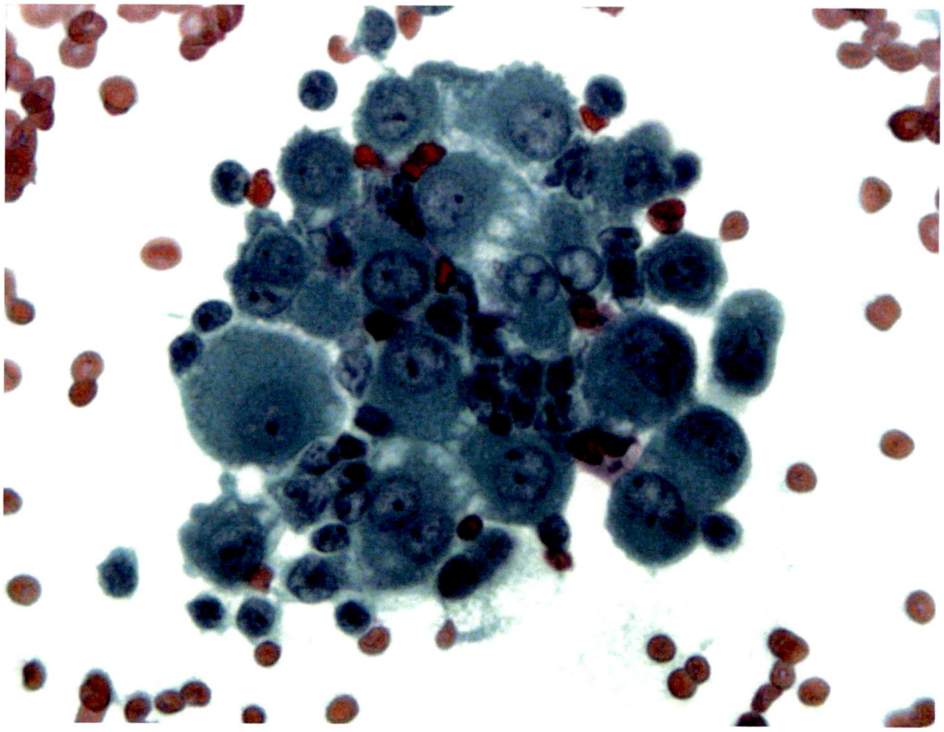

Q-41. What is the diagnosis of this pleural effusion specimen?
(a) Metastatic adenocarcinoma
(b) Reactive mesothelial cells
(c) Mesothelioma
(d) Metastatic serous carcinoma of the ovary

Fig. 2.42

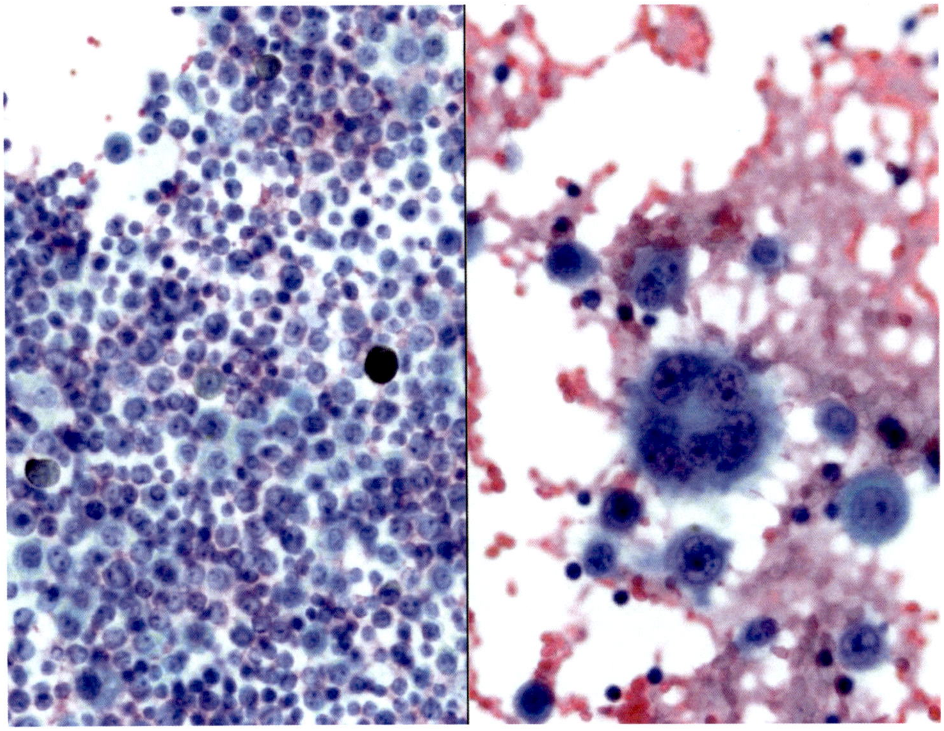

Q-42. Which one of the following diagnoses is correct?
(a) Metastatic poorly differentiated adenocarcinoma of the lung
(b) Metastatic small cell lung carcinoma
(c) Metastatic melanoma
(d) Lymphoma

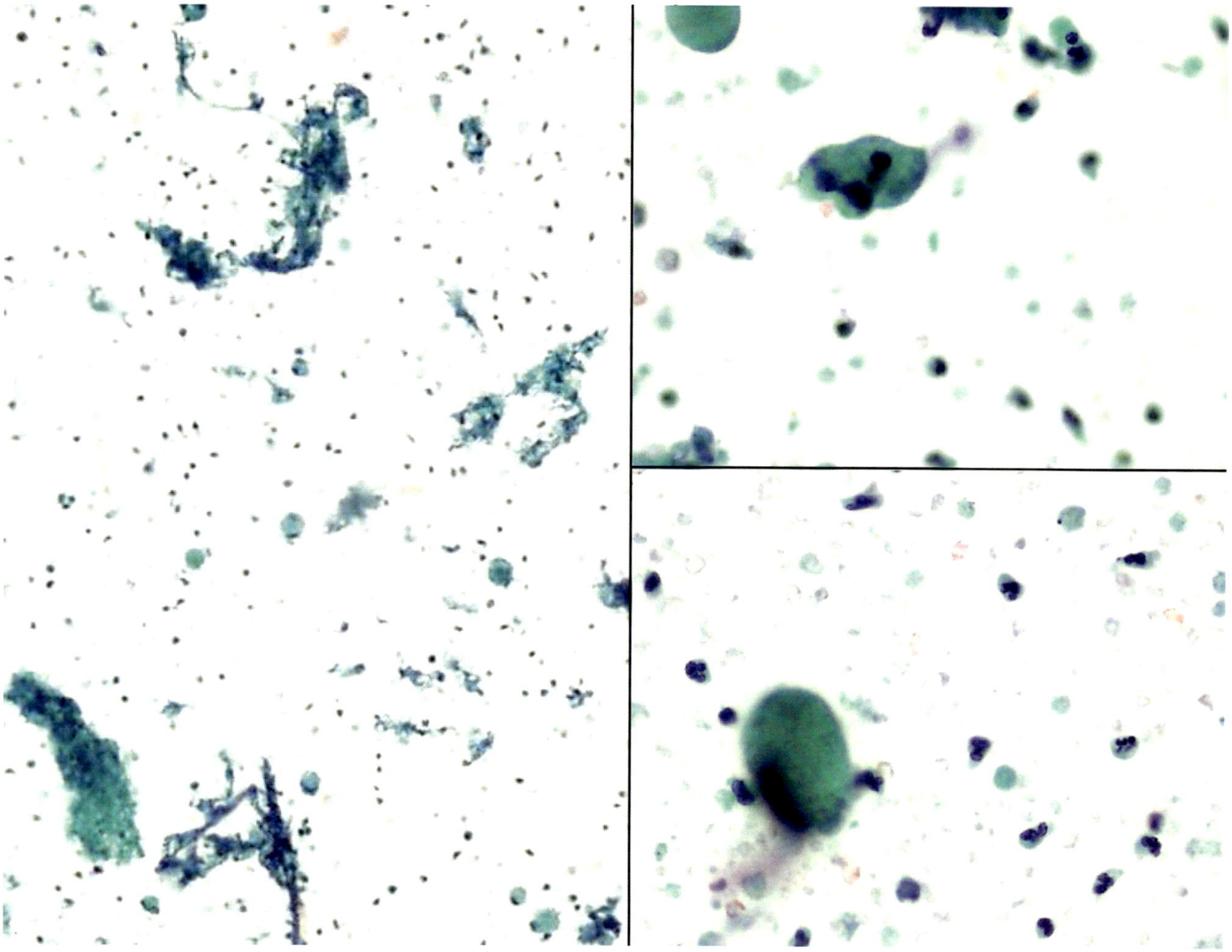

Fig. 2.43

Q-43. Pleural effusion was found in a patient with rheumatoid arthritis. What is the diagnosis of this pleural effusion?
(a) Rheumatoid pleuritis
(b) Reactive mesothelial cells
(c) Lymphocytosis
(d) Lymphoma

Fig. 2.44

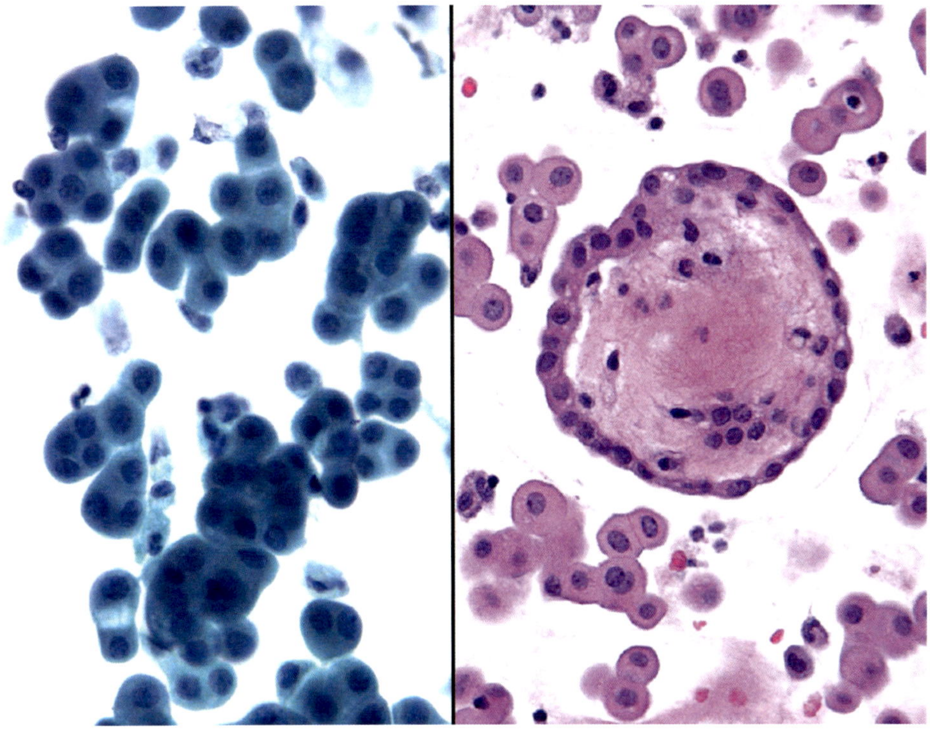

Q-44. What is the diagnosis of this cytological specimen?
(a) Metastatic adenocarcinoma
(b) Mesothelioma
(c) Reactive mesothelial cells
(d) Metastatic serous carcinoma of the ovary

Fig. 2.45

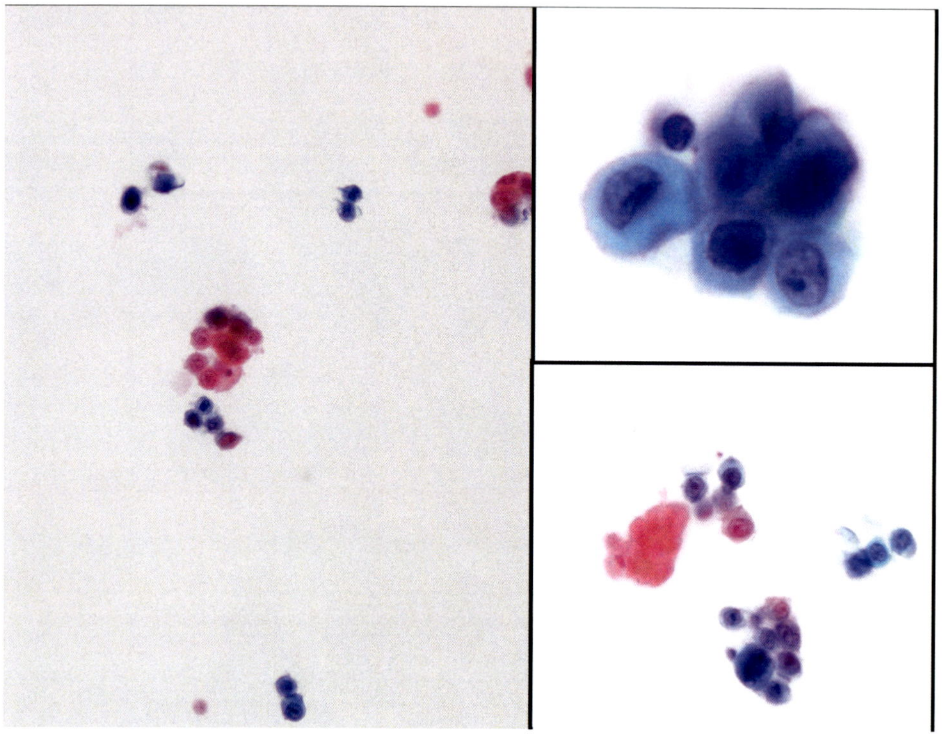

Q-45. What is the diagnosis of this pleural effusion specimen?
(a) Metastatic adenocarcinoma
(b) Mesothelioma
(c) Reactive mesothelial cells
(d) Metastatic squamous cell carcinoma

Fig. 2.46

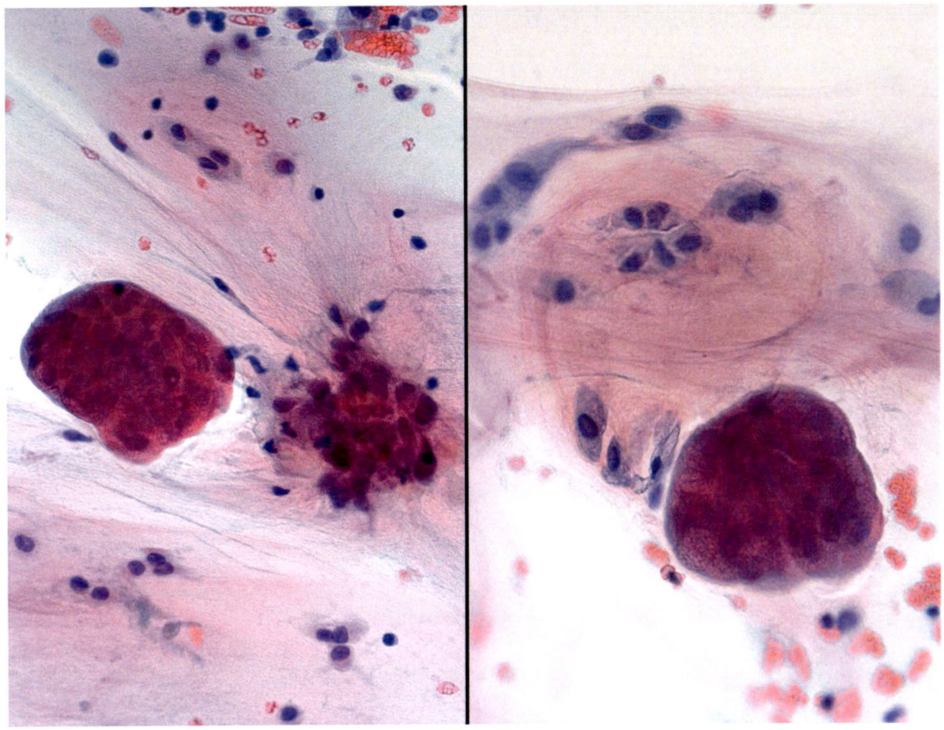

Q-46. A paracentesis was performed in a 46-year-old female patient with abdominal pain and distension. What is the diagnosis of cytological findings?

(a) Metastatic adenocarcinoma
(b) Mesothelioma
(c) Reactive mesothelial cells
(d) Pseudomyxoma peritonei

Fig. 2.47

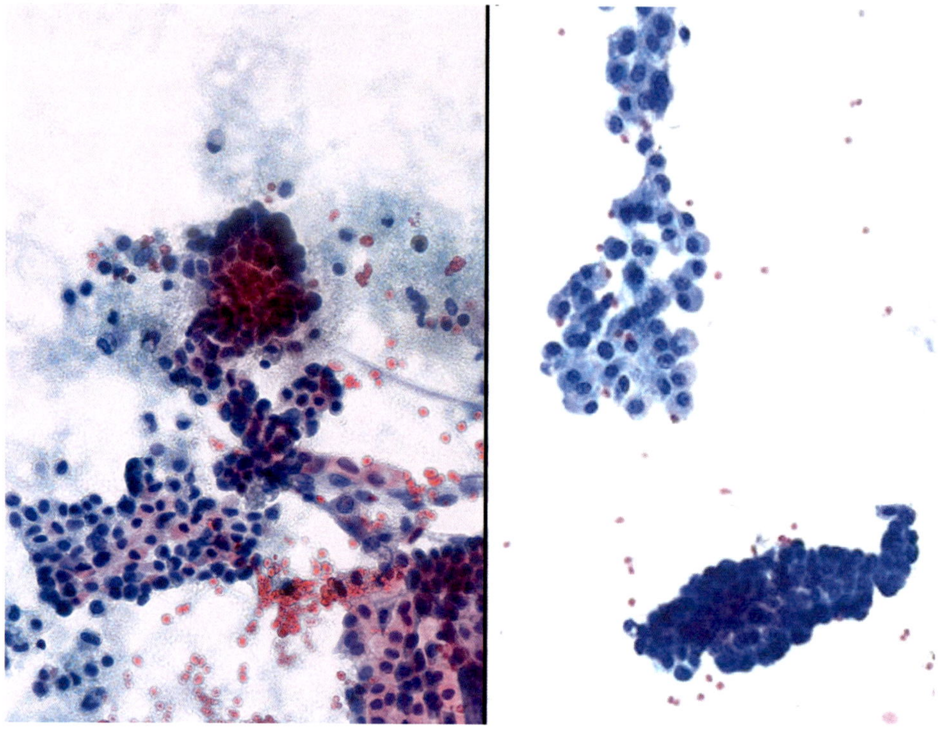

Q-47. What is the diagnosis of this pleural effusion specimen?

(a) Metastatic adenocarcinoma
(b) Reactive mesothelial cells
(c) Mesothelioma
(d) Metastatic serous carcinoma of the ovary

Fig. 2.48

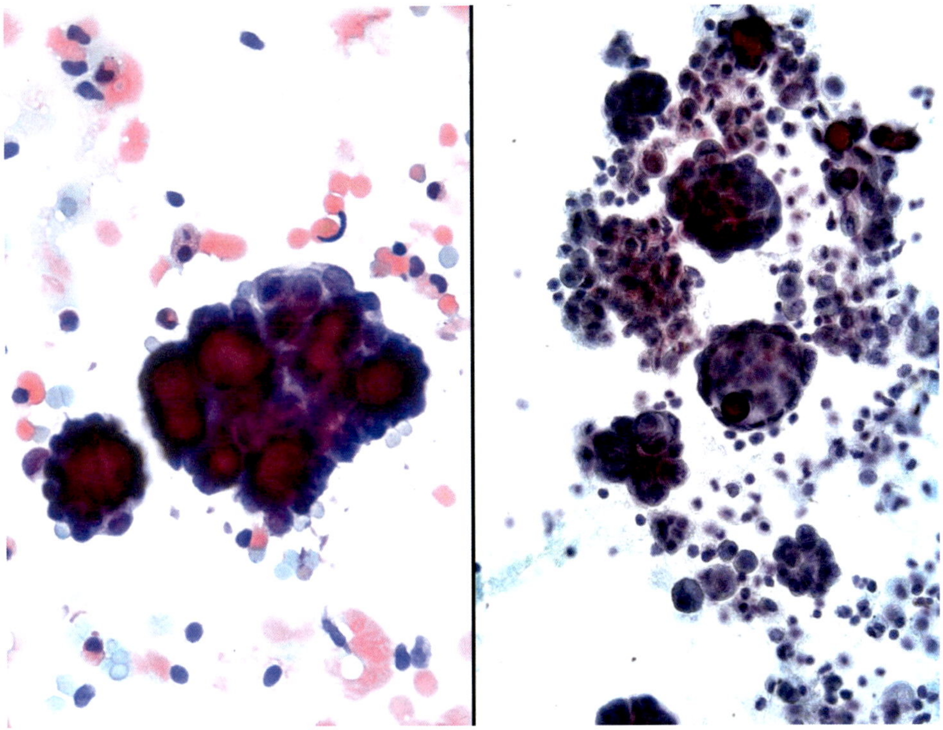

Q-48. In this ascites specimen, what is the correct diagnosis?
(a) Metastatic serous carcinoma
(b) Mesothelial cell hyperplasia
(c) Endosalpingiosis
(d) Metastatic squamous cell carcinoma

Fig. 2.49

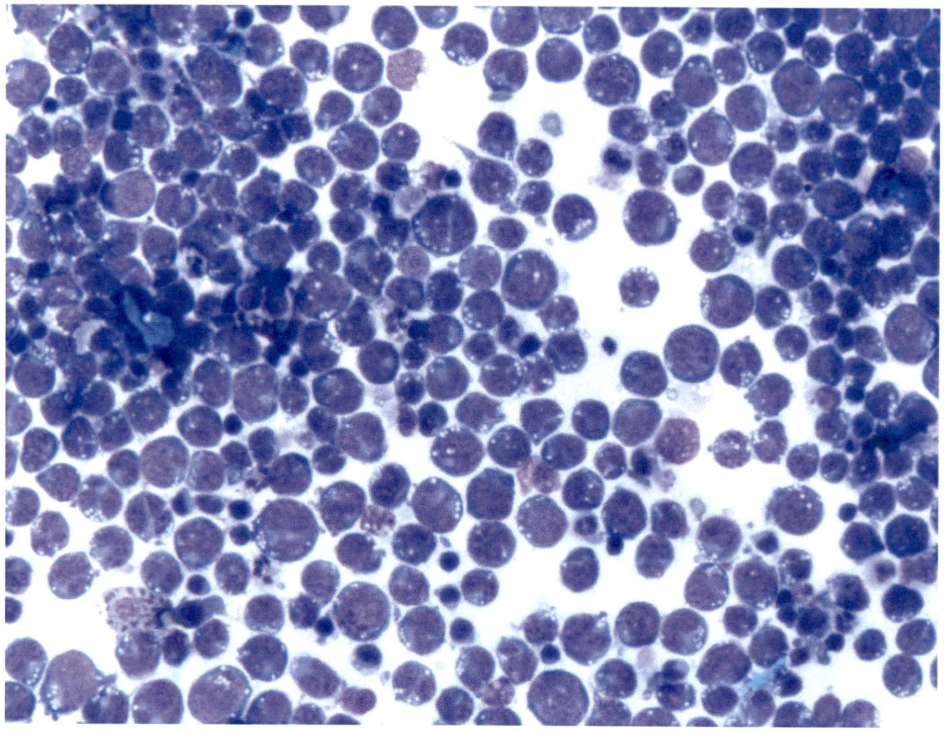

Q-49. What is the diagnosis of this pleural effusion from a 66-year-old male with HIV infection?
(a) Diffuse large B cell lymphoma
(b) Hodgkin lymphoma
(c) Burkitt lymphoma
(d) Lymphocytic pleural effusion

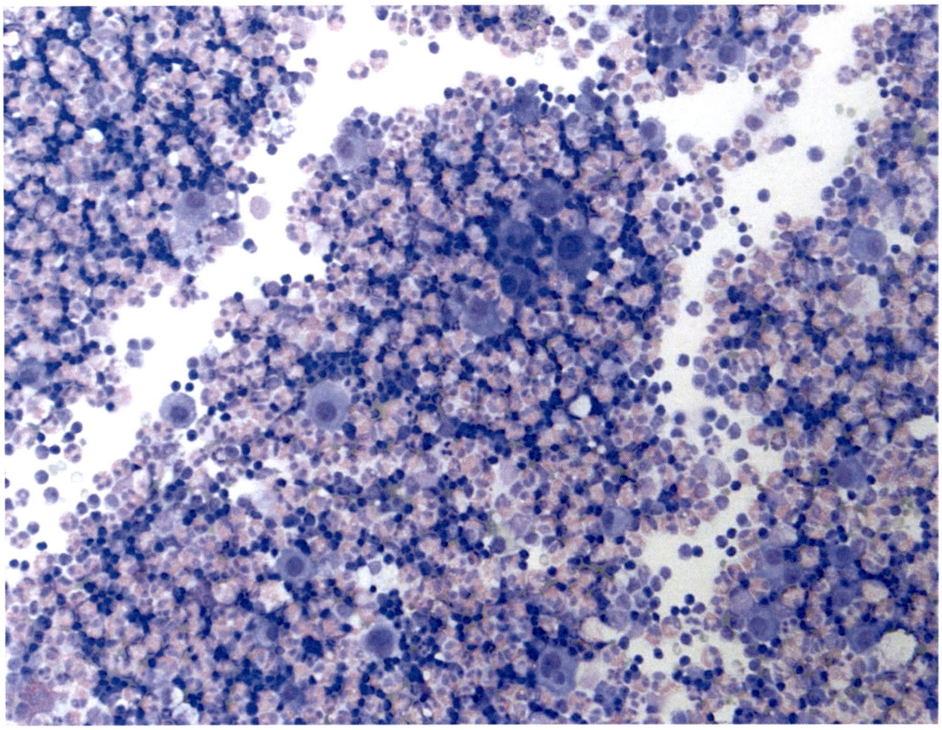

Fig. 2.50

Q-50. What is the correct diagnosis of this pleural effusion?
(a) Diffuse large B cell lymphoma
(b) Hodgkin lymphoma
(c) Eosinophilic pleural effusion
(d) Lymphocytic pleural effusion

2.2 Text-Based Questions 51–100

Q-51. In a pleural effusion, all of the following features are seen in reactive mesothelial cells, except:
(a) Scattered individual "atypical" mesothelial cells
(b) A spectrum of cellular changes, ranging from "normal" to "atypical" mesothelial cells
(c) Variation in nuclear size, binucleation, and multinucleation
(d) Numerous large three-dimensional cellular clusters

Q-52. Which panel of immunohistochemical markers is the most useful in the differential diagnosis of mesothelioma from a metastatic adenocarcinoma of the lung?
(a) AE1/AE3, CK7, TTF1, calretinin, Ki67, WT1, and P53
(b) BerEP4, Napsin A, TTF1, calretinin, WT1, and P53
(c) AE1/AE3, CK7, CK20, TTF1, calretinin, and Ki67
(d) BerEP4, Napsin A, TTF1, calretinin, and Ki67

Q-53. Which one of the following is the most useful feature for separating reactive mesothelial cells (reactive atypia) from a well-differentiated lung adenocarcinoma?
(a) Two- or three-dimensional clusters of cells with nuclear variations
(b) "Window" between atypical cells
(c) Normal to low N/C ratio
(d) Binucleation and/or multinucleation

Q-54. An ultrasound-guided thoracentesis was performed on a 65-year-old male smoker who has a right pleural effusion and a right lower pleura-based mass. The cytospin smear reveals numerous large clusters of epithelioid cells with well-defined cell borders, large nuclei and prominent nucleoli, and intercellular "windows." What is the most likely diagnosis?
(a) Reactive mesothelial cells
(b) Well-differentiated adenocarcinoma of the lung
(c) Poorly differentiated carcinoma
(d) Mesothelioma

Q-55. All of the following features can be seen in a squamous cell carcinoma, except:
(a) Smudgy chromatin
(b) Dense cytoplasm
(c) Prominent nucleoli
(d) Shared cell borders

Q-56. Radiation- and chemotherapy-induced mesothelial changes include all of the following, except:
(a) Cytomegaly with proportionate nuclear enlargement
(b) Multinucleation and a vesicular chromatin pattern
(c) Prominent nucleoli
(d) Hyperchromatic nucleoli and clumped chromatin

Q-57. A 60-year-old male patient presents with left pleural effusion. An ultrasound-guided thoracentesis was performed. On cytology smear and cell block section, lymphoid population and rare mesothelial cells were identified. Which of the following features is considered an "abnormal" lymphoid population?
(a) Polymorphous population of lymphocytes
(b) "Lacunar" space on cell block section
(c) Monomorphous population of lymphocytes
(d) Lymphoglandular bodies

Q-58. On a scant effusion specimen, which of the following tumors is most likely to be mistaken for "reactive mesothelial cells"?
(a) Adenocarcinoma with lepidic growth pattern (bronchoalveolar carcinoma)
(b) Poorly differentiated squamous cell carcinoma
(c) Basaloid carcinoma
(d) Small cell carcinoma

Q-59. The differential diagnosis of eosinophils in pleural effusion (eosinophilic pleural effusion) includes all of the following, except:
(a) Repeat tap (thoracentesis)
(b) Renal transplantation
(c) Mesothelioma
(d) Tuberculosis

Q-60. Fluid cytology is more sensitive than a "blind" serosal biopsy for the detection of serosal malignancy.
(a) True
(b) False

Q-11. The most common cause of eosinophilic pleural effusion is:
(a) Blood in the pleural space (hemothorax)
(b) Lung cancers
(c) Air in the pleural space (pneumothorax)
(d) Tuberculosis

Q-62. Which of the following irritation/trauma induces a rapid development of eosinophilic pleural effusion in hours?
(a) Blood in the pleural space (hemothorax)
(b) Air in the pleural space (pneumothorax)
(c) Pleural biopsy
(d) Repeat thoracentesis

Q-63. The most common cause of eosinophilic ascites is:
(a) Metastatic colon cancers
(b) Metastatic lung cancers
(c) Blood in the peritoneal space
(d) Cirrhosis

Q-64. Metastatic squamous cell carcinomas in the fluid cytology can be distinguished from metastatic adenocarcinomas based on the presence of the following features, except:
(a) Keratinization
(b) Mucin production (cytoplasmic mucin)
(c) Pseudoacinar arrangement of tumor cells
(d) Prominent nucleoli

Q-65. A thoracentesis was performed on a 65-year-old male smoker who presented with a right upper lobe infiltration and pleural effusion. On the cytological preparation, large sheets and tight clusters of atypical epithelioid cells are identified; some of them have "signet ring" cell features. The differential diagnoses include:
(a) Metastatic adenocarcinoma of the lung
(b) Reactive mesothelial cell hyperplasia
(c) A metastatic adenocarcinoma from the stomach
(d) All of the above

Q-66. Cytological features of so-called neuroendocrine tumors may include all of the following, except:
(a) Fine chromatin pattern (so-called "salt-and-pepper" pattern)
(b) Inconspicuous or small nucleoli
(c) Scant cytoplasm
(d) Nuclear grooves

Q-67. Which type of mucin is commonly seen in mesothelioma?
(a) Neutral
(b) Acid (simple or non-sulfated
(c) Acid (simple, mesenchymal)
(d) Acid (complex or sulfated, epithelial)

Q-68. Which type of mucin stain is more specific to demonstrate mucopolysaccharide substances in tissues (i.e., mucin in adenocarcinoma)?
(a) Colloidal iron
(b) Alcian blue
(c) PAS (Periodic acid–Schiff)
(d) Mucicarmine

Q-69. A cytological smear of ascites reveals numerous two-dimensional clusters and/or sheets of spindle cells; the differential diagnosis of the lesion includes all of the following, except:
(a) Spindle cell carcinoma
(b) Sarcomatoid mesothelioma
(c) Metastatic melanoma
(d) Poorly differentiated adenocarcinoma

Q-70. Which feature is not seen in a small cell carcinoma?
(a) Paranuclear blue bodies in the cytoplasm
(b) The size of tumor cells are two- to threefold of mature lymphocytes
(c) Abundant cytoplasm
(d) Nuclear crowding and molding

Q-71. Which of the following cytological features is helpful in the differential diagnosis of large cell neuroendocrine tumor from a poorly differentiated adenocarcinoma in a pleural effusion specimen?
(a) Fine (salt-and-pepper) chromatin pattern
(b) Three-dimensional and/or pseudoacinar arrangements of tumor cells
(c) Lacy cytoplasm with vacuolization
(d) Dispersed tumor cells with markedly atypia and enlargement

Q-72. A 50-year-old female developed chronic cough and shortness of breath. The chest x-ray showed bilateral small opaque infiltrates and left pleural effusion. The ultrasound-guided thoracentesis was performed. A large amount of fluid is obtained. The initial evaluation of the specimen revealed scattered clusters of atypical epithelioid cells, and a metastatic adenocarcinoma was suspected. What is the next step of action?
(a) Repeat thoracentesis in few weeks
(b) Make cell block as usual
(c) Core biopsy the lung lesions
(d) Do nothing

Q-73. An HIV-positive patient developed pleural and pericardial effusion. The cytological preparation of the effusion reveals numerous atypical lymphoid cells. A primary effusion lymphoma is suspected. Which of the following cytological features can be seen in primary effusion lymphoma?

(a) Individual large lymphocyte with enlarged round nuclei
(b) Coarse chromatin and prominent nucleoli
(c) Abundant basophilic cytoplasm on the Diff-Quik stain
(d) All of the above

Q-74. In a malignant ascites specimen, tumor cells were found to have "intranuclear inclusions." Which one of the following tumors is the more likely to have an "intranuclear inclusion" in a fluid cytology?
(a) Renal cell carcinoma
(b) Urothelial cell carcinoma
(c) Colonic adenocarcinoma
(d) Hepatocellular carcinoma

Q-75. A stage 3 lung cancer patient developed a pleural effusion. A thoracentesis was performed, and the cytological examination confirmed the diagnosis of metastatic adenocarcinoma of the lung. The oncologist asked you to send specimen for molecular studies of *EGFR* and *KRAS* mutations. What is the next step of action?
(a) Tell the clinician to obtain tumor tissue from primary tumor.
(b) Biopsy specimen is needed for molecular studies.
(c) Prepare cell blocks and make sure that they have adequate tumor cells.
(d) It is not necessary to do molecular study on metastatic lung adenocarcinoma.

Q-76. In cytological preparation from ascites, the finding of psammoma bodies is suggestive of which of the following diagnoses?
(a) Ovarian carcinoma
(b) Mesothelial cell hyperplasia
(c) Endosalpingiosis
(d) All of the above

Q-77. Which of the features is not seen in a metastatic squamous cell carcinoma in fluid specimens?
(a) Large nuclei with smudgy chromatin
(b) Nuclei with variation in size and shape
(c) Pyknotic nuclei
(d) Cytokeratin formation

Q-78. An HIV-positive patient developed a lymphomatous effusion. The differential diagnosis should include all of the following, except:
(a) Burkitt's or Burkitt's-like lymphoma (BL)
(b) Diffuse large B-cell lymphoma (DLBCL)
(c) Peripheral T-cell non-Hodgkin lymphoma (NHL)
(d) Primary effusion lymphoma (PEL)

Q-79. A paracentesis was performed on a patient with ascites. On the cell block preparation, it revealed three-dimensional clusters of tall columnar cells with hyperchromatic nuclei, coarse chromatin, prominent nucleoli, irregular nuclear membrane, and feathering cytoplasm. Which one is the most likely primary site of the tumor?
(a) Breast
(b) Lung
(c) Colon
(d) Renal

Q-80. Which of the following cytological features is most useful in the separation of a poorly differentiated adenocarcinoma from a small cell carcinoma in fluid cytology specimen?
(a) Prominent nucleoli
(b) Fine or coarse chromatin pattern
(c) Tumor necrosis
(d) Organoid and/or rosette arrangement of tumor cells

Q-81. A patient who had malignant history of desmoplastic/spindle cell melanoma developed ascites. In cytological preparations, scattered "atypical spindle cells" were identified. Which of the following options is the best one in the differential diagnosis of a metastatic desmoplastic/spindle cell melanoma?
(a) Using unstained slides to perform IHC markers S100, HMB45, and melanin A
(b) Making cell block to perform IHC markers S100, HMB45, and melanin A
(c) Making cell block to perform IHC marker of melanin A only
(d) Making cell block to perform IHC marker of S100 only

Q-82. A female patient with a breast mass developed a pleural effusion. All of the following features can be seen in a metastatic breast carcinoma, except:
(a) Prominent nucleoli
(b) Intracytoplasmic lumina (magenta body)
(c) Three-dimensional cell clusters
(d) Naked nuclei

Q-83. On a cell block preparation, which one of the following positive stains indicates a mesothelioma, but not a metastatic adenocarcinoma of the lung?
(a) Mucicarmine
(b) Periodic acid–Schiff (PAS)
(c) Hyaluronic acid–alcian blue
(d) Cytokeratin

Q-84. In a cytological preparation of a pleural effusion from a patient who has breast cancer, the diagnosis of metastatic breast carcinoma is made. The characteristic cytological features include all of the following, except:
- (a) Hyperchromatic nuclei and prominent nucleoli
- (b) Intranuclear inclusion
- (c) Three-dimensional cell clusters with smooth border
- (d) Bipolar nuclei

Q-85. A fluid cytological preparation characteristic of a metastatic small cell carcinoma includes all of the following, except:
- (a) Hyperchromatic nuclei and prominent nucleoli
- (b) Scant cytoplasm
- (c) Three-dimensional cell clusters with nuclear molding
- (d) Individual tumor cells with fine chromatin

Q-86. In a fluid cytological preparation, the differential diagnosis of lymphocytic effusion includes which of the following?
- (a) Tuberculosis
- (b) Metastatic carcinoma
- (c) Small lymphocytic lymphoma/chronic lymphocytic leukemia
- (d) All of the above

Q-87. In a fluid cytological preparation, characteristics of a metastatic small cell carcinoma were found. Which of the following IHC markers has better sensitivity for detection of small cell carcinomas?
- (a) TTF1
- (b) Synaptophysin
- (c) Chromogranin A
- (d) CD56

Q-88. TTF1 is always positive in small cell lung carcinomas (SCLCs). It can be used to distinguish the origin of the tumor, i.e., pulmonary versus extrapulmonary origin. True or false?
- (a) True
- (b) False

Q-89. Which of the following tumors has a weak punctate ("dotlike") labeling for cytokeratins, including AE1/AE3 and CAM 5.2?
- (a) Lung adenocarcinoma
- (b) Small cell lung carcinoma
- (c) Metastatic colonic adenocarcinoma to the lung
- (d) Prostate adenocarcinoma

Q-90. The patient with a mediastinal mass has presented with a left pleural effusion. On the cytospin, the specimen reveals "atypical small blue cells." The main differentiation diagnosis of the pleural effusion is small cell lung carcinoma versus lymphoma. Of the following tests/markers, which one is the most useful for the differential diagnosis?
- (a) Immunostains of TTF1 and BerEP4
- (b) Immunostains of AE1/AE3 and TTF1
- (c) Immunostains of CD20 and CD5
- (d) Immunostains of synaptophysin, chromogranin, CD56, and CD45

Q-91. A fluid cytological preparation characteristic of "benign" nuclear enlargements and/or reactive nuclear changes in mesothelial cells includes all of the following, except:
- (a) Large nuclei in a cell with normal N/C ratio
- (b) Irregular nuclear membrane and hyperchromasia
- (c) Two-dimensional cell clusters with intercellular "window"
- (d) Prominent nucleoli

Q-92. Which one of the following procedures has the highest sensitivity in the diagnosis of malignant pleural lesions as well as malignant effusion?
- (a) Thoracentesis
- (b) CT-guided transthoracic needle biopsy
- (c) "Blind" transthoracic needle biopsy
- (d) Ultrasound-guided transthoracic needle biopsy

Q-93. In a patient with pleural effusion, a cytological specimen is routinely obtained by thoracentesis or ultrasound- and/or CT-guided thoracentesis. Which one of the procedures has the highest specificity in the diagnosis of malignant pleural effusion?
- (a) Thoracentesis
- (b) CT-guided transthoracic thoracentesis
- (c) "Blind" transthoracic needle biopsy
- (d) Ultrasound-guided thoracentesis

Q-94. In a malignant fluid specimen, the appearance of two- and three-dimensional tumor cell clusters is only seen in adenocarcinomas but not in squamous cell carcinomas. True or false?
- (a) True
- (b) False

Q-95. Pleural effusion was found in a patient with rheumatoid arthritis. The diagnostic features of rheumatoid pleuritis include:
- (a) Multinucleated giant cells
- (b) Characteristic "granular" debris

(c) Scattered lymphocytes
(d) All of the above

Q-96. Which type of cells is usually not present in a rheumatoid pleuritis?
(a) Multinucleated giant cells
(b) Lymphocytes
(c) Mesothelial cells
(d) Clusters of histiocytes

Q-97. Charcot–Leyden crystals can be found in:
(a) Asthma
(b) Eosinophilic effusion
(c) Allergic sinusitis
(d) All of the above

Q-98. All of these statements/descriptions of the lupus erythematosus (LE) cell are correct in lupus pleuritis, except:
(a) The characteristic cell is the lupus erythematosus (LE) cells.
(b) LE cells contain denatured nuclear material with a glassy and homogeneous appearance.
(c) LE cells can be identified in the majority of lupus pleuritis patients.
(d) LE cells contain nuclear material with visible chromatin structures, such as coarse chromatin granules.

Q-99. In a fluid specimen, which one of the following features is indicative of a malignant effusion?
(a) Numerous large clusters of cells
(b) Lacunae spaces on cell block preparation
(c) Presence of "second population" cells
(d) All of the above

Q-100. The finding of clear spaces (lacunae) either around individual cells or around clusters of cells is characteristic of malignant effusion. True or false?
(a) True
(b) False

2.3 Answers and Discussion of Image-Based Questions 1–50

A-1. **(c) Collagen ball**

The finding of a collagen ball in peritoneal washing specimens is not uncommon. Collagen balls are composed of collagen which is covered with a thin layer of benign mesothelial cells. One study has shown that collagen balls were found in 1.6 % of peritoneal washings and 5.8 % of pelvic washings, respectively. Collagen balls are a nonspecific finding and most probably originate on the surface of the ovary. It can be found in benign conditions and/or from detached fragments of a papillary ovarian neoplasm. Common differential diagnoses of collagen balls include metastatic mucinous adenocarcinomas, papillary serous carcinomas of the ovary, and mesotheliomas. In all these malignant lesions, tumor cells reveal high N/C ratio, hyperchromatic nuclei, irregular nuclear membrane, and prominent nucleoli.

A-2. **(a) Lupus erythematosus (LE) cells**

The lupus erythematosus (LE) cell is a neutrophil or macrophage that has phagocytized (engulfed) the denatured nuclear material (hematoxylin body) of another cell. Denatured nuclear material in the neutrophil/macrophage has a glassy and homogeneous appearance; it may push the nuclei to the peripheral location. In contrast, tart cells contain ingested nuclei with a visible chromatin rather than homogeneous appearance. Reactive mesothelial cells have "windows" between cells, and mucin-producing cells, such as a mucin-producing adenocarcinoma, have cytoplasmic vacuole and lacy cytoplasm.

A-3. **(d) Metastatic breast lobular carcinoma**

The diagnosis of this pericardial effusion is metastatic breast carcinoma. In fluid preparation, metastatic breast carcinoma may reveal several patterns. Tumor cells of metastatic ductal carcinoma may form three-dimensional "cannon ball" clusters. In cases of poorly differentiated (high-grade) ductal carcinomas, specimens consist of predominantly dispersed individual cells, whereas in metastatic lobular carcinomas, tumor cells are predominantly presented as dispersed individual cells. The size of tumor cells is relatively smaller than metastatic adenocarcinomas from the lung and/or GI tract. The presence of intracytoplasmic lumina, so-called magenta bodies, is also one of the characteristics of a metastatic breast carcinoma. In metastatic adenocarcinomas of the lung, columnar tumor cells are arranged in three-dimensional or acinar/papillae clusters, with high N/C ratio, prominent nucleoli, lacy cytoplasm, and cytoplasmic vacuolization. The size of tumor cells is larger than those in breast carcinomas. Reactive mesothelial cells have "windows" between cells. Metastatic melanomas reveal dispersed large tumor cells with prominent nucleoli, binucleation, and cytoplasmic melanin pigments.

A-4. **(c) Ewing's sarcoma**

Ewing's sarcoma is a malignant small, round, blue cell tumor. It predominantly involves males and usually presents in childhood or early adulthood, with a peak between 10 and 20 years of age. The tumor can occur anywhere in the body but most commonly in the pelvis and proximal long tubular bones. The cytological preparations reveal dispersed individual small blue cells with two types of tumor cells (tigroid appearance), i.e., tumor cells with pale nuclei and fine chromatin, and degenerated tumor cells with hyperchromatic nuclei and smudged chromatin. Nuclear molding is common. The cytoplasm is scant and with vacuolization. Ewing's sarcoma cells are positive for CD99 and MIC2 and negative for CD45. The most common translocation, present in approximately 90 % of Ewing's sarcoma cases, is t(11;22)(q24;q12). Other translocations are at t(21;22) and t(7;22). The differential diagnosis includes lymphoma, alveolar rhabdomyosarcoma, desmoplastic small round cell tumor, small cell carcinoma, and others.

A-5. **(d) Mesothelioma**

The cytological finding of mesotheliomas reveals numerous three-dimensional clusters with scalloped (knobby) edges, characteristic of mesotheliomas. Tumor cells have round centrally placed nuclei, coarse chromatin, prominent nucleoli, dense cytoplasm with peripheral "halo," and intercellular "windows." Reactive mesothelial cells show a spectrum of changes ranging from normal to markedly atypical cells. In adenocarcinoma and poorly differentiated carcinoma, tumor cells form three-dimensional clusters with smooth edges. They have hyperchromatic nuclei, irregular nuclear membrane, prominent nucleoli, scant cytoplasm, and without intercellular "windows." In addition, immunostains of mesothelial cell markers (calretinin, GLUT-1, D2-40, WT1, P53) and adenocarcinoma markers (TTF, Napsin A, BerEP4, B72.3, CEA, CD15) may be helpful in the differential diagnosis. Metastatic melanomas have large dispersed tumor cells with large nuclei, prominent nucleoli, and cytoplasmic melanin pigments.

A-6. **(d) Metastatic rhabdomyosarcoma**
Rhabdomyosarcoma is commonly seen in children ages one to five and in adolescents. It is also seen in adults but is rare. The most common anatomic locations for the tumor include the head, neck, and genitourinary tract. Several different histological subtypes of rhabdomyosarcoma exist, each of which has different clinical and morphological characteristics. Prognosis and clinical behavior of the tumor also partially depend on histological subtype. The most common subtypes are embryonal rhabdomyosarcoma and alveolar rhabdomyosarcoma. The cytology sample consists predominantly of dispersed cells. The tumor cells are intermediate in size and admixed with scattered large bizarre cells. Tumor cells reveal hyperchromatic nuclei, prominent nucleoli, and dense cytoplasm (indicative of muscle differentiation). MyoD1 and myogenin are positive for tumor cells.

A-7. **(d) Lymphomatous effusion most consistent with malignant lymphoma**
Monomorphous population of lymphocytes is usually seen in lymph proliferative disorders and/or lymphomas, particularly with the presence of apoptosis. It represents a monoclonal proliferation of lymphoma cells. Other cytological features of lymphoma include discohesive tumor cells with hyperchromatic nuclei, clumped (soccer-ball-like) chromatin, irregular nuclear membrane, nucleoli, and scant cytoplasm. In small cell carcinomas, tumor cells form clusters or dispersed individual cells. Nuclear crowding and molding are common. Metastatic poorly differentiated adenocarcinomas reveal clusters of large tumor cells with hyperchromatic nuclei, coarse chromatin, prominent nucleoli, and cytoplasmic vacuoles. Metastatic melanomas reveal dispersed individual large tumor cells with eccentrically located nuclei, prominent nucleoli, and cytoplasmic melanin pigment.

A-8. **(b) Metastatic small cell lung carcinoma**
In small cell carcinomas, tumor cells form two- or three-dimensional clusters or dispersed individual cells and reveal hyperchromatic nuclei, fine granular (salt-and-pepper) chromatin, and scant cytoplasm. In addition, nuclear crowding, molding, apoptotic body, and mitotic figures are common features. The background of the smear may also reveal "blue stripes" (indicative of breakdown of nuclear material). In adenocarcinomas, tumor cells form acini and/or three-dimensional clusters and reveal hyperchromatic nuclei, vesicular or coarse chromatin, prominent nucleoli, and vacuolated cytoplasm (indicative of mucin production). In lymphoma, tumor cells are discohesive with clumped chromatin and scant cytoplasm. Lymphoglandular bodies may be identified in the background of the smear. Metastatic melanoma reveals large discohesive tumor cells with prominent nucleoli and cytoplasmic pigment.

A-9. **(b) Mesothelial cell hyperplasia**
The specimen reveals clusters of reactive mesothelial cells with psammoma bodies. Reactive mesothelial cells may show nuclear atypia; however, the normal or low N/C ratio is usually maintained. The findings of reactive atypia represent a spectrum of cellular changes that range from normal to markedly atypical. Psammoma bodies can be found in both benign and malignant conditions. Reactive mesothelial changes can be caused by a variety of conditions, such as chemotherapy and radiation therapy, inflammation, chronic irritation, and others. In mesothelioma, tumor cells form numerous three-dimensional clusters. An intercellular "window" can be seen in both reactive mesothelial cells and mesothelioma. In ovarian serous carcinomas, tumor cells form three-dimensional or papillary clusters with hyperchromatic nuclei, irregular nuclear membranes, prominent nucleoli, and coarse chromatin. In mesotheliomas, tumor cells form numerous three-dimensional clusters with hyperchromatic nuclei, irregular nuclear membranes, and coarse chromatin.

A-10. **(d) Lymphocytosis (lymphocytic effusion)**
Lymphocytosis (lymphocytic effusion) is the condition in which most of nucleated cells are lymphocytes. It is a nonspecific finding and can be caused by a variety of diseases, such as tuberculosis, infections, lymphoma, and other malignancies. In malignancy, lymphocytic effusion is caused by the obstruction of lymphatic outflow by the tumor or peritumoral lymphocytic reaction. Repeat tap and cytological evaluation may increase the chance of finding tumor cells. In lymphoma, particularly in small lymphocytic lymphoma/chronic lymphocytic leukemia, tumor cells reveal hyperchromatic nuclei with clump chromatin. Flow cytometry and immunostain of B-cell markers may help in the diagnosis. Other causes, such as status postcoronary artery bypass, may also induce a lymphocytic effusion. In benign lymphocytosis, lymphocytes reveal euchromatic nuclei with evenly distributed chromatin and inconspicuous nucleoli.

A-11. **(c) Metastatic melanoma**
In metastatic melanoma, tumor cells are usually arranged in loosely cohesive clusters or dispersed individual cells. Nuclei of tumor cells are eccentrically

located and highly variable in size with finely to coarsely granular chromatin and single prominent cherry-red nucleoli. The cytoplasm tends to be abundant and may or may not contain melanin pigment. The N/C ratio may not be high. Melanin pigment appears coarsely granular and dark brown on the Papanicolaou stain. Other characteristic features include plasmacytoid appearance, binucleation, and intranuclear inclusions. The differential diagnosis of malignant melanoma in effusion includes poorly differentiated carcinoma and sarcoma.

A-12. (**d**) **Mesothelioma**
The cytological findings of mesothelioma include that tumor cells form numerous three-dimensional clusters with scalloped (knobby) edges. Tumor cell has round or oval centrally placed nuclei, coarse chromatin, prominent nucleoli, dense cytoplasm with peripheral "halo," and intercellular "windows." Reactive mesothelial cells show a spectrum of changes ranging from normal to markedly atypical cells. In adenocarcinomas and poorly differentiated carcinomas, tumor cells form three-dimensional clusters with smooth edges. Tumor cells reveal hyperchromatic nuclei, irregular nuclear membrane, prominent nucleoli, and lacy or vacuolated cytoplasm, without intercellular "windows." Immunostains of mesothelial cell markers (calretinin, D2-40, WT1, P53) and adenocarcinoma markers (TTF, Napsin A, BerEP4, B72.3, CEA, CD15) may be helpful in the differential diagnosis. Metastatic melanomas have dispersed tumor cells with large nuclei, prominent nucleoli, and cytoplasmic melanin pigments.

A-13. (**c**) **Metastatic melanoma**
The diagnosis is a metastatic melanoma. Prominent cherry-red nucleoli and intranuclear pseudoinclusions are common findings in metastatic melanomas. Nuclei of tumor cells are eccentrically located (plasmacytoid appearance) and highly variable in size with finely to coarsely granular chromatin. The cytoplasmic melanin pigment is in dark brown color on the Papanicolaou stain. Another characteristic feature is the presence of binucleated cells. The differential diagnosis of intranuclear pseudoinclusions in malignant tumors includes papillary thyroid carcinoma, breast carcinoma, lung adenocarcinoma, meningioma, and others.

A-14. (**a**) **Metastatic squamous cell carcinoma**
The diagnosis is metastatic squamous cell carcinoma. In fluid cytology, tumor cells of metastatic squamous cell carcinomas may be rounded up and form loose clusters. In squamous cell carcinomas, tumor cells have enlarged nuclei, smudgy chromatin, and dense cytoplasm. In nonkeratinizing squamous cell carcinomas, prominent nucleoli may be present and can be confused with an adenocarcinoma. Squamous carcinoma cells have distinct cell borders due to the production of cytokeratin. In contrast, cytoplasm of adenocarcinoma is lacy and vacuolated.

A-15. (**b**) **Reactive mesothelial cells**
In reactive mesothelial cells, nuclear atypia can be quite striking; however, the normal or low N/C ratio is usually maintained in reactive atypia. The findings of reactive atypia represent a spectrum of cellular changes that range from normal to markedly atypical. Reactive mesothelial changes (reactive atypia) can be caused by a variety of conditions, such as chemotherapy and radiation therapy, inflammation, chronic irritation, and others. In mesothelioma, tumor cells form numerous three-dimensional clusters. An intercellular "window" can be seen in both reactive mesothelial cells and mesothelioma.

A-16. (**d**) **Metastatic signet ring cell carcinoma**
The diagnosis is metastatic signet ring cell carcinoma. The differential diagnosis of so-called "signet ring" cells in effusion cytology is broad, including both benign and malignant conditions. Benign reactive mesothelial cells may have "signet ring" cell features. A careful evaluation of the nuclear features is important for distinguishing benign from malignant lesions. Both metastatic adenocarcinomas of the lung and stomach can present "signet ring" cell morphology. The nuclear features of a carcinoma include large nuclei, hyperchromatic chromatin, irregular nuclear member, and large prominent nucleoli. The immunostains of TTF1, Napsin A, and CDX2 may help in the differential diagnosis of lung adenocarcinoma from stomach carcinoma. In a metastatic lung adenocarcinoma, TTF1 and Napsin A are usually positive, but CDX2 is negative.

A-17. (**a**) **Metastatic papillary renal cell carcinoma**
Papillary renal cell carcinoma is the second most common carcinoma of the renal tubules and has been characterized genetically. There are two histomorphologic types. Type 1 tumor consists of papillae and tubular structures covered by small cells with pale cytoplasm and characterized by small oval nuclei with inconspicuous nucleoli, frequent glomeruloid papillae, foamy macrophages in papillary cores, and psammoma bodies. Type 2 tumor consists of papillae covered by large cells with abundant eosinophilic cytoplasm and characterized by pseudostratification

and large spherical nuclei with prominent nucleoli and psammoma bodies, but it is uncommon to see foamy macrophages in papillary cores. Type 2 tumors are larger, more common in patients younger than age 40, and more frequent in stage 3 and 4 tumors. The reactivity of cytokeratin 7 is specific for papillary renal cell carcinomas.

A-18. **(a) Metastatic adenocarcinoma of the lung**
Metastatic adenocarcinomas of the lung may have a variety of appearances. In lung adenocarcinomas, particularly well-differentiated adenocarcinomas, tumor cells form acinar/papillary arrangements, or three-dimensional clusters. Tumor cells are intermediate or large in size and have hyperchromatic nuclei with coarse granular chromatin, prominent nucleoli, and vacuolated or clear cytoplasm. An intercellular "window" characteristic of mesothelial cells is not seen in adenocarcinomas. Small cell carcinomas have fine granular (salt-and-pepper) chromatin, nuclear crowding, and molding.

A-19. **(d) CD56**
This is a small cell lung carcinoma. CD56 is considered to be the most sensitive neuroendocrine marker for small cell lung carcinoma. Approximately 25 % of small cell lung carcinomas are negative for both synaptophysin and chromogranin A, but most of these tumors are positive for CD56. The reactivities for synaptophysin and chromogranin A are typically weak in small cell lung carcinomas. TTF1 is expressed by thyroid and pulmonary cells and is positive in approximately 70–80 % of small cell lung carcinomas. Still, 10 % of small cell lung carcinomas are negative for all three commonly used neuroendocrine markers, synaptophysin, chromogranin A, and CD56.

A-20. **(b) Neuron-specific enolase (NSE), synaptophysin, S100, and glial fibrillary acidic protein (GFAP)**
The diagnosis is a metastatic neuroblastoma. Neuroblastoma is the most common solid cancer in infancy and early childhood. Nearly half of neuroblastoma cases occur in children younger than two years. The tumor derives from primitive sympathetic neural precursors and most frequently involves the adrenal glands, neck, chest, abdomen, and pelvis. The great majority of cases are sporadic. About 1–2 % of cases run in families. N-myc oncogene amplification is a common finding in neuroblastoma. Other genetic abnormalities include activation of *HRAS*, chromosome deletion or allelic loss at 1p, aberrant expression of *TRKA* and *TRAB*, and others. In histology sections, tumor cells typically reveal as small, round and blue cells with Homer–Wright rosettes. In fluid cytology, the specimen is cellular and consists of discohesive small cells with hyperchromatic nuclei and inconspicuous nucleoli. Necrotic debris is common. The chromatin is finely granular and has "salt-and-pepper" appearance. Rosettes may be seen on cell block preparation. A variety of immunohistochemical stains are used to distinguish neuroblastomas from other tumors, such as rhabdomyosarcomas, Ewing's sarcoma, lymphoma, and Wilms' tumor. Neuroblastomas are immunoreactive for neuron-specific enolase (NSE), synaptophysin, S100, and glial fibrillary acidic protein (GFAP). Cytogenetic studies may demonstrate alterations of chromosome 1.

A-21. **(c) Metastatic hepatocellular carcinoma**
In metastatic hepatocellular carcinoma, particularly a poorly differentiated tumor, numerous pleomorphic dispersed individual cells with hyperchromatic nuclei, prominent nucleoli, and dense granular cytoplasm are revealed. The identification of cytoplasmic bile pigment or lipofuscin pigment is helpful. In poorly differentiated adenocarcinoma, tumor cells have acinar arrangements with vesicular chromatin and lacy cytoplasm. In poorly differentiated squamous cell carcinomas, tumor cells have smudged nuclei and cytoplasmic keratin. In reactive mesothelial cells, cells reveal reactive atypia.

A-22. **(c) Metastatic colonic adenocarcinoma**
A metastatic colonic adenocarcinoma has characteristic cytological features, such as tall columnar "picket fence" appearance, hyperchromatic pencil-shaped nuclei, coarse chromatin, and prominent nucleoli. The presence of "dirty" necrosis can be seen in both cytospin smear and cell block sections. In breast carcinomas, tumor cells form tight three-dimensional "cannon ball" clusters. The size of tumor cells is smaller than colon adenocarcinomas; they may have intranuclear inclusions. Both reactive mesothelial cells and mesotheliomas have intercellular "windows," and the edge of the cell cluster is knobby (scalloped appearance).

A-23. **(d) Metastatic mucinous adenocarcinoma of the lung**
Cytological features of mucinous adenocarcinomas include three-dimensional clusters and acinar and papillary groups. Tumor cells reveal large round- or oval-shaped nuclei, coarse chromatin, irregular nuclear membrane, and prominent nucleoli. The cytoplasm

of tumor cells is vacuolated (indicative of mucin production). Mucinous material can be seen in the background of cytospin smears and cell block preparation. In true papillary adenocarcinoma, numerous papillary structures could be identified. A metastatic colonic adenocarcinoma has hyperchromatic pencil-shaped nuclei and tumor necrosis. Reactive mesothelial cells reveal an intercellular "window" and reactive atypia.

A-24. (**d**) **Metastatic squamous cell carcinoma**
In metastatic squamous cell carcinomas, the cytological features of tumor cells include large nuclei with smudgy chromatin, nuclei with variation in size and shape, and dense cytoplasm (indicative of cytokeratin formation). In well-differentiated tumors, cytokeratin stains orangeophilic on the Papanicolaou method. Tumor cells are usually rounded up in the fluid specimens. The formation of two- and three-dimensional tumor cell clusters is not uncommon, particularly in poorly differentiated squamous cell carcinomas. In addition, prominent nucleoli can be seen in poorly differentiated squamous cell carcinomas and should not be confused with poorly differentiated adenocarcinomas.

A-25. (**b**) **Primary effusion lymphoma**
Primary effusion lymphoma (PEL) is a rare HIV-associated non-Hodgkin lymphoma (NHL) that accounts for approximately 4 % of all HIV-associated NHL. In PEL, tumor cells are large and have hyperchromatic round nuclei, prominent nucleoli, and varying amounts of cytoplasm. The cells show a range of appearances, from immunoblastic (round nuclei with central prominent nucleoli) to plasmablastic (eccentric nuclei with abundant cytoplasm, sometimes containing a perinuclear clearing) to anaplastic (very large round or polygonal cells with bizarre, pleomorphic nuclei). Anaplastic forms may also contain multinucleated and/or Reed–Sternberg-like cells. Immunophenotypically, PEL cells reveal a "null" lymphocyte phenotype (i.e., CD45 is expressed), but routine B-cell (including surface and cytoplasmic immunoglobulin, CD19, CD20, CD79a) and T-cell (CD3, CD4, CD8) markers are negative.

A-26. (**d**) **Hodgkin lymphoma**
The cytology reveals scattered large atypical cells with binucleation and prominent nucleoli (Reed–Sternberg cells) in a background of mixed inflammatory cells, and findings are characteristic of Hodgkin lymphoma. Classic Hodgkin lymphoma is a monoclonal lymphoid neoplasm (in most instances derived from B cells) composed of mononuclear Hodgkin and multinucleated Reed–Sternberg cells residing in an infiltrate containing a variable mixture of nonneoplastic small lymphocytes, eosinophils, neutrophils, histiocytes, and plasma cells. Large tumor cells (Reed–Sternberg cells) are positive for CD30 and CD15. In SLL/CLL, it consists of monomorphous small lymphocytes.

A-27. (**c**) **Reactive mesothelial cells**
The specimen consists of epithelioid cells and inflammatory cells. The epithelioid cells are reactive mesothelial cells, and some of them show signet ring cell morphology. The finding of signet ring cell morphology is not uncommon in reactive mesothelial cells. A careful evaluation of the nuclear features is important for distinguishing benign from malignant conditions. The nuclear features of a signet ring cell carcinoma include large nuclei, hyperchromatic chromatin, irregular nuclear member, and large prominent nucleoli. All these features are absent in benign reactive mesothelial cells with signet ring morphology.

A-28. (**b**) **Metastatic squamous cell carcinoma**
In metastatic squamous cell carcinomas, the cytological features of tumor cells include large nuclei with smudgy chromatin, nuclei with variation in size and shape, and dense cytoplasm (indicative of cytokeratin formation). In well-differentiated tumors, cytokeratin stains orangeophilic on the Papanicolaou method. Tumor necrosis may be found in the smear and cell block preparation, too.

A-29. (**d**) **Metastatic serous carcinoma**
The diagnosis is metastatic serous carcinoma. The specimen reveals large papillary clusters of malignant cells and psammoma bodies. Psammoma bodies can be found in both benign and malignant conditions. In serous carcinomas, tumor cells form three-dimensional or papillary clusters with hyperchromatic nuclei, irregular nuclear membrane, prominent nucleoli, and coarse chromatin. Reactive mesothelial cells reveal a spectrum of reactive changes and intercellular "windows" and the presence of psammoma bodies. In colonic adenocarcinomas, tumor cell forms numerous three-dimensional clusters with hyperchromatic elongated nuclei and tumor necrosis. In squamous cell carcinomas, tumor cells are arranged in loose clusters or dispersed individual cells with variable shaped nuclei and dense cytoplasm with cytokeratin formation. Psammoma bodies are not seen in these two types of carcinomas.

A-30. **(c) Reactive mesothelial cells**
Reactive cellular changes can happen in a variety of settings, such as radiation therapy and chemotherapy. Reactive mesothelial cells may form cohesive sheets and/or two-dimensional clusters of cells. These cells can be larger in size and have enlarged nuclei, but the normal N/C ratio is maintained. The differential diagnosis of reactive mesothelial cells includes mesotheliomas and carcinomas, particularly mesotheliomas. In mesotheliomas, tumor cells form three-dimensional clusters with knobby edges. They have hyperchromatic nuclei, irregular nuclear membranes, and prominent nucleoli.

A-31. **(b) Calretinin, TTF, and BerEP4**
The cytological preparation shows a metastatic adenocarcinoma. In pleural effusion, the most common metastatic adenocarcinoma is from the lung. In lung adenocarcinomas, tumor cells form three-dimensional clusters with smooth edges and without intercellular "windows." They have hyperchromatic nuclei, irregular nuclear membrane, prominent nucleoli, and scant cytoplasm. The immunostains of calretinin (negative), TTF1 (positive), and BerEP4 (positive) would confirm the diagnosis of a metastatic adenocarcinoma of the lung.

A-32. **(a) Metastatic mucinous adenocarcinoma**
The diagnosis is metastatic mucinous adenocarcinoma. As seen in adenocarcinomas, tumor cells form three-dimensional clusters. They have hyperchromatic nuclei, irregular nuclear membrane, and prominent nucleoli. The striking cytological feature of mucinous adenocarcinomas is the cytoplasm vacuoles and clear cytoplasm (indicative of cytoplasmic mucin production). Reactive mesothelial cells form sheets or loose clusters; they have dense cytoplasm and intercellular "windows." Metastatic melanomas reveal dispersed large tumor cells with prominent nucleoli and cytoplasmic melanin pigment. In metastatic small cell carcinomas, tumor cells have fine granular (salt-and-pepper) chromatin, nuclear crowding, and molding.

A-33. **(c) Reactive mesothelial cells**
The specimen consists of small clusters of cuboid cells with lumen formation and dispersed individual cells, characteristic of reactive mesothelial cells. Reactive mesothelial cell may be larger in size and have enlarged nuclei, but the normal N/C ratio is maintained. Multinucleation and prominent nucleoli may be also seen. In mesothelioma, tumor cells form numerous large clusters with hyperchromatic nuclei, clumped chromatin, and irregular nuclear membrane. In colonic adenocarcinoma, tumor cells form three-dimensional clusters with elongated nuclei and tumor necrosis. In serous carcinomas, tumor cells have papillary arrangements, hyperchromatic nuclei, irregular nuclear membrane, prominent nucleoli, scant cytoplasm, and without intercellular "windows."

A-34. **(b) Metastatic dysgerminoma**
The diagnosis is a metastatic dysgerminoma. Dysgerminoma of the ovary and its counterpart seminoma of the testis present as discohesive clusters and single cells that resemble enlarged mesothelial cells, although their cytoplasm is generally scant and clear. The nuclei are large and round with coarse chromatin and prominent nucleoli. The tumor cells have abundant clear cytoplasm. The background may contain numerous lymphocytes. But, the "tigroid' appearance that is so characteristic of seminomas/dysgerminoma on fine-needle aspiration specimens (owing to the abundance of glycogen from disruption of the delicate cytoplasm) is not apparent in fluid specimens. The differential diagnosis includes poorly differentiated carcinoma, melanoma, anaplastic large cell lymphoma, and epithelioid mesothelioma. The tumor cells of dysgerminoma are positive for periodic acid–Schiff (PAS) stain, placental alkaline phosphatase (PLAP), CD117, and OCT4, but usually negative for cytokeratin (CAM5.2 and/or AE1/AE3) and epithelial membrane protein (EMA).

A-35. **(c) Reactive mesothelial cells**
Reactive mesothelial cells can form cohesive sheets and/or two-dimensional clusters of cells. These cells can be larger in size and have enlarged nuclei, but the normal N/C ratio is maintained. Multinucleation and prominent nucleoli are common. Intercellular "windows" are the feature of mesothelial cells. The differential diagnosis of reactive mesothelial cells includes mesothelioma and carcinoma, particularly a well-differentiated adenocarcinoma. In adenocarcinomas, tumor cells form three-dimensional clusters with smooth edges. They have hyperchromatic nuclei, irregular nuclear membrane, prominent nucleoli, scant cytoplasm, and without intercellular "windows." In mesothelioma, tumor cells form numerous large three-dimensional clusters.

A-36. **(c) Reactive mesothelial cells**
See answer of Q-35.

A-37. (**b**) **Reactive mesothelial cells**
See answer of Q-35.

A-38. (**c**) **Endometriosis**
The diagnosis of this pelvic washing specimen is endometriosis. Endometriosis is typically seen during the reproductive years; it has been estimated that endometriosis occurs roughly in 10 % of women. The most common location is the ovary. On a fluid specimen, benign columnar cells (endometrial glands), hemosiderin-laden macrophages, spindle cells (endometrial stroma), and debris are common findings. The specimen can be quite bloody. Older lesions may display no glands but hemosiderin deposits.

A-39. (**b**) **Reactive mesothelial cells**
Reactive mesothelial cells may form sheets and/or cohesive clusters of cells. These cells can be larger in size and have enlarged nuclei, but the normal N/C ratio is maintained. Multinucleation and prominent nucleoli are common. In mesotheliomas, tumor cells form numerous large three-dimensional clusters. Tumor cells have hyperchromatic nuclei, irregular nuclear membrane, prominent nucleoli, scant cytoplasm, and intercellular "windows." In adenocarcinomas, tumor cells form three-dimensional clusters with smooth edges. They have hyperchromatic nuclei, irregular nuclear membrane, prominent nucleoli, vacuolated cytoplasm, and without intercellular "windows."

A-40. (**a**) **Metastatic adenocarcinoma of the lung**
The diagnosis is a metastatic adenocarcinoma of the lung. The specimen reveals many variably sized three-dimensional clusters and scattered psammoma bodies, characteristic of lung adenocarcinoma. In adenocarcinomas, tumor cells form three-dimensional clusters with smooth edges. They have hyperchromatic nuclei, irregular nuclear membrane, prominent nucleoli, vacuolated cytoplasm, and without intercellular "windows." In benign conditions such as mesothelial cell hyperplasia and endosalpingiosis, the presence of psammoma bodies is a common finding. In ovarian serous carcinomas, tumor cells form three-dimensional or papillary clusters with hyperchromatic nuclei, irregular nuclear membranes, prominent nucleoli, and coarse chromatin. In mesotheliomas, tumor cells form numerous three-dimensional clusters with hyperchromatic nuclei, irregular nuclear membranes, and coarse chromatin.

A-41. (**b**) **Reactive mesothelial cells**
Reactive mesothelial cells show a spectrum of changes, including sheets and/or cohesive clusters of cells, and they are larger in size with enlarged nuclei, but the normal N/C ratio is maintained. Multinucleation and prominent nucleoli are common. In mesotheliomas, tumor cells form numerous large three-dimensional clusters. Tumor cells have hyperchromatic nuclei, irregular nuclear membrane, prominent nucleoli, and scant cytoplasm. In adenocarcinomas and serous carcinomas, tumor cells form three-dimensional or papillary clusters with smooth edges. They have hyperchromatic nuclei, irregular nuclear membrane, prominent nucleoli, vacuolated cytoplasm, and without intercellular "windows."

A-42. (**c**) **Metastatic melanoma**
The diagnosis is a metastatic melanoma. In metastatic melanomas, tumor cells are usually arranged in loosely cohesive clusters or dispersed individual cells. Nuclei of tumor cells are eccentrically located and highly variable in size with finely to coarsely granular chromatin and single prominent cherry-red nucleoli. The cytoplasm tends to be abundant and may or may not contain melanin pigment. The N/C ratio may not be high. Melanin pigment appears coarsely granular and dark brown on the Papanicolaou stain. Other characteristic features include plasmacytoid appearance, multinucleation, binucleation, and intranuclear inclusions. The differential diagnosis of malignant melanomas in effusion includes poorly differentiated carcinoma, lymphoma, and sarcoma.

A-43. (**a**) **Rheumatoid pleuritis**
The diagnosis is rheumatoid pleuritis. The rheumatoid pleuritis occurs in approximately 2–3 % of patients with rheumatoid arthritis. The pleural effusion can be unilateral or bilateral. Cytological features include abundant granular debris, multinucleated giant cells, and scattered lymphocytes. The presence of granular debris is characteristic of rheumatoid pleuritis. Granular debris is amorphous material and forms variable sized green- or pink-red-colored clumps by the Papanicolaou stain. It is believed that the amorphous material is different from fibrin. Diagnosis of rheumatoid pleuritis relies on the characteristic cytological findings in an exudative pleural fluid.

A-44. (**c**) **Reactive mesothelial cells**
The diagnosis is reactive mesothelial cells. The specimen consists of small clusters of cuboid cells

with lumen formation and dispersed individual cells characteristic of reactive mesothelial cells. Reactive mesothelial cells may be larger in size and have enlarged nuclei, but the normal N/C ratio is maintained. In mesotheliomas, tumor cells form numerous three-dimensional clusters with hyperchromatic nuclei, clumped chromatin, and irregular nuclear membrane. In adenocarcinomas, tumor cells form three-dimensional clusters with hyperchromatic nuclei, irregular nuclear membrane, prominent nucleoli, and scant cytoplasm, and without intercellular "windows."

A-45. (**d**) **Metastatic squamous cell carcinoma**

The diagnosis is a metastatic squamous cell carcinoma. When a squamous cell carcinoma involves serosal surfaces and/or tumor cells shed into the fluid, tumor cells may be rounded up in the fluid and with less "squamous" features. Tumor cells of squamous cell carcinomas form loose clusters or dispersed individual cells, whereas tumor cells of adenocarcinoma form three-dimensional clusters or pseudoacinar arrangements. Tumor cells of squamous cell carcinomas have hyperchromatic nuclei, smudgy chromatin, and dense cytoplasm (indicative of cytokeratin formation). Tumor cells of adenocarcinomas have vesicular nuclei, coarse chromatin, and vacuolated cytoplasm (indicative of mucin production). The presence of prominent nucleoli can be seen in both adenocarcinomas and poorly differentiated squamous cells carcinomas.

A-46. (**d**) **Pseudomyxoma peritonei**

The diagnosis is pseudomyxoma peritonei. Pseudomyxoma peritonei is a condition caused by the production of abundant mucin or gelatinous material by tumor cells, which fills the abdominal cavity. The mucin or gelatinous material stains blue-green or purple color with the Papanicolaou method. This disease is most commonly caused by an appendiceal primary cancer, mucinous tumors of the ovary, and other gastrointestinal cancers. The primary tumor appears to arise from the MUC2-producing goblet cells in the appendix. The *KRAS* (P53) gene mutations have also be identified in the tumor cells. Cytological findings of pseudomyxoma peritonei include viscous, mucoid fluid that is difficult to smear (thick), free-floating columnar epithelial cells or goblet-like cells, occasional papillae, or fibrovascular cores. Since the majority of these tumors in pseudomyxoma peritonei are low-grade malignancy/borderline tumors, it is recommended to be called mucinous tumors unless there is surgical pathology confirmation of a mucinous carcinoma.

A-47. (**b**) **Reactive mesothelial cells**

The diagnosis is reactive mesothelial cells. Reactive mesothelial cells show a spectrum of changes, including sheets and/or cohesive clusters of cells; they are larger in size with enlarged nuclei, but the normal N/C ratio is maintained. Multinucleation and prominent nucleoli are common. In mesotheliomas, tumor cells form numerous large three-dimensional clusters. Tumor cells have hyperchromatic nuclei, irregular nuclear membrane, prominent nucleoli, and scant cytoplasm. In adenocarcinomas and serous carcinomas, tumor cells form three-dimensional or papillary clusters with smooth edges. They have hyperchromatic nuclei, irregular nuclear membrane, prominent nucleoli, vacuolated cytoplasm, and without intercellular "windows."

A-48. (**a**) **Metastatic serous carcinoma**

The diagnosis is metastatic serous carcinoma. The specimen reveals clusters of atypical epithelial cells and psammoma bodies. Psammoma bodies are round collections of calcium which is covered with a thin layer of benign mesothelial cells. It stains purple in color with the Papanicolaou method. Psammoma bodies can be found in both benign and malignant conditions. In benign conditions such as mesothelial cell hyperplasia and endosalpingiosis, the presence of psammoma bodies is a common finding. In malignant conditions such as ovarian serous carcinoma and mesothelioma, numerous psammoma bodies can be identified in specimens. In ovarian serous carcinoma, tumor cells form three-dimensional or papillary clusters with hyperchromatic nuclei, irregular nuclear membrane, prominent nucleoli, and coarse chromatin. In mesothelioma, tumor cell forms numerous three-dimensional clusters with hyperchromatic nuclei, irregular nuclear membrane, and coarse chromatin. Tumor cells of squamous cell carcinomas have hyperchromatic nuclei, smudgy chromatin, and dense cytoplasm (indicative of cytokeratin formation); however, psammoma bodies are not seen in squamous cell carcinomas.

A-49. (**c**) **Burkitt lymphoma**

Burkitt lymphoma accounts for 30–50 % of childhood lymphoma. It is a highly aggressive B-cell lymphoma and has three main clinical variants: the endemic, the sporadic, and the immunodeficiency-associated variants. The endemic variant occurs in African and Asian children, commonly involves the jaw or other facial bone and distal ileum, and is associated with Epstein–Barr virus (EBV) infection. The sporadic variant (also known as "non-African") occurs in the United States and is not associated with the EBV and involves the ileocecal region. The immunodeficiency-associated Burkitt lymphoma occurs in adults and is usually associated with HIV infection or immunocompromised patients. All three variants have similar morphology. The tumor consists of intermediate-sized cells with round nuclei, coarse chromatin, multiple nucleoli, and scant cytoplasm. The cytoplasmic vacuolization is a striking feature of the tumor. Numerous tingible body macrophages, apoptosis, and mitoses can be seen. The "starry sky" appearance seen under low power is due to scattered tingible body macrophages. The tumor cells are positive for B-cell markers (CD20, CD22, CD19) as well as CD10 and BCL6, but generally negative for BCL2 and TdT. The *c-myc* gene is commonly involved (80 % of t(8;14), 15 % of t(2;8), and 5 % of t(8;22)).

A-50. **(c) Eosinophilic pleural effusion**

Eosinophilic pleural effusion (EPF) is defined as a nucleated cell count containing more than 10 % eosinophils in the effusion specimen. It is estimated that approximately 10 % of exudative pleural effusions are eosinophilic. The mechanism of the development of EPF is still not fully understood. One hypothesis is that stimulation of pleural mesothelial cells by injury (such as trauma, air, and blood) leads to the production of cytokines, chemokines, and adhesion molecules that induce the accumulation of eosinophils. The most common causes of EPF are pleural irritation or trauma (i.e., hemothorax, pneumothorax, thoracic surgery) and malignancy. Other causes include infections (i.e., bacteria, fungi, mycobacteria, parasites, and viruses) and certain medications. EPF also occurs idiopathic in 8–35 % of patients.

2.4 Answers and Discussion of Text-Based Questions 51–100

A-51. (**d**) **Numerous large three-dimensional cellular clusters**

Mesothelial cells may undergo reactive changes in a variety of clinical settings such as with acute and chronic inflammations. The so-called "reactive" mesothelial cells can have markedly nuclear atypia, including nuclear enlargement and variation, multinucleation, and prominent nucleoli. These findings represent a spectrum of cellular changes that range from normal to atypical in reactive mesothelial cells. Variation in nuclear size, binucleation, and multinucleation can be also found in malignant mesothelial cells. Reactive cells may form two- and three-dimensional cellular clusters or sheets of cells; however, the cellular cluster usually contains less number of cells than that of mesothelioma. In contrast, in mesotheliomas, tumor cells form "large" three-dimensional clusters with more than 20–50 cells.

A-52. (**b**) **BerEP4, Napsin A, TTF1, Calretinin, WT1, and P53**

Mesothelioma is positive for calretinin, P53, and WT1, whereas, adenocarcinoma of the lung is positive for TTF, BerEP4, CEA, B72.3, and CD15. Among the so-called adenocarcinoma markers, BerEP4 has the membrane staining pattern; Napsin A is a relative specific marker for lung adenocarcinoma with a cytoplasmic staining pattern; and TTF1 has nuclear staining pattern whereas, among mesothelioma cell markers such as calretinin, WT1, and P53, calretinin has the nuclear staining pattern and relatively high sensitivity. Cytokeratin markers, including AE1/AE3 and CK7, are positive for both epithelial and mesothelial cells. CK20 and Ki67 play no roles in the differential diagnosis of mesothelioma and adenocarcinoma. The combination of BerEP4, Napsin A, TTF1, calretinin, WT1, and P53 will provide a critical differential diagnosis for adenocarcinoma and mesothelioma.

A-53. (**b**) **"Window" between atypical cells**

Reactive mesothelial changes (reactive atypia) can be caused by a variety of conditions, such as chemotherapy and radiation therapy, inflammation, chronic irritation, and others. In reactive mesothelial cells, nuclear atypia can be quite striking, and the normal or low N/C ratio is usually maintained in reactive atypia. These findings represent a spectrum of cellular changes that range from normal to atypical. The reactive cells may form two- or three-dimensional small clusters or sheets of cells. The cellular arrangement may be confused with an adenocarcinoma. Variation in nuclear size, binucleation, and multinucleation can be found in both reactive mesothelial cells and adenocarcinoma. The most characteristic finding of mesothelial cells is the presence of "window" between cells.

A-54. (**d**) **Mesothelioma**

Pleural mesothelioma is the most common form of the tumor, accounting for roughly 70 % of mesothelioma cases. An individual may be at risk to develop mesothelioma if he or she was exposed to asbestos. Pleural effusion is the common clinical presentation of mesothelioma. The cytological findings of mesothelioma include that tumor cells form numerous three-dimensional clusters with scalloped (knobby) edges. High-power view reveals that tumor cell has round centrally placed nuclei, coarse chromatin, prominent nucleoli, dense cytoplasm with peripheral "halo," and intercellular "windows." Reactive mesothelial cells show a spectrum of changes ranging from normal to markedly atypical cells. In adenocarcinoma and poorly differentiated carcinoma, tumor cells form three-dimensional clusters with smooth edges. They have hyperchromatic nuclei, irregular nuclear membrane, prominent nucleoli, scant cytoplasm, and without intercellular "windows." In addition, immunostains of mesothelial cell marker (calretinin, D2-40, WT1, P53) and adenocarcinoma markers (TTF, Napsin A, BerEP4, B72.3, CEA, CD 15) should be performed to aid in the differential diagnosis.

A-55. (**d**) **Shared cell borders**

In squamous cell carcinomas, tumor cells have enlarged nuclei, smudgy chromatin, and dense cytoplasm. In poorly differentiated squamous cell carcinoma, prominent nucleoli may be present and can be confused with an adenocarcinoma. Squamous carcinoma cells have distinct cell borders due to the production of cytokeratin; therefore, shared cell borders are not a feature of squamous cell carcinomas. It is more often seen in an adenocarcinoma.

A-56. (**d**) **Hyperchromatic nucleoli and clumped chromatin**

Reactive mesothelial cell changes are commonly seen in patients with radiation therapy and chemotherapy. The main differential diagnosis of reactive mesothelial cells includes mesothelioma and carcinoma, particularly a well-differentiated adenocarcinoma. Reactive mesothelial cell may form cohesive sheets and two- and three-dimensional clusters. These cells can be larger in size and have enlarged nuclei, but the normal N/C ratios are maintained. Multinucleation and prominent nucleoli are common. However, hyperchromatic nuclei, clumped chromatin, and irregular nuclear membrane are not features seen in reactive atypia. The presence of these features indicates malignant lesions. In adenocarcinomas, tumor cells form three-dimensional clusters with smooth edges. They have hyperchromatic nuclei, irregular nuclear membranes, prominent nucleoli, lacy and vacuolated cytoplasm, and without intercellular "windows."

A-57. (c) **Monomorphous population of lymphocytes**
Monomorphous population of lymphocytes is usually seen in lymph proliferative disorders and/or lymphomas, particularly in small lymphocytic lymphomas/chronic lymphocytic leukemia (SLL/CLL). It represents a monoclonal proliferation of lymphoma cells. Other cytological features of SLL/CLL include discohesive tumor cells with hyperchromatic nuclei, clumped (soccer-ball-like) chromatin, irregular nuclear membrane, inconspicuous nucleoli, and scant cytoplasm. Polymorphous population of lymphocytes is the feature of reactive lymphoid population. The presence of lacunar space (i.e., malignant cells are situated in an empty space) on the cell block section is a feature of malignancy such as metastatic adenocarcinoma and melanoma. Lymphoglandular bodies can be seen in both reactive lymphocytes and lymphoma cases.

A-58. (a) **Adenocarcinoma with lepidic growth pattern (bronchoalveolar carcinoma)**
Adenocarcinoma with lepidic growth pattern (formerly bronchoalveolar carcinoma) is considered a well-differentiated adenocarcinoma. It can be difficult to distinguish from reactive mesothelial cells, particularly in a scant specimen. In a well-differentiated adenocarcinoma, tumor cells are arranged in two- or three-dimensional clusters. They may also form a honeycomb-like arrangement. Tumor cells are intermediate in size and have round hyperchromatic nuclei, vesicular chromatin, small nucleoli, and foamy cytoplasm. However, no "window" is identified between tumor cell clusters. Reactive mesothelial cells may form cohesive sheets and/or two-dimensional clusters. These cells can be larger in size and have enlarged nuclei, but the normal N/C ratios are maintained. Multinucleation and prominent nucleoli are common. Hyperchromatic nuclei, clumped chromatin, and irregular nuclear membrane are not features seen in reactive mesothelial cells. In a poorly differentiated squamous cell carcinoma, tumor cells have smudgy chromatin and dense cytoplasm with or without cytokeratin formation. In basaloid carcinoma and small cell carcinoma, tumor cells are relatively small in size with hyperchromatic nuclei, nuclear molding and crowding, and scant cytoplasm.

A-59. (b) **Renal transplantation**
Pleural fluid eosinophilia, also called eosinophilic pleural effusion (EPF), is defined as a nucleated cell count containing more than 10 % eosinophils in the effusion specimen. It is estimated that approximately 10 % of exudative pleural effusions are eosinophilic. The mechanism of the development of EPF is still not fully understood. One hypothesis is that stimulation of pleural mesothelial cells by injury (such as trauma, air, and blood) leads to the production of cytokines, chemokines, and adhesion molecules that induce the accumulation of eosinophils. The most common causes of EPF are pleural irritation or trauma (i.e., hemothorax, pneumothorax, thoracic surgery) and malignancy. Other causes include infections (i.e., bacteria, fungi, mycobacteria, parasites, and viruses) and certain medications. EPF also occurs idiopathic in 8–35 %of patients. Although it was common decades ago, the development of EPF in the setting of tuberculosis is now considered rare. Renal transplantation has no direct connection to EPF.

A-60. (a) **True**
The sensitivity of fluid cytology for detecting malignancy is approximately 60–70 %, whereas the sensitivity of "blind" biopsy is less than 50 %. The reason fluid cytology has a higher sensitivity is that it may provide more diagnostic cells. The sensitivity of fluid cytology and the detection rate of malignancy may be further increased when multiple specimens are examined from a clinically suspicious patient.

A-61. (c) **Air in the pleural space (pneumothorax)**
Common causes of EPF are pleural irritation or trauma (i.e., hemothorax, pneumothorax, thoracic surgery), malignancy, infections (i.e., bacteria, fungi, mycobacteria, parasites, and viruses), and certain medications. The reported frequency of pleural malignancy in patients with EPF ranges from 6 to 40 %. Among the malignancies associated with EPF, lung cancer is the most common one. EPF also occurs idiopathic in 8–35 % of patients. In many case studies, pneumothorax, particularly the spontaneous

pneumothorax, is the most common cause of EPF and accounts for more than 50 % of cases.

A-62. **(b) Air in the pleural space (pneumothorax)**
Pneumothorax, particularly the spontaneous pneumothorax, is the most common cause of EPF. An intense eosinophilic pleuritis occurs within hours after air entry into the pleural space. In contrast to the rapid development of EPF after spontaneous pneumothorax, hemothorax-induced EPF appears typically by the tenth day, with the development of a peripheral blood eosinophilia days later. Pleural space hemorrhage may contribute to the development of PFE in the setting of thoracic surgery, thoracotomy, chest trauma, benign asbestos pleural effusion, and pulmonary infarction. The thoracic surgery and biopsy may also result in EPF which typically occurs within 30 days after the procedure, particularly when the pleura has been excised, such as internal mammary grafting. Repeated thoracentesis has been suggested as a cause of EPF; it develops within days but not in hours after the procedure.

A-63. **(d) Cirrhosis**
The most common cause of eosinophilic ascites is cirrhosis. Other causes of eosinophilic effusion include peritoneal irritation or trauma, malignancy, infections (i.e., bacteria, fungi, mycobacteria, parasites, and viruses), and idiopathic. A rare cause of development of eosinophilic ascites is eosinophilic gastroenteritis, which has been increasingly reported recently. It should be included in the differential diagnosis of eosinophilic ascites.

A-64. **(d) Prominent nucleoli**
When squamous cell carcinoma involves serosal surfaces and/or tumor cells shed into the fluid, the distinction of squamous cell carcinoma and adenocarcinoma can be difficult in some cases, since tumor cells may be rounded up in the fluid and with less "squamous" features. Tumor cells of squamous cell carcinoma form loosely clusters or dispersed individual cells, whereas tumor cells of adenocarcinoma form three-dimensional clusters or pseudoacinar arrangements. In general, tumor cells of squamous cell carcinoma have hyperchromatic nuclei, smudgy chromatin, and dense cytoplasm (indicative of cytokeratin formation). Tumor cells of adenocarcinoma have vesicular nuclei, coarse chromatin, and vacuolated cytoplasm (indicative of mucin production). The presence of prominent nucleoli can be seen in both adenocarcinoma and poorly differentiated squamous cells carcinoma.

A-65. **(d) All of the above**
The differential diagnosis of so-called "signet ring" cells in effusion cytology is broad, including both benign and malignant conditions. In benign reactive mesothelial cells, they can have "signet ring" cell features. Both metastatic adenocarcinomas of the lung and stomach can present "signet ring" cell morphology. A careful evaluation of the nuclear features is important for distinguishing benign from malignant lesions. The nuclear features of a carcinoma include large nuclei, hyperchromatic chromatin, irregular nuclear member, and large prominent nucleoli. The immunostains of TTF1, Napsin A, and CDX2 may help in the differential diagnosis of lung adenocarcinoma from stomach carcinoma. In a metastatic lung adenocarcinoma, TTF1 and Napsin A are usually positive, but CDX2 is negative. However, in cases of metastatic mucinous adenocarcinoma of the lung, stains of TTF and CDX2 may not help, since the TTF may be negative and CDX2 may be focally positive in the mucinous adenocarcinoma.

A-66. **(d) Nuclear grooves**
Neuroendocrine tumors (NET) are a spectrum of neoplasms, arising from various neuroendocrine cells. NETs are most often located in the intestine and the lungs. Although NETs have different embryological origin, they have common phenotypic characteristics. For example, tumors show immunoreactivity for neuroendocrine markers, including chromogranin, synaptophysin, CD56, and neuron-specific enolase (NES) and may secrete various peptides and hormones. Cytological features of NET are characterized by fine granular chromatin (salt-and-pepper chromatin) pattern, inconspicuous nucleoli, and scant cytoplasm. Mitosis may be rare or abundant depending on the differentiation of the tumor. Nuclear crowding and molding are often seen in small cell carcinoma; however, nuclear groove is not a feature of neuroendocrine tumors. The World Health Organization (WHO) classifies neuroendocrine tumors into three main categories: (1) well-differentiated neuroendocrine tumors with benign behavior, (2) well-differentiated (low-grade) neuroendocrine carcinomas with low-grade malignant behavior, and (3) poorly differentiated (high-grade) neuroendocrine carcinomas with aggressive clinical course, such as the large cell neuroendocrine and small cell carcinomas. In addition, cellular proliferative rate (Ki67 labeling) has been considered as a useful marker for the classification of the tumor.

A-67. **(c) Acid (simple, mesenchymal)**
Mucin can be produced by both epithelial cells and stroma. Neutral mucin can be found in glands of the GI tract and in the prostate, and they stain with PAS but not with alcian blue, colloidal iron, mucicarmine, or metachromatic dyes. There are several types of acid mucins. Acid mucin (simple or non-sulfated) is the typical mucin of epithelial cells containing sialic acid, and they stain with PAS, alcian blue at pH 2.5, colloidal iron, and metachromatic dyes. They resist hyaluronidase digestion. Acid mucin (simple, mesenchymal) contains hyaluronic acid and does not stain with PAS, but does stain with alcian blue at pH 2.5, colloidal iron, and metachromatic dyes. They digest with hyaluronic acid and can be found in sarcomas and mesotheliomas. Acid mucin (complex, or sulfated, epithelial) is found in adenocarcinomas; PAS is usually positive; alcian blue is positive at pH 1, and colloidal iron, mucicarmine, and metachromatic stains are also positive. They resist the digestion with hyaluronidase. Finally, acid mucin (complex, connective tissue) are found in stromal tissue such as cartilage and bone, and they are PAS negative but do stain selectively with alcian blue at pH 0.5.

A-68. **(d) Mucicarmine**
There are a variety of mucin stains. In the colloidal iron stain, iron particles are stabilized in ammonia and glycerin and are attracted to acid mucopolysaccharides. It requires formalin fixation. Phospholipids and free nucleic acids may also stain. The actual blue color comes from a Prussian blue reaction. The tissue can be predigested with hyaluronidase to provide more specificity. In alcian blue stain, the pH of the stain can be adjusted to improve the specificity. In PAS stain, both glycogen and mucins are stained, but the tissue can be predigested with diastase to remove glycogen. In mucicarmine stain, epithelial mucins are stained. It is the most specific mucin stain for adenocarcinoma, but its sensitivity is low. The most sensitive mucin stain is PAS, but its specificity is poor. Colloidal iron stains are unpredictable. Alcian blue stains are simple, but have a lot of background staining.

A-69. **(d) Poorly differentiated adenocarcinoma**
The differential diagnosis of spindle cells in fluid cytology is broad, including spindle cell carcinoma, sarcomatoid mesothelioma, melanoma, and all other tumors with spindle cell morphology. Therefore, careful review of the patient's malignant history is extremely important, and it may help to narrow down the differential diagnosis. The spindle cell appearance is not the feature of a poorly differentiated adenocarcinoma. The cytological features of a poorly differentiated adenocarcinoma include three-dimensional clusters, acinar and papillary groups, or honeycomb-like sheets of epithelial cells. Tumor cells have large round- or oval-shaped hyperchromatic nuclei, coarse chromatin, irregular nuclear membrane, and prominent nucleoli. The cytoplasm of tumor cells is feathery and foamy. Cytoplasmic vacuolization (indicative of mucin production) can be seen.

A-70. **(c) Abundant cytoplasm**
In small cell carcinomas, tumor cells are relatively small, and they are two- to threefold in size of mature lymphocytes; however, in small cell carcinoma large cell variant, the size of tumor cells can be much larger. Tumor cells show scant cytoplasm and high N/C ratio, large nuclei with fine chromatin (salt-and-pepper) pattern, nuclear crowding and molding, and paranuclear blue bodies in the cytoplasm. The nucleoli are inconspicuous in small cell carcinomas. Abundant cytoplasm is not a feature seen in small cell carcinoma. It can be seen in carcinoid and large cell neuroendocrine tumor.

A-71. **(a) Fine granular (salt-and-pepper) chromatin pattern**
The World Health Organization (WHO) classification recognizes four major types of lung neuroendocrine tumors: typical carcinoid, atypical carcinoid, small cell lung cancer (SCLC), and large cell neuroendocrine carcinoma (LCNEC). The classification is based on morphology, mitotic rate, and the absence or presence of necrosis. Ki-67 (MIB1) labeling is also play an important role in the diagnosis and classification of these tumors. In histological section, the characteristics of LCNEC include three features: high-grade nuclei, neuroendocrine morphology, and positive neuroendocrine IHC markers. In cytological preparations, LCNEC typically reveals as dispersed individual cells or loosely formed clusters. The size of cells is usually larger than those of SCLC. Tumor cell has prominent nucleoli, fine rather than coarse granular chromatin (seen in adenocarcinoma), and more markedly cytological pleomorphism, whereas the reactivities for synaptophysin and chromogranin may be weak in small cell lung carcinoma. Tumor cells have coarse granular rather than fine chromatin and lacy or vacuolated cytoplasm. In difficult cases, diagnosis of LCNEC versus a poorly differentiated adenocarcinoma depends on IHC staining of

neuroendocrine markers. Although LCNEC are positive for neuroendocrine markers, 10–20 % of non-small cell lung cancers label for neuroendocrine markers. Therefore, the differential diagnosis of these two tumors should be based on the combination of cytomorphology and IHC study.

A-72. (**b**) **Make cell block as usual**
Making a cell block preparation is important in fluid cytology, particularly in cases with atypical epithelial cells and/or suspicious metastatic carcinomas. In such cases, IHC study is usually helpful in the differential diagnosis. Repeat tap and biopsy of the lung lesion are not necessary. The main differential diagnosis is reactive mesothelial cells versus adenocarcinoma. Reactive mesothelial cells show a spectrum of changes ranging from normal to markedly atypical cells. In adenocarcinomas, tumor cells form three-dimensional clusters with smooth edges. They have hyperchromatic nuclei, irregular nuclear membrane, prominent nucleoli, scant cytoplasm, and without intercellular "windows." In addition, immunostains of mesothelial cell marker (calretinin, D2-40) and adenocarcinoma markers (TTF, Napsin A, BerEP4, B72.3, CEA, CD15) may help in the differential diagnosis.

A-73. (**d**) **All of the above**
Primary effusion lymphoma (PEL) is a rare HIV-associated non-Hodgkin lymphoma (NHL) that accounts for approximately 4 % of all HIV-associated NHL. PEL has a unique clinical predilection for arising in body cavities such as the pleural space, pericardium, and peritoneum. There is an evidence of human herpesvirus (HHV)-8 infection in patients. The exact oncogenic mechanisms of HHV-8 have not been clearly defined. Treatment is usually with combination CHOP (cyclophosphamide, doxorubicin, vincristine, and prednisone) chemotherapy and antiretroviral therapy (if HIV positive). The prognosis for PEL is poor, with a median survival time of around 6 months. The diagnosis of PEL requires cytomorphological analysis of effusion specimen, immunophenotypic and molecular tests, and virologic criteria (i.e., previously infection with HHV-8). The diagnosis is usually made on a cytological preparation (e.g., liquid-based preparation, cytospin, cell block) of the effusion fluid. Morphologically, tumor cells are large and have round to irregular nuclei, prominent nucleoli, and varying amounts of cytoplasm. The cells show a range of appearances, from immunoblastic (round nuclei with central prominent nucleoli) to plasmablastic (eccentric nuclei with abundant cytoplasm, sometimes containing a perinuclear clearing) to anaplastic (very large round or polygonal cells with bizarre, pleomorphic nuclei). Anaplastic forms may also contain multinucleated and/or Reed–Sternberg-like cells. Immunophenotypically, PEL cells reveal a "null" lymphocyte phenotype (i.e., CD45 is expressed), but routine B-cell (including surface and cytoplasmic immunoglobulin, CD19, CD20, CD79a) and T-cell (CD3, CD4, CD8) markers are negative. Instead, various markers of lymphocyte activation (CD30, CD38, CD71, human leukocyte antigen DR) and plasma cell differentiation (CD138) are usually displayed. Molecular studies have provided evidence that immunoglobulin gene rearrangements and somatic mutation have occurred in PEL cells. Cytogenetic analysis has revealed complex karyotypes but no common chromosomal abnormality in PEL.

A-74. (**d**) **Hepatocellular carcinoma**
"Intranuclear inclusions" have been described in a variety of malignant tumors, such as papillary thyroid carcinoma, lung adenocarcinoma, meningioma, hepatocellular carcinoma, and others. It has not been found in renal cell carcinomas. The cytological features of renal cell carcinomas (clear cell renal cell carcinomas) include loosely cohesive clusters and/or scattered individual tumor cells. They have slightly enlarged round nuclei with or without nucleoli depending on the Fuhrman grade of the tumor. The background of smears can be bloody with vascular structures, best seen on cell block preparations. Tumor cells also have abundant vesicular cytoplasm and cytoplasmic vacuoles. The N/C ratio is usually in normal range.

A-75. (**c**) **Prepare cell blocks and make sure that it have adequate tumor cells**
Currently *EGFR*, *KRAS*, and other mutations are routinely tested in non-small cell lung cancer patients. Any type of formalin-fixed and paraffin-embedded specimen, including cell block preparations, can be used for these molecular and mutational analyses. For any type of specimens, the presence of adequate tumor cells is crucial and necessary to be confirmed prior to sending the specimen for molecular tests. In lung adenocarcinoma, the *EGFR* and *KRAS* mutational rates are 10–15 and 15–20 % in the United States. EGFR mutation is associated with a good response to tyrosine kinase inhibitors therapy, whereas *KRAS* mutation is associated with a resistance to tyrosine kinase inhibitor therapy in lung cancer patients. It is not necessary to obtain tissue

from primary tumor; molecular studies can be performed using tissue from a metastatic tumor.

A-76. (**d**) **All of the above**
Psammoma body can be found in both benign and malignant conditions. In benign conditions such as mesothelial cell hyperplasia and endosalpingiosis, the presence of psammoma body is a common finding. In malignant conditions such as ovarian serous carcinoma and mesothelioma, numerous psammoma bodies can be identified in ascites specimens.

A-77. (**c**) **Pyknotic nuclei**
In a fluid specimen, tumor cells of metastatic squamous cell carcinoma are usually rounded up and form loosely clusters. The cytological features of tumor cells include large nuclei with smudgy chromatin, nuclei with variation in size and shape, and dense cytoplasm (indicative of cytokeratin formation), except the feature of pyknotic nuclei. Pyknotic nuclei are usually seen reactive and/or benign squamous cells. Finally, prominent nucleoli can be seen in poorly differentiated squamous cell carcinomas and should not be confused with poorly differentiated adenocarcinomas. Tumor cells of adenocarcinoma have vesicular nuclei, coarse chromatin, and vacuolated cytoplasm.

A-78. (**a**) **Burkitt's or Burkitt's-like lymphoma (BL)**
The most common histological types of AIDS-related non-Hodgkin lymphoma (ARL) include Burkitt's or Burkitt's-like lymphoma (BL), diffuse large B-cell lymphoma (DLBCL) (including the subtypes immunoblastic (including most cases of PCNSL) and centroblastic lymphoma), plasmablastic lymphoma (including oral cavity involved and multicentric Castleman's disease [MCD] associated), and primary effusion lymphoma (PEL). Among them, BL rarely presents as a lymphomatous effusion. BL tumor cells are positive for the characteristic c-myc gene rearrangement and show no evidence of HHV-8 infection. Peripheral T-cell NHLs presenting with an effusion can usually be distinguished by routine immunohistochemistry for T-cell markers or T-cell receptor (TCR) gene rearrangement studies. Because of similar morphology, T-cell anaplastic large cell lymphoma may also be confused for PEL in some cases; immunohistochemical staining for anaplastic lymphoma kinase in addition to the TCR gene rearrangement studies may be helpful in these cases. Both DLBCL and PEL can have similar cytomorphology. In DLBCL, tumor cells are positive for Epstein–Barr virus, but negative for HHV-8. In PEL, tumor cells are negative for Epstein–Barr virus, but positive for HHV-8.

A-79. (**c**) **Colon**
A metastatic colonic adenocarcinoma has these classic cytological features. Tumor cells showed tall columnar "picket fence" appearance, hyperchromatic pencil-shaped nuclei, coarse chromatin, and prominent nucleoli. The presence of "dirty" necrosis is usually not as apparent as seen in histological sections. In breast carcinomas, tumor cells form tight three-dimensional "cannon ball" clusters. The size of tumor cells is smaller than that of colon adenocarcinomas; they may have intranuclear inclusion. Renal cell carcinomas usually reveal a centrally located nuclei and clear cytoplasm. Lung adenocarcinomas may have a variety of morphological features. The finding of tall columnar cells favors a colonic primary rather than the lung primary; IHC stain of TTF, Napsin A, CK7, CK20, and CDX2 may aid to the differential diagnosis in difficult cases.

A-80. (**a**) **Prominent nucleoli**
The presence of prominent nucleoli is not the feature seen in small cell carcinomas. All other features can be seen in both adenocarcinoma and small cell carcinoma. In adenocarcinomas, tumor cells form acini and/or three-dimensional clusters and reveal hyperchromatic nuclei, vesicular or coarse chromatin, prominent nucleoli, and vacuolated cytoplasm (indicative of mucin production). All neuroendocrine tumors share many cytological features, such as fine granular (salt-and-pepper) chromatin and acini/rosette arrangements of tumor cells. In addition, in small cell carcinomas, nuclear crowding and molding are common features. Tumor necrosis can be seen in both adenocarcinoma and small cells carcinoma.

A-81. (**b**) **Making cell block to perform IHC markers S100, HMB45, and melanin A**
Metastatic melanoma to serosal cavities, including pleural, pericardial, and peritoneal cavities, is not uncommon. Tumor cells are usually rounded up in a fluid specimen and may or may not produce melanin pigment, particularly in desmoplastic/spindle cell melanoma (no pigment production). The cytological features of a metastatic melanoma include individual large cells with prominent nucleoli, intranuclear inclusion, cytoplasmic pigment, binucleation, and the presence of plasmacytoid cells. In desmoplastic/spindle cell melanoma, tumor cells reveal bizarre nuclei and prominent nucleoli. Immunomarkers S100, HMB45, and MelanA/Mart1 are helpful in the

differential diagnosis. S100 stains nuclei and cytoplasm with 90 % sensitivity but not specific. HMB45 stains cytoplasm; it is more specific but less sensitive than S100; only 20 % of desmoplastic/spindle cell melanomas are immunoreactive with HMB45. MelanA/Mart1 stains cytoplasm, and is a sensitive marker, but it also stains steroid-producing cells in the ovary, testis, and adrenal cortex; it is also negative in desmoplastic/spindle cell melanoma. Although unstained cytospin slides can be used for IHC study, cell block preparation provides better results. The combination of S100, HMB45 and melanin A may result in the best immunopattern in the differential diagnosis of melanomas.

A-82. (**d**) **Naked nuclei**
The presence of naked nuclei is not the feature seen in metastatic breast carcinoma. In pleural effusion cytology, tumor cells of metastatic breast carcinoma form tight three-dimensional "cannon ball" clusters. The size of tumor cells is relatively smaller than that of metastatic adenocarcinoma from the lung and/or GI tract. The presence of intracytoplasmic lumina, so-called magenta body, is also one of the characteristics of metastatic breast carcinoma. Magenta bodies are variably sized red-to-purple perinuclear inclusions seen by the Diff-Quik stains. The prominent nucleoli are a common cytological feature seen in a variety of adenocarcinomas. Naked nuclei can be seen in metastatic melanoma and hepatocellular carcinoma.

A-83. (**c**) **Hyaluronic acid–alcian blue**
Both mesothelioma and adenocarcinoma produce mucins. In adenocarcinomas, tumor cells are positive for mucicarmine, PAS, and cytokeratin. Similarly, in mesotheliomas, particularly in epithelial mesotheliomas, tumor cells may also be positive for mucicarmine, PAS, and cytokeratin. Studies have shown that mucicarmine and PAS stains were usually eradicated or reduced in intensity by pretreatment of the tissue sections with hyaluronidase, suggesting that hyaluronic acid was responsible for the positive mucin reactions in mesothelioma. Therefore, hyaluronic acid–alcian blue stain is a characteristic feature of a mesothelioma rather than an adenocarcinoma. In alcian blue stain, the pH of the stain can be adjusted to improve the specificity.

A-84. (**d**) **Bipolar nuclei**
The presence of bipolar nuclei is not the feature seen in metastatic breast carcinoma. In pleural effusion cytology, tumor cells of metastatic breast carcinoma form tight three-dimensional "cannon ball" clusters. The size of tumor cells is relatively smaller than that of metastatic adenocarcinoma from the lung and/or GI tract. The presence of intracytoplasmic lumina (magenta body) is also one of the characteristics of metastatic breast carcinoma.

A-85. (**a**) **Hyperchromatic nuclei and prominent nucleoli**
The presence of prominent nucleoli is not the feature seen in small cell carcinomas. All other features can be seen in small cell carcinoma. In small cell carcinomas, tumor cells form three-dimensional clusters or dispersed individual cells and reveal hyperchromatic nuclei, fine granular (salt-and-pepper) chromatin, and scant cytoplasm. In addition, nuclear crowding, molding, apoptotic body, and mitotic figures are common features. The background of the smear may also reveal "blue strips" (indicative of breakdown nuclear material). In adenocarcinomas, tumor cells form acini and/or three-dimensional clusters and reveal hyperchromatic nuclei, vesicular or coarse chromatin, prominent nucleoli, and vacuolated cytoplasm (indicative of mucin production).

A-86. (**d**) **All of the above**
Lymphocytic effusion is the effusion in which almost all nucleated cells are lymphocytes. In the cytological preparation, it reveals small lymphocytes. In tuberculosis, the identification of eosinophils is important; it may be suggestive of the diagnosis. The diagnosis of tuberculosis can be confirmed by microbiology culture or pleural biopsy. Malignancy is the common cause of lymphocytic effusion. It may be caused by the obstruction of lymphatic outflow by the tumor or peritumoral lymphocytic reaction. Repeat tap and cytological evaluation may increase the chance of finding tumor cells. Small lymphocytic lymphoma/chronic lymphocytic leukemia may cause lymphocytic effusion, particularly in a patient with peripheral lymphocytosis. Flow cytometry and immunostain of B-cell markers may help in the diagnosis. Other causes, such as status for post coronary artery bypass may also induce a lymphocytic effusion.

A-87. (**d**) **CD56**
CD56 is considered to be the most sensitive neuroendocrine marker for small cell lung carcinoma, whereas the reactivities for synaptophysin and chromogranin A are typically weak in small cell lung carcinoma. Approximately 25 % of small cell lung

carcinomas are negative for both synaptophysin and chromogranin A, but most of these tumors are positive for CD56. Still, 10 % of small cell lung carcinomas are negative for all three commonly used neuroendocrine markers. The frequency of neuroendocrine marker negativity in small cell lung carcinoma is even higher in small biopsy and cytology specimens, in which focal reactivity may not be represented on the smear due to the nature of the specimen and the heterogeneity of the tumor. If the cytomorphology is classic for small cell carcinomas, the lack of supporting immunohistochemical stains should not serve as evidence against the diagnosis. TTF1 is positive for both small cell lung carcinoma and lung adenocarcinomas.

A-88. (**b**) **False**

TTF1 (thyroid transcription factor 1) is expressed by thyroid and pulmonary cells and is positive in approximately 70–80 % of small cell lung carcinomas. TTF1 is usually used to identify the pulmonary (and/or thyroid) origin of metastatic adenocarcinomas. In contrast to adenocarcinomas, TTF1 in small cell carcinomas cannot be used to distinguish the origin of the tumor, i.e., pulmonary versus extrapulmonary origin. In addition to lung small cell carcinomas, the expression of TTF1 has been found to occur in 20–80 % of small cell carcinomas of various sites, including the prostate, bladder, cervix, and gastrointestinal tract.

A-89. (**b**) **Small cell lung carcinoma**

Both adenocarcinomas and small cell carcinomas are cytokeratin positive. The weak punctate ("dotlike") labeling pattern for cytokeratins, including both AE1/AE3 and CAM 5.2, is the feature commonly seen in small cell lung carcinomas. In contrast, a strong circumferential labeling of tumor cells is characteristic of a non-small cell lung carcinoma, particularly an adenocarcinoma. However, this feature may be seen in other high-grade carcinomas. Although all resected small cell carcinomas are cytokeratin positive, some tumors may show weak and minimal reactivity. Thus, on small biopsy and/or cytology specimens, a subset of small cell carcinomas may appear cytokeratin negative. In the absence of confirmatory markers, it is important to exclude the possibility of lymphoma, basaloid squamous cell carcinoma, and other small round blue cell tumors. If the cytomorphology is classic for small cell carcinomas, the lack of supporting immunohistochemical stains should not serve as evidence against the diagnosis.

A-90. (**d**) **Immunostains of synaptophysin, chromogranin, CD56, and CD45**

An important differential diagnosis of small cell lung carcinoma is lymphoma. In small cell carcinomas, tumor cells form three-dimensional clusters or dispersed individual cells and reveal hyperchromatic nuclei, fine granular (salt-and-pepper) chromatin, and scant cytoplasm. In addition, nuclear crowding, molding, apoptotic body, and mitotic figures are common features. The background of the smear may also reveal "blue strips" (indicative of breakdown of nuclear material). Positive immunostains of synaptophysin, chromogranin and CD56, and negative stain of CD45 may confirm the diagnosis. In lymphomas, tumor cells are discohesive and dispersed throughout the smear. The finding of a "lymphoglandular body" is characteristic of lymphoma. The chromatin of lymphoma cells are coarse granular, and they may have prominent nucleoli. Flow cytometry and immunostain of lymphoma markers may help in the diagnosis. Immunomarkers of AE1/AE3, TTF, and BerEP4 are best used for carcinomas, particularly adenocarcinoma. CD20 and CD5 may stain background lymphocytes in the smear of a small cell carcinoma.

A-91. (**b**) **Irregular nuclear membrane and hyperchromasia**

Reactive cellular changes can happen in a variety of settings, such as radiation and chemotherapy. Reactive mesothelial cell may form cohesive sheets and/or two-dimensional clusters of cells. These cells can be larger in size and have enlarged nuclei, but the normal N/C ratio is maintained. Multinucleation and prominent nucleoli are common. Intercellular "windows" are a feature of mesothelial cells. However, hyperchromatic nuclei, clumped chromatin, and irregular nuclear membranes are not features seen in reactive atypia. The presence of these features indicates malignant lesions. The differential diagnosis of reactive mesothelial cells includes mesothelioma and carcinoma, particularly a well-differentiated adenocarcinoma. In adenocarcinomas, tumor cells form three-dimensional clusters with smooth edges. They have hyperchromatic nuclei, irregular nuclear membranes, prominent nucleoli, scant cytoplasm, and without intercellular "windows."

A-92. (**b**) **CT-guided transthoracic needle biopsy**

The most common primary malignant lesions involving the pleural cavity are mesotheliomas and lymphomas. Malignant pleural effusion is a condition in which cancer causes an abnormal accumulation of fluid between the thin layers of pleura lining the outside of the lung and the wall of the chest cavity. Lung cancer and breast cancer account for about 50–65 % of malignant pleural effusions. Among these procedures, blind transthoracic needle biopsy has the sensitivity of less than 50 %; thoracentesis cytology has a sensitivity of 60 %; ultrasound-guided transthoracic needle biopsy has a sensitivity of 73 %; and a CT-guided transthoracic needle biopsy has a sensitivity of 87 %.

A-93. **(d) Ultrasound-guided thoracentesis**
The ultrasound-guided thoracentesis has a specificity of 100 % for distinguishing malignant pleural effusions from other causes of pleural effusion, based on the presence of visible pleural lesions (i.e., metastases), pleural thickening greater than 1 cm, pleural nodularity, diaphragmatic thickening greater than 7 mm, and an echogenic swirling pattern visible in the pleural fluid.

A-94. **(b) False**
Cytological features of adenocarcinomas include three-dimensional clusters, acinar and papillary groups, or honeycomb-like sheets of tumor cells. Tumor cells reveal large round- or oval-shaped nuclei, coarse chromatin, irregular nuclear membrane, and prominent nucleoli. The cytoplasm of tumor cells is feathery and foamy (indicative of mucin production). Squamous cell carcinomas account for 30–40 % of non-small cell lung cancers. In metastatic squamous cell carcinomas, the cytological features of tumor cells include large nuclei with smudgy chromatin, nuclei with variation in size and shape, and dense cytoplasm (indicative of cytokeratin formation). Tumor cells are usually rounded up in the fluid specimens. The formation of two- and three-dimensional tumor cell clusters is not uncommon, particularly in poorly differentiated squamous cell carcinomas. In addition, prominent nucleoli can be seen in poorly differentiated squamous cell carcinomas and should not be confused with poorly differentiated adenocarcinomas.

A-95. **(d) All of the above**
The rheumatoid pleuritis may occur in approximately 2–3 % of patients with rheumatoid arthritis. The pleural effusion can be unilateral or bilateral. Cytological features include abundant granular debris, multinucleated giant cells, and scattered lymphocytes. The presence of granular debris is characteristic of the rheumatoid pleuritis. Granular debris are amorphous material and form variable sized green- or pink-red-colored clumps by the Papanicolaou stain. It is believed that the amorphous material is different from fibrin. Diagnosis of rheumatoid pleuritis relies on the characteristic cytological findings in an exudative pleural fluid.

A-96. **(c) Mesothelial cells**
The diagnosis features of a rheumatoid pleuritis rely on the characteristic cytological findings of the exudative pleural fluid, which contains elongated and giant multinucleated histiocytes in a sea of amorphous granular material. The absence of mesothelial cells is also characteristic of the disease.

A-97. **(d) All of the above**
Charcot–Leyden crystal is a needle-shaped crystal. They vary in size and may be as large as 50 μm in length. They consist of lysophospholipase, an enzyme synthesized by eosinophils, and are produced from the breakdown of these cells. It was first described by Friedrich Albert von Zenker in 1851. The finding of Charcot–Leyden crystals in pathology specimen is indicative of a disease involving eosinophilic inflammation or proliferation, such as in allergic reactions, parasitic infections, and eosinophilic effusions.

A-98. **(d) LE cells contain nuclear material with visible chromatin structures, such as coarse chromatin granules**
The lupus pleuritis may occur in one third of lupus patients. The finding of LE cells in the fluid cytological preparations is characteristic and can be identified in the majority of cases. The LE cell was discovered in bone marrow by Hargraves et al. in 1948. The LE cell is a neutrophil or macrophage that has phagocytized (engulfed) the denatured nuclear material (hematoxylin body) of another cell. Denatured nuclear material in the neutrophil/macrophage has a glassy and homogeneous appearance; it may push the nuclei to the peripheral location. The hematoxylin body may be green, blue, or purple in color with the Papanicolaou stain and magenta color with the Diff-Quik stains. Cells contain nuclear material with visible chromatin structures (i.e., coarse chromatin pattern) are the so-called Tart cells; they are not LE cells.

A-99. **(d) All of the above**
In effusion as well as ascites and pericardial effusion, the presence of a second population of cells, numerous large clusters of cells, and lacunae spaces on cell block preparation is characteristic of a malignant

effusion. The cellularity in a malignant effusion may be markedly increased. Numerous tumor cell clusters are seen in the specimen. In addition to mesothelial cells, metastatic tumor cells represent a second cellular component in the fluid specimen. Lacuna is the empty space surrounding the tumor cell cluster on the cell block preparation. It has been reported that lacunae have been identified in 75 % of malignant effusions, particularly in adenocarcinomas.

A-100. (**b**) **False**

Lacuna is the empty space surrounding the tumor cell cluster on the cell block preparation. It is an artifact and has been found in 75 % of malignant effusions. The finding of lacunae at low magnification is helpful for identifying suspicious cells. Although it is a common finding in a malignant effusion, lacunae can also be seen in benign conditions. Therefore, evaluation of cells at high magnification is necessary to confirm the diagnosis of a malignant effusion.

Reading List

Abadi MA, Zakowski MF. Cytologic features of sarcoma in fluids. Cancer Cytopathol. 1998;84:71–6.

Bibbo M, Wood MD, Fitzpatrick BT. Peritoneal washings and ovary. In: Bibbo M, Wilbur D, editors. Comprehensive cytopathology. 3rd ed. Philadelphia: Saunders/Elsevier; 2008.

Cagle PT. Pleural histology. In: Light RW, Lee YCG, editors. Pleural disease: an international textbook. London, England: Arnold Publishers; 2003. p. 249–55.

Cibas ES. Peritoneal washings. In: Cibas ES, Ducatman BS, editors. Cytology: diagnostic principles and clinical correlates. Philadelphia: Saunders/Elsevier; 2009.

DeMay RM. The art and science of cytopathology, exfoliative cytology, vol. 1. 2nd ed. Chicago: ASCP Press; 2012.

Ellis CL, Burroughs F, Michael CW, Li QK. Cytology of metastatic renal medullary carcinoma in pleural effusion. A study of two cases. Diagn Cytopathol. 2009;37:843–8.

Gupta S, Sodhani P, Jain S. Cytomorphological profile of neoplastic effusions: an audit of 10 years with emphasis on uncommonly encountered malignancies. J Cancer Res Ther. 2012;8:602–9.

Henderson DW, Reid G, Kao SC, van Zandwijk N, Klebe S. Challenges and controversies in the diagnosis of mesothelioma: Part 1. Cytology-only diagnosis, biopsies, immunohistochemistry, discrimination between mesothelioma and reactive mesothelial hyperplasia, and biomarkers. J Clin Pathol. 2013;66(10):847–53.

Jing X, Li QK, Bedrossian U, Michael CW. Morphologic and immunmocytochemical performances of effusion cell blocks prepared using three different methods. Am J Clin Pathol. 2013;139:177–82.

Khalbuss WE, Yang H, Lian Q, Elhosseiny A, Pantanowitz L, Monaco SE. The cytomorphologic spectrum of small-cell carcinoma and large-cell neuroendocrine carcinoma in body cavity effusions: a study of 68 cases. Cytojournal. 2011;8:18.

Khalbuss WE, Monaco SE, Pantanowitz L. Chapter 9. Serous effusions. In: The ASCP quick compendium (QC) of cytopathology. Chicago: ASCP Press; 2013. p. 128–59.

Li Q, Bavikatty N, Michael CW. The role of immunohistochemistry in the distinguishing squamous cell carcinoma from mesothelioma and adenocarcinoma in pleural effusion. Semin Diagn Pathol. 2006;23:15–9.

Longatto-Filho A, Bisi H, Bortolan J, Granja NV, Lombardo V. Cytologic diagnosis of metastatic sarcoma in effusions. Acta Cytol. 2003;47:317–8.

Nauen D, Li QK. Cytological diagnosis of metastatic glioblastoma in the pleural effusion of a lung transplant patient. Diagn Cytopathol. 2014;42(7):619–23.

Stoll LM, Johnson MW, Gabrielson E, Askin F, Clark DP, Li QK. The utility of Napsin-A in the identification of primary and metastatic lung adenocarcinoma among cytologically "poorly differentiated carcinoma". Cancer Cytopathol. 2010;118:441–9.

Tong LC, Ko HM, Saieg MA, Boerner S, Geddie WR, da Cunha SG. Subclassification of lymphoproliferative disorders in serous effusions: a 10-year experience. Cancer Cytopathol. 2013;121:261–70.

Wheeler YR, Burroughs F, Li QK. Fine needle aspiration of a well-differentiated papillary mesothelioma in the hernia sac: case report and review of literature. Diagn Cytopathol. 2009;37:748–54.

Wojcik EM, Naylor B. "Collagen balls" in peritoneal washings. Prevalence, morphology, origin and significance. Acta Cytol. 1992;36(4):466–70.

3 Cerebrospinal Fluid (CSF) Cytology

Marilyn M. Bui, Ehab A. ElGabry, and Walid E. Khalbuss

Contents

3.1 Image-Based and Text-Based Questions 201

3.2 Answers and Discussion of Image-Based and Text-Based Questions 230

Reading List 239

M.M. Bui, MD, PhD. (✉)
Department of Anatomic Pathology, Moffitt Cancer Center (MCC), 12902 Magnolia Drive, Tampa, FL 33612, USA
e-mail: marilyn.bui@moffitt.org

E.A. ElGabry, MD.
University of Pittsburgh Medical Center (UPMC)-Shadyside, 5150 Centre Avenue; POB2, Suite 201, Pittsburgh, PA 15232, USA
e-mail: drgabry2013@gmail.com

W.E. Khalbuss, MD, PhD, FIAC.
Department of Pathology, GE Clarient Diagnostic Services, 31 Columbia, Aliso Viejo, California, 92656, USA
e-mail: Walid.khalbuss@ge.com

W.E. Khalbuss, Q.K. Li (eds.), *Diagnostic Cytopathology Board Review and Self-Assessment*, DOI 10.1007/978-1-4939-1477-7_3, © Springer Science+Business Media New York 2015

Table 3.1 CSF cytology: basic information

CSF is produced by the choroid plexus and reabsorbed by the arachnoid granulations into the venous system
CSF functions as a protective cushion for the entire CNS, collects waste products, circulates nutrients, and provides a stable ionic concentration for the CNS
Conditions that can be diagnosed by CSF cytology include primary tumors of the CNS or metastatic cancers, infectious diseases, inflammatory diseases or other immune responses, and bleeding within the brain or skull
Normal CSF smear is hypocellular or acellular which may show rare mononuclear cells (lymphocytes, monocytes) and few RBCs
Other components seen in CSF samples include neutrophils (traumatic), squamous cells, choroid plexus cells, ependymal cells, brain tissue, (neuropile) cartilage (chondrocytes), bone and soft tissue fragments (adipose tissue and muscle), bone marrow elements, and capillaries
Plasma cells in CSF are abnormal and may be seen in benign inflammatory conditions such as Lyme disease, or neoplastic conditions

Table 3.2 Cytomorphology of common malignancies in the CSF

Adenocarcinoma: Isolated large cells or small clusters; cells with abundant vacuolated, ill-defined cytoplasm, eccentric large nuclei, and prominent nucleoli
Small cell carcinoma: Single cells or clusters of small cells with nuclear molding, karyorrhexis, mitoses, marked pleomorphism, and inconspicuous nucleoli
Leukemia/lymphoma: Dispersed cells, atypical large hematopoietic cells (larger than normal lymphocytes), scant cytoplasm stains dark blue with Diff-Quik, irregular nuclear contours, abnormal immature chromatin, and multiple or prominent nucleoli
Melanoma: Large dyscohesive dispersed cells, binucleation, dusty cytoplasm with melanin pigment, cytoplasmic blebs, intranuclear inclusions, and prominent or giant nucleoli

3.1 Image-Based and Text-Based Questions

Fig. 3.1

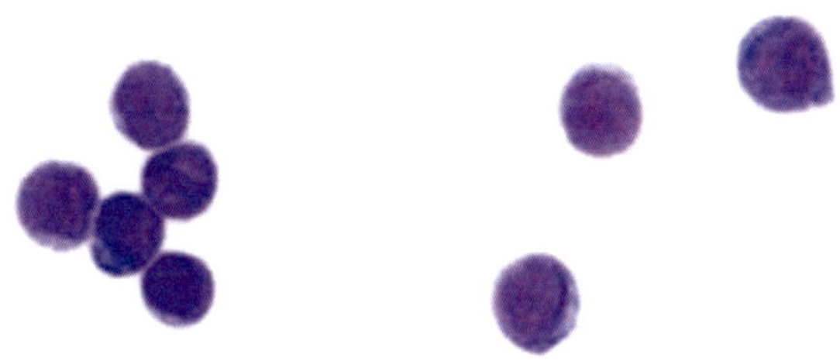

Q-1. A 28-year-old man was diagnosed with mixed type acute leukemia on bone marrow biopsy and aspiration two months ago. There was no CNS involvement at diagnosis. Now he complains of a headache for a day with roaring in his right ear. His CSF is examined on cytospin slide with DQ preparation under high-power field (×20). Flow cytometry demonstrates blasts which phenotypically express CD34, CD33, CD19, CD10, TdT, and MPO. CD34 + cells make up 38.6 % of gate population and approximately 8.62 % of total cells. What is the diagnosis?
(a) Acute leukemia
(b) Diffuse large B-cell lymphoma
(c) Hodgkin lymphoma
(d) Plasmacytoma

Q-2. Which answer regarding CNS involvement of leukemia is correct?
(a) CNS testing is useful for both the diagnosis and monitoring of the intrathecal chemotherapy effect.
(b) Acute lymphoblastic leukemia (ALL) is more common in adults than in children.
(c) Leukemic involvement of CNS presenting with large number of blasts in the CSF denotes significant parenchymal involvement.
(d) More than half of the leukemia patients present with CNS involvement at initial diagnosis.

Fig. 3.3

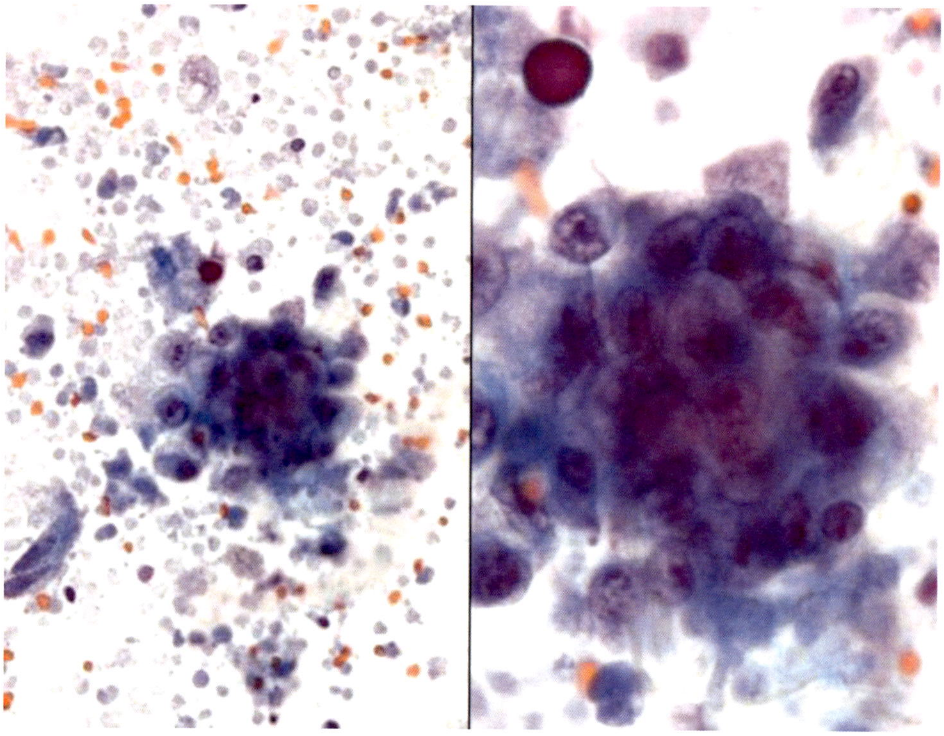

Q-3. A 69-year-old woman has a right temporal brain mass with cystic changes. Differential diagnosis includes neoplasm vs. abscess. Tumor cyst fluid cytology is examined on cytospin slide with PAP stain using medium power (left, ×40) and high power (right, ×100). What is the diagnosis?
(a) Acute inflammation
(b) Small cell carcinoma
(c) Chronic inflammation
(d) Metastatic adenocarcinoma

Fig. 3.4

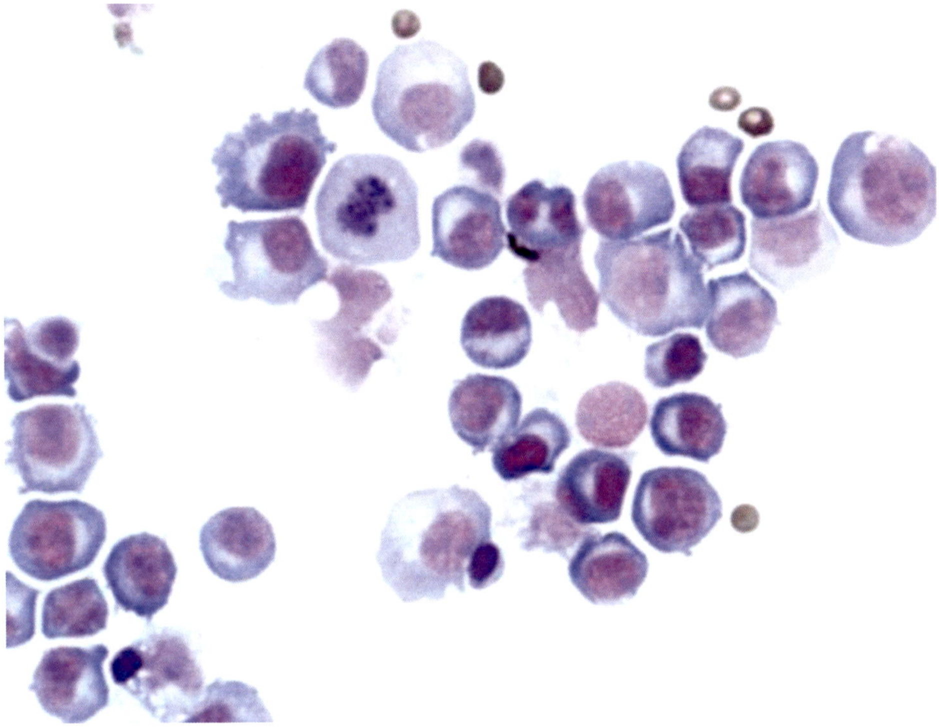

Q-4. A 58-year-old man has a history of autologous stem cell transplant for multiple myeloma. He also has a history of renal insufficiency, hypogonadism, and BK virus cystitis. The patient presents with new CNS symptoms. Examination of CNS specimen on DQ satin with high power (×60) reveals the following cells. What is the diagnosis?

(a) Melanoma
(b) Myeloma
(c) Inflammation
(d) Multiple sclerosis

Fig. 3.5

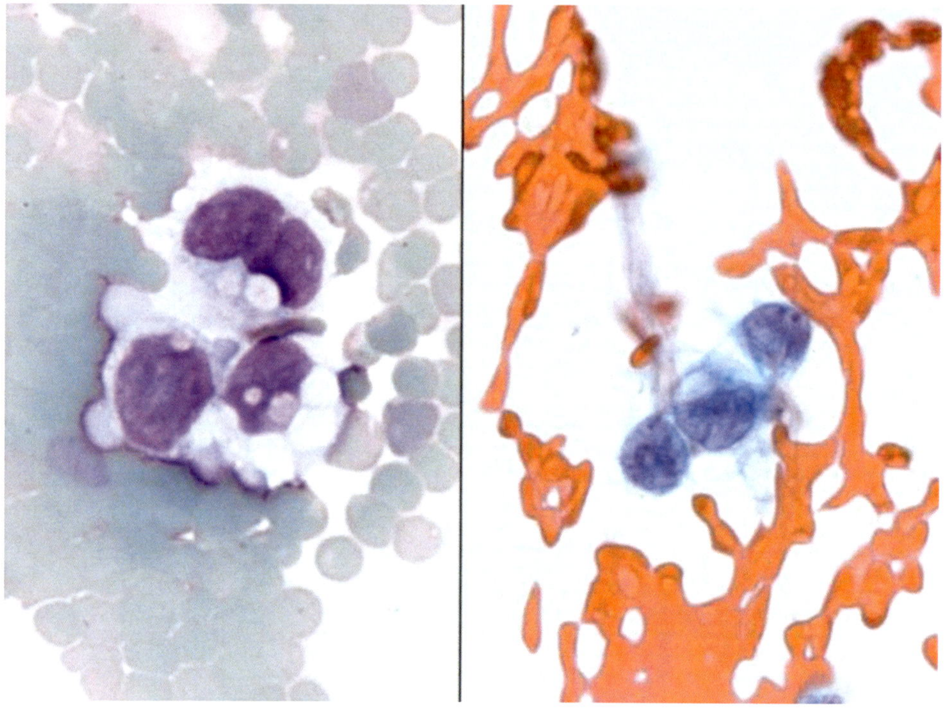

Q-5. A 67-year-old woman was seen by the neuro-oncology service for the evaluation of metastatic breast cancer with leptomeningeal spread of disease. She had a history of lobular carcinoma with focal pleomorphic features. The CSF is examined on DQ- and PAP-stained slides under high power (×100). What is the diagnosis?
(a) Atypical ependymal cells
(b) Metastatic melanoma
(c) Small cell carcinoma
(d) Metastatic adenocarcinoma of the breast

Fig. 3.6

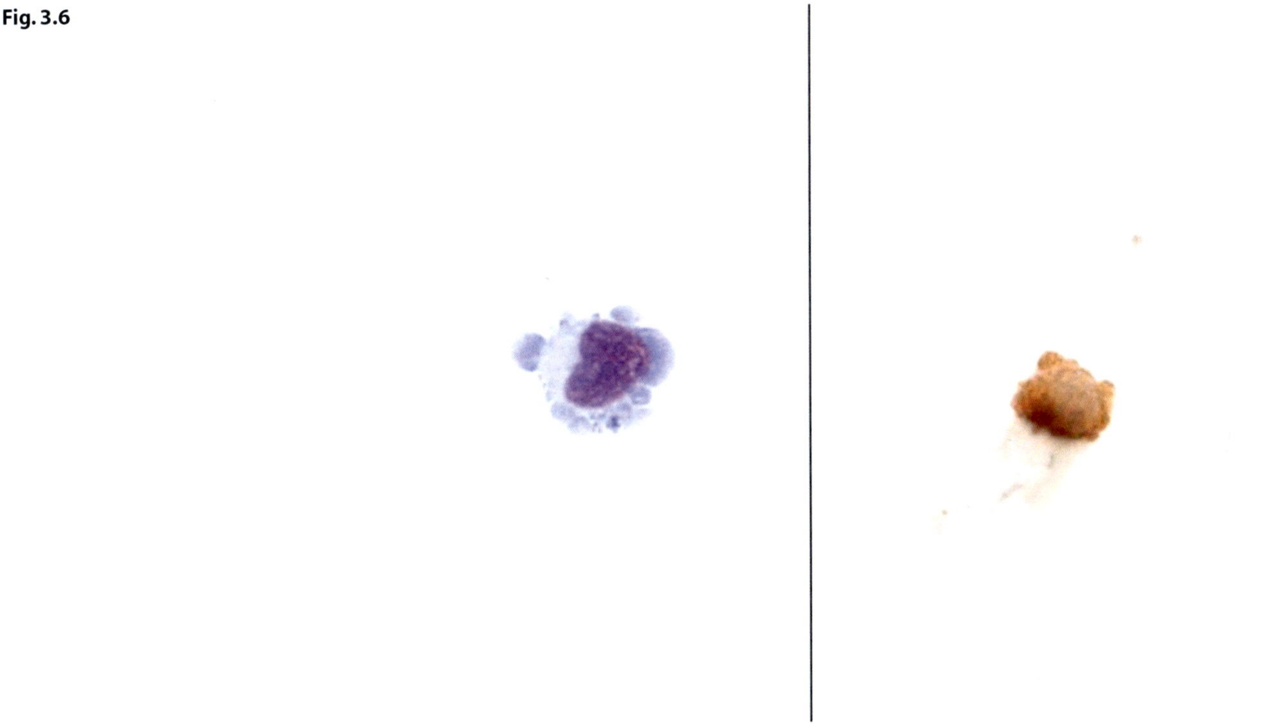

Q-6. A 50-year-old female has a history of stage 4 melanoma with predominant CNS disease. The patient has had whole brain radiotherapy as well as multiple prior treatments including Temodar and ipilimumab. Most recently the patient had an Ommaya reservoir placed with obstruction of flow. Hence, a repeat CSF sample is done. CSF cytology is examined by DQ stain (left) and S-100 immunostain (right) under high magnification (×100). What is the diagnosis?

(a) Metastatic adenocarcinoma
(b) Metastatic melanoma
(c) Lymphoma
(d) Small cell carcinoma

Fig. 3.7

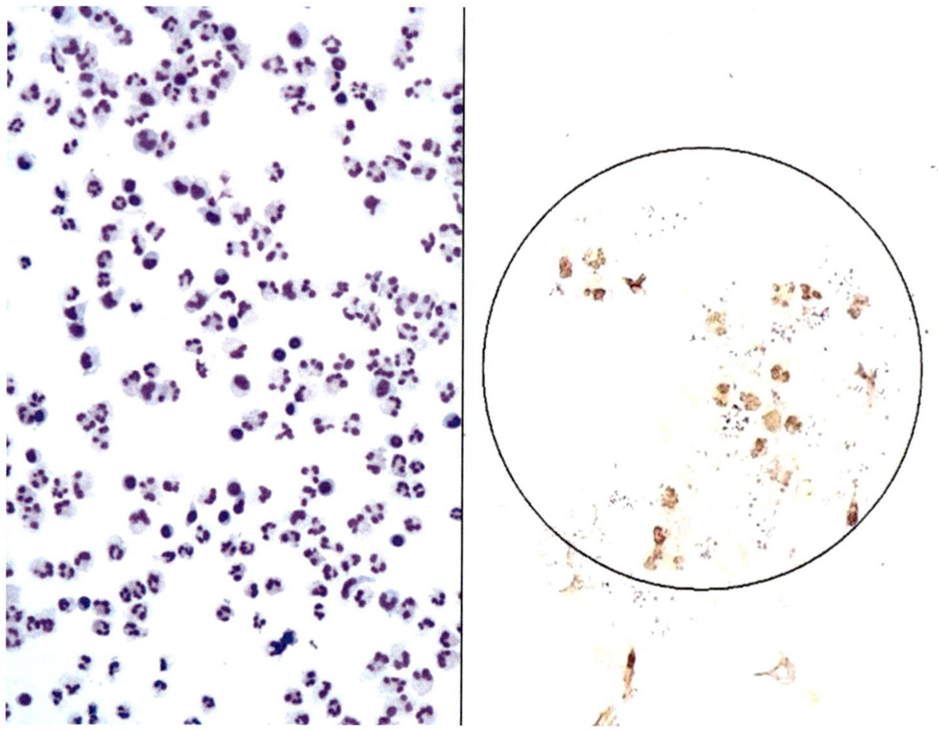

Q-7. A 44-year-old female with a history of non-small cell lung cancer developed leptomeningeal disease. She underwent placement of an Ommaya reservoir and began intrathecal chemotherapy. After her third dose of therapy, the patient stated having fevers as well as lethargy, fatigue, drainage from the Ommaya reservoir site. CSF tap was performed and was positive for Staphylococcus; accordingly the patient was placed on antibiotics. Per the recommendation of the Infectious Disease physician, the Ommaya was removed. After completing her antibiotic therapy and craniospinal radiation therapy, she came to the neuro-oncologist for follow-up visit. CSF tap was performed (DQ stain, left, ×10, right × 100). What is the diagnosis?
(a) Acute bacterial meningitis
(b) Metastatic adenocarcinoma
(c) Nondiagnostic
(d) Small cell carcinoma

Q-8. What is true about acute bacterial meningitis?
(a) Acute bacterial meningitis is not a life-threatening condition and does not need to be reported to the treating clinical team to render prompt treatment.
(b) Neonatal acute bacterial meningitis is caused by *Haemophilus influenzae* in 60–70 % of cases.
(c) Cytological examination of CSF showing predominantly neutrophils with the presence of intracellular or extracellular bacteria is diagnostic for acute bacterial meningitis.
(d) Haemophilus vaccine is effective against *meningococci*.

Q-9. A 75-year-old man with 50-year smoking history has not seen a physician for 20 years. He seeks medical attention in an Emergency Department because of headache, fever, meningismus, and altered mental status. His CNS cytology reveals numerous neutrophils and few large atypical epithelioid cells. All the following can cause neutrophilic pleocytosis except:
(a) Acute bacterial meningitis
(b) Cytomegalovirus radiculopathy
(c) Metastatic carcinoma
(d) Aseptic meningitis

Q-10. A CSF cytology reveals blood elements only. No lymphocytes or monocytes are seen. What is the diagnosis?
(a) Unsatisfactory
(b) Negative for malignancy
(c) Positive for malignancy
(d) Atypical

Q-11. A 58-year-old female has B-cell acute lymphoblastic leukemia (Philadelphia chromosome positive) with CNS involvement. She received induction intrathecal chemotherapy. The PAP stain of CSF reveals mainly red blood cells with rare lymphocytes and monocytes. No blasts are seen. What is the diagnosis?
(a) Unsatisfactory due to peripheral blood contamination
(b) Negative for malignancy
(c) Positive for malignancy
(d) Atypical

Q-12. A CSF cytology reveals few benign lymphocytes and monocytes. There are no red blood cells in the background. What is the diagnosis?
(a) Unsatisfactory
(b) Negative for malignancy
(c) Positive for malignancy
(d) Atypical

Q-13. Which statement is correct regarding the components of CSF?
(a) Macrophages, plasma cells, and eosinophils are a normal finding of CSF.
(b) Hypercellular benign lymphocytes are a normal finding of CSF.
(c) Ependymal cells, choroid plexus, brain fragments, and megakaryocytes are common normal elements in CSF.
(d) Neutrophils are a normal finding if there is contamination from peripheral blood.

Fig. 3.14

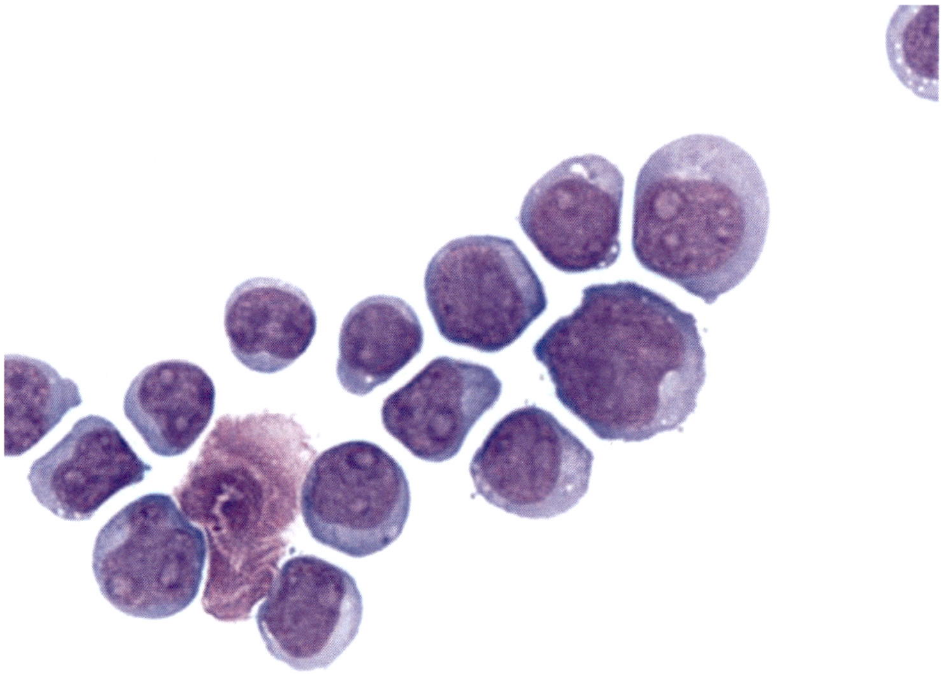

Q-14. A 49-year-old male with history of gastric lymphoma diagnosis now presents with headache. This is his finding in CNS cytology (DQ stain, ×100) after lumbar puncture. What is the diagnosis?
(a) Chronic inflammation
(b) Diffuse large B-cell lymphoma
(c) Small cell carcinoma
(d) Metastatic carcinoma

Q-15. Which statement is correct?
(a) The most common malignancy in CSF is metastatic carcinoma, followed by melanoma, and leukemia/lymphoma.
(b) Meningioma is more likely to involve CNS than glioma and medulloblastoma.
(c) Most frequent leukemia in CSF is not acute lymphoblastic leukemia.
(d) Acute myeloid leukemia is more common in CSF than acute lymphoblastic leukemia.

Fig. 3.16

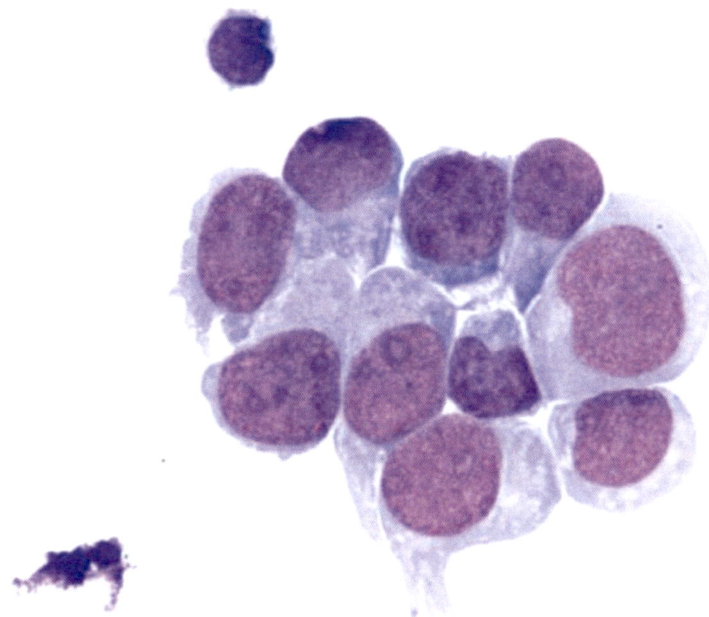

Q-16. This CSF was obtained from a 19-year-old female with anaplastic large cell lymphoma. What are the cytomorphological features supporting the diagnosis of CNS involvement by anaplastic large cell lymphoma?
(a) Hypercellular specimen with large number of mature lymphocytes
(b) Large immature lymphocytes with abundant cytoplasm and pleomorphic horseshoe-shaped nuclei
(c) Medium-sized immature lymphocytes with round nuclei of clumped chromatin and deeply basophilic cytoplasm with abundant lipid vacuoles
(d) Large epithelioid cells with intracytoplasmic mucin

Fig. 3.17

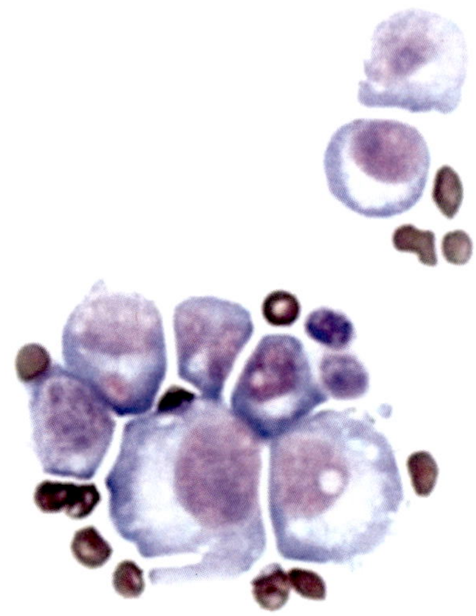

Q-17. A 68-year-old female with a histology of stage III IgG lambda multiple myeloma status post stem cell transplant recently presented with nausea and vomiting. Subsequently, the patient got hospitalized to assess CNS involvement. CSF cytology is shown here (DQ, ×60). What is the diagnosis?
(a) Metastatic adenocarcinoma
(b) Ependymoma
(c) Multiple myeloma
(d) Chronic inflammation

Q-18. What is the most commonly identified fungus in cerebrospinal fluid specimens?
(a) *Candida albicans*
(b) *Histoplasma capsulatum*
(c) *Blastomyces dermatitidis*
(d) *Cryptococcus neoformans*

Q-19. A hypercellular CSF specimen that is predominantly mature lymphocytes may be related to:
(a) Acute bacterial meningitis
(b) Multiple sclerosis
(c) Chronic, subacute, or viral meningitis
(d) Lymphoma or leukemia involvement of CNS

Q-20. What is the most common neuronal element seen in CSF specimens that has vacuolated and pigmented cytoplasm with small, eccentric, and vesicular nuclei:
(a) Leptomeningeal cells
(b) Ependymal cells
(c) Neurons
(d) Nucleus pulposus cells

Q-21. All of the following are proper indications for CSF cytology except:
(a) Meningitis
(b) Metastatic neoplastic disease
(c) Monitoring intrathecal chemotherapy
(d) Neurosyphilis

Q-22. What is the ideal amount of CSF necessary for proper cytological evaluation of patients with suspected CNS malignancy?
(a) 1 ml
(b) 3 ml
(c) 5 ml
(d) 10 ml

Q-23. If lymphoma is suspected, what is the best CSF cytology preparation?
(a) Alcohol-fixed Papanicolaou-stained slides
(b) Air-dried Wright-stained slides
(c) Alcohol-fixed DQ-stained slides
(d) Air-dried Papanicolaou-stained slides

Fig. 3.24

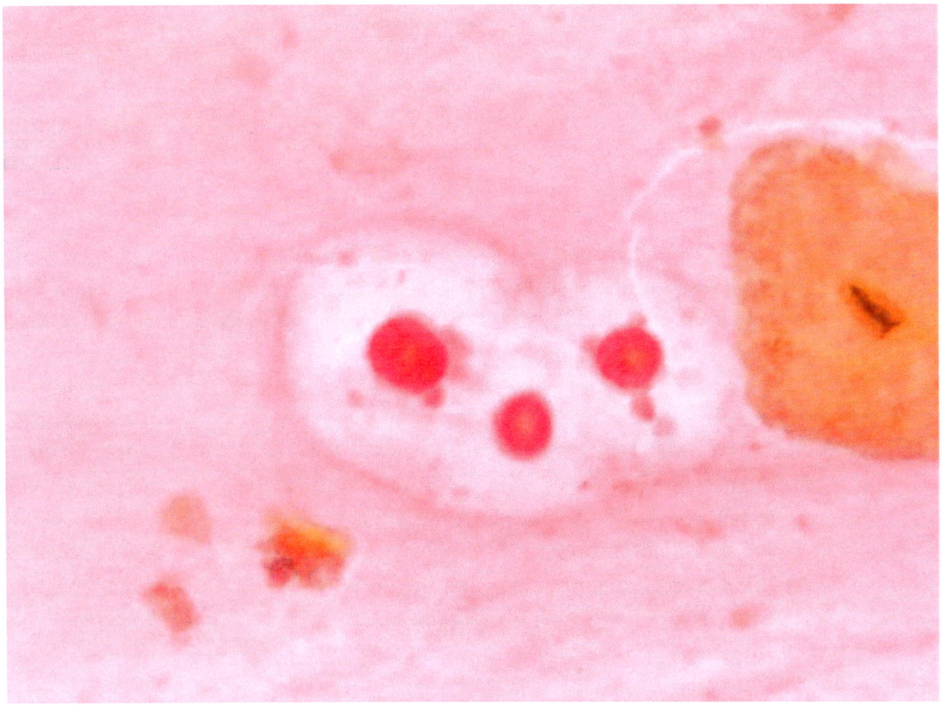

Q-24. This mucin stain reveals round yeast-like structures (5–10 μm in diameter) with distinctive mucinous capsules (positive for mucicarmine stain). What is the organism?
(a) *Candida albicans*
(b) *Histoplasma capsulatum*
(c) *Blastomyces dermatitidis*
(d) *Cryptococcus neoformans*

Q-25. All of the following statements are correct, except:
(a) CSF is positive for malignant cells in about 60 % of specimens from patients with leptomeningeal involvement of their tumor.
(b) The sensitivity depends on multiple factors including the number of specimens examined, the volume and freshness of the specimen, and the extent of leptomeningeal or ventricular involvement by tumor.
(c) A CNS tumor will not result in a positive CSF unless it invades into a ventricle or the subarachnoid spaces.
(d) False-positive diagnoses are estimated at 10 %.

Q-26. The most common cause of a false-positive diagnosis is overdiagnosis of:
(a) Lymphoma or leukemia
(b) Metastatic carcinoma
(c) Primary CNS neoplasm
(d) Metastatic sarcoma

Q-27. What is occasionally seen in benign CSF of neonates that mimics a small cell malignancy such as medulloblastoma?
(a) Immature cells of germinal matrix origin
(b) Lymphoid cells
(c) Choroid plexus/ependymal cells
(d) Histiocytes

Q-28. CSF macrophages are common findings in all of the following except:
(a) Subarachnoid or intraventricular hemorrhage
(b) Multiple sclerosis
(c) Therapy changes
(d) Tuberculosis meningitis

Q-29. The most commonly encountered cancers in CSF are:
(a) Metastatic carcinoma
(b) Metastatic melanoma
(c) CNS lymphoma
(d) CNS malignancy

Q-30. Which statement is correct regarding CSF specimens?
(a) Primary lymphoma is more common than secondary lymphoma.
(b) Primary CNS tumors are more common than metastatic tumors.
(c) Lymphoblastic lymphoma leukemia and Burkitt lymphoma more commonly involve CNS than Hodgkin lymphoma and small lymphocytic lymphoma.

(d) Most common adult primary CNS tumors include anaplastic astrocytoma, glioblastoma multiforme, primary CNS lymphoma, and medulloblastoma.

Q-31. Which of the following statements is incorrect?
(a) CSF is an ultrafiltrate of plasma produced by ependyma.
(b) CSF flows from the ventricles to the subarachnoid space which is lined by leptomeninges.
(c) CSF is reabsorbed by the arachnoid granulations into venous system.
(d) The CSF cycle renews 10–12 times daily.

Q-32. Which is not a normal function of CSF?
(a) A protective cushion for CNS
(b) A mechanism to circulate nutrients and provide a stable ionic concentration for CNS
(c) Provide extra space in case of brain hemorrhage or bleeding
(d) A waste collection venue for CNS

Q-33. What is the most important diagnostic role of CSF cytology in patients with neurologic symptoms?
(a) Brain hemorrhage or bleeding
(b) Leptomeningeal metastasis
(c) Infectious diseases include meningitis and encephalitis
(d) Multiple sclerosis

Q-34. Which statement is true?
(a) The total volume of CSF in children is 100 ml.
(b) The ideal volume for CSF cytological examination is 3 ml.
(c) The total volume of CSF in adult is approximately 100 ml.
(d) Approximately 500 ml CSF is produced daily in adults.

Q-35. CSF is most commonly obtained from the following locations:
(a) Intervertebral space at L3–L4 or L4–L5
(b) Cisterna magna at the base of the brain
(c) Lateral ventricle
(d) Ommaya reservoir

Q-36. Which of the following is not appropriate collection procedure for CSF cytology?
(a) The fresh fluid should be prepared less than 1 h.
(b) For delayed preparation, the fluid should be refrigerated at 4 °C.
(c) If delayed preparation is more than 48 h, equal volume of 50 % ethanol is added for preservation.
(d) If delayed preparation is more than 48 h, the specimen should be kept frozen.

Q-37. Which statement is not correct regarding CSF preparation?
(a) Peripheral blood contamination is best detected on alcohol-fixed slides.
(b) Cytocentrifugation can yield good-quality air-dried and alcohol-fixed slides.
(c) CSF is most commonly prepared by centrifugation (cytospin).
(d) Hematopoietic cells are best evaluated using air-dried DQ-/Wright-stained slides.

Q-38. Which statement regarding the accuracy of CSF cytology for meningeal malignancy is true?
(a) The sensitivity is approximately 90 %.
(b) The sensitivity is not related to the site from which the sample is obtained.
(c) The false-positive rate is approximately 2–3 %.
(d) The specificity is 90 %.

Q-39. What is the diagnosis for a CSF specimen that contains only a small number of mature lymphocytes and monocytes?
(a) Negative
(b) Unsatisfactory
(c) Atypical
(d) Positive

Q-40. Blasts are identified in CSF cytology specimen in a patient with history of leukemia. Which of the following is diagnostic for CNS involvement of the leukemia, not peripheral blood contaminant?
(a) There are red blood cells identified in the CSF.
(b) There are no red blood cells identified in the CSF.
(c) There are no red blood cell identified in the CSF, and the cell count is similar to the blood.
(d) There are no red blood cell identified in the CSF, and the cell count is different from the blood.

Fig. 3.41

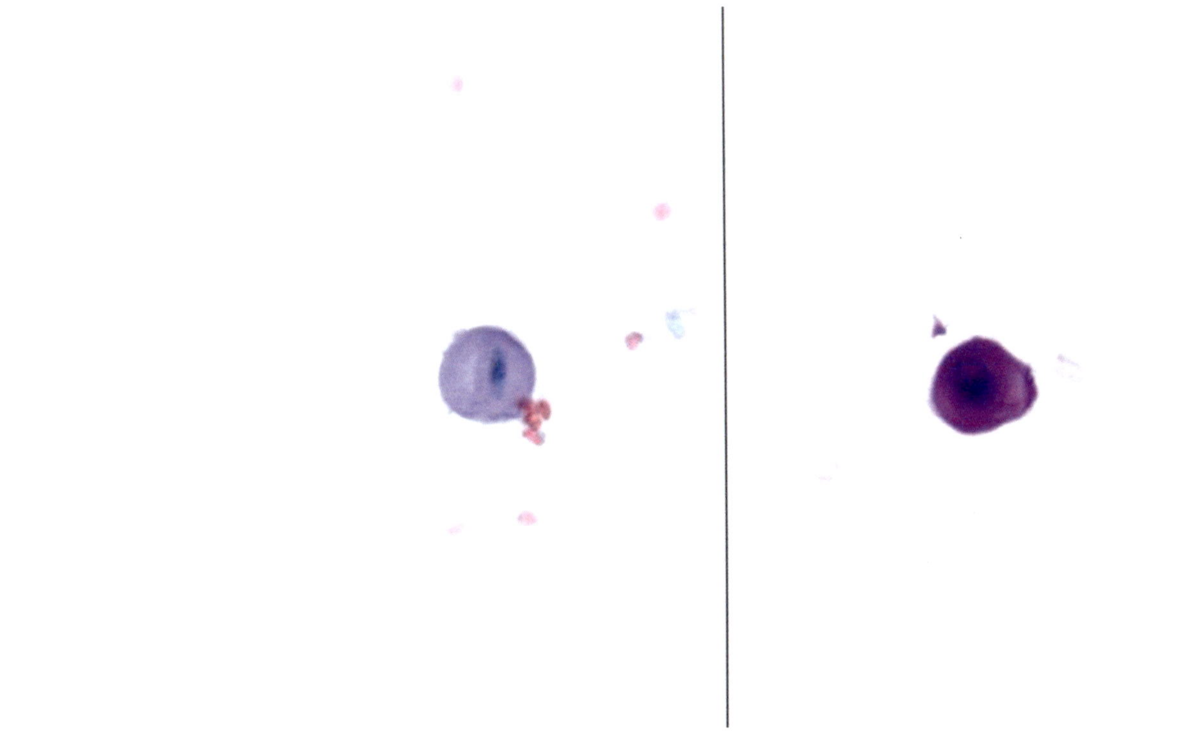

Q-41. This cell in a CSF specimen represents which of the following?
(a) Squamous cell
(b) CMV-infected cell
(c) Chondrocyte
(d) Foreign material

Fig. 3.42

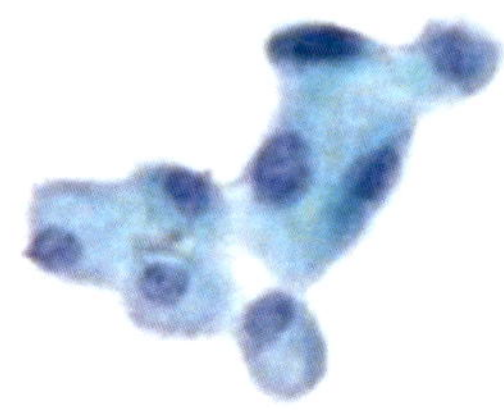

Q-42. These cells in a CSF specimen represent which of the following?
(a) Macrophages
(b) Adenocarcinoma
(c) Ependymal cells
(d) Neurons

Fig. 3.43

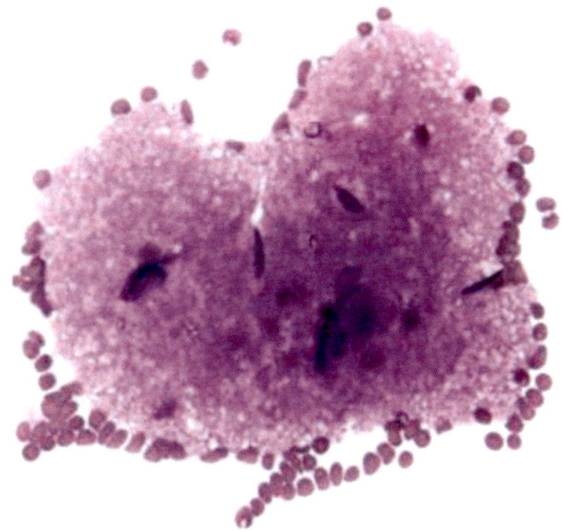

Q-43. The bluish material in this CSF specimen represents which of the following?
(a) Brain tissue
(b) Granuloma
(c) *Pneumocystis carinii*
(d) Histiocytes

Fig. 3.44

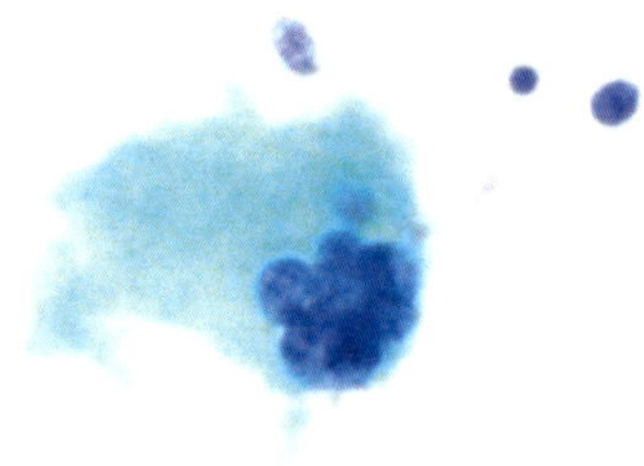

Q-44. This cell in a CSF specimen represents which of the following?
(a) Histiocyte
(b) Osteoclast
(c) Megakaryocyte
(d) Carcinoma

Fig. 3.45

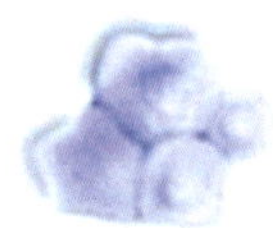

Q-45. These structures in a CSF specimen represent which of the following?
(a) Corpora amylacea
(b) *Cryptococcus neoformans*
(c) Starch granules
(d) Talc

Q-46. Which statement is not correct?
(a) CSF cytology is mainly used to diagnose CNS primary tumor at initial presentation.
(b) Primary CNS tumor includes lymphoma.
(c) Primary CNS tumor includes atypical teratoid/rhabdoid tumor.
(d) Primary CNS tumor includes germ cell tumor.

Q-47. Which tumor is most commonly diagnosed by CSF cytology?
(a) Pineoblastoma
(b) Ependymoma
(c) Astrocytoma and glioblastoma multiforme
(d) Medulloblastoma

Q-48. Which is true regarding lymphoma in to CNS?
(a) The most common type of primary CNS lymphoma is Hodgkin lymphoma.
(b) Non-primary CNS lymphomas are mostly low-grade lymphomas (DLBL).
(c) Tprimary CNS DLBL is EBV positive in immunocompetent Pahent.
(d) Large B-cell lymphoma cells exhibit extreme nuclear irregularity.

Fig. 3.49

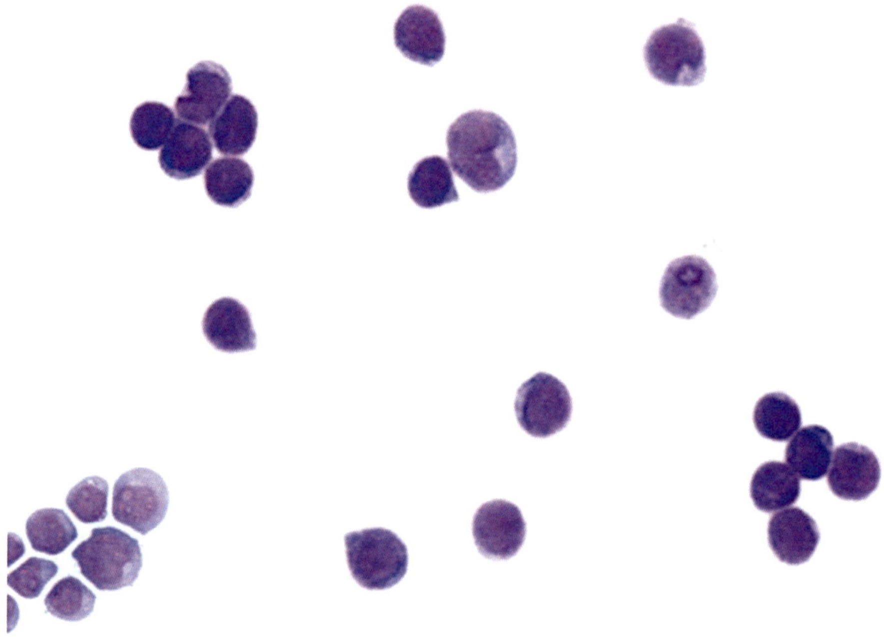

Q-49. A 50-year-old female with history of diffuse large B-cell lymphoma, stage 4A, is status post chemotherapy. Her CSF specimen reveals the following (DQ stain, ×60). Which infections agent is associated with this Condition?

(a) HIV
(b) CMV
(c) EBV
(d) Herpes

Q-50. Which of the following primary CNS tumors exhibit large cell morphology?

(a) Glioblastoma multiforme
(b) Medulloblastoma
(c) Pineoblastoma
(d) Primitive neuroectodermal tumors (PNETs)

Fig. 3.51

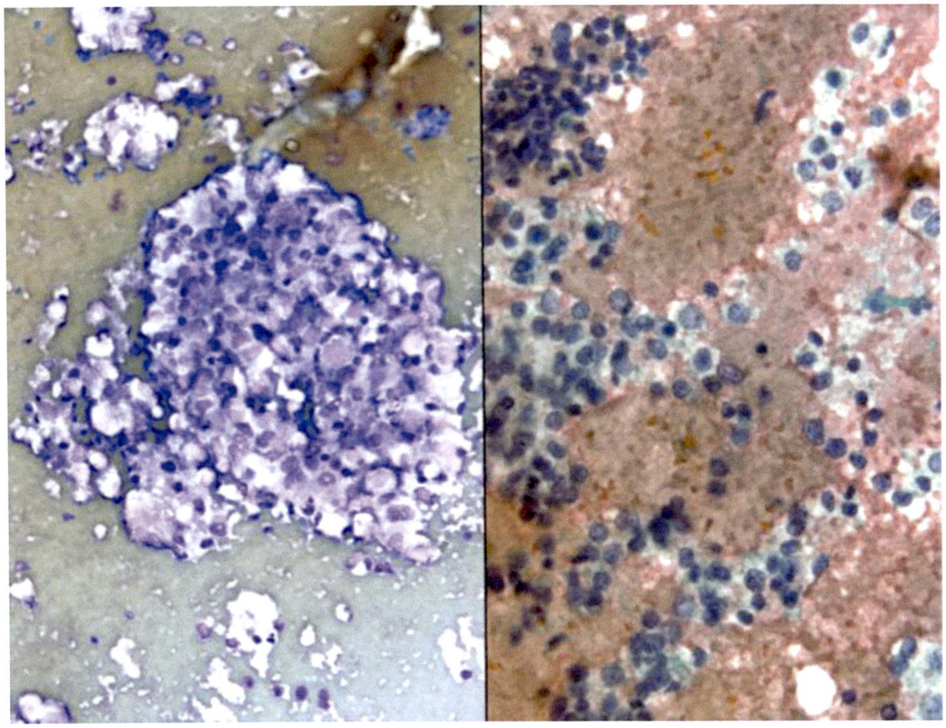

Q-51. The cells in this CSF specimen represent which of the following?
(a) Low-grade astrocytoma
(b) High-grade astrocytoma
(c) Medulloblastoma
(d) Lymphoma

Q-52. All the following lesions may cytologically resemble medulloblastoma except:
(a) Small cell carcinoma
(b) Neuroblastoma
(c) Retinoblastoma
(d) Melanoma

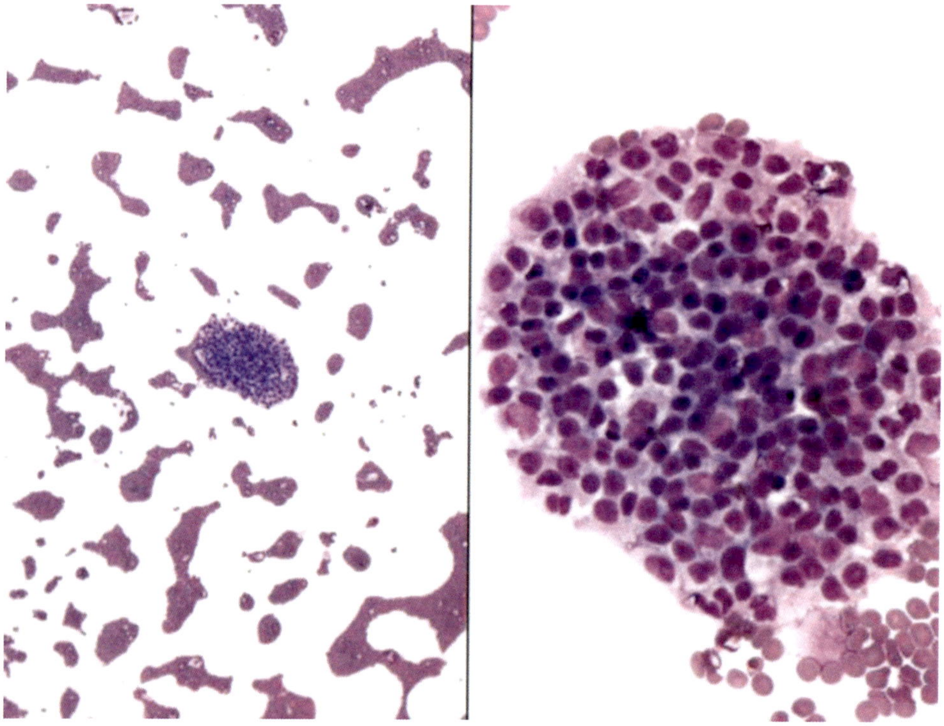

Fig. 3.53

Q-53. The cells shown in this CSF specimen represent which of the following?
(a) Medulloblastoma
(b) Melanoma
(c) Carcinoma
(d) Astrocytoma

Q-54. Which immunostains are helpful in the diagnosis of medulloblastoma on CSF cellblock?
(a) Cytokeratin positive/neuroendocrine markers positive
(b) GFAP positive/neuroendocrine markers positive
(c) Cytokeratin negative/neuroendocrine markers positive/high proliferation index of Ki-67
(d) Neuroendocrine markers positive/high proliferation index of Ki-67

Q-55. An adolescent patient has a history of a germ cell tumor. His CSF cytology shows large polygonal cells with round nuclei, prominent nucleoli, and coarse chromatin. The background is composed of mature lymphocytes. What is the diagnosis?
(a) Hodgkin lymphoma
(b) Germinoma
(c) Diffuse large B-cell lymphoma
(d) Melanoma

Q-56. Which of the following cytomorphological features is most important in the diagnosis of melanoma involving CSF?
(a) Large, dispersed cells; some are plasmacytoid.
(b) Binucleation, some with intranuclear cytoplasmic inclusion
(c) Dusty cytoplasm or melanin pigment
(d) Prominent macronucleoli

Q-57. Which of the following statements is correct?
(a) Medulloblastoma is the most common primary CNS tumor detected by CSF cytology in adult.
(b) Astrocytoma is the most common primary CNS tumor detected by CSF cytology in children.
(c) Medulloblastoma is usually located in the cerebellum.
(d) Ependymoma is usually located in the fourth ventricle.

Q-58. Macrophages in CSF are not associated with:
(a) Multiple sclerosis
(b) Acute meningitis
(c) Subarachnoid and intraventricular hemorrhage
(d) Malignancy

Q-59. A CSF specimen shows few plasma cells. Which of the statements regarding plasma cells in CSF is correct?
- (a) It is indicative of myeloma.
- (b) It is an abnormal but nonspecific finding in CSF.
- (c) It is indicative of cerebral infarction.
- (d) It is indicative of CMV radiculopathy.

Q-60. Which of the following is not a differential diagnosis of eosinophils in CSF?
- (a) Toxoplasma meningoencephalitis
- (b) *Coccidioides immitis*
- (c) Rocky Mountain spotted fever
- (d) Ventriculoperitoneal shunts

Q-61. Which of the statements regarding Mollaret meningitis is false?
- (a) Mollaret meningitis is a form of recurrent aseptic meningitis.
- (b) It is related to herpes simplex viruses 1 and 2.
- (c) CSF cytology shows predominant lymphocytes.
- (d) Mollaret cells are characteristic of but not specific for Mollaret meningitis.

Q-62. Which of the following is a false statement about fungal meningitis caused by *Cryptococcus neoformans*?
- (a) This is mostly seen in patients with a debilitated or immunocompromised state.
- (b) *Cryptococcus* usually appears as round yeast forms measuring from 1 to 2 microns with a refractive center.
- (c) A mucin stain will highlight the narrow neck budding.
- (d) *Cryptococcal* antigen can often be detected in the CSF.

Fig. 3.63

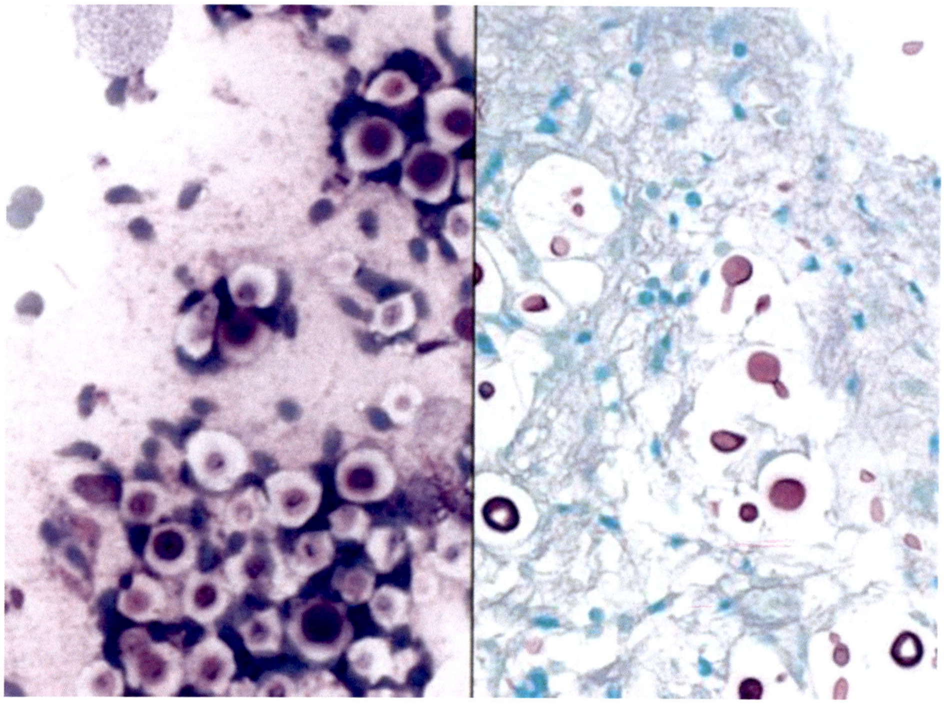

Q-63. What structures do these images represent from a CSF specimen?
(a) Starch granules
(b) Artifact
(c) *Cryptococcus neoformans*
(d) *Histoplasma capsulatum*

Fig. 3.64

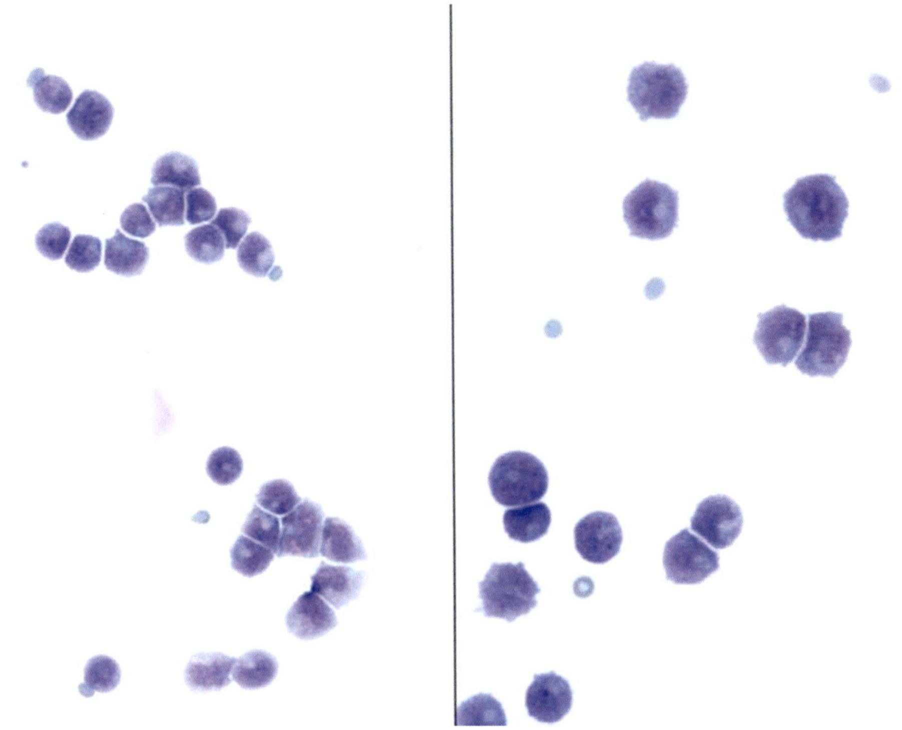

Q-64. What is false regarding this neoplasm involving CSF?
(a) It is less common in the CSF than acute lymphoblastic leukemia.
(b) The Diff-Quik stain is the ideal stain for AML specimens.
(c) The blasts are large cells with round or highly irregular nucleus, fine immature chromatin, and prominent nucleoli.
(d) They are blasts.

Q-65. A 65-year-old woman has a history of breast cancer and lung cancer. She recently presented with hemiparesis. Her CSF cytology reveals loose clusters of cells with hyperchromatic nuclei, irregular nuclear membranes, macronucleoli, and dense squamoid cytoplasm. What is the most likely primary site/type of tumor that involves her CSF?
(a) Lung/adenocarcinoma
(b) Breast/adenocarcinoma
(c) Lung/squamous cell carcinoma
(d) Breast/squamous cell carcinoma

Fig. 3.66

Q-66. Hemosiderin-laden macrophages (siderophages) are an indication of the following condition:
(a) Melanoma
(b) Tuberculous meningitis
(c) Intracranial hemorrhage
(d) Megakaryocytes

Q-67. What percentage of CSF specimens are negative?
(a) 90 %
(b) 80 %
(c) 70 %
(d) 60 %

Q-68. A CSF specimen is obtained from a premature neonate. It reveals rare clusters of small immature cells adjacent to hemosiderin-laden macrophages. They are molded to one another. What are these cells most likely to be?
(a) Medulloblastoma
(b) Ependymal cells
(c) Glial cells
(d) Germinal matrix

Q-69. Plasma cells within the CSF may be associated with all of the following except:
(a) Cerebral infarction
(b) Lyme disease
(c) Multiple sclerosis
(d) Syphilis

Q-70. Which of the following diagnoses reflect a rare form of aseptic meningitis that is associated with herpes simplex virus and presents with recurring attacks of fever, headache, and neck stiffness?
(a) Lymphocytic choriomeningitis
(b) Mollaret meningitis
(c) Acute bacterial meningitis
(d) Aseptic meningitis

Q-71. A CSF specimen shows eosinophilia (>80 % eosinophils). Which of the following is associated with eosinophilia?
(a) Cysticercosis
(b) Toxoplasmosis
(c) Ventriculoperitoneal shunts
(d) Tuberculosis

Q-72. Which of the following choices describe the most common malignancies that are associated with CNS metastases?
(a) Squamous cell carcinoma and sarcoma
(b) Lung cancer, breast cancer, and melanoma
(c) Melanoma and lymphoma
(d) Lung cancer, gastric cancer, breast cancer, and melanoma

Q-73. A CSF cytospin reveals a cellular specimen composed of a monomorphic population of large cells with high N:C ratio, fine chromatin, and prominent

nucleoli, and cytoplasmic granules in a background of abundant red blood cells. This likely represents which of the following?
(a) Melanoma involving the CSF
(b) Plasma cell myeloma
(c) Leukemic cells involves CSF
(d) Peripherally circulating leukemic cells within CSF

Q-74. What is the most common primary CNS neoplasm encountered in CSF cytology?
(a) Meningioma and ependymoma
(b) Medulloblastoma and high-grade astrocytoma
(c) Ependymoma and lymphoma
(d) Germ cell tumor and astrocytoma

Q-75. A patient presents with headache. His medical history included "a blood malignancy." The CSF cytology reveals numbers of atypical lymphoid cells. What is the most appropriate ancillary study for this specimen?
(a) Microbiological culture
(b) Immunohistochemistry
(c) Fungal stain
(d) Flow cytometry

Q-76. A CSF cytology is suggestive of infection of *Cryptococcus neoformans*. What is the best ancillary test to confirm the diagnosis?
(a) Fungal stain
(b) Mucin stain
(c) *Cryptococcus* testing
(d) Immunocytochemistry

Fig. 3.77

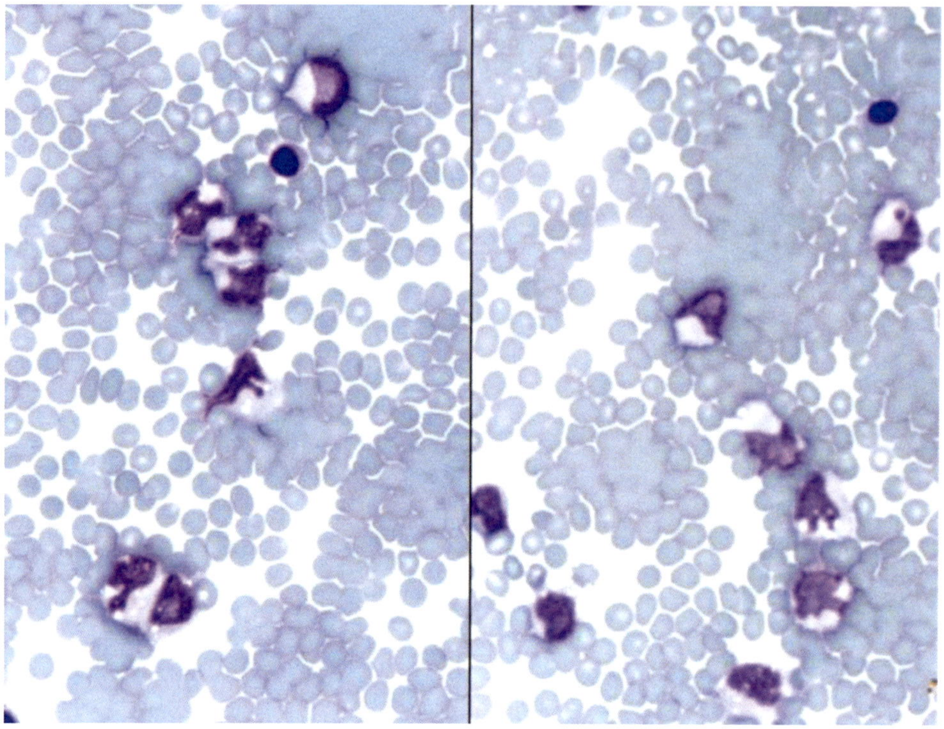

Q-77. Which of the following is the most likely diagnosis in this CSF (image above) from a patient who presented with recurring attacks of fever, headache, and neck stiffness?

(a) Lymphocytic choriomeningitis
(b) Lymphoma
(c) Acute bacterial meningitis
(d) Mollaret meningitis

Fig. 3.78

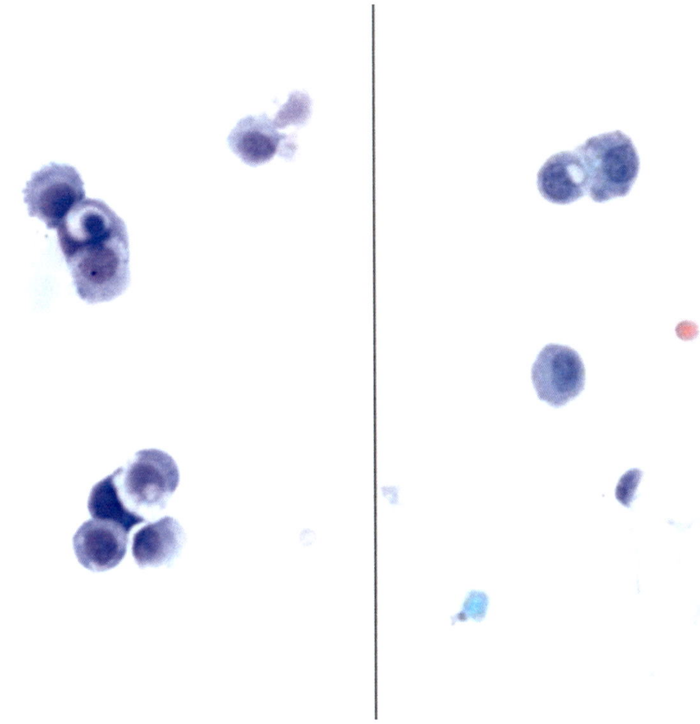

Q-78. What is the most likely diagnosis in this CSF specimen?
(a) Adenocarcinoma
(b) Lymphoma
(c) Squamous cell carcinoma
(d) Ependymal cells

Fig. 3.79

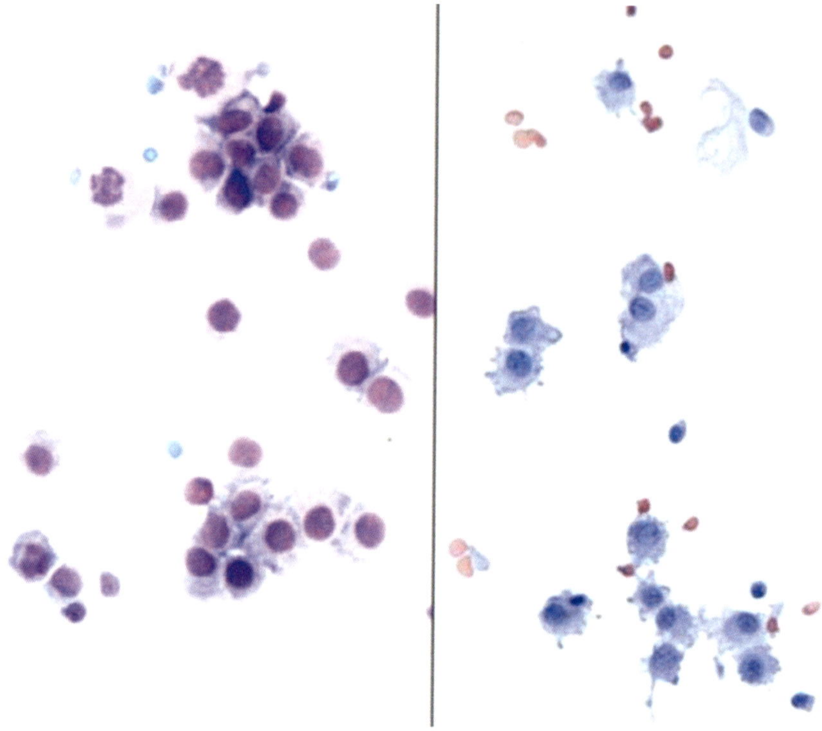

Q-79. What is the most likely diagnosis in this CSF specimen from patient who has history of melanoma?
(a) Adenocarcinoma
(b) Lymphoma
(c) Melanoma
(d) Atypical lymphocytes

Fig. 3.80

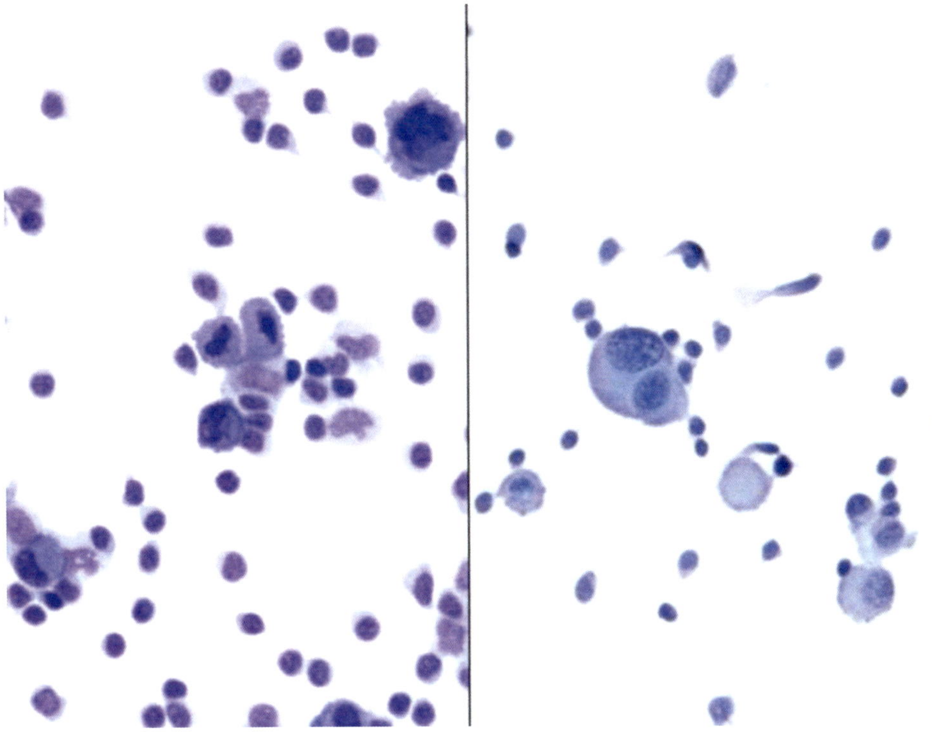

Q-80. What is the most likely diagnosis in this CSF specimen with large cells and lymphocytosis?
(a) Adenocarcinoma
(b) Lymphoma
(c) Melanoma
(d) Atypical lymphocytes vs. aseptic meningitis

3.2 Answers and Discussion of Image-Based and Text-Based Questions

A-1. **Answer Key: (a). Acute leukemia**
Cytospin preparation demonstrates a predominance of immature myeloid cells admixed with monocytes and occasional granulocytes. There is no background of peripheral blood contamination. Blasts are medium in size and show lacy or immature chromatin, irregular nuclei, and prominent nucleoli. There is moderate amount of cytoplasm; some contain cytoplamic vacuoles. In conjunction, the clinical history, flow cytometry result, and the overall morphological and immunophenotypical findings are consistent with B-myeloid leukemia. For acute myeloid leukemia, characteristic morphological features can be recognized with a DQ stain. CSF testing for leukemia involvement is for both initial diagnosis and relapse.

A-2. **Answer Key: (a) CNS testing is useful for the diagnosis (initial diagnosis and relapse) and monitoring of the intrathecal chemotherapy effect.**
Only 5 % of leukemia patients exhibit CNS involvement at initial diagnosis. More than 50 % of leukemia patients will develop CNS involvement without prophylaxis. Acute lymphoblastic leukemia (ALL) is more common in children than in adults. Although in most cases, a large number of blasts can be detected in CSF, leukemic involvement of the CNS has little or no parenchyma involvement. Therefore, CNS testing is useful for the initial diagnosis of CNS involvement, relapse, and monitoring of the intrathecal chemotherapy effect.

A-3. **Answer Key: (d). Metastatic adenocarcinoma**
In a female patient, the most common carcinoma is breast cancer but the most common fatal cancer is lung cancer. Both cancers may involve CNS at end stage causing meningeal carcinomatosis. The most common types of lung carcinoma metastasis to CNS are small cell carcinoma and adenocarcinoma. Squamous cell carcinomas of the lung rarely metastasize to the CNS.

Adenocarcinoma cells in CSF are dysplastic epithelioid cells arranged in single cells or 3-D clusters. Detection of mucinous vacuoles is diagnostic; additional features include vacuolated cytoplasm and prominent nucleoli. Cellblock (not shown here) reveals a moderdely differentiated adenocarcinoma. Immunostains of the cellblock (not shown here) reveal that tumor cells are positive for CK7 and TTF-1, supporting the diagnosis of metastatic adenocarcinoma of the lung.

A-4. **Answer Key: (b). Myeloma**
The specimen is hypercellular with individually dispersed highly atypical plasmacytoid cells. The cells have eccentrically located nuclei with distinct perinuclear hofs (melanoma cells lack this feature), some with prominent nucleoli. The chromatin is coarsely clumped. The cytoplasm is abundant. Binucleation and mitotic activity are seen. These features are characteristic for myeloma.

Normal plasma cells are not seen in the CSF except in inflammatory CNS diseases such as viral infections and neurosyphilis. Plasmacytosis with immature forms can be seen in patients with multiple sclerosis and cerebral cysticercosis. Therefore, the presence of atypical plasma cells alone does not make the diagnosis of meningeal myeloma.

Multiple myeloma uncommonly involves the meninges and manifests in CNS. Clinical history, bone marrow, serological, and flow cytometry studies are warranted to confirm meningeal myeloma. On the other hand, primary CNS myeloma without bone marrow or serological findings has been reported, whereby cytological examination of CSF with flow cytometry study has proven very useful in establishing a definitive diagnosis.

A-5. **Answer Key: (d). Metastatic adenocarcinoma of the breast consistent with lobular carcinoma**
Breast cancer patients can develop meningeal carcinomatosis. The tumor cells may be single or in groups. The presence of intracytoplasmic mucin is the hallmark of metastatic adnenocarcinema However, adenocarcinoma of the lung and breast may be morphologically similar. Compared to ductal carcinoma which may be larger in size with abundant and vacuolated cytoplasm, open chromatin, and prominent nucleoli, lobular carcinoma may have smaller cells with hyperchromatic nuclei and scant cytoplasm. Clinical history and/or immunocytochemical studies of the cytospin slides or cellblock are helpful in confirming the diagnosis.

A-6. **Answer Key: (b). Metastatic melanoma**
The cytomorphology of CSF melanoma includes large single cells with eccentric nuclei, intranuclear cytoplasmic inclusions, and macronucleoli. The cytoplasm is usually abundant with blebs (projections) with epithelioid appearance; however, the cytoplasm is dusty. Binucleation and/or multinucleation is commonly seen. The hallmark feature of melanoma is the presence of melanin pigment; however, it is not commonly seen. The main differential diagnosis is metastatic adenocarcinoma. Clinical history and/or immunocytochemical studies of the cytospin slides or cellblock are helpful in confirming the diagnosis.

A-7. **Answer Key**: (**a**). **Acute bacterial meningitis**
Increased neutrophils in the CSF of immunocompetent patients raises the possibility of acute meningitis. Immunocompromised status and/or instrumentation increases the risk of acute meningitis. Other differential diagnoses of neutrophils include peripheral blood contamination and toxoplasma meningoencephalitis. This case has numerous neutrophils and bacteria seen within the neutrophils, which is consistent with an acute meningitis.

A-8. **Answer Key**: (**c**). **Cytological examination of CSF is diagnostic for acute bacterial meningitis when it is predominantly neutrophils with the presence of intracellular or extracellular bacteria**.
Acute bacterial meningitis is a life-threatening condition that needs to be reported to the treating clinical team for prompt treatment. Cytological examination of CSF is diagnostic for acute bacterial meningitis when it is predominantly neutrophils with the presences of intracellular or extracellular bacteria. In neonatal acute bacterial meningitis is caused by beta-hemolytic *Streptococci* and enteric gram-negative bacilli in 60–70 % of cases. In patients older than two months and less than ten years, *Haemophilus influenzae*, *meningococci, or pneumococci* cause 90 % of cases of acute bacterial meningitis. Haemophilus vaccine is effective against *Haemophilus influenzae*.

A-9. **Answer Key**: (**d**). **Aseptic meningitis**
Predominant neutrophils with the presence of intracellular or extracellular bacteria on cytological examination are diagnostic for acute bacterial meningitis. Other reasons for neutrophilic pleocytosis include fungal infection, cytomegalovirus radiculopathy, early-stage viral meningitis, cerebral abscess, CNS hemorrhage, cerebral infarct, and concurrent high-grade malignancy. The presence of large atypical epithelioid cells warrants further investigation. This patient is at high risk of developing metastatic carcinoma. The most common cancers to metastasize to case of leptomeninges include lung cancer, breast cancer, and melanoma.

A-10. **Answer Key**: (**a**). **Unsatisfactory**
CSF reporting terminologies include "unsatisfactory, negative for malignancy, atypical, suspicious, or positive." Blood is a common contaminant. Neutrophils, if accompanied by red blood cells, should not necessarily be interpreted as acute meningitis. Leukemic blast contamination from peripheral blood should not be interpretal as leukemic involvement of the meninges. Traumatic taps consist predominantly of red blood cells. Since alcohol fixation lyses red blood cells, air-dried preparations are best for detection of red blood cells.

A-11. **Answer Key**: (**a**). **Unsatisfactory due to peripheral blood contamination**
The primary role of CSF cytology is to assess circulating malignant cells in CSF pathways. Blood is a common contaminant. Neutrophils, if accompanied by red blood cells should not be necessarily interpreted as acute meningitis. Leukemic blast contamination from peripheral blood should not be confused with leukemia involving the meninges. If the specimen contains mainly red blood cells, it is consistent with a traumatic tap. The specimen is unsatisfactory due to peripheral blood contamination.

A-12. **Answer Key**: (**b**). **Negative for malignancy**
Normal CSF contains less than 10 cells/ mm^3. Normal CSF cytology is composed of only small number of mature lymphocytes and monocytes. Benign lymphocytes have round, deeply basophilic nuclei with clumped chromatin. There is a scant rim of basophilic cytoplasm at the periphery. Increased cellularity of mature lymphocytes is associated with viral meningitis and other inflammatory or infectious conditions. in leukemia or lymphoma the tumors cells are hypercellular and look abnormal. Monocytes are larger than lymphocytes with moderate amount of cytoplasm and folded, kidney bean-shaped hypochromatic nuclei. Other normal elements that can be rarely identified include choroid plexus/ependymal cells, brain fragments, germinal matrix, chondrocytes, and bone marrow. Neutrophils are a normal finding if there is contamination from peripheral blood.

A-13. **Answer Key**: (**d**). **Neutrophils are a normal finding if there is contamination from peripheral blood**.
Typically, normal CSF should contain a small number of benign lymphocytes and monocytes. Neutrophils are a normal finding if there is contamination from peripheral blood. Macrophages, plasma cells, and eosinophils are abnormal findings in CSF. Other rarely identified normal elements include choroid plexus/ependymal cells, brain fragments, germinal matrix, chondrocytes, and bone marrow.

A-14. **Answer Key**: (**b**). **Diffuse large B-cell lymphoma**
The DQ stain reveals a hypercellular specimen with sheets of abnormal lymphoid cells. The cells are dispersed and large with high N/C ratios, irregular nuclear contours, immature chromatin, and prominent nucleoli. The cytoplasm is deeply basophilic. The most common malignancy in CSF is leukemia/lymphoma, followed by metastatic carcinoma (breast and lung) and melanoma. Most lymphomas that involve the leptomeninges are high grade, such as diffuse large B-cell lymphoma, Burkitt lymphoma, and anaplastic T-cell lymphoma.

A-15. **Answer Key**: (**a**). **The most common malignancy in CSF is metastatic carcinoma, followed by melanoma, and leukemia/lymphoma.**
The most common malignancies in CSF are metastatic carcinoma (breast and lung), and melanoma, followed by leukemia/lymphoma. Most leukemia in CSF is acute lymphoblastic leukemia (ALL), especially in children. Acute myeloid leukemia (AML) is more common in adults than children, but it is less common than ALL. Medulloblastoma is more likely to involve CNS than glioma and meningioma.

A-16. **Answer Key**: (**b**). **Immature large lymphocytes with abundant cytoplasm and pleomorphic horseshoe-shaped nuclei**
Anaplastic large cell lymphoma is a T-cell lymphoma which is CD30 and ALK positive immunochemically. The cells are usually large with abundant cytoplasm and pleomorphic eccentric horseshoe-shaped (kidney-shaped) nuclei. Nucleoli are present. Burkitt lymphoma is composed of medium-sized tumor cells with round nuclei of clumped chromatin and deeply basophilic cytoplasm with abundant lipid vacuoles. Mitotic activity is frequent. Large epithelioid cells with intracytoplasmic mucin are diagnostic for metastatic adenocarcinoma.

A-17. **Answer Key**: (**c**). **Multiple myeloma**
The specimen is hypercellular with individually dispersed highly atypical plasma cells. The cells have eccentrically located nuclei with distinct perinuclear hofs, some with prominent nucleoli. The chromatin is coarsely clumped. The cytoplasm is abundant. Binucleation and mitotic activity are seen. These features are characteristic for myeloma. Multiple myeloma uncommonly involves the meninges and CNS. Clinical history, bone marrow, serological, and flow cytometry studies are warranted to confirm meningeal myeloma.

A-18. **Answer Key**: (**d**). ***Cryptococcus neoformans***
Cryptococcus neoformans is the most frequent cause of fungal meningitis. The organism enters the body through the respiratory system and disseminates to the CNS hematogenously. It is frequently seen in immunocompromised patients. The diagnostic features to identify are the presence of single, yeastlike structures (5–10 μm in diameter) with distinctive mucinous capsules (positive for mucicarmine stain) and teardrop buddings. Differential diagnosis includes starch crystals (with Maltese cross birefringence). *Cryptococcus* exhibits teardrop (narrow-necked) buddings, which can be distinguished from other types of budding yeast: *Blastomyces dermatitidis* (large 8–12 μm in diameter with broad-based budding) and *Histoplasma capsulatum* (1–5 μm).

A-19. **Answer Key**: (**c**). **Chronic, subacute or viral meningitis**
Hypercellular CSF specimens represent a pathologic process. Acute bacterial meningitis is associated with neutrophilic infiltration. Culture of the CSF should be performed to specify the etiology of the infection. Plasma cell infiltrate is related to multiple sclerosis, neurosyphilis, viral infections, sarcoidosis, or sclerosing panencephalitis. Lymphocytic infiltration can be seen in chronic inflammation, subacute inflammation, viral infection, tuberculous infection, and also lymphoma or leukemia involving the CNS.

A-20. **Answer Key**: (**a**). **Leptomeningeal cells**
Leptomeningeal cells are derived from the pia-arachnoid layers of the brain covering. They resemble mesothelial cells or monocytes. They are the most common neuronal element seen in CSF specimens that have vacuolated and pigmented cytoplasm with small, eccentric, and vesicular nuclei. Other rarely identified normal elements include choroid plexus/ependymal cells, brain fragments, germinal matrix, chondrocytes, and bone marrow.

A-21. **Answer Key**: (**d**). **Neurosyphilis**
The clinical indications to order lumbar punctures for the evaluation of CSF include change of neurologic status such as headache, especially associated with fever, change of consciousness and weakness, or monitoring patients with seizure disorder and cancer. CSF can be submitted to the clinical pathology laboratory for cells counts, microbiology, and clinical chemistries and/or to the cytology laboratory. The above diseases are appropriate indications for CSF cytology except neurosyphilis.

A-22. **Answer Key**: (**d**). **10 ml**
Most CSF specimens are obtained by lumbar puncture through the intervertebral space at L3–L4 or L4–L5. When indicated it can be aspirated from the cisterna magna at the base of the brain or lateral ventricle. In patients undergoing intrathecal chemotherapy for meningeal metastases, fluid can be drawn from as Ommaya reservoir. The minimal volume submitted for CSF cytology is 1 ml, but 3 ml or more is preferable. If CNS malignancy is suspected, at least 10 ml of CSF for cytological evaluation is ideal.

A-23. **Answer Key**: (**b**). **Air-dried Wright-stained slides**
CSF fluid should be collected fresh and delivered to the cytology laboratory as quickly as possible.

Refrigeration at 4 °C for less than 24-h storage or transport is required to prevent cellular deterioration. However, if delay is more than 48 h, the sample can be preserved by adding equal volume of 50 % ethanol. Lymphoid cells are best evaluated on air-dried preparations and Wright-stained slides are ideal. However, it is advisable to prepare both air-dried Wright-stained slides and alcohol-fixed Papanicolaou-stained slides. The most common ways to prepare CSF specimens are cytocentrifugation, membrane filtration, or thin layer preparation.

A-24. **Answer Key**: (**d**). ***Cryptococcus neoformans***
The primary role of CSF cytology is to assess circulating malignant cells in CSF pathways. Although a specific diagnosis of some benign diseases (such as *Cryptococcus neoformans*) can be made cytologically, the cause of aseptic, viral, or tuberculous meningitis (manifested by pleocytosis, i.e., increase numbers of lymphocytes) is best identified by other clinical and laboratory methods. The thick mucopolysaccharide capsule of *Cryptococci* can be stained readily with mucicarmine, alcian blue, and colloidal iron satins. *Cryptococci* exhibit teardrop (thin-necked) buddings, which can be distinguished from other types of budding yeast: *Blastomyces dermatitidis* (large 8–12 μm in diameter with broad-based budding) and *Histoplasma capsulatum* (1–5 μm).

A-25. **Answer Key**: (**d**). **False-positive diagnoses are estimated at 10%**
The specificity of CSF is high. The false-positive diagnoses are estimated at 2–3 %. The statements from A to C are correct. Cytological examination of CSF for meningeal malignancy is moderately sensitive and highly specific.

A-26. **Answer Key**: (**a**). **Lymphoma or leukemia**
The most common cause of a false-positive diagnosis is overdiagnosis of lymphoma or leukemia, particularly in patients with herpes zoster meningitis, cryptococcal meningitis, Lyme disease, and viral meningitis. Diagnostic yield is greatly enhanced by the use of ancillary studies, cellblock preparations, and flow cytometry.

A-27. **Answer Key**: (**a**). **Immature cells of germinal matrix origin**
Choroid plexus and ependymal cells are seen in less than 0.5 % CSF specimen. Small, immature cells of germinal matrix origin are commonly seen in premature neonates. These benign cells are beneath the ependyma in the wall of the lateral ventricles and exfoliate when there is a subependymal hemorrhage thus are often accompanied by hemosiderin-laden macrophages. They are frequently clustered and molded to one another, mimicking a small cell malignancy.

A-28. **Answer Key**: (**d**). **Tuberculosis meningitis**
Macrophages have abundant, vacuolated cytoplasm that sometimes contains pigments, organisms, and ingested cells. Macrophages are most commonly associated with chronic meningitis, subarachnoid or intraventricular hemorrhage, cerebral infarction, postsurgical inflammation, multiple sclerosis, malignancy, and posttreatment inflammation. Tuberculosis meningitis may be associated with increased plasma cells; however, this finding is not diagnostic of TB meningitis.

A-29. **Answer Key**: (**a**). **Metastatic carcinoma**
Metastatic tumors are more frequently seen in CSF than primary CNS tumors. The latter only account for 6 % of the all positive CSF samples. Cytological examination of CSF is the diagnostic procedure of choice for the diagnosis of metastatic malignancy. In most cases, the malignant cells are obviously different from normal CSF cells (lymphocytes and monocytes). The most common cancers in CSF are lung cancer, breast cancer, melanoma, and lymphoma. Adenocarcinomas are the most common. Unlike lung and stomach carcinoma, it is uncommon for primary breast carcinoma to be occult. Primary CNS malignancy including CNS lymphoma are rare.

A-30. **Answer Key**: (**c**). **Lymphoblastic lymphoma and Burkitt lymphoma more commonly involve CNS than Hodgkin lymphoma and small lymphocytic lymphoma**.
Primary lymphomas arise in the CNS. Secondary involvement of the meninges occurs in approximately 4 % of the patients with lymphoma. Lymphoblastic and Burkitt lymphoma have high affinity for CNS; on the other hand, Hodgkin and small lymphocytic lymphoma are almost never seen in CSF. A definitive diagnosis is greatly benefited by lymphoid marker studies, flow cytometry, or cellblock. In adults, the most common CNS tumors in CSF are anaplastic astrocytomas, glioblastoma multiforme, and primary CNS lymphoma. In children, medulloblastoma is the most common.

A-31. **Answer Key**: (**d**). **The above cycle renews 10–12 times daily**.
CSF is an ultrafiltrate of plasma produced by ependyma. CSF flows from the ventricles to the subarachnoid space which is lined by leptomeninges. CSF is

reabsorbed by the arachnoid granulations into venous system. The total volume of CSF in adults is approximately 150 ml. Daily production of CSF is 500 ml. This means the CSF cycle renews three to four times daily.

A-32. **Answer Key**: (**c**). **Provide extra space in case of brain hemorrhage or bleeding**
The normal functions of CSF include providing a protective cushion, nutrient circulation, and a stable ionic concentration for CNS; It is not able to provide space for brain hemorrhage or bleeding, which is a pathologic condition.

A-33. **Answer Key**: (**b**). **Leptomeningeal metastasis**
CSF cytological examination is a crucial diagnostic test for evaluating a wide variety of treatable yet potentially fatal diseases and conditions affecting the CNS. These conditions include hemorrhage or bleeding of the brain, malignancies (primary tumors of the CNS or metastasis), infectious diseases (fungal, viral, bacterial, and tuberculosis meningitis) or encephalitis, and other immunological diseases such as Guillain-Barré syndrome, sarcoidosis, and multiple sclerosis. Identification of malignancy is the primary and most important utility of CSF cytology. The diagnosis of other diseases is heavily dependent on other non-cytological tests including cell counts, flow cytometry, chemical analysis, immunological and serological testing, molecular testing, and microbiological culture.

A-34. **Answer Key**: (**d**). **Approximately 500 ml CSF is produced daily in adult**.
The total volume of CSF in the adult is approximately 150 ml. The total volume of CSF in the children is approximately 10–60 ml. The minimum volume for CSF cytological examination is 1 ml; the preferable volume is 3 ml. In cases of malignancy, the ideal volume would be 10 ml. Approximately 500 ml CSF is produced daily (0.35 ml/min) in adults.

A-35. **Answer Key**: (**a**). **Intervertebral space at L3–L4 or L4–L5**
CSF is most commonly obtained by lumbar puncture through the intervertebral space at the L3–L4 or L4–L5. When indicated it can be obtained from the cisterna magna at the base of the brain, lateral ventricle, and Ommaya reservoir.

A-36. **Answer Key**: (**d**). **If delayed preparation is more than 48 h, the specimen should be kept frozen**.
For optimal cell preservation, the fresh CSF specimen should be delivered to the laboratory in less than one hour for immediate preparation. This helps to avoid a false-negative diagnosis due to degeneration of important diagnostic material. For delayed preparation, the fluid should be refrigerated at 4 °C. If the delay is more than 48 h, equal volume of 50 % ethanol is added. The specimen should never be frozen.

A-37. **Answer Key**: (**a**). **Peripheral blood contamination is best detected on alcohol-fixed slides**.
CSF is most commonly prepared by centrifugation (cytospin). Both air-dried and alcohol-fixed slides can be prepared. Air-dried slides can be prepared for Diff-Quik/Wright stain and alcohol-fixed slides for Papanicolaou stain. Air-dried DQ-stained slides can detect any nucleated cells and red blood cells due to peripheral blood contamination. It is superior in detecting hematopoietic malignancy. Alcohol fixation lyses blood.

A-38. **Answer Key**: (**c**). **The false-positive rate is approximately 2–3 %**.
CSF cytology for meningeal malignancy is considered a moderately sensitive and highly specific test. The sensitivity is approximately 60 % and is dependent on the number of specimens examined, volume obtained, extent of leptomeningeal involvement, and the site of the sampling. Multiple specimens, 10 ml specimens, disseminated leptomeningeal diseases, and the site close to the tumor will increase the sensitivity. The specificity is approximately 97–98 %. The false-positive result (approximately 2–3 %) is mainly due to overdiagnosis of lymphoma and leukemia.

A-39. **Answer Key**: (**a**). **Negative**
Normal CSF cytology is composed of only a small number of mature lymphocytes and monocytes. Benign lymphocytes have round, deeply basophilic nuclei with clumped chromatin. There is a scant rim of basophilic cytoplasm at the periphery. Increased cellularity of mature lymphocytes is associated with viral meningitis and other inflammatory or infectious conditions. Lymphocytes in leukemia or lymphoma are hypercellular and look abnormal. Monocytes are larger than lymphocytes with a moderate amount of cytoplasm and folded, kidney bean-shaped, and hypochromatic nuclei. Occasional neutrophils are considered normal in concentrated specimens. However, increased neutrophils accompanied by red blood cells indicate peripheral blood contamination.

A-40. **Answer Key**: (**d**). **There are no red blood cells identified in the CSF, and the cell count is different from the blood**.
In patients with a history of leukemia, blast contamination from peripheral blood should not be interpreted

as evidence of leukemic involvement of the meninges. If the specimen contains mainly red blood cells, it is consistent with a traumatic tap. If there are no red blood cells identified in the CSF and both peripheral blood and CSF cell counts are similar, that may indicate peripheral blood contamination with lysed (undetectable) blood. The absence of CSF red blood cells and a CSF cell count that is different from the blood may indicate leptomeningeal involvement with leukemia. The use of flow cytometry should be implemented to further lymphoma of classification.

A-41. **Answer Key**: (**c**). **Chondrocyte**
Chondrocytes are rare in CSF specimens and are contaminants picked up as the needle is advanced through the nucleus pulposus of the intravertebral disk. Chondrocytes have chondroid or myxoid cytoplasm with a ringlike condensation of the cytoplasm and a clear space (lacuna space) surrounding their round nucleus. Chondrocytes should be easily recognized and should not be confused with squamous cells, CMV-infected cells, or vegetable cells.

A-42. **Answer Key**: (**c**). **Ependymal cells**
Ependymal cells are rare normal elements in of CSF. Ependymal and choroid plexus cells are morphologically similar on CSF cytology. They are round or columnar cells with abundant cytoplasm and bland round nuclei. They can be single or form small clusters. They do not have malignant features.

A-43. **Answer Key**: (**a**). **Brain tissue**
Brain tissue including glial cells and neurons can be introduced by a CNS tap. The neuropil has a characteristic fibrillar appearance with astrocytes (larger nuclei) and oligodendroglial cells (small and dark nuclei).

A.44. **Answer Key**: (**c**). **Megakaryocyte**
The presence of hematopoietic elements from one of the three cell liniages is a useful morphological clue that the sample has been contaminated with marrow elements such as megakaryocytes. Megakaryocytic cells from bone marrow may mimic poorly differentiated adenocarcinoma, multinucleated giant cells in granuloma, and osteoclasts.

A-45. **Answer Key**: (**d**). **Talc**
Corpora amylacea are spherical transparent proteinaceous structures that are commonly seen in the brain of the elderly and may occasionally be seen in the CSF. Corpora amylacea have a laminated appearance. Starch granules from powdered surgical gloves may contaminate the CSF. The particles show a Maltese cross configuration upon polarization. *Cryptococcus* is smaller than starch granules, often shows budding or a mucous capsule, and does not polarize. Talc is crystal-like structure with areas of central clearing.

A-46. **Answer Key**: (**a**). **CSF cytology is mainly used to diagnose CNS primary tumor at initial presentation**.
CSF cytology is an important test for the diagnosis of leptomeningeal involvement of primary CNS tumor and to monitor tumor recurrence. The common primary CNS tumors detected by CNS cytology include medulloblastoma, glioblastoma multiforme, ependymoma, oligodendroglioma, and astrocytoma. Less common primary CNS tumors include choroid plexus tumor, germ cell tumor, germinoma, pineoblastoma, primitive neuroectodermal tumors (PNETs), and atypical teratoid /rhabdoid tumor. Lymphoma can also present as a primary CNS tumor. However, it is rare in general population and more commonly seen in immunocompromised patients. It is essential to correlate with appropriate clinical information when using CSF to diagnose primary CNS tumor. The main utility of CNS cytology is to confirm a previously characterized CNS neoplasm by histology, not initial diagnosis.

A-47. **Answer Key**: (**d**). **Medulloblastoma**
The common primary CNS tumors detected by CNS cytology include medulloblastoma (50 % in children; cerebellum location), glioblastoma multiforme (14 % in adults; cerebral location), ependymoma (12 % in children; fourth ventricle location, in young adults; spinal cord location), oligodendroglioma (12 % in adults; cerebral location), and astrocytoma (7 % in adults; cerebral location). Less common primary CNS tumors include choroid plexus tumors (in children and forth ventricle location), germ cell tumors and germinoma (in children/adolescents; pineal, suprasellar location), pineoblastoma (2 % in children and pineal location), primitive neuroectodermal tumors (PNETs), atypical teratoid/rhabdoid tumors (in children; wide range in location), craniopharyngioma, hemangioblastoma, and sarcoma.

A-48. **Answer Key**: (**c**). **The most common type of primary lymphoma is diffuse large B-cell lymphoma**.
Lymphoma can present as a primary CNS tumor. It involves the brain parenchyma and involves the leptomeninges in 8 %. It is rare in the general population. It is more commonly seen in immunocompromised

patients such as HIV/AIDS patients and organ transplant recipients. It is associated with Epstein-Barr virus (EBV). The most common type of primary lymphoma is large B-cell lymphoma. Non-primary CNS lymphomas are mostly high-grade lymphomas including large B cell, T cell, Burkitt, and lymphoblastic. Primary CNS, DLBL is EBVpositive only in immunocopmpromised patients .

A-49. **Answer Key**: (**c**). **EBV**
These are abnormal lymphoid cells. The cells are dispersed and large with high N/C ratios, irregular nuclear contours, immature chromatin, and prominent nucleoli. This is compatible with the patient's history of diffuse large B-cell lymphoma. It is associated with Epstein-Barr virus (EBV).

A-50. **Answer Key**: (**a**). **Glioblastoma multiforme**
Gliomas (astrocytoma and glioblastoma multiforme) are the most commonly encountered primary CNS malignancies in adults. They may arise from the cerebrum, cerebellum, brainstem, or spinal cord. They may also spread to the ventricles and subarachnoid space.

They arrange from low to high grade. Glioblastoma multiforms is the most poorly differentiated astrocytoma (grade IV). The cytology is usually cellular and shows isolated cells and small clusters of large cells with hyperchromatic and pleomorphic nuclei. The isolated cells have long, hairlike cytoplasmic processes. All the other tumors have small blue round cell morphology.

A-51. **Answer Key**: (**b**). **High-grade astrocytoma**
Glioblastoma multiform is the most poorly differentiated astrocytoma (Who grade IV, high grade). The cytology is usually cellular and shows isolated cells and small clusters of large cells with hyperchromatic and pleomorphic nuclei. The nuclear contours are markedly irregular. The cells have long, hairlike cytoplasmic processes indicating glial origin. These features are consistent with high-grade astrocytoma.

A-52. **Answer Key**: (**d**). **Melanoma**
Medulloblastoma is a poorly differentiated small cell tumor that arises in the cerebellum. It invades the adjacent fourth ventricle or meninges with 25 % of patients having positive CSF cytology. The cells are single and in clusters; they are small to medium sized, with scant cytoplasm, hyperchromatic nuclei, and nuclear molding that closely resembles small cell carcinoma. The cells exhibit neuroendocrine markers, occasional positivity for GFAP, negativity for cytokeratin, and sometimes high Ki-67 prohifertion index. Medulloblastoma should be differentiated from other small blue cell tumors that can also be seen in the CSF such as metastatic neuroblastoma, retinoblastoma, pineoblastoma, and primitive neuroectodermal tumors (PNETs). The age, tumors location patient, and immunohistochemical studies can aid in the diagnosis.

A-53. **Answer Key**: (**a**). **Medulloblastoma**
Medulloblastoma is a poorly differentiated small cell tumor. The cells are seen in single and cluster arrangements; they are small to medium sized, with scant cytoplasm, hyperchromatic nuclei, and nuclear molding that closely resembles small cell carcinoma. Medulloblastoma should be differentiated from other small blue cell tumors that can also be seen in the CSF such as metastatic neuroblastoma, retinoblastoma, pineoblastoma, and primitive neuroectodermal tumors (PNETs).

A-54. **Answer Key**: (**c**). **Cytokeratin negative /neuroendocrine markers positive high/Ki-67 prohifertion index**
Medulloblastoma is a poorly differentiated small cell tumor. Medulloblastoma should be differentiated from other small blue cell tumors that can also be seen in the CSF such as metastatic small cell carcinoma, neuroblastoma, retinoblastoma, pineoblastoma, and primitive neuroectodermal tumors (PNETs). Medulloblastoma cells express neuroendocrine markers, occasional positivity for GFAP, negativity for cytokeratin, and sometimes high Ki-67.

A-55. **Answer Key**: (**b**). **Germinoma**
Germ cell tumors occur rarely in children and adolescents patients. The tumor is usually located in the pineal gland or suprasellar region. CSF cytology shows a dual population of cells. Large polygonal cells with round nuclei, prominent nucleoli, and coarse chromatin and background is composed of mature lymphocytes.

A-56. **Answer Key**: (**c**). **Dusty cytoplasm or melanin pigment**
All the above features are seen in melanoma. However, the most specific feature for a melanoma diagnosis is melanin pigment in malignant cells.

A-57. **Answer Key**: (**d**). **Ependymoma is usually located in the fourth ventricle**.
The common primary CNS tumors detected by CNS cytology include medulloblastoma (50 % in children; cerebellum location), glioblastoma multiforme (14 %

in adults; cerebral location), ependymoma (12 % in children; fourth ventricle location, in young adults; spinal cord location), oligodendroglioma (12 % in adults; cerebral location), astrocytoma (7 % in adults; cerebral location).

A-58. **Answer Key**: (**b**). **Acute meningitis**
Macrophages in CSF are an abnormal finding. They are associated with malignancy, therapy-related changes, chronic meningitis, subarachnoid hemorrhage, intraventricular hemorrhage, cerebral infarction, and multiple sclerosis.

A-59. **Answer Key**: (**b**). **Plasma cells are an abnormal but nonspecific finding in CSF**.
Plasma cells are an abnormal but nonspecific finding in CSF. They are associated with viral meningitis, Lyme disease, tuberculosis, syphilis, cysticercosis, and multiple sclerosis. However, macrophages are associated with cerebral infarction, neutrophils are associated with CMV radiculopathy, abnormal/dysplastic plasma cells are seen in myeloma, and red blood cells and neutrophils are seen in peripheral blood contamination.

A-60. **Answer Key**: (**a**). **Toxoplasma meningoencephalitis**
A large number of eosinophils in CSF are suggestive of a parasite infection. Other considerations include ventriculoperitoneal shunts, infection of *Coccidioides immitis*, and Rocky Mountain spotted fever. Toxoplasma meningoencephalitis is associated with increased neutrophils in CSF.

A-61. **Answer Key**: (**c**). **CSF cytology shows predominant lymphocytes**.
Mollaret meningitis is a rare form of recurrent aseptic meningitis that may be related to herpes simplex viruses 1 and 2. Cytological findings are nonspecific and may show a predominance of monocytes (Mollaret cells). They have deep nuclear clefts that impart a footprint-like morphology to the nucleus. They are characteristic of but not specific for Mollaret meningitis. They can be seen in sarcoidosis and Behcet diseases.

A-62. **Answer Key**: (**b**). ***Cryptococcus* usually appears as round yeast forms measuring from 1 to 2 microns with a refractive center**.
The most frequent causes of fungal meningitis are *Cryptococcus neoformans*, *Candida*, and *Coccidioides immitis*. This is mostly seen in patients with a debilitated or immunocompromised state such as diabetes mellitus, lymphoma/leukemia, organ transplant recipients, and patients with HIV/AIDS. Cryptococcus is a ubiquitous organism found in the soil. It usually enters the body through the respiratory system and disseminates to the CNS hematogenously. *Cryptococcus* can be seen intracellularly within a variety of cells. *Cryptococcus* usually appears as round yeast forms measuring from 5 to 10 microns with a refractive center. A mucin stain will highlight the narrow neck budding (string-of-pearls appearance). *Cryptococcal* antigen can often be detected in the CSF providing a valuable aid to the diagnosis.

A-63. **Answer Key**: (**c**). ***Cryptococcus neoformans***
Cryptococcus can be seen intracellularly within a variety of cells. *Cryptococcus* usually appears as round yeast forms measuring from 5 to 10 microns with a refractive center. A PAS stain highlights the narrow neck budding. Mimickers of *Cryptococcus* include air bubbles, water droplets, starch granules, red blood cells, and other fungal organisms such as *Blastomyces dermatitidis* (more uniform in sizes, 8–12 microns) and *Histoplasma capsulatum* (small and uniform in size, 1–5 micron).

A-64. **Answer Key**: (**d**). **The Diff-Quik stains is the ideal stain for AML specimens**.
This is an acute myeloid leukemia (AML). AML is less common in the CSF than acute lymphoblastic leukemia (ALL). It is more common in adults than in children. The most common subtype of AML to involve the CNS is acute myelomonocytic leukemia (AML M4) at the time of clinical presentation. The blasts in AML will show large cells (larger than lymphocytes), with round or highly irregular nucleus, fine immature chromatin, prominent nucleoli, occasional azurophilic granules, and occasional mature granulocytes the ideal stain for AML specimens Wright- Gimsa Stain.

A-65. **Answer Key**: (**c**). **Lung/squamous cell carcinoma**
Lung cancer and breast cancer are common in women and commonly metastatic to the brain. Although adenocarcinoma is the most common type, in this case, the morphological description is that of a squamous cell carcinoma.

A-66. **Answer Key**: (**c**). **Intracranial hemorrhage**
Hemosiderin pigments are gold and refractile. Hemosiderin-laden macrophages (siderophages) are as indication of intracranial or intraventricular hemorrhage. Melanin pigments are dark and black. Most importantly, melanoma cells have characteristic features that can be differentiated from benign macrophages. Tuberculosis meningitis is associated with increased plasma cells. Megakaryocytes are large cells

with multinucleation and coarse-appearing chromatin. They can be from bone marrow or blood. However, they lack any pigments.

A-67. **Answer Key**: (**a**). **90 %**
The primary role of CSF cytology is to diagnose malignant involvement of CNS. Malignancy involving the CNS is reported in 10 % patients. Thus, the CSF specimens are reported negative in 90 % of cases.

A-68. **Answer Key**: (**d**). **Germinal matrix**
Germinal matrix is composed of benign small immature cells that are beneath the ependyma in the wall of the lateral ventricles. They exfoliate where there is subependymal and intraventricular hemorrhage. They are often clustered and molded to one another, mimick medulloblastoma.

A-69. **Answer Key**: (**a**). **Cerebral infarction**
Benign plasma cells are an abnormal but nonspecific finding in CSF. They are associated with viral meningitis, Lyme disease, tuberculosis, syphilis, cysticercosis, and multiple sclerosis. However, macrophages are associated with cerebral infarction.

A-70. **Answer key**: (**b**). **Mollaret meningitis**
Mollaret meningitis is a rare form of recurrent aseptic meningitis that may be related to herpes simplex viruses 1 and 2. The clinical presentation includes recurring attacks of fever, headache, and neck stiffness. Cytological findings may show a predominance of monocytes (Mollaret cells). They have deep nuclear clefts that impart a footprint-like morphology to the nucleus. They are characteristic of but not specific for Mollaret meningitis. They can be seen in sarcoidosis and Behcet diseases.

A-71. **Answer Key**: (**c**). **Ventriculoperitoneal shunts**
A large number of CSF eosinophils are usually suggestive of a parasite infection; other considerations include ventriculoperitoneal shunts, *Coccidioides immitis* infection, and Rocky Mountain spotted fever. Cerebral cysticercosis is caused by larvae of the tapeworm *Taenia solium*. Tuberculosis and cysticercosis are associated with plasmacytosis. Toxoplasma meningoencephalitis is associated with increased neutrophils in CSF.

A-72. **Answer Key**: (**b**). **Lung cancer, breast cancer, and melanoma**
See also A29, A52, and A65

A-73. **Answer Key**: (**d**). **Peripherally circulating leukemic cells within CSF**
The above described cytomorphology represents myeloid blasts. The background of red blood cells indicates peripheral blood contamination.

A-74. **Answer Key**: (**b**). **Medulloblastoma and high-grade astrocytoma**
The common primary CNS tumors detected by CNS cytology include medulloblastoma (50 % in children and cerebellum location), glioblastoma multiforme (14 % in adults and cerebral location), ependymoma (12 % in children and fourth ventricle location, in young adults and spinal cord location), oligodendroglioma (12 % in adults and cerebral location), and astrocytoma (7 % in adults and cerebral location). Less common primary CNS tumors include choroid plexus tumor (in children and forth ventricle location), germ cell tumor and germinoma (in children/adolescents and pineal, suprasellar location), pineoblastoma (2 % in children and pineal location), primitive neuroectodermal tumors (PNETs), atypical teratoid /rhabdoid tumors (in children and wide range in location), craniopharyngioma, hemangioblastoma, and sarcoma.

A-75. **Answer Key**: (**d**). **Flow cytometry**
Atypical lymphocytes can be seen in lymphomas/leukemias as well as infectious processes. However, his medical history indicates CNS involvement of a lymphoma/leukemia. Flow cytometry is the most appropriate next ancillary study.

A-76. **Answer Key**: (**b**). **Mucin stain**
The most frequent cause of fungal meningitis is *Cryptococcus neoformans*. This is mostly seen in patients with a debilitated or immunocompromised state such as diabetes mellitus, lymphoma/leukemia, organ transplant recipients, and patients with HIV/AIDS. *Cryptococcus* can be seen intracellularly within a variety of cells. *Cryptococcus* usually appears as round yeast forms measuring from 5 to 10 microns with a refractive center. A mucin stain will highlight the narrow neck budding (string-of-pearls appearance). *Cryptococcal* antigen can also be detected in the CSF, providing a valuable aid to the diagnosis.

A-77. **Answer key**: (**d**). **Mollaret meningitis**
Mollaret meningitis is a rare form of recurrent aseptic meningitis that may be related to herpes simplex viruses 1 and 2. The clinical presentation includes recurring attacks of fever, headache, and neck stiffness. Cytological findings may show a predominance of monocytes (Mollaret cells). They have deep nuclear clefts that impart a footprint-like morphology to the nucleus. They are characteristic of but not specific for

Mollaret meningitis. They can be seen in sarcoidosis and Behcet diseases.

A-78. **Answer Key**: (**a**). **Adenocarcinoma**

This patient has history of lung adenocarcinoma. Adenocarcinoma is the most common type of carcinoma seen in the CSF. In a female patient, the most common carcinoma is breast cancer but the most common fatal cancer is lung cancer. Both cancers involve the CNS at end stage, causing meningeal carcinomatosis. The most common types of lung carcinoma metastasis to CNS are small cell carcinoma and adenocarcinoma. Squamous cell carcinoma of the lung rarely metastasizes to the CNS.

Adenocarcinoma cells in CSF are dysplastic epithelioid cells arranged in single cells or 3-D clusters. Detection of mucinous vacuoles is diagnostic; additional features include vacuolated cytoplasm and prominent nucleoli. Immunostains, if needed, can be done on a smear or cellblock and would show positive staining for CK7 and TTF-1, supporting the diagnosis of metastatic adenocarcinoma of the lung.

A-79. **Answer Key**: (**c**). **Melanoma**

This patient has history of melanoma. The cytomorphology of CSF melanoma includes large single cells with eccentric nuclei, intranuclear cytoplasmic inclusions, and macronucleoli. The cytoplasm is dusty and usually abundant with occasional blebs (cytoplasmic projections) and with an epithelioid appearance. Binucleation and/or multinucleation is commonly seen. The hallmark feature of melanoma is the presence of melanin pigment; however, it is not commonly seen. The main differential diagnosis is metastatic adenocarcinoma. Melanoma can be a primary from leptomeninges (very rare). Clinical history and/or immunocytochemical studies of the cytospin slides or cellblock are helpful in confirming the diagnosis. Immunostains, if needed, can be done on a smear or cellblock and would show positive staining for S-100, HMB45, and melan A, supporting the diagnosis of metastatic melanoma.

A-80. **Answer Key**: (**a**). **Adenocarcinoma**

This patient has history of breast adenocarcinoma. Adenocarcinoma is the most common type of carcinoma seen in the CSF. In a female patient, the most common carcinoma is breast cancer. Breast carcinoma involves the CNS at end stage, causing meningeal carcinomatosis. Adenocarcinoma cells in CSF are dysplastic epithelioid cells arranged in single cells or 3-D clusters. Lymphocytosis can be present in the background. Detection of mucinous vacuoles is helpful. Additional features include large cells and prominent nucleoli. Immunostains, if needed, can be done on a smear or cellblock and would show positive staining for pan-CK, ER, and mammaglobulin, supporting the diagnosis of metastatic adenocarcinoma of the breast.

Reading List

Ali SZ. Chapter 23. Central nervous system. In: Demay RM, editor. The art and science of cytopathology. Chicago: ASCP Press; 2011. p. 1438–65.

Bigner SH, Carter AL. Chapter 16. Central nervous system. In: Bibbo M, Wilbur DC, editors. Philadelphia: Sauders Elsevier: 2008. p. 439–54.

Cibas ES. Chapter 4. Cerebrospinal fluid. In: Cibas ES, Ducatman BS, editors. Cytology diagnostic principles and clinical correlates. Philadelphia: Saunders Elsevier; 2009. p. 171–95.

Demay RM. Chapter 6. Cerebrospinal fluid. In: Demay RM, editor. The art and science of cytopathology. Chicago: ASCP Press; 2011. p. 490–525.

Geisinger KR, Stanley MW, Raab SS, Silverman JF, Abati A. Chapter 13. Cerebrospinal fluid. In: Geisinger KR, Stanley MW, Raab SS, Silverman JF, Abati A, editors. Modern cytopathology. Philadelphia: Churchill Livingstone; 2004. p. 313–33.

Melamed M. Chapter 27. Cerebrospinal and miscellaneous fluids. In: Koss LG, Melamed MR, editors. Koss' diagnostic cytology and its histopathologic bases. Philadelphia: Lippincott Williams & Wilkins; 2006. p. 1023–55.

Thyroid Fine-Needle Aspiration

4

Reda S. Saad, Jan F. Silverman, and Walid E. Khalbuss

Contents

4.1 **Image-Based Questions 1–44** 245

4.2 **Text-Based Questions 45–50** 289

4.3 **Answers and Discussion of Image-Based Questions 1–44** 290

4.4 **Answers and Discussion of Text-Based Questions 45–50** 302

Reading List 303

Table 4.1 Thyroid nodules and risk factors

• Thyroid nodules are usually detected by palpation in 4–7 % of adults in the United States
• Although a thyroid nodule raises the suspicion of cancer, fewer than 5 % are malignant
• The malignancy rate for nodules occurring in children is twofold higher than in adult patients. Clinical factors reported to be associated with increased risk of malignancy include head and neck irradiation, family history of medullary carcinoma or MEN2, extremes of age, male sex, a growing or fixed nodule, firm/hard consistency, cervical lymphadenopathy, and persistent hoarseness, dysphonia, dysphagia, or dyspnea
• Given the high prevalence of thyroid nodules and the impracticality of surgically excising all nodules, FNA provides a relative risk of malignancy from which the clinicians can plan their management decisions, i.e., surgery vs. clinical follow-up
• Using FNA as screening test for thyroid nodules decreases the percentage of patients requiring thyroid surgery from 67 to 43 % with doubling or tripling the incidence of malignancy detected at thyroidectomy

R.S. Saad, MD, PhD, FRCPC (✉)
Medical Director and Chief, Department of Laboratory Medicine
Chatham-Kent Health Alliance, 1030 Ouellette Avenue, Windsor, ON N8W 1L9, Canada

Director, Cytology Section, Windsor Regional Hospital,
137 Brian Drive, Toronto, ON M2J 3Y8, Canada
e-mail: reda.saad@wrh.on.ca

J.F. Silverman, MD
Department of Pathology, Allegheny General Hospital,
320 E North Ave, Pittsburgh, PA 15212, USA

W.E. Khalbuss, MD, PhD, FIAC
Department of Pathology, GE Clarient Diagnostic Services,
31 Columbia, Aliso Viejo, California, 92656, USA
e-mail: Walid.khalbuss@ge.com

W.E. Khalbuss, Q.K. Li (eds.), *Diagnostic Cytopathology Board Review and Self-Assessment*,
DOI 10.1007/978-1-4939-1477-7_4, © Springer Sciencc+Business Media New York 2015

Table 4.2 Methods for assessing thyroid nodules

- Ultrasound (US) is recommended as the initial test for patients with palpable thyroid nodules, for high-risk patients even with normal examination, and for those with adenopathies suggestive of a malignant lesion. Significant numbers of nodules are incidentally discovered, during the work-up of metastatic disease unrelated to the thyroid
- The prevalence of cancer appears to be similar in palpable and nonpalpable thyroid nodules, with microinvasive papillary carcinomas being increasingly diagnosed at earlier stages
- FNA can be avoided in patients who have a hyperfunctioning ("hot") nodule (about 5 % of all nodules), confirmed by a radionuclide thyroid scan, since a hot thyroid nodule is rarely malignant

Table 4.3 Aspiration technique and slide preparation in thyroid FNA

- US guidance permits the operator to be certain that the nodule of interest is aspirated to reduce the number of unsatisfactory specimens. It is recommended for nonpalpable nodules, nodules that have a significant cystic component (>25 %), and nodules that previously yielded an unsatisfactory sample. In multinodular goiter palpable nodules, FNA sampling should be focused on lesions with suspicious US features rather than on larger or clinically dominant nodules
- Nodules less than 1 cm are usually not aspirated unless they have sonographically suspicious features (e.g., microcalcifications) or patients with high-risk history. When cystic lesion is aspirated, the volume, color, and presence of blood should be recorded. If there is a residual mass after aspiration, it should be reaspirated
- The patient should be placed in a supine position with the neck extended; a pillow under the patient's neck is helpful. Local dermal anesthesia may be used, but not recommended. Palpation should be performed as the patient swallows. After selection of the area for the aspiration, the overlaying skin is sterilized by an alcohol pad. A fine (22–27-gauge) needle can be used for most thyroid nodules because the thyroid gland is vascular. During the puncture, the patient is instructed to remain immobile, holding his/her breath. The gland is immobilized against the trachea with one hand as the aspiration is done rapidly and gently, moving back and forth several times for short distances in one channel and maintaining a negative pressure (5–10 mL suction) until blood appears at the cone of the needle. If suction is used, it should be released before the needle is withdrawn from the nodule. Sampling without suction has been reported to yield better results than conventional FNA. If US guidance is used, the needle should not pass through gel, which obscures cytomorphology. The number of passes needed to ensure adequacy varies depending on the nature of the lesion and the experience of the operator, usually three to five times. The central zones should be avoided because they often have regressive changes
- Slides are prepared by expelling and smearing the cells on a slide. Smears can be alcohol fixed and Papanicolaou stained or air-dried and stained with a Romanowsky-type stain. Alternatively, or as an adjunct to smears, the needle is rinsed and the resulting cell suspension used for thin layer or cell block preparations

Table 4.4 Complications of thyroid FNA

- No specific contraindications to thyroid FNA have been reported. Nonetheless, special care should be taken in patients with infectious fever, persistent cough, or bleeding disorders, in children and incapacitated adults, in whom it is difficult to ensure immobility of the neck. Subcutaneous hematoma can be prevented by applying local pressure after the puncture. Other complications, such as abscesses, postaspiration thyrotoxicosis, acute thyroid swelling, delayed swelling of the perithyroid soft tissue, tracheal injury, or damage to the recurrent laryngeal nerve or blood vessels, are uncommon
- Seeding of neoplastic cells along the needle track after aspiration biopsy have been reported both in experimental animals and in humans with the most frequent being papillary carcinoma, followed by follicular carcinoma and anaplastic carcinoma. The incidence of seeding along the needle track is calculated to be ten times lower than that for hepatocellular carcinoma or pancreatic adenocarcinoma and probably is related to the low degree of malignancy of thyroid carcinomas and also to the frequent use of postoperative radioiodine treatment

Table 4.5 Accuracy of thyroid FNA

- Sensitivity of thyroid FNA ranges from 65 to 98 %, and specificity ranges from 72 to 100 %
- The false-positive rate varies from 0 to 7 %. The majority of false-positive diagnoses are due to overinterpretation of repair, hyperplastic papillae, and reactive nuclear changes as features of papillary carcinoma. If the lesion is diagnosed as suspicious for malignancy, the percentage of patients who undergo unnecessary surgery ranges from 15 to 40 %
- False negative rates range from 1 to 11 % and are predominately due to inadequate sampling or improper preparation of the smear and, to a lesser degree, to interpretation error or to the presence of dual pathology. Excluding these causes, the most common errors are due to the presence of a cystic component, hiding occult, and small size carcinomas. Large multinodular goiters may represent an important source of false negatives because 10 % of these cases may show a micropapillary carcinoma on surgical resection

Table 4.6 Thyroid diagnostic categories and risk of malignancy (%)

- Nondiagnostic (1–4 %)
- Benign/Negative (0–3 %)
- Atypical (AUS/FLUS) (5–15 %)
- Follicular neoplasm or suspicious for follicular neoplasm (15–30 %)
- Hurthle cell neoplasm or suspicious for Hurthle cell neoplasm (25–45 %)
- Suspicious for malignancy (60–75 %)
- Malignant (97–99 %)

NCI National Cancer Institute, *PSC* Papanicolaou Society of Cytopathology

Table 4.7 Role of repeat FNA in thyroid

- Indications for repeat FNA of thyroid nodules include follow-up of benign nodules, enlarging nodules, nodules larger than 4 cm, recurrent cyst, and an initial unsatisfactory/nondiagnostic FNA. Repeat conventional (free-hand) FNA in patients with initial unsatisfactory specimens results in an adequate sample in approximately 50 % of cases. Conversely, repeat US-guided FNA of previously nondiagnostic biopsies can lead to a definitive diagnosis in up to 90 % of cases. This is especially helpful in small nodules less than 1.5 cm and complex cystic lesions, where needles can target the more solid component. On the other hand, repeated US-FNA has led to a more definitive diagnosis in 80 % of "indeterminate for follicular neoplasm" diagnoses with follow-up surgical resection
- Repeat FNA in patients with initial benign cytologic diagnoses increases the sensitivity for detecting malignancy from 82 to 90 %

Table 4.8 Management of the thyroid nodule

- The first approach in the study of thyroid nodules should be TSH measurement. If serum TSH is subnormal, a radionuclide thyroid scan should be obtained. Because functioning nodules (hot nodules) rarely harbor malignancy, no additional cytological evaluation is necessary. In patients with cold as well as those with high or normal TSH levels, a thyroid US should be performed. Taking into account the US results, a decision is made about whether FNA directly or assisted by US should be done
- It is difficult to indicate which the most appropriate surgical approach is for patients with suspicious lesions; total thyroidectomy may be excessive, but simple lobectomy may fall short in a large tumor. The selection of the most appropriate procedure should be based on the following findings: gross invasion, tumor size, adherence to neck structures, and palpable nodules in the other lobe. Intraoperative surgical biopsy is not useful because its sensitivity in detecting signs of malignancy is extremely limited. Hamburger and Hamburger have found that in patients with FNA, frozen section results influenced the surgical approach in less than 1 % of the cases
- If the cytologic results are benign, no further immediate diagnostic studies are required; however, cytologically benign but clinically suspicious lesions should be excised. Surgery is indicated in benign lesions with neck disfigurements and local symptoms. Some authors advocate performing a second or even a third FNA several months later to confirm the test, whereas others do not recommend a repeat FNA if the first yielded adequate tissue, provided that the nodule was less than 2 cm and has been stable in size during a year of follow-up. Thyroid incidentalomas should be followed by US in 6–12 months and regularly thereafter. The natural history of the benign conditions is not fully understood, with two reports finding that most nodules became smaller in size, 38 % disappeared, and 23 % increased in size; in those subjected to surgery, there was a malignancy rate of 4.5 %
- Thyroid nodules in children should be managed as in adults (clinical evaluation, serum TSH, US, and FNA). Management in pregnant women should be the same as that for the nonpregnant patient, with the exception that a radionuclide scan is contraindicated. If a nodule discovered early in pregnancy yields a malignant FNA cytology result, it should be monitored sonographically; if it grows substantially by 24 weeks gestation, surgery should be performed at that point. If it remains stable by midgestation or if it is diagnosed in the second half of pregnancy, surgery may be done after delivery

Table 4.9 Ancillary studies

- Ancillary studies, especially immunohistochemistry, may prove valuable in the differential diagnosis of thyroid tumors, provided a cell block or liquid-based preparation is used. New technologies have been developed, but both planimetry and DNA quantitation present overlapping values in benign and malignant lesions. The diagnosis of malignancy should be established based on the cytomorphologic features
- Only a few studies describing the utilization of molecular tests on thyroid FNA specimens have been reported. Papillary carcinoma shows three mutation groups (*RET/PTC*, *RAS*, and *BRAF*) that appear to be functionally similar and mutually exclusive. RET/PTC rearrangements have been reported to be useful as ancillary tests to confirm the diagnosis of malignancy. Detection of a $BRAF^{V600E}$ mutation has proved potentially useful in the diagnosis of suspicious cases of papillary carcinoma in cytology specimen. On the other hand, BRAF mutations, which are common in the classic variant of papillary carcinoma, have been associated with poor prognosis. In follicular adenoma and follicular carcinomas, the most distinctive molecular features are the high prevalence of *RAS* and *PAX8-PPARγ* rearrangements. *RAS* mutations are also commonly activated in nodular goiter and papillary carcinoma and do not provide any useful information from a diagnostic standpoint
- Other genetic and/or epigenetic alterations that play a role in the pathogenesis of papillary carcinomas are TRK rearrangements, which are present in about 20 % of the cases. *MYC* is overexpressed in aggressive malignant differentiated tumors, and *TP53* is almost consistently mutated in poorly differentiated and anaplastic carcinomas. In medullary carcinoma, both familial and sporadic, several specific mutations for *RET* proto-oncogene have been described

Table 4.10 Selective immunohistochemical stains in the differential diagnosis of thyroid tumors

- *Papillary carcinoma, follicular neoplasm:* Thyroglobulin +, TTF1 +
- *Histiocytes and cyst-lining cells:* CD68+, cytokeratin-
- *Endocrine tumors:* Chromogranin+, synaptophysin+, thyroglobulin-, calcitonin+(medullary carcinoma), PTH+(parathyroid adenoma), S-100+ (sustentacular cells in paraganglioma)
- *Metastatic carcinoma:* TTF1+, mCEA+, and thyroglobulin- (lung), GCFP+, mammoglobin+(breast), ER/PR+(breast, ovary), PLAP+(germ cell tumor), HepParl+ (liver), PSA+(prostate), S100+ and HMB 45+ (melanoma), CD10+, EMA+, RCA+, TTF1-, thyroglobulin- (renal cell carcinoma)

EMA Epithelial membrane antigen, *ER/PR* Estrogen/progesterone receptor, *GCFP* Gross cystic fluid protein, *PLAP* Placental like alkaline phosphatase, *PSA* Prostate specific antigen, *PTH* Parathyroid hormone, *RCA* Renal cell antigen, *TTF1* Thyroid transcription factor-1

Table 4.11 Hyalinizing trabecular tumor

- Aspirates from these tumors are easily confused with papillary carcinoma and medullary carcinoma. Cytologic clues to the diagnosis include a whirling, parallel array of elongated cells; amorphous hyaline material that is not amyloid; cytoplasmic "yellow bodies" (which stain light green with the Papanicolaou stain); and a perinucleolar clear zone that are mainly identified by histologic, not cytologic, examination. The follicular cells have a low nucleocytoplasmic ratio and are arranged singly and in cohesive aggregates radially oriented around lumpy polymorphous extracellular material that stains green and pink with Pap and diff-quick stains, respectively. The molecular findings reveal the characteristic RET/PTC rearrangement of papillary carcinoma
- Hyalinizing trabecular tumor is a rare tumor of follicular cell origin, well circumscribed and sometimes encapsulated, formed of solid nests or trabeculae of polygonal or oval cells separated by connective tracks with hyalinization of the perivascular stroma. Tumoral cells are similar to those of papillary carcinoma because they contain cytoplasmic nuclear inclusions and nuclei with longitudinal folds. In its pure form, hyalinizing trabecular tumor almost always has a favorable prognosis

Table 4.12 Thyroid tumors with clear cell features

- Metastatic renal cell carcinoma
- Follicular adenoma
- Follicular carcinoma
- Papillary carcinoma, i.e., columnar cell variant
- Medullary carcinoma
- Paraganglioma
- Parathyroid adenoma
- Histiocytes and cyst-lining cells
- Salivary gland type cancers, i.e., mucoepidermoid carcinoma
- Other metastatic cancers, i.e., lung, head and neck, breast, liver, germ cell tumor

Table 4.13 Malignancies metastatic to the thyroid gland

- Kidney
- Lung
- Breast
- Colon
- Melanoma
- Direct extension from upper aerodigestive tract, i.e., squamous carcinoma, adenoid cystic carcinoma

4.1 Image-Based Questions 1–44

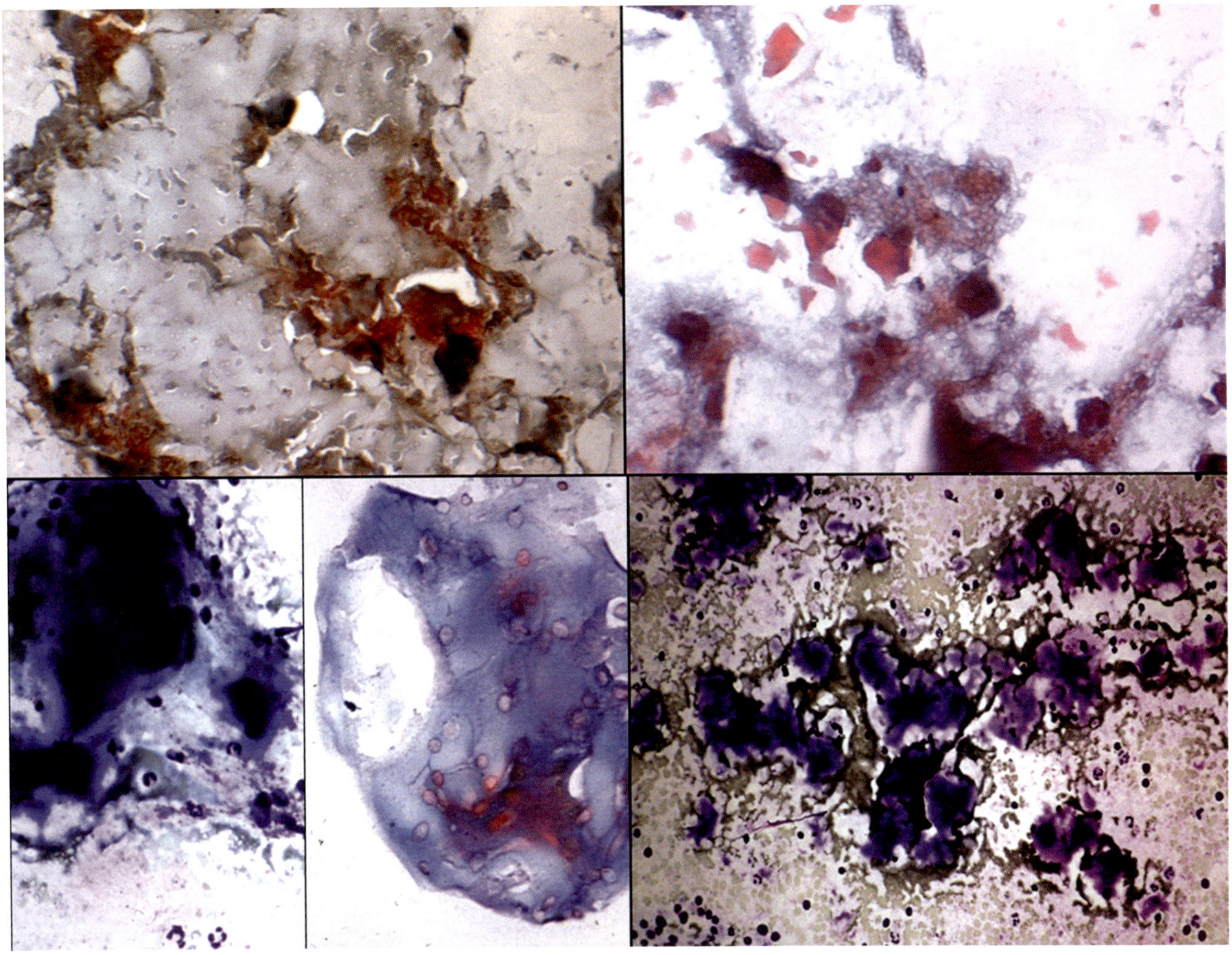

Fig. 4.1

Q-1. This aspirate is from a 49-year-old woman who complains of neck fullness. She has noticed gradual painless enlargement of her thyroid gland for more than 1 year. Laboratory studies of thyroid function shows normal free T4 and TSH levels. Ultrasound examination shows a multiple thyroid nodules with a prominent nodule measuring 4.0 cm and showing complexity of architecture. US-guided FNA of the nodule is performed. Which of the following is the most likely diagnosis?

(a) Benign, colloid nodule
(b) Follicular neoplasm
(c) Benign, lymphocytic (Hashimoto) thyroiditis
(d) Unsatisfactory specimen
(e) Malignant, medullary carcinoma with amyloid

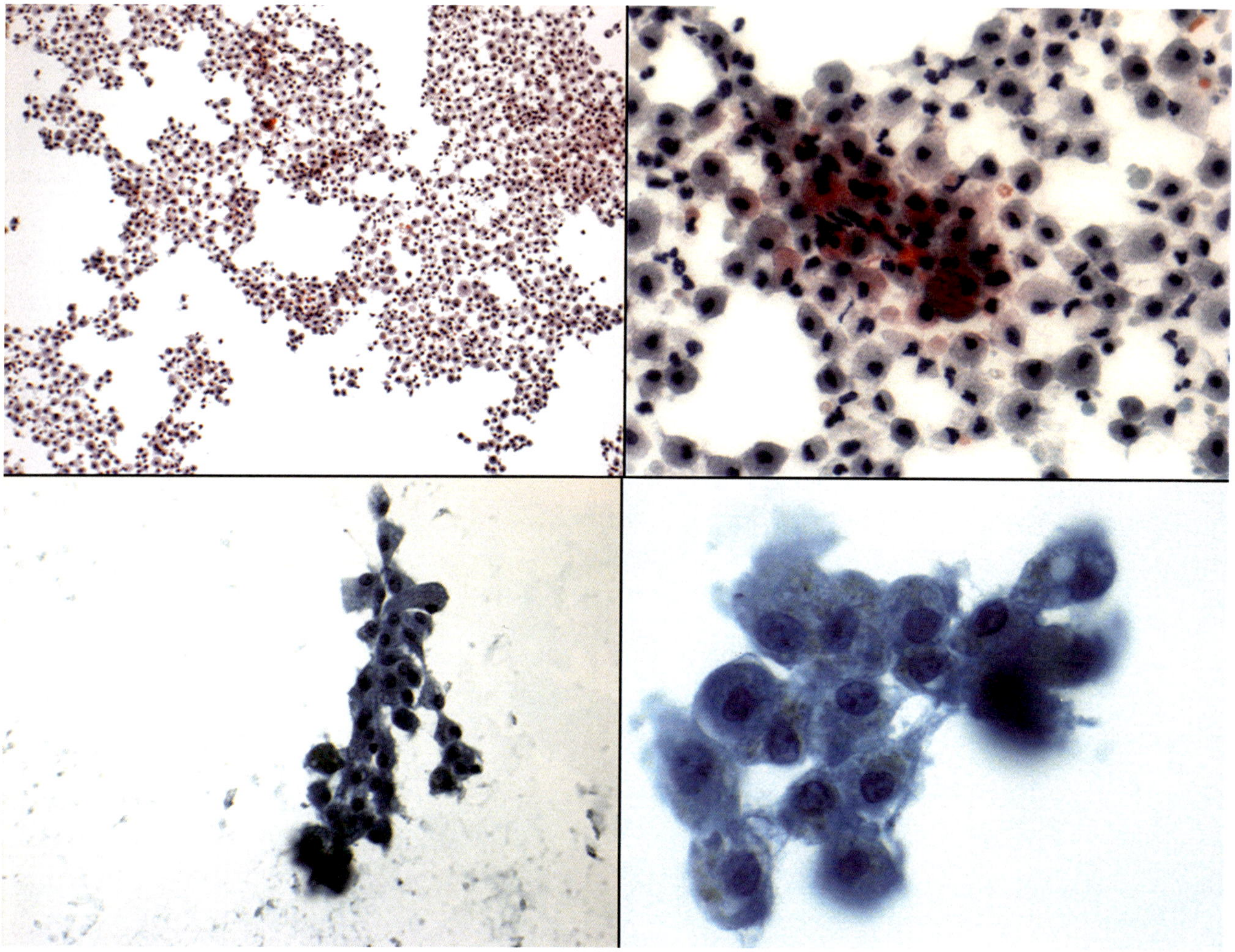

Fig. 4.2

Q-2. This aspirate is from a 56-year-old woman who complains of neck fullness. Physical examination shows multiple painless thyroid nodules. Laboratory studies of thyroid function show normal free T4 and TSH levels. Ultrasound examination shows a large prominent nodule measuring 3.5 cm. US-guided FNA of the thyroid nodule is done. Which of the following is the most likely diagnosis?

(a) Benign, colloid nodule
(b) Benign; adenomatous goiter
(c) Nondiagnostic, cyst fluid only
(d) Lymphocytic thyroiditis
(e) Negative for malignancy

Fig. 4.3

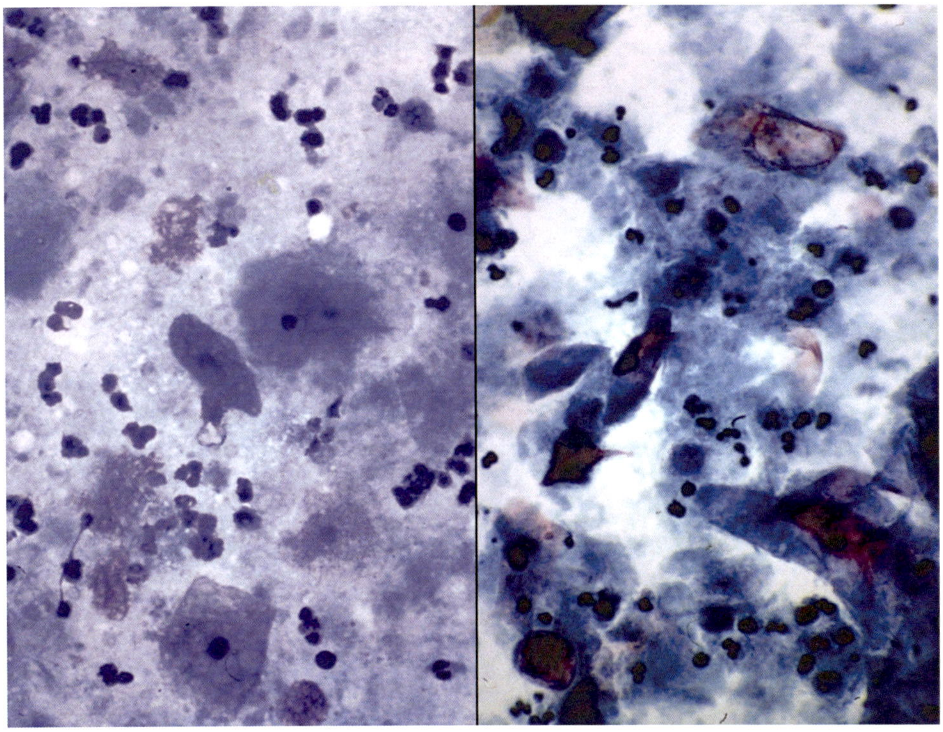

Q-3. This aspirate is from a 35-year-old man who complains of lateral neck nodule. Physical examination shows a painless lateral right neck nodule, but not moving with swallowing. Laboratory studies of thyroid function shows normal free T4 and TSH levels. Ultrasound examination shows a cystic lesion measuring 2.8 cm. US-guided FNA is performed. Which of the following is the most likely diagnosis?

(a) Benign, colloid nodule
(b) Branchial cleft cyst
(c) Benign, thyroid colloid cyst
(d) Benign, lymphocytic thyroiditis
(e) Nondiagnostic, unsatisfactory specimen

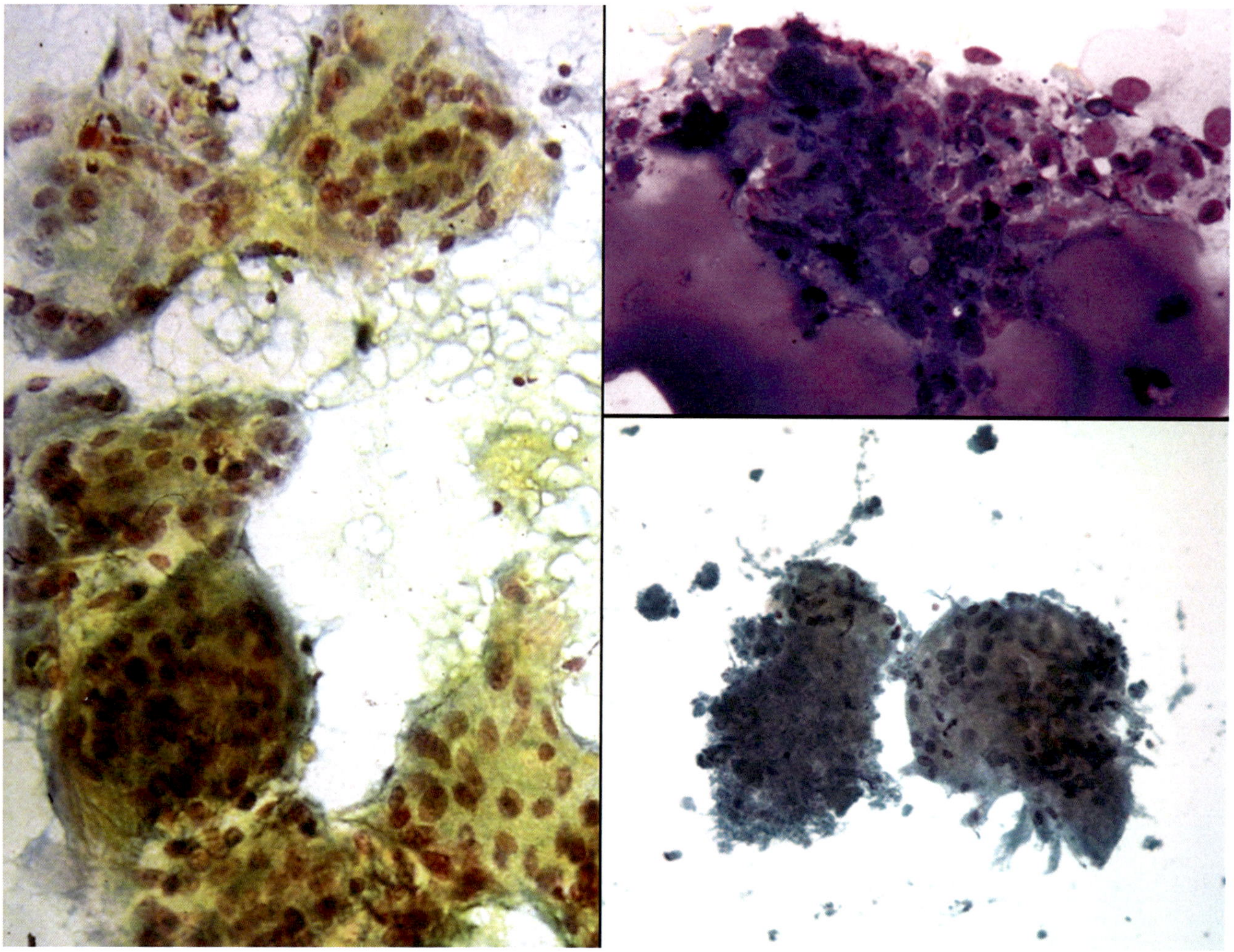

Fig. 4.4

Q-4. This aspirate is from a 37-year-old woman who presents with difficulty swallowing and a feeling of fullness in her neck for the past 2 weeks. She is recovering from a mild upper respiratory tract infection 1 month ago. Palpation of her diffusely enlarged thyroid elicits pain. Laboratory studies show an increased serum free T4 level and a decreased TSH level. US-guided FNA is performed. Which of the following is the most likely diagnosis?

(a) Medullary carcinoma
(b) Benign, subacute granulomatous (de Quervain) thyroiditis
(c) Benign, multinodular goiter
(d) Benign, Hashimoto thyroiditis
(e) Benign, toxic thyrotoxicosis (Grave's disease)

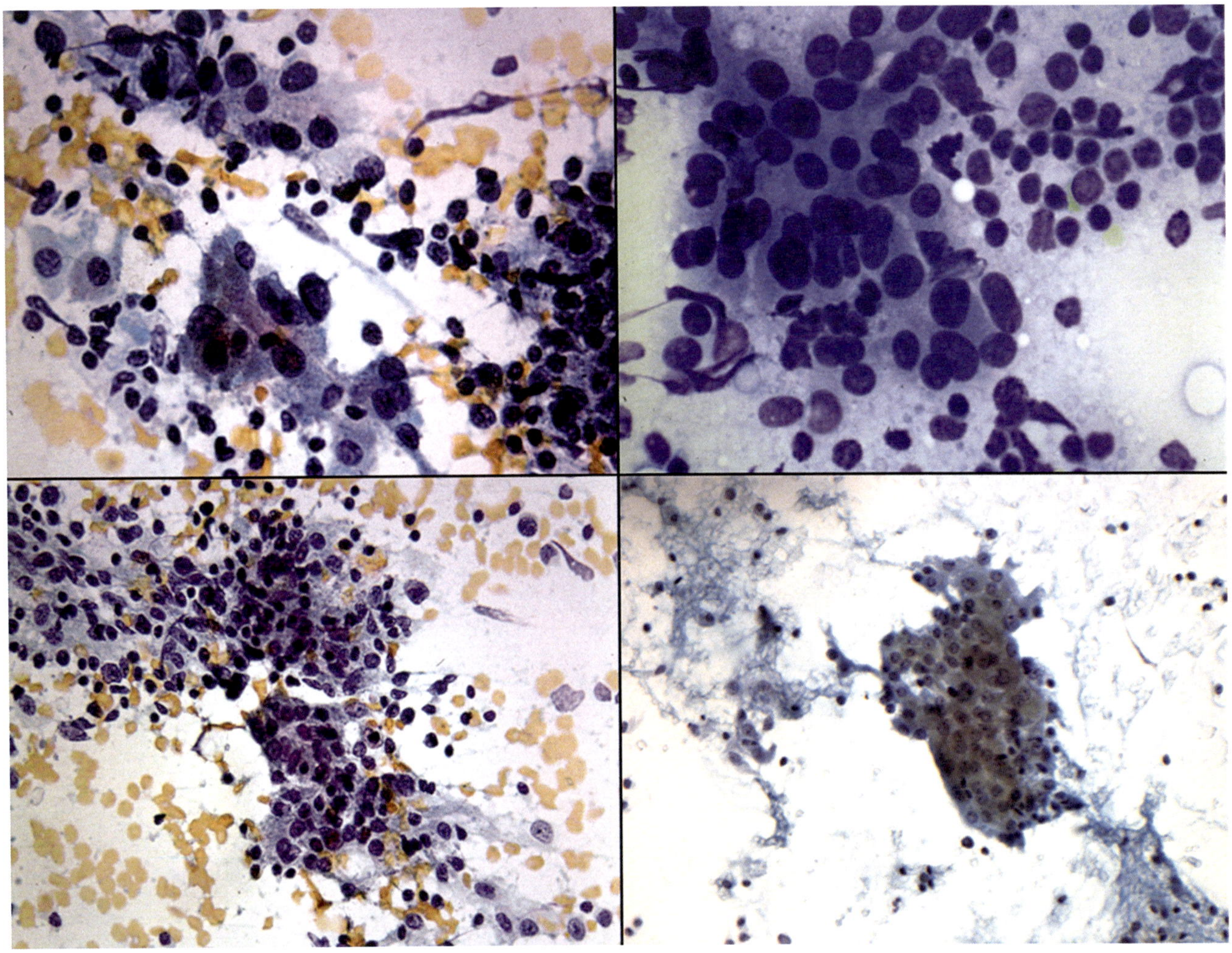

Fig. 4.5

Q-5. This aspirate is from a 61-year-old woman who has experienced a feeling of fullness in her neck for the past year. She complains of loss of energy, easy fatigue, and difficulty concentrating at work. On physical examination, the thyroid gland is diffusely large with a feeling of one thyroid nodule. The gland is not tender on palpation. She has dry, coarse skin and alopecia. US-guided FNA of the thyroid nodule is performed. Which of the following is the most likely the diagnosis?

(a) Hurthle cell neoplasm
(b) Subacute granulomatous (de Quervain) thyroiditis
(c) Benign, acute thyroiditis
(d) Atypical (FLUS/AUS), radiation atypia
(e) Benign, chronic lymphocytic (Hashimoto) thyroiditis

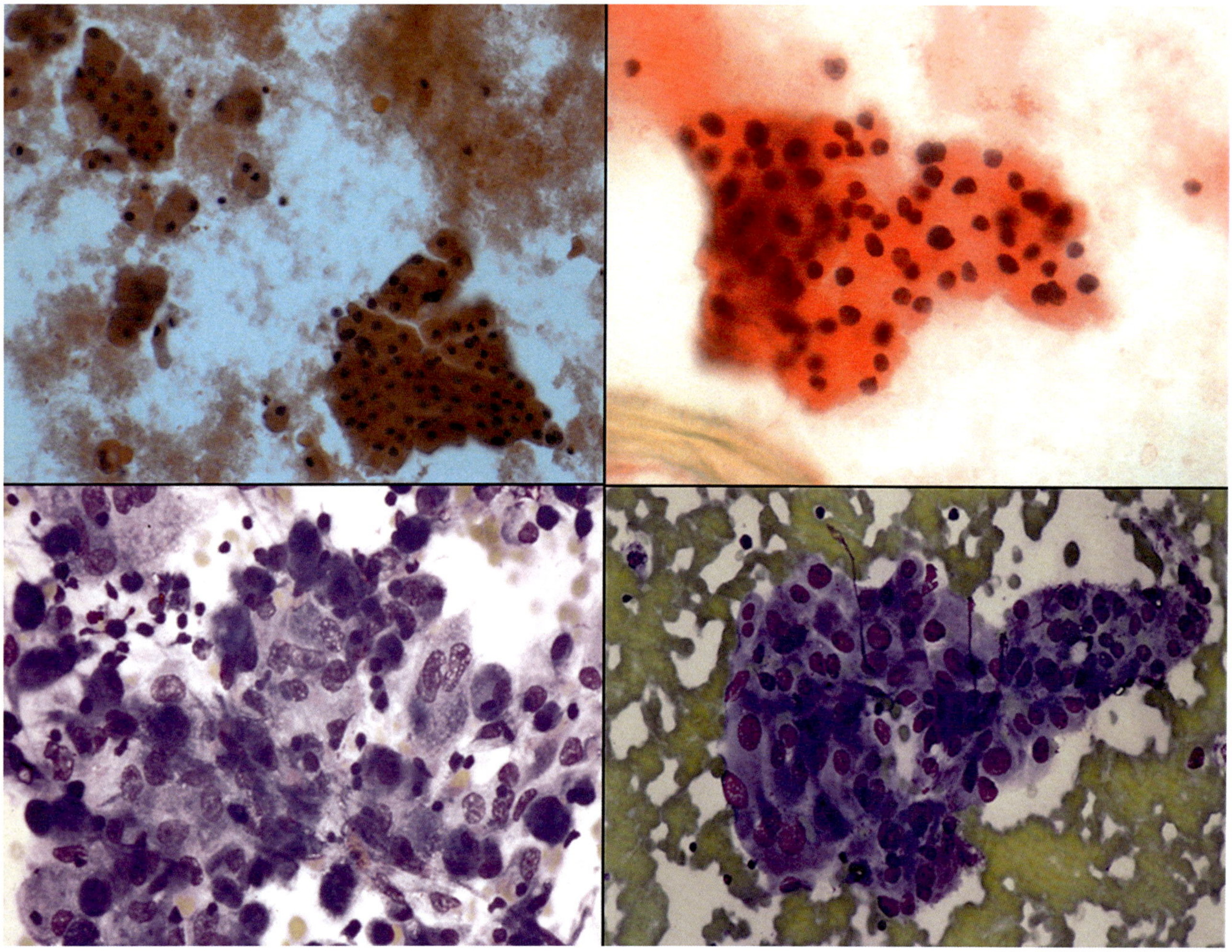

Fig. 4.6

Q-6. This aspirate is from a 76-year-old woman who complains of neck fullness. Physical examination shows diffusely enlarged thyroid gland with a thyroid nodule. Laboratory studies of thyroid function show normal free T4 with low TSH levels. Ultrasound examination shows a large prominent nodule measuring 3.0 cm. US-guided FNA of the thyroid nodule is performed. Which of the following is the most likely diagnosis?
(a) Benign colloid nodule
(b) Benign, multinodular goiter
(c) Benign, Hurthle cell metaplasia in background of lymphocytic thyroiditis
(d) Hurthle cell neoplasm
(e) Malignant, papillary thyroid carcinoma

Fig. 4.7

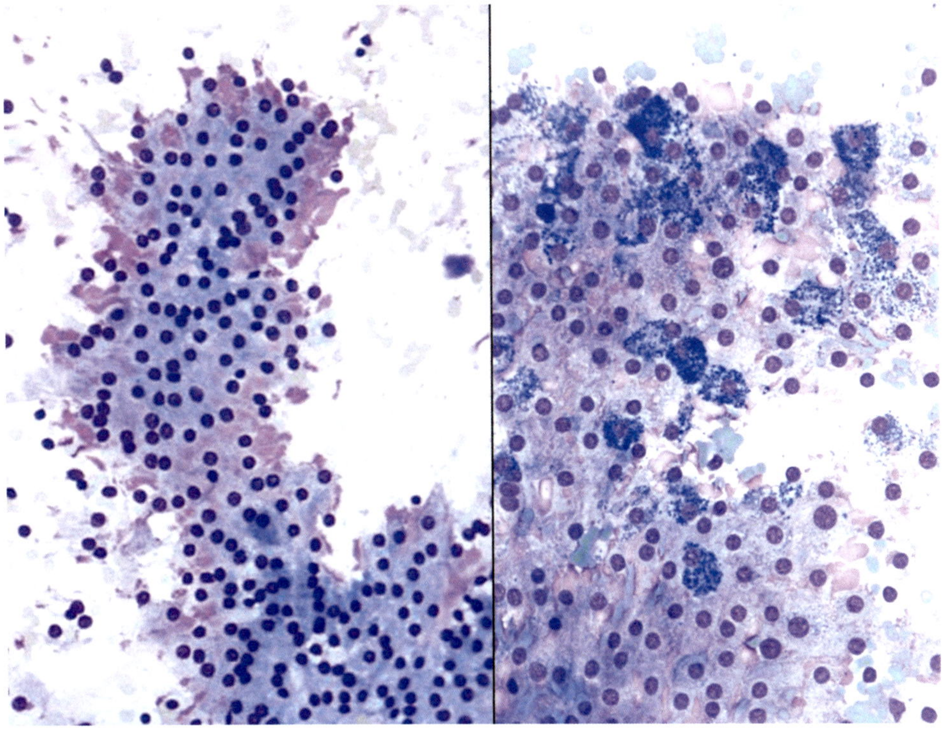

Q-7. This aspirate is from a 22-year-old woman who has experienced increasing fatigue and weight loss in spite of increasing her appetite over the past 4 months. She complains of increasing anxiety and nervousness with no apparent changes in her job or lifestyle. She now has diarrhea. Physical examination shows a diffusely enlarged thyroid gland with vague nodularity. The clinician decides to do US-guided FNA of the thyroid gland to confirm the benign diagnosis. Later, a radionuclide scan of the thyroid shows a diffuse increase in radioactive iodine uptake. Which of the following is the most likely diagnosis?

(a) Irradiation effect
(b) Toxic diffuse hyperplasia (Graves' disease)
(c) Colloid nodule
(d) Multinodular goiter
(e) Papillary carcinoma

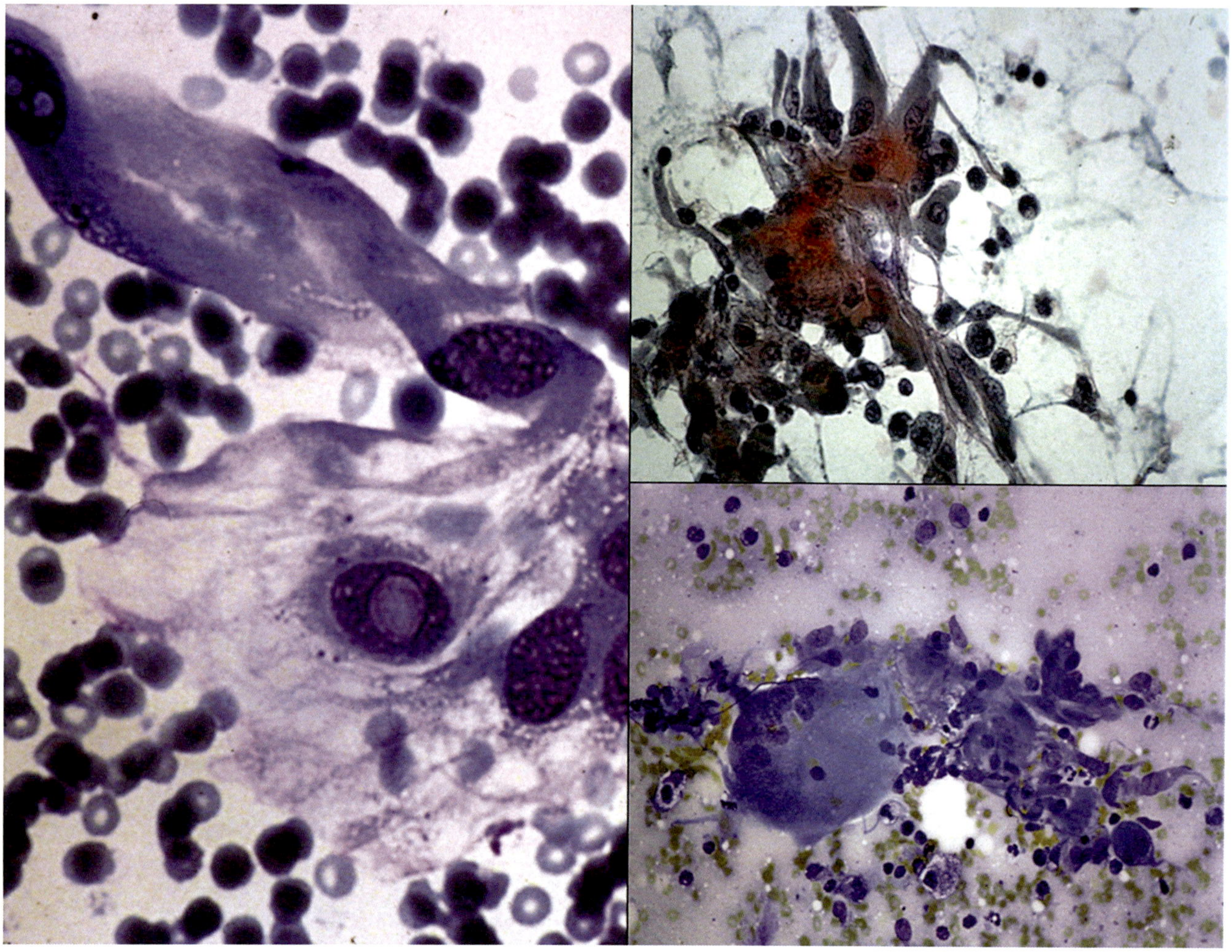

Fig. 4.8

Q-8. This aspirate is from an 80-year-old man who has history of tongue squamous cell carcinoma. The patient has past history of receiving radiotherapy for his neck lymph nodes. Now he comes with sense of neck fullness. Physical examination shows diffusely enlarged thyroid gland with thyroid nodule. Ultrasound examination shows a prominent thyroid nodule measuring 2.5 cm. US-guided FNA of the thyroid nodule is performed to exclude the presence of malignancy. Which of the following is the most likely diagnosis?

(a) Metastatic renal cell carcinoma
(b) Metastatic squamous cell carcinoma
(c) Benign, radiation changes
(d) Hurthle cell neoplasm.
(e) Malignant, papillary carcinoma

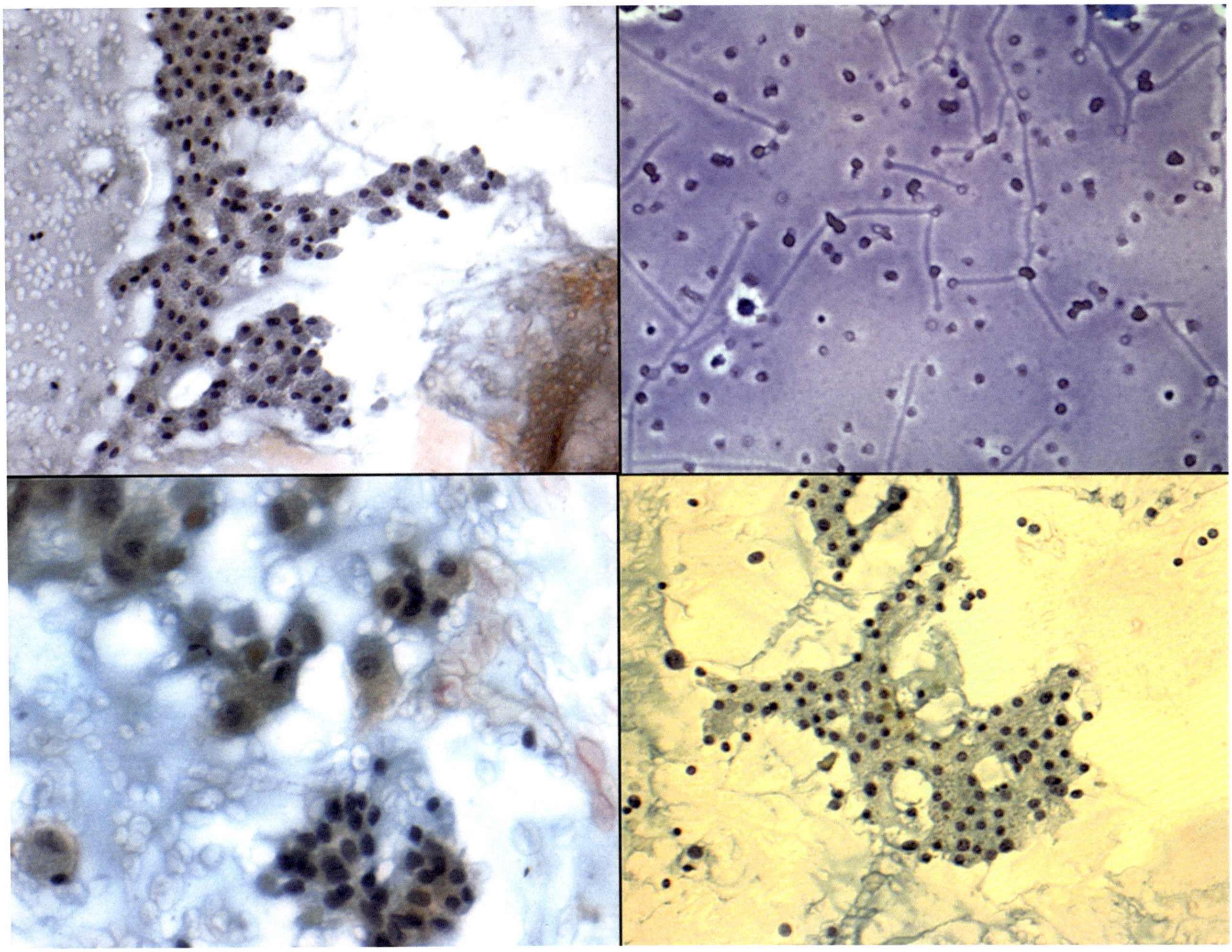

Fig. 4.9

Q-9. This aspirate is from a 47-year-old woman who complains of neck fullness. Physical examination shows multiple painless thyroid nodules. Laboratory studies of thyroid function show normal free T4 and TSH levels. Ultrasound examination shows a large prominent nodule measuring 3.5 cm. US-guided FNA is performed. Which of the following is the most likely diagnosis?

(a) Hurthle cell neoplasm
(b) Nondiagnostic, cyst fluid only
(c) Benign, lymphocytic thyroiditis
(d) Benign colloid nodule
(e) Benign, hyperplastic thyroid nodule

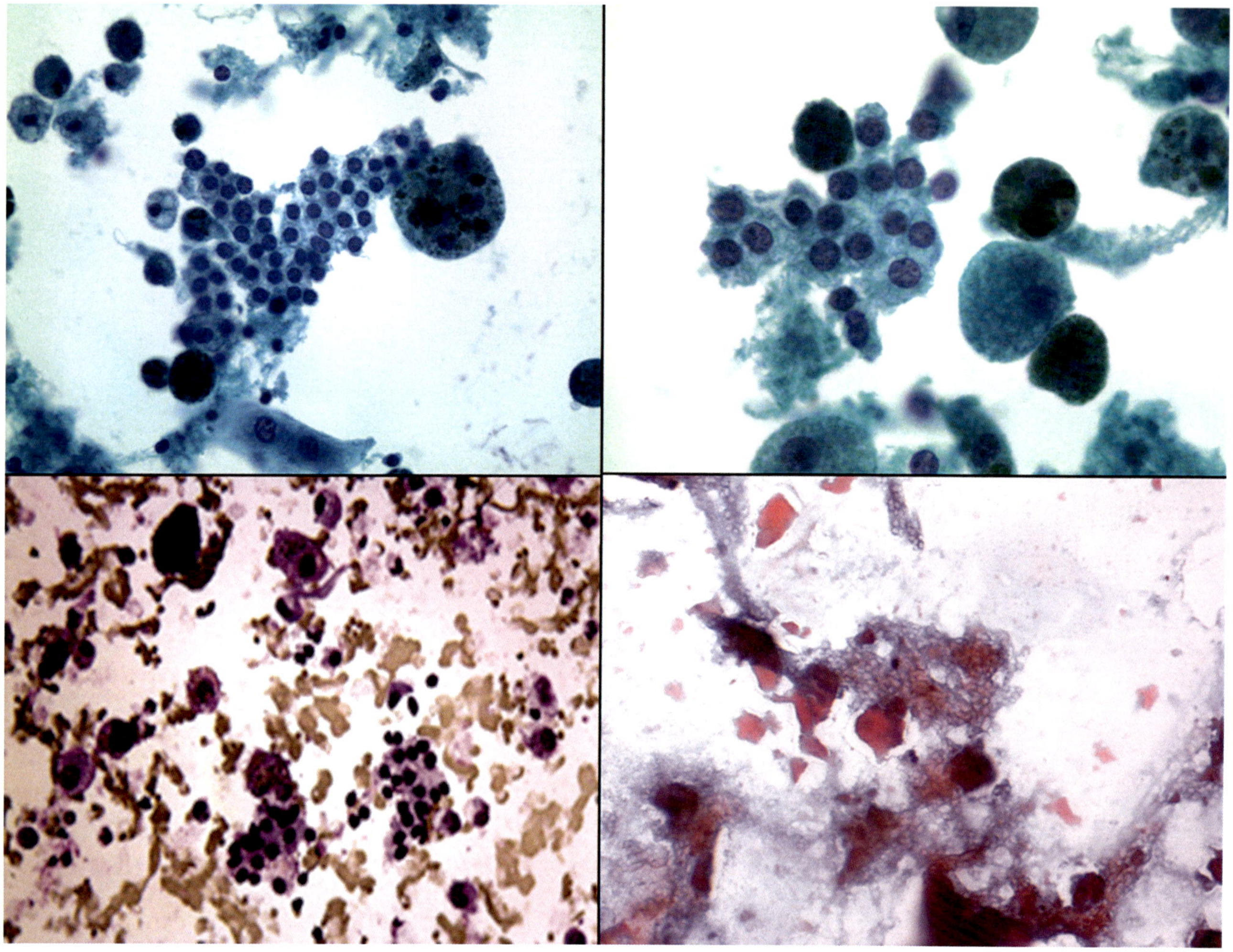

Fig. 4.10

Q-10. This aspirate is from a 56-year-old woman who complains of neck fullness. Physical examination shows multiple painless thyroid nodules. Laboratory studies of thyroid function show normal free T4 and TSH levels. Ultrasound examination shows a large prominent nodule measuring 3.5 cm. US-guided FNA of the thyroid nodule is performed. Which of the following is the most likely diagnosis?

(a) Hurthle cell neoplasm
(b) Benign colloid nodule
(c) Nondiagnostic, cyst fluid only
(d) Benign, lymphocytic thyroiditis
(e) Benign, hyperplastic thyroid nodule

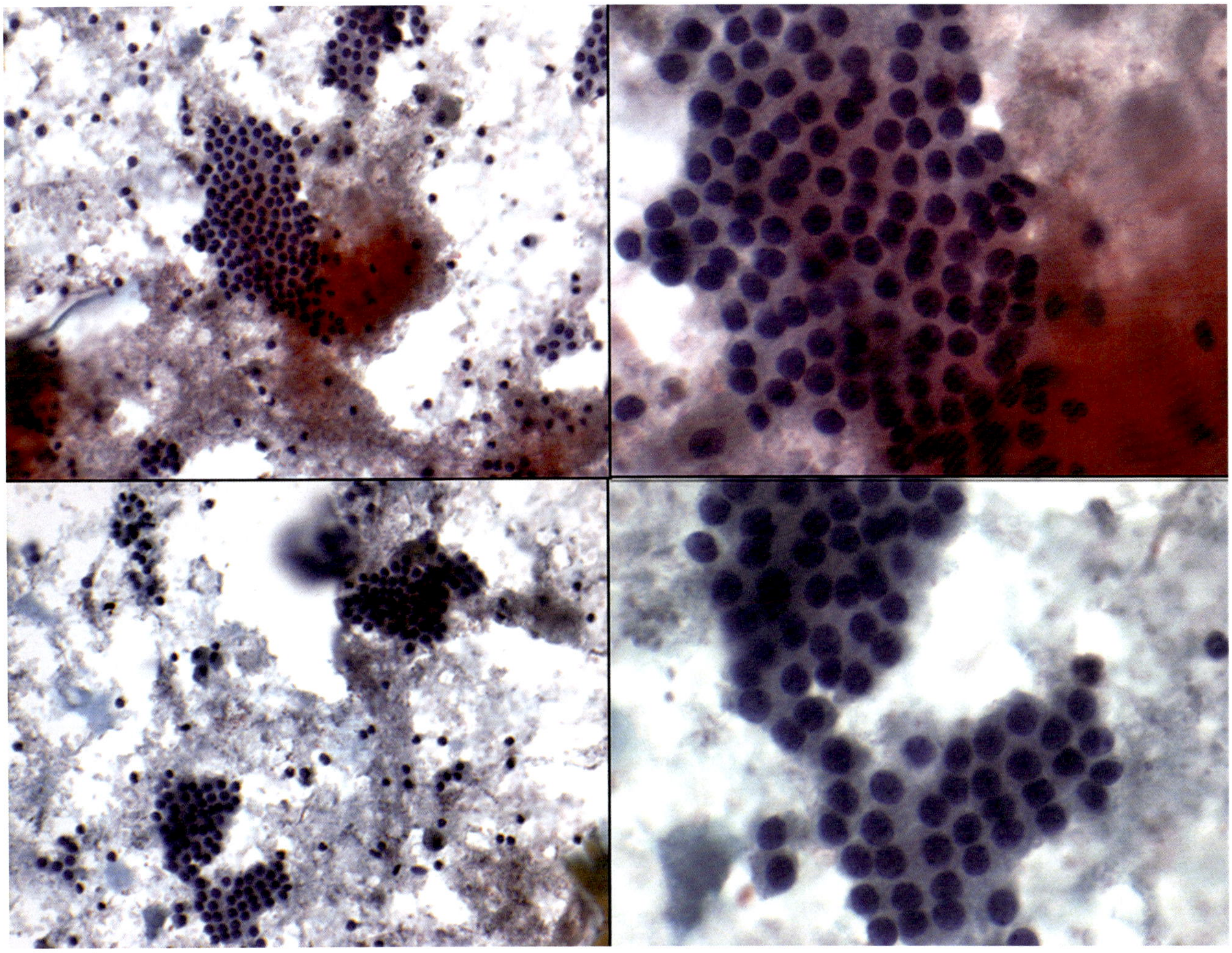

Fig. 4.11

Q-11. This aspirate is from a 45-year-old woman who complains of neck fullness. Physical examination shows multiple painless thyroid nodules. Laboratory studies of thyroid function show normal free T4 and TSH levels. Ultrasound examination shows a large prominent nodule measuring 3.5 cm. US-guided FNA of the thyroid nodule is performed. Which of the following is the most likely diagnosis?

(a) Hurthle cell neoplasm
(b) Benign colloid nodule
(c) Nondiagnostic, cyst fluid only
(d) Benign, lymphocytic thyroiditis
(e) Benign, hyperplastic (adenomatoid) nodule

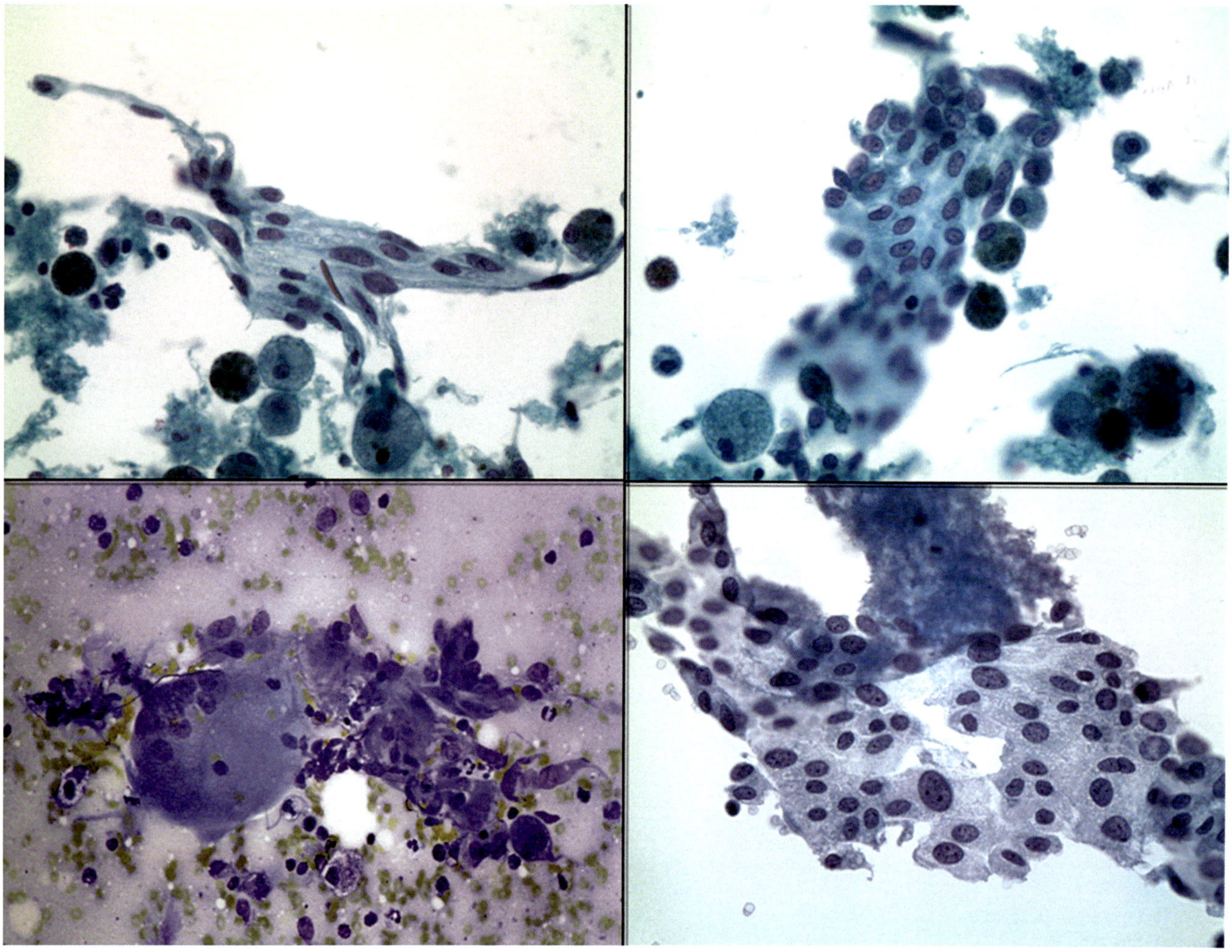

Fig. 4.12

Q-12. This aspirate is from a 55-year-old woman who complains of neck fullness. Physical examination shows multiple painless thyroid nodules with some showing cystic changes. Laboratory studies of thyroid function shows normal free T4 and TSH levels. Ultrasound examination shows a large prominent nodule measuring 4.0 cm. US-guided FNA of the thyroid nodule is performed. Which of the following is the most likely diagnosis?

(a) Benign, reactive atypia/cyst-lining
(b) Malignant, papillary thyroid carcinoma
(c) Malignant, anaplastic carcinoma
(d) Benign, lymphocytic thyroiditis
(e) Benign, hyperplastic nodule

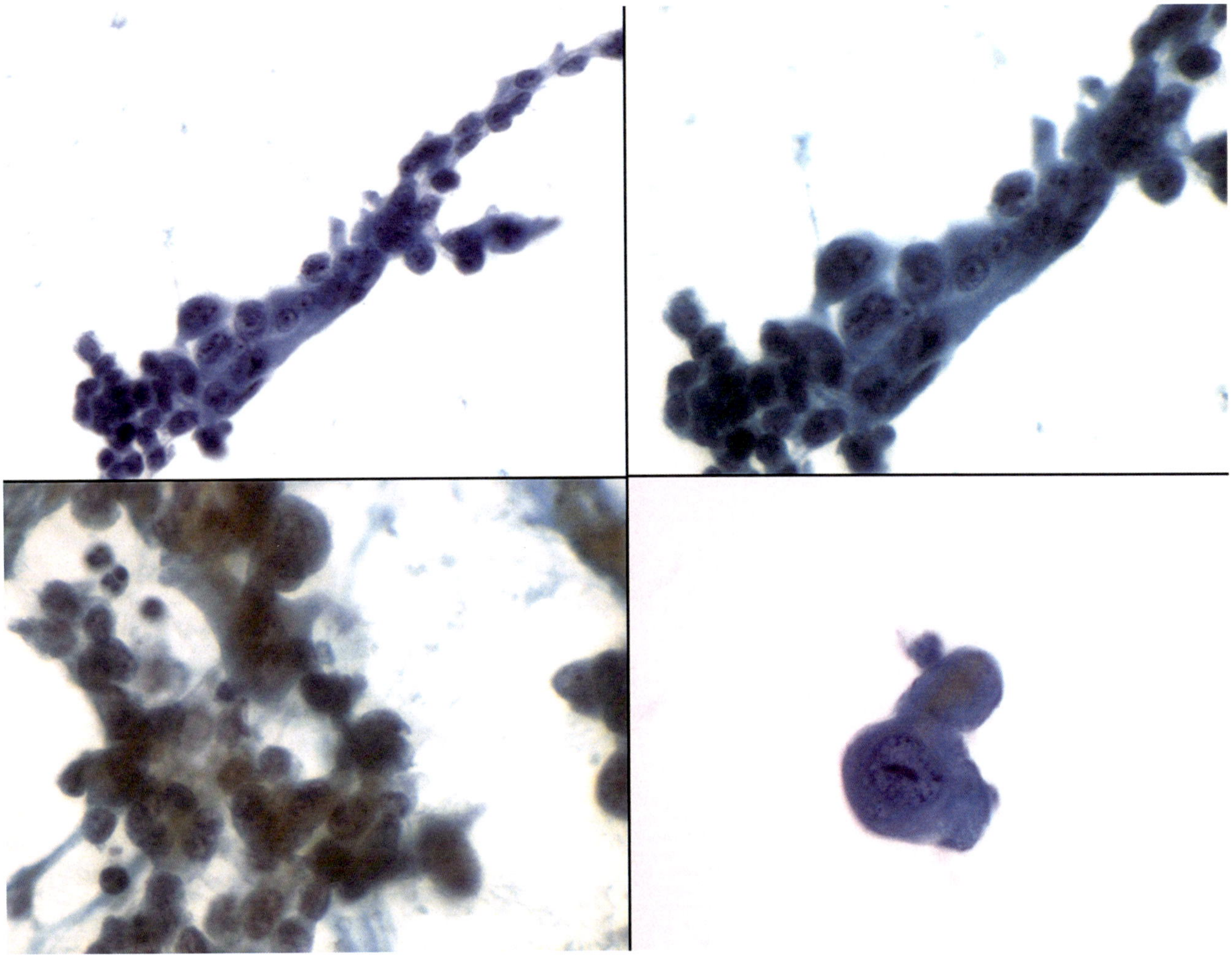

Fig. 4.13

Q-13. This aspirate is from a 55-year-old man who noticed a nodule in his neck. Physical examination shows a painless thyroid nodule, 2.0 cm in greatest dimension. Laboratory studies of thyroid function shows normal free T4 and TSH levels. Ultrasound examination shows a large prominent nodule with complex architecture, suspicious for thyroid cancer. US-guided FNA of the thyroid nodule is performed. Which of the following is the most likely diagnosis?

(a) Hurthle cell neoplasm
(b) Benign, colloid nodule
(c) Nondiagnostic, cyst fluid only
(d) Atypical cells of undetermined significance (AUS/FLUS)
(e) Benign, hyperplastic (adenomatoid) nodule

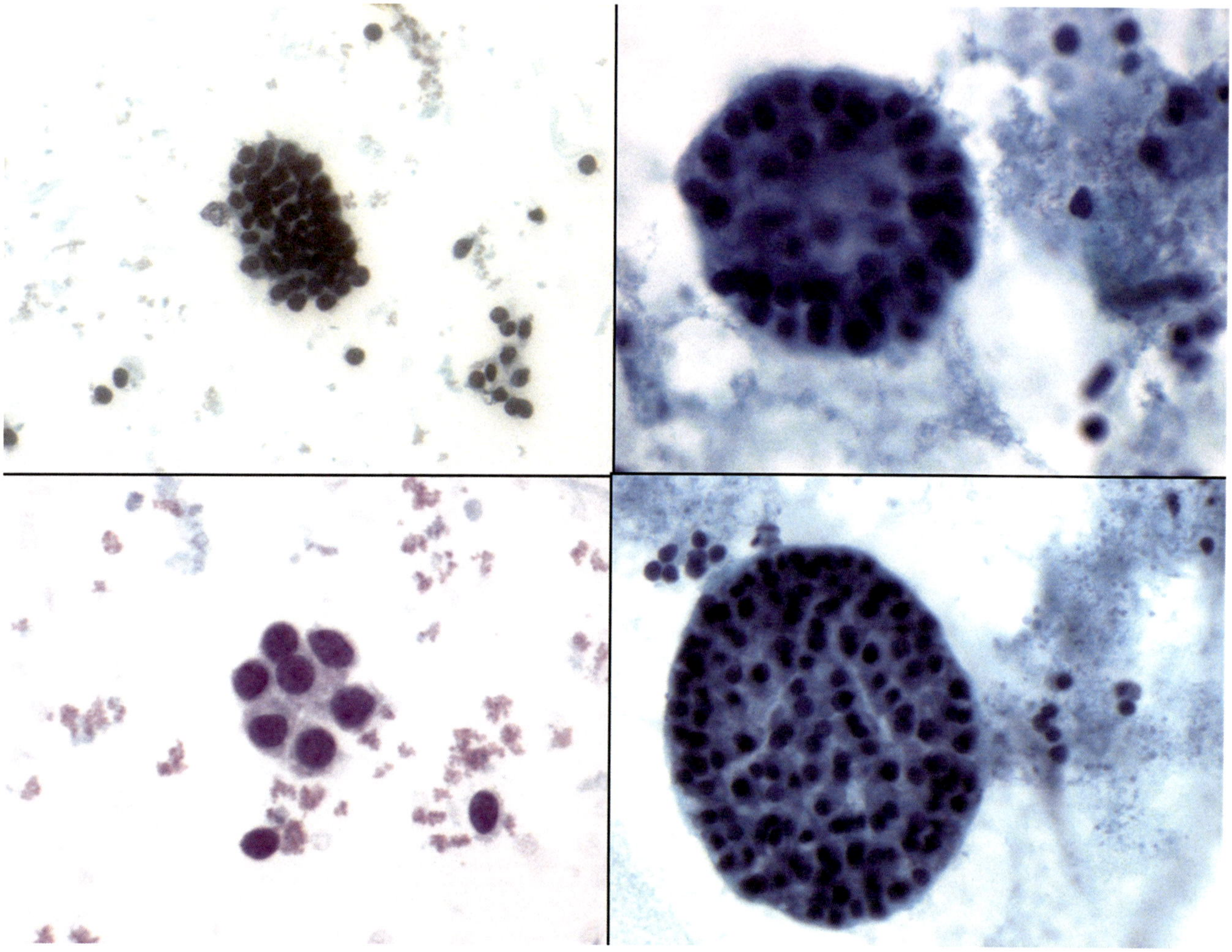

Fig. 4.14

Q-14. A 49-year-old woman complains of neck fullness. She has noticed gradual painless enlargement of her thyroid gland for more than 1 year. Physical examination demonstrates diffuse enlargement of the thyroid gland. Laboratory studies of thyroid function show normal free T4 and TSH levels. Ultrasound examination shows a prominent nodule measuring 4.0 cm with complexity of architecture. There is background of multinodular goiter. US-guided FNA of the thyroid nodule is performed. Which of the following is the most likely diagnosis?

(a) Papillary carcinoma
(b) Follicular neoplasm
(c) Benign, hyperplastic/adenomatoid nodule
(d) Medullary carcinoma
(e) Lymphocytic thyroiditis

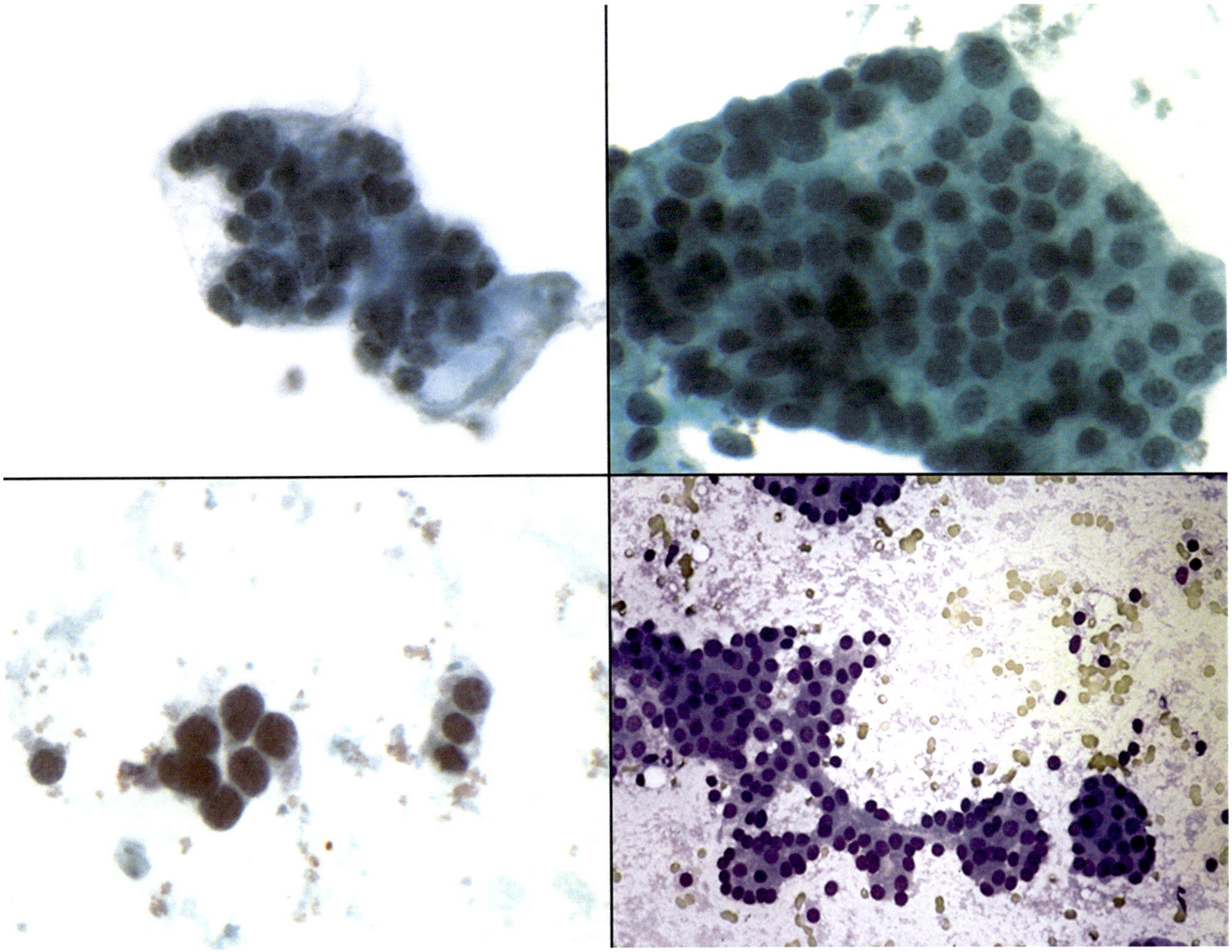

Fig. 4.15

Q-15. A 47-year-old man visits his physician because he noticed a "lump" in his neck 3 weeks ago. His past history is unremarkable. On physical examination, there is a 3-cm nodule in the right lobe of the thyroid gland. Laboratory studies of thyroid function shows normal free T4 and TSH levels. US-guided FNA of the thyroid nodule is performed. What is the most appropriate diagnosis of this lesion?

(a) Papillary carcinoma
(b) Follicular neoplasm
(c) Medullary carcinoma
(d) Benign, lymphocytic thyroiditis
(e) Benign, hyperplastic (adenomatoid) nodule

Fig. 4.16

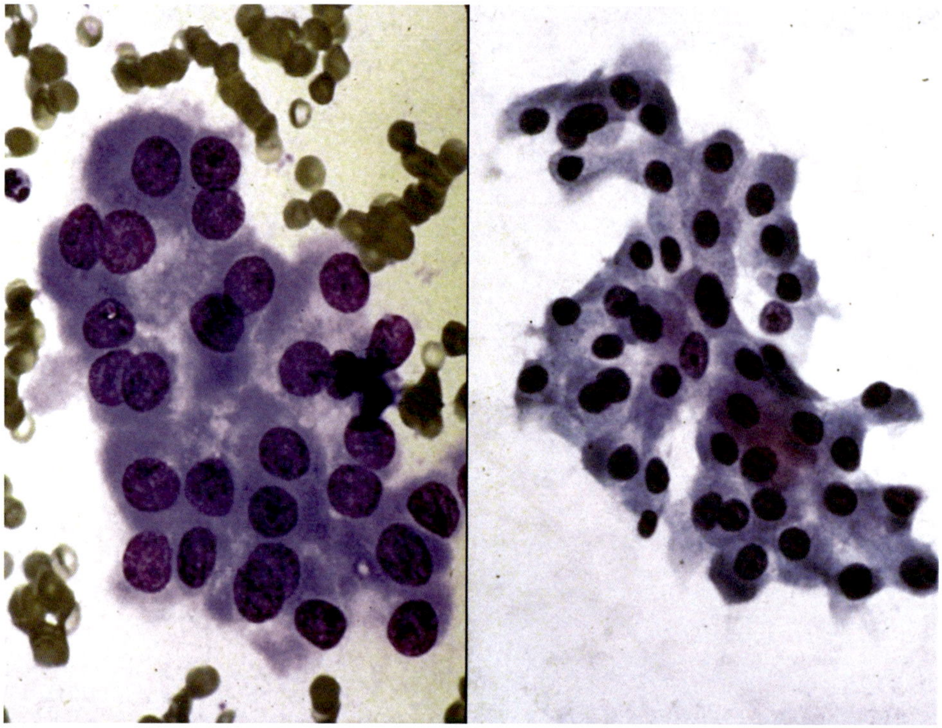

Q-16. This aspirate is from a 65-year-old woman who noticed a nodule in her neck. Physical examination shows a painless thyroid nodule, measuring 2.0 cm. Laboratory studies of thyroid function show normal free T4 and TSH levels. The nodule is cold on scan. Ultrasound examination shows a large prominent nodule. US-guided FNA of the thyroid nodule is performed. Which of the following is the most likely diagnosis?

(a) Hürthle cell neoplasm
(b) Benign colloid nodule
(c) Benign, hyperplastic/adenomatoid nodule
(d) Follicular neoplasm
(e) Papillary carcinoma

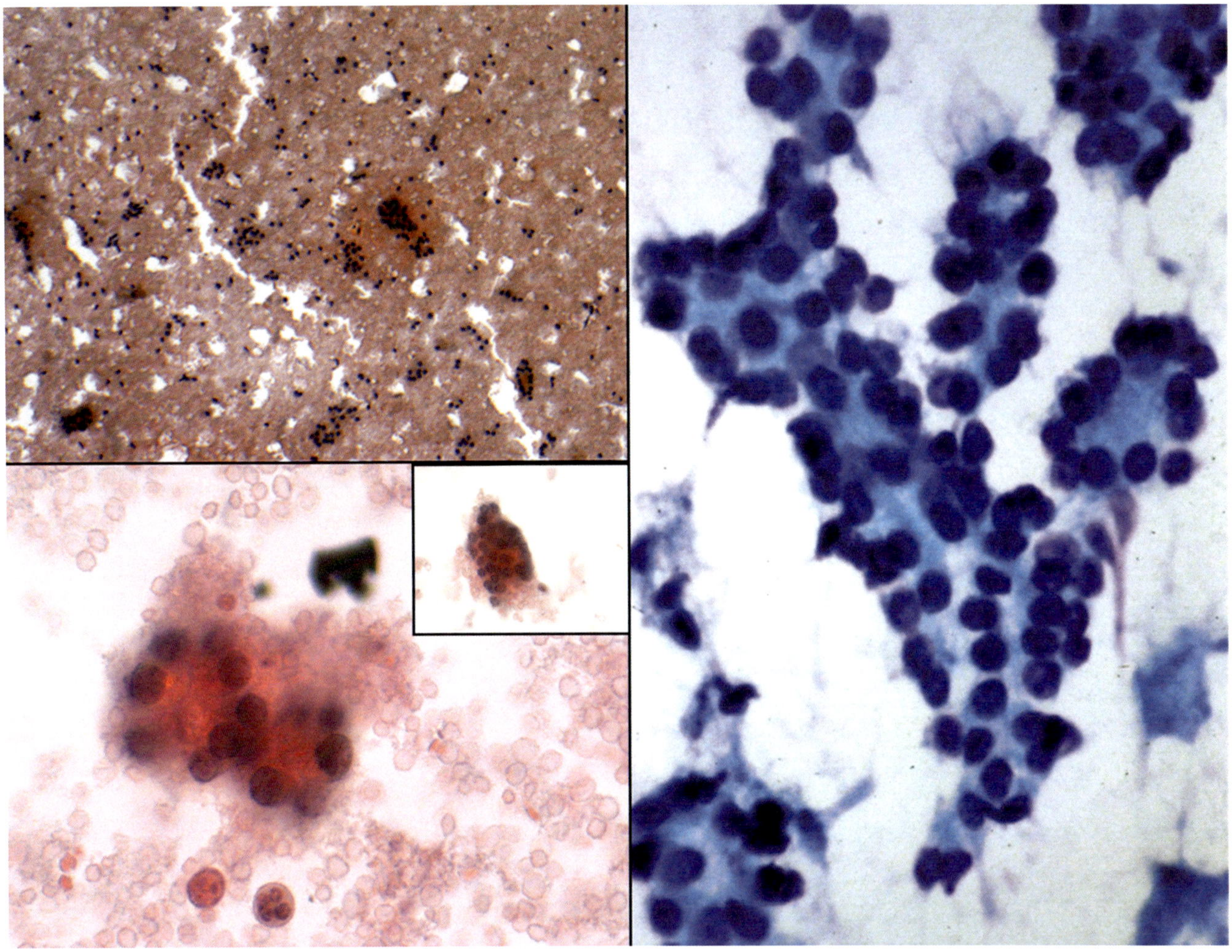

Fig. 4.17

Q-17. A 60-year-old woman has felt a lump on the right side of her neck for several months. On physical examination, she has a firm 3-cm mass in the right lobe of the thyroid gland. There is no palpable lymphadenopathy. Laboratory studies show normal TSH and T4 levels. A fine-needle aspiration biopsy is performed. Which of the following is the most likely diagnosis?

(a) Anaplastic carcinoma
(b) Medullary carcinoma
(c) Granulomatous thyroiditis
(d) Benign, Hashimoto thyroiditis
(e) Follicular neoplasm

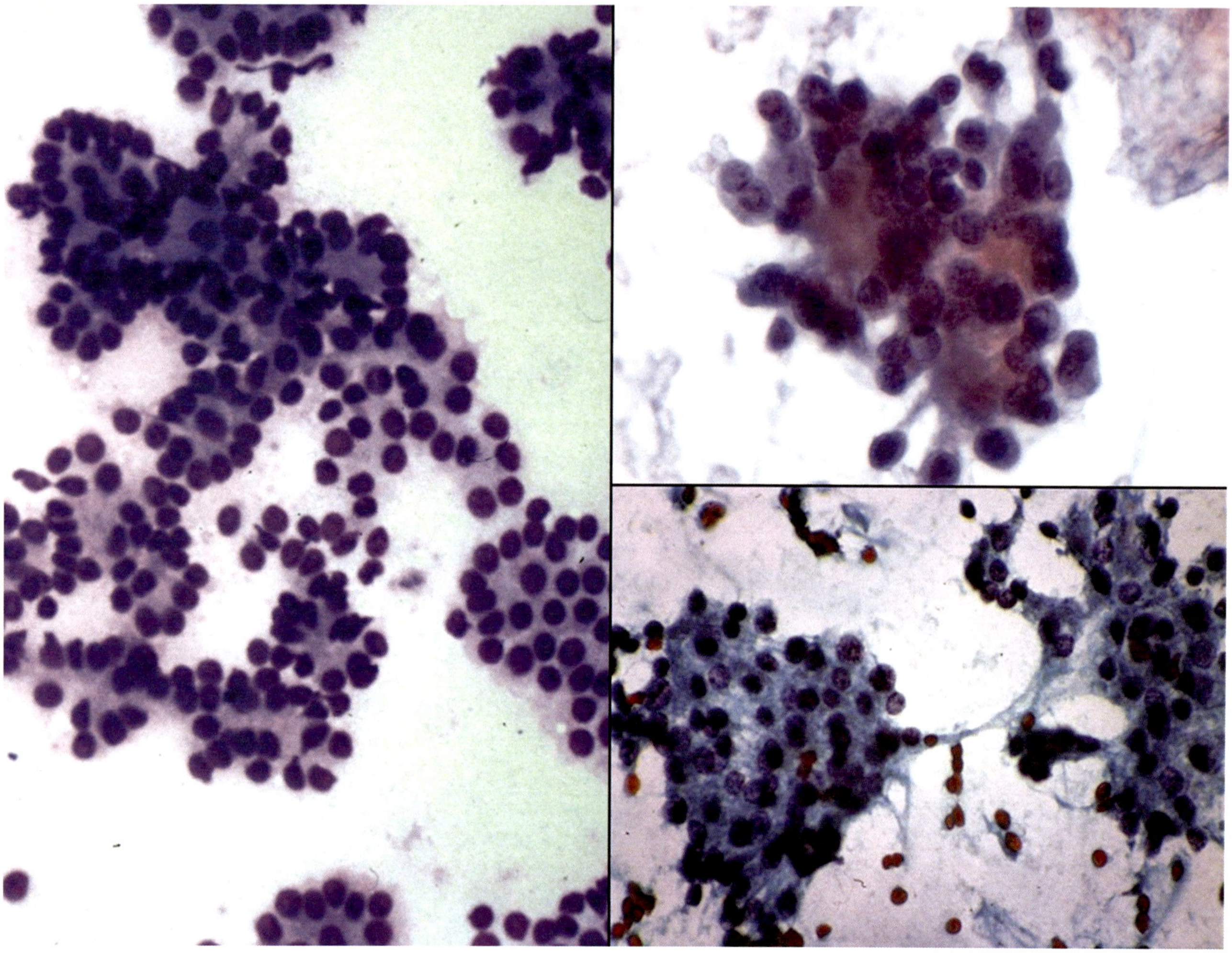

Fig. 4.18

Q-18. This aspirate is from a 60-year-old woman who has felt a "lump" on the right side of her neck for several months. On physical examination, she has a firm 3-cm mass in the right lobe of the thyroid gland. There is no palpable lymphadenopathy. Laboratory studies show normal TSH and T4 levels. Seven months later, she visits her physician again because of pain in the right hip. A radiograph shows a fracture of the right femur with an area of lytic bone destruction. FNA for both thyroid nodule and femur lesion is performed. Which of the following is the most likely diagnosis?

(a) Anaplastic carcinoma
(b) Follicular neoplasm, favoring follicular carcinoma
(c) Granulomatous thyroiditis
(d) Follicular neoplasm
(e) Medullary carcinoma

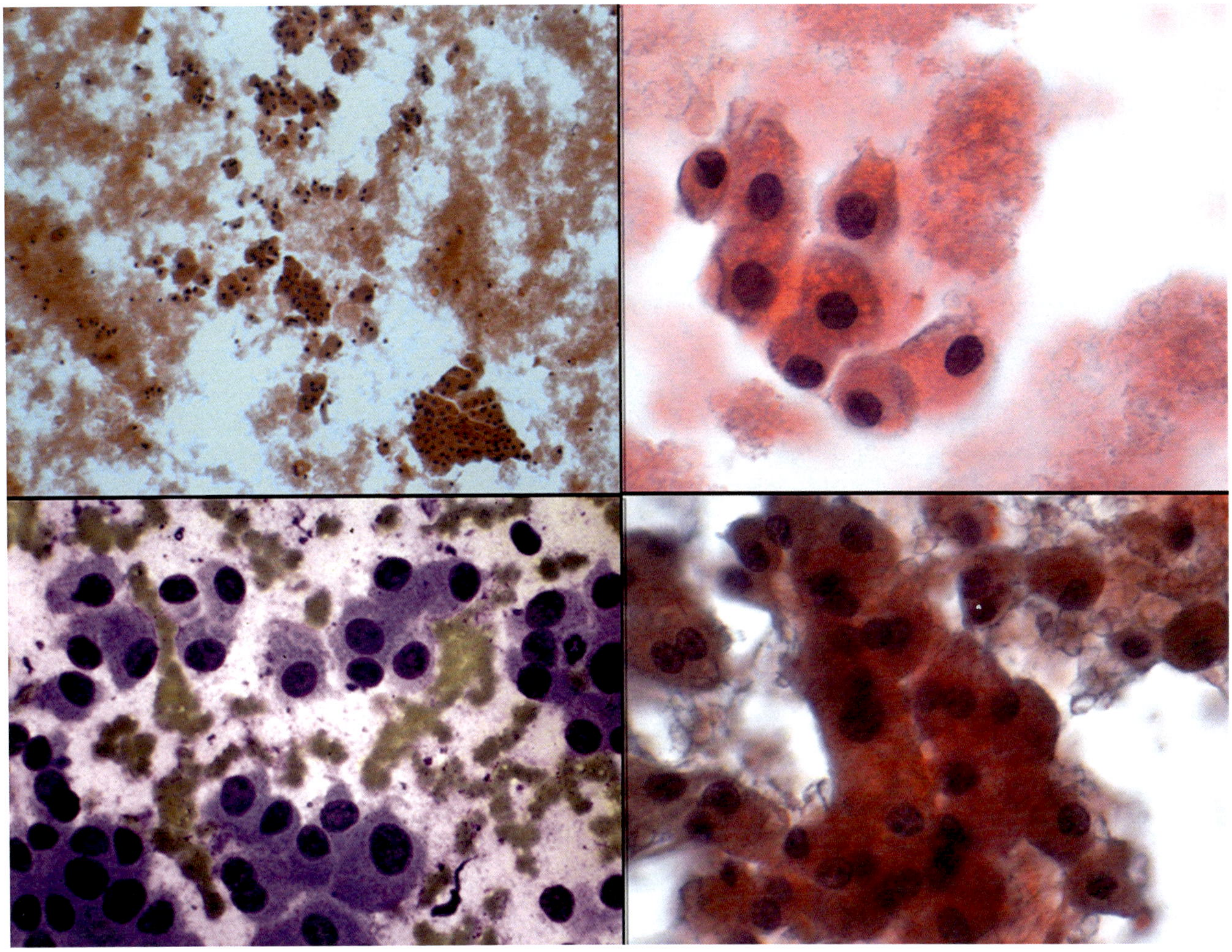

Fig. 4.19

Q-19. A 62-year-old woman presents with a "lump" on right side of her neck for several months. On physical examination, she has a firm 2.5-cm mass in the isthmus lobe of the thyroid gland. There is no palpable lymphadenopathy. Laboratory studies show normal TSH and T4 levels. US-guided FNA of the thyroid nodule is performed. Which of the following is the most likely diagnosis?

(a) Anaplastic carcinoma
(b) Follicular neoplasm
(c) Benign, granulomatous thyroiditis
(d) Benign, Hashimoto thyroiditis
(e) Hurthle cell neoplasm

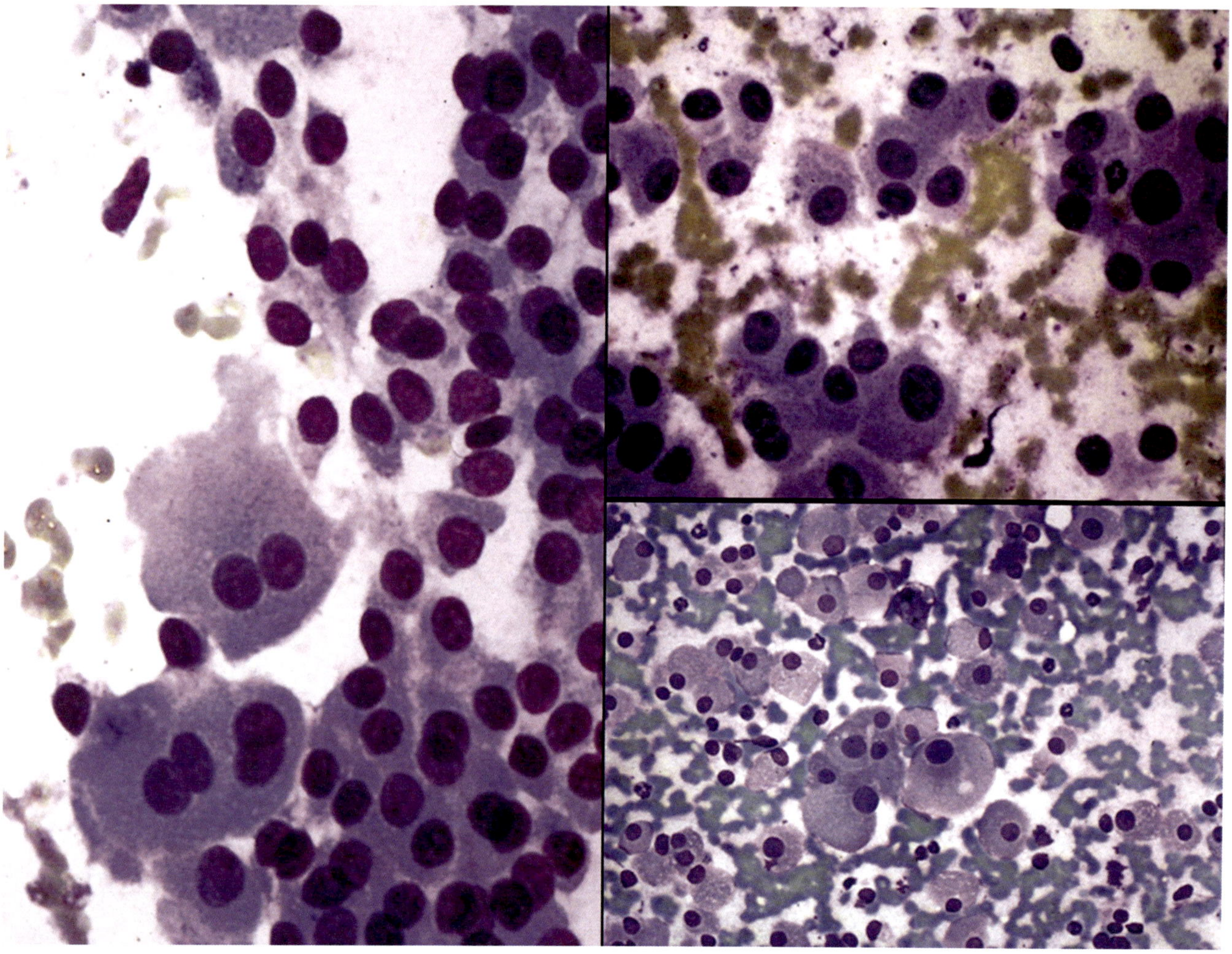

Fig. 4.20

Q-20. This aspirate is from a 62-year-old man who has felt a "lump" on the left side of his neck. Physical examination reveals a firm 3-cm nodule in the left lobe of the thyroid gland. There is no palpable lymphadenopathy. Laboratory studies show normal TSH and T4 levels. Five months later, he presents with pain in his right hip. A radiograph shows a fracture of the right femur with an area of lytic bone destruction. A radioiodine scan shows uptake localized to the region of the fracture. FNA for both thyroid nodule and femur lesion is performed. Which of the following is the most likely diagnosis?

(a) Anaplastic carcinoma
(b) Hurthle cell metaplasia
(c) Granulomatous thyroiditis
(d) Medullary carcinoma
(e) Hürthle cell neoplasm favoring Hurthle cell carcinoma

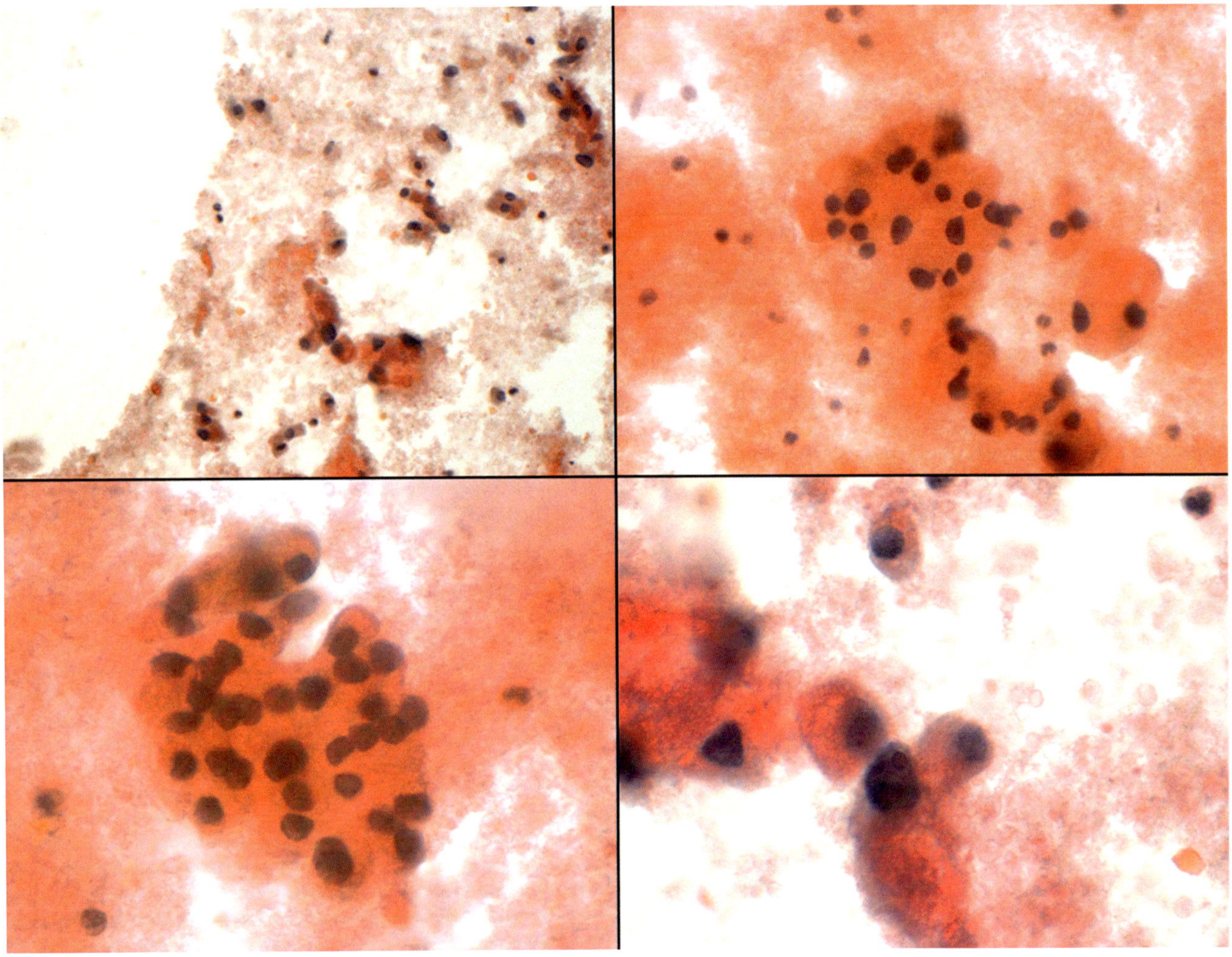

Fig. 4.21

Q-21. This aspirate is from a 53-year-old woman who has felt a "lump" on the left side of his neck. Physical examination reveals a firm 3.0-cm nodule in the left lobe of the thyroid gland. There is no palpable lymphadenopathy. Laboratory studies show normal TSH and T4 levels. FNA of the thyroid is performed. Which of the following is the most likely diagnosis?

(a) Anaplastic carcinoma
(b) Hürthle cell Carcinoma
(c) Benign, Hurthle cell metaplasia
(d) Benign, granulomatous thyroiditis
(e) Medullary carcinoma

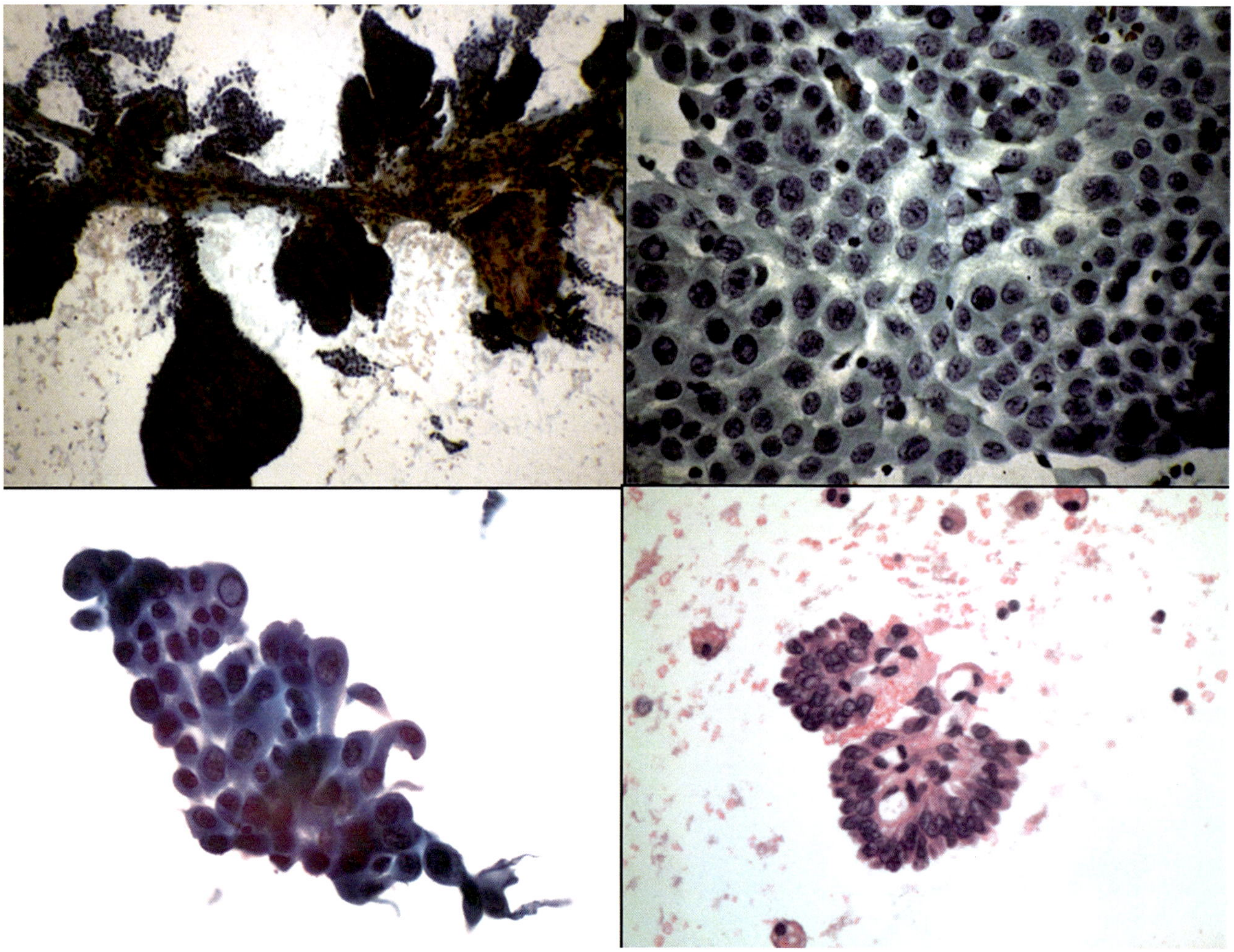

Fig. 4.22

Q-22. A 45-year-old man presents to his physician because of "lump" on the left side of his neck. Physical examination shows a nontender nodule on the left lobe of the thyroid gland. A cervical lymph node is enlarged and nontender. Laboratory thyroid studies show no thyroid autoantibodies in his serum, and the T4 and TSH levels are normal. US-guided FNA of thyroid nodule is performed. Which of the following is the most likely diagnosis?

(a) Malignant, anaplastic carcinoma
(b) Benign, Hurthle cell metaplasia
(c) Malignant, papillary thyroid carcinoma
(d) Malignant, medullary carcinoma
(e) Malignant, Hurthle cell carcinoma

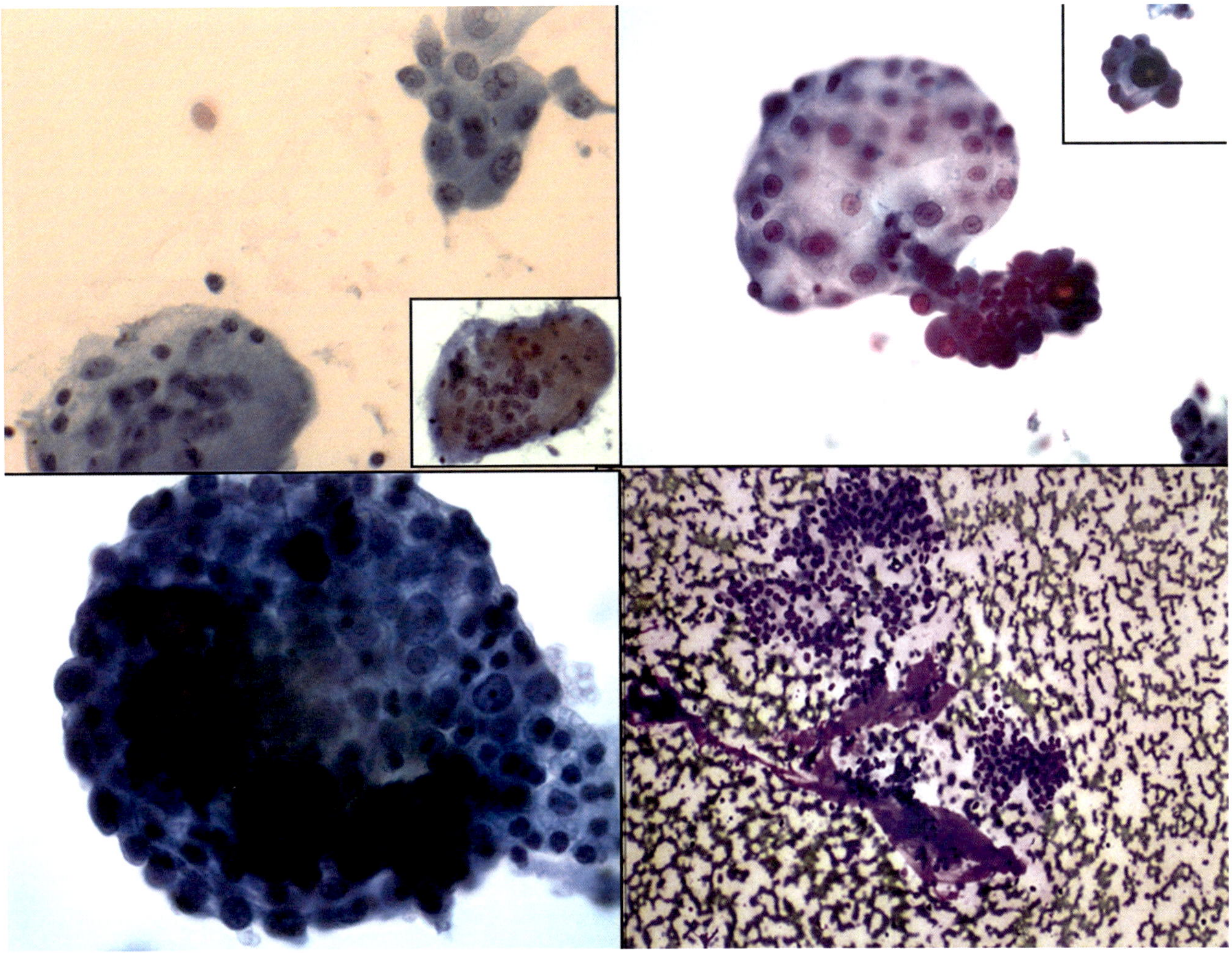

Fig. 4.23

Q-23. A 45-year-old female presents with a nodule on the right lobe of her thyroid. Physical examination shows a nontender nodule on the right lobe of the thyroid gland. Laboratory thyroid studies show no thyroid autoantibodies in his serum, and the T4 and TSH levels are normal. US-guided FNA of the thyroid nodule is performed. Which of the following is the most likely diagnosis?

(a) Malignant, anaplastic carcinoma
(b) Hurthle cell metaplasia
(c) Malignant, papillary thyroid carcinoma
(d) Malignant, medullary carcinoma
(e) Malignant, Hurthle cell carcinoma

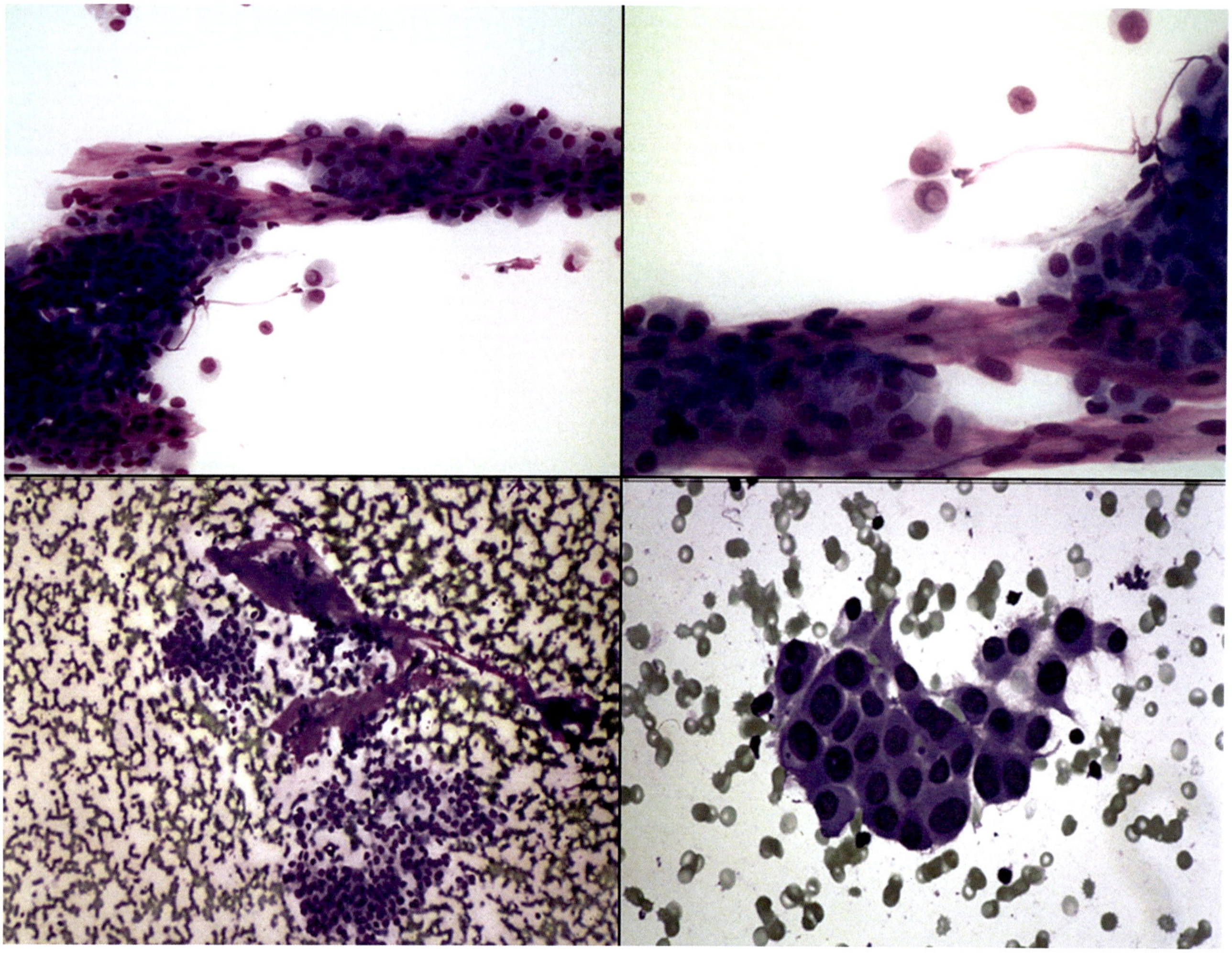

Fig. 4.24

Q-24. A 50-year-old man presents with neck mass on the left side. Physical examination shows a nontender nodule on the left lobe of the thyroid gland, 2.5 cm. A cervical lymph node is enlarged and nontender. Laboratory thyroid studies show no thyroid autoantibodies in his serum, and the T4 and TSH levels are normal. US-guided FNA of the thyroid nodule is performed. Which of the following is the most likely diagnosis?

(a) Anaplastic carcinoma
(b) Benign, Hurthle cell metaplasia
(c) Medullary carcinoma
(d) Hurthle cell neoplasm
(e) Papillary carcinoma

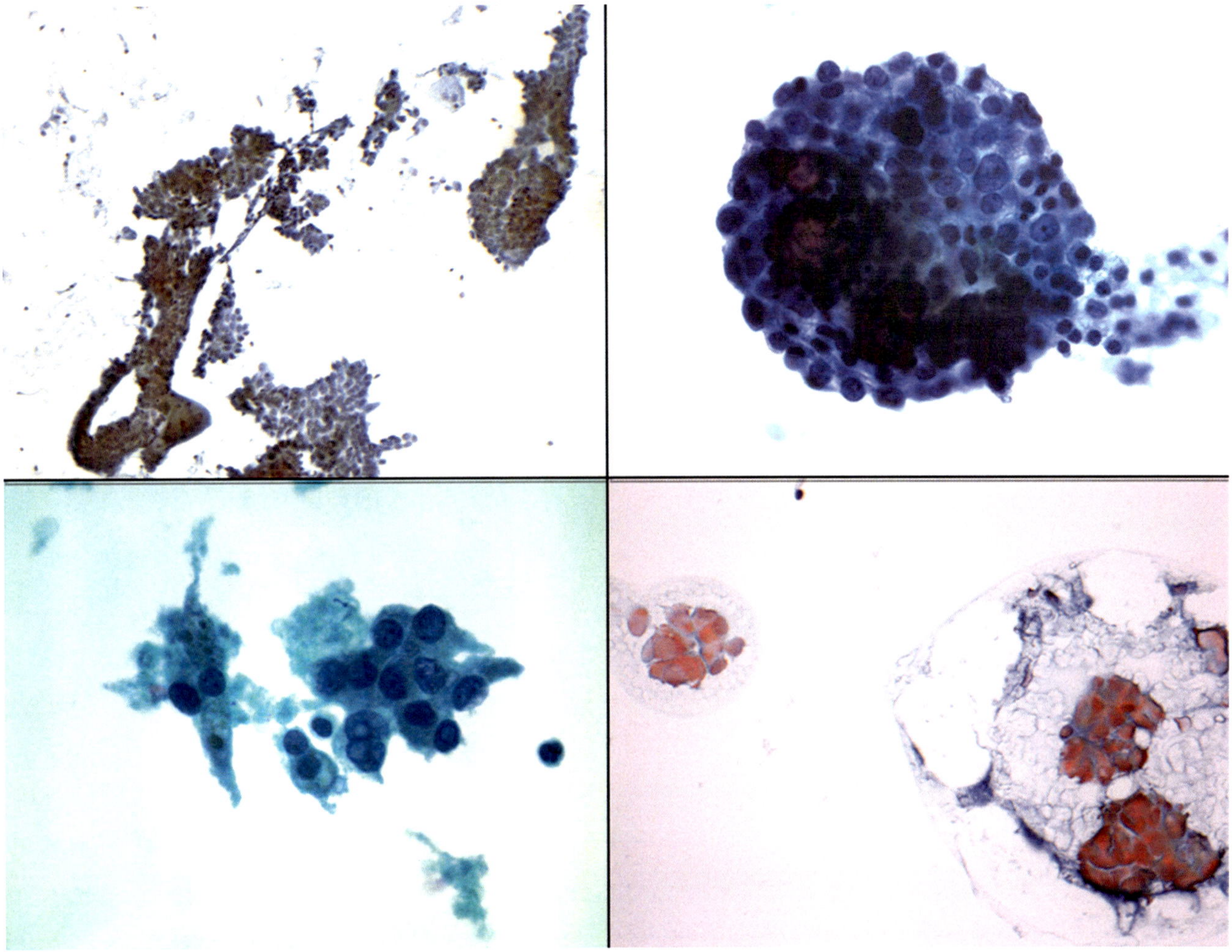

Fig. 4.25

Q-25. A 55-year-old man presents with large mass on right side of his thyroid. Physical examination shows a nontender nodule on the right lobe of the thyroid gland. A cervical lymph node is enlarged and nontender. Laboratory thyroid studies show no thyroid autoantibodies in his serum, and the T4 and TSH levels are normal. US-guided FNA of the thyroid nodule is performed. ThinPrep smear was prepared. Which of the following is the most likely diagnosis?

(a) Malignant, anaplastic carcinoma
(b) Malignant, papillary thyroid carcinoma
(c) Hurthle cell metaplasia
(d) Malignant, medullary carcinoma
(e) Hurthle cell neoplasm

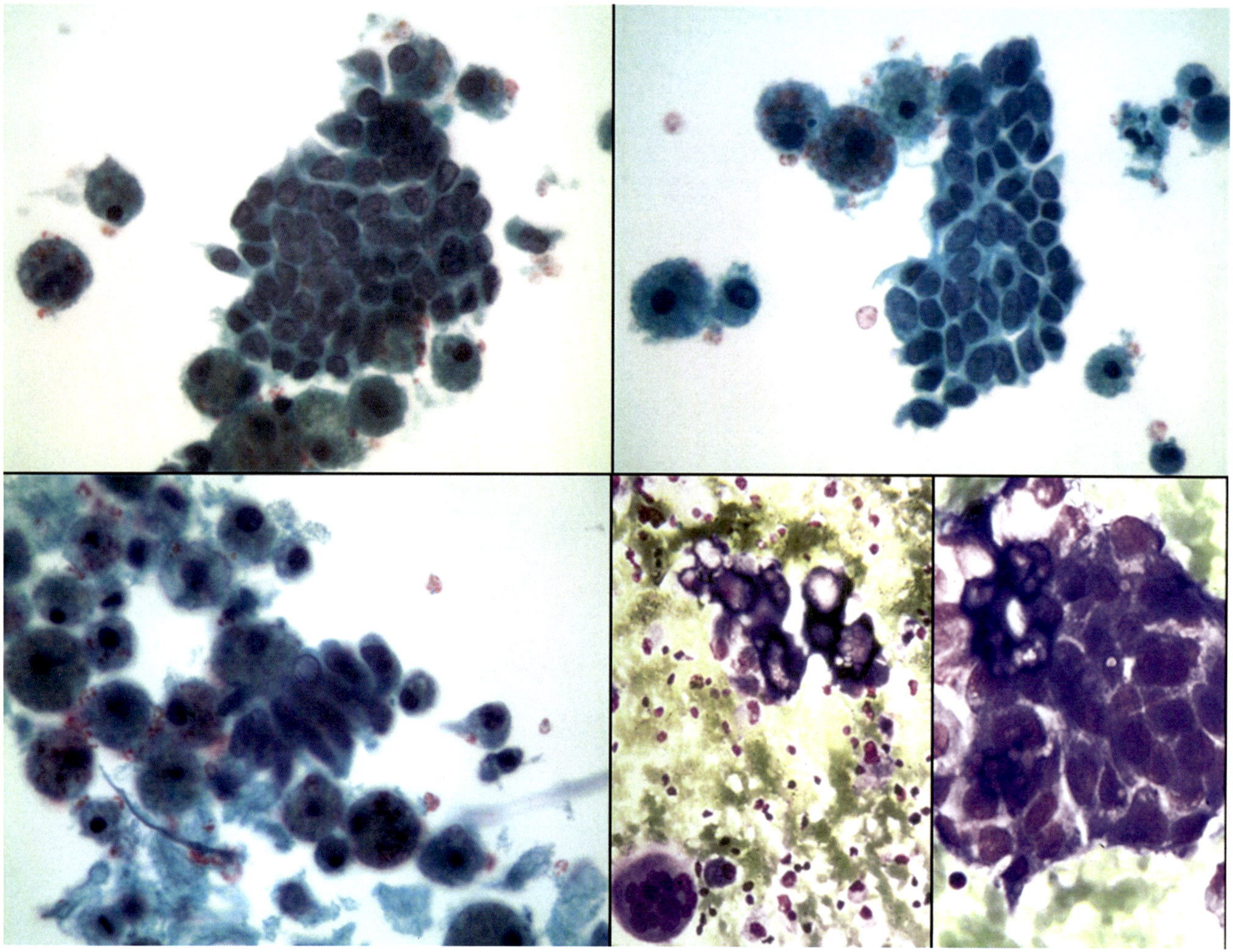

Fig. 4.26

Q-26. This aspirate is from a 65-year-old woman who presents to his physician because of "lump" on the left side of her neck. Physical examination shows a nontender nodule on the left lobe of the thyroid gland. Laboratory thyroid studies show normal free T4 and TSH levels. Ultrasound examination shows a cystic lesion with complex architecture. US-guided FNA of the thyroid nodule is performed. Which of the following is the most likely diagnosis?

(a) Malignant, anaplastic carcinoma
(b) Benign, Hashimoto thyroiditis with Hurthle cell metaplasia
(c) Cystic papillary carcinoma
(d) Nondiagnostic, cyst fluid content
(e) Hurthle cell neoplasm

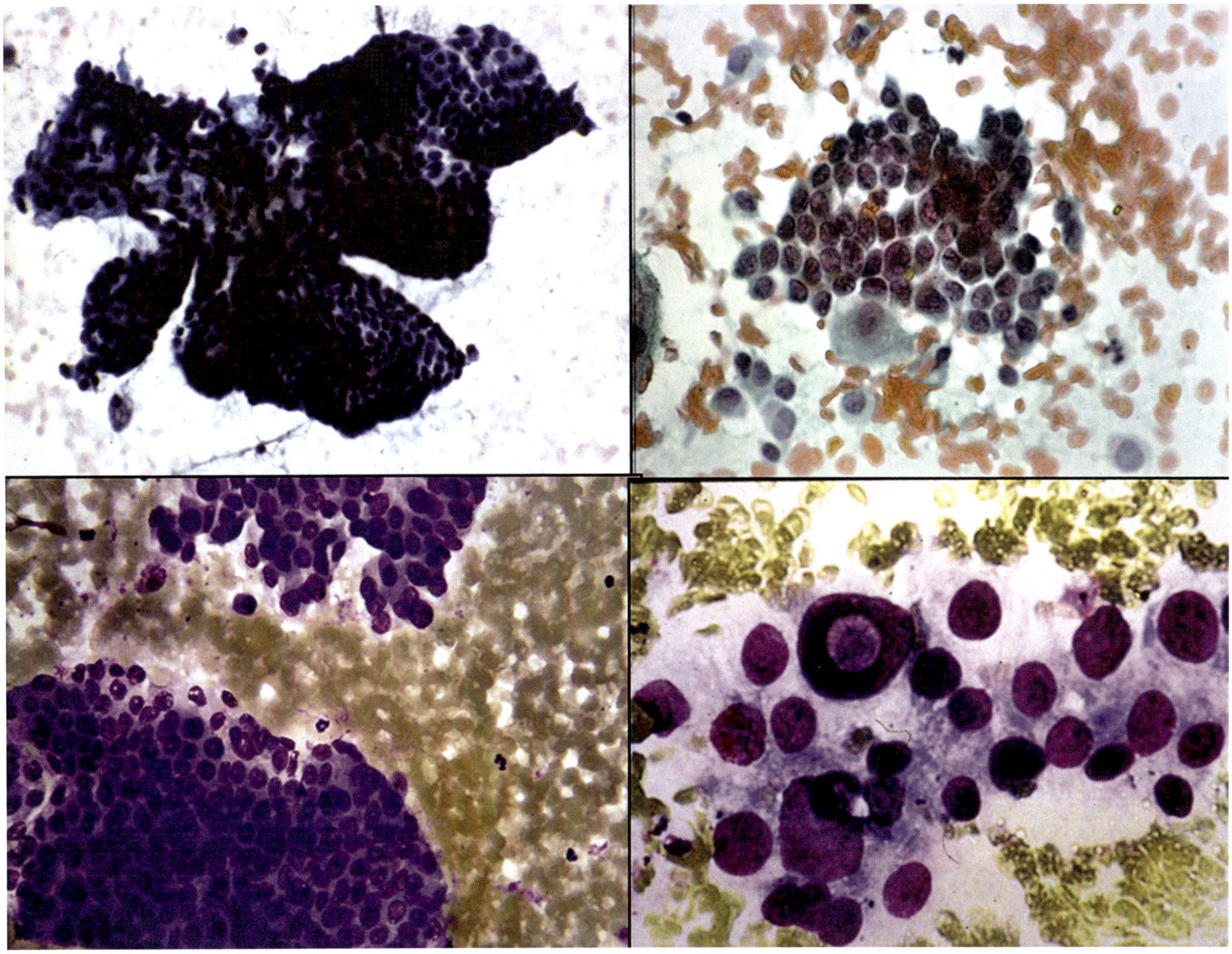

Fig. 4.27

Q-27. A 50-year-old man presents to his physician because of "lump" on the left side of his neck. Physical examination shows a nontender enlarged cervical lymph node. Laboratory thyroid studies show normal free T4 and TSH levels. A fine-needle aspiration biopsy of the cervical lymph node is performed. Which of the following is the most likely diagnosis?

(a) Metastatic anaplastic carcinoma
(b) Reactive lymphoid hyperplasia
(c) Metastatic medullary carcinoma
(d) Metastatic papillary thyroid carcinoma
(e) Metastatic Hurthle cell carcinoma

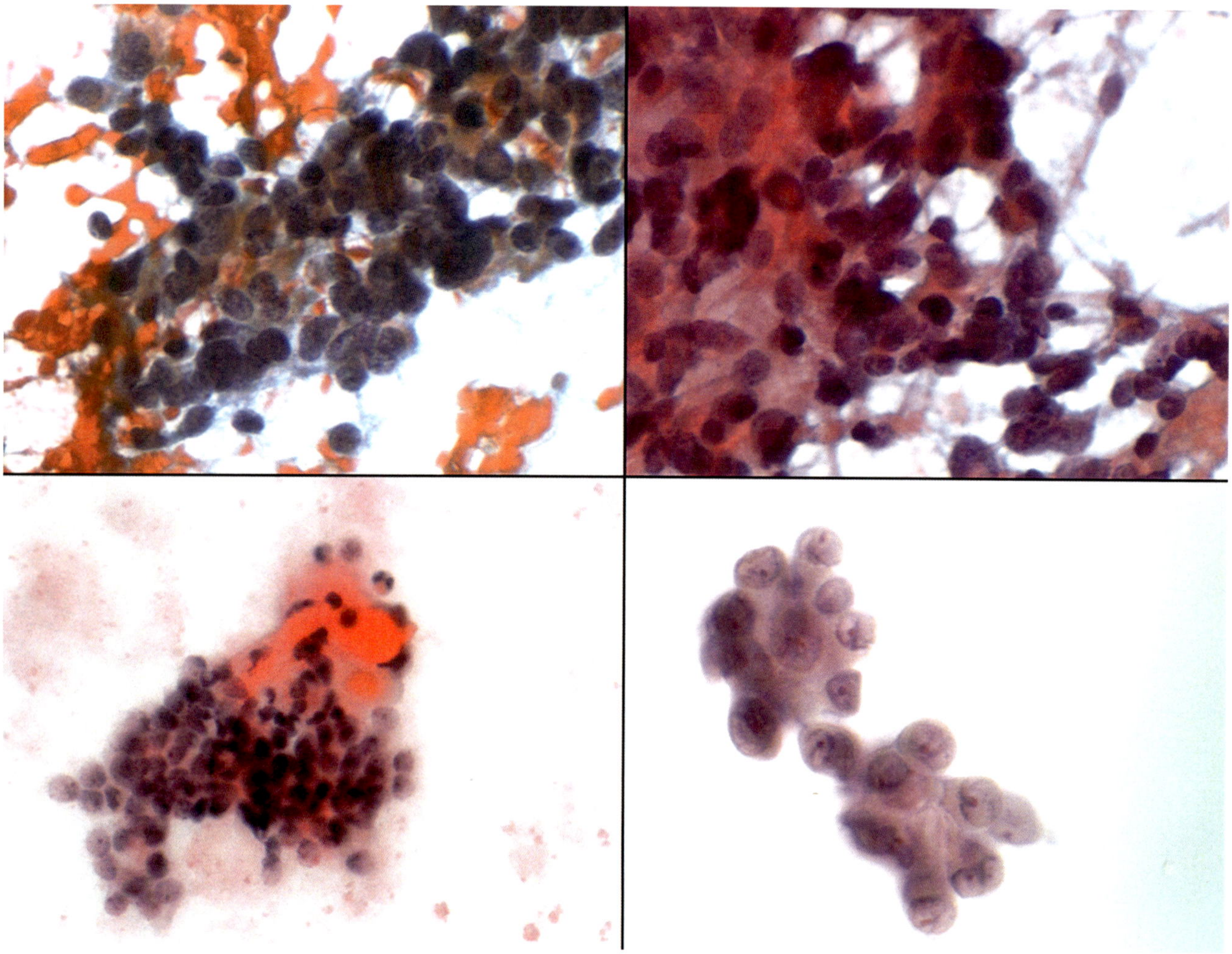

Fig. 4.28

Q-28. This aspirate is from a 42-year-old man who presents to his physician because of "lump" on the left side of his neck. Physical examination shows a nontender nodule on the left lobe of the thyroid gland. Laboratory thyroid studies show normal free T4 and TSH levels. Ultrasound examination shows a cystic lesion with complex architecture. US-guided FNA of the thyroid nodule is performed. Which of the following is the most likely diagnosis?

(a) Malignant, anaplastic carcinoma
(b) Suspicious for papillary carcinoma
(c) Malignant, medullary carcinoma
(d) Follicular carcinoma
(e) Hurthle cell neoplasm

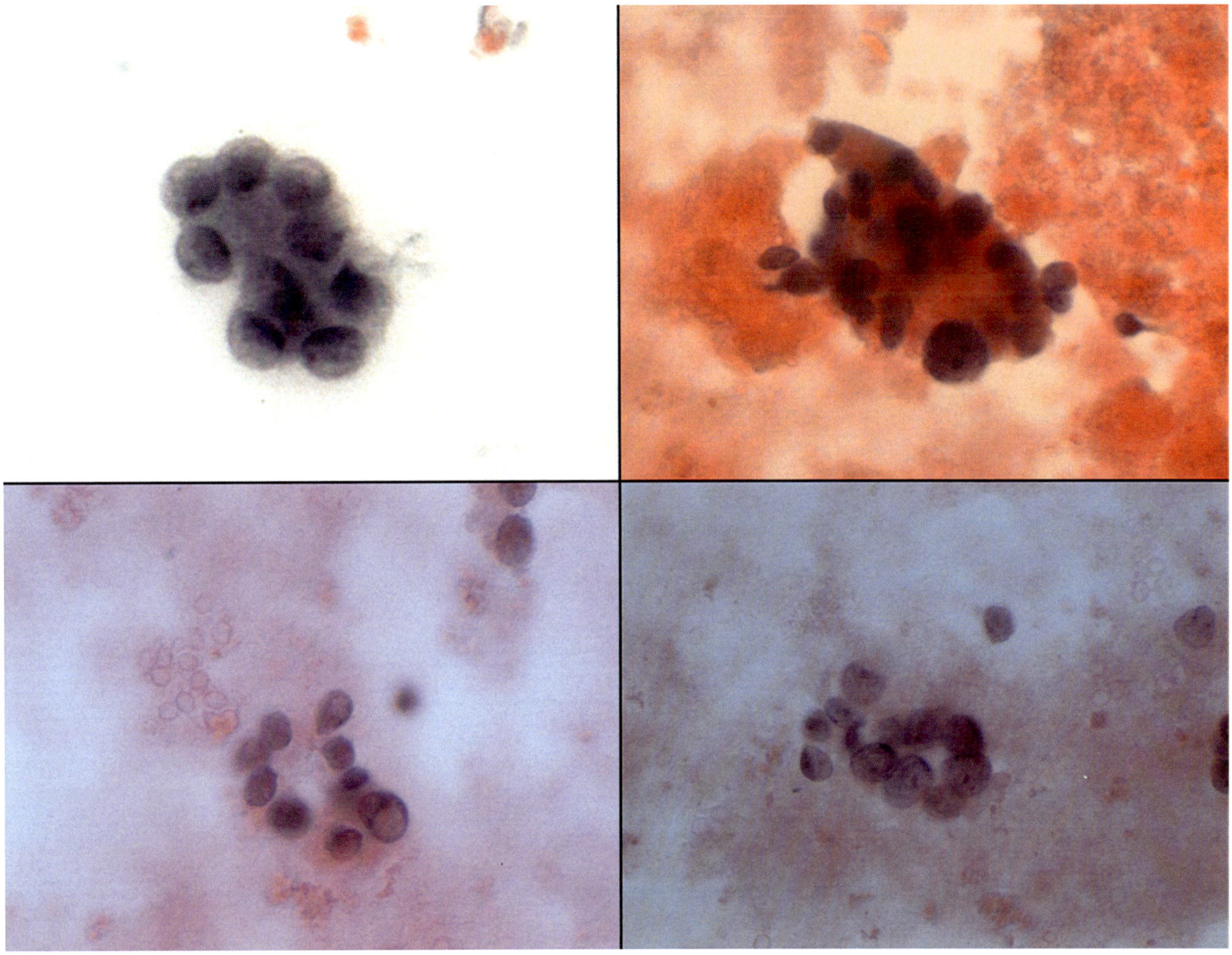

Fig. 4.29

Q-29. A 38-year-old man feels a small thyroid nodule on the left side of his neck. Physical examination reveals a firm, painless, 2.5-cm cervical lymph node. The thyroid gland is not enlarged. A chest radiograph is unremarkable with normal laboratory studies. Fine-needle aspiration biopsy of the cervical lymph node is performed. Which of the following is the most likely diagnosis?

(a) Papillary carcinoma (Follicular variant)
(b) Medullar carcinoma
(c) Follicular carcinoma
(d) Hurthle cell neoplasm
(e) Anaplastic carcinoma

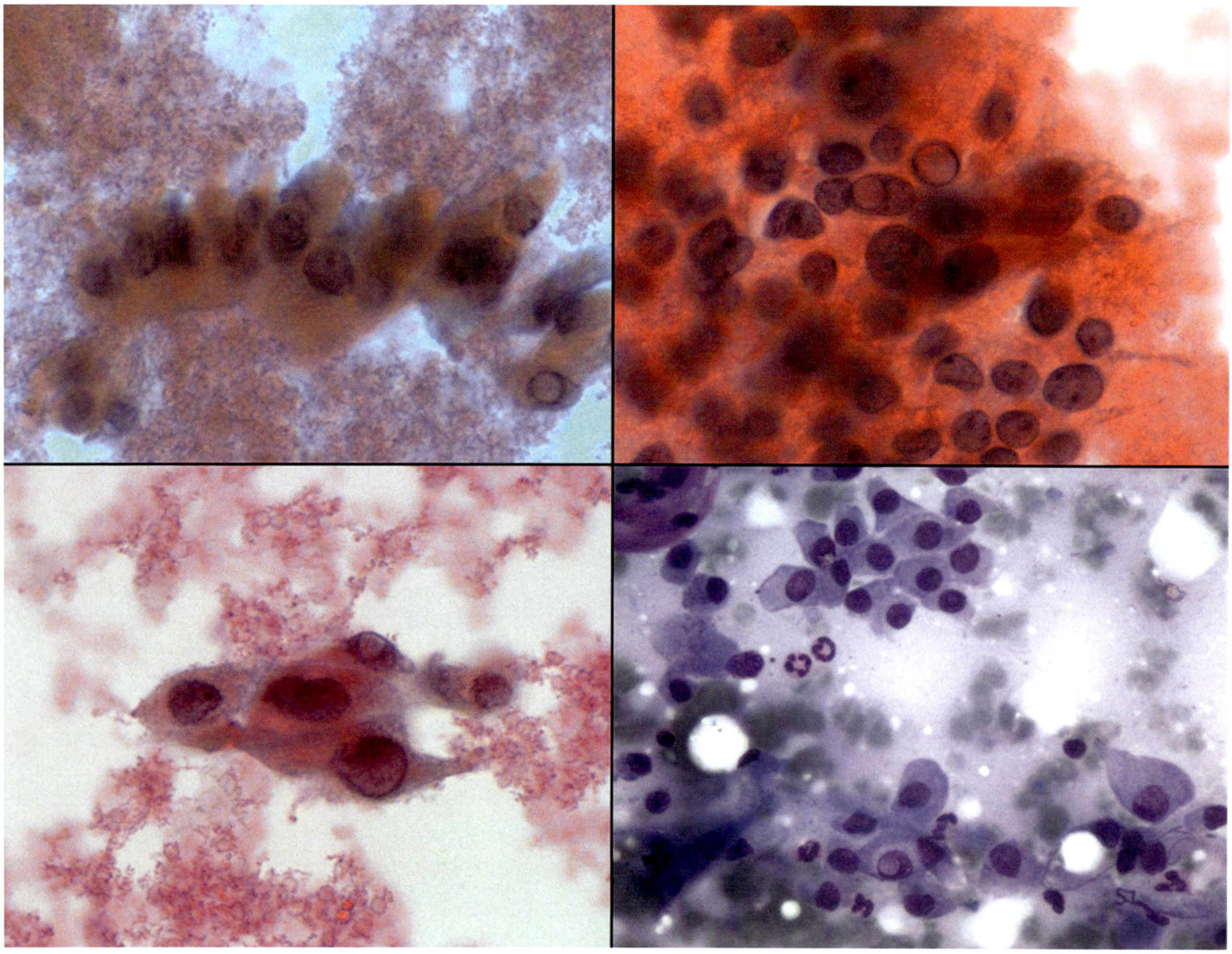

Fig. 4.30

Q-30. A 63-year-old man feels a thyroid nodule on the left side of his neck. Physical examination reveals a firm, painless, 2.5- cm thyroid nodule. The thyroid gland is not enlarged. A chest radiograph is unremarkable with normal laboratory studies. US-guided FNA of the thyroid nodule is performed. Which of the following is the most likely diagnosis?

(a) Papillary thyroid carcinoma, oncocytic variant
(b) Medullar carcinoma
(c) Follicular carcinoma
(d) Hurthle cell carcinoma
(e) Anaplastic carcinoma

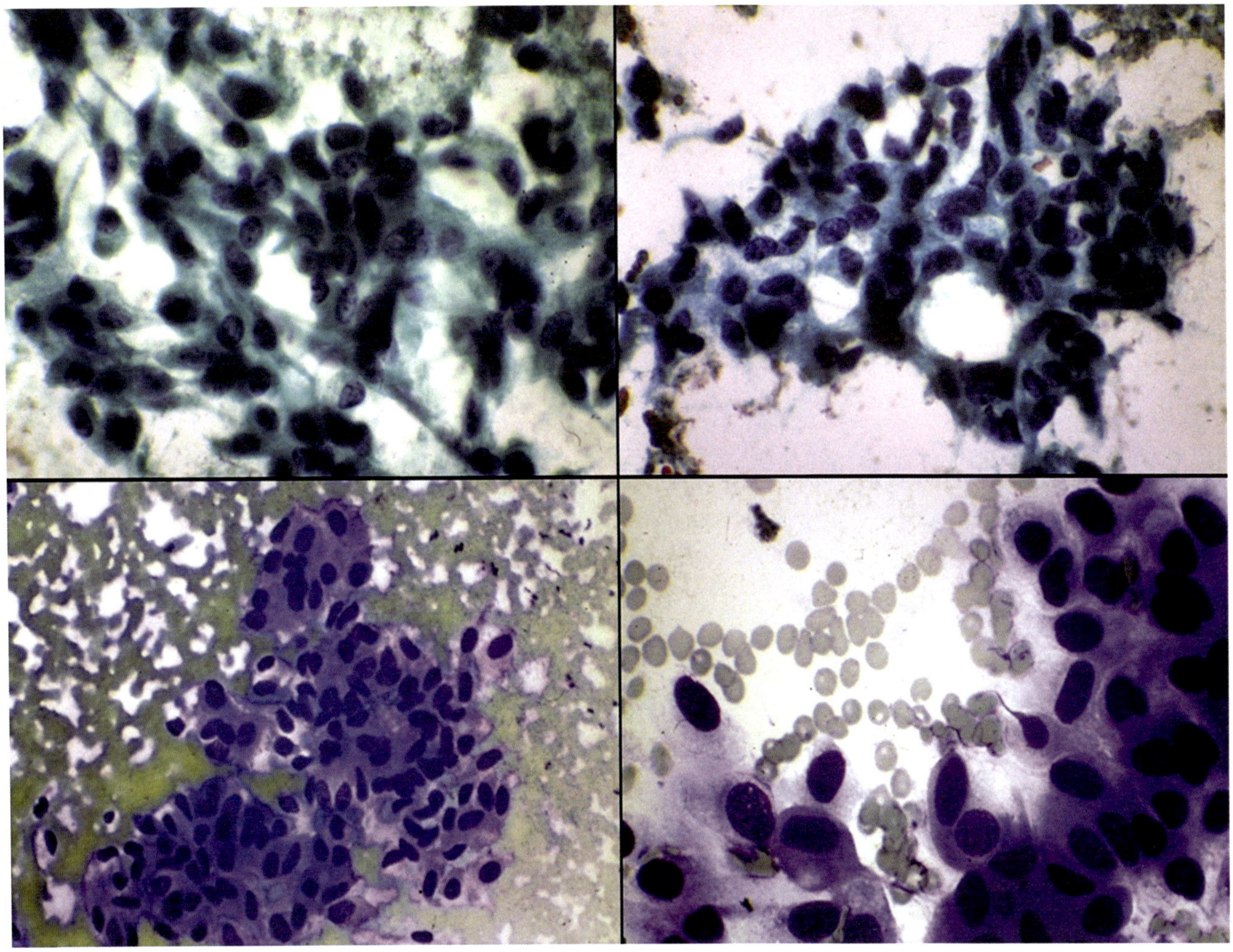

Fig. 4.31

Q-31. This aspirate is from a 37-year-old man who presents with a single, firm mass within the thyroid gland. Patient has a family history of thyroid tumor affecting his father when he was 32 years of age. Ultrasound examination reveals a solid thyroid mass, suspicious for malignancy. FNA is performed. Which of the following is the most likely diagnosis?

(a) Follicular neoplasm
(b) Papillary thyroid carcinoma
(c) Squamous cell carcinoma
(d) Medullary carcinoma
(e) Benign, nodular goiter

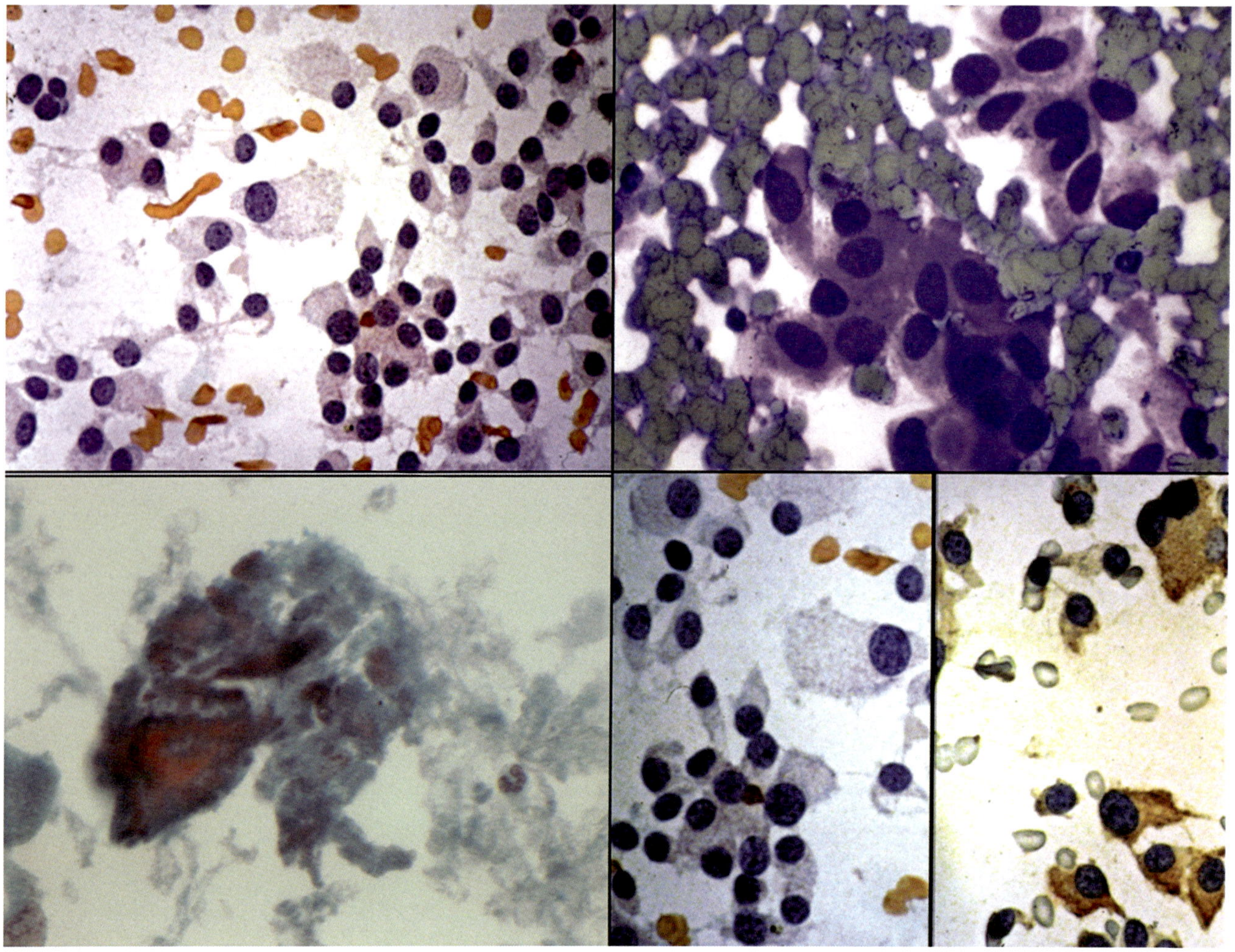

Fig. 4.32

Q-32. A 65-year-old man presents to his physician because of "lump" on the left side of his neck. Physical examination shows vague thyroid enlargement but no nodule can be identified. A cervical lymph node is enlarged and nontender. Laboratory thyroid studies show no thyroid autoantibodies in his serum, and the T4 and TSH levels are normal. A fine-needle aspiration biopsy of the cervical lymph node was performed. Which of the following is the most likely diagnosis?

(a) Metastatic anaplastic carcinoma
(b) Benign, reactive lymphoid hyperplasia
(c) Metastatic medullary carcinoma
(d) Metastatic papillary carcinoma
(e) Metastatic Hurthle cell Carcinoma

Fig. 4.33

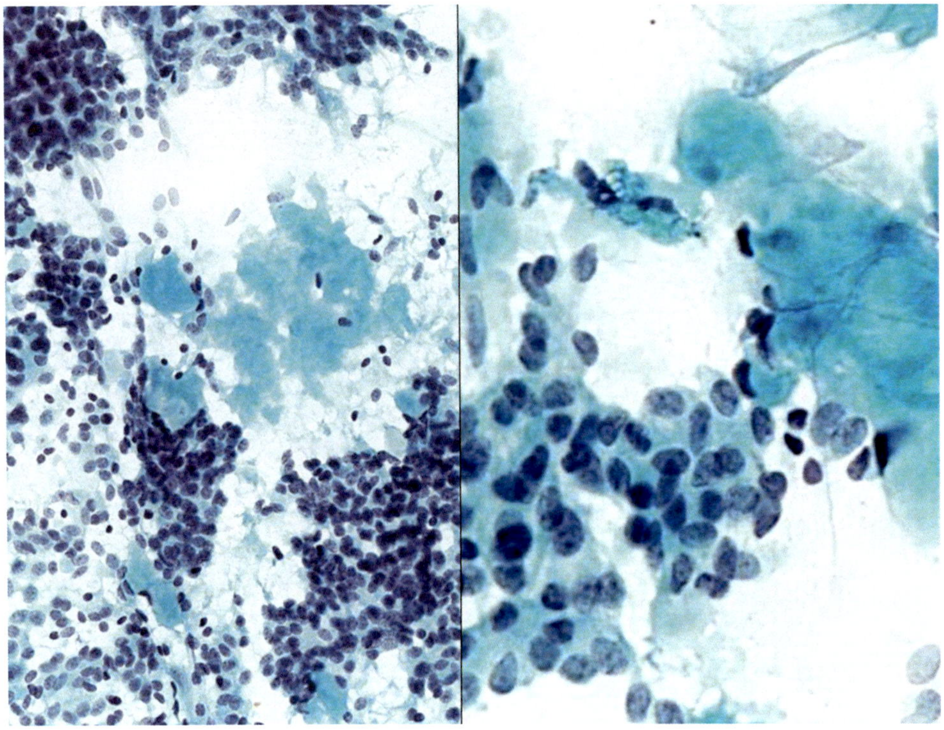

Q-33. This aspirate is from a 30-year-old woman who presents with a single left thyroid nodule. Patient has a family history of thyroid tumor. Ultrasound examination reveals a solid thyroid mass, suspicious for malignancy. FNA is performed. Which of the following is the most likely diagnosis?

(a) Follicular neoplasm
(b) Papillary thyroid carcinoma
(c) Suspicious for medullary carcinoma
(d) Squamous cell carcinoma
(e) Anaplastic carcinoma

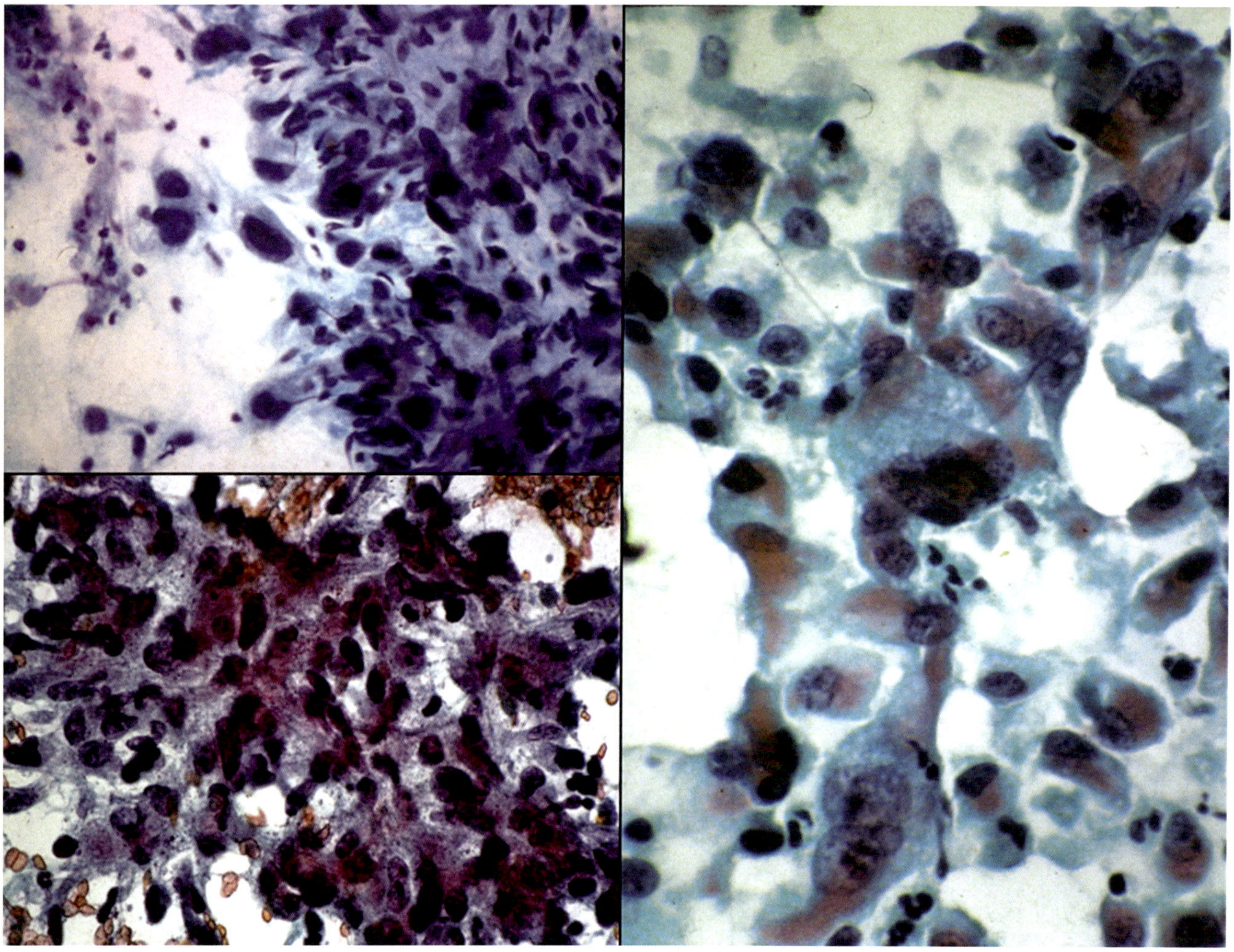

Fig. 4.34

Q-34. A 76-year-old man with no previous illnesses sees his physician because he has had progressive hoarseness, shortness of breath, and stridor for the past 3 weeks. On physical examination, he has a firm, large, tender mass involving the entire right thyroid lobe. CT scan shows that this mass extends posterior to the trachea and into the upper mediastinum. Cervical lymph nodes were enlarged and X-ray shows multiple pulmonary metastases on chest radiograph. A fine-needle aspiration biopsy of the thyroid mass is performed. Which of the following neoplasms is the most likely diagnosis?

(a) Non-Hodgkin lymphoma
(b) Follicular carcinoma
(c) Medullary carcinoma
(d) Papillary carcinoma
(e) Anaplastic carcinoma

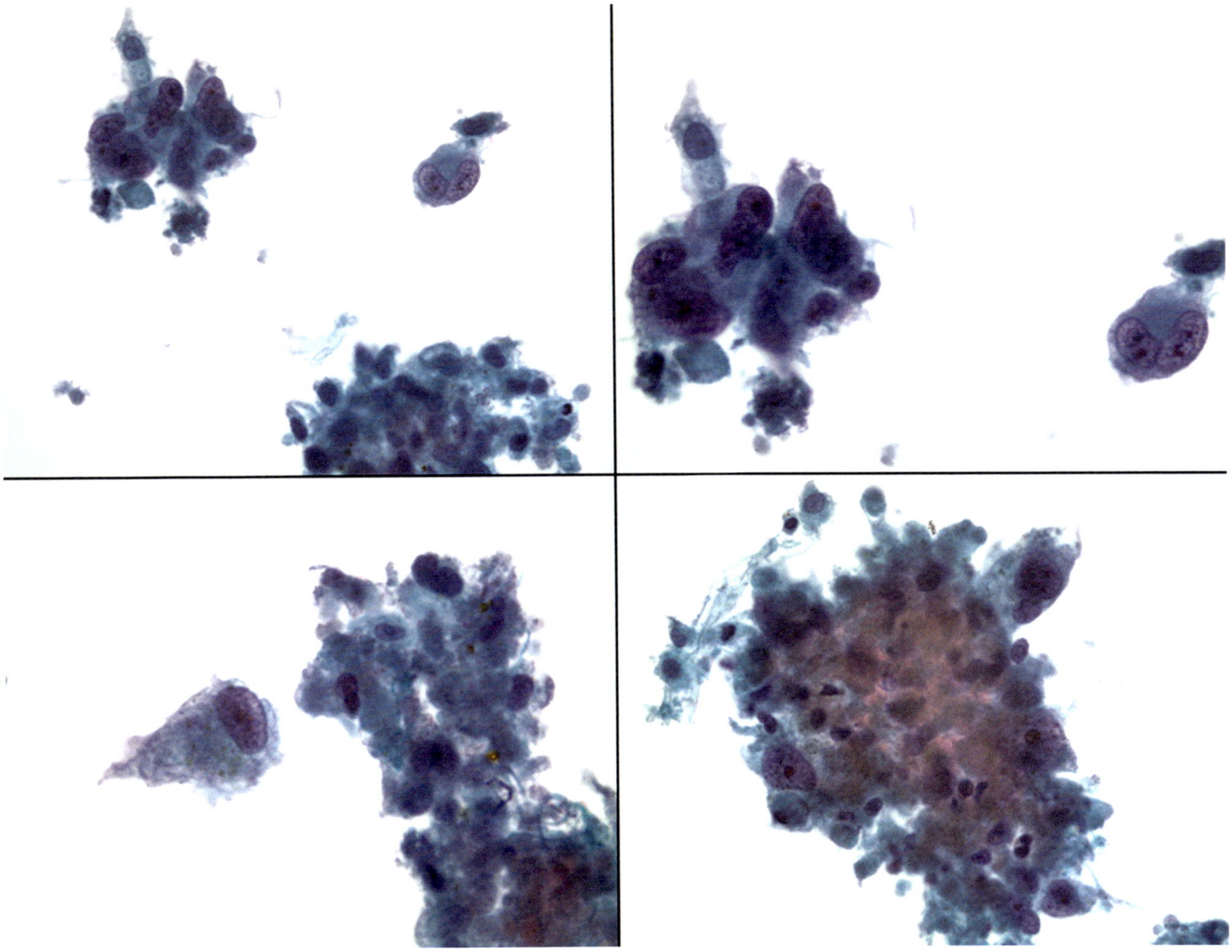

Fig. 4.35

Q-35. A 63-year-old man presents with thyroid mass and progressive hoarseness. On physical examination, he has a firm, large, painless mass involving the left thyroid lobe. CT scan shows that this mass extends posterior to the trachea. A fine-needle aspiration biopsy of the mass is performed. Which of the following neoplasms is most likely to be present in this patient?

(a) Large cell lymphoma
(b) Hurthle cell carcinoma
(c) Anaplastic carcinoma
(d) Papillary carcinoma
(e) Medullary carcinoma

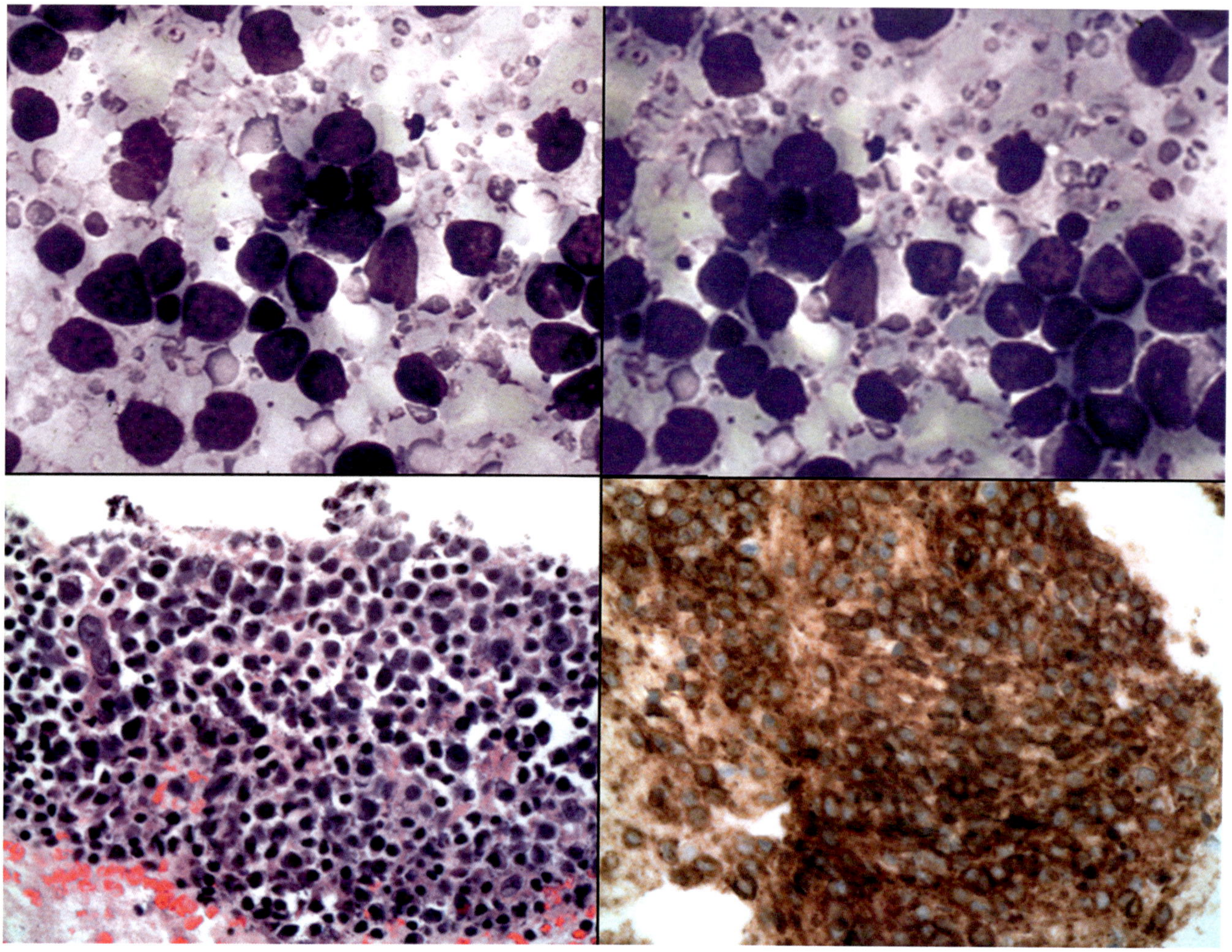

Fig. 4.36

Q-36. A 70-year-old woman feels a diffuse enlargement of his thyroid gland with sense of fullness and compression. Physical examination reveals a diffuse painless thyroid enlargement. A chest radiograph is unremarkable with normal laboratory studies. A fine-needle aspiration biopsy of the thyroid is performed. Which of the following is the most likely diagnosis?

(a) Papillary carcinoma (follicular variant)
(b) Medullary carcinoma
(c) Follicular carcinoma
(d) Large cell lymphoma
(e) Anaplastic carcinoma

Fig. 4.37

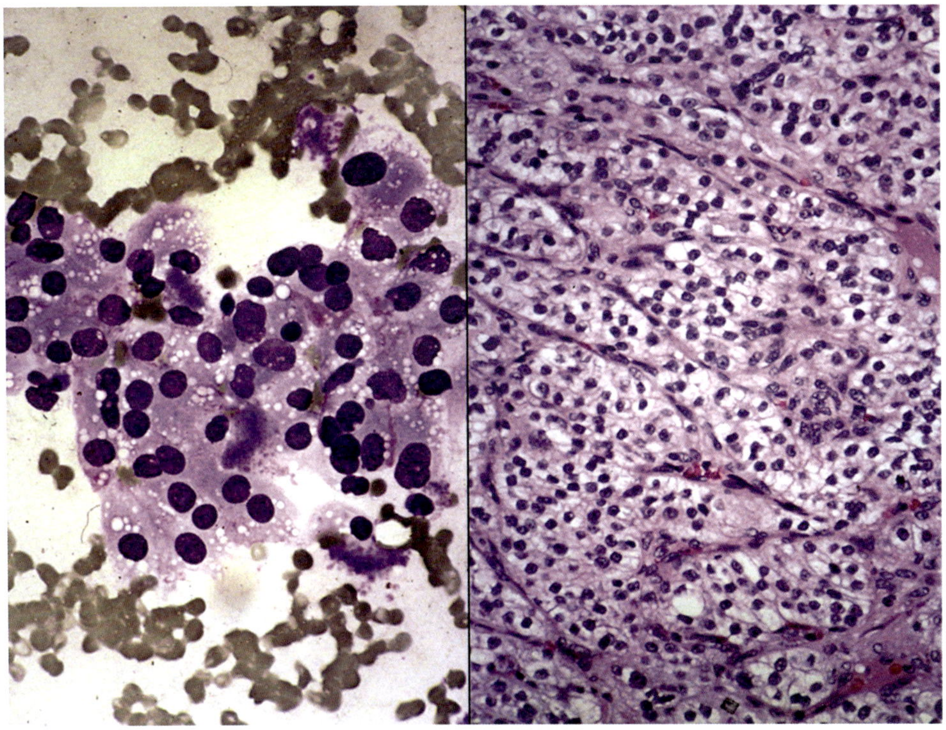

Q-37. A 55-year-old man feels a thyroid nodule on the left side of his neck. Physical examination reveals a firm, painless, 2.5-cm thyroid nodule. Patient has past history of renal carcinoma which was treated by nephrectomy. A chest radiograph is unremarkable with normal laboratory studies. US-guided FNA of the thyroid nodule is performed. Which of the following is the most likely diagnosis?

(a) Papillary carcinoma
(b) Medullary carcinoma
(c) Metastatic renal cell carcinoma
(d) Metastatic squamous cell carcinoma
(e) Hurthle cell neoplasm

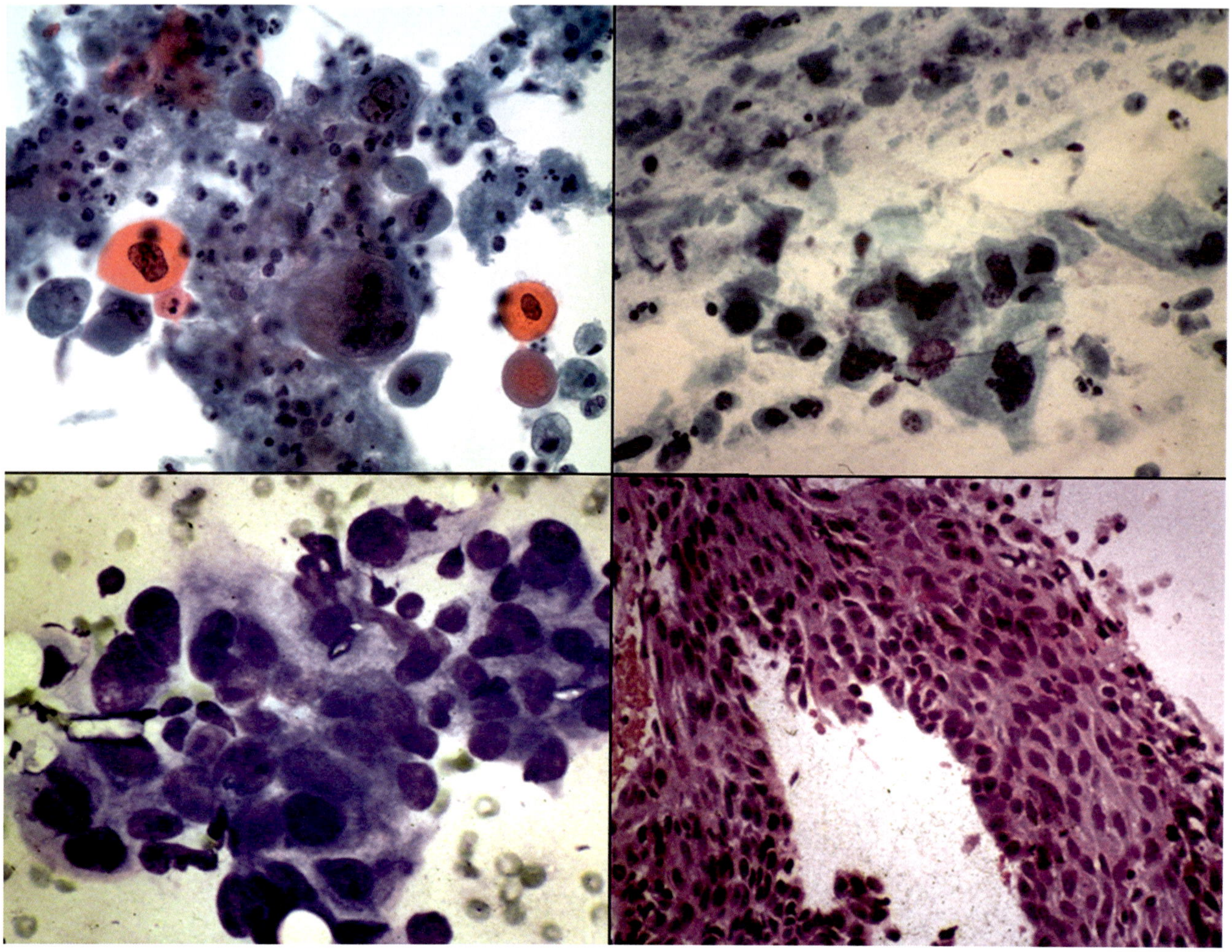

Fig. 4.38

Q-38. A 55-year-old man feels a thyroid nodule on the left side of his neck. Physical examination reveals a firm, painless, 2.5-cm thyroid nodule. Patient has past history of heavy smoking for many years. A fine-needle aspiration biopsy of the thyroid nodule is performed. Which of the following is the most likely diagnosis?
(a) Papillary carcinoma
(b) Medullary carcinoma
(c) Metastatic renal cell carcinoma
(d) Metastatic squamous cell carcinoma
(e) Hurthle cell neoplasm

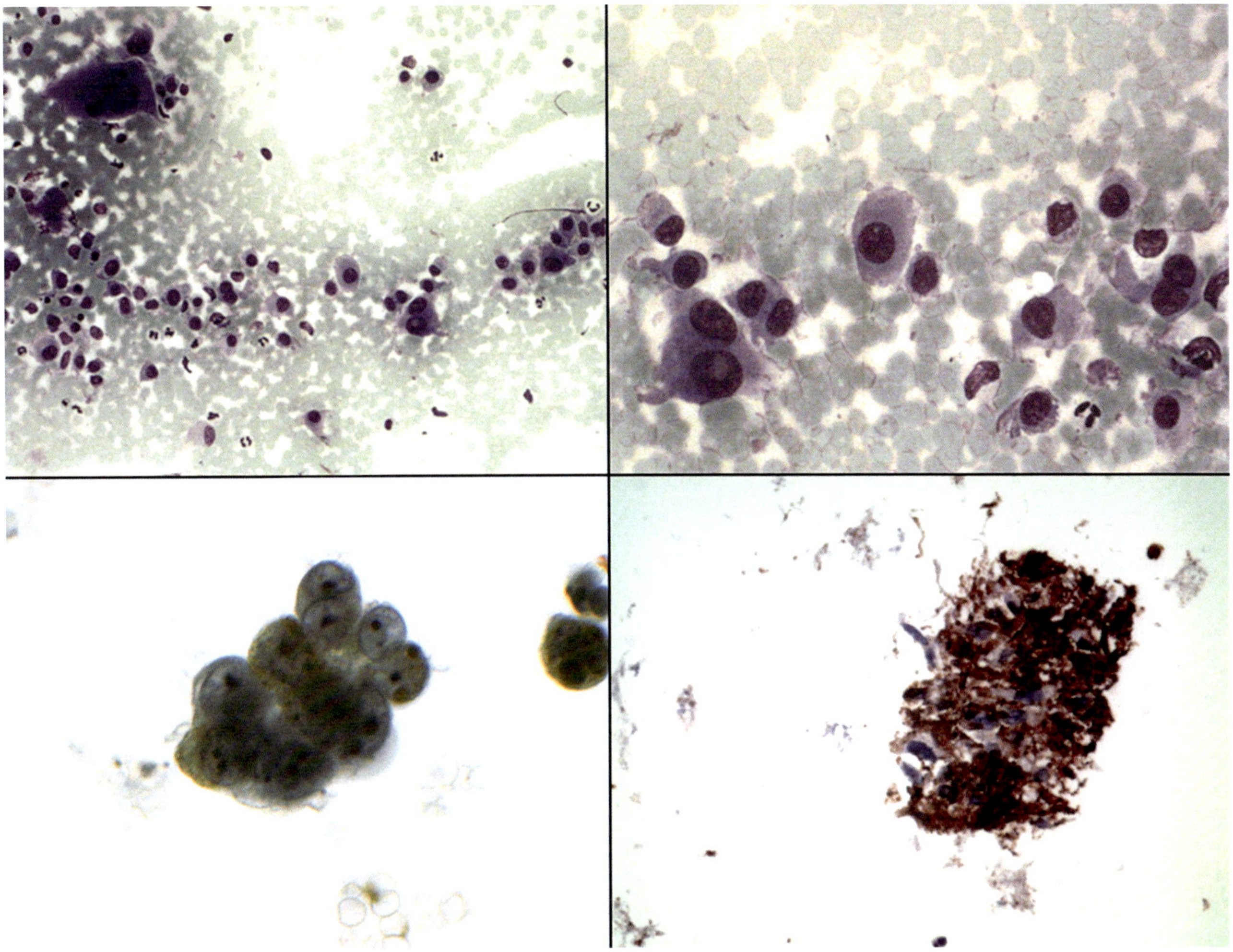

Fig. 4.39

Q-39. A 55-year-old man feels a thyroid nodule on the left side of his neck. Physical examination reveals a firm, painless, 3.0-cm thyroid nodule. Patient has past history of skin melanoma 8 months ago. US-guided FNA of the thyroid nodule is performed. Which of the following is the most likely diagnosis?
(a) Papillary carcinoma
(b) Metastatic melanoma
(c) Metastatic renal cell carcinoma
(d) Metastatic squamous cell carcinoma
(e) Hurthle cell neoplasm

Fig. 4.40

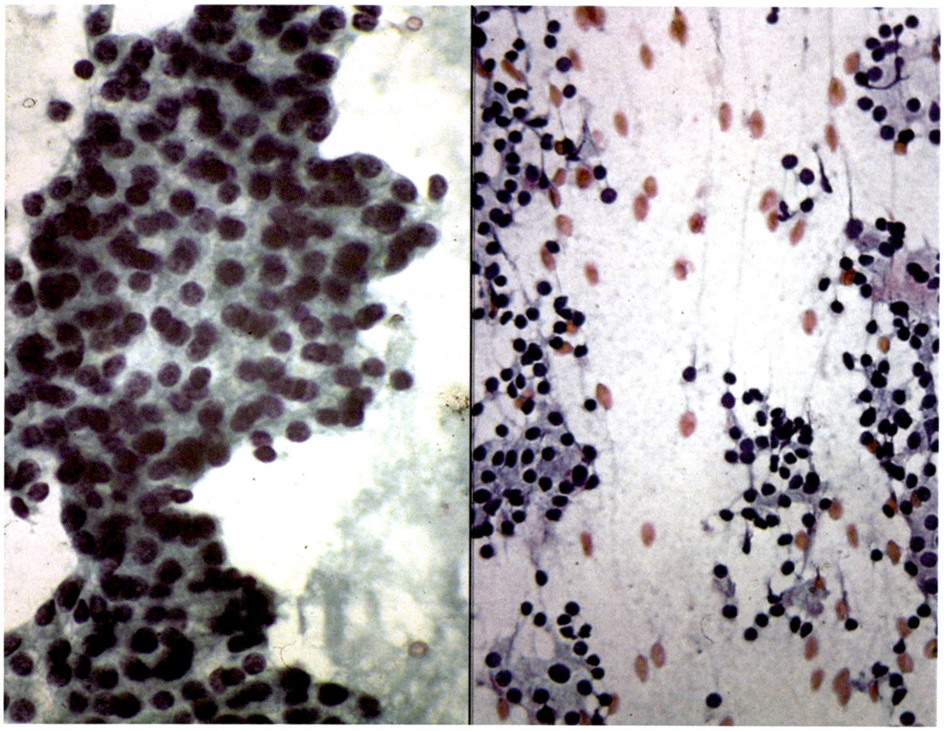

Q-40. A 45-year-old woman feels a thyroid nodule on the left side of her neck. Physical examination reveals a firm, painless, 1.5-cm thyroid nodule. Laboratory thyroid studies show normal free T4 and TSH levels. Patient has a history of kidney stones. US-guided FNA of the nodule is performed. Which of the following is the most likely diagnosis?

(a) Colloid nodule
(b) Hyperplastic thyroid nodule
(c) Papillary carcinoma
(d) Follicular neoplasm
(e) Parathyroid adenoma

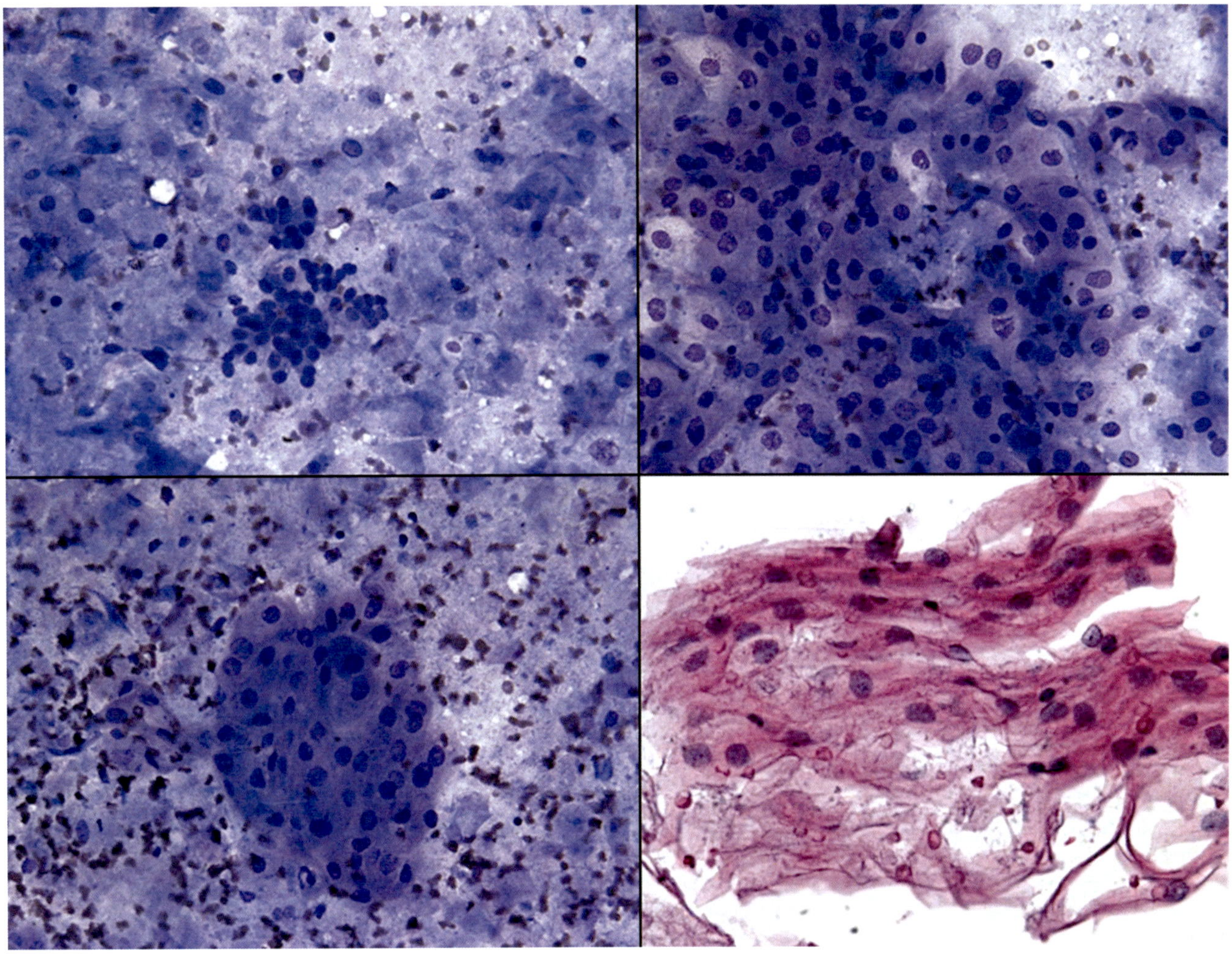

Fig. 4.41

Q-41. This aspirate is from a 27-year-old man who complains of a 3-cm right cystic thyroid nodule. Laboratory studies of thyroid function show normal free T4 and TSH levels. Ultrasound examination shows a 3-cm cystic/solid lesion. US-guided FNA is performed. Which of the following is the most likely diagnosis?

(a) Benign, colloid nodule
(b) Benign, thyroid colloid cyst
(c) Benign, lymphocytic thyroiditis
(d) Nondiagnostic, unsatisfactory specimen
(e) Benign, intrathyroidal branchial cleft cyst

Fig. 4.42

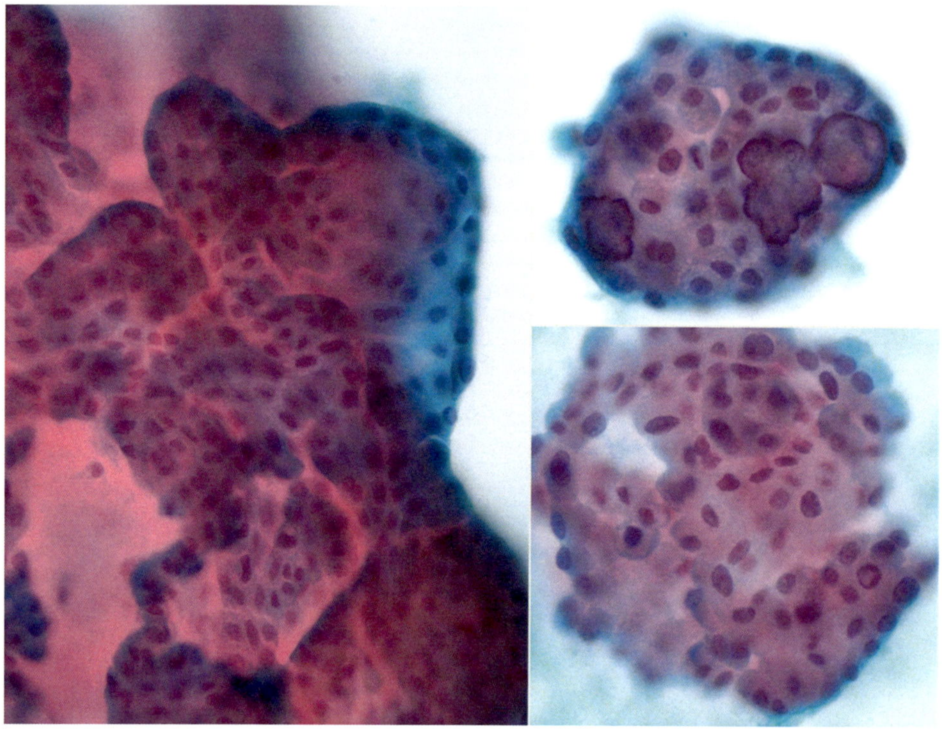

Q-42. A 21-year-old young woman presents with a nontender left thyroid nodule. A cervical lymph node is enlarged and nontender. Laboratory thyroid studies show normal free T4 and TSH levels. US-guided FNA of thyroid nodule is performed. Which of the following is the most likely diagnosis?

(a) Malignant, papillary thyroid carcinoma
(b) Malignant, anaplastic carcinoma
(c) Benign, Hurthle cell metaplasia
(d) Malignant, medullary carcinoma
(e) Malignant, Hurthle cell carcinoma

Fig. 4.43

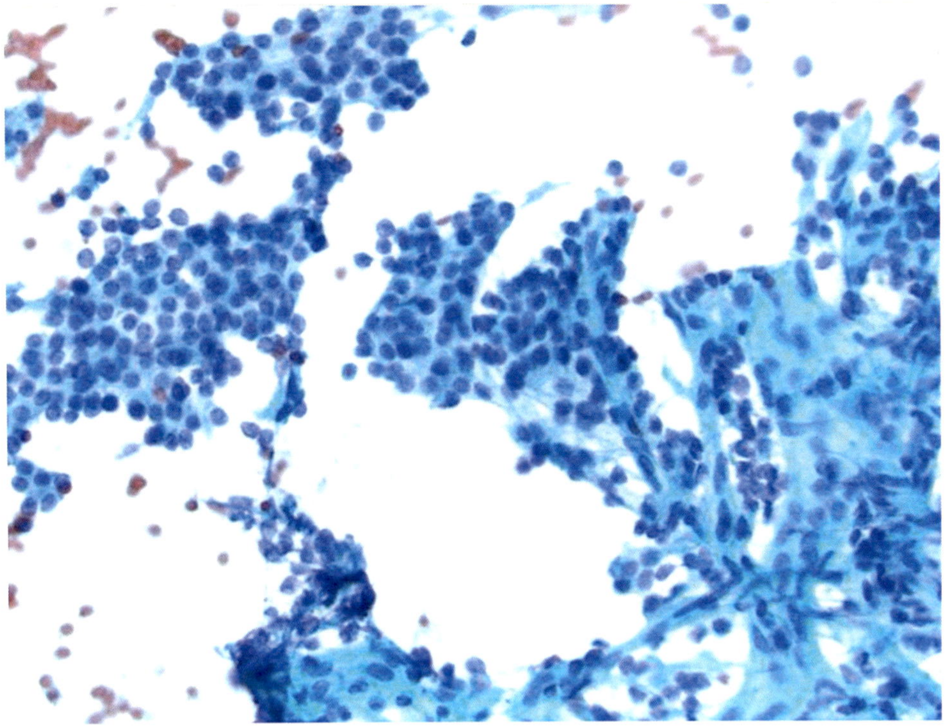

Q-43. A 38-year-old woman presented with a thyroid nodule on the left side of her neck. Physical examination reveals a firm, painless 2-cm thyroid nodule. Laboratory thyroid studies show normal free T4 and TSH levels. US-guided FNA of the nodule is performed. Which of the following is the most likely diagnosis?

(a) Benign, colloid nodule
(b) Benign, hyperplastic thyroid nodule
(c) Papillary carcinoma
(d) Follicular carcinoma
(e) Parathyroid adenoma/hyperplasia

Fig. 4.44

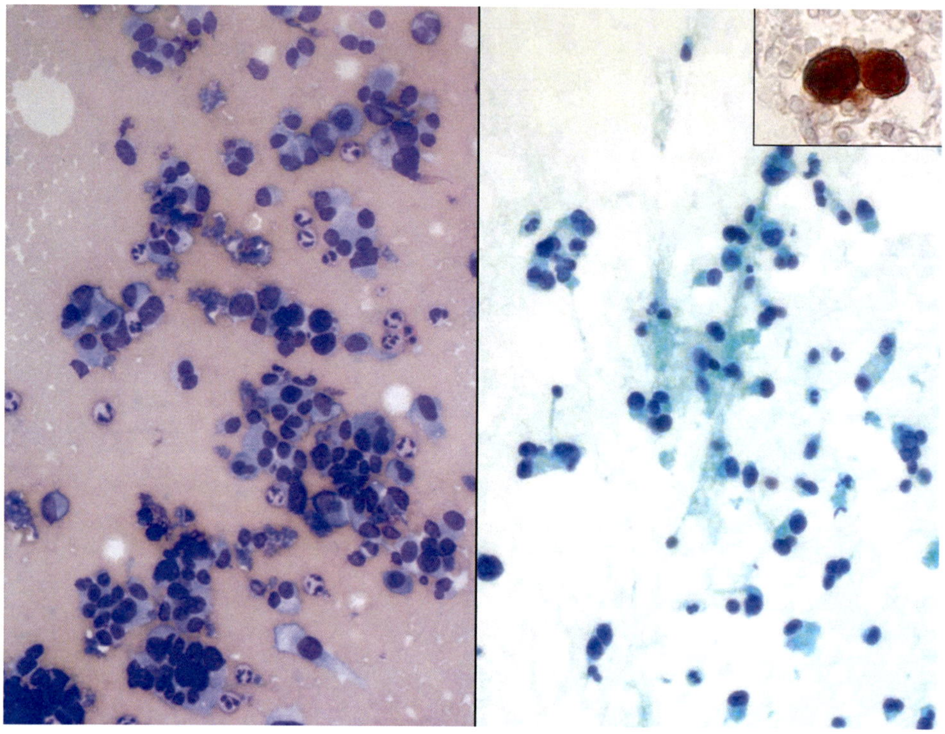

Q-44. The most likely immunostain in this case (insert) is:

(a) TTF-1
(b) Calcitonin.
(c) PTH
(d) Thyroglobulin
(e) CD138

4.2 Text-Based Questions 45–50

Q-45. All of the following are correct about insular/poorly differentiated carcinoma of the thyroid except:
(a) The smears are usually highly cellular and composed of monomorphic appearing small follicular cells, occurring singly and in clusters.
(b) The neoplastic cells show scant delicate cytoplasm with round hyperchromatic nuclei, coarsely granular chromatin, and mild to moderate nuclear irregularities.
(c) Many naked nuclei are often present in the background. Microfollicles as well as infrequent grooves and inclusions can be seen, mimicking follicular neoplasm and PTC. Colloid is scant.
(d) Although foci of necrosis are common in histologic sections, necrosis is generally not appreciated on cytologic preparations.
(e) It is a rare aggressive malignancy and accounts for 4–7 % of thyroid carcinoma and the disease is slightly more frequent in men and young adult. Metastases to regional lymph nodes are uncommon.

Q-46. Which is true about malignant lymphoma of the thyroid?
(a) The smears usually show a monomorphic cell with eccentric nuclei.
(b) The differential diagnosis includes lymphoid hyperplasia, lymphocytic thyroiditis, and papillary thyroid carcinoma.
(c) Primary thyroid lymphoma represents approximately 15 % of all thyroid tumors.
(d) Diffuse large B-cell lymphoma and extranodal marginal zone B-cell lymphoma are the most common types.
(e) The tumor presents as a firm cervical mass of rapid growth that in a third of the cases is accompanied by compressive symptoms (hoarseness, dyspnea, dysphagia, and obstruction of the vena cava).

Q-47. Which is true about anaplastic thyroid carcinoma?
(a) The cells can be arranged as large clusters.
(b) Tumor cells can be monotonous or columnar.
(c) The nuclei are large, pleomorphic with irregular nuclear membranes, coarse and irregular chromatin clumping, and macronucleoli.
(d) Intranuclear inclusions are rarely seen.
(e) Anaplastic carcinoma/undifferentiated carcinoma (UC) represents more than 5 % of all thyroid carcinomas.

Q-48. Which is true about psammoma bodies in thyroid FNA?
(a) Psammoma bodies are basophilic calcified material.
(b) It is seen in 80 % of papillary thyroid carcinoma.
(c) Psammoma bodies are specific for papillary thyroid carcinoma.
(d) Psammoma bodies can be seen in benign conditions and in Hürthle cell neoplasms.
(e) Psammoma bodies and dystrophic calcification are the same.

Q-49. All of the following thyroid FNA are considered satisfactory except:
(a) A thyroid FNA with abundant of colloid with no follicular or Hurthle cells seen
(b) A thyroid FNA with lymphoid tissue and no follicular or Hurthle cells seen
(c) Hypocellular smears with few atypical cells showing large, pleomorphic nuclei with irregular nuclear membranes, coarse and irregular chromatin clumping, and macronucleoli
(d) Predominance of histiocytes, cholesterol clefts, and cellular debris
(e) Smears with colloid and only six sheet of Hurthle cells and no follicular cells

Q-50. The management of thyroid FNA with an initial diagnosis of nondiagnostic/unsatisfactory should be repeated within:
(a) One year
(b) One week
(c) Two week
(d) Three weeks
(e) Two to three months

4.3 Answers and Discussion of Image-Based Questions 1–44

A-1. (**a**) **Benign thyroid nodule**.

The images represent thyroid FNA with abundance of colloid with rare clusters of follicular cells (less than six clusters). Aspirates with large amounts of colloid are considered adequate for interpretation even when they contain less the six groups of follicular cells. Thyroid FNA is considered adequate for evaluation if it contains a minimum of six groups of well-visualized follicular cells, with at least ten cells per group, preferably on a single slide. However, exceptions to this requirement apply to three special circumstances: (1) Solid nodules with cytologic atypia. A sample that contains significant cytologic atypia is never considered nondiagnostic. It is mandatory to report any significant atypia as atypical (FLUS or AUS) or other abnormal category. A minimum number of follicular cells in these circumstances is not required. (2) Solid nodules with inflammation (lymphocytic/Hashimoto thyroiditis, thyroid abscess, or granulomatous thyroiditis) may contain only numerous inflammatory cells with no follicular cells. Such cases are interpreted as benign and not as nondiagnostic and a minimum number of follicular cells is not required. (3) Colloid nodules. Specimens that consist of abundant thick colloid are considered benign and a minimum number of follicular cells is not required if easily identifiable colloid is seen.

A-2. (**c**) **Nondiagnostic, cyst fluid only** (**cystic nodules**)

The images show the findings of thyroid cyst. Thyroid cyst fluid may be clear yellow, hemorrhagic, or dark brown. Specimens that consist of cyst contents (macrophages and inflammatory cells) without follicular cells are problematic, as up to 20 % of papillary carcinomas may show only cystic change. At the 2007 Bethesda Conference, it was decided that cyst fluid cases should be considered nondiagnostic, but that they create a separate subcategory called "Cyst Fluid Only" (CFO). Cystic nodules represent from 15 to 25 % of all thyroid nodules, and most are seen as a consequence of ischemia in a nodular goiter or in follicular cell neoplasms. The highest proportion of nondiagnostic specimens occurred in cystic lesions. The incidence of malignancy varies widely from 5 to 51 % of nondiagnostic specimens, depending on the selection criteria for surgical treatment, with papillary carcinoma being most common. In a study that analyzed them separately from other insufficient specimens, the risk of malignancy for a CFO sample was 4 %. Taking into account the incidence of malignancy among these nodules, follow-up evaluation is mandatory and a second or third aspiration, preferably using US guidance, should be done.

Occasional follicular cells with degenerative nuclear (smudging or hyperchromasia) or cytoplasmic (vacuolization) changes can be seen. In some aspirates, nuclei can demonstrate fine pale chromatin and grooves, mimicking papillary carcinoma, and may lead to false-positive diagnosis. The origin of these cells is still debated. Nassar et al. have reported that these cells stained for macrophages marker (CD-68 positive), while Faquin et al. demonstrated that these are reactive follicular cells (cytokeratin and thyroglobulin positive). In addition, lining cells from benign cysts often show reparative features, with dense cytoplasm, distinct cell borders, and prominent nucleoli. The mixture of these atypical reparative cells with benign-looking follicular cells is a clue favoring benignancy rather than malignancy. In addition, cystic papillary thyroid carcinoma often lacks the repair-like spindle morphology and shows other cytologic and nuclear features of papillary carcinoma.

Features associated with benign cysts include complete drainage of the cyst with no residual mass, no recurrence, and absence of cytologic atypia. If the nodule is almost entirely cystic, with no worrisome sonographic features, an endocrinologist might proceed as if this were a benign result. After evacuating any thyroid cyst, a new evaluation must be made, and any residual mass must be reaspirated under ultrasound guidance to rule out thyroid cancer.

A-3. (**b**) **Branchial cleft cyst**

The images represent the cytologic features of branchial cleft cyst. Branchial cyst usually presents in the lateral neck and can be confused with salivary/thyroid neoplasms. Aspiration of these squamous-lined cyst yields proteinaceous debris with nucleated and anucleated squamous cells, occasional columnar cells, lymphocytes, and germinal center fragments. If the cyst fluid is scant, aspirates may mimic epidermal inclusion cyst. When atypia is prominent, well-differentiated squamous cell carcinoma should be excluded. The presence of numerous anucleated squamous supports a branchial cleft cyst; however, excision should be recommended.

Other cystic lesions of the neck should be considered in the differential diagnosis such as thyroglossal, parathyroid cysts, and cystic lymph node metastases of papillary carcinoma. Clear-colorless fluid, however, should suggest a parathyroid cyst and trigger submitting cyst fluid for parathyroid hormone measurements.

A-4. **(b) Benign, subacute granulomatous (de Quervain) thyroiditis**

The images represent the cytologic findings of subacute thyroiditis. FNA is often painful, preventing adequate sampling. The key cytologic features of thyroiditis of de Quervain are presence of multinucleated giant cells; epithelioid histiocytes admixed with lymphocytes; and neutrophils, frequent degenerated follicular cells and dirty background with cellular debris, naked distorted nuclei, and colloid. Multinucleated giant cells are usually numerous with bizarre, angular shapes and more than 100 nuclei. Cytoplasm is densely granular with occasional colloid droplets, in contrast to the frothy cytoplasm typical of the multinucleated cells in multinodular goiter nodules with cystic degeneration. The degenerated follicular cells contain frequent intracytoplasmic dark-blue granules that correspond to lysosomal debris. In advanced stages, the aspirates contain scant inflammatory cells and reactive fibroblasts.

Subacute (de Quervain) thyroiditis is a rare disease and affects frequently middle-aged patients after a respiratory infection. It is characterized by painful enlargement of the thyroid gland with early, transient hypothyroidism and usually resolves spontaneously in the course of 2 or 3 months.

A-5. **(e) Chronic lymphocytic (Hashimoto) thyroiditis**:

The images show the cytomorphologic features of lymphocytic (Hashimoto) thyroiditis (HT). The aspirate is usually cellular, with numerous dispersed, polymorphic lymphoid populations, often intimately admixed with the follicular cells. Follicular cells occasionally demonstrate reactive changes and atypia, including nuclear grooves and nuclear enlargement. In our experience, HT is one of the most common causes of false-positive diagnosis for papillary carcinoma. Therefore, the diagnostic threshold for papillary thyroid carcinoma should be raised in the presence of lymphocytic thyroiditis and only considered when nuclear features of papillary carcinoma are diffusely present in a population of cells devoid of infiltrating lymphocytes.

HT is an autoimmune disease that usually affects middle-aged women. It is the most common form of noniatrogenic hypothyroidism. The disease usually results in a diffuse, painless goiter with or without nodularity. The diagnosis of HT is usually confirmed clinically by serologic tests for one or more of a variety of circulating autoantibodies; the most common are anti-thyroglobulin and antithyroid peroxidase. Clinically, HT may present as a thyroid nodule. This nodule can be originated by a nonneoplastic proliferation of follicular/Hurthle cells, extensive fibrosis, heavy focal lymphoid infiltrate, or true neoplasm in 17–22 % of the patients. The most common malignancy is papillary carcinoma.

Although the presence of a lymphoid infiltrate is an important clue for the diagnosis of HT, it can be seen in other entities, such as inflammation (tuberculosis), Graves' disease, lymphoepithelial lesions, papillary carcinoma, and lymphoma. FNA of benign lymphoepithelial lesion is characterized by scant cellularity of the epithelial component and predominance of the lymphoid component. The squamous and mucinous epithelial component may show degenerative changes, but without significant atypia.

A-6. **(c) Benign, Hurthle cell metaplasia in background of lymphocytic thyroiditis**

The images represent the cytologic findings of Hurthle cell nodule associated with HT. Aspirates from HT with a predominance of the epithelial component may be confused with Hürthle cell tumors or with papillary carcinoma. However, in Hürthle cell neoplasms, the oncocytic cells show a uniform appearance, more prominent nucleoli, and a more dyshesive pattern and usually lack the lymphocytic component. Papillary thyroid carcinoma (PTC) variants, such as Warthin-like, tall cell, and oncocytic types, arising in a background of lymphocytic thyroiditis should also be considered in the differential diagnosis. The absence of nuclear and other cytologic features of papillary carcinoma and the presence of inflammatory infiltrate may aid in resolving the problem. In a patient with a history of HT, a nodule is more likely to represent Hürthle cell hyperplasia rather than neoplasm. If the inflammatory infiltrate is the main feature, the cytologic picture may simulate a malignant lymphoma. In these circumstances, flow cytometry, immunohistochemistry, or molecular analysis are necessary to confirm clonality.

A-7. **(b) Toxic diffuse hyperplasia (Graves' disease)**

The images represent the cytologic findings of toxic diffuse hyperplasia (Graves' disease). The key cytologic features of Graves' disease are bloodstained smear with little or no colloid, numerous pale follicular cells dispersed or arrayed in cluster, and discrete to moderate anisonucleosis with marginal cytoplasmic vacuoles. The follicular cells are commonly arranged in flat sheets and have foamy delicate cytoplasm with distinctive flame (flare) cells, because of their irregular and radiating appearance. Flame cells are best appreciated on Diff-Quick stain and represent marginal cytoplasmic vacuoles with red to pink frayed edges, due to expansion of endoplasmic reticulum caused by the low pressure in the syringe during FNA. Flame cells, however, are not specific and may be encountered in other thyroid conditions. Prominent microfollicular architecture, significant nuclear overlapping and crowding, and considerable cell pleomorphism are occasionally seen. Hurthle cells (oncocytes) and lymphocytes may be found in the background. Sometimes the follicular cells display focal nuclear chromatin clearing, but other diagnostic nuclear features of papillary carcinoma are absent. The reported incidence of carcinoma in Graves' disease is 5 % of cases, of which papillary carcinoma is the most common.

The usefulness of FNA in Graves' disease is limited because the diagnosis is generally made on the basis of clinical features and laboratory data. Occasionally, however, thyroid nodules develop and prompt FNA. The cytologic features of Graves' disease are nonspecific, and clinical correlation is needed for a definitive diagnosis.

Graves' disease is an autoimmune disorder, typically characterized by diffuse goiter, hyperthyroidism, and exophthalmos. It is the most common cause of thyroid hyperfunction and usually affects middle-aged women. Glandular enlargement and hyperfunction are initiated by at least two immunoglobulin G (IgG) antibodies: thyroid-stimulating immunoglobulin (TSI) and thyrotropin-binding inhibitor immunoglobulin (TBII).

A-8. (**c**) **Benign, radiation changes**

The images show the cytologic features of radiation changes such as enlarged follicular cells with normal nuclear-to-cytoplasmic ratio, cytoplasmic vacuolization, marked nuclear atypia, hyperchromasia, and smudged nuclei with pseudoinclusions. Nuclei vary greatly in size, with dark, coarsely granular chromatin and eosinophilic prominent nucleoli. Cytoplasm is abundant and eosinophilic, suggestive of Hürthle cell change.

The differential diagnosis includes follicular carcinoma, papillary carcinoma, and undifferentiated (anaplastic) carcinoma. Both external radiation to the neck and systemic administration of radioactive iodine (^{131}I) can cause long-term morphologic changes in the thyroid gland. In addition, external radiation has been associated with an increased risk of thyroid cancer. External radiation is used in low doses to treat a variety of benign conditions and in high doses for malignancies like Hodgkin lymphoma. Radioactive iodine is administered to treat hyperthyroidism.

A-9. (**d**) **Benign colloid**

The images show abundant colloid material and low number of follicular cells. Watery colloid often forms a "thin membrane/cellophane" coating or film and is difficult to recognize in Papanicolaou and Diff-Quik-stained specimens. It can also be confused with serum in bloody specimens. Colloid may also disappear completely in thin-layer liquid-based preparations. Helpful clues are the recognition of cracking and folding in colloid, as well as its tendency to surround follicular cells, whereas serum accumulates at the edges of the slide and around platelets, fibrin, and blood clots. Dense colloid is easy to recognize and has a hyaline quality, with folds imparting a "crazy pavement" appearance and/or cracks.

Colloid nodule aspiration usually shows few follicular cells and may result in a cytologically unsatisfactory specimen. We do not restrict ourselves to the number of follicular cells mentioned in the adequacy section when aspirates are predominately cystic or contain abundant colloid, as the presence of few benign follicular cells (3–4 groups) is sufficient to issue a diagnosis of benign/colloid nodule in these situations. However, we usually add to our diagnosis that colloid nodule is suggested if clinically benign and recommend repeat ultrasound and FNA in 6 months.

Benign colloid nodules are usually encountered in patients with multinodular goiter (MNG). MNG affects over 500 million people, especially in people with low dietary iodine. In the United States, despite iodine supplementation, the prevalence of MNG is roughly 4–7 %. MNG have 2 types of nodules (aspirates): hypocellular (colloid) nodules and hypercellular (hyperplastic) nodules. *Hypocellular (colloid) nodules* are the most common nodules.

A-10. (**b**) **Benign colloid nodule**

The aspirate demonstrates the cytologic findings of benign colloid nodule. The smears are hypocellular and consist of abundant colloid material and low number of follicular cells. Follicular cells are predominantly arranged in honeycomb configuration of the evenly spaced thyroid cells with rare follicle formation. During the FNA, most large macrofollicles break into fragments, forming flat sheets arranged in honeycomb sheets. The nuclei are more or less homogeneous, about the size of a red blood cell (7–9 μ), oval or round, centrally located with finely granular chromatin, and small or inconspicuous nucleoli. The cytoplasm is pale and poorly delimited and may have small blue-black granules that are of no diagnostic significance. Isolated cells have marked cytoplasmic fragility and often appear as bare, hyperchromatic nuclei that may simulate lymphocytes. Tissue fragments (microbiopsies) may be sparse or absent. Oncocytic (Hurthle) cells admixed with the usual follicular cells may be observed. The number of macrophages present in the background usually coincides with the extent of cystic degeneration. Focal reparative changes such as the presence of spindle cells and cells with tissue culture medium appearance can be seen. Microfollicles are usually absent or rare finding.

A-11. (e) **Benign, hyperplastic (adenomatoid) nodule**
The images represent the cytologic features of hyperplastic (adenomatoid) nodule. The aspirates are hypercellular with less colloid than seen in colloid nodules. Smears show abundant benign follicular cells arranged in honeycomb appearance and admixed with Hürthle cells in up to 50 % of cases. Macrophages with foamy or hemosiderin-laden cytoplasm, including multinucleated giant cells, are often present and are a nonspecific finding indicating cystic degeneration.

The distinction between a benign hypercellular nodule and papillary carcinoma depends primarily on careful examination of nuclear features. The large, pale nuclei of cyst-lining cells may bear a resemblance to the cells of papillary carcinoma, but missing other nuclear features characteristic of papillary carcinoma. Hürthle cells can be seen but admixed with ordinary follicular cells arranged in macrofollicles, which is a benign finding. By contrast, Hürthle cell neoplasms yield an exclusive population of oncocytic cells. Occasionally FNA is comprised predominantly of microfollicles which can be misinterpreted as follicular neoplasm. Hyperplastic nodule and follicular adenoma can be indistinguishable by FNA. However, both receive the same treatment. Early reports on the application of immunohistochemistry for galectin-3 and MIB-1 appeared promising, but subsequent studies showed overlapping results and were not conclusive.

A-12. (a) **Benign, reactive atypia/cyst-lining cyst**
Focal reparative changes are observed, especially in cystic lesions, including cyst-lining cells with enlarged nuclei, finely granular chromatin, and a squamoid- or spindle-shaped ("tissue-culture cell") appearance. However, if the cyst-lining cells show marked atypia due to the presence of nuclear grooves, prominent nucleoli, elongated nuclei and cytoplasm, and/or intranuclear cytoplasmic inclusions in an otherwise predominantly benign-appearing sample, then, it may better be categorized as atypical (AUS or FLUS).

A-13. (d) **Atypical cells of undetermined significance (AUS/FLUS)**
The images represent the cytologic findings of atypical cells of undetermined significance. Some thyroid FNAs are not easily classified into the benign, suspicious, or malignant categories. Such cases represent the "indetermined" category and in the Bethesda System are reported as atypical cells of undetermined significance (AUS/FLUS). An AUS/FLUS diagnosis represents 3–7 % of thyroid FNAs. The recommended management is clinical correlation and a repeat FNA at an appropriate interval (6 months). Examples include a sparsely cellular specimen but one that shows a predominance of microfollicles or a case with rare but atypical cells that might represent cyst-lining cells but whose atypia extends beyond the usual.

Resection reveals malignancy in population of patients with repeatedly AUS results or patients with worrisome clinical or sonographic findings. In this selected population, 20–25 % of patients with AUS prove to have cancer after surgery.

A-14. (c) **Benign, hyperplastic/adenomatoid nodule**
The images represent the cytologic findings of hyperplastic adenomatoid nodule. Smears are usually cellular with colloid present. If the amount of colloid is small/scanty or no colloid present and nuclear overlapping is present, then, it should be categorized as follicular neoplasm. Follicular lesions of the thyroid represent the most problematic area in thyroid FNA cytology. Clearly, one of the most difficult problems in thyroid cytology is distinguishing hyperplastic nodule with little colloid from follicular neoplasm with some colloid. On surgical resection, they can be hyperplastic nodules, follicular adenoma, follicular carcinoma, or follicular variant of papillary carcinoma. Aspirates from hyperplastic thyroid nodule are cellular and contain colloid. Microfollicular structures can be seen. However, follicular cells are arranged mainly in flat sheets with a honeycomb configuration. The nuclei are uniform in appearance with smooth contour and approximate the size of RBCs. There is minimal nuclear overlapping and crowding. Although presence of colloidal material is indicative of a benign lesion, some papillary and follicular carcinomas may contain abundant colloid. *Nodules with papillary hyperplasia* yield follicular cells arranged in papillary structures. Special attention is required to avoid mistaking papillary hyperplasia for papillary carcinoma because nuclear features of papillary carcinoma are not present.

A-15. **(b) Follicular neoplasm**

Synonymous: Suspicious for follicular neoplasm = follicular neoplasm

The images represent the cytologic findings of follicular neoplasm. The purpose of this diagnostic category is to identify a nodule that might be a follicular carcinoma and triage it for surgical excision. The majority of cases in this suspicious category turn out to be follicular adenoma or hyperplastic nodules of multinodular goiter, both of which are more common than follicular carcinoma. About 15–30 % of cases turn to be malignant. As previously mentioned, the mere presence of microfollicles is not diagnostic of follicular neoplasm (FN), as microfollicles may be focally seen in 5–10 % of hyperplastic nodules. Although degenerative changes are often associated with hyperplastic nodule, they may be found in up to 30 % of FN. Low cellularity may be encountered in aspirates of FN due to poor biopsy technique or due to a macrofollicular architecture yielding abundant colloid and scant follicular cells. Some of them are highly vascular, yielding abundant blood and rare follicular groups.

Several studies have evaluated the variability in reporting and diagnosing FN and cellular hyperplastic nodules. Some pathologists apply the terms "follicular lesion" and FN interchangeably, while others require more stringent criteria for the diagnosis of FN. For example, the proportion of microfollicles needed to establish a FN diagnosis has ranged in the literature from none to predominant. A wide range of interobserver variability (fair to substantial) has been reported, even within the same institution. Carpi et al. have shown that the preoperative use of large-needle biopsy may show a mixed pattern of micro- and macrofollicles in 50 % of cases, with very low probability to be neoplastic.

Marked cellularity alone does not qualify the nodule for this category. If the sample is cellular but mostly macrofollicular (intact spheres and flat fragments), a benign interpretation is appropriate. A suspicious interpretation is rendered when the majority of the follicular cells are arranged in (microfollicles or crowded trabeculae/synchial pattern). If nuclear features of papillary carcinoma (nuclear grooves, pseudoinclusions, etc.) are present, the case should be reported as suspicious for papillary carcinoma.

A-16. **(a) Hürthle cell neoplasm**

Synonymous: Suspicious for Hurthle cell neoplasm = Hurthle cell neoplasm

The images represent the cytologic features of Hurthle cell neoplasm. The aspirate is composed exclusively of Hürthle cells. Smears demonstrate often isolated cells with abundant granular eosinophilic cytoplasm, resulting from accumulation of mitochondria. Groups, with crowded and syncytium-like pattern, can be seen. A large nucleolus is more typical of neoplastic than hyperplastic Hürthle cells. Colloid can be present, but abundant lymphocytes and normal follicular cells are absent. Basophilic structures with concentric lamellae, indistinguishable from psammoma bodies, are seen in some cases. The purpose of this diagnostic category is to identify a nodule that might be a Hürthle cell carcinoma (HC) and triage it for surgical excision.

Hürthle cells can be a component of HT when they are admixed with numerous lymphoid cells. Similarly, they can be seen admixed with macrofollicles and colloid, a heterogeneous mixture in MNG. Macronucleoli are usually absent. Macrophages can sometimes be confused with Hürthle cells, and vice versa, particularly with liquid-based preparations, in which the usually granular cytoplasm of Hürthle cells appears microvacuolated. But the pseudovacuolization of Hürthle cells in liquid-based preparations is fine and does not have the coarsely vacuolated appearance of macrophage cytoplasm. In addition, Hürthle cells generally lack hemosiderin and are more polygonal, rather than rounded like macrophages.

Variants of papillary carcinoma (tall cell and oncocytic) can be excluded by the absence of nuclear features diagnostic of papillary carcinoma. Because Hürthle cell tumors can have clear cell features, mimicking metastatic renal cell carcinoma, a clinical history of renal cell carcinoma can alert the cytopathologist to this possibility and should be provided on the requisition. Immunohistochemistry for thyroglobulin and TTF-1 is helpful because renal cell carcinoma is negative for these markers.

A-17. **(e) Follicular neoplasm**

The images represent the cytologic features of follicular neoplasm category. FNAs of follicular neoplasm (FN) are typically highly cellular with little or no colloid. Follicular cells are arranged in microfollicles and/or syncytial fragments, involving greater than 50–75 % of the cellular groups. Microfollicles are defined as groups of cells (6–12 cells) arranged in a ring or rosette-like configuration and often display a repetitive pattern. The syncytial groups exhibit a three-dimensional appearance with loss of cell borders.

The amount of colloid in the background is a very important feature of neoplastic lesions since large pools of colloid are usually seen in benign hyperplastic/adenomatoid nodules or in normo- and macrofollicular adenomas. The presence of abundant blood in the smears rather than being related to poor technique may be of help in the cytodiagnosis because follicular neoplasms are highly vascularized. The nuclei are uniform, slightly enlarged, round with smooth contour, but usually demonstrate prominent overlapping and crowding. The chromatin is finely to coarsely granular, and nucleoli are infrequent. The cytoplasm is pale with poorly defined border and no paravacuolar granules or oxyphilic changes. Significant nuclear atypia may or may not be present and characterized by nuclear enlargement that is greater than twice the size of red blood cells, coarse and clumped chromatin, and prominent enlarged nucleoli. Although large nuclei are more likely to be seen in carcinomas, small nuclei do not rule out malignancy. Nuclei of different sizes are more common in hyperplastic goiter and adenomas than in carcinomas.

A-18. (**b**) **Follicular neoplasm, favoring follicular carcinoma**

The images represent the cytologic findings of follicular carcinoma. There is no morphometric, cytometric data or even immunocytochemistry permit differentiation of adenomas and well-differentiated (minimally invasive) follicular carcinomas. Distinction of follicular carcinoma from adenoma on cytologic features (even histology) is difficult if not impossible, since histologic confirmation is needed to demonstrate the presence of capsular and/or vascular space invasion. The diagnosis of carcinoma is rendered in this case because of the presence of metastatic disease.

Some studies have reported several cytologic features to predict high cancer risk (40–60 % cancer risk) such as an enlarged nuclei (at least twice the size of RBC), marked nuclear atypia including significant nuclear pleomorphism and irregularity, significant nuclear overlapping, and predominance of microfollicular structures (involving > 75 % of thyroid clusters). Most follicular carcinomas (>90 %) have prominent microfollicular architecture. However, the mere presence of microfollicles is not equated with neoplasia, since they can be seen in hyperplastic nodule. Microfollicles lacking nuclear overlap and mixed with abundant colloid had a 0 % chance of harboring cancer. The issue of nuclear atypia and its relationship to malignancy has been the subject of debate. The presence of microfollicles without cytologic atypia has a low cancer risk (6 %), while the presence of atypia increases the cancer risk to 44 %, most of which represented follicular variant of papillary carcinoma.

A-19. (**e**) **Oncocytic (Hürthle cell) neoplasm**

The images represent the cytologic features of Hürthle cell neoplasm category. FNA usually render highly cellular aspirates with scant colloid and rare to absent lymphocytes. The oncocytes are arranged mainly in large and small clusters and isolated single cells. Occasional microfollicles may be seen. The cells show uniform appearance and have abundant granular cytoplasm with well-defined border, round to oval nuclei, and granular chromatin. The nuclei show prominent cherry-red nucleoli. Cytologic atypia may be observed in oncocytic lesions, including nuclear enlargement and pleomorphism.

The main differential diagnosis includes oncocytic nodule in association with a nodular goiter or lymphocytic thyroiditis. A mixture of Hürthle cells with benign thyroid follicular cells and colloid favors nodular goiter, while a prominent lymphoid cell component favors lymphocytic thyroiditis. In medullary carcinoma, the nuclei typically have a "salt and pepper" chromatin, but may show pleomorphism with prominent nucleoli and scattered stripped atypical nuclei. Silver and Busseniers called attention to the presence of prominent vascularity and intracytoplasmic lumina as characteristic features of Hürthle cell neoplasms. In contrast, Elliot et al. have confirmed the lack of significance of intracytoplasmic lumina as a differentiating feature between neoplastic and nonneoplastic Hürthle cell lesions. Hürthle cells may occasionally contain nuclear cytoplasmic inclusions and should not be considered a papillary carcinoma in absence of other nuclear features. Hürthle cells arranged in papillary clusters may occasionally be found; however, nuclear features of papillary carcinoma are absent.

A-20. (**e**) **Hürthle cell neoplasm favoring Hürthle cell carcinoma**

The images represent the cytologic features of the Hürthle cell carcinoma. Similar to FN, there is no morphometric, cytometric data, cytological or even immunocytochemistry permit differentiation of adenomas and well-differentiated (minimally invasive) Hürthle cell carcinomas, since histologic confirmation is needed to demonstrate the presence of capsular and/or vascular space invasion. The diagnosis of Hürthle cell carcinoma was rendered in this case because of the presence of metastatic carcinoma to the bone of right hip.

Some cytologic features may help in establishing the diagnosis of Hurthle cell carcinoma. Nuclear membrane irregularities, nuclear cytoplasmic inclusions, and multiple nucleoli or a cherry-red macronucleolus have been suggested. Nonetheless, using several of these criteria, the diagnostic precision reaches only 60 %, since 67 % of the adenomas and 25 % of nonneoplastic Hürthle cell metaplasias were found to fulfill the cytologic criteria for malignancy. Ordinary follicular cells are usually fairly scarce or absent; their presence in large numbers is a favoring feature of nodular goiter. Hürthle cell tumors constitute 5 % of thyroid tumors and are associated with nodal metastases in 30 % of cases.

A-21. **(b) Hürthle cell carcinoma**

The images represent the cytologic features of the Hürthle cell carcinoma in ThinPrep smear. Nuclear membrane irregularities, nuclear cytoplasmic inclusions, and multiple nucleoli or a cherry-red macronucleolus have been suggested as cytologic criteria to diagnose Hurthle cell carcinoma. However, similar to FN, there is no morphometric, cytometric data, cytological or even immunocytochemistry permit differentiation of adenomas and Hürthle cell carcinomas, since histologic confirmation is needed to demonstrate the presence of capsular and/or vascular space invasion. Using several of these criteria, the diagnostic precision reaches only 60 %, since 67 % of the adenomas and 25 % of nonneoplastic Hürthle cell metaplasias were found to fulfill the cytologic criteria for malignancy. Ordinary follicular cells are usually fairly scarce or absent; their presence in large numbers is a favoring feature of nodular goiter.

A-22. **(c) Malignant, papillary thyroid carcinoma**

The images represent the cytologic features of classic papillary carcinoma (PTC) category. Smears show distinctive architectural and cytologic features. Architectural features include the presence of papillary and tightly cohesive three-dimensional syncytial clusters of neoplastic cells. In other cases, there are large tissue fragments with prominent vascular networks and frequent digitiform projections (complex papilla). The tips of the papillae may appear as spherical cellular fragments (CAPS) with palisaded and overlapping nuclei. Many of the neoplastic groups demonstrate prominent nuclear crowding and overlapping. In most cases, the cytoplasm has a thick "metaplastic" consistency, with well-defined borders.

Nuclear features are the most important diagnostic clues for PTC. The diffuse presence of nuclear grooves, nuclear enlargement, and finely granular (powdery) chromatin must be present, before a definitive diagnosis is rendered. Nuclei are oval and large in size mimicking "bag of potato." The ground glass appearance of the nuclei seen in histologic sections is an artifact of formalin fixation and is not recognized in cytologic preparations. Nucleoli are often small and peripherally situated against a thickened nuclear membrane. Nuclear grooves may traverse the entire longitudinal axis of the nucleus or may appear as invaginations of the nuclear membrane. Intranuclear pseudoinclusions, which are also distinctive of PTC, are not present in all cases. However, they can be seen in more than 5 % of the cells in 90 % of cases. The inclusions usually have sharp margins and should reflect the color of the cytoplasm of that cell (not just a clear hole in the nucleus). Cell block can be helpful in definitive diagnosis of papillary carcinoma.

Papillary thyroid carcinoma (PTC) is the most common thyroid malignancy, accounting for 80 % of all thyroid cancers in the United States. It can occur at any age, but most patients are between 20 and 50 years old with a female-to-male ratio of 4:1. It is the most common pediatric thyroid malignancy. PTC presents as a solitary nodule or a distinct nodule within a nodular goiter. PTC can be partially or entirely cystic in up to 10 % of cases. In more than 50 % of the patients, regional cervical lymph nodes are affected at the time of surgery. Cervical lymphadenopathy resulting from a metastatic tumor can be the initial presentation in some cases.

A-23. **(c) Malignant, papillary thyroid carcinoma**

The images represent the other cytologic features of classic papillary carcinoma (PTC) category. In addition to the previous distinctive architectural and cytologic features, other features can be seen.

Psammoma bodies are a useful diagnostic feature, identified in only about 50 % of PTC and less frequent on cytologic preparations. Psammoma bodies are not specific and can also be seen in MNG and Hürthle cell neoplasms. However, the presence of psammoma bodies should raise the suspicion of PTC, especially in a cystic background. Psammoma bodies should not be confused with the nonlaminated dystrophic calcification that sometimes is observed in benign thyroid lesions.

A proportion of cases may show multinucleated giant cells, the presence of which should increase awareness about the possibility of PTC and invoke a more thorough search for diagnostic nuclear features. The colloid in papillary carcinoma is scant but fairly characteristic; it is thick (chewing gum colloid) and appears as threads of irregular thickness or dense blobs. Sometimes follicular cells may show degenerative changes, such as cytoplasmic microvacuolization (resembling macrophages).

A-24. (**e**) **Papillary thyroid carcinoma**
The images represent the cytologic features of classic papillary carcinoma (PTC) category in air-dried preparation (Diff-Quick stain). Although distinctive architectural features of papillary carcinoma can be seen, nuclear details are usually not appreciated. However, nuclei are usually large and oval. Intranuclear inclusion can be identified. Cytoplasm is dense and thick (squamoid in nature).

The colloid in papillary carcinoma is fairly characteristic, particularly in air-dried preparation; it is thick (chewing gum colloid) and appears as threads of irregular thickness or dense blobs. Psammoma bodies are a useful diagnostic feature. Although they are not specific and can also be seen in other conditions, their presence should raise the suspicion of PTC, especially in a cystic background. Psammoma bodies should not be confused with the nonlaminated dystrophic calcification that sometimes is observed in benign thyroid lesions.

A-25. (**b**) **Malignant, papillary thyroid carcinoma**
The images represent the cytologic features of classic papillary carcinoma (PTC) category in ThinPrep smears. Smears show distinctive architectural and cytologic features. Architectural features include the presence of papillary and tightly cohesive three-dimensional syncytial clusters of neoplastic cells. Large tissue fragments with prominent vascular networks and frequent digitiform projections (complex papilla) were seen. The tips of the papillae may appear as spherical cellular fragments (CAPS) with palisaded and overlapping nuclei. Powdery chromatin nature of nuclei with inconspicuous nucleoli, irregular nuclear membranes, and abundant nuclear grooves are seen in the cells. Intranuclear pseudoinclusions can be seen. The inclusions usually have sharp margins and should reflect the color of the cytoplasm of that cell (not just a clear hole in the nucleus). Cytologic classification is accurate in over 90 % of classic PTC, but is much less reproducible in other PTC variants.

A-26. (**c**) **Cystic papillary thyroid carcinoma**
The images represent the cytologic findings of papillary carcinoma associated with cystic changes. In cystic PTC or lymph node metastases of papillary carcinoma, aspiration yields abundant brown or bloody fluid with numerous hemosiderin-laden macrophages and occasional follicular neoplastic cells with characteristic nuclear findings and sometimes psammoma bodies.

PTC accounts for the most common cystic neoplasm of the thyroid. FNA is unable to establish a diagnosis of malignancy in 50 % of entirely cystic PTC. This is mainly due to scant cellularity and presence of abundant foamy macrophages, blood, and reparative changes. The hallmark for diagnosing PTC, however, is based on its distinctive nuclear features.

Few cases of papillary carcinoma arising in a thyroglossal cyst have been diagnosed by FNA. Previously described cytologic features are useful in the diagnosis of papillary carcinoma, except squamous metaplasia, because squamous cells are a common component of the nonneoplastic thyroglossal cyst.

A-27. (**d**) **Metastatic papillary thyroid carcinoma**
The images represent the cytologic findings of metastatic papillary carcinoma. Smears shows the characteristic features of papillary carcinoma, admixed with lymphocytic background. PCs are immunoreactive for keratins, thyroglobulin, and TTF-1.

A-28. (**b**) **Suspicious for papillary thyroid carcinoma**
The images represent the cytologic features of "suspicious for papillary carcinoma" category. The majority of PTCs are straightforward to diagnose, because most or all of the nuclear and architectural features previously described are clearly identifiable and widespread. It is important to note that there is no single feature that is diagnostic of PTC and that a definitive diagnosis should be based on a constellation of cytologic features. If only one or two characteristic features of PTC are present, or present only focal, or if the sample is sparsely cellular, a malignant diagnosis cannot be made with certainty. Such cases are best classified as "suspicious for papillary carcinoma." It is important to recognize "suspicious for PTC" as a distinct and separate category, and not to lump it with other "indeterminate" or "follicular neoplasm" diagnoses, due to its substantially greater association with malignancy on surgical follow-up. "Suspicious for PTC" has been reported to show PTC on histologic resection in approximately 75 %, while it is 10–30 % with indeterminate or FN diagnoses. With such a high risk of malignancy, clinicians and patients may consider total thyroidectomy as an alternative management option to lobectomy.

Several studies have attempted to determine the most sensitive cytologic criteria for diagnosing PTC and found nuclear inclusions, nuclear grooves, papillary structures, and metaplastic cytoplasm, when present in combination, to be the most reliable cytologic features. The coexistence of longitudinal folds and nuclear inclusions in the same nucleus is very improbable. Some authors showed that the presence of more than three enlarged nuclei with intranuclear cytoplasmic inclusion in a single aspirate is almost pathognomonic for PTC.

Care must be taken not to overinterpret nonspecific findings as malignant or suspicious for PTC. None of the features mentioned before is diagnostic of PTC by itself, and therefore a diagnosis (or even suspicion) of PTC cannot be made on the basis of a single finding. If a well-sampled nodule has the characteristics of a benign follicular nodule, but a few grooves are present, they have little significance and can be ignored. The same applies to psammoma bodies, which can be also seen in MNG. Nuclear pallor not accompanied by other nuclear changes can result from a technical staining problem. Mimickers of intranuclear pseudoinclusions as a result of a fixation artifact or overlying red blood cells can be seen.

A-29. (a) **Papillary thyroid carcinoma (Follicular variant)**

The images represent the cytologic features of follicular variant of papillary carcinoma category. The *follicular variant of PTC (FVPC)* is by far the most common of papillary carcinoma subtypes. The smears consist predominately of follicular structures, admixed with flat syncytial sheets. Cells demonstrate large nuclei and fine powdery chromatin and nuclear grooves, specific cytologic nuclear features for the diagnosis of FVPC. Fulciniti et al. emphasized the importance of nuclear grooves and nucleoli over intranuclear inclusions in the diagnosis of FVPC. The predominance of microfollicles in some cases can lead to misclassification as follicular neoplasm. However, careful high power examination of the nuclei and recognition of the nuclear features of PTC in these cases will usually establish the diagnosis of FVPC. FVPC is the second to sampling error as the most common cause of false negative diagnoses in thyroid FNA.

A-30. (a) **Papillary thyroid carcinoma, oncocytic variant**

The images represent the cytologic features of oncocytic variant of papillary carcinoma. Smears are characterized by large tumor cells with abundant dense granular cytoplasm, well-defined cytoplasmic borders, eccentric nuclei, and nuclear features of PTC.

Other PTC variants: The *tall-cell variant of papillary carcinoma* shows, elongated to tall cells with distinct cell borders, cyanophilic and eosinophilic cytoplasm, and a high nucleocytoplasmic ratio. The nuclear features of PTC, in tall cell variant, are often diffuse and extensive, compared to classic PTC. Often, the nuclei contain numerous inclusions, imparting a soap-bubble appearance. *Columnar cell variant of PTC* demonstrates columnar cells with ill-defined cell borders, delicate cytoplasm with focal vacuolization/clearing, nuclear pseudostratification, and oval to elongated hyperchromatic nuclei. Architecturally, it may resemble colonic adenocarcinoma.

Diffuse sclerosing papillary carcinoma is a relatively common lesion that affects one or both thyroid lobes and consists of multiple foci of papillary carcinoma immersed in a fibrous stroma with lymphoid infiltration. The smears show a dense lymphocytic inflammatory component together with a monolayer of squamous metaplastic cells and numerous psammoma bodies. Cases with marked stromal lymphocytic infiltrate are also called the Warthin-like variant.

A-31. (d) **Medullary thyroid carcinoma**

The images represent the cytologic features of medullary carcinoma (MTC). MTC is notorious for its variable cytologic appearances, ranging from a monomorphic to a pleomorphic cell population. Typically, medullary carcinoma presents mostly as dyscohesive cells. The neoplastic cells may have a plasmacytoid-, spindle-, epithelioid-, or carcinoid-like appearance, but often a mixture of different cell types is encountered in the same specimen. Binucleated or multinucleated cells are sometimes seen. The cytoplasm has a delicate lacy quality and may show pink cytoplasmic granules. The nuclei are round to oval, with fine to coarse chromatin (salt and pepper), and have small or inconspicuous nucleoli. Occasional intranuclear inclusions are appreciated in some cases. Variable amount of amyloid may be present in the background. Amyloid has an appearance similar to thick colloid, but is confirmed with Congo red stain, which shows apple-green dichroism with polarized light. Immunocytochemical stains for calcitonin and neuroendocrine markers such as chromogranin and Synaptophysin and antigen (CEA) are positive, but negative for thyroglobulin.

Medullary thyroid carcinoma (MTC) constitutes 5–10 % of all thyroid carcinomas. It does not show a sex or age association. About 80–90 % of MTC are sporadic and occur in adults with a mean age of 50 years. The rest occur in children in association with genetic syndromes like multiple endocrine neoplasia (MEN2) syndromes with a dominant autosomal inheritance. Serum calcitonin levels are elevated in most patients and help establish the diagnosis.

A-32. (c) **Metastatic medullary carcinoma**
The images represent the cytologic features of metastatic medullary carcinoma. Up to 50 % of patients with MTC present with regional node metastases, and therefore, MTC should be considered in the differential diagnosis of patients with a positive neck node and an unknown primary. MTC is notorious for its variable cytologic appearances, ranging from a monomorphic to a pleomorphic cell population.

The differential diagnosis of medullary carcinoma includes Hürthle cell tumor, hyalinizing trabecular tumor, papillary carcinoma, anaplastic carcinoma, and metastatic neoplasms, particularly malignant melanoma. However, oncocytic neoplasm usually has cells with well-defined borders, in contrast to ill-defined wispy cytoplasmic borders of medullary carcinoma. Oncocytic tumors show prominent nucleoli and lack the neuroendocrine chromatin pattern. MTC may display intranuclear inclusions, but other diagnostic nuclear features of PTC are absent. Spindle cell melanoma are included in the differential diagnosis of predominately spindle medullary carcinoma, while plasmacytoma and melanoma may be confused with plasmacytoid medullary carcinoma. The most characteristic findings to support the diagnosis of medullary carcinoma are abundant isolated cells with marked variations in size and form, plasmacytic-like cells, and presence of metachromatic cytoplasmic granules. Positive staining for calcitonin in cell blocks is helpful in confirming the cytologic diagnosis of MTC.

A-33. (c) **Suspicious for medullary thyroid carcinoma**
The images represent the cytologic features suspicious for medullary carcinoma (MTC) with amyloid deposit present. MTC is notorious for its variable cytologic appearances, ranging from a monomorphic to a pleomorphic cell population. Typically, medullary carcinoma presents mostly as dyscohesive cells. The neoplastic cells may have a plasmacytoid-, spindle-, epithelioid-, or carcinoid-like appearance, but often a mixture of different cell types is encountered in the same specimen. Binucleated or multinucleated cells are sometimes seen. The cytoplasm has a delicate lacy quality and may show pink cytoplasmic granules. The nuclei are round to oval, with fine to coarse chromatin (salt and pepper), and have small or inconspicuous nucleoli. Occasional intranuclear inclusions are appreciated in some cases. Variable amount of amyloid may be present in the background. Amyloid has an appearance similar to thick colloid, but is confirmed with Congo red stain, which shows apple-green dichroism with polarized light. Positive diagnosis of medullary carcinoma requires elevated serum calcitonin or positive immunocytochemical stains for calcitonin and neuroendocrine markers such as chromogranin and Synpatophysin and CEA are positive, but negative for thyroglobulin. Serum calcitonin levels are elevated in most patients and help establish the diagnosis.

A-34. (e) **Anaplastic carcinoma/undifferentiated carcinoma**
The images represent the cytologic features of anaplastic carcinoma. The cytologic appearance is variable, reflecting the diversity of histologic patterns. Three basic types of anaplastic cells (fusiform, giant, and squamous) can coexist in different proportions, but the predominance of any one lacks prognostic significance. The nuclear features are unmistakably malignant. The cells can be arranged as large loose fragments, small clusters, or isolated cells. Tumor cells can be spindle-shaped or epithelioid, with squamoid features. Nuclei are hyperchromatic and vary widely in size and shape. Extremely large, pleomorphic, and bizarrely shaped cells are seen. Some FNAs contain numerous osteoclast-type multinucleated giant cells. The nuclear features are unmistakably malignant. The nuclei are large, pleomorphic with irregular nuclear membranes, coarse and irregular chromatin clumping, and macronucleoli. Intranuclear inclusions are common, and mitotic figures may be numerous. Abundant necrosis may be present in the background.

Anaplastic carcinoma/undifferentiated carcinoma (UC) represents less than 5 % of all thyroid carcinomas. It is the most aggressive thyroid neoplasm: more than 90 % of patients die within a year of diagnosis.

A-35. (c) **Anaplastic carcinoma**
The images represent the cytologic features of anaplastic carcinoma. The cytologic smears are hypercellular and consist of anaplastic cells. The cells can be arranged as large loose fragments, small clusters, or isolated cells. Extremely large, pleomorphic, and bizarrely shaped cells are seen. Some FNAs contain numerous osteoclast-type multinucleated giant cells. Abundant necrosis may be present in the background.

The differential diagnosis of anaplastic carcinoma includes medullary carcinoma, sarcoma, and metastatic carcinoma to the thyroid. Sarcomas can be excluded with an immunohistochemical panel that includes cytokeratins, muscle markers (desmin, Myo-D1, myogenin), and vascular markers (CD31, CD34).

Metastatic carcinoma and medullary carcinoma are probably the most important consideration. Anaplastic carcinomas are usually reactive for keratins, but are negative for thyroglobulin and TTF-1. The distinction rests heavily on clinical correlation, imaging studies, and immunohistochemistry; UC is ultimately a diagnosis of exclusion.

A-36. **(d) Large cell lymphoma**

The images represent the cytologic findings of large cell lymphoma. FNA cytology of thyroid lymphoma is similar to its lymph node counterpart. The smears have a monomorphic lymphoid appearance and show many lymphoglandular bodies in the background. Diffuse large B-cell lymphoma and extranodal marginal zone B-cell lymphoma are the most common types. Flow cytometry and/or immunocytochemistry are necessary for establishing a definitive diagnosis, particularly in patients with no previous history. Differential diagnosis includes lymphoid hyperplasia and lymphocytic thyroiditis, both of which are characterized by a polymorphic population of lymphoid cells.

Primary thyroid lymphoma represents approximately 5 % of all thyroid tumors and 2.5–7 % of all extrathyroid lymphomas. Non-Hodgkin lymphoma is by far the most common type, with Hodgkin disease representing a rarity in the thyroid. Because 15 % of patients with systemic malignant lymphomas present with thyroid involvement, systemic disease must be excluded before diagnosing primary thyroid lymphoma. The tumor presents as a firm cervical mass of rapid growth that in a third of the cases is accompanied by compressive symptoms (hoarseness, dyspnea, dysphagia, and obstruction of the vena cava).

A-37. **(c) Metastatic renal cell carcinoma**

The images represent the cytologic features of metastatic renal cell carcinoma. Smears show single cells and sheets with moderate to abundant finely vacuolated/clear cytoplasm and frayed cytoplasmic borders. Nuclear to cytoplasmic ratios may range from low to high, and nucleoli may or may not be prominent. Occasionally, vascularized epithelial fragments are seen. Metastatic renal cell carcinoma should first be excluded, when a neoplasm displays prominent clear cell change.

Cellular proliferations with clear cell features raise the possibility of primary and secondary thyroid neoplasms. Follicular neoplasm (adenoma or carcinoma) may show clear cell features; however, these changes are usually focal, and there is often an associated prominent microfollicular architecture and/or syncytial arrangement and pronounced nuclear overlap and crowding. Clustering of histiocytes and cyst-lining cells may at times raise the possibility of neoplasia; however, these aspirates are of scant cellularity and show spindling and degenerative changes. Granular renal cell carcinoma can cytologically mimic oncocytic neoplasm. Again, the utilization of immunohistochemical stains such as calcitonin, chromogranin, kappa, lambda, cytokeratin, thyroglobulin, and TTF-1 may be helpful in the work-up of renal cell carcinoma. Finally, other metastatic cancers from such sites as lung, head and neck, breast, and liver, as well as germ cell tumors, may show prominent clear cell features and should be considered in the differential diagnosis. Detailed clinical history is crucial. Clear cell carcinoma may appear as synchronic or metachronic disease, even after a long latency period.

In clinical practice, the incidence of metastatic carcinoma amounts to 5.7–7.5 % in preoperative FNA thyroid masses, but in postmortem examination, it ranges from 1.25 to 24.5 %. Metastasis to the thyroid can present as multiple small nodules or as a solitary tumor mass mimicking a primary neoplasm. The majority are produced by contiguous spread of primary neoplasms of the pharynx, larynx, and upper third of the esophagus. In addition, the thyroid is subject to hematogenously disseminated disease in the advanced stages of carcinoma of the breast, lung, and kidney; melanoma; leukemia; and lymphoma. In some cases, metastasis to the thyroid can present after long time from the detection of primary cancer, especially renal cell carcinoma. Breast and lung cancers are the most common primary tumors seen in autopsy studies, while the kidney is the most common site reported in surgical series. Melanoma and colon cancers do not infrequently metastasize to the thyroid. Metastasis should be suspected when the microscopic features appear alien to those neoplasms more commonly encountered in the thyroid. Michelow and Leiman reported 21 cases of metastases to the thyroid gland, in which only five patients had a known history of malignancy.

A-38. **(d) Metastatic squamous cell carcinoma**

The images represent the cytologic findings of metastatic squamous cell carcinoma. Although the appearance of a thyroid nodule in the case of disseminated tumoral disease usually is suggestive of metastatic disease, this is not always so. Approximately 71 % of the thyroid nodules in patients with extrathyroid cancer turn to be benign lesions, metastatic tumors in 17 %, and primary malignant tumors in 6 %.

A-39. (b) **Metastatic melanoma**

The images represent the cytologic findings of metastatic melanoma. Although the appearance of a thyroid nodule in the case of disseminated tumoral disease usually is suggestive of metastatic disease, this is not always so. Approximately 71 % of the thyroid nodules in patients with extrathyroid cancer turn to be benign lesions, metastatic tumors in 17 %, and primary malignant tumors in 6 %.

In recent years, the cytologic characteristics of unusual thyroid lesions have been described. Among the very unusual thyroid lesions, there have been cases of ectopic lingual thyroid, mucoepidermoid carcinoma, synovial sarcoma, neural tumors (schwannoma and malignant peripheral nerve sheath tumor), intrathyroid parathyroid adenoma, squamous cell carcinoma, thymoma, Langerhans histiocytosis, and liposarcoma. Among the extrathyroid lesions initially interpreted as cold nodules, cases of lipoma and thymoma have been reported.

A-40. (e) **Parathyroid adenoma**

Parathyroid adenomas and the rare parathyroid carcinoma can be mistaken clinically for thyroid nodules. Smears are cellular, composed of cohesive sheets, ribbon-like cords, and occasional microacini. Nuclei are round and have a coarsely granular chromatin pattern; nucleoli are small. Cytoplasm is moderately abundant and granular. Isolated cells and naked nuclei can be present. Focal nuclear pleomorphism is seen, but it is not prominent. Colloid is absent.

Parathyroid adenomas are frequently mistaken cytologically for a follicular lesion of the thyroid. Most patients with a parathyroid adenoma have hypercalcemia, which is a clue to the correct diagnosis. Immunohistochemistry for thyroglobulin and parathyroid hormone can be helpful if a nonthyroid origin is suspected.

A-41. (e) **Benign, intrathyroidal branchial cleft cyst**

The images represent the cytologic features of intrathyroidal branchial cleft cyst. Branchial cyst usually presents in the lateral neck and can be presented also as intrathyroid cyst. Aspiration of these cysts shows in addition to follicular cells or colloid, squamous cells and proteinaceous debris with nucleated and anucleated squamous cells, occasional columnar cells, lymphocytes, and germinal center fragments. If the cyst fluid is scant, aspirates may mimic epidermal inclusion cyst. When atypia is prominent, well-differentiated squamous cell carcinoma should be excluded. The presence of numerous anucleated squamous supports a branchial cleft cyst; however, excision should be recommended.

Other cystic lesions of the thyroid should be considered in the differential diagnosis such as thyroglossal, parathyroid cysts, and cystic metastases of papillary carcinoma. Clear-colorless fluid, however, should suggest a parathyroid cyst and trigger submitting cyst fluid for parathyroid hormone measurements.

A-42. (a) **Malignant, papillary thyroid carcinoma**

The images represent the cytologic features of papillary carcinoma (PTC) category with psammoma bodies. Smears show distinctive architectural and cytologic features. Architectural features include the presence of papillary and tightly cohesive three-dimensional syncytial clusters of neoplastic cells. In other cases, there are large tissue fragments with prominent vascular networks and frequent digitiform projections (complex papilla). The tips of the papillae may appear as spherical cellular fragments (CAPS) with palisaded and overlapping nuclei. Many of the neoplastic groups demonstrate prominent nuclear crowding and overlapping. In most cases, the cytoplasm has a thick "metaplastic" consistency, with well-defined borders. Basophilic structures with concentric lamellae, indistinguishable from psammoma bodies, are seen in some cases. Psammoma bodies are a useful diagnostic feature, identified in only about 50 % of PTC and less frequent on cytologic preparations. Psammoma bodies are not specific and can also be seen in MNG and Hürthle cell neoplasms. However, the presence of psammoma bodies should raise the suspicion of PTC, especially in a cystic background. Psammoma bodies should not be confused with the nonlaminated dystrophic calcification that sometimes is observed in benign thyroid lesions.

A-43. (e) **Parathyroid adenoma/hyperplasia**

Parathyroid adenomas and the rare parathyroid carcinoma can be mistaken clinically for thyroid nodules. Smears are cellular and composed of cohesive sheets, ribbon-like cords, and occasional microacini. Nuclei are round and have a coarsely granular chromatin pattern; nucleoli are small or prominent. Cytoplasm is moderately abundant and granular. Isolated cells and naked nuclei can be present. Focal nuclear pleomorphism is seen, but it is not prominent. Colloid is absent. Prominent vascular structures may be seen. Parathyroid adenomas are frequently mistaken cytologically for a follicular lesion of the thyroid. Most patients with a parathyroid adenoma have hypercalcemia, which is a clue to the correct diagnosis. Immunohistochemistry for thyroglobulin and parathyroid hormone can be helpful if a nonthyroid origin is suspected.

A-44. **(b) Calcitonin**
The images represent the cytologic features of medullary carcinoma. MTC has variable cytologic appearances, ranging from a monomorphic to a pleomorphic cell population. Typically, medullary carcinoma presents mostly as dyscohesive plasmacytoid cells. The neoplastic cells may have a plasmacytoid-, spindle-, epithelioid-, or carcinoid-like appearance, but often a mixture of different cell types is encountered in the same specimen. Binucleated or multinucleated cells are sometimes seen. The cytoplasm has a delicate lacy quality and may show pink cytoplasmic granules. The nuclei are round to oval, with fine to coarse chromatin (salt and pepper), and have small or inconspicuous nucleoli. Occasional intranuclear inclusions are appreciated in some cases. Variable amount of amyloid may be present in the background. Amyloid has an appearance similar to thick colloid, but is confirmed with Congo red stain, which shows apple-green dichroism with polarized light.

4.4 Answers and Discussion of Text-Based Questions 45–50

A-45. **(e) It is a rare aggressive malignancy and accounts for 4–7 % of thyroid carcinoma and the disease is slightly more frequent in men and young adult. Metastases to regional lymph nodes are uncommon**.
The images represent the cytologic features of insular (poorly differentiated carcinoma). FNA smears are usually highly cellular and composed of monomorphic appearing small follicular cells, occurring singly and in clusters. The neoplastic cells show scant delicate cytoplasm with round hyperchromatic nuclei, coarsely granular chromatin, and mild to moderate nuclear irregularities. Many naked nuclei are often present in the background. Microfollicles as well as infrequent grooves and inclusions can be seen, mimicking follicular neoplasm and PTC. Colloid is scant. Although foci of necrosis are common in histologic sections, necrosis is generally not appreciated on cytologic preparations. A helpful clue to the aggressive nature of this tumor is the presence of increased mitotic activity and individual cell necrosis. In our experience, a definitive diagnosis of insular carcinoma cannot be established by FNA.

The differential diagnosis is broad. The presence of intranuclear inclusions and grooves in many of these tumor cells suggests a PTC, but the prominence of isolated cells is unusual and might suggest PDC. Focal nuclear pleomorphism, if present, raises the possibility of an undifferentiated (anaplastic) carcinoma. Metastatic carcinoma is also in the differential diagnosis. Immunohistochemistry and clinical history may be definitive for solving the problem.

A-46. **(d) Diffuse large B-cell lymphoma and extranodal marginal zone B-cell lymphoma are the most common types**
The images represent the cytologic findings of large cell lymphoma. FNA cytology of thyroid lymphoma is similar to its lymph node counterpart. The smears have a monomorphic lymphoid appearance and show many lymphoglandular bodies in the background. Diffuse large B-cell lymphoma and extranodal marginal zone B-cell lymphoma are the most common types. Flow cytometry and/or immunocytochemistry is necessary for establishing a definitive diagnosis, particularly in patients with no previous history. Differential diagnosis includes lymphoid hyperplasia and lymphocytic thyroiditis, both of which are characterized by a polymorphic population of lymphoid cells. Primary thyroid lymphoma represents approximately 5 % of all thyroid tumors and 2.5–7 % of all extrathyroid lymphomas. Non-Hodgkin lymphoma is by far the most common type, with Hodgkin disease representing a rarity in the thyroid. Because 15 % of patients with systemic malignant lymphomas present with thyroid involvement, systemic disease must be excluded before diagnosing primary thyroid lymphoma.

A-47. **(c) The nuclei are large, pleomorphic with irregular nuclear membranes, coarse and irregular chromatin clumping, and macronucleoli**.
The cytologic appearance of anaplastic thyroid carcinoma is variable, reflecting the diversity of histologic patterns. Three basic types of anaplastic cells (fusiform, giant, and squamous) can coexist in different proportions, but the predominance of any one lacks prognostic significance. The nuclear features are unmistakably malignant. The cells can be arranged as large loose fragments, small clusters, or isolated cells. Tumor cells can be spindle-shaped or epithelioid, with squamoid features. Nuclei are hyperchromatic and vary widely in size and shape. Extremely large, pleomorphic, and bizarrely shaped cells are seen. Some FNAs contain numerous osteoclast-type multinucleated giant cells. The nuclear features are unmistakably malignant. The nuclei are large, pleomorphic with irregular nuclear membranes, coarse and irregular chromatin clumping, and macronucleoli. Intranuclear inclusions are common, and mitotic figures may be numerous. Abundant necrosis may be

present in the background. Therefore, the presence of rare pleomorphic cells associated with necrosis, in an elderly patient, should raise the possibility of anaplastic carcinoma and trigger additional studies. The cytoplasm can be densely granular or contain tiny vacuoles. Tumor cells may be accompanied by an inflammatory component rich in neutrophils and may show neutrophilic cannibalism.

Anaplastic carcinoma/undifferentiated carcinoma (UC) represents less than 5 % of all thyroid carcinomas. It is the most aggressive thyroid neoplasm: more than 90 % of patients die within a year of diagnosis.

A-48. **(d) Psammoma bodies can be seen in benign conditions and in Hürthle cell neoplasms.**
Psammoma bodies are basophilic structures with concentric lamellae, indistinguishable from psammoma bodies, seen in some cases. Psammoma bodies are a useful diagnostic feature, identified in only about 50 % of PTC and less frequent on cytologic preparations. Psammoma bodies are not specific and can also be seen in MNG and Hürthle cell neoplasms. However, the presence of psammoma bodies should raise the suspicion of PTC, especially in a cystic background. Psammoma bodies should not be confused with the nonlaminated dystrophic calcification that sometimes is observed in benign thyroid lesions.

A-49. (d) Predominance of histiocytes, cholesterol clefts, and cellular debris should be considered nondiagnostic cyst fluid only. Abundant of colloid with rare or no clusters of follicular cells should be adequate for benign (satisfactory thyroid FNA) diagnosis. Aspirates with large amounts of colloid are considered adequate for interpretation even when they contain less the six groups of follicular cells. Thyroid FNA is considered adequate for evaluation if it contains a minimum of six groups of well-visualized follicular cells, with at least ten cells per group, preferably on a single slide. However, exceptions to this requirement apply to three special circumstances: (1) Solid nodules with cytologic atypia. A sample that contains significant cytologic atypia is never considered nondiagnostic. It is mandatory to report any significant atypia as atypical (FLUS or AUS) or other abnormal category. (2) Solid nodules with inflammation (lymphocytic/Hashimoto thyroiditis, thyroid abscess, or granulomatous thyroiditis) may contain only numerous inflammatory cells with no follicular cells. Such cases are interpreted as benign and not as nondiagnostic (3) Colloid nodules. Specimens that consist of abundant thick colloid are considered benign and if easily identifiable colloid is seen.

A-50. **(e) Two to three months**
Indications for repeat FNA of thyroid nodules include follow-up of benign nodules, enlarging nodules, nodules larger than 4 cm, recurrent cyst, and an initial unsatisfactory/nondiagnostic FNA. Repeat thyroid FNA, without image-guided, in patients with initial unsatisfactory specimens results in an adequate sample in approximately 50 % of cases. However, repeat US-guided FNA of previously nondiagnostic biopsies can lead to a definitive diagnosis in up to 90 % of cases. This is especially helpful in small nodules less than 1.5 cm and complex cystic lesions, where needles can target the more solid component. On the other hand, repeated US-FNA has led to a more definitive diagnosis in 80 % of "indeterminate for follicular neoplasm" diagnoses with follow-up surgical resection. Repeat FNA in patients with initial benign cytologic diagnoses increases the sensitivity for detecting malignancy from 82 to 90 %. Two to three months interval is recommended to prevent false-positive interpretations due to reactive/reparative changes. US-guided FNA with immediate, onsite adequacy evaluation is preferred for repeat aspiration after an initial nondiagnostic diagnosis.

Reading List

Castro MR, Gharib H. Continuing controversies in the management of thyroid nodules. Ann Intern Med. 2005;142(11):926–31.

Cibas ES. Thyroid. In: Cibas ES, Ducatman BS, editors. Cytology: diagnostic principles and clinical correlates. 3rd ed. Edinburgh: Saunders/Elsevier; 2009.

Cichón S, Anielski R, Konturek A, et al. Metastases to the thyroid gland: seventeen cases operated on a single clinical center. Langenbecks Arch Surg. 2006;391:581–7.

Galera-Davidson H, González-Cámpora R. Thyroid. In: Bibbo M, Wilbur DC, editors. Comprehensive cytopathology. 3rd ed. NJ, USA: Saunders/Elsevier; 2009.

Gharib H, Papini E, Valcavi R, Baskin HJ, Crescenzi A, Dottorini ME, Duick DS, Guglielmi R, Hamilton CR Jr, Zeiger MA, Zini M; AACE/AME Task Force on Thyroid Nodules. American Association of Clinical Endocrinologists and Associazione Medici Endocrinologi medical guidelines for clinical practice for the diagnosis and management of thyroid nodules. Endocr Pract. 2006;12(1):63–102.

Guarda LA, Peterson CE, Hall W, et al. Anaplastic thyroid carcinoma. Cytomorphology and clinical implications of fine needle aspiration. Diagn Cytopathol. 1991;7:63–7.

Khalbuss WE, Monaco SE, Pantanowitz L. Chapter 15. Thyroid. In: In the ASCP quick compendium (QC) of cytopathology. Chicago: ASCP Press; 2013. p. 314–39.

Koss LG, Melamed MR. Thyroid cytology. In: Koss LG, Melamed MR, editors. Koss' diagnostic cytology and its histopathologic bases, vol. 2, set (Hardcover). NY, USA: Lippincott Williams & Wilkins; 2005

Luze T, Totsch M, Banger LI, et al. Fine needle aspiration cytodiagnosis of anaplastic carcinoma and malignant haemangioendothelioma of the thyroid in an endemic goiter area. Cytopathology. 1990;1:305–10.

Michelow PM, Leiman G. Metastases to the thyroid gland: diagnosis by aspiration cytology. Diagn Cytopathol. 1995;13:209–13.

NCI thyroid fine needle aspiration state of the science conference. Review and conclusions document. In: http://thyroidfna.cancer.gov/pages/conclusions/, ed. http://thyroidfna.cancer.gov/pages/conclusions/. 2007.

Papanicolaou Society of Cytopathology recommendations for thyroid fine needle aspiration. Diagnostic terminology and criteria for the cytologic diagnosis of thyroid lesions. www.papsociety.org/guidelines.html. 2006.

Lymph Node Cytopathology

5

Matthew A. Smith and Walid E. Khalbuss

Contents

5.1 **Image-Based Questions 1–34 (Some Images Have More Than One Question)** 306

5.2 **Text-Based Questions 35–101** 334

5.3 **Answers and Discussion of Image-Based Questions 1–34** 341

5.4 **Answers and Discussion of Text-Based Questions 35–101** 345

Reading List 352

M.A. Smith, MD
Department of Pathology, University of Pittsburgh Medical Center-Shadyside, Pittsburgh, PA, USA

W.E. Khalbuss, MD, PhD, FIAC (✉)
Department of Pathology, GE Clarient Diagnostic Services, 31 Columbia, Aliso Viejo, California, 92656, USA
e-mail: walid.khalbuss@ge.com

W.E. Khalbuss, Q.K. Li (eds.), *Diagnostic Cytopathology Board Review and Self-Assessment*, DOI 10.1007/978-1-4939-1477-7_5, © Springer Science+Business Media New York 2015

5.1 Image-Based Questions 1–34 (Some Images Have More Than One Question)

Fig. 5.1

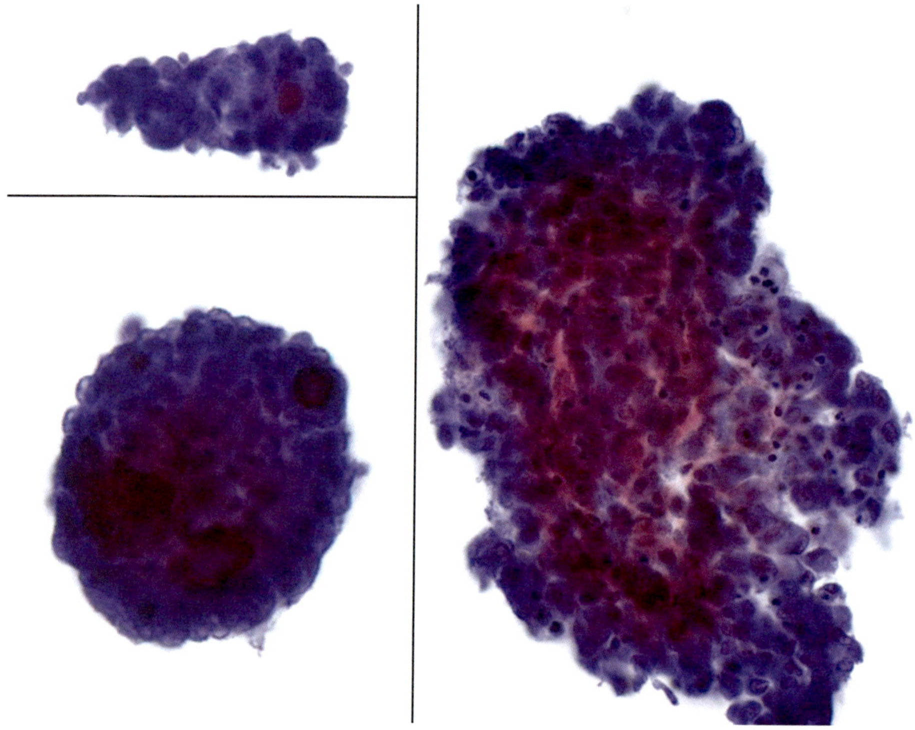

Q-1. A 26-year-old nonsmoker female undergoes FNA of an enlarged cervical lymph node. The following are reprehensive images from ThinPrep preparation (Pap stain). Given the age of the patient and the cytomorphology, what are the most likely diagnosis and the appropriate stain to confirm the diagnosis?
(a) Reactive lymphocytes and histiocytes (LCA and CD68)
(b) Metastatic lung adenocarcinoma (TTF1)
(c) Metastatic carcinoma (Pan CK, AE1/AE3)
(d) Lymphoma (CD20 and CD3)
(e) Metastatic papillary thyroid carcinoma (TTF1 and thyroglobulin)

Fig. 5.2

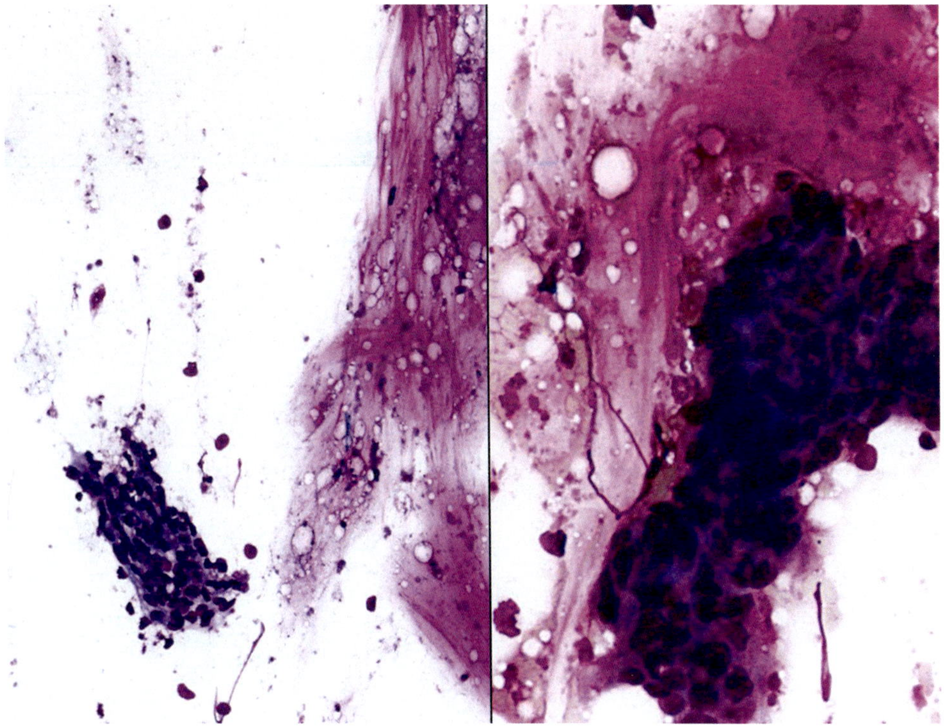

Q-2. A 47-year-old female with a history of a colonic mass found to have cervical lymphadenopathy. She underwent FNA of one of the enlarged lymph node. Representative images from DQ-stained smear are below. The most likely diagnosis is:
(a) Reactive hyperplasia
(b) Metastatic melanoma
(c) Metastatic mucinous adenocarcinoma
(d) Posttransplant lymphoproliferative disorder
(e) Diffuse large B-cell lymphoma

Fig. 5.3

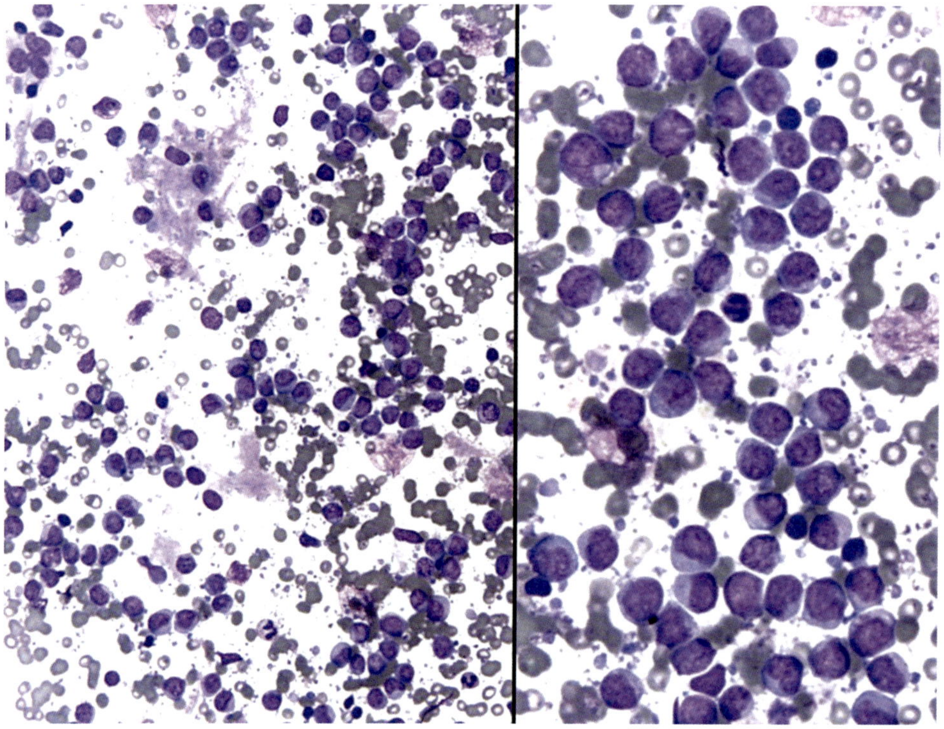

Q-3. A 55-year-old male presents with an enlarged lymph node. A FNA of the lymph node demonstrates atypical lymphocytes seen in these images (DQ stain). The cells are positive for CD20 and CD10, while negative for CD5 and CD23. These cells are most likely to demonstrate which of the following translocation?

(a) t(11;14)
(b) t(14;18)
(c) t(8:14)
(d) t(8;22)
(e) t(2;5)

Fig. 5.4

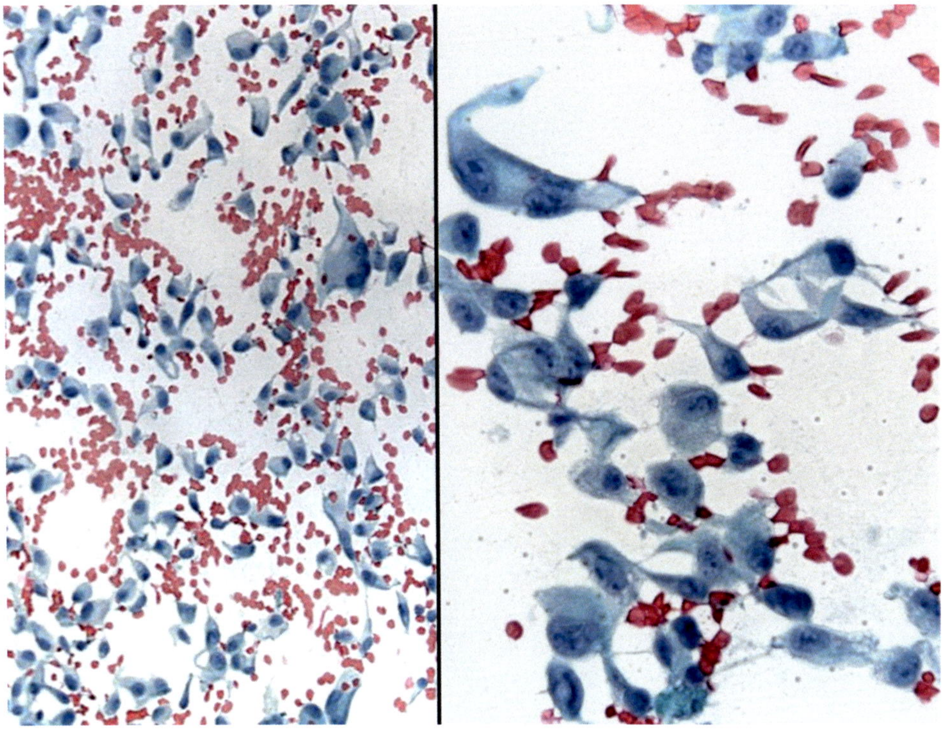

Q-4. FNA of lymph node shows cells seen in these images (Pap stain). The patient is a 24-year-old male with previous diagnosis of malignancy. The best immunostain to confirm the diagnosis in this case is:
(a) CD138
(b) CK 5
(c) Melan-A
(d) CD3
(e) OCT 3/4

Fig. 5.5

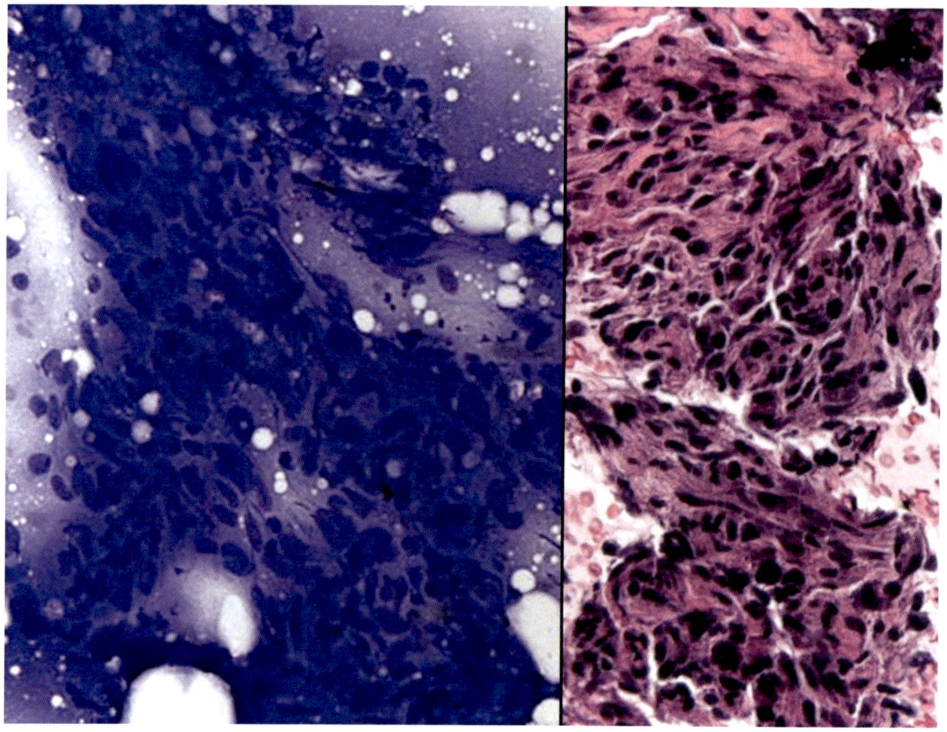

Q-5. A 57-year-old female with a history of a previously treated retroperitoneal mass presents new-onset lymphadenopathy. A FNA is performed and demonstrates the cell pictured. The most likely diagnosis is:

(a) Sarcoma
(b) Melanoma
(c) Lymphoma
(d) Carcinoma
(e) Infection

Fig. 5.6

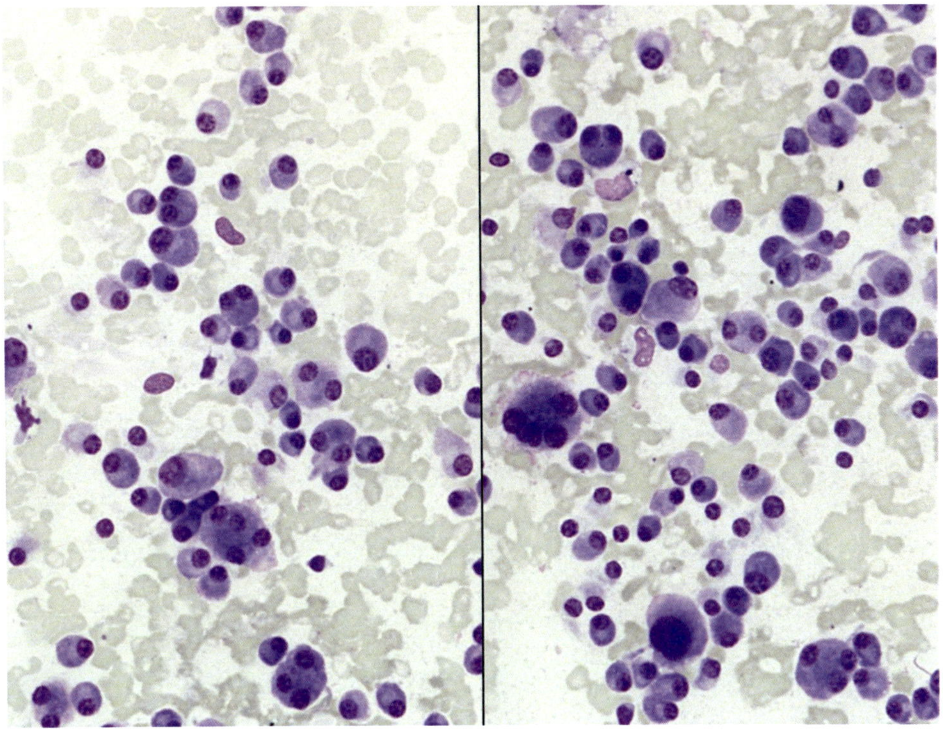

Q-6. The neoplasm that is presented in these images most likely be positive for:
(a) CD138
(b) CK 5
(c) Melan-A
(d) CD3
(e) OCT 3/4

Fig. 5.7

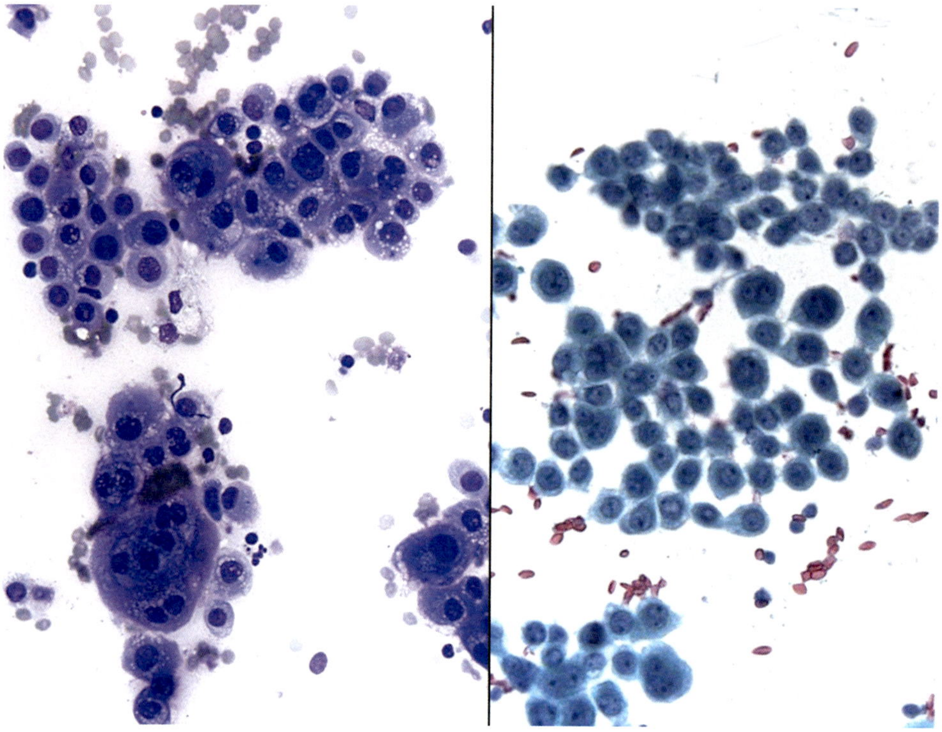

Q-7. This patient presented with pleural thickening and cervical lymphadenopathy. The pictured proliferation will most likely demonstrate positivity for:
(a) WT1 and calretinin
(b) Caldesmon and HMB45
(c) CK 7 and mucicarmine
(d) CD10 and PAX8
(e) CD68 and CD168

Fig. 5.8

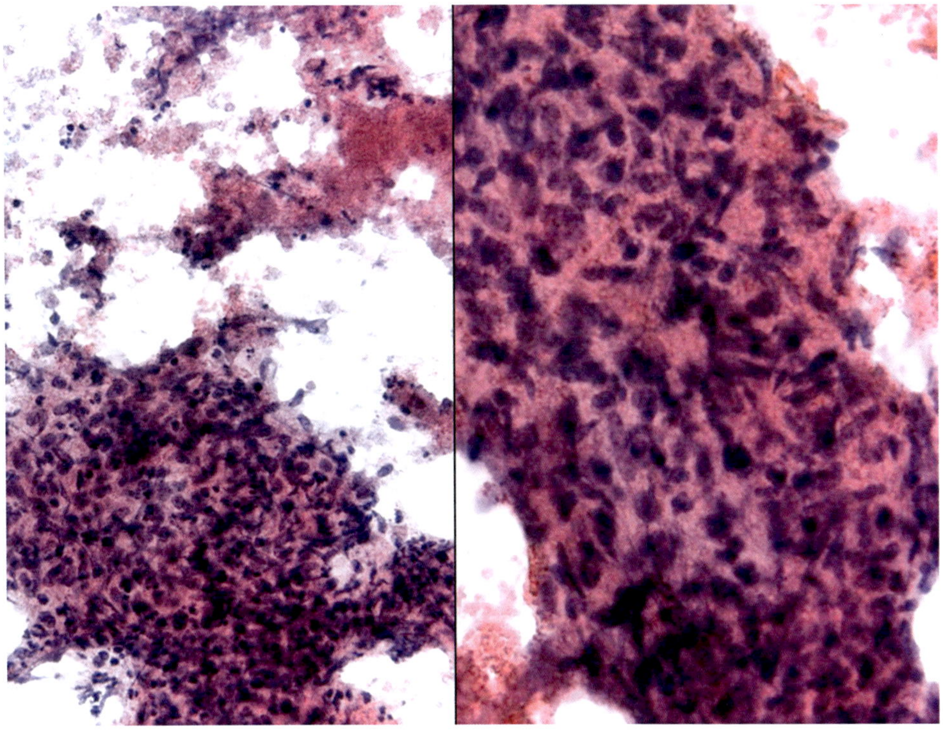

Q-8. The above findings are demonstrated during an on-site evaluation of a lymph node. The most appropriate next step is:

(a) Request additional material for cell blocks
(b) Request additional material for flow cytometry
(c) Request additional material for molecular studies
(d) Request additional material for culture
(e) Request additional material for research

Fig. 5.9

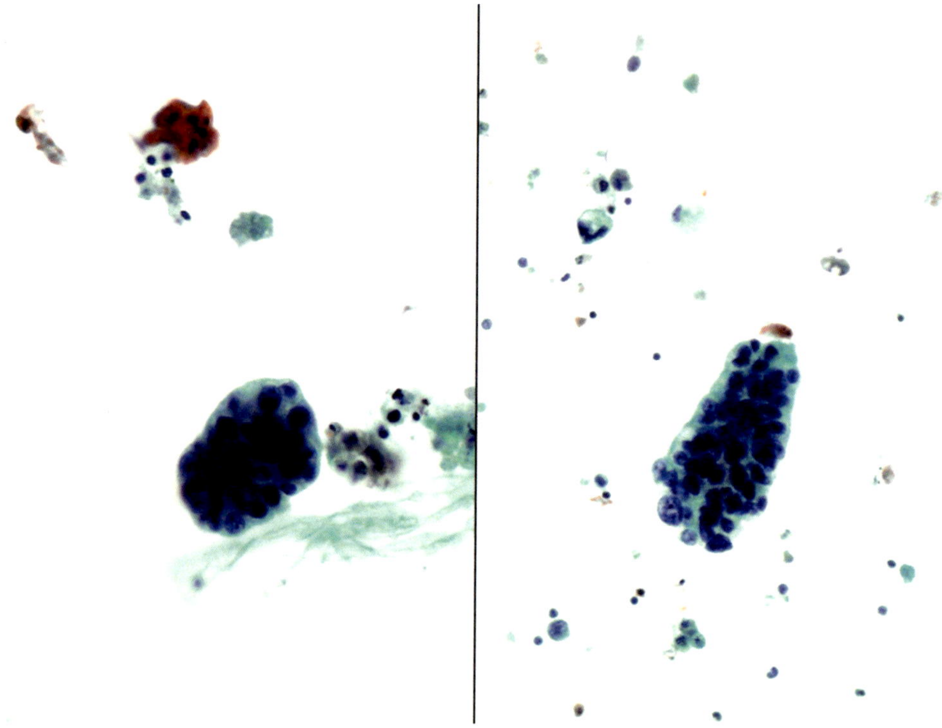

Q-9. A 57-year-old female presents with an enlarged paraesophageal lymph node demonstrating the above findings. The most likely diagnosis is:

(a) Adenocarcinoma
(b) Squamous cell carcinoma
(c) Glomus cell tumor
(d) Small cell carcinoma
(e) Adenosquamous carcinoma

Figs. 5.10 and 5.11

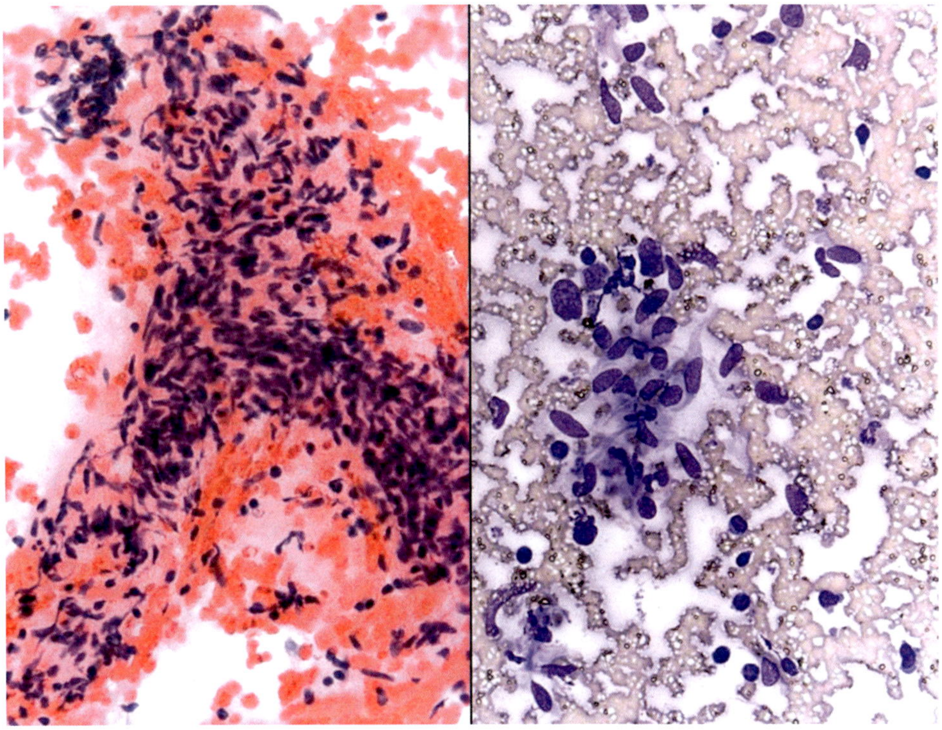

Q-10. A 27-year-old male with history of HIV/AIDS presents with an enlarged right supraclavicular lymph node. A FNA of the lymph node is pictured. What is the best confirmatory stain?

(a) HTLV-1
(b) HCV
(c) CMV
(d) EBV
(e) HHV-8

Q-11. In the previously described case, the differential diagnosis includes all of the following except:

(a) Angiosarcoma
(b) Reactive lymphadenopathy
(c) Melanoma
(d) Hemangioma
(e) Intranodal myofibroblastoma

Figs. 5.12 and 5.13

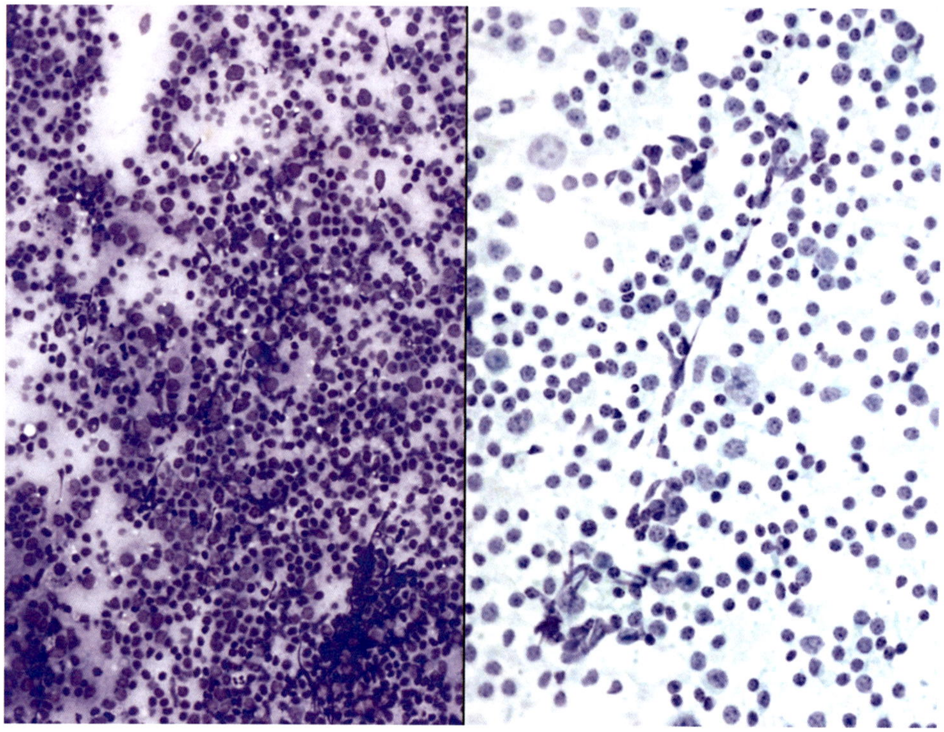

Q-12. A 22-year-old male with a history of malaise, mild fevers, and occasional headaches presents with several enlarged lymph nodes. Based on the image, the most likely diagnosis is:

(a) Reactive viral lymphadenopathy
(b) Toxoplasmosis
(c) Castleman disease
(d) Tuberculosis lymphadenitis
(e) Cat scratch disease

Q-13. The most useful finding to substantiate the diagnosis in the previous image is:

(a) Necrosis
(b) Granuloma
(c) Plasma cell proliferation
(d) Infiltrating neutrophils
(e) Mixed inflammatory response

Figs. 5.14 and 5.15

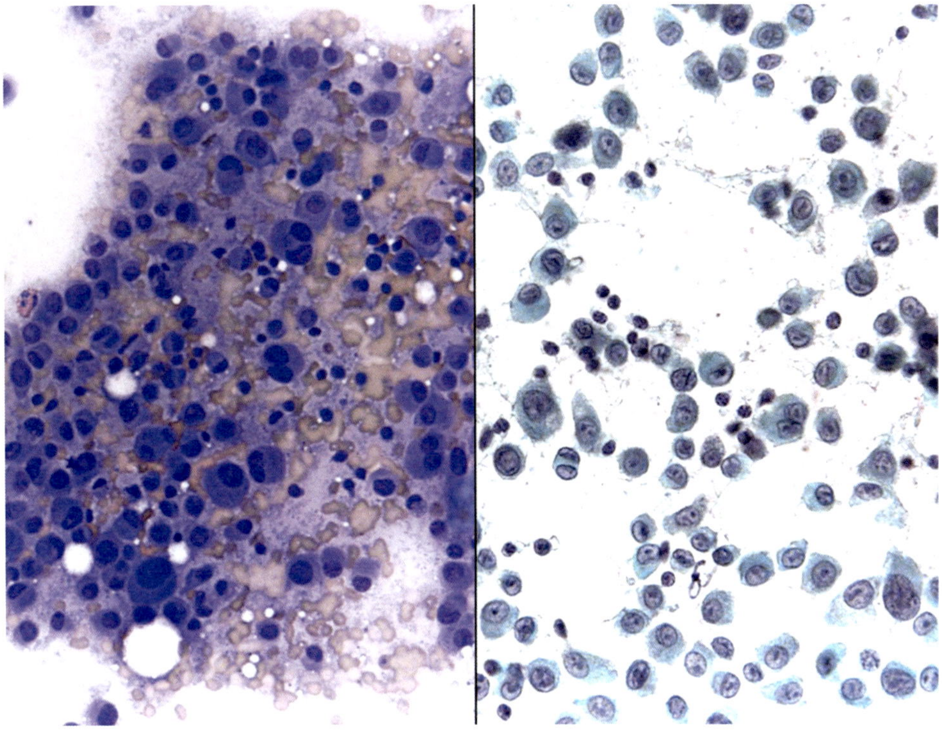

Q-14. A 53-year-old male presents with an enlarged axillary lymph node. Based on the above image, the stain most likely to confirm the diagnosis is:
(a) CD138
(b) LCA
(c) Cytokeratin 7
(d) Melan-A
(e) Cytokeratin 20

Q-15. The previous image demonstrates a proliferation of large, atypical cells with scattered melanin pigment. The cell demonstrates a plasmacytoid morphology and occasional binucleation. The differential diagnosis includes all of the following except:
(a) Multiple myeloma
(b) Hodgkin lymphoma
(c) Metastatic melanoma
(d) Diffuse large B-cell lymphoma
(e) Small cell carcinoma

Fig. 5.16

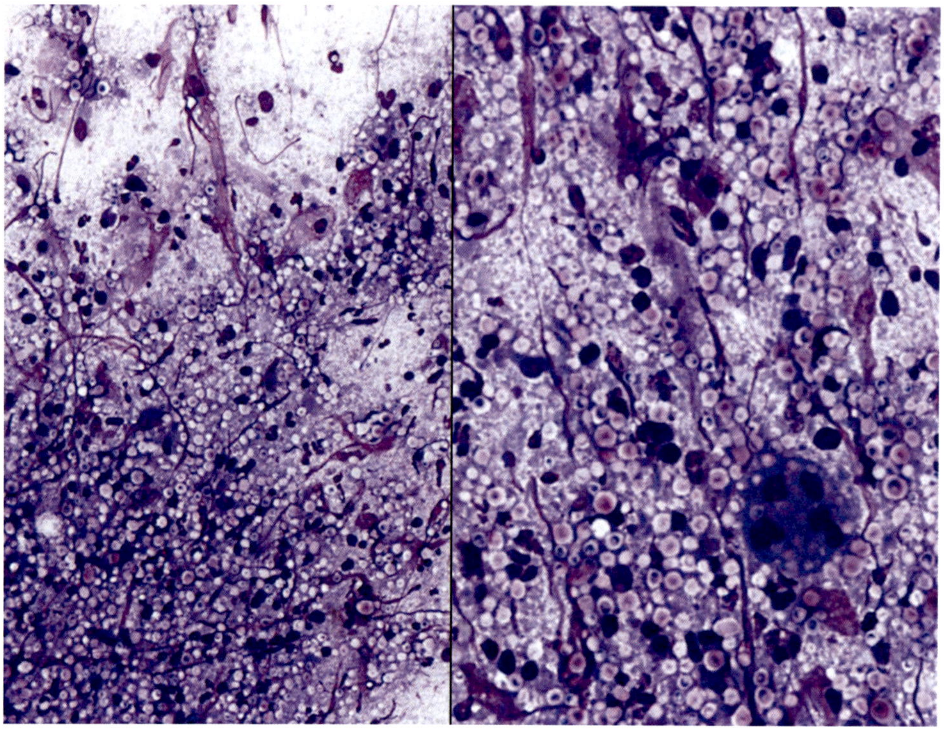

Q-16. An immunocompromised patient presents with lymphadenopathy and the pictured findings. The most likely diagnosis is:

(a) Reactive lymphadenopathy
(b) *Cryptococcus neoformans*
(c) Trypanosoma cruzi
(d) Leishmaniasis
(e) Fat emboli

Fig. 5.17

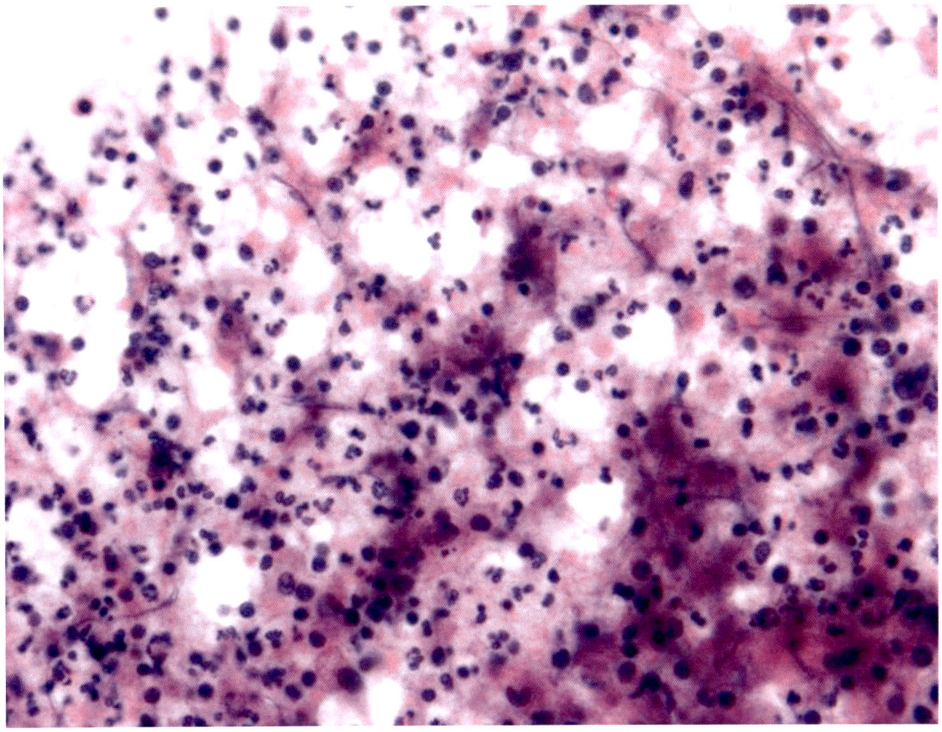

Q-17. This is the lymph node FNA from a 7-year-old girl with an enlarged neck lymph node. What is the best preliminary diagnosis and triage of the specimen?

(a) Suspicious for lymphoma; collect material for flow cytometry.
(b) Suspicious for leukemia; collect material for flow cytometry.
(c) Small round blue cell tumor; collect material for cell block and immunostains.
(d) Acute suppurative lymphadenitis; collect material for microbial cultures.
(e) Process additional material for cell block.

Fig. 5.18

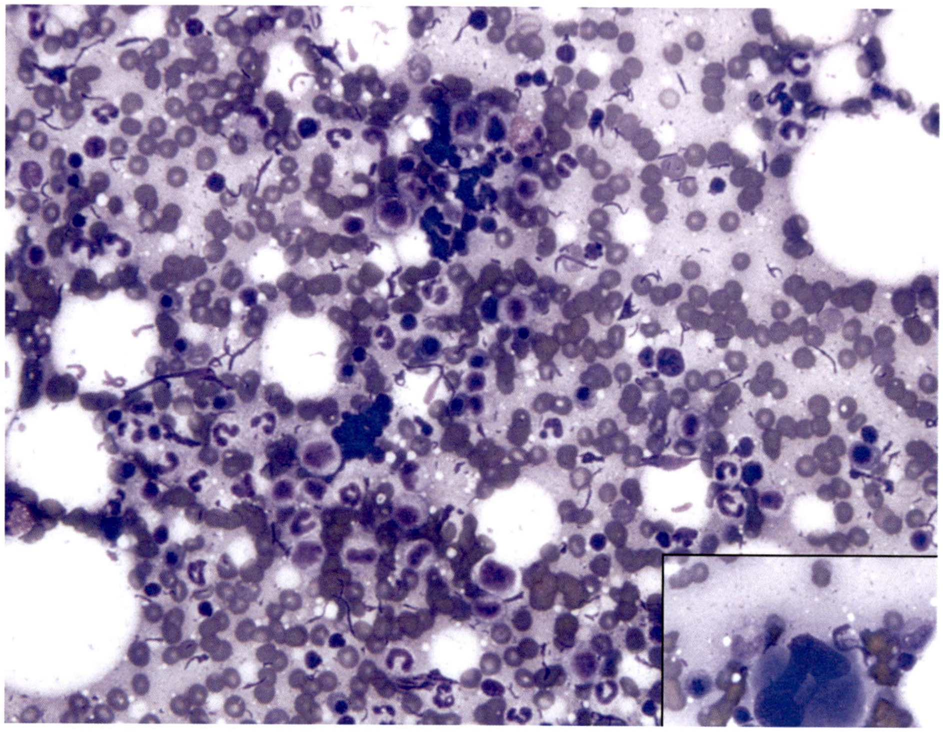

Q-18. A 42-year-old female with a retroperitoneal mass undergoes an FNA. The mass demonstrates adipocytes with bone marrow hematopoietic elements including erythrocytes and megakaryocytes. Which of the following is true regarding myelolipomas?

(a) HMB45 positive
(b) HMB45 negative
(c) Are small in size
(d) Are not incidental findings
(e) Are common

Fig. 5.19

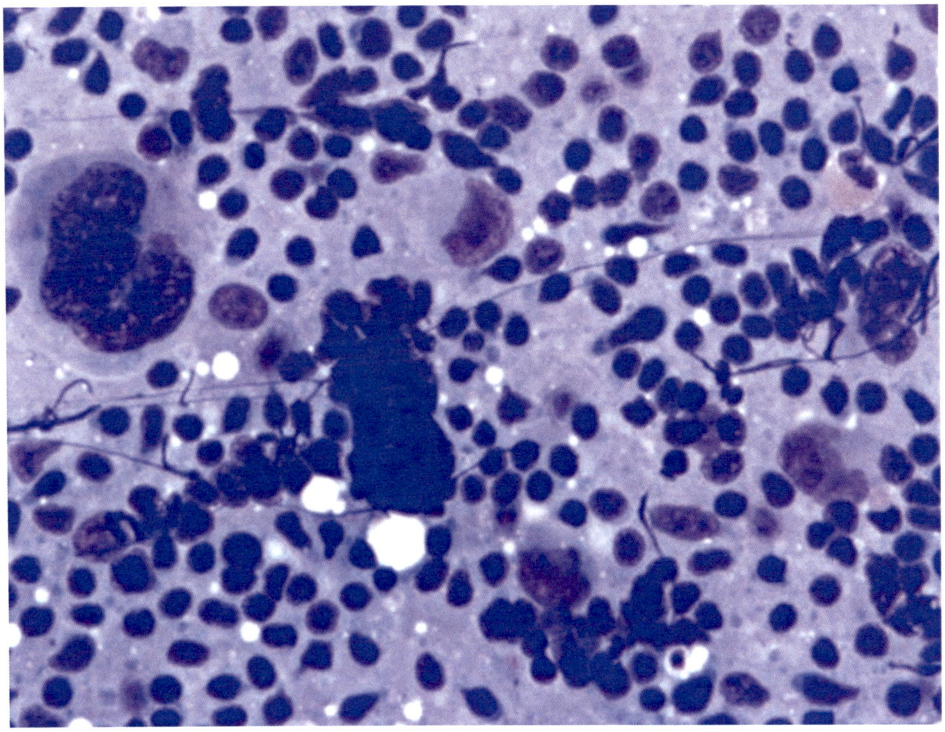

Q-19. A 39-year-old male undergoes a biopsy of a persistently enlarged cervical lymph node. The FNA demonstrates mixed inflammation with rare large, irregular cells with binucleation and prominent nuclei. Which of the following is true regarding classical Hodgkin lymphoma?

(a) It is usually CD30−, CD15−.
(b) CD45 is usually positive.
(c) Sclerosis is uncommon.
(d) EBV stains LMP-1 in Reed-Sternberg cells.
(e) It typically presents in young children.

Fig. 5.20

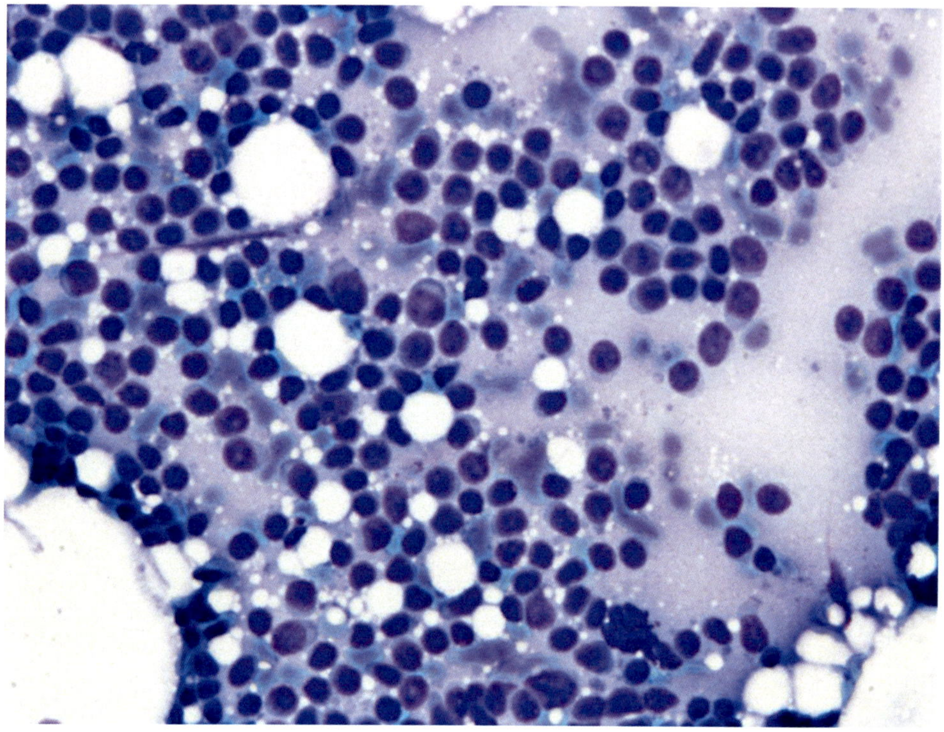

Q-20. An FNA of an enlarged lymph node is performed. The neoplasm consists of small lymphocytes with mature chromatin and minimal cytoplasm. Immunohistochemical stains demonstrate CD5 and CD23 positivity. Which of the following morphological features would not be consistent with the diagnosis?

(a) Clumped chromatin
(b) Plasmacytoid appearance
(c) Increased prolymphocytes
(d) Prominent nucleoli
(e) Minimal cytoplasm

Fig. 5.21

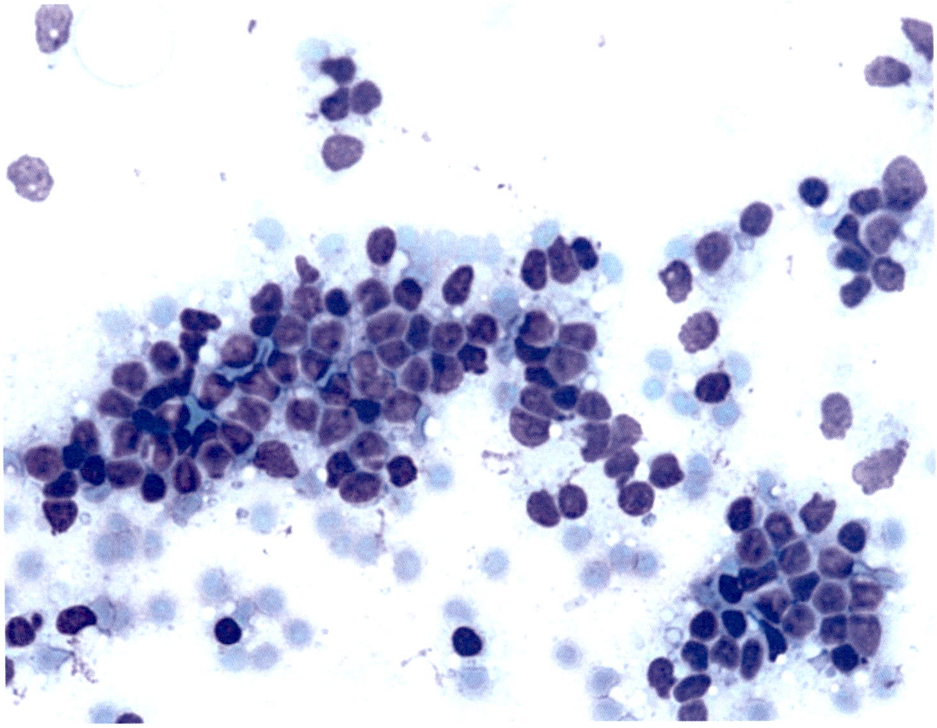

Q-21. The above FNA demonstrates a proliferation of small to medium-sized lymphoid cells with mature chromatin with a suggestion of clustering. Immunohistochemical stains in the suspicious cells are positive for CD10, Bcl-2, and Bcl-6. They are negative for CD5. Which of the following is true regarding follicular lymphoma?

(a) The translocation pattern genes are Bcl-6 and Bcl-2.
(b) Grading is based on the number of centroblasts.
(c) It is the second most common small cell lymphoma.
(d) Ki-67 proliferation index does not help in grading.
(e) Nuclear irregularities are uncommon.

Fig. 5.22

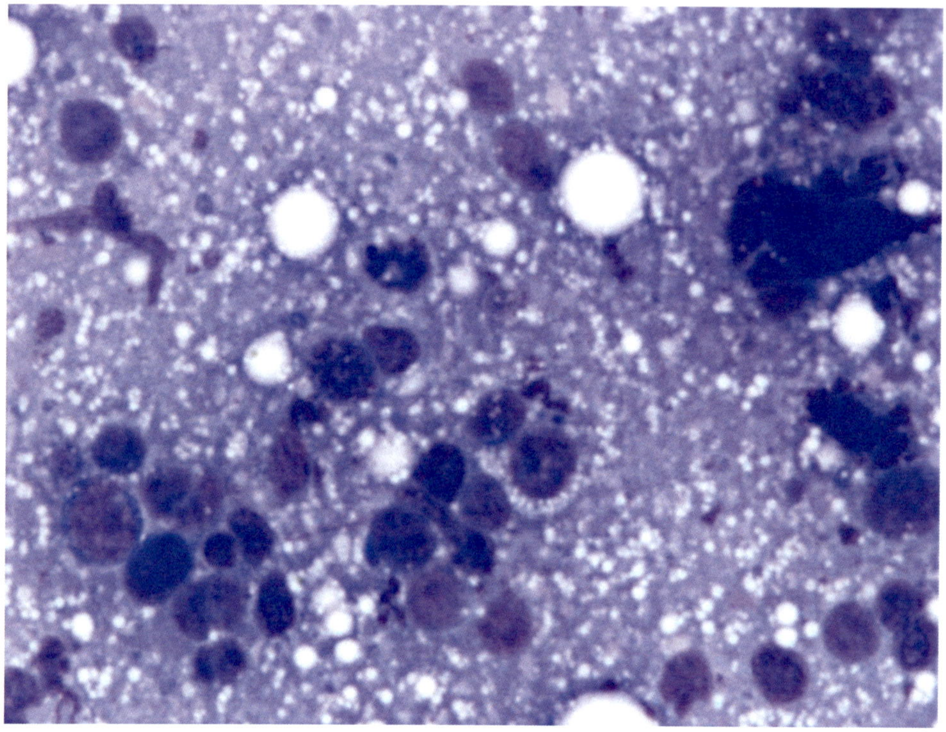

Q-22. A 7-year-old male presents with a rapidly enlarging mandibular lesion demonstrated in the following image composed of medium to large cells with smooth chromatin and multiple conspicuous nucleoli. There are occasional cytoplasmic vacuoles. The cells demonstrate a t(8;14) translocation. The most likely diagnosis is:

(a) Follicular lymphoma
(b) Anaplastic large cell lymphoma
(c) Burkitt lymphoma
(d) Blastic plasmacytoid dendritic cell neoplasm
(e) Multiple myeloma

Fig. 5.23

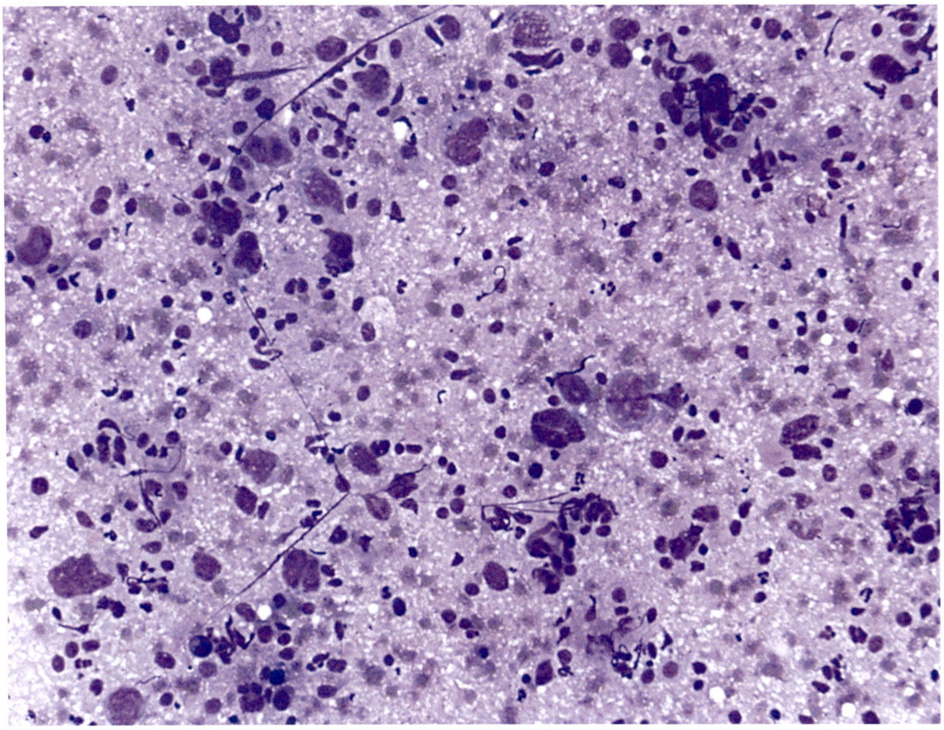

Q-23. An FNA of an axillary neoplasm demonstrates the following image consisting of large cells with large atypical nuclei occasionally in hallmark or donut shapes. The neoplastic cells are positive for CD30 and ALK and negative for CD15. Which of the following is true regarding the proliferation?

(a) ALK positivity confers a better prognosis.
(b) It is associated with EBV.
(c) Characteristic cells have prominent red nucleoli with binucleation.
(d) The t(2:5) translocation partners are ALK and Bcl-2.
(e) It typically presents in elderly.

Figs. 5.24 and 5.25

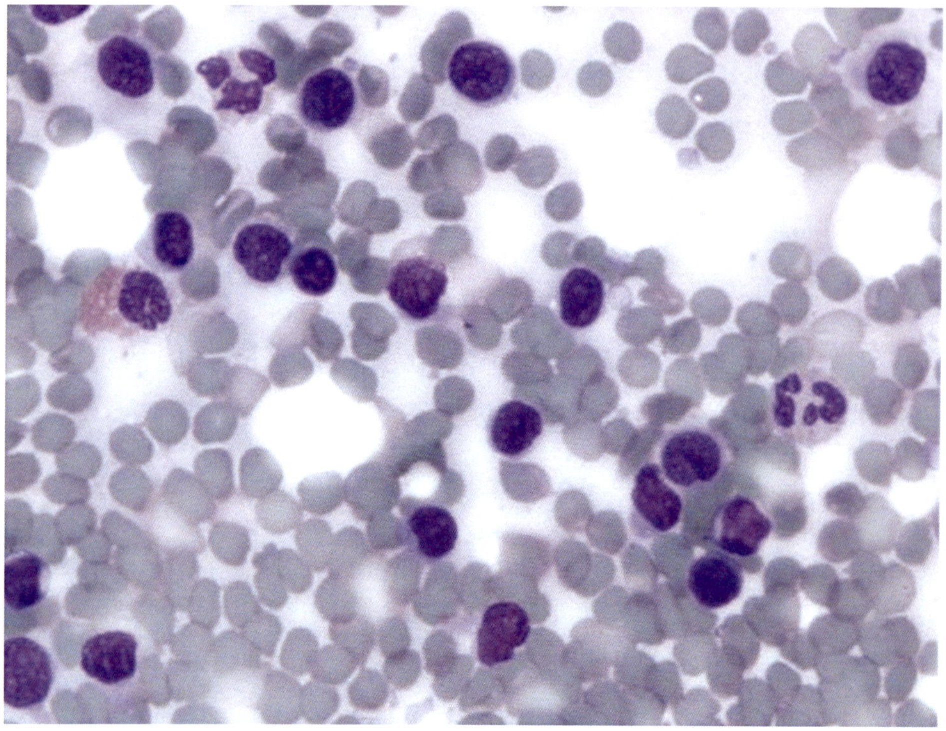

Q-24. A 56-year-old man presents with a localized rash with skin thickening and generalized lymphadenopathy. A fine-needle aspiration of an inguinal lymph node demonstrates a discohesive population of intermediate size cells with prominent pleomorphism including nuclear contour irregularities, prominent nucleoli, and variable chromatin patterns. The cells of interest are positive for CD2 and CD7 and negative for CD20. A biopsy of the skin lesion will most likely demonstrate:

(a) Lichen sclerosis
(b) Mycosis fungoides
(c) Actinic keratosis
(d) Folliculitis
(e) Dermatofibrosarcoma protuberans

Q-25. Based on the previous image and findings, the cells of interest are mostly likely:

(a) CD4+/CD8+/CD34−
(b) CD4+/CD8−/CD34−
(c) CD4−/CD8−/CD34−
(d) CD4+/CD8+/CD34+
(e) CD4+/CD8−/CD34+

Fig. 5.26

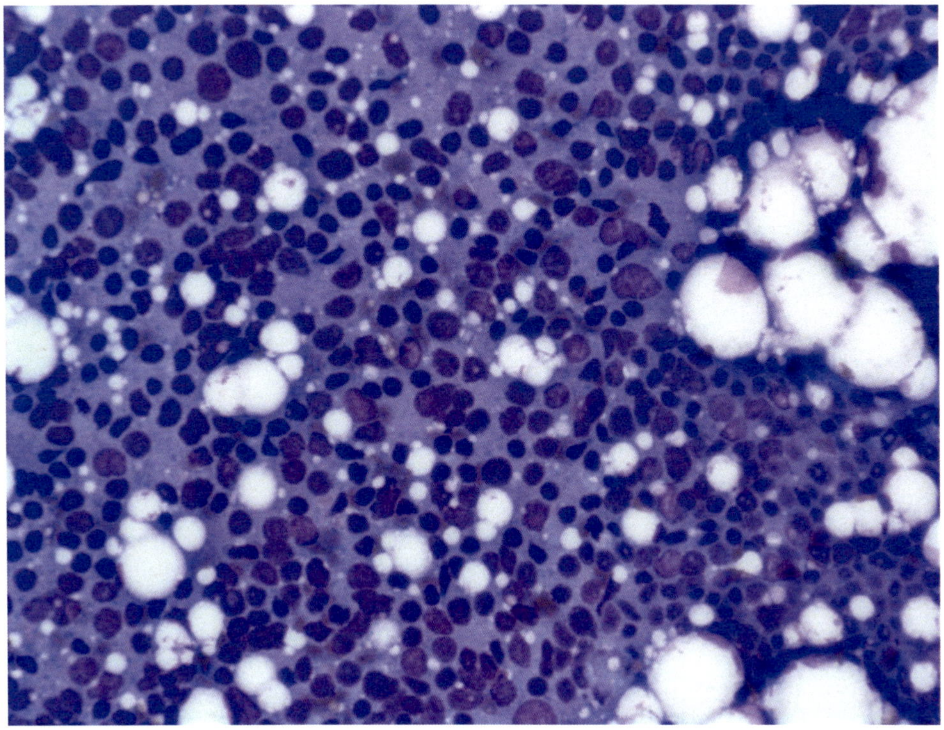

Q-26. An FNA of an enlarged lymph node demonstrates the pictured findings including a proliferation of small to medium cells, with mild nuclear pleomorphism and irregularity, inconspicuous nucleoli, and minimal cytoplasm. The cells are positive for CD20, CD5, and Bcl-2 and negative for CD10 and CD23. Which is true regarding Mantle cell lymphoma?

(a) It rarely demonstrates a t(11;14) translocation.
(b) The blastoid variant is usually cyclin D1 negative.
(c) Cyclin D1 is specific to mantle cell lymphoma.
(d) The cells are usually intermediate to large.
(e) Bcl-1 is usually positive.

Figs. 5.27 and 5.28

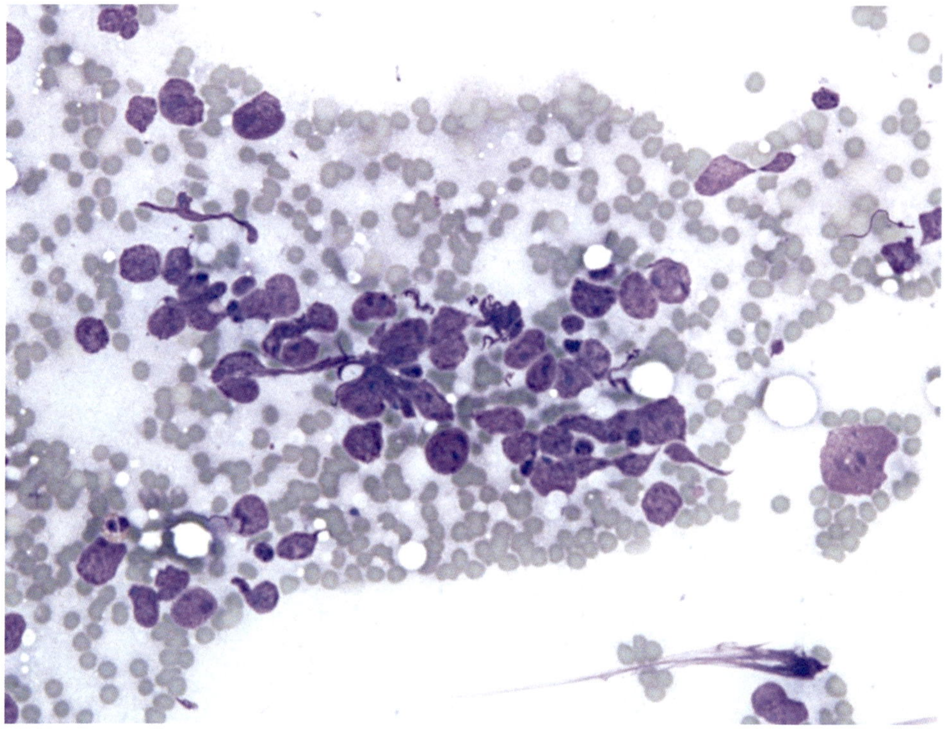

Q-27. An FNA of an enlarged lymph node is pictured above and demonstrates a proliferation of large cells with extremely irregular nuclear contours and increased nuclear to cytoplasmic ratios. The cells are discohesive but focally clustered. There are prominent nucleoli and scattered lymphoglandular bodies are present. Which is true regarding diffuse large B-cell lymphoma?

(a) Germinal center phenotype has a worse prognosis.
(b) Germinal center phenotype has a better prognosis.
(c) CD10 negativity is considered specific for non-germinal center type.
(d) Non-germinal center phenotype has a better prognosis.
(e) FOXP1 is not useful for determining germinal center type.

Q-28. If the cells in the previous FNA demonstrated CD5 positivity, what would be the most appropriate subsequent immunohistochemical stain to order?

(a) CD20
(b) CD138
(c) TdT
(d) Cyclin D1
(e) Ki-67

Fig. 5.29

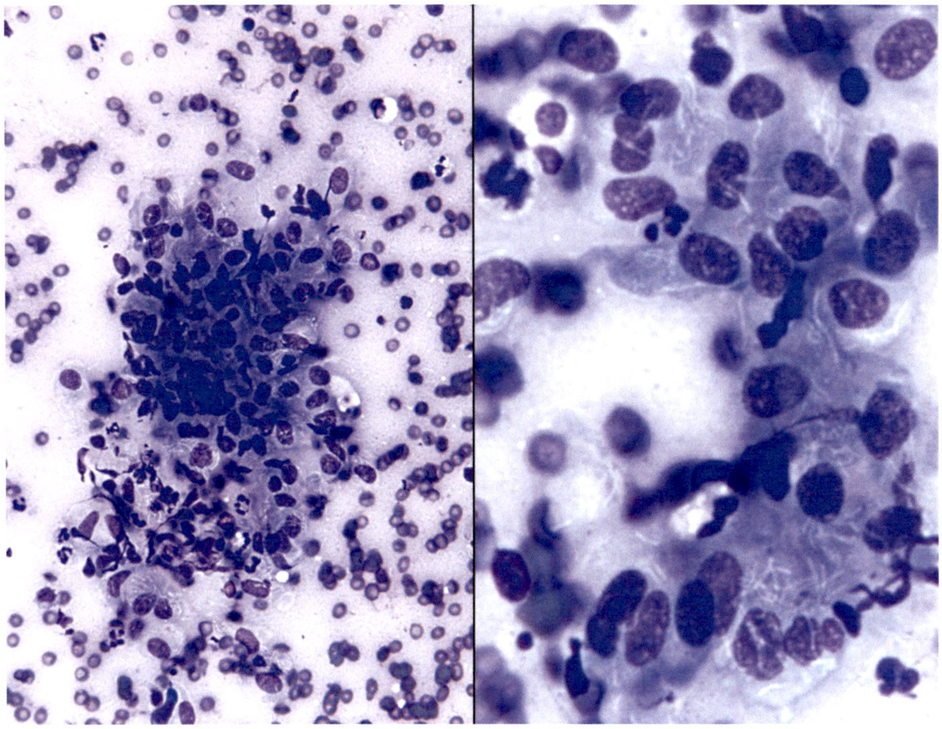

Q-29. What is the most appropriate additional ancillary test after flow cytometry for the above sample?
(a) Culture
(b) Acid-fast stain
(c) Cytochemical stains
(d) Cut levels on the cell block
(e) Viral PCR on the specimen

Figs. 5.30 and 5.31

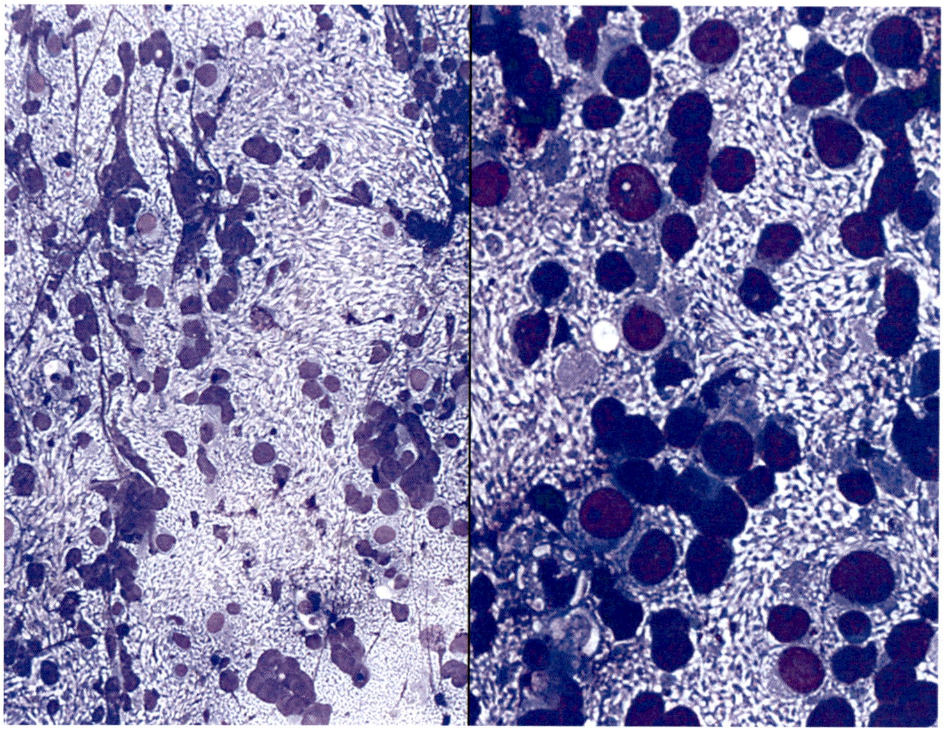

Q-30. The pictured findings are most consistent with which diagnosis?
(a) Diffuse large B-cell lymphoma
(b) Seminoma
(c) Reactive lymphadenopathy
(d) Sarcoidosis
(e) Metastatic melanoma

Q-31. The differential diagnosis of the above lesion includes all of the following except:
(a) Metastatic melanoma
(b) Metastatic squamous cell carcinoma
(c) Poorly differentiated small cell carcinoma
(d) Anaplastic large cell lymphoma
(e) Metastatic prostate carcinoma

Fig. 5.32

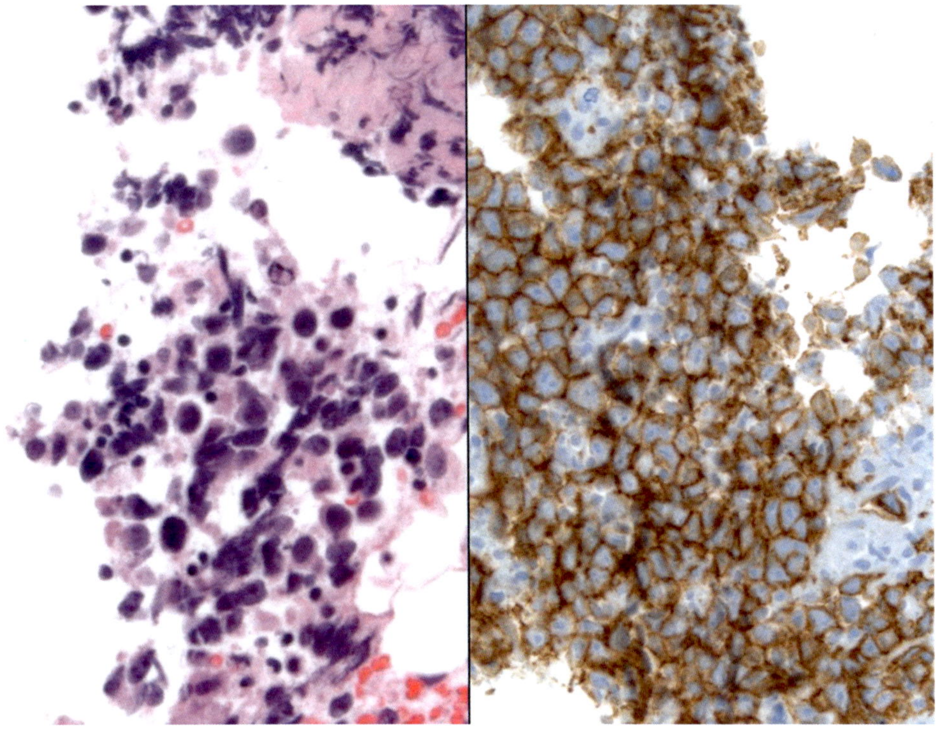

Q-32. These images of cell block and immunostain of c-Kit corresponding to case seen in Q-30. Which of the following stains is most likely to confirm the above diagnosis?
(a) PLAP
(b) Melan-A
(c) Congo red
(d) Grocott
(e) CK 20

Fig. 5.33

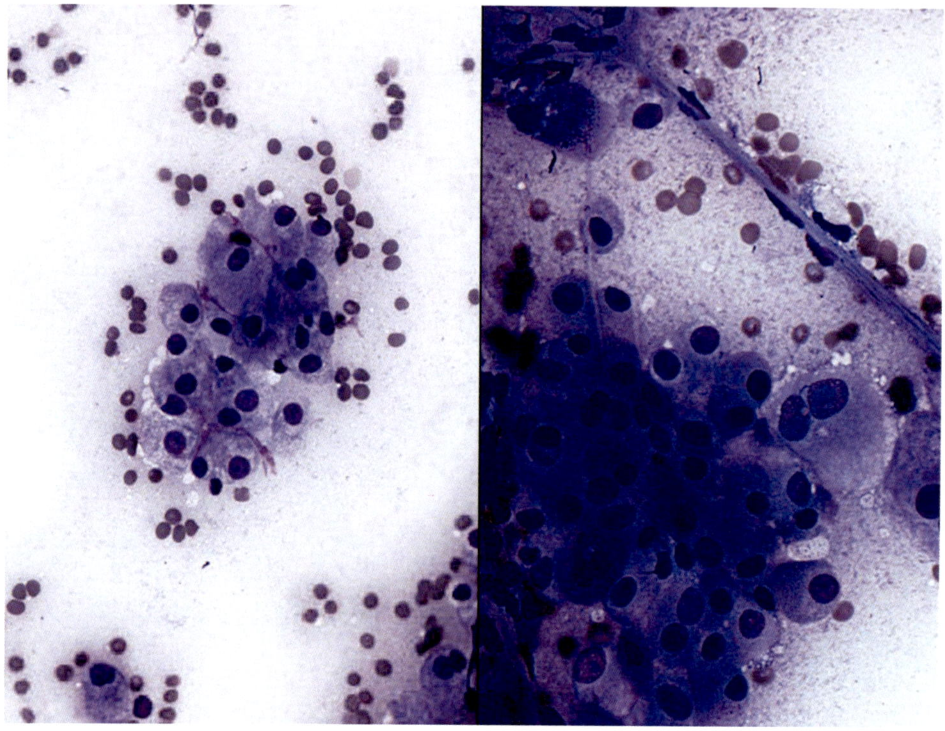

Q-33. A 65-year-old female with a history of a renal mass undergoes an FNA of an axillary lymph node. Which of the following is the most likely diagnosis?
(a) Metastatic renal cell carcinoma
(b) Metastatic thyroid carcinoma
(c) Metastatic ovarian carcinoma
(d) Plasma cell neoplasm
(e) Metastatic liposarcoma

Fig. 5.34

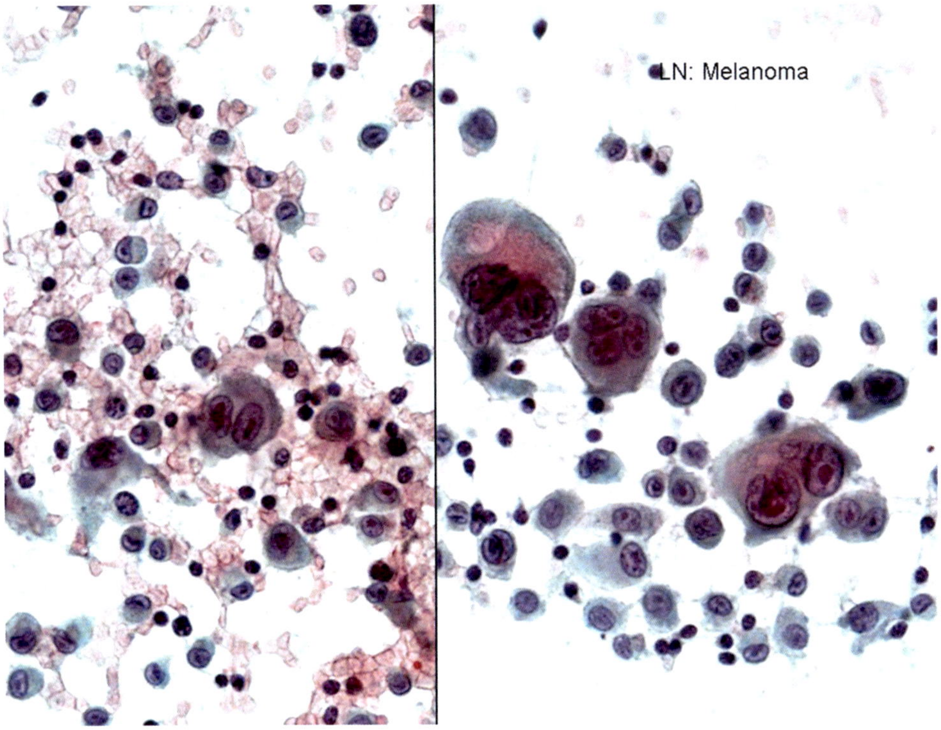

Q-34. The images depict a predominant of single large markedly pleomorphic plasmacytoid cells with giant nucleoli. Which is the most likely diagnosis of this case?

(a) Plasmacytoma
(b) Kimura disease
(c) Non-Hodgkin lymphoma (NHL)
(d) Metastatic melanoma
(e) Giant cell tumor of bone

5.2 Text-Based Questions 35–101

Q-35. Which of the following is true regarding sarcoidosis?
(a) It typically presents in a single organ system.
(b) Asteroid bodies are more common than Schaumann bodies.
(c) Hamazaki-Wesenberg bodies may mimic fungi.
(d) Granulomas are typically necrotizing.
(e) Infectious etiologies do not need to be ruled out.

Q-36. Which of the following is true regarding Mycobacterium avium infections?
(a) It is the second most common infections in patient with AIDS.
(b) It rarely presents with granulomas.
(c) Negative images of rod-shaped organisms are not seen.
(d) Using auramine O does highlight the organism.
(e) Positive acid-fast staining is specific to mycobacterium.

Q-37. Which of the following is false regarding the t(2;5) translocation in lymphoma cases?
(a) It is present in many anaplastic large cell lymphomas.
(b) The translocation partner genes are ALK and PMN.
(c) It is seen in other neoplasms.
(d) It is present in primary cutaneous ALCL.
(e) It is the most frequent, but not the sole translocation seen in ALCL.

Q-38. Which of the following is true regarding Burkitt lymphoma?
(a) The most common translocation is t(2;8).
(b) The cells are positive for CD20, CD23, and Bcl-2.
(c) The Ki-67 proliferation index is low.
(d) It affects immunocompromised patients.
(e) It most commonly involves the orbit.

Q-39. Hematolymphoid malignancies are the #1 cause of malignant effusions in which patient population?
(a) Older men (age 60+)
(b) Older women (age 60+)
(c) Middle-age women
(d) Middle-age men
(e) Children/adolescents

Q-40. The most helpful morphologic feature to support reactive lymphoid hyperplasia (and exclude lymphoma) is which of the following?
(a) Germinal center cells
(b) Lymphoglandular bodies
(c) Plasma cells
(d) Histiocytes
(e) Heterogeneity of the lymphoid population

Q-41. Which of the following *cannot* be reliably distinguished from reactive lymphoid hyperplasia by FNA?
(a) Castleman disease
(b) Dermatopathic lymphadenopathy
(c) HIV-associated lymphadenopathy
(d) Toxoplasma lymphadenitis
(e) All of the above

Q-42. Lymphomas in patients receiving rituximab-containing chemotherapy are most likely to lose which marker?
(a) CD19
(b) CD20
(c) CD38
(d) CD10
(e) CD23

Q-43. A 28-year-old man with a history of AIDS presents for FNA with new-onset cervical lymphadenopathy. The most likely diagnosis is:
(a) Reactive lymphoid hyperplasia
(b) Kaposi sarcoma
(c) Tuberculosis
(d) *Cryptococcus neoformans*
(e) Non-Hodgkin lymphoma

Q-44. An FNA specimen demonstrates multiple acid-fast bacilli staining positive for the Ziehl-Neelsen technique intermixed with a mixed population of lymphocytes and histiocytes including foamy multinucleated cells with perinuclear vesicles. The most likely etiologic agent is;
(a) Tuberculosis
(b) Lepra bacilli
(c) Cat scratch disease
(d) Suppurative lymphadenitis
(e) Actinomyces

Q-45. An FNA of a lymph node from a 7-year-old male who was scratched by a cat demonstrates suppurative lymphadenitis including stellate microabscesses. The best method to confirm the diagnosis is:
(a) Special silver stains
(b) Immunohistochemistry on the cell block
(c) Cultures
(d) Papanicolaou stain alone
(e) Molecular testing

Q-46. A 25-year-old, Asian, male with an enlarged right cervical lymph node undergoes an FNA which demonstrates abundant karyorrhexis, small to medium histiocytes with irregular, angulated nuclear contours, abundant cytoplasmic debris, and plasmacytoid monocytes. The most appropriate therapeutic intervention is:
(a) Lymph node biopsy
(b) Lymph node excision
(c) Neck dissection
(d) Watch and wait
(e) Antibiotics

Q-47. Flow cytometry performed on a lymph node FNA demonstrates an atypical population of CD19+, CD5+, CD23+, kappa-restricted lymphocytes. Which chromosomal abnormality portends a more aggressive phenotype?
(a) 13q14 deletion
(b) 17p deletion
(c) 17q addition
(d) Trisomy 12
(e) 11p deletion

Q-48. A 42-year-old male recently returned from Brazil and presented with lymphadenopathy. A FNA demonstrates lymphocytes with admixed histiocytes containing cytoplasm expanded by small round cells with large nuclei, thin membranes, and small rod-shaped structures. The most likely diagnosis is:
(a) Histoplasmosis
(b) Leishmaniasis
(c) Toxoplasmosis
(d) Acute promyelocytic leukemia
(e) Plasmodium vivax malaria

Q-49. A 12-year-old male presents with fevers, night sweats, and malaise. An FNA of a lymph node is performed which demonstrates abundant small lymphocytes and large histiocytes with abundant cytoplasm containing occasional lymphocytes. The most likely diagnosis is:
(a) Leishmaniasis
(b) Acute myelocytic leukemia
(c) Reactive lymphoid hyperplasia
(d) Rosai-Dorfman disease
(e) Kikuchi lymphadenitis

Q-50. A FNA of a cervical lymph node demonstrates a mixed population of lymphocytes admixed with a minority population of large cell with irregular multilobated nuclei. Immunohistochemical stains are positive for CD20, EMA, and CD45 and negative for CD30 and CD15. The most likely diagnosis is:
(a) Nodular-sclerosing Hodgkin lymphoma
(b) Lymphocyte-depleted Hodgkin lymphoma
(c) Nodular lymphocyte-predominant Hodgkin lymphoma
(d) Lymphocyte-rich Hodgkin lymphoma
(e) Mixed-cellularity Hodgkin lymphoma

Q-51. The most common variant of Hodgkin lymphoma in developing countries is:
(a) Nodular sclerosing
(b) Lymphocyte depleted
(c) Nodular lymphocyte predominant
(d) Lymphocyte predominant
(e) Mixed cellularity

Q-52. A lymph node FNA demonstrates a proliferation of mixed sized lymphocytes positive for CD19, CD20, CD10, Bcl-6, and Bcl-2. The atypical cells are negative for CD5. The most likely molecular finding is:
(a) t(14;18)
(b) t(11;14)
(c) t(8;22)
(d) t(2;5)
(e) t(x;18)

Q-53. Which small cell lymphoma generally lacks transformed lymphocytes?
(a) Mantle cell lymphoma
(b) CLL/SLL
(c) Follicular lymphoma
(d) Hodgkin lymphoma
(e) Anaplastic large cell lymphoma

Q-54. A lymph node FNA demonstrates a predominant population of small lymphocytes including a dominant population of centrocytes and few centroblasts. Immunohistochemical stains demonstrate a population of CD5 negative and CD20 and 10 positive cells. FISH studies are most likely to demonstrate which finding?
(a) t(14;18)(q32;q31)
(b) t(14;18)(p32;p31)
(c) t(14;18)(q32;p31)
(d) t(11;14)
(e) t(8;14)

Q-55. Mucosa-associated lymphoid tissue lymphoma is associated with which of the following:?
(a) Rheumatoid arthritis
(b) Pseudogout
(c) Helicobacter pylori chronic gastritis
(d) Ocular melanoma
(e) Chronic bronchiolitis

Q-56. Which type of Burkitt lymphoma is most likely to demonstrate Epstein-Barr virus positivity?
(a) None, EBV is not associated with Burkitt lymphoma.
(b) Endemic type.
(c) Immunodeficiency related.
(d) Sporadic.
(e) Diffuse T-cell predominant.

Q-57. A 43-year-old man with a history of AIDS presents with a rapidly enlarging inguinal lymph node. FNA of the lymph node demonstrated a proliferation of CD5−, CD10+, Bcl-6+, c-Myc positive, large B cells with extensive apoptosis and tingible body macrophages. The expected Ki-67 proliferation index is:
(a) 0 %
(b) 10 %
(c) 45 %
(d) 70 %
(e) 95 %

Q-58. Which of the following T-cell lymphomas is most likely to demonstrate a characteristic translocation?
(a) Precursor T-cell lymphoblastic lymphoma
(b) Anaplastic large cell lymphoma
(c) Angioimmunoblastic T-cell lymphoma
(d) Mycosis fungoides
(e) Extranodal NK/T-cell lymphoma, nasal type

Q-59. A child is diagnosed with precursor T-cell lymphoblastic lymphoma. Which of the following is true of the disease?
(a) Usually presents above the diaphragm.
(b) Is associated with superior vena cava thrombosis.
(c) Is easily distinguished immunophenotypically from thymoma.
(d) Smears rarely demonstrate lymphoblasts.
(e) TdT positivity is rarely demonstrated.

Q-60. Which virus is commonly associated with the development of post-transplant lymphoproliferative disorders (PTLD)?
(a) CMV
(b) HPV
(c) HTLV-1
(d) EBV
(e) HIV

Q-61. A useful finding that helps distinguish between recurrent lymphoma and PTLD is:
(a) Large, atypical cells
(b) Positive EBV immunohistochemical stains in a minority of cells
(c) High mitotic rate
(d) Lymphoglandular bodies
(e) Positive EBV immunohistochemical stains in a majority of cells

Q-62. Which neoplasm may demonstrate lymphoglandular bodies?
(a) Nasopharyngeal carcinoma
(b) Granular cell tumor
(c) Melanoma
(d) Ovarian papillary serous carcinoma
(e) Medullary carcinoma

Q-63. Anaplastic large cell lymphoma may be confused with carcinoma because of which of the following features?
(a) Many lymphoglandular bodies
(b) Discohesiveness
(c) EMA positivity
(d) Monomorphism
(e) Paucity of spindled cells

Q-64. Cluster designation 163 positivity is characteristic of which histiocytic neoplasm?
(a) Langerhans cell histiocytosis
(b) Langerhans cell sarcoma
(c) Histiocytic sarcoma
(d) Interdigitating dendritic cell sarcoma
(e) Follicular dendritic cell sarcoma

Q-65. A 43-year-old male presents with an enlarging axillary mass and recent allergic dermatitis. A fine-needle aspiration of the axillary mass demonstrates many CD1a positive grooved cells and scattered pigment laden macrophages. The most likely diagnosis is:
(a) Langerhans cell histiocytosis
(b) Dermatopathic lymphadenopathy
(c) Langerhans cell sarcoma
(d) Myeloid sarcoma
(e) Interdigitating dendritic cell sarcoma

Q-66. A FNA is performed on a perihilar lymph node and demonstrates a population of small to medium-sized cells with salt and pepper chromatin, nuclear molding, and some degeneration. The immunohistochemical stain most likely to be positive is:
(a) CD3
(b) CD20
(c) CD56
(d) Melanin
(e) Oct4

Q-67. A FNA of a left axillary lymph node demonstrates a proliferation of large cells with prominent nucleoli and occasional binucleated forms mixed with scattered small lymphocytes. There are scatted pigmented cells and necrotic debris. Immunohistochemical stains demonstrate S100, HMB45, and Melan-A positivity. The most appropriate molecular test is:
(a) KRAS
(b) BRAF
(c) BRD4-NUT
(d) t(2:5)
(e) t(14;18)

Q-68. A useful technique to improve adequacy in lymph node FNA is:
(a) A single pass at the periphery of the lesion
(b) Using a smaller gauge needle
(c) Applying anesthetic creams prior to the procedure
(d) Performing multiple passes in different locations
(e) Not stabilizing the lymph node prior to aspiration

Q-69. A monocytoid proliferation in a lymph node FNA suspicious for infectious mononucleosis is best confirmed by which method?
(a) Monospot test
(b) Clinical history
(c) Urine screen
(d) Breath test
(e) Molecular testing

Q-70. Which of the following morphologic features is most useful in identifying metastatic colorectal carcinoma?
(a) Intranuclear inclusions
(b) Signet ring cells
(c) Columnar cells and necrosis.
(d) Brown pigment
(e) Nuclear molding

Q-71. A 31-year-old female with a history of fevers underwent a FNA of an enlarged lymph node. A sample is sent for flow cytometric analysis. The generally accepted minimum number of events to ensure diagnostic accuracy is:
(a) 500 events
(b) 5,000 events
(c) 10,000 events
(d) 30,000 events
(e) 50,000 events

Q-72. Which of the following does not suffer from loss of important architectural changes for diagnosis on an FNA specimen?
(a) Progressively transformed germinal centers
(b) Castleman disease
(c) CLL/SLL
(d) Nodular lymphocyte-predominant Hodgkin lymphoma
(e) Vascular transformation of lymph node sinuses

Q-73. Which of the following is not part of the differential diagnosis for sarcoidosis?
(a) Melanoma
(b) Infection
(c) Foreign body reactions
(d) Dendritic lymphocyte aggregates
(e) Spindle-cell neoplasm

Q-74. Which of the following is not a feature of Kikuchi lymphadenitis?
(a) Necrotic debris
(b) Small phagocytic histiocytes
(c) Cytoplasmic tingible body macrophages
(d) Extensive neutrophilic infiltrate
(e) Absence of neutrophilic infiltrate

Q-75. Which of the following diagnoses are not in the differential diagnosis of infectious mononucleosis?
(a) Mantle cell lymphoma
(b) Reactive lymphoid hyperplasia
(c) Large cell lymphoma
(d) Hodgkin lymphoma
(e) Immunoblastic lymphoma

Q-76. Which of the following is not useful for differentiating anaplastic large cell lymphoma from classical Hodgkin lymphoma?
(a) Number of malignant cells relative to lymphocytes
(b) Morphology of the malignant cells
(c) Staining pattern of epithelial membrane antigens
(d) Molecular studies
(e) Staining pattern of ALK

Q-77. Which of the following small lymphomas is generally considered the most aggressive?
(a) CLL/SLL
(b) Lymphoplasmacytic
(c) Mantle cell lymphoma
(d) Marginal zone/mucosal-associated lymphoid tissue lymphoma
(e) Follicular lymphoma

Q-78. An 18-year-old male presents with a rapidly enlarging mandibular mass. A fine-needle aspiration demonstrates a starry-sky pattern of with extensive necrosis and composed of medium-sized lymphocytes with occasional vacuoles. The cells are positive for c-Myc. The most common translocation in these lymphomas is:
(a) t(8;14)
(b) t(2;5)
(c) t(2;8)
(d) t(8;22)
(e) t(9;22)

Q-79. The c-Myc proto-oncogene is located on which chromosome?
(a) 14
(b) 22
(c) 8
(d) 2
(e) 9

Q-80. In addition to Burkitt lymphoma, c-Myc rearrangement may also be seen in which neoplasm?
(a) Multiple myeloma
(b) CLL/SLL
(c) Mantle cell lymphoma
(d) Hodgkin lymphoma
(e) Castleman disease

Q-81. All of the following may mimic Bartonella lymphadenitis except:
(a) *Chlamydia trachomatis*
(b) *Yersinia enterocolitica*
(c) *Francisella tularensis*
(d) Pyogenic cocci
(e) Epstein-Barr virus

Q-82. Which of the following is true regarding T-cell lymphoblastic lymphoma?
(a) Most frequent in elderly males
(b) Usually present with low leukocyte count
(c) Comprise the majority of lymphoblastic lymphomas
(d) Never present in mediastinum
(e) Generally grow slowly

Q-83. A 47-year-old female presents with an enlarged axillary lymph node and a history of malaise and fevers. A fine-needle aspiration demonstrates small lymphocytes and numerous, irregular, cleaved lymphocytes with few tingible body macrophages. Immunohistochemical stains highlight the lymphocytes with CD10 and Bcl-6 and negative for CD5, CD23, and cyclin D1. Molecular studies for translocation 14;18 are positive. Which of the following diagnoses is most likely?
(a) Follicular lymphoma
(b) CLL/SLL
(c) MCL
(d) MZL
(e) DLBCL

Q-84. An enlarged neck mass in a patient with a history of a thigh mass undergoes a FNA. The FNA demonstrates large cells with eosinophilic cytoplasm, eccentric nuclei, and scattered mitoses in a background of unremarkable small lymphocytes. The stains most likely to confirm the diagnosis are:
(a) Desmin, myogenin, CD138, and SMA
(b) CD138, wide-spectrum cytokeratin, CD5, CD45
(c) HMB45, SMA, Melan-A, wide-spectrum cytokeratin
(d) CD99, vimentin, wide-spectrum cytokeratin
(e) PLAP, CA-125, WT-1

Q-85. Which molecular abnormality is most common in CLL/SLL?
(a) Trisomy 12
(b) del 11q22-23
(c) del 13q14.3
(d) del 17p13
(e) del 6q21

Q-86. A FNA of an enlarged pelvic lymph node demonstrates dispersed large cleaved and non-cleaved cells. There are irregular nuclear profiles with occasional nuclear protrusions. There are occasional cytoplasmic vacuoles and the cells are discohesive. The differential diagnosis includes all the following except:
(a) DLBCL
(b) Metastatic melanoma
(c) Small cell carcinoma
(d) Seminoma
(e) Pulmonary adenocarcinoma

Q-87. A specimen submitted for flow cytometric analysis suspicious for plasmacytoma is most likely to demonstrate which of the following immunophenotypic findings?
(a) Surface kappa restriction, normal lambda
(b) Surface lambda restriction, normal kappa

(c) Cytoplasmic kappa restriction, normal lambda
(d) Equal cytoplasmic kappa and lambda
(e) Negativity for surface and cytoplasmic kappa and lambda

Q-88. Which cell population is most fragile and least likely to be accurately characterized on a flow cytometry sample that has been excessively delayed?
(a) CD20-positive cells
(b) CD138-positive cells
(c) CD3-positive cells
(d) CD13-positive cells
(e) CD56 positive cells

Q-89. A patient presents with a gastric mass composed of a proliferation of lymphocytes consistent with a gastric mucosal-associated lymphoid tissue lymphoma. Special chemical stains highlight corkscrew-shaped organisms in the epithelium. What is the best next step in therapy?
(a) Start triple therapy.
(b) Gastric resection.
(c) Perform a breath urease test.
(d) Watch and wait.
(e) Perform an endoscopic mucosal resection.

Q-90. A patient with an enlarged spleen undergoes a perisplenic lymph node FNA. This demonstrates multiple medium lymphocytes with asymmetric cytoplasmic buds but lacking cytoplasmic clearing. Imaging of the spleen revealed diffuse enlargement. Which immunophenotype is consistent with splenic marginal zone lymphoma?
(a) CD103+, CD25+, CD23−
(b) CD20+, CD79+, CD38+
(c) CD20−, CD79+, CD138+
(d) CD5+, CD23+, CD43+
(e) CD5+, CD23−, CD10−

Q-91. Which immunophenotype is consistent with hairy cell leukemia?
(a) CD103+, CD25+, CD23−
(b) CD20+, CD79+, CD38+
(c) CD20−, CD79+, CD138+
(d) CD5+, CD23+, CD43+
(e) CD5+, CD23−, CD10−

Q-92. Fine-needle aspiration of lymphoma and metastases is least sensitive for which of the following?
(a) Non-Hodgkin lymphoma
(b) Hodgkin lymphoma
(c) Metastatic melanoma
(d) Infections
(e) Metastatic carcinoma

Q-93. Which of the following lymphomas is least likely in adults?
(a) Diffuse large B cell
(b) Small lymphocytic leukemia/chronic lymphocytic lymphoma
(c) Follicular lymphoma
(d) Endemic Burkitt lymphoma
(e) Anaplastic large cell lymphoma

Q-94. A FNA of an enlarge lymph node demonstrates grape bunch-like clusters of cells with minimal cytoplasm and composed of cells ranging in size from 25 to 150 um in diameter consistent with Warthin-Finkeldey cells. These are associated with all of the following except:
(a) Measles
(b) Systemic lupus erythematosus
(c) Kimura disease
(d) Hodgkin lymphoma
(e) Metastatic melanoma

Q-95. Which of the following is not associated with sinus histiocytosis?
(a) Exogenous lipids
(b) Rosai-Dorfman disease
(c) Kikuchi disease
(d) Whipple disease
(e) Hodgkin lymphoma

Q-96. A patient with a history of systemic lupus erythematosus undergoes a FNA that demonstrates medium-sized cells with bright pink eosinophilic, hyaline-appearing bodies along with intermixed plasma cells. The eosinophilic material is composed of which of the following?
(a) Denatured RNA and immunoglobulin
(b) Denatured DNA and immunoglobulin
(c) Immunoglobulin only
(d) Amyloid
(e) Calcium

Q-97. A 61-year-old man presents with an enlarged lymph node, bone pain, hypercalcemia, and a monoclonal gammopathy. A FNA of the lymph node demonstrates many plasma cells including occasional cells with strong metachromatic staining in the peripheral cytoplasm. The cells are referred to as which of the following?
(a) Dutcher bodies
(b) Flame cells

(c) Russell bodies
(d) Lymphoglandular bodies
(e) Mott cells

Q-98. Which of the following is true regarding pediatric nodal marginal zone lymphoma?
(a) It has a poor prognosis.
(b) It most commonly presents in the groin.
(c) It is predominantly in females.
(d) It has the same immunophenotype as in adults.
(e) It is easy to differentiate from reactive conditions.

Q-99. The most common mutation associated with ALK-positive large B-cell lymphoma is:
(a) t(2;5)(p23;35)
(b) t(2;17)(p23;q23)
(c) Cryptic insertion of 3'ALK into 4q22-24
(d) t(5;17)
(e) t(9;22)(q34;p11.2)

Q-100. Which of the following is the most common B-cell lymphoma in adults?
(a) Diffuse large B-cell lymphoma (DLBCL)
(b) Follicular lymphoma
(c) CLL/SLL
(d) Mantle cell lymphoma
(e) MALT lymphoma

Q-101. The most common mature T-cell lymphoma in adults is:
(a) Peripheral T-cell lymphoma NOS
(b) Angioimmunoblastic lymphoma
(c) Extranodal natural killer/T-cell lymphoma
(d) Hepatosplenic T-cell lymphoma
(e) ALK+ anaplastic large cell lymphoma

5.3 Answers and Discussion of Image-Based Questions 1–34

A-1. (**e**) **Metastatic papillary thyroid carcinoma** (**TTF1 and thyroglobulin**)
The FNA demonstrates cohesive clusters of cells with increased nuclear to cytoplasmic ratios and nuclear irregularities suggestive of a metastatic carcinoma. Psammoma bodies are also present. Given the age of the patient, the location of the lymph node, and the cytomorphology features, this is most suggestive of metastatic papillary thyroid carcinoma. To confirm thyroid carcinoma, a positive thyroglobulin and TTF1 would be most useful. TTF-1, while positive in papillary thyroid carcinoma, like AE1/AE3, may be positive in a variety of other carcinomas. Calretinin is primarily used to identify mesothelial cells and LCA "common leukocyte antigen" is used to highlight lymphocytes.

A-2. (**c**) **Metastatic mucinous adenocarcinoma**
The history of a colon mass combined with the FNA findings of abundant mucin with scattered clusters of large, atypical cells with prominent nucleoli and increased nuclear to cytoplasmic ratios is most likely metastatic mucinous adenocarcinoma. A reactive hyperplastic lymph node should not demonstrate any mucin. Metastatic melanoma, PTLD, and DLBCL typically do not have abundant mucin production.

A-3. (**b**) **t**(**14**;**18**)
The t(14;18) translocation is seen in follicular lymphoma. The FNA demonstrates a proliferation of small to medium lymphocytes, primarily small cleaved centrocytes with occasional larger centroblasts. Many cells demonstrate characteristic extensive nuclear contour irregularities. The chromatin is coarse and nucleoli are inconspicuous. Follicular cell lymphoma usually is CD20+, CD10+, CD5−, and CD23−.

A-4. (**c**) **Melan-A**
The above FNA demonstrates a moderately cellular smear with dusty cytoplasm. These cells are dispersed as single cells with occasional aggregates. They are epithelioid with occasional binucleation. The cells have finely dispersed chromatin and prominent nucleoli. These features are most compatible with metastatic melanoma. Melan-A, along with S100 and HMB45, is positive in melanoma. Melanoma is notorious for presenting in a variety of forms and mimicking many neoplasms. CD138 is positive in plasma cells, CK 5 in squamous cell carcinoma and other carcinomas, CD3 in T lymphocytes, and OCT3/4 in intratubular germ cell neoplasia.

A-5. (**a**) **Sarcoma**
The FNA demonstrates a proliferation of spindled cells with many bizarre forms and intermixed necrosis. The history of a previous retroperitoneal mass and the morphologic findings support the diagnosis of a metastatic sarcoma. Melanoma may present with spindled cells and can be difficult to differentiate from sarcoma; however, the clinical history is supportive of a sarcoma. A lymphoma will be predominantly lymphocytes. Carcinomas tend to form clusters and also demonstrate epithelioid morphology. Soft tissue infections may cause reactive changes in the mesenchymal cells, but, generally, not proliferations to the degree demonstrated in the FNA.

A-6. (**a**) **CD138 is positive in plasma cells**.
The image demonstrates a proliferation of plasma cells with eccentric nuclei, clockface chromatin, and perinuclear hoffs suggesting a diagnosis of multiple myeloma/plasmacytoma. CK 5 is a basic, high-molecular-weight cytokeratin typically positive in squamous cell carcinoma. Melan-A is positive in melanoma. CD3 is positive in T lymphocytes. OCT3/4 is positive in germ cell neoplasia.

A-7. (**a**) **WT-1 and calretinin**
The image demonstrates a proliferation of mesothelial cells with large nuclei and nuclear contour irregularities. The cells have areas of clearing between cytoplasmic borders known as windows and are characteristic of mesothelial cells. The distinction between reactive mesothelial cells and a malignant mesothelioma can be difficult. In addition, differentiating between an adenocarcinoma and mesothelioma is challenging. Immunohistochemical stains may be useful. Mesothelial cells are positive for WT-1 and calponin. Caldesmon is seen in soft tissue neoplasm. HMB45 is a marker for melanoma and angiomyolipomas. CD7 and mucicarmine positivity would be seen in an adenocarcinoma. CD10 and PAX8 positivity is seen in clear cell renal cell carcinoma. CD68 and CD168 highlight macrophages/histiocytes.

A-8. (**d**) **Request additional material for culture**.
The FNA demonstrates multinucleated giant cells with a background of mixed lymphoplasmacytic inflammation. The differential diagnosis would

include infection, sarcoidosis, foreign body reaction, and certain malignancies such as Hodgkin lymphoma and seminoma. Flow cytometry would not be particularly helpful for the possible malignancies in the differential diagnosis. Tissue for cell blocks may or may not be useful and is not as sensitive as culture for infectious etiologies. Tissue for molecular studies will not likely be helpful. Acquiring tissue for research purpose should be performed after adequate material for diagnosis is acquired.

A-9. (**e**) **Adenosquamous carcinoma**
The fine-needle aspiration demonstrates two populations of malignant cells in clusters. There are keratinized cells with dense cytoplasm, large nuclei, single cells with pleomorphism, and irregularly dispersed chromatin. In addition, there are clusters of large cells with cytoplasmic mucin, prominent nucleoli, round enlarged nuclei, and occasional cytoplasmic vacuoles. The findings of both features of adenocarcinoma and squamous cell carcinoma support a diagnosis of adenosquamous carcinoma. Glomus cell tumors usually behave in a benign manner and are found in the extremities and skin. Small cell carcinomas are usually less cohesive and composed of smaller cells frequently demonstrating molding.

A-10. (**e**) **HHV-8**
The FNA specimen demonstrates abundant atypical spindle cells and erythrocytes in a patient with a history of HIV/AIDS. These findings are most suggestive of Kaposi sarcoma. Kaposi sarcoma is related to infection with HHV-8 in patients with HIV/AIDS. HHV-8 immunohistochemical stains would confirm the diagnosis. HTLV-1 is the causative agent of adult T-cell lymphoma/leukemia, HCV is associated with hepatocellular carcinoma, and CMV is not associated with neoplasms but demonstrates characteristic nuclear and cytoplasmic inclusions. Finally, EBV is associated in varying degrees with the three types of Burkitt lymphoma, associated with many B-cell lymphomas in immunosuppressed individuals, extranodal NK/T-cell lymphoma, and two pediatric lymphomas but not Kaposi sarcoma.

A-11. (**b**) **Reactive lymphadenopathy**
The differential diagnosis for Kaposi sarcoma includes angiosarcoma, melanoma (spindle-cell type), hemangioma, and intranodal myofibroblastoma. All of these possible diagnoses may demonstrate proliferations of spindled cells or vessels that may mimic Kaposi sarcoma. Reactive lymphadenopathy presents with a mixed lymphocytic inflammatory pattern and spindled cell are uncommon.

A-12. (**a**) **Viral lymphadenopathy**
The image depicts a mixed inflammatory infiltrate including small lymphocytes, centrocytes, and a mixture of other mature lymphoid cells. A large collection of neutrophils or granulomas is lacking. The lack of neutrophils makes a diagnosis of toxoplasmosis or cat scratch disease unlikely. The lack of granulomas makes tuberculosis lymphadenitis unlikely. A diagnosis of Castleman disease on FNA typically cannot be made reliably.

A-13. (**e**) **Mixed inflammatory response**
The findings of necrosis, granulomas, predominantly plasma cell proliferation, or infiltrating neutrophils would suggest a diagnosis other than viral lymphadenopathy.

A-14. (**d**) **Melan-A**
The image depicts classic findings of metastatic melanoma including prominent nucleoli, binucleation, enlarged size and nuclear to cytoplasmic ratio, and black pigment. Melanoma will be positive for Melan-A. CD138 highlights plasma cells and LCA are positive in lymphoid cells, CK 7 in certain epithelial cells, and cytokeratin in certain epithelial cells.

A-15. (**c**) **Small cell carcinoma**
Small cell carcinoma typically presents as small cells, with minimal cytoplasm and occasional to abundant nuclear molding with characteristic chromatin. While melanoma is considered a frequent mimicker of a variety of neoplasms, when melanoma is the primary consideration for a neoplasm, it is important to consider other lesions that may demonstrate similar appearances and remember that the melanin pigment is not always present. The differential diagnosis for melanoma includes multiple myeloma (due to the plasmacytoid nature of some of the cells), Hodgkin lymphoma, and diffuse large B-cell lymphoma among others.

A-16. (**b**) ***Cryptococcus neoformans***
The FNA demonstrates a diffuse infiltrate of round yeast-like forms, which are variable in size with occasional indentations and demonstrate narrow-based budding. There is mild inflammation. These findings, in conjunction with the patient's immunocompromised status, support a diagnosis of

Cryptococcus lymphadenitis. Reactive lymphadenopathy typically does not demonstrate a specific organism, otherwise it would be further classified. *Trypanosoma and Leishmania* have different morphologies and presentations. Fat emboli may resemble the circular nature of *Cryptococcus*; however, it is typically seen within vessels and is associated with trauma to the bone marrow.

A-17. **(d) Acute suppurative lymphadenitis; collect material for microbial cultures.**
The inflammatory infiltrate is primarily composed of neutrophils consistent with acute suppurative lymphadenitis. In such cases, it is helpful to collect/submit material for cultures, as this may help identify the etiologic organism. Immunohistochemical stains, flow cytometry, and the cell block would be of minimal value.

A-18. **(b) HMB45 negative**
Myelolipomas are uncommon neoplasms occurring in and around the adrenal gland. They may grow very large and are often incidental findings. In contrast to angiomyolipomas, they are HMB45 negative but do include adipocytes.

A-19. **(d) EBV stains LMP-1 in Reed-Sternberg cells**
Classical Hodgkin lymphoma (CHL) usually demonstrates CD30 and frequently CD15 positivity with CD45 negativity. Sclerosis is common and it typically presents in a bimodal distribution, the first 15–35 years old and the second peak later in life. When EBV in situ staining is performed, it stains LMP-1 in Reed-Sternberg cells, which is a protein involved in antiapoptotic activity.

A-20. **(d) Prominent nucleoli**
CLL/SLL is characterized as a mature B-cell lymphoma/leukemia composed of small cells, clumped mature chromatin, variable plasmacytoid appearance (eccentric nuclei and plasmacytoid rim demonstrates in image), and minimal cytoplasm occasionally demonstrating increased numbers of prolymphocytes and paraimmunoblasts. Prominent nucleoli are not typically seen in the CLL/SLL cells and are usually identified in other lymphoid malignancies, often higher grade or more immature types.

A-21. **(b) Grading is based on the number of centroblasts**
The grading system for follicular lymphoma is based on the number of centroblasts per high-power field: grade I, 0–5 centroblasts per hpf; grade II, 6–15 centroblasts per hpf; and grade III, >15 centroblasts per hpf. Grade 3 is split into 3A and 3B with 3A demonstrating centrocytes while 3B is solid sheets of centroblasts. Cases are usually reported as either low grade (grades 1–2) or high grade (grade 3). It is important to grade follicular lymphomas as cases with higher grades have demonstrated worse clinical outcomes and higher rates of progression to diffuse large cell lymphoma. The Ki-67 proliferation index can be used as supportive evidence of the grade, as it usually correlates with the grade. The t(14;18) translocation involves Bcl2, but not Bcl6. Nuclear irregularities are common and follicular lymphoma is generally the most common small cell lymphoma.

A-22. **(c) Burkitt lymphoma**
The clinical description in combination with the morphology and translocation is most supportive of a Burkitt lymphoma diagnosis. While the other answer choices may demonstrate similar findings, they less frequently present in children, do not demonstrate the translocations, or have different cytologic morphology.

A-23. **(a) ALK positivity confers a better prognosis.**
The findings of the large atypical cells with hallmark and donut-shaped nuclei that are CD30 and ALK positive are suggestive of anaplastic large cell lymphoma (ALCL). ALCLs have better outcomes when ALK positive. They are not associated with EBV and typically do not show prominent red nucleoli with binucleation (like melanoma); the t(2;5) translocation partner genes are ALK and NPM. It typically presents in the first three decades of life.

A-24. **(b) Mycosis fungoides**
The descriptions of a discohesive population of intermediates size cells that are positive for CD2 and CD7 while negative for CD20 suggest a T-cell lymphoproliferative disorder. Combined with the dermatologic presentation, it is most suspicious for mycosis fungoides. Lichen sclerosis, actinic keratosis, folliculitis, and DFSP may demonstrate varying degrees of inflammation, but disseminated proliferation of lymphoid cells is not seen.

A-25. **(a) CD4+/CD8−/CD34−**
Mycosis fungoides is the most likely diagnosis. These typically present with an increased CD4 population. CD8 positivity is rare. CD34 should highlight epithelial and lymphoblast cells, which would be unlikely to be part of this proliferation. Dual-positive or dual-negative CD4/CD8 is

uncommon in mycosis fungoides and is more often seen in immature proliferations such as angioimmunoblastic lymphoma.

A-26. (e) **Bcl-1 is usually positive**.
Bcl-1 is the alternate name for cyclin D1 and typically positive in mantle cell lymphoma. Mantle cell lymphomas are positive for the t(11;14) translocation, the blastoid variant is usually cyclin D1 positive, the cells are usually small to medium in size, and cyclin D1 is not specific to mantle cell lymphoma and may also be seen in carcinomas, parathyroid neoplasms, multiple myeloma, and hairy cell leukemia.

A-27. (b) **Germinal center phenotype has a better prognosis**.
The germinal center phenotype (CD10+ or Bcl6+ and MUM1−) has a better prognosis than non-germinal center phenotype (CD10−, Bcl6−, MUM+). CD10 negativity alone is not considered specific for non-germinal center phenotype. If CD10 is negative, then additional stains for Bcl6 and MUM1 should be performed. A newer marker, FOXP1, has been recommended as an addition to the three-stain algorithm for determining germinal center type and has shown improved accuracy.

A-28. (d) **Cyclin D1**
The above cell are suggestive of a diffuse large B-cell lymphoma and would be supported by an appropriate immunophenotype (CD20+, CD19+, CD10+/−, CD5−, increase Ki-67 and surface immunoglobulin positive). In the event of CD5 positivity, the possibility of a blastoid mantle cell lymphoma should be entertained. The most useful stain to investigate this possibility is cyclin D1. In addition, molecular testing for the t(11;14)(CCND1-IGH) rearrangement would be useful. CD20 may be lost in DLBCL treated with rituximab but are usually otherwise positive. CD138 would highlight a plasma cell neoplasm and marginal zone lymphoma. Tdt is a marker of cell immaturity and seen primarily in lymphoblastic neoplasms. Ki-67 proliferation index would not help further differentiate the type of malignancy.

A-29. (b) **Acid-fast stain**
The image demonstrates a proliferation of small lymphocytes concerning for lymphoma. In addition, close examination of the lymphocytes demonstrates rod-shaped negative images. Morphologically and based on the negative staining, these are concerning for mycobacterium and would best be evaluated with an acid-fast stain.

A-30. (b) The image depicts a loosely cohesive proliferation of medium-sized cells with a tigroid background. These findings are most consistent with metastatic seminoma.

A-31. (e) **Metastatic prostate carcinoma**
While the tigroid background is typical of seminomas, this is not the only diagnosis that may present with this background. In addition, the cytomorphology may also be present in melanoma, small cell carcinoma, and ALCL. Prostate carcinoma is cohesive and demonstrates glandular morphology.

A-32. (a) **PLAP**
Seminomas typically stain positive with PLAP, c-Kit, and OCT3/4. Melan-A is positive in melanoma, Congo red is used for amyloid, Grocott is a silver stain that highlights fungal walls, and CK 20 stains many carcinomas.

A-33. (a) **Metastatic renal cell carcinoma**
The proliferation demonstrated in the image represents a lymph node involved by metastatic renal cell carcinoma. When dealing with metastatic disease, clinical history and examination are often the most helpful clue. In cases lacking history or where the history is not concordant with the findings in the FNA specimen, immunohistochemical stains of a cell block are often the most useful ancillary tool.

A-34. (d) **Metastatic melanoma**
Metastatic melanoma is frequently discohesive or presents in loose clusters, epithelioid, often binucleated with prominent nuclei, plasmacytoid morphology, and dusty cytoplasm. Melanoma may demonstrate cytoplasmic pigment and intranuclear inclusions. Plasmacytoma or NHL are small- to medium-sized cells and rarely shows large cells with giant nucleoli. Giant cell tumor of bone is a low-grade malignancy and shows cytologically bland cells and very rare causes metastatic disease.

5.4 Answers and Discussion of Text-Based Questions 35–101

A-35. (c) **Hamazaki-Wesenberg bodies may mimic fungi**.
Hamazaki-Wesenberg bodies are highlighted by GMS and acid-fast stains and may be misinterpreted as fungi. Schaumann bodies are more common than asteroid bodies and sarcoidosis typically presents in multiple organ systems with non-necrotizing granulomas. Any granulomatous presentation needs to include investigation of an infectious etiology.

A-36. (d) **Auramine O may highlight the organism**.
Mycobacterium avium often presents with granulomas and may present as negative images of the organisms and they typically stain positive with acid-fast stains. Auramine O highlights mycobacterium and is now the most common infection in patients with AIDS. Acid-fast staining, while it does highlight mycobacterium, may also highlight nocardia, cryptosporidium, and Cyclospora.

A-37. (a) **It is present in primary cutaneous ALCL**.
Typical ALCLs presenting in lymph nodes and other sites frequently demonstrate the t(2;5) translocation. In contrast, cutaneous ALCL does not demonstrate the translocation. The t(2;5) does include the partner genes ALK and PMN is seen in other neoplasms (inflammatory myofibroblastic tumor) and is the most frequent translocation seen in ALCL.

A-38. (d) **It affects immunocompromised patients**.
There are three forms of Burkitt lymphoma, endemic, sporadic, and immunodeficiency associated. The most common translocation is the t(8;14); the cells are usually positive for CD20, CD19, CD10, and BCL-6, while the Ki-67 proliferation index approaches 100 %. It most commonly involves the abdomen, mandible, gonads, kidneys, salivary glands, breasts, and lymph nodes.

A-39. (e) **Children and adolescents**.
In adult men and women, the most likely source of a malignant effusion is an occult primary neoplasm such as lung, breast, or colorectal carcinoma.

A-40. (e) **Heterogeneity of the lymphoid population**.
The differentiation between lymphoid hyperplasia and lymphoma can be difficult. All of the features may help suggest a lymphoid population is benign. Several lymphoid malignancies consistently demonstrate heterogeneity, which makes classification difficult and includes: follicular lymphoma, MALT lymphoma, T-cell-rich large B-cell lymphoma, and Hodgkin lymphoma.

A-41. (e) **All of the above**
Each diagnosis listed demonstrates features similar to reactive lymphoid hyperplasia and cannot be reliably classified.

A-42. (b) **CD20**
Many patients are treated with Rituxan (rituximab) chemotherapy for CD20+ lymphoma. This chemotherapy targets CD20-positive B cells and the CD20 receptor. As a result, residual and recurrent B-cell lymphomas, status post therapy often lack this marker. The other markers may be modified after chemotherapy; however, this is not seen as frequently as the loss of CD20.

A-43. (a) **Reactive lymphoid hyperplasia**.
Patients with AIDS are prone to many opportunistic infections including tuberculosis and *Cryptococcus neoformans*. In addition, these patients may develop Kaposi sarcoma or non-Hodgkin lymphoma. However, the most frequent cause of lymphadenopathy in AIDS patients is reactive lymphoid hyperplasia.

A-44. (a) **Lepra bacilli**
The described foamy cells are the classic Virchow cells with vacuoles containing multiple bacilli. Cat scratch disease, actinomyces, and suppurative lymphadenitis contain primarily neutrophils. Tuberculosis contains acid-fast bacilli and histiocytes, but not with the Virchow cell morphology.

A-45. (e) **Molecular testing**
All of the other techniques may demonstrate the organism (*Bartonella henselae*); however, they are unreliable. Molecular techniques, serologic testing, or immunofluorescence are more reliable alternatives to confirming the suspicion of cat scratch disease.

A-46. (d) **Watch and wait**
The findings and clinical history are typical of Kikuchi lymphadenitis. It is characterized by extensive karyorrhexis, histiocytes with sharply angulated nuclei, and plasmacytoid monocytes. Clinical intervention including antibiotics is unnecessary in these cases as the lymphadenopathy is self-limited and will resolve without intervention.

A-47. (**b**) **17p deletion**
The 17p deletion in CLL/SLL is associated with a more aggressive course. An 11q deletion is also aggressive, not 11p. The 13q14 deletion phenotype has a better prognosis. The 17q addition is not a common known mutation. Trisomy 12 has an intermediate phenotype.

A-48. (**b**) **Leishmaniasis**
The description of the histiocytic intracytoplasmic amastigotes is consistent with leishmanial infection. The rod-shaped structure is the kinetoplast. Visceral leishmaniasis is caused by *Leishmania donovani* and is endemic to parts of Africa and South America. The amastigotes may be found within histiocytes or outside upon rupture of the cells.

A-49. (**d**) **Rosai-Dorfman disease**
Rosai-Dorfman disease, also known as sinus histiocytosis with massive lymphadenopathy, most frequently occurs in children and adolescents. Clinically it frequently presents with symptoms similar to lymphoma and leukemia including fevers, night sweats, malaise, and joint pain. Cytologically, the characteristic finding in addition to abundant lymphocytes is lymphocytes transgressing through histiocytes (emperipolesis). The histiocytes are S100 and CD68 positive. The alternate answer choices do not typically demonstrate emperipolesis.

A-50. (**c**) Nodular lymphocyte-predominant Hodgkin lymphoma usually presents in patients between 30 and 50 years of age and classically demonstrates CD20-, EMA-, and CD45-positive L&H (popcorn) cells, which are CD30 negative and often CD15 negative. Compared to Reed-Sternberg cells in classical forms of Hodgkin lymphoma, L&H cells usually have a single irregular or multinucleated nucleolus with extreme irregularities, hence the popcorn cell description. The other choices are subcategories of classical-type Hodgkin lymphoma, which usually demonstrate CD30 and CD15 positivity and are characterized by the Reed-Sternberg cell.

A-51. (**e**) **Mixed cellularity** is the most common subtype of Hodgkin lymphoma in the developing world. In the developed world, nodular-sclerosing variant is the most common subtype. Overall, the classical subtypes comprise 95 % of cases worldwide.

A-52. (**a**) The **t(14;18)** translocation is classically found in follicular cell lymphoma and characteristically positive for B-cell markers and follicular center markers Bcl-6 and Bcl-2. The t(14;18) translocation represents a Bcl-2 gene rearrangement. Translocation t(11;14) is typically found in mantle cell lymphoma, t(8;22) Ewing sarcoma, t(2;5) anaplastic large cell lymphoma, and t(x;18) in synovial sarcoma.

A-53. (**a**) Unlike the other small cell lymphomas (follicular lymphoma, CLL/SLL) mantle cell typically lacks transformed lymphocytes. Hodgkin lymphoma and anaplastic large cell lymphomas typically are not considered small cell lymphomas.

A-54. (**a**) **A. t(14;18)(q32;q31)**
The cytologic and immunohistochemical findings suggest follicular lymphoma. The translocation partners for follicular lymphoma are both found on the long arms of chromosomes 14 and 18. This translocation results in rearrangement of the Bcl-2 gene. The t(11;14) is found in mantle cell lymphoma and t(8;18) in Burkitt lymphoma.

A-55. (**c**) MALT lymphomas are associated with several chronic autoimmune conditions including Sjögren disease, H. pylori chronic gastritis, and Hashimoto thyroiditis. The most frequent site is the gastric mucosa. MALT lymphomas frequently demonstrate the t(11;18) translocation.

A-56. (**b**) The endemic form of Burkitt lymphoma is most likely to demonstrate EBV positivity. The endemic form is found in patients from Africa and less frequently in the Middle East and Asia. The endemic form is rare in the United States. Burkitt lymphoma commonly presents in young children, frequently in the mandible or abdomen.

A-57. (**e**) **95 %**
The cytomorphologic and immunohistochemical findings suggest a Burkitt lymphoma, immunodeficiency-related type. Burkitt lymphoma is known to demonstrate a very high proliferation index approaching 100 %, as such a value greater than 70 % is expected.

A-58. (**b**) **Anaplastic large cell lymphoma** frequently demonstrates a t (2;5)(p23;q35) translocation. The translocation results in expression of the ALK protein from the fusion of the ALK gene with the nucleophosmin gene. ALCL is among the more common T-cell lymphomas. ALCL usually demonstrates positivity for T-cell markers: however, occasionally they are negative for T-cell markers and are given the null designation. In the classic form, the neoplastic cells are large with extensive pleomorphism. Many cells may demonstrate a horseshoe-shaped nucleus, known as a "horseshoe" cell. The tumor cells are positive for CD30. Usually tingible body macrophages are absent and lymphoglandular bodies are rare.

A-59. (**a**) Precursor T-cell lymphoblastic lymphoma is a common lymphoma of childhood. Clinically, it most frequently presents as an anterior compartment mediastinal mass. Due to its location, the mass may place pressure on adjacent structures and induce symptoms that mimic other diagnoses including acute bronchitis and superior vena cava thrombosis. Smears are usually hypercellular and composed of large lymphoblasts with inconspicuous nucleoli, fine chromatin, and increased nuclear to cytoplasmic ratios. The cell may demonstrate molding. Immunophenotypically, the lymphoblasts are characteristically TdT positive. The distinction from thymoma is made by cytomorphology and clinical history, as both neoplasms demonstrate immature immunophenotypes.

A-60. (**d**) **EBV**.
A large percentage of PTLDs are associated with concomitant EBV infection. It is thought that Epstein-Barr virus induces the monoclonal or polyclonal proliferations. Human papilloma virus (HPV) is associated with squamous cell carcinomas. Human T-cell lymphoma virus 1 (HTLV-1) is associated with Kaposi sarcoma. Human immunodeficiency virus (HIV) has not been directly implicated in the development of a neoplasm.

A-61. (**e**) **Positive EBV immunohistochemical stains in a majority of cells**.
Recurrent lymphomas may take many forms and have a variety of characteristics. It is often useful to compare to the previous material or report to confirm morphological and immunohistochemical similarities. Findings such as large atypical cells, high mitotic rate, and lymphoglandular bodies do not specifically help distinguish between PTLD and recurrent lymphoma. A small number of EBV positive cells are not a reliable indicator of PTLD as this may be seen in a variety of settings. True EBV-related PTLD demonstrates EBV positivity in the majority of cells.

A-62. (**a**) **Nasopharyngeal carcinoma** and seminoma are two neoplasms that may mimic diffuse large B-cell lymphoma. Other neoplasms may mimic DLBCL, including melanoma, epithelioid carcinoma, and poorly differentiated carcinomas. Nasopharyngeal carcinoma occurring in a lymph node will frequently demonstrate lymphoglandular bodies. Lymphoglandular bodies are fragments of lymphocytes and are accepted as markers of lymphoid tissue and may be seen in the background in tumors involving lymph nodes or intermixed in malignant lymphoid populations.

A-63. (**c**) Anaplastic large cell lymphoma (ALCL) may be confused with carcinoma for several reasons. These neoplasms usually have a paucity of lymphoglandular bodies, are cohesive or frequently clustered, demonstrate EMA positivity (which is generally a marker of epithelial derivation), are pleomorphic, small lymphocytes, and may be rare and often ALCL contains spindled cells.

A-64. (**c**) **Histiocytic sarcoma**, formerly known as true histiocytic lymphoma, may be nodal or extranodal and is characterized by CD68 and CD163 positivity with CD1a, CD30, and keratin negativity. They are composed of sheets of large cells with abundant eosinophilic cytoplasm. Langerhans cell histiocytosis and Langerhans cell sarcoma demonstrate S100 and CD1a positivity. Interdigitating dendritic cell sarcoma shows S100 positivity and follicular dendritic cell sarcoma is positive for CD23, CD21, and CD35.

A-65. (**b**) **Dermatopathic lymphadenopathy** is a frequent mimic of Langerhans cell histiocytosis. Both may demonstrate CD1a grooved Langerhans cells. Dermatopathic lymphadenopathy is seen as a result of a recent dermatologic infection or reaction and results from Langerhans cell from the skin migrating to lymph nodes and includes surrounding pigment laden macrophages. Langerhans cell histiocytosis usually also has a population of eosinophils. On surgical excision, Langerhans cells in LCH are usually in the interfollicular zones, while in dermatopathic lymphadenopathy, they are usually located in the sinuses and peripheral node.

A-66. (**c**) The description is of a small cell carcinoma. Small cell carcinomas may demonstrate some similarities in their cell size to a lymphocytic proliferation. The characteristic features of nuclear molding and salt and pepper chromatin are seen in small cell carcinoma. In addition to being positive for neuroendocrine markers including CD56, chromogranin, and synaptophysin, it is also positive for cytokeratins. CD3 and CD20 are positive in lymphoid proliferations. Melanin is positive in melanoma and Oct4 is seen in germ cell tumors.

A-67. (**b**) **BRAF** testing in metastatic melanoma/stage IV melanoma is important to help aid in therapy. Currently, signal transduction therapeutics (vemurafenib) is available for patients with the BRAF V600E mutation. These have been shown to help prolong survival in patients with metastatic disease. KRAS may be mutated in melanoma but is rare and not currently an approved therapeutic target. The BRD4-NUT and BRD3-NUT translocations are seen in NUT midline carcinoma. The t(2;5) translocation is important in identifying anaplastic large cell lymphoma; however, the immunohistochemical studies in this case support a diagnosis of melanoma. The t(14;18) translocation is seen in follicular lymphoma.

A-68. (**d**) Performing multiple passes with the needle helps improve sampling by evaluating multiple areas of the lymph node and acquiring more material. Applying anesthetic creams may help decrease the pain associated with the technique for the patient, but will not directly improve adequacy. Lymph nodes should be stabilized while performing the aspiration; otherwise, they may move and inhibit proper sampling. Large gauge needles provide more tissue but are more painful for the patient and result in more bleeding. Gauges are counterintuitive in that the higher the number, the smaller the needle.

A-69. (**a**) The Monospot test is an agglutination test developed in 1968, using the principle that horse erythrocytes are more likely to react than sheep erythrocytes to the presence of heterophile antibodies produced in response to infection by Epstein-Barr virus. Clinical history is not highly specific for infectious mononucleosis; currently there is neither urine test for EBV antibodies nor a breath test. Molecular testing could be performed for the presence of EBV, but this does not determine whether an immune response has occurred, leading to the infectious mononucleosis manifestations.

A-70. (**c**) **Tall columnar cells**
Colorectal adenocarcinoma commonly includes tall columnar cells often with mucin production and gland formation. Signet ring cells are characteristic of gastric adenocarcinoma. Intranuclear pseudoinclusions are frequently seen in papillary thyroid carcinoma. Brown pigment may be either hemosiderin or melanin in metastatic melanoma. Nuclear molding is seen in small cell carcinoma and herpes simplex infections.

A-71. (**c**) **10,000 events.**
The generally accepted minimum number of events to be confident in flow cytometric results is 10,000. This number is based on statistical calculations and the clinical implications of diagnoses requiring a low enough coefficient of variation for a subpopulation of cells comprising 5 % of the sample.

A-72. (**c**) **CLL/SLL** is a lymphoid proliferation of small mature B-lineage lymphocytes with mature clumped chromatin. The architectural findings in CLL/SLL are not necessary diagnostic and usually the most useful additional information is the immunophenotype of the proliferation (CD5 and CD23+ B cells). Progressively transformed germinal centers, Castleman disease, nodular lymphocyte-predominant Hodgkin lymphoma, and vascular transformation of the lymph node sinuses, either all rely on or are substantially supported by architectural findings.

A-73. (**a**) **Melanoma**
Sarcoidosis demonstrates granulomas usually composed of epithelioid histiocytes and variable nonspecific findings such as asteroid bodies (starlike eosinophilic shapes in histiocytes). Sarcoid is commonly a diagnosis of exclusion; once other etiologies with similar morphologic findings are excluded. Entities demonstrating similar granulomatous reactions includes: infections, foreign body reactions, dendritic lymphocytic aggregates, and spindle-cell neoplasms. All of these may have a proliferation of histiocytes. Melanoma typically does not demonstrate a granulomatous reaction unless presenting in the setting of another concurrent process. Immunohistochemical stains for Melan-A and HMB45 would help confirm the diagnosis of melanoma if there is a concern.

A-74. (**d**) **Extensive neutrophilic infiltrate**
Kikuchi lymphadenitis is a reactive process that typically demonstrates necrotic debris, small phagocytic histiocytes, tingible body macrophages, and minimal to no neutrophilic inflammation. A reactive lymph node with a neutrophilic infiltrate would not only make the diagnosis of Kikuchi lymphadenitis unlikely but would raise suspicion for alternate diagnoses including cat scratch disease, *Francisella*, *Yersinia*, and *Chlamydia*.

A-75. (a) **Mantle cell lymphoma**

Infectious mononucleosis can mimic many neoplasms. It is caused by EBV and seen frequently in adolescents. Lymph nodes may be tender and splenomegaly is a frequent finding. Aspirates usually demonstrate a mix of small lymphocytes, plasmacytoid lymphocytes, centroblasts, and immunoblasts. In addition, there is an increase in large cells, which may mimic large cell lymphoma, Hodgkin lymphoma, or immunoblastic lymphoma. The mixed inflammation is similar to reactive lymphoid hyperplasia. The proliferations can be differentiated from infectious mononucleosis by the polyclonality of IM.

A-76. (b) **Morphology of malignant cells**

Anaplastic large cell lymphoma (ALCL) and classical Hodgkin lymphoma may have very similar appearances. ALCL usually has a higher number of malignant cells compared to an alternate composition in classical Hodgkin lymphoma. EMA is typically negative in classical HL (positive in NLPHL) and positive in ALCL. Molecular studies may demonstrate t(2;5) seen in ALCL and not HL. Finally, ALK immunohistochemical stains are positive in most ALCLs and negative in HL.

A-77. (c) **Mantle cell**

When comparing the aggressiveness of small lymphomas, Mantle cell lymphoma is considered the most aggressive. In comparison, small lymphocytic, follicular, marginal zone/MALT, and lymphoplasmacytic are considered indolent. Of these lymphomas, marginal zone/MALT lymphoma is the only one considered regularly curable, while follicular lymphomas are rarely cured.

A-78. (a) **t(8;14)**

The c-Myc immunohistochemical stain is positive in Burkitt lymphoma, which has an associated t(8;14) translocation and has presentation both clinically and morphologically similar to the described patient. A subset of Burkitt lymphomas demonstrate the t(2:8) or t(8;22) translocations, but they occur much less frequently than the t(8;14) translocation. Rarely, diffuse large B-cell lymphomas may be positive for c-Myc. However, they typically demonstrate Bcl-2 gene rearrangement or abnormalities in 3q27. Translocation t(2;5) is typically seen in anaplastic large cell lymphoma and t(9;22) translocation is seen in chronic myelogenous leukemia and acute lymphoblastic leukemia.

A-79. (c) **8**

C-Myc was first discovered in Burkitt lymphoma and is located on chromosome 8 and acts as a transcription factor involved in gene regulation. The c-Myc translocation occurs from band 8q24 to the IG heaving chain 14q32. Occasionally it occurs at the 22q11 lambda or 2p12 kappa light chain loci. C-Myc has also been identified in diffuse large B-cell lymphoma and multiple myeloma.

A-80. (a) **Multiple myeloma**

The c-Myc rearrangement may be seen in a variety of lymphoid neoplasms including Burkitt lymphoma, multiple myeloma, and diffuse large B-cell lymphoma. In Burkitt lymphoma, the c-Myc positivity is a common finding, while it is uncommon in diffuse large B-cell lymphoma and multiple myeloma.

A-81. (e) **EBV**

The differential diagnosis of a fine-needle aspiration with findings including neutrophilic infiltrate consistent with a suppurative lymphadenitis includes: *Chlamydia trachomatis*, *Yersinia enterocolitica*, *Francisella tularensis*, *Bartonella henselae*, and pyogenic cocci. Clinical history and cultures are frequently necessary to confirm a diagnosis or further classify the etiology of suppurative lymphadenitis. Bartonella frequently demonstrates palisading histiocytes and stellate abscesses, which may help lend weight to cat scratch diagnosis. Epstein-Barr-related lymphadenitis may present as infectious mononucleosis or in relation to a neoplastic process. These typically lack a prominent neutrophilic component.

A-82. (c) **Comprise the majority of lymphoblastic lymphomas**

T-cell lymphoblastic lymphoma most frequently occurs in children. B-cell lymphoblastic lymphomas are also frequent in children, however, more common than T-cell lymphoblastic lymphomas, in adults. The leukocyte count is typically elevated. The neoplastic process frequently presents in the mediastinum and may be included in the differential diagnosis with thymomas. They usually grow rapidly and comprise the majority of lymphoblastic lymphomas.

A-83. (a) **Follicular lymphoma**

The cytologic features of a small lymphocytic proliferation with irregular cleaved lymphocytes and few tingible body macrophages suggests a small lymphocyte lymphoma and provides nonspecific findings in favor of follicular lymphoma. The immunophenotype is characteristic of follicular lymphoma and confirmed by the t(14;18) translocation. CLL/SLL is typically positive for CD5 and CD23, mantle cell is CD5 positive and has the t(11;14) translocation, and marginal zone lymphoma is usually negative for CD5, CD23, Bcl-6, and CD10 and does not demonstrate (14;18). Finally, diffuse large B cell may demonstrate CD10 and Bcl-6 positivity and also may have the t(14;18) translocation, but morphologically is comprised of larger cells with a higher proliferation index.

A-84. (**a**) **Desmin, myogenin, CD138, and SMA**
The history of a thigh mass, coupled with the description of large eosinophilic cytoplasm and eccentric nuclei suggests rhabdoid morphology, likely rhabdomyosarcoma. Confirming a diagnosis of rhabdomyosarcoma is best done with positivity for desmin and myogenin. CD138 should be negative and rule out a plasma cell neoplasm and smooth muscle actin would be positive in a leiomyosarcoma. HMB45 and Melan-A would confirm a melanoma, cytokeratins are positive in epithelial neoplasms; CD99 can be seen in a variety of more immature and spindled neoplasms; vimentin highlights mesenchymal elements, but is not specific; PLAP is useful to confirm yolk sac tumors; CA-125 is positive in ovarian neoplasms; and WT-1 will highlight mesothelial cells and mullerian tumors in general.

A-85. (**c**) **del 13q14.3**
CLL/SLL may demonstrate several abnormalities molecular abnormalities. The most common abnormality is the deletion of 13q14.3 (approximately 50 % of cases), while approximately 20 % of cases demonstrate trisomy 12. Additional less frequent cytogenetic abnormalities are deletions of 11q22-23, 17p13, and 6q21.

A-86. (**e**) **Pulmonary adenocarcinoma**
The FNA description highlights the cell size (large) and shape (cleaved and non-cleaved) and cytoplasmic characteristics (vacuoles) with a lymphoid appearance. These findings suggest a lymphoid malignancy, but additional neoplasms may demonstrate similar morphology. Metastatic melanoma is frequently discohesive or presents in loose clusters, epithelioid, often binucleated with prominent nuclei and may demonstrate cytoplasmic black pigment. Small cell carcinoma is characterized by smaller cells that are often discohesive and have a lymphoid appearance but usually demonstrate molding. Testicular and mediastinal seminomas frequently metastasize to lymph nodes and typically have macronucleoli and abundant cytoplasm occurring in a tigroid background. The most likely process given the findings is diffuse large B-cell lymphoma. Pulmonary adenocarcinoma presents as medium to large cells clustered in three-dimensional sheets with prominent nucleoli and occasional cytoplasmic vacuoles.

A-87. (**c**) **Cytoplasmic kappa restriction, normal lambda**
Clonal proliferation of plasma cells is seen in mature neoplasms. Over the course of their maturity, plasma cells transition form surface to cytoplasmic expression of immunoglobulins. Normal plasma cell population will present with a kappa to lambda ratio of 2–4 kappa to 1 lambda. In malignant plasma cell proliferations, there is usually a predominance of either kappa or lambda and it is found cytoplasmically. This is important as a clonal plasma cell population may not be identified immunophenotypically if cell lysis procedures that can characterize cytoplasmic expression are not performed.

A-88. (**b**) **CD138-positive cells**
CD138-positive cells are primarily plasma cells. Plasma cells are more fragile than most other cell types. Due to their fragility, plasma cells may be hard to characterize in general, and when a sample is not rapidly processed, the cells will most likely degrade to a degree that prevents accurate evaluation.

A-89. (**a**) **Start triple therapy**
Triple therapy consists of a regimen of amoxicillin, clarithromycin, and omeprazole to eradicate *Helicobacter pylori* and/or Helmenii from the stomach. Both organisms are associated with gastric MALT lymphomas and have led to a complete response. If this therapy fails, the next step would include gastric resection. It would be inappropriate to watch and wait, perform the urease breath test, or perform an endoscopic mucosal resection.

A-90. (**b**) **B. CD20+, CD79+, CD38+**
Splenic marginal zone lymphoma has a typically nonspecific immunophenotype. In contrast, hairy cell leukemia is positive for CD103 and CD25, while negative for CD23. Plasma cell neoplasms are typically CD20– but CD79+ and CD138+ and have typical plasmacytoid morphology. CLL/SLL is positive for CD5 and CD23, while mantle cell lymphoma is positive for CD5, but negative for CD23 and CD10.

A-91. (**a**) **CD103+, CD25+, CD23–**
Hairy cell leukemia is positive for CD103 and CD23, while negative for CD23. Splenic marginal zone lymphoma has a typically nonspecific immunophenotype. Plasma cell neoplasms are typically CD20–, but CD79+ and CD138+ and have typical plasmacytoid morphology. CLL/SLL is positive for CD5 and CD23, while mantle cell lymphoma is positive for CD5, but negative for CD23 and CD10.

A-92. (**b**) **Hodgkin lymphoma**
Based on various studies there is a range of sensitivities and specificities for FNA of lymph nodes depending on the underlying character of a lesion. In general, the lowest sensitivities are seen in Hodgkin lymphoma, likely due to the mixed inflammatory infiltrate and frequently the paucity of malignant cells in addition to difficulties with flow cytometric analysis for characterizing Hodgkin lymphoma. The low ends of sensitivity ranges are higher for non-Hodgkin lymphoma and metastatic disease.

A-93. (**a**) **Burkitt lymphoma**
Endemic and sporadic Burkitt lymphoma typically present in younger patients. Immunodeficiency-associated Burkitt lymphoma may be more frequent in young adults depending on the HIV/AIDS demographics of a population. CLL/SLL, DLBCL, follicular lymphoma, and ALCL are more common in adults.

A-94. (**a**) **Metastatic melanoma**
Warthin-Finkeldey cells are described as grape bunch-like clusters of cells with minimal cytoplasm of variable size. These cells are classically associated with vaccination for measles. In addition, they have been demonstrated in systemic lupus erythematosus, Kimura disease, and Hodgkin lymphoma. They have not classically been associated with metastatic melanoma.

A-95. (**e**) **Hodgkin lymphoma**
Sinus histiocytosis on FNA or touch imprint is characterized by increased benign histiocytes in loose clusters or individually. They usually contain foamy cytoplasm. The intermixed cells are composed of mixed maturity lymphocytes and plasma cells. Of the listed diseases, Hodgkin lymphoma is classically not associated with sinus histiocytosis. All of the other entities may demonstrate increased sinus histiocytes.

A-96. (**b**) **Denatured DNA and immunoglobulin**
Systemic lupus erythematosus (SLE) lymphadenopathy on FNA typically demonstrate a mixed pattern with small lymphocytes, plasma cells, tingible body macrophages, and transformed cells. There may be background karyorrhexis. A characteristic feature of SLE material is lupus erythematosus (LE) cells. These are brightly eosinophilic cells with a hyalinized appearance hematoxylin bodies. The hematoxylin bodies contain denatured DNA and immunoglobulin.

A-97. (**b**) **Flame cells**
The description of plasma cell leukemia and cells with strong metachromatic staining in the peripheral cytoplasm is characteristic of flame cells. These cells have been associated with IgA secretion. Dutcher bodies are intranuclear and contain immunoglobulin, while Russell bodies are intracytoplasmic and also contain immunoglobulin. Lymphoglandular bodies are fragments of lymphocytes cytoplasm. Finally, Mott cells are plasma cell with abundant Russell bodies formed from immunoglobulin that cannot be eliminated.

A-98. (**c**) **It has the same immunophenotype as in adults**.
Pediatric nodal marginal zone lymphoma typically has the same immunophenotype as adult nodal marginal zone lymphomas, which is typically nonspecific and may mimic other neoplasms. They have an excellent prognosis, commonly present in the head and neck lymph nodes, predominantly in males (20:1), and may be difficult to distinguish from reactive conditions. In addition, they may require IGH clonal rearrangement studies.

A-99. (**b**) **t(2;17)(p23;q23)**
In contrast to anaplastic large cell lymphoma, which most frequently demonstrates the t (2:5) translocation, ALK-positive LBCL most commonly demonstrates the t(2;17) translocation. This is responsible for clathrin-ALK fusion protein. The cryptic insertion of 3′ ALK into 4q22–24 has been rarely reported. The t(5:17) translocation is not a common translocation and the t(9;22) translocation is seen in chronic myelogenous leukemia.

A-100. (**a**) **DLBCL**
Among adults, DLBCL is the most common B-cell lymphoma. The second most common is follicular lymphoma, followed by CLL/SLL, MALT lymphoma, and mantle cell lymphoma.

A-101. (a) **Peripheral T-cell lymphoma NOS**

The most common mature T-cell lymphoma subtype is peripheral T-cell lymphoma NOS followed by angioimmunoblastic lymphoma. Extranodal NK/T-cell lymphoma makes up about 10 % of case followed by much less frequent anaplastic large cell lymphoma, ALK+, and hepatosplenic T-cell lymphoma.

Reading List

Caraway NP, Katz RL. Chapter 31. Lymph nodes. In: Koss LG, Melamed MR, editors. Koss' diagnostic cytology and its histopathologic bases. 5th ed. Philadelphia: Lippincott Williams & Wilkins; 2006. p. 1186–228.

DeMay RM. Chapter 13. Lymph nodes. In: DeMay RM, editor. The art & science of cytopathology. 2nd ed. Chicago: ASCP Press; 2012. p. 966–1031.

Khalbuss WE, Monaco SE, and Pantanowitz L. Chapter 13. Lymph nodes. In: The ASCP quick compendium of cytopathology. IL, USA: ASCP Press; 2013. p 259–91.

Monaco SE, Pantanowitz L, Khalbuss WE. Cytopathology of nonneoplastic and infectious lymphadenopathy. In: Cualing HD, Bhargava P, Sandin RL, editors. Nonneoplastic hematopathology and infections. NJ, USA: Wiley- Blackwell; 2012. p 481.

Pambuccian SE, Bardales RH. Lymph node cytopathology. New York: Springer; 2011.

Wakely PE, Cibas ES. Chapter 11. Lymph nodes. In: Cibas ES, Ducatman BS, editors. Cytology diagnostic principles & clinical correlates. 3rd ed. Philadelphia: Saunders Elsevier; 2009. p. 319–57.

Young NA, Al-Saleem T. Chapter 24. Lymph nodes: cytomorphology & flow cytometry. In: Bibbo M, Wilbur DC, editors. Comprehensive cytopathology. 3rd ed. Philadelphia: Saunders Elsevier; 2008. p. 671–711.

Salivary Gland Fine-Needle Aspiration

6

Abdelmonem Elhosseiny and Walid E. Khalbuss

Contents

6.1 **Image-Based Questions 1–45** 354

6.2 **Text-Based Questions 46–65** 399

6.3 **Answers and Discussion of Image-Based Questions 1–45** 401

6.4 **Answers and Discussion of Text-Based Questions 46–65** 407

Reading List 408

A. Elhosseiny, MD (✉)
Department of Pathology, Fletcher Allen Health Care, University of Vermont, 111 Colchester Avenue, Burlington, VT 05405, USA
e-mail: abdel.elhosseiny@vtmednet.org

W.E. Khalbuss, MD, PhD, FIAC
Department of Pathology, GE Clarient Diagnostic Services, 31 Columbia, Aliso Viejo, California, 92656, USA
e-mail: Walid.khalbuss@ge.com

W.E. Khalbuss, Q.K. Li (eds.), *Diagnostic Cytopathology Board Review and Self-Assessment*, DOI 10.1007/978-1-4939-1477-7_6, © Springer Science+Business Media New York 2015

6.1 Image-Based Questions 1–45

Fig. 6.1

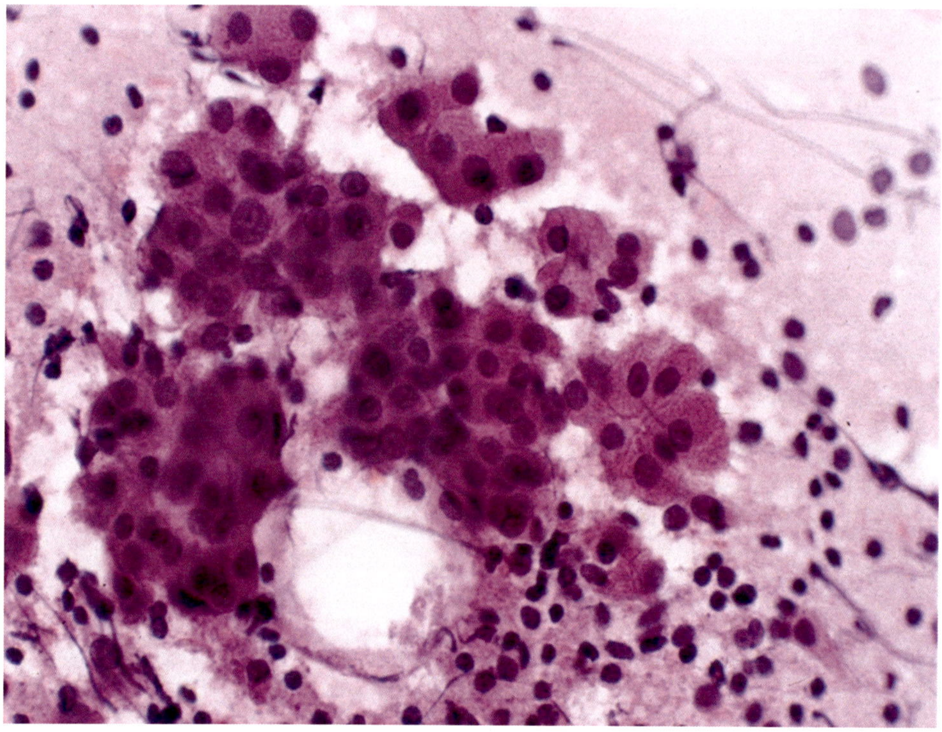

Q-1. A 45-year-old male has a 6-month history of a 3.5 cm cystic mass in the right parotid. FNA of parotid mass.
(a) Pleomorphic adenoma (mixed tumor)
(b) Warthin tumor
(c) Low grade mucoepidermoid carcinoma
(d) Acinic cell carcinoma
(e) Oncocytoma

Fig. 6.2

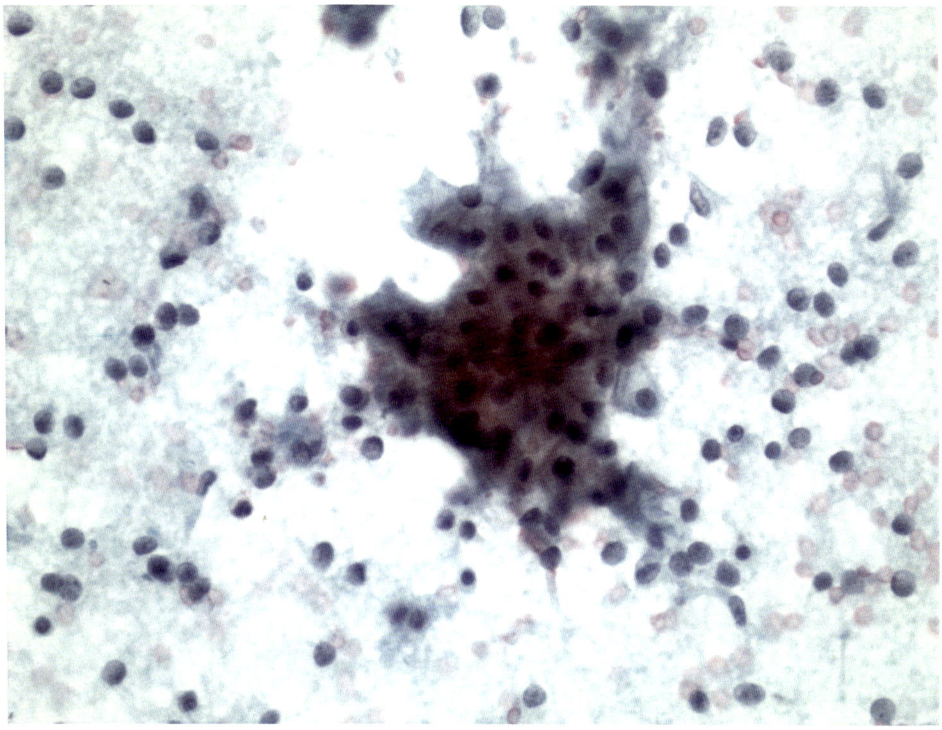

Q-2. A 3-cm parotid mass in a 50-year-old male. Mass was noted 3 months earlier. FNA of parotid mass.

(a) Pleomorphic adenoma (mixed tumor)
(b) Adenoid cystic carcinoma
(c) Warthin tumor
(d) Acinic cell carcinoma
(e) Oncocytoma

Fig. 6.3

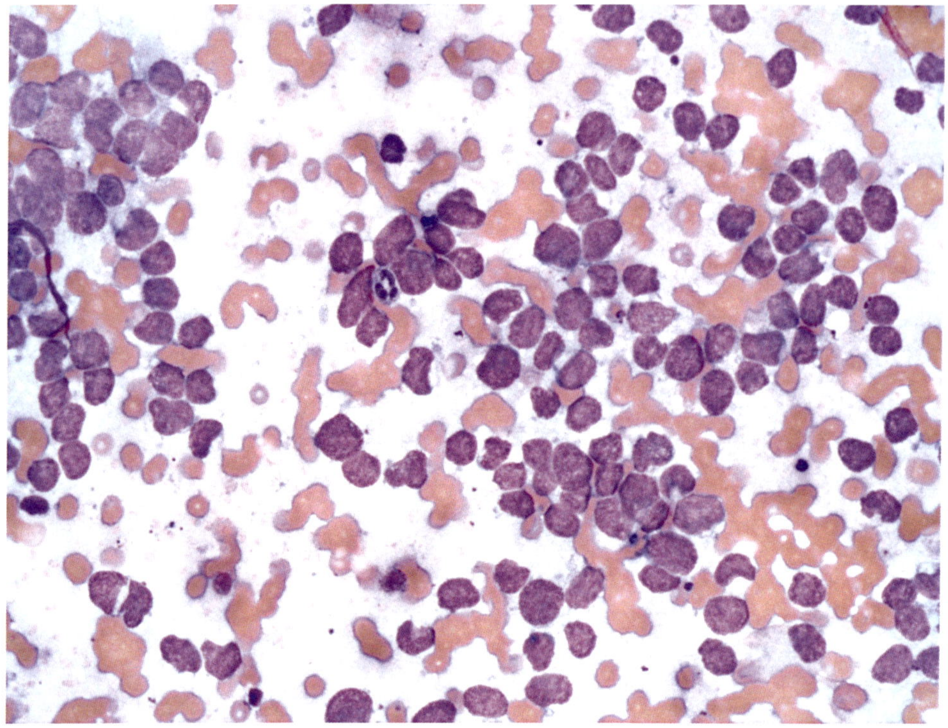

Q-3. Parotid mass in a 72-year-old male. FNA of the mass.
(a) Reactive intraparotid lymph node
(b) Lymphoma
(c) Melanoma
(d) Neuroendocrine carcinoma
(e) Acinic cell carcinoma

Fig. 6.4

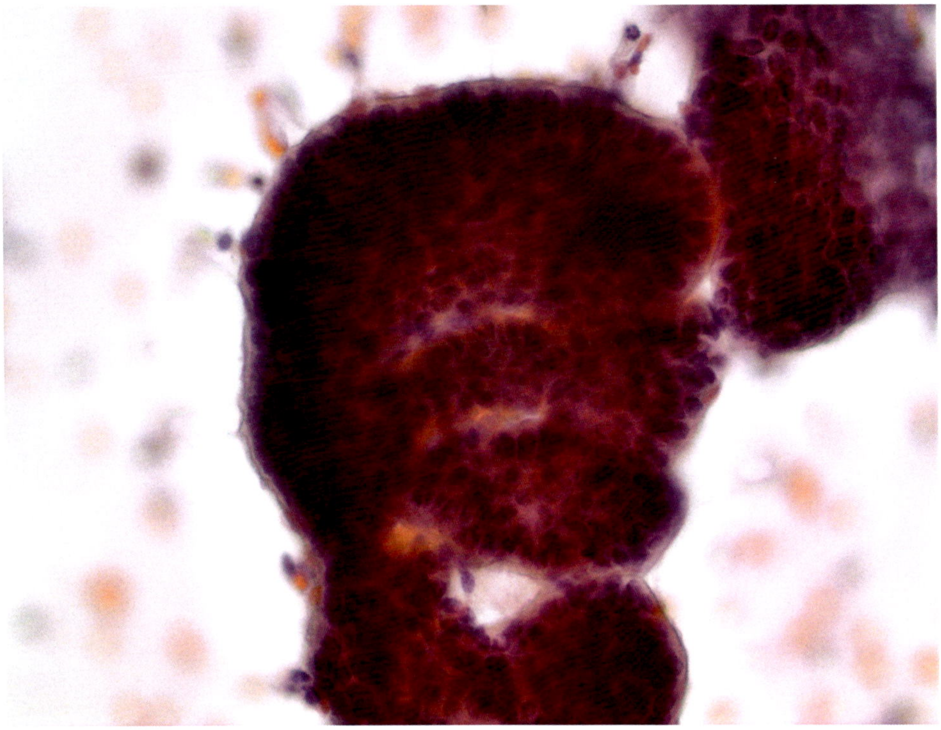

Q-4. Mass in the left submandibular in a 49-year-old female. Mass is slowly growing and not painful. FNA of mass.

(a) Adenoid cystic carcinoma
(b) Pleomorphic adenoma
(c) Polymorphous low grade adenocarcinoma
(d) Basal cell adenoma/adenocarcinoma
(e) Metastatic basaloid squamous carcinoma

Fig. 6.5

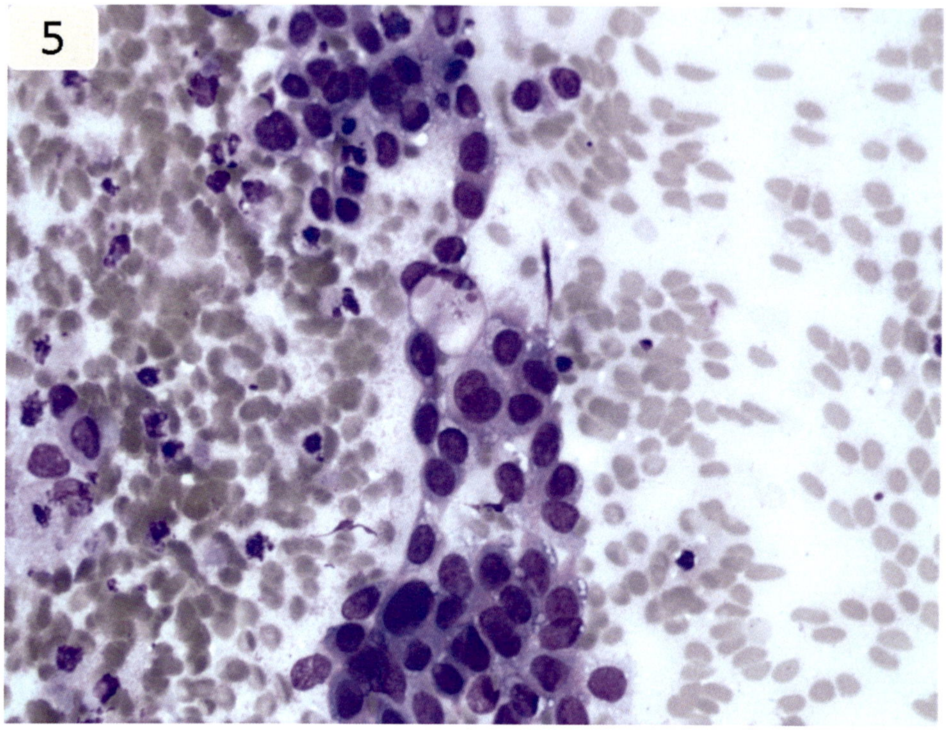

Q-5. A submandibular mass in a 73-year-old male. FNA of the mass.

(a) Pleomorphic adenoma
(b) Warthin tumor
(c) Mucoepidermoid carcinoma
(d) Acinic cell carcinoma
(e) Polymorphous low grade adenocarcinoma

Fig. 6.6

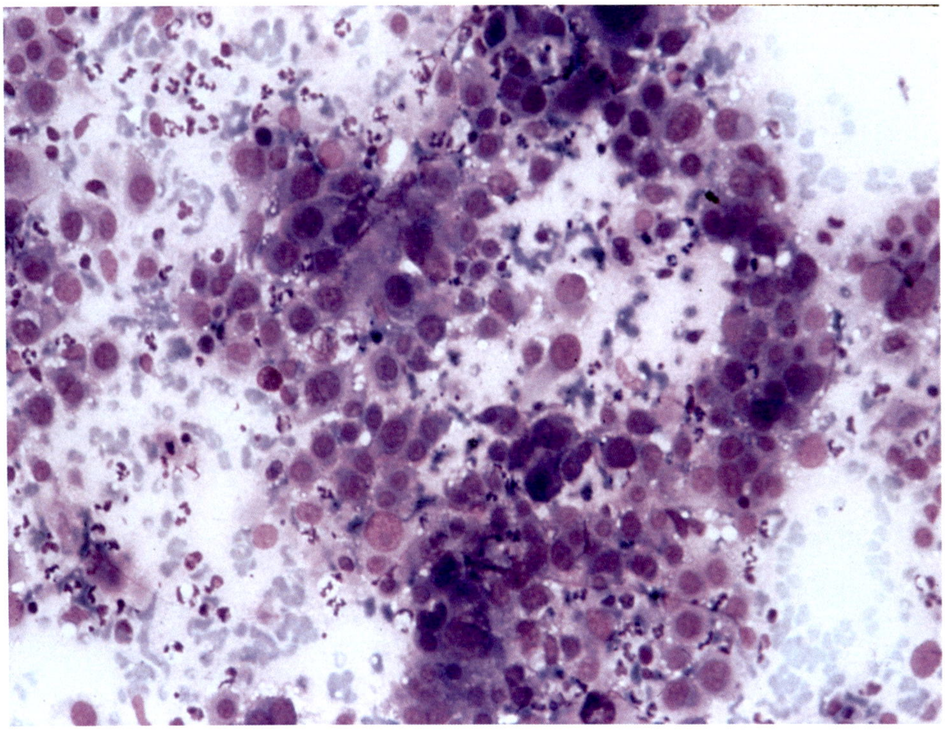

Q-6. A 69-year-old male has a 5-cm mass in the left parotid. Mass is increasing in size but not painful. FNA of parotid mass.

(a) Low grade mucoepidermoid carcinoma
(b) Oncocytoma
(c) Salivary duct carcinoma
(d) Adenoid cystic carcinoma
(e) Acinic cell carcinoma

Fig. 6.7

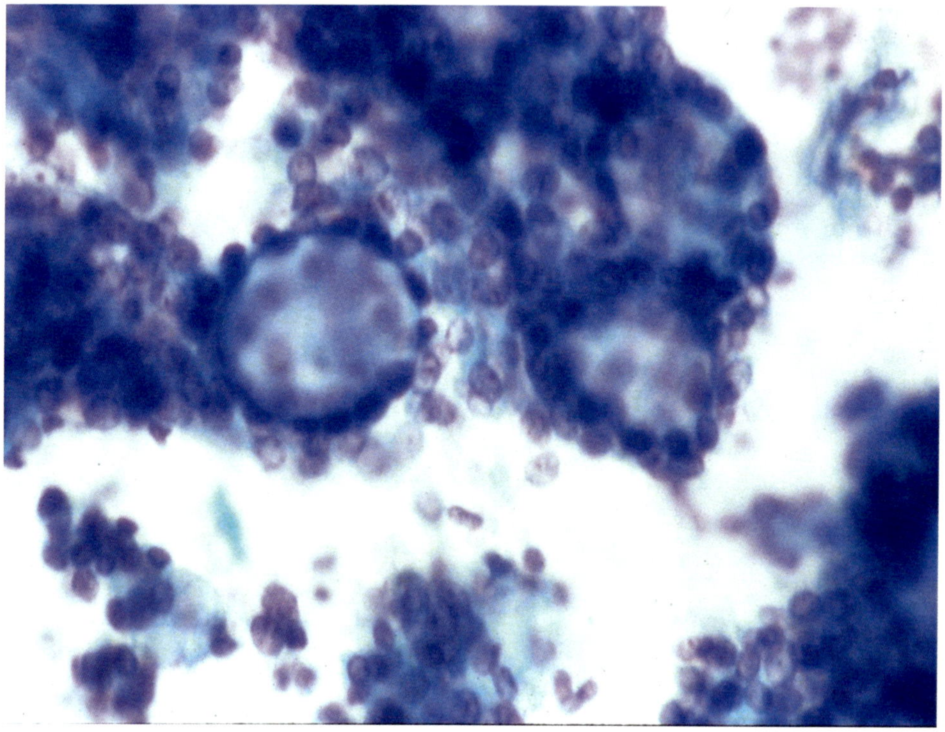

Q-7. A 60-year-old female presents with a 2.5-cm painful mass in the right parotid. FNA of parotid mass.
(a) Pleomorphic adenoma
(b) Adenoid cystic carcinoma
(c) Basal cell adenoma/adenocarcinoma
(d) Acinic cell carcinoma
(e) Oncocytoma

Fig. 6.8

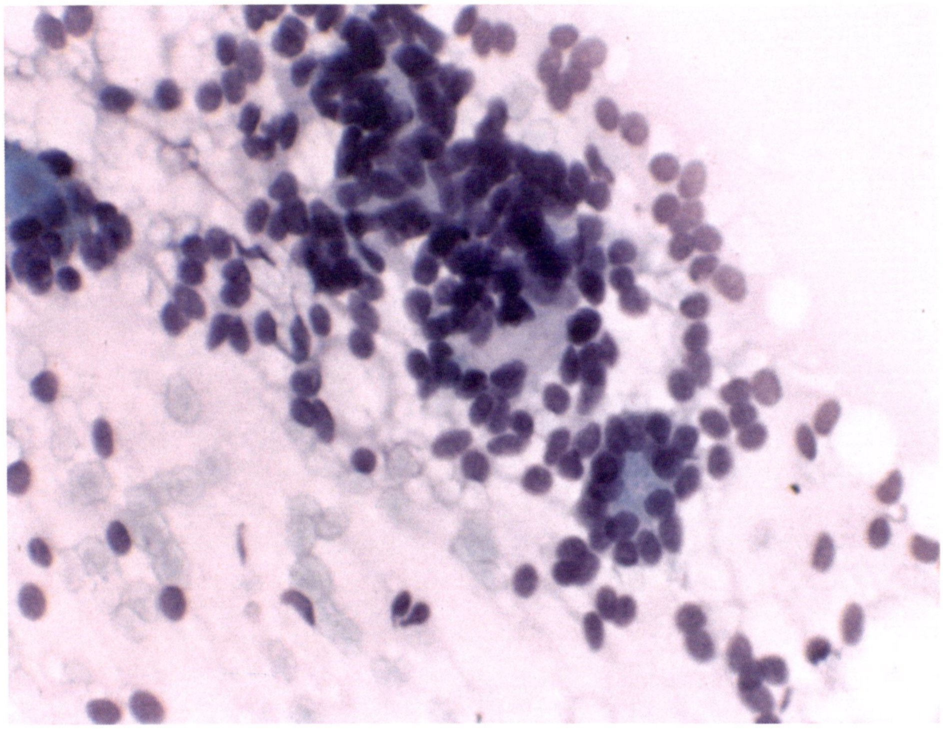

Q-8. A 65-year-old male presents with a slow growing 2-cm mass in the left submandibular gland. FNA of submandibular mass.

(a) Adenoid cystic carcinoma
(b) Basal cell adenoma/adenocarcinoma
(c) Pleomorphic adenoma
(d) Epithelial myoepithelial carcinoma
(e) Polymorphous low grade adenocarcinoma

Fig. 6.9

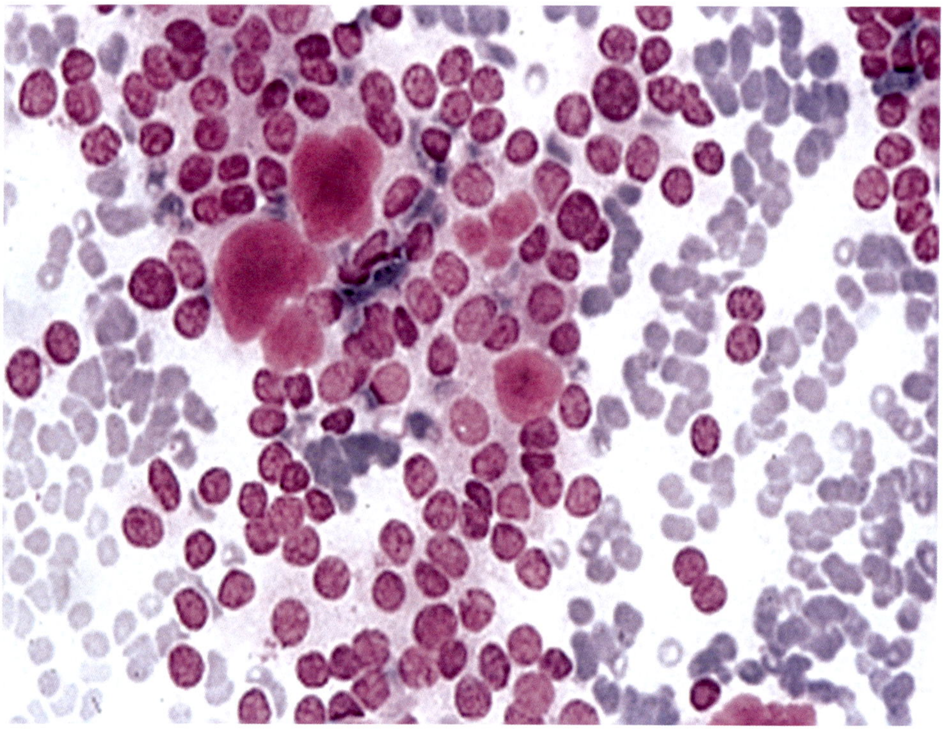

Q-9. A 57-year-old male with a 1.5 cm-nodule in the hard palate of 3-month duration. FNA of hard palate mass.
(a) Adenoid cystic carcinoma
(b) Basal cell adenoma/adenocarcinoma
(c) Epithelial myoepithelial carcinoma
(d) Carcinoma expleomorphic adenoma
(e) Polymorphous low grade adenocarcinoma

Fig. 6.10

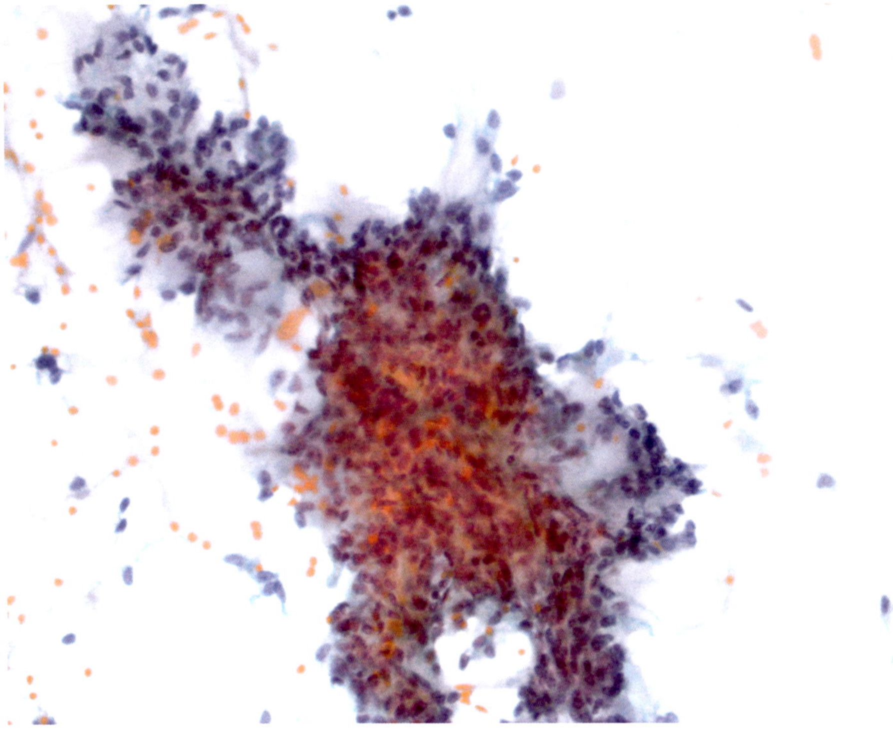

Q-10. A43-year-old female presents with a 1.5-cm mass lifting her left ear lobe. FNA of the mass.

(a) Spindle cell lipoma
(b) Schwannoma
(c) Pleomorphic adenoma (mixed tumor)
(d) Acinic cell carcinoma
(e) Polymorphous low grade adenocarcinoma

Fig. 6.11

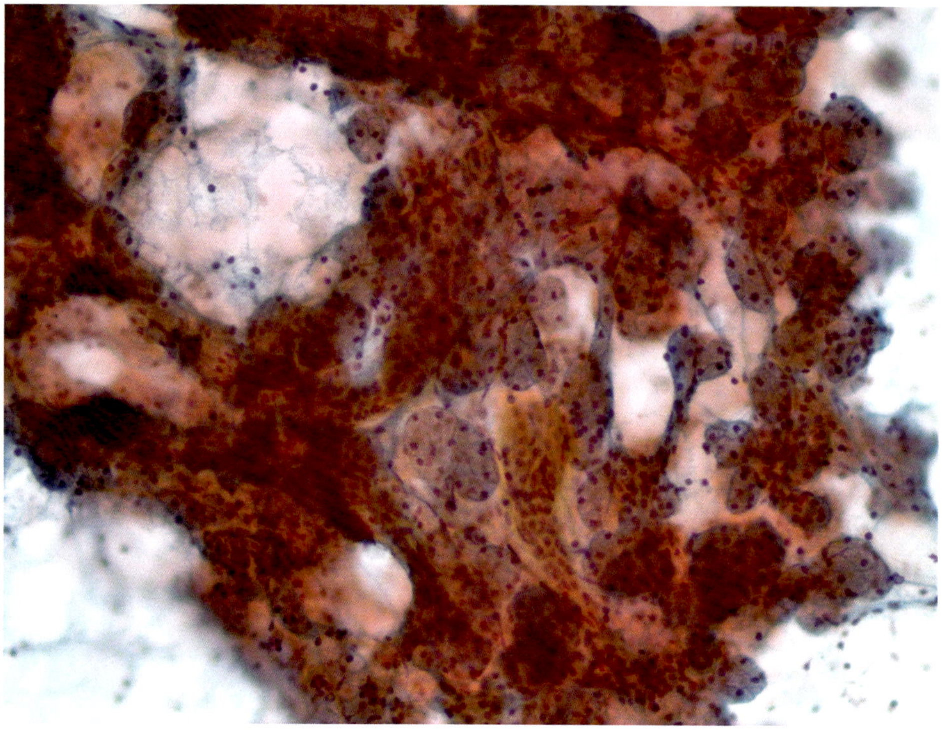

Q-11. A 50-year-old male presents with mild enlargement of the right parotid. FNA of right parotid.

(a) Pleomorphic adenoma (mixed tumor)
(b) Acinic cell carcinoma
(c) Benign acini
(d) Low grade mucoepidermoid carcinoma
(e) Adenoid cystic carcinoma

Fig. 6.12

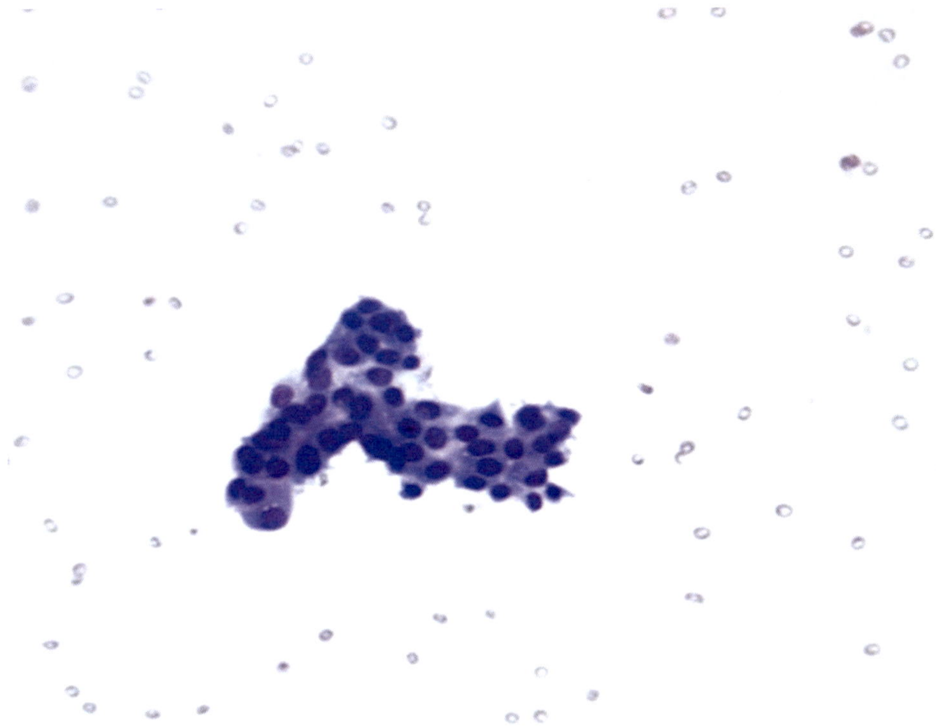

Q-12. This is an aspirate of a slightly enlarged left submandibular gland from a 57-year-old male.
(a) Benign duct epithelium
(b) Low grade mucoepidermoid carcinoma
(c) Pleomorphic adenoma (mixed tumor)
(d) Acinic cell carcinoma
(e) Warthin tumor

Fig. 6.13

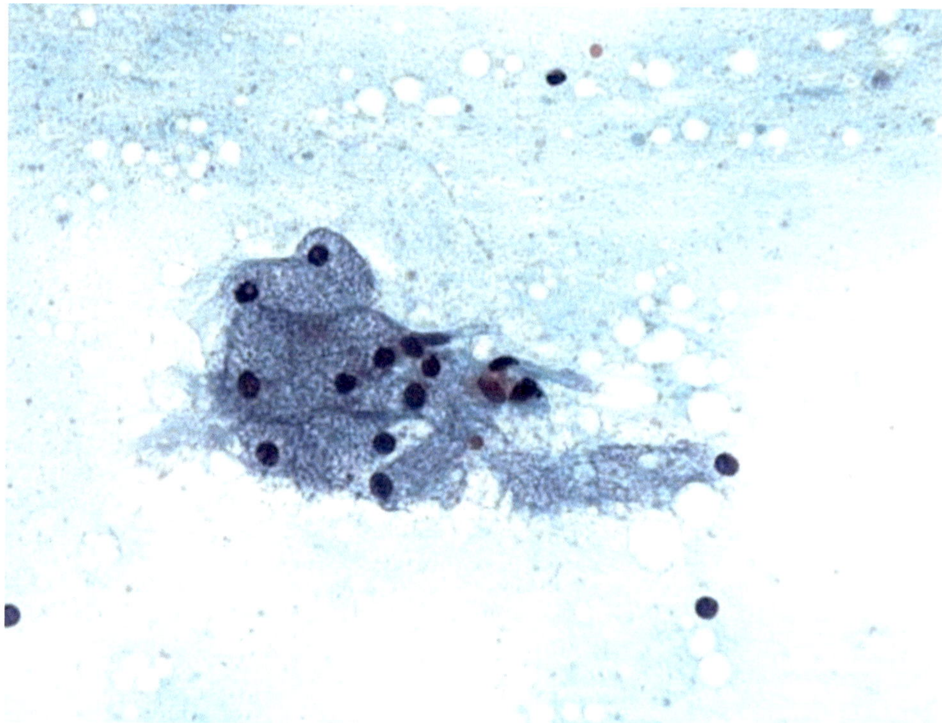

Q-13. FNA of an enlarged right parotid gland in a 67-year-old female.
(a) Metastatic renal cell carcinoma
(b) Low grade mucoepidermoid carcinoma
(c) Clear cell acinic cell carcinoma
(d) Pleomorphic adenoma (mixed tumor)
(e) Sebaceous differentiation

Fig. 6.14

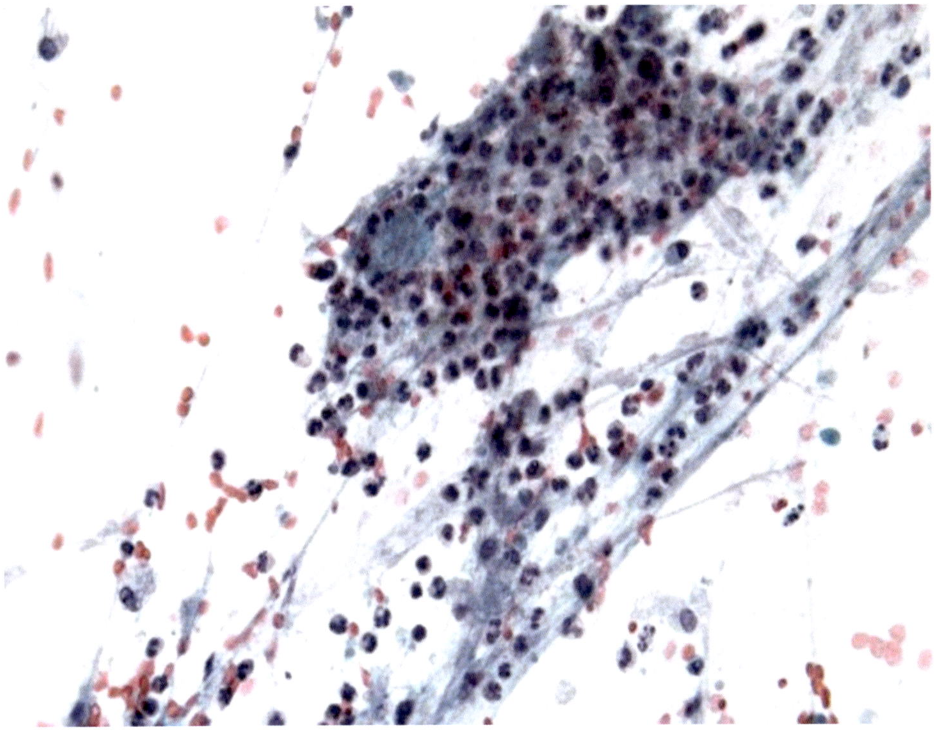

Q-14. Aspirated from an enlarged and tender right parotid mass in a 37-year-old female.
(a) Warthin tumor
(b) Low grade lymphoma
(c) Acute sialadenitis
(d) Chronic sialadenitis
(e) Sialometaplasia

Fig. 6.15

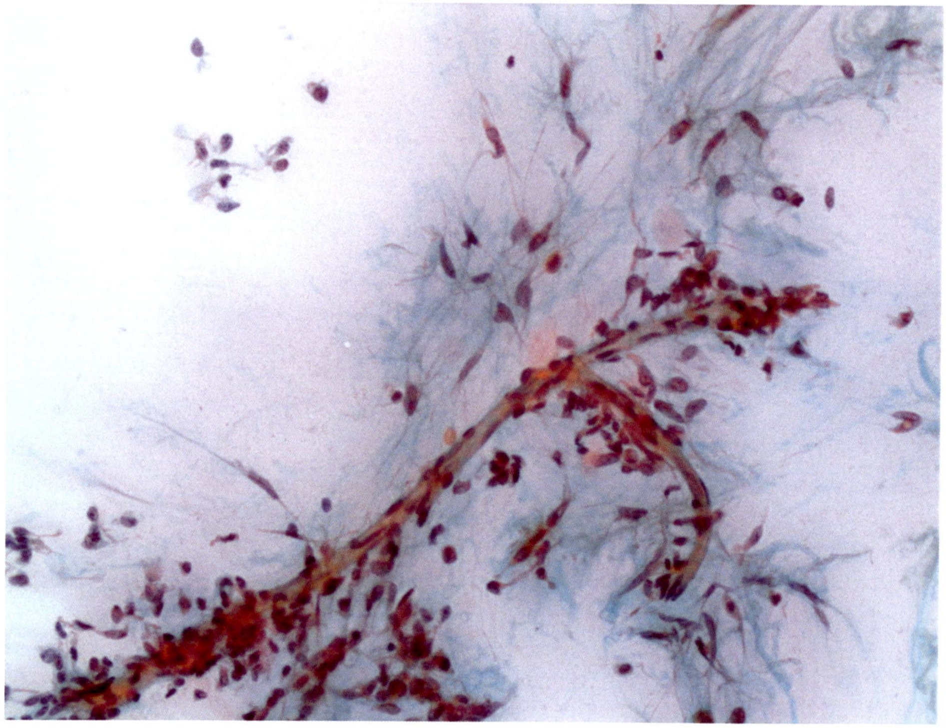

Q-15. This submandibular aspirate is most likely representative of…

(a) Low grade mucoepidermoid carcinoma
(b) Pleomorphic adenoma (mixed tumor)
(c) Acinic cell carcinoma
(d) Myxoid lipoma
(e) Hamartoma

Fig. 6.16

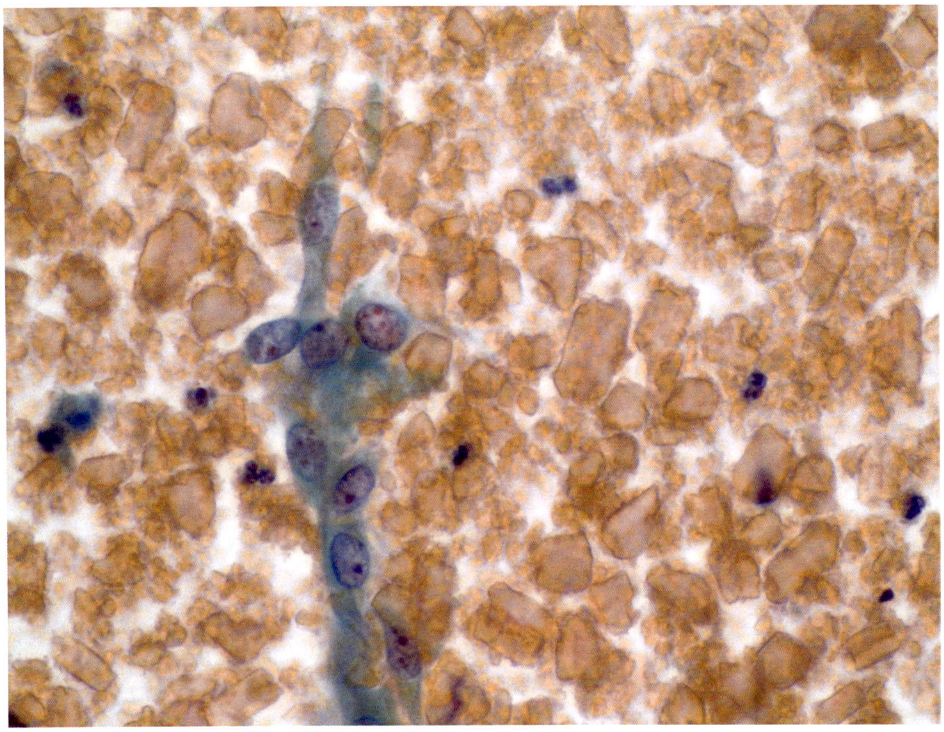

Q-16. This is an aspirate of right parotid mass of a 32-year-old male. The most likely diagnosis is…

(a) Chronic sialadenitis
(b) Pleomorphic adenoma (mixed tumor)
(c) Nondiagnostic aspirate
(d) Acinic cell carcinoma
(e) Warthin tumor

Fig. 6.17

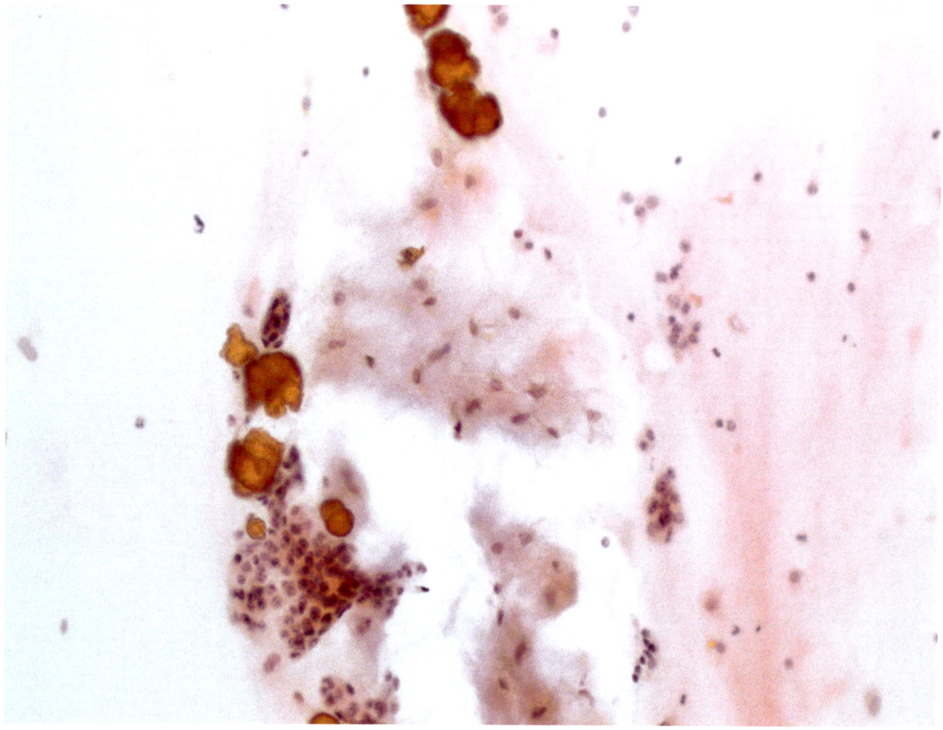

Q-17. A 56-year-old male presented with a 2.5-cm mass in the left submandibular gland. FNA of the mass.

(a) Low grade mucoepidermoid carcinoma
(b) Acinic cell carcinoma
(c) Chronic sialadenitis with crystalloid formation
(d) Pleomorphic adenoma (mixed tumor)
(e) Benign salivary component

Fig. 6.18

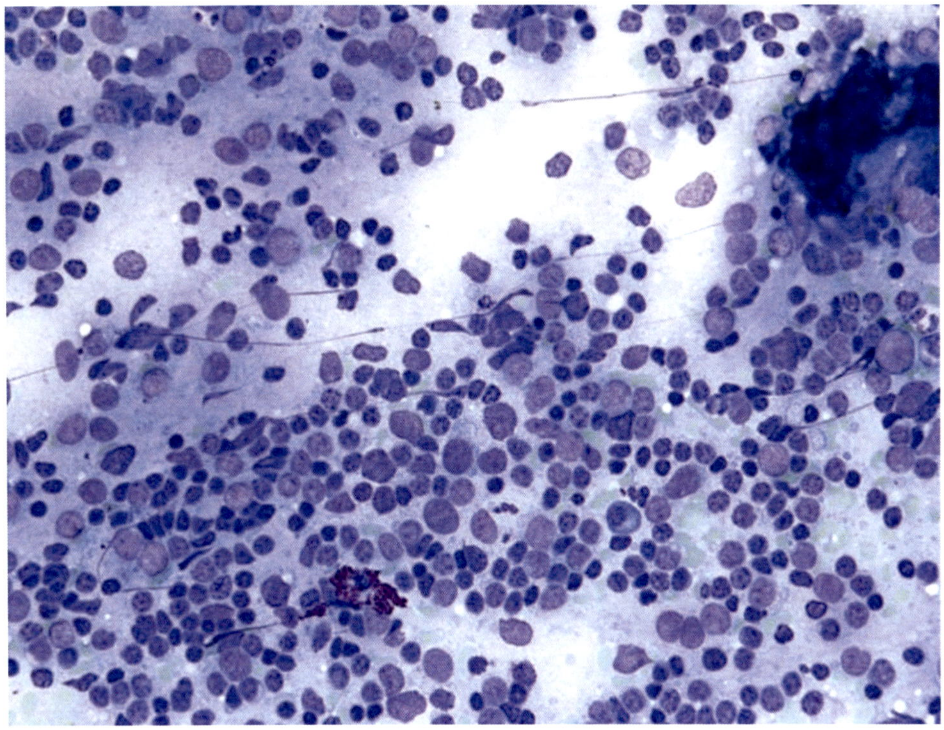

Q-18. FNA of a right parotid enlargement in a 49-year-old female.

(a) Warthin tumor
(b) Acinic cell carcinoma
(c) Chronic sialadenitis
(d) Pleomorphic adenoma (mixed tumor)
(e) Benign intra-parotid lymph node

Fig. 6.19

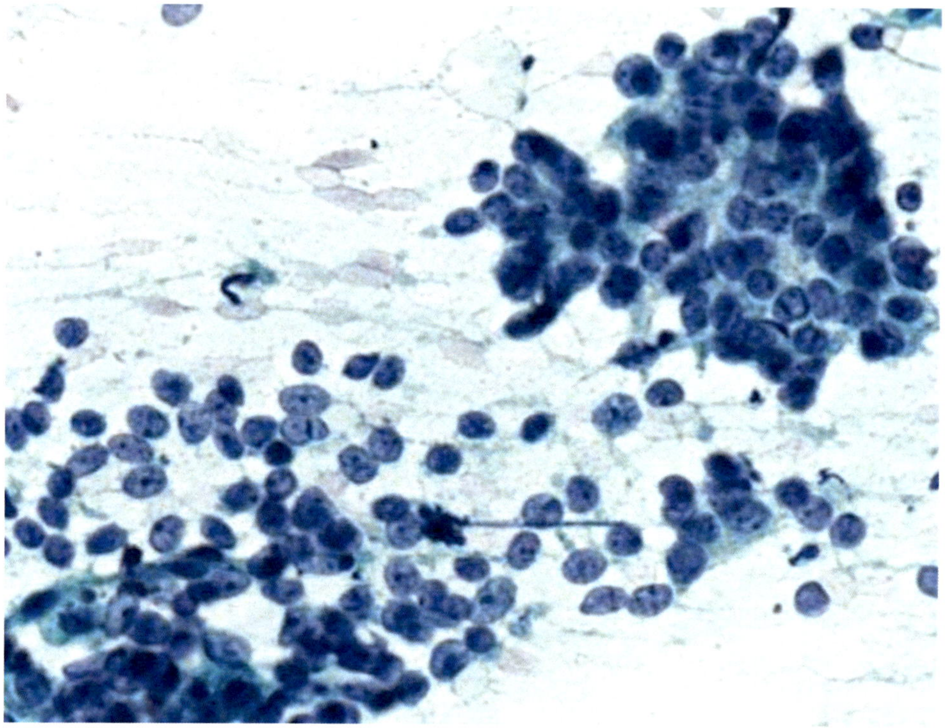

Q-19. This aspirate is from a submandibular mass in a 76-year-old female. What is the most likely diagnosis?
(a) Adenoid cystic carcinoma
(b) Basal cell adenoma/adenocarcinoma
(c) Pleomorphic adenoma (mixed tumor)
(d) Warthin tumor
(e) Basaloid neoplasm

Fig. 6.20

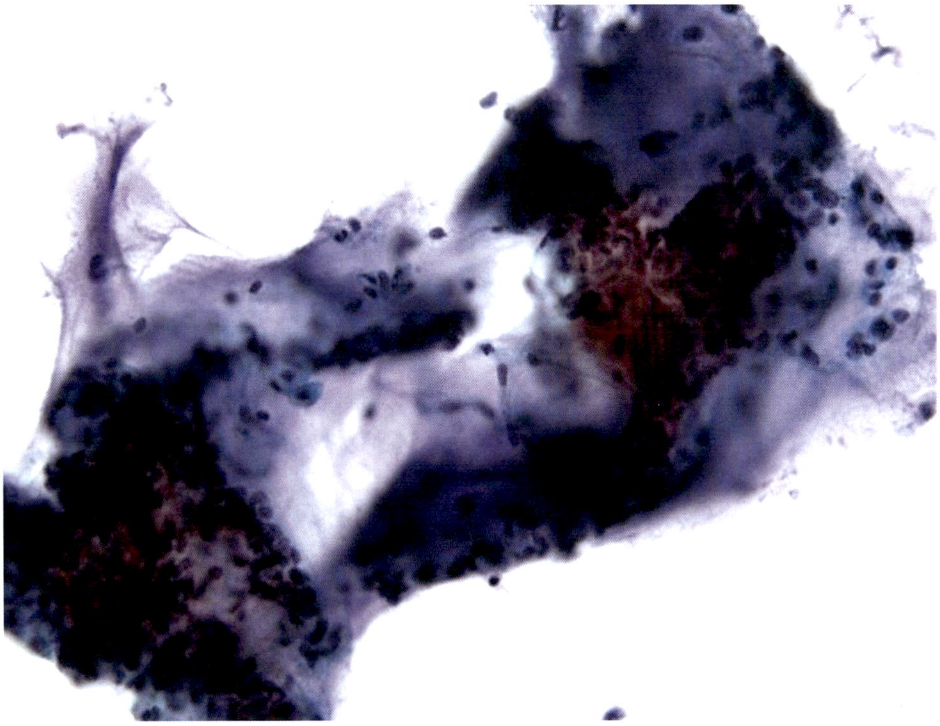

Q-20. A 17-year-old male presented with a right parotid mass. FNA of parotid mass.
(a) Pleomorphic adenoma
(b) Warthin tumor
(c) Mucocele
(d) Low grade mucoepidermoid carcinoma
(e) Chronic sialadenitis

Fig. 6.21

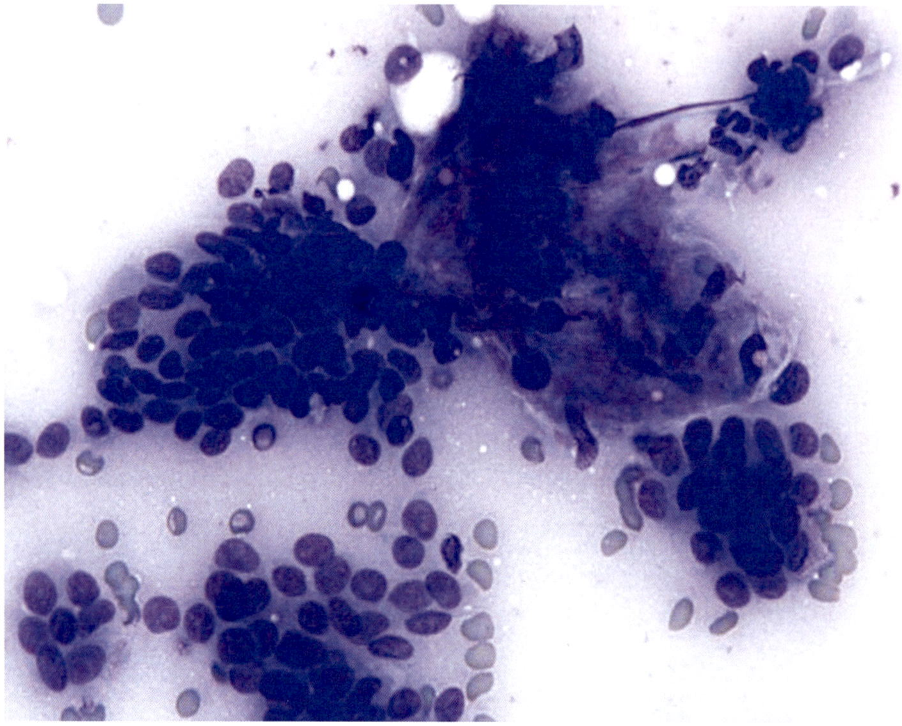

Q-21. This 58-year-old female presented with a slowly enlarging nodule in the hard palate. FNA of palate nodule.

(a) Adenoid cystic carcinoma
(b) Pleomorphic adenoma (mixed tumor)
(c) Acinic cell carcinoma
(d) Warthin tumor
(e) Polymorphous low grade adenocarcinoma

Fig. 6.22

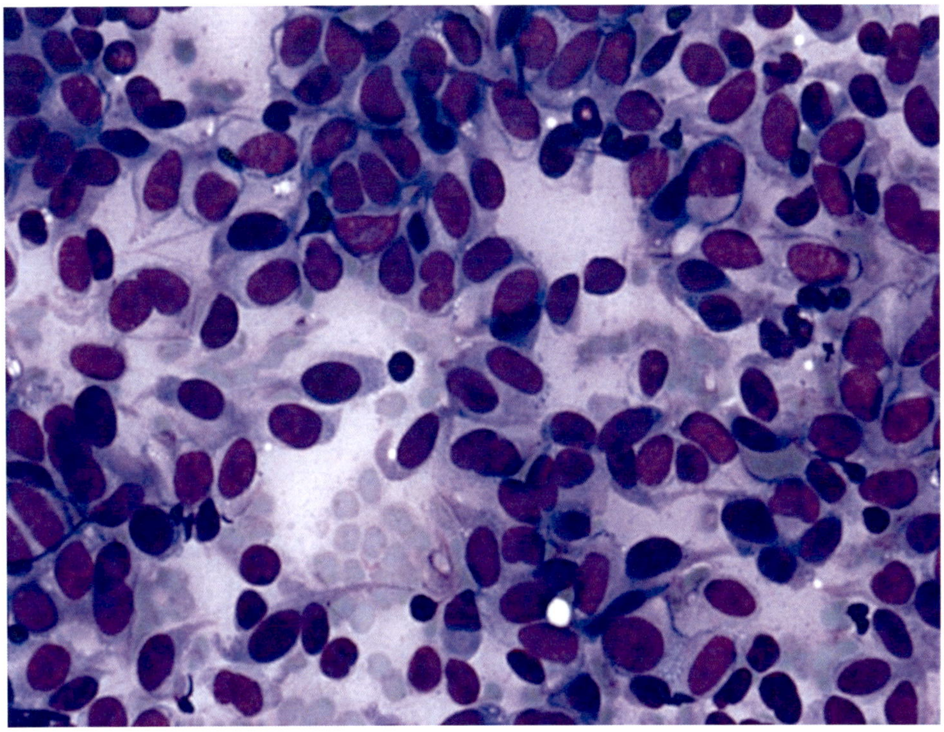

Q-22. An aspirate from a left parotid mass in a 69-year-old male. Patient had a malignant tumor of skin. What is the most likely diagnosis?

(a) Metastatic squamous cell carcinoma
(b) Metastatic spindle cell melanoma
(c) Salivary duct carcinoma
(d) Cellular pleomorphic adenoma
(e) Acinic cell carcinoma

Fig. 6.23

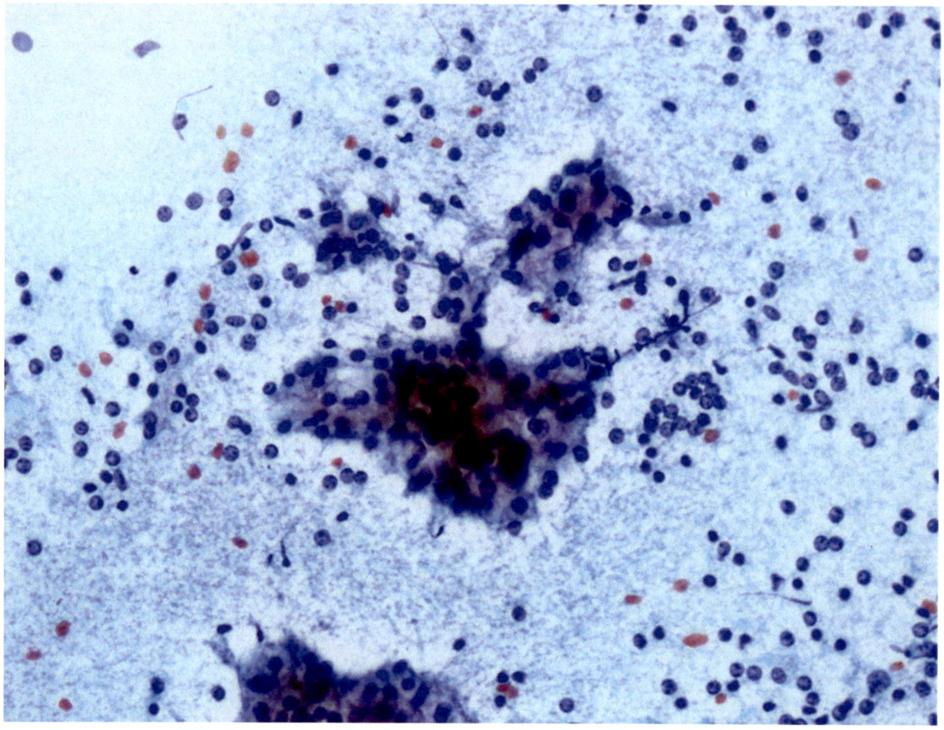

Q-23. A 58-year-old male with a slowly enlarging mass in the right submandibular. FNA submandibular mass.

(a) Pleomorphic adenoma (mixed tumor)
(b) Warthin tumor
(c) Acinic cell carcinoma
(d) Low grade mucoepidermoid carcinoma
(e) Benign intra-parotid lymph node

Fig. 6.24

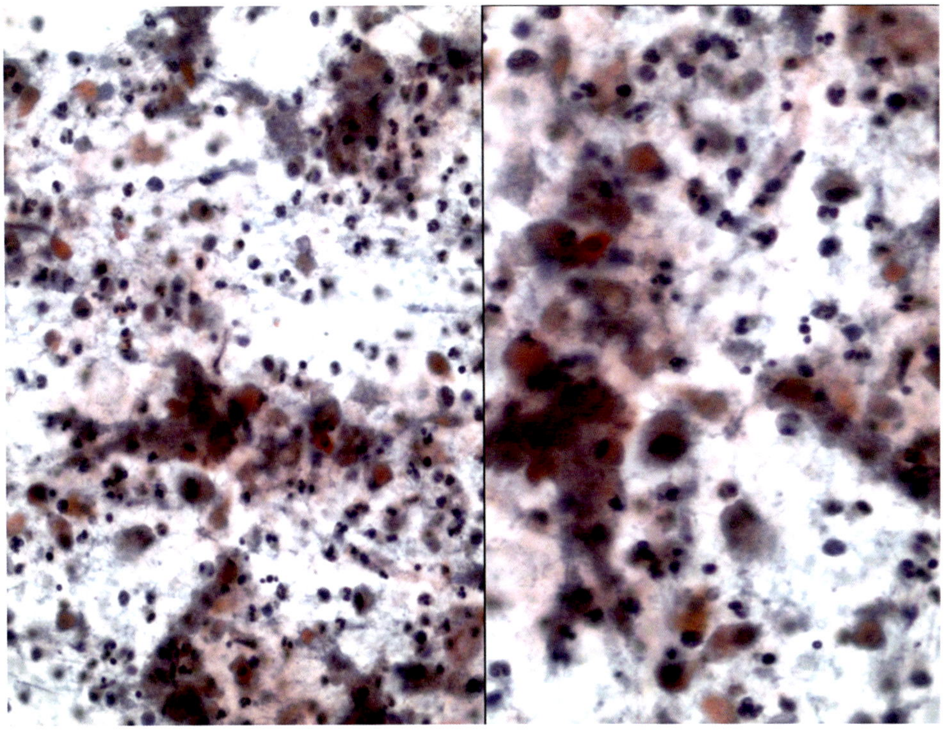

Q-24. A 74-year-old male presented with a 3.5 cm cystic mass in the right parotid. Mass was noted present for many years. FNA parotid mass.

(a) Acinic cell carcinoma
(b) Metastatic squamous cell carcinoma
(c) Warthin tumor
(d) High grade mucoepidermoid carcinoma
(e) Chronic sialadenitis

Fig. 6.25

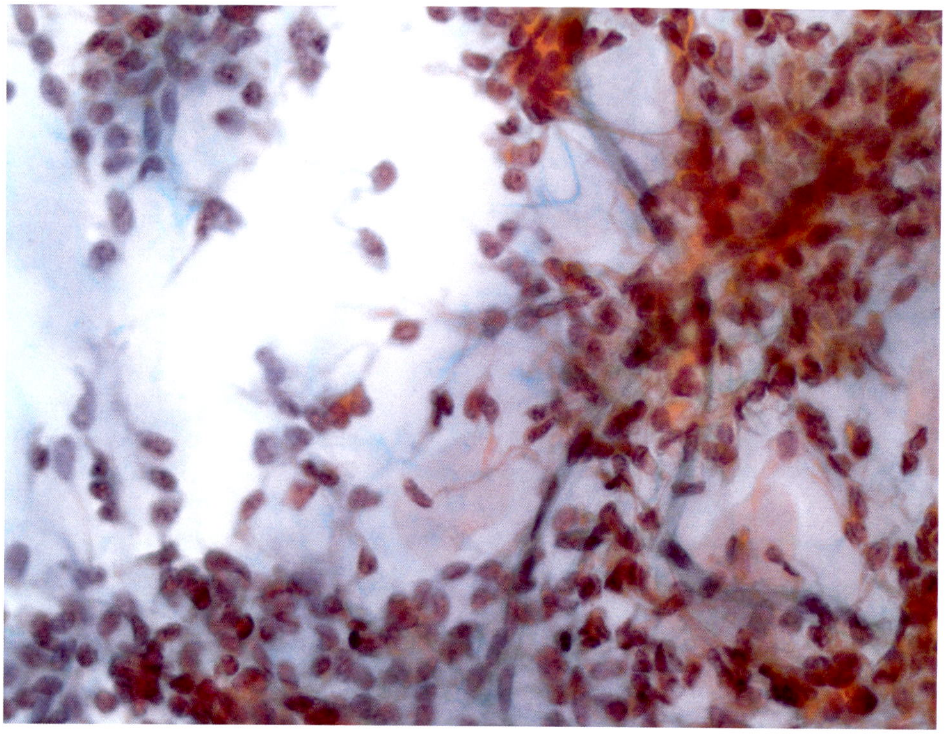

Q-25. Which of the following is *not true* regarding this tumor?

(a) It is the most common tumor of salivary glands
(b) It may contain tyrosine-rich crystalloids
(c) It may occasionally contain cystic area
(d) It may contain squamous or oncocytic cells
(e) If untreated, it commonly undergo sarcomatous changes

Fig. 6.26

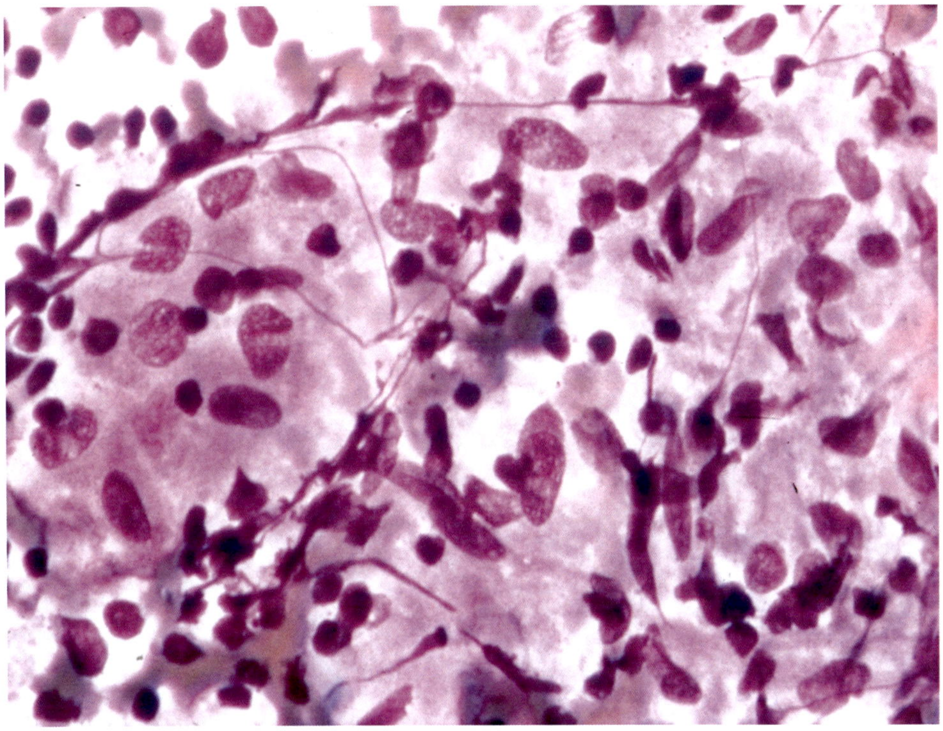

Q-26. A 55-year-old male presented with an enlarged left parotid of few months duration. FNA of parotid mass.

(a) Granulomatous sialadenitis
(b) Mucocele
(c) Cellular pleomorphic adenoma
(d) Acinic cell carcinoma
(e) Warthin tumor

Fig. 6.27

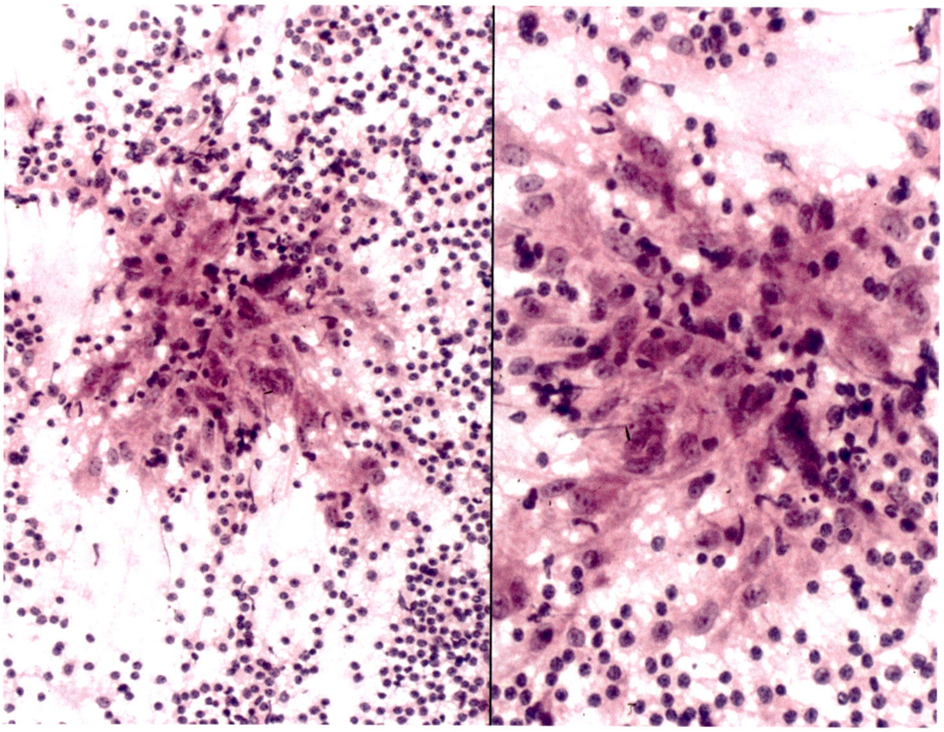

Q-27. Parotid swelling in a 58-year-old female of several months duration. FNA of parotid mass.

(a) Acinic cell carcinoma
(b) Metastatic renal cell carcinoma
(c) Mucoepidermoid carcinoma
(d) Warthin tumor
(e) Lymphoepithelial sialadenitis

Fig. 6.28

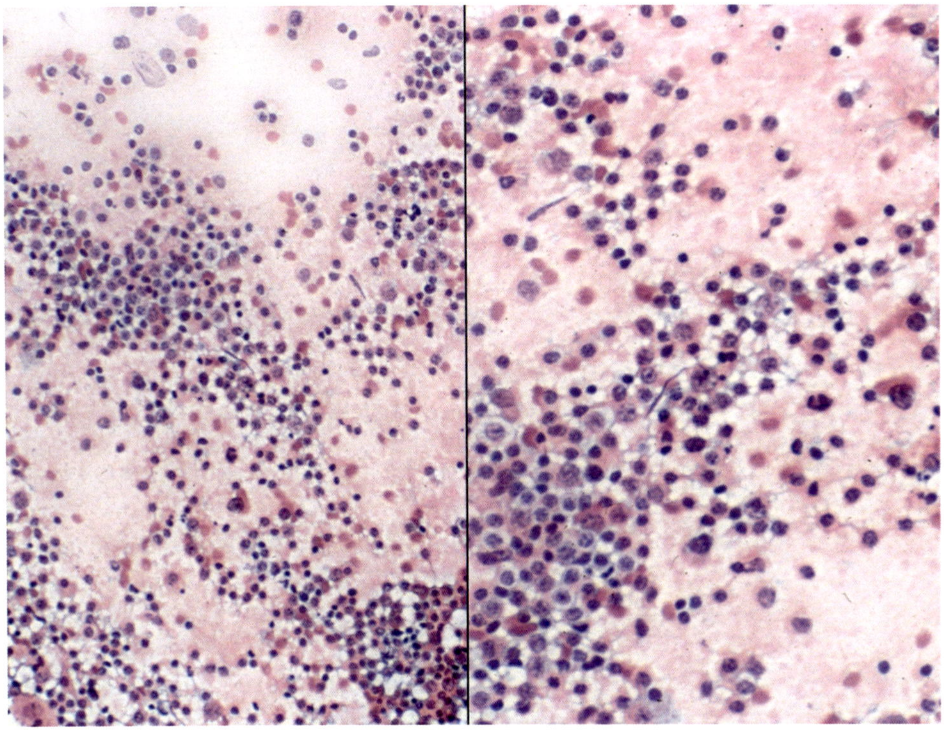

Q-28. A 45-year-old HIV positive presented with a cystic mass in his left parotid. FNA of cystic parotid mass.

(a) Lymphoepithelial cyst
(b) Warthin tumor
(c) Lymphoepithelial sialadenitis
(d) Low grade mucoepidermoid carcinoma
(e) Benign intra-parotid lymph node

Fig. 6.29

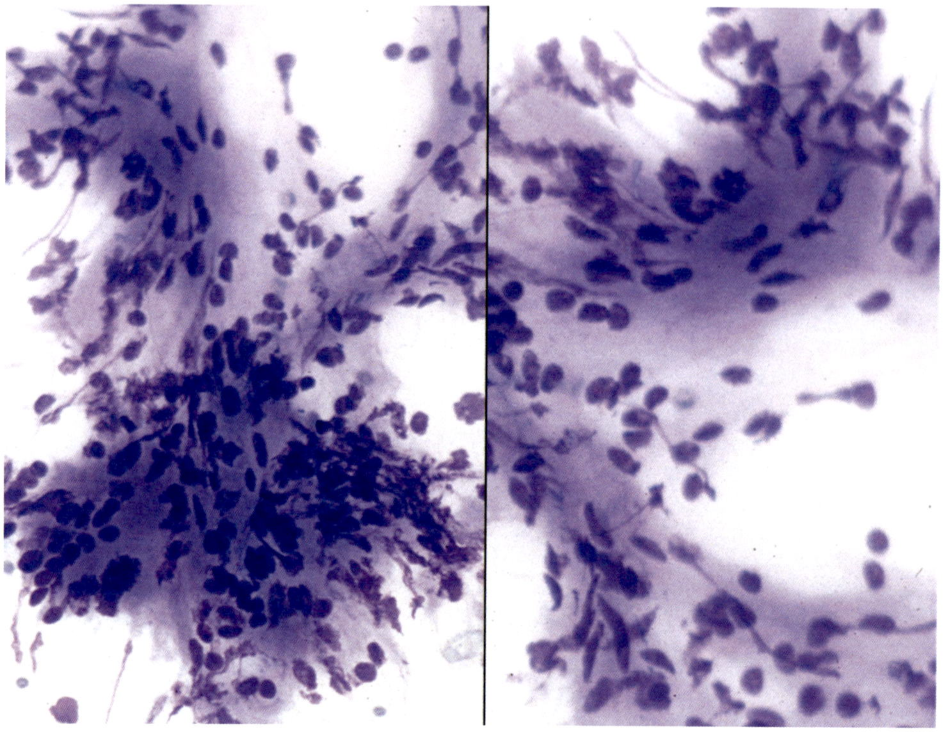

Q-29. A 55-year-old male reported to the ENT clinic because of a swelling in the right parotid region. FNA of right parotid mass.

(a) Myoepithelioma
(b) Schwannoma
(c) Myoepithelial predominant pleomorphic adenoma
(d) Nodular fasciitis
(e) Fibromatosis

Fig. 6.30

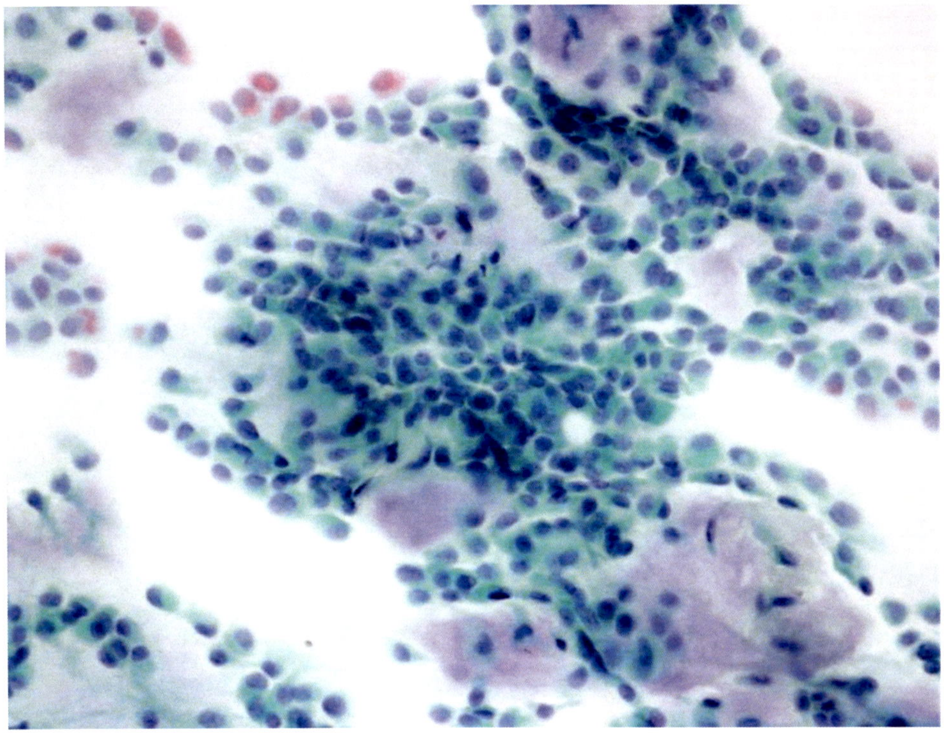

Q-30. FNA of a 2-cm parotid mass in a 45-year-old female.
FNA of the parotid mass.
(a) Low grade mucoepidermoid carcinoma
(b) Pleomorphic adenoma
(c) Warthin tumor
(d) Acinic cell carcinoma
(e) Myoepithelioma

Fig. 6.31

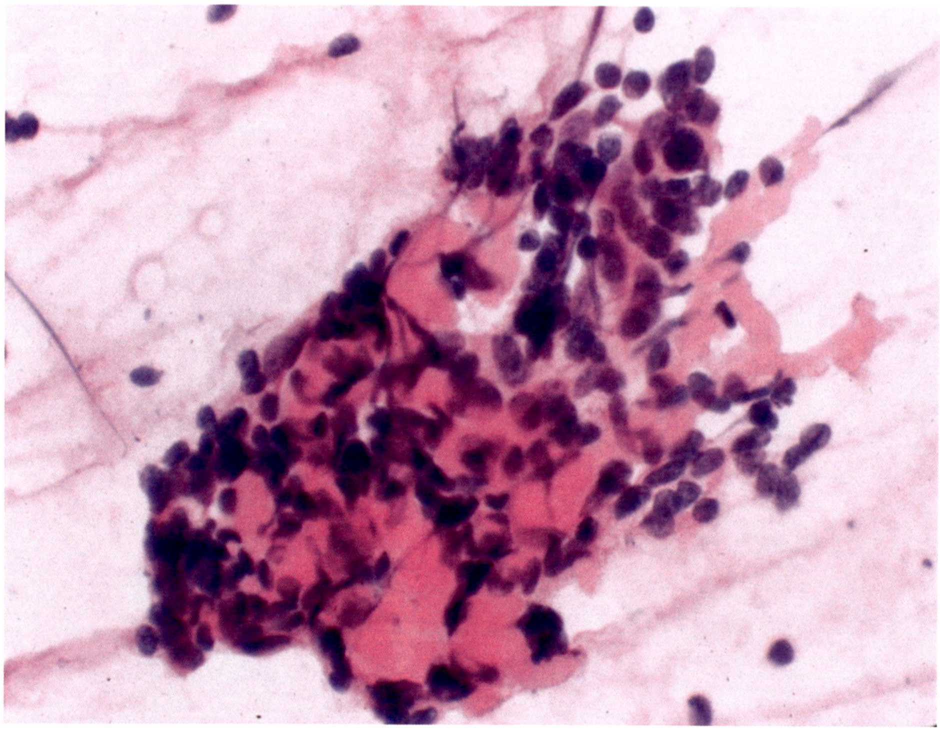

Q-31. A 47-year-old female presented with a 2-cm mass in the left submandibular gland. FNA of submandibular mass.

(a) Warthin tumor
(b) Basal cell adenoma/adenocarcinoma
(c) Pleomorphic adenoma
(d) Epithelial myoepithelial carcinoma
(e) Polymorphous low grade adenocarcinoma

Fig. 6.32

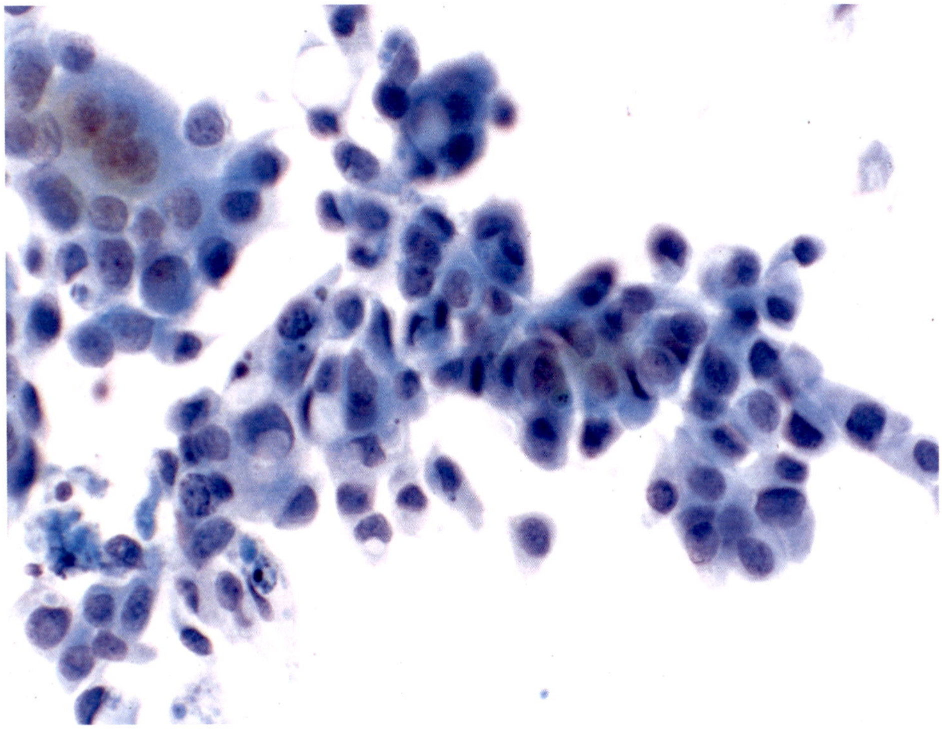

Q-32. A 65-year-old male presented with a right parotid mass of few months duration. FNA of parotid mass.

(a) Pleomorphic adenoma
(b) Adenoid cystic carcinoma
(c) Basal cell adenoma/adenocarcinoma
(d) Mucoepidermoid carcinoma
(e) Metastatic squamous cell carcinoma

Fig. 6.33

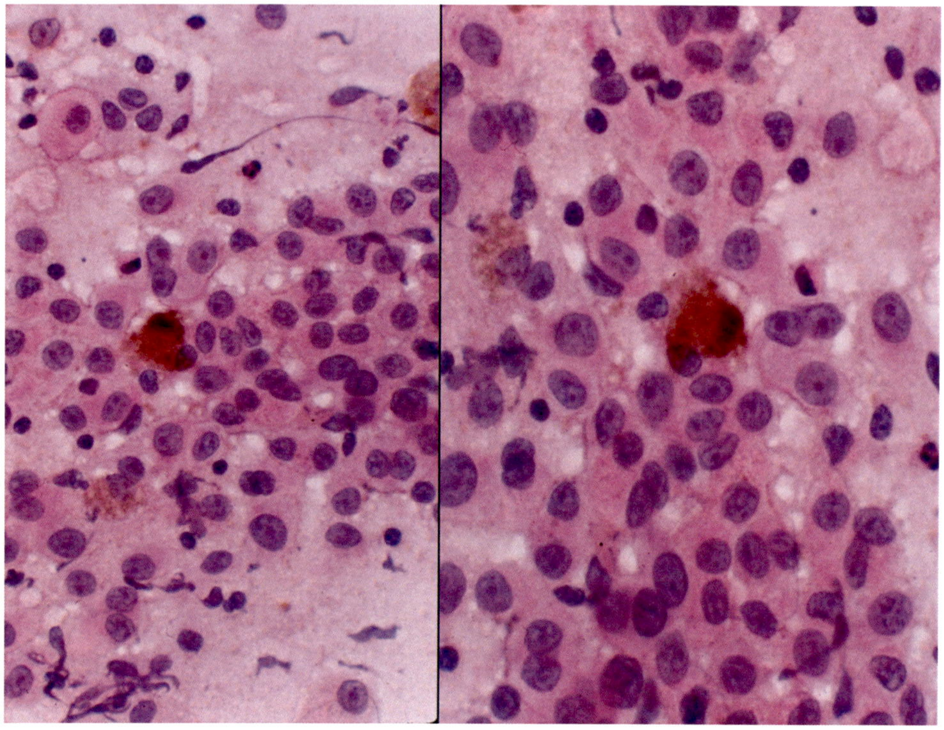

Q-33. A 78-year-old male with history of prior malignancy in the skin of the neck presented with a right parotid mass. FNA of parotid mass.

(a) Metastatic melanoma
(b) Mucocele
(c) Low grade mucoepidermoid carcinoma
(d) Oncocytoma
(e) Lymphoma, diffuse large B-type

Fig. 6.34

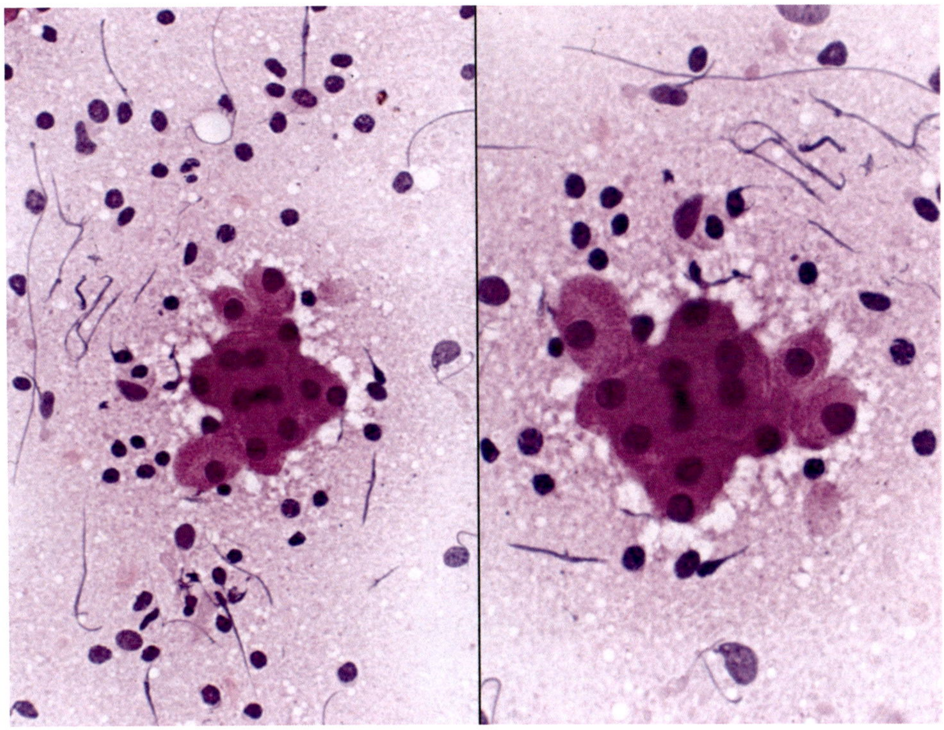

Q-34. Cystic mass left parotid in a 48-year-old female. FNA of cystic parotid mass
(a) Acinic cell carcinoma
(b) Warthin tumor
(c) Oncocytoma
(d) Pleomorphic adenoma with oncocytic metaplasia
(e) Oncocytic mucoepidermoid carcinoma

Fig. 6.35

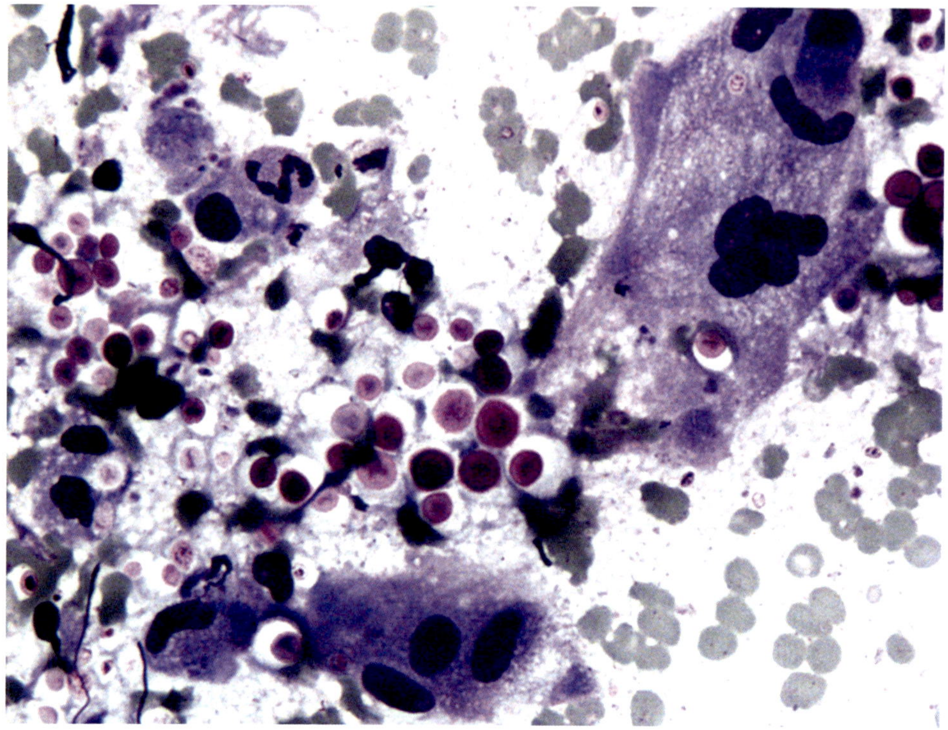

Q-35. Parotid mass in a 38-year-old male. FNA of parotid mass.

(a) Pleomorphic adenoma
(b) Adenoid cystic carcinoma
(c) Chronic sialadenitis
(d) Sarcoidosis
(e) Cryptococcus sialadenitis

Fig. 6.36

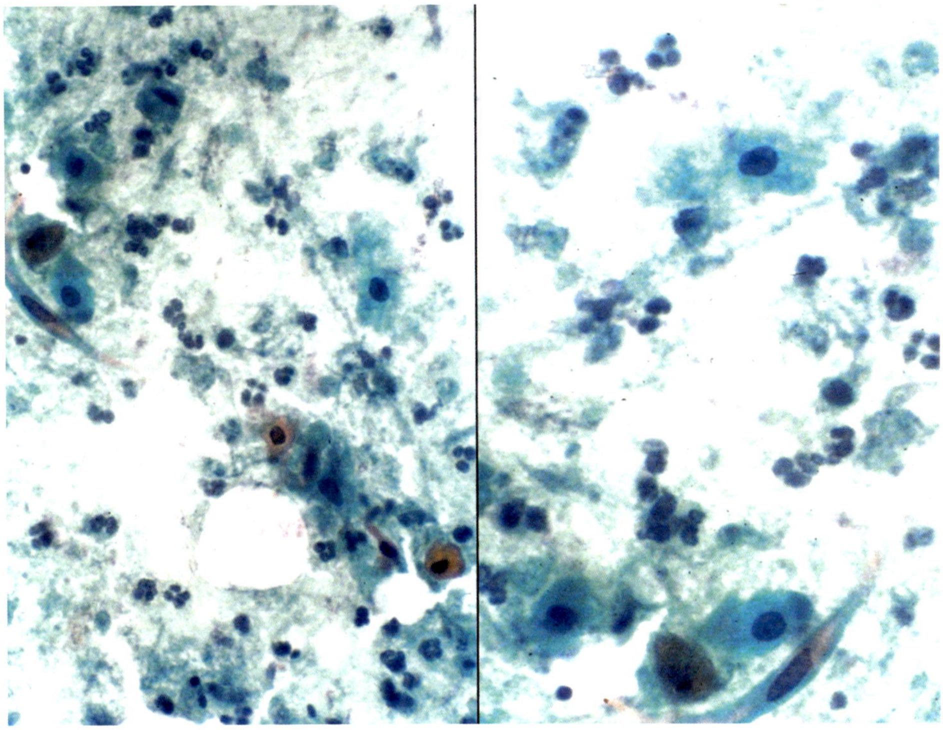

Q-36. Cystic parotid mass in a 50-year-old female. FNA of parotid cystic mass.
(a) Mucoepidermoid carcinoma
(b) Metastatic squamous carcinoma
(c) Cystic pleomorphic adenoma
(d) Chronic sialadenitis
(e) Warthin tumor with squamous metaplasia

Fig. 6.37

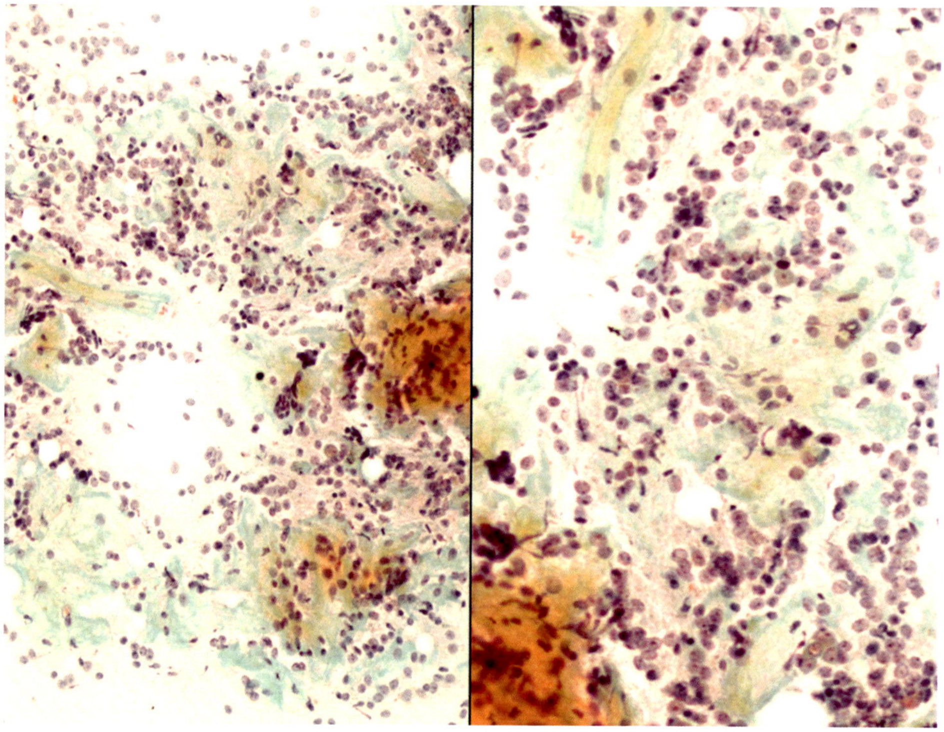

Q-37. Parotid mass in a 69-year-old male. Mass was present for many years but recently enlarging. FNA of parotid mass.

(a) Pleomorphic adenoma
(b) Mucoepidermoid carcinoma
(c) Carcinoma expleomorphic adenoma
(d) Warthin tumor
(e) Myoepithelioma

Fig. 6.38

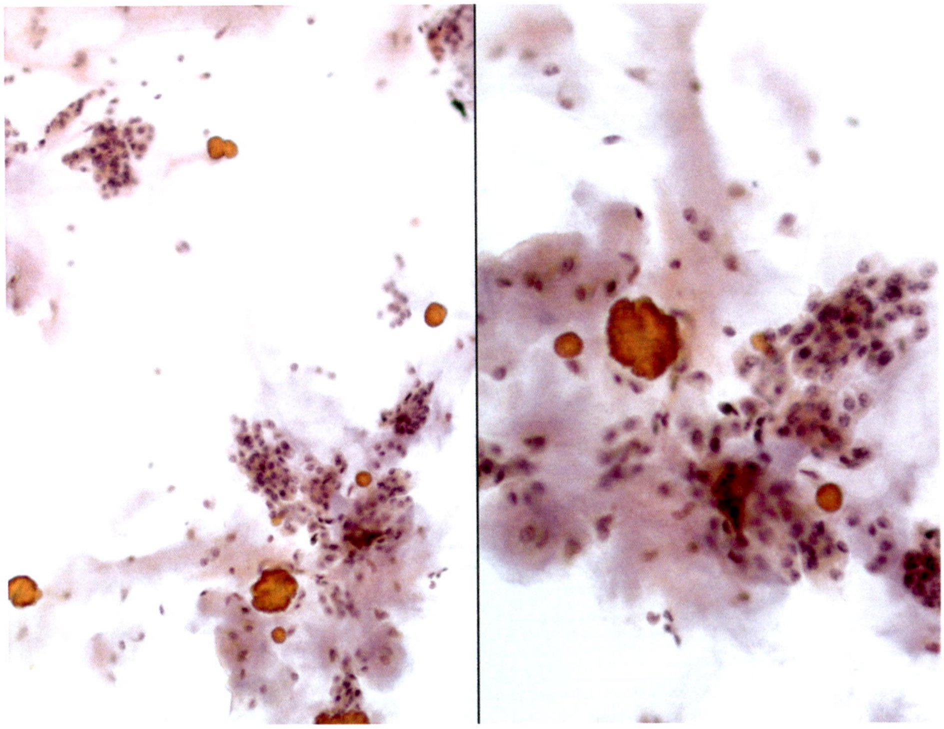

Q-38. Parotid mass in a 45-year-old female. FNA of parotid mass.

(a) Pleomorphic adenoma with amylase crystalloid
(b) Pleomorphic adenoma with tyrosine rich crystalloids
(c) Chronic sialadenitis
(d) Mucoepidermoid carcinoma, low grade
(e) Acinic cell carcinoma with crystalloids

Fig. 6.39

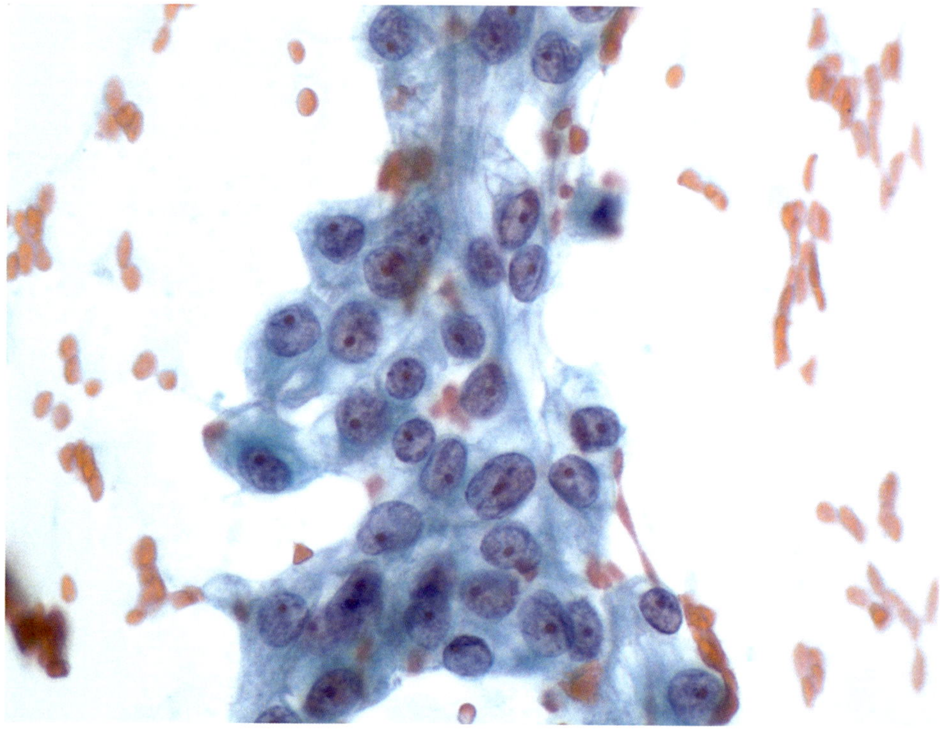

Q-39. A 45-year-old male presents with a mass in the left parotid gland. Five years ago patient had left nephrectomy due to carcinoma. FNA parotid mass.

(a) Pleomorphic adenoma
(b) Mucoepidermoid carcinoma, low grade
(c) Myoepithelioma
(d) Acinic cell carcinoma
(e) Metastatic renal cell carcinoma

Fig. 6.40

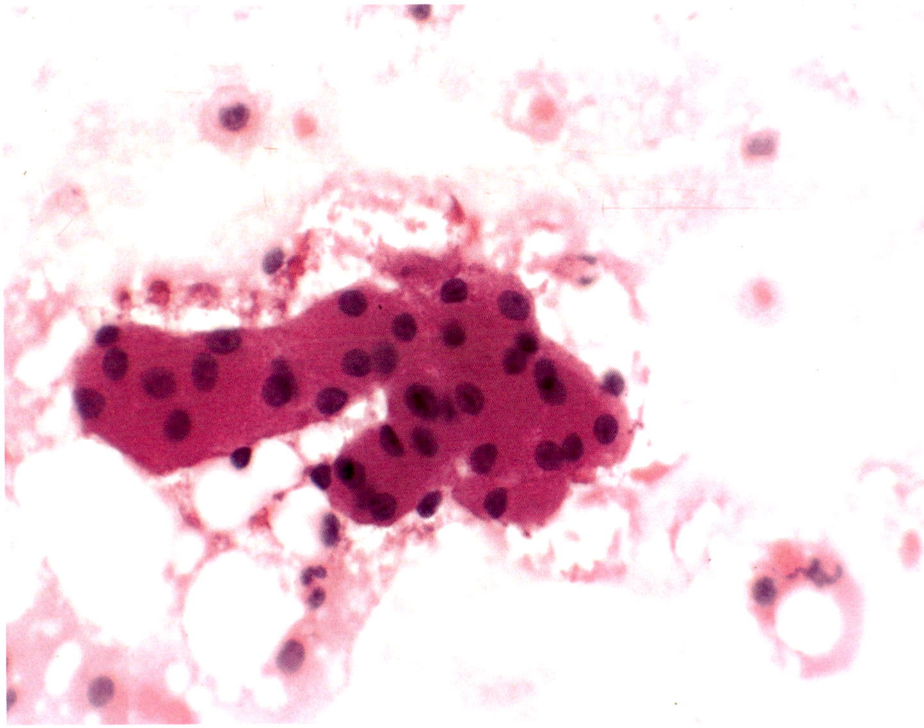

Q-40. Left parotid mss in a 43-year-old male. FNA of parotid mass.
(a) Warthin tumor
(b) Oncocytic mucoepidermoid carcinoma
(c) Myoepithelioma
(d) Pleomorphic adenoma with an oncocytic component
(e) Oncocytoma

Fig. 6.41

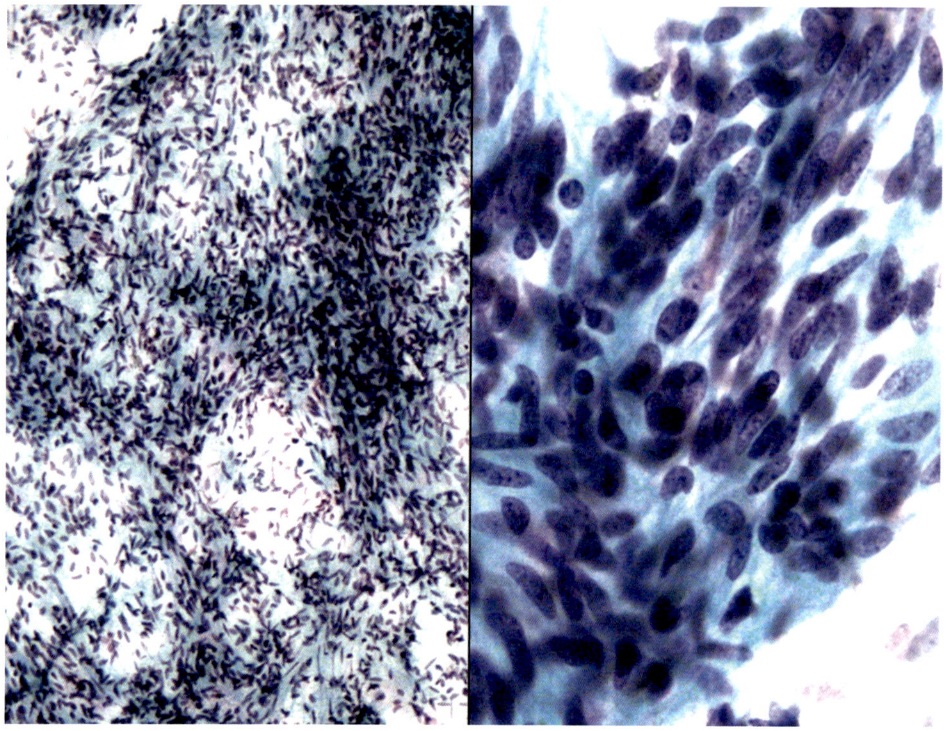

Q-41. A 11-year-old female presents with a mass in the left parotid gland. She has history of embryonal rhabdomyosarcoma in the head and neck region. FNA parotid mass.

(a) Pleomorphic adenoma
(b) inflammatory pseudotumor
(c) Metastatic rhabdomyosarcoma
(d) Mucoepidermoid carcinoma
(e) Myoepithelioma

Fig. 6.42

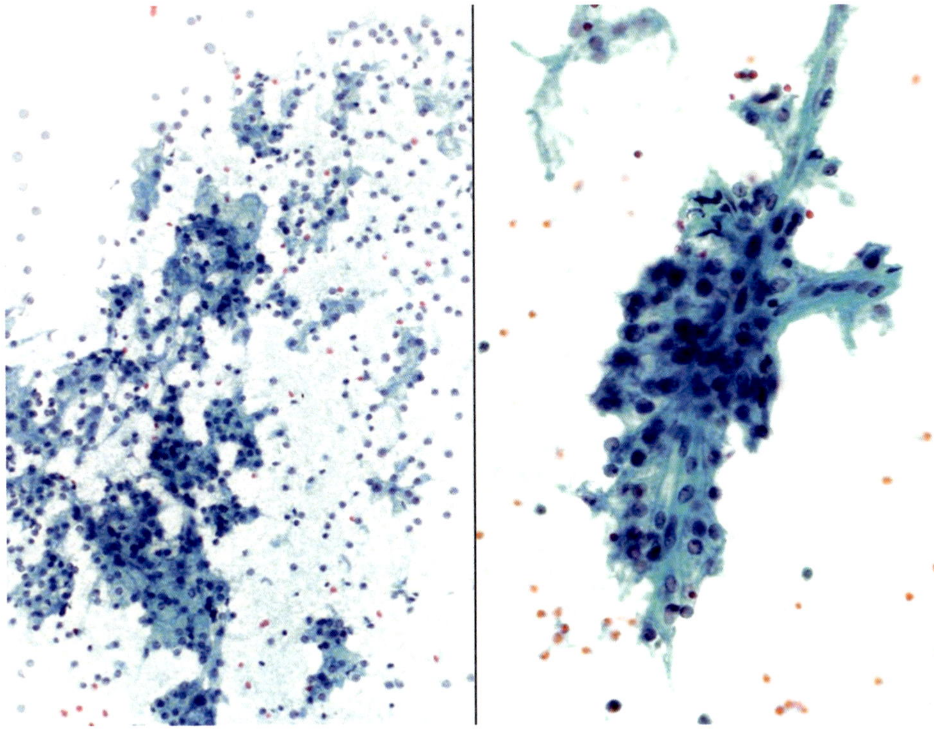

Q-42. A 66-year-old male presented with 2-cm parotid mass. FNA of parotid mass was performed. Representative images are seen below. What is the most likely diagnosis?
(a) Pleomorphic adenoma (mixed tumor)
(b) Acinic cell carcinoma
(c) Warthin tumor
(d) Low grade mucoepidermoid carcinoma
(e) Benign intra-parotid lymph node

Fig. 6.43

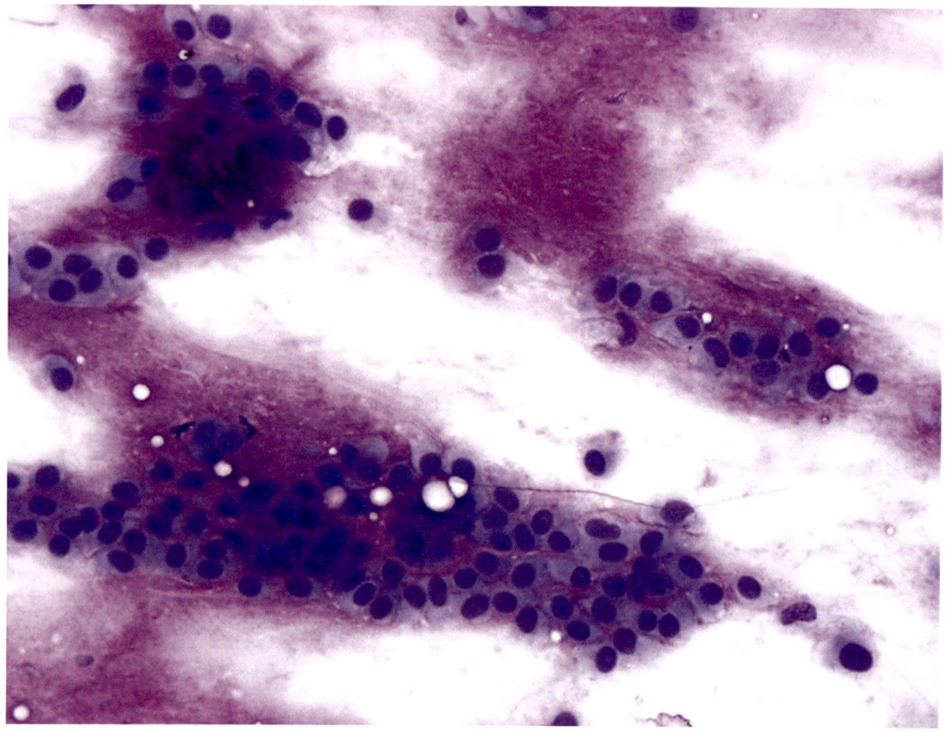

Q-43. A 37-year-old female presented with 3-cm parotid mass. FNA of parotid mass was performed. Representative image is seen below. What is the most likely diagnosis?

(a) Pleomorphic adenoma (mixed tumor)
(b) Acinic cell carcinoma
(c) Warthin tumor
(d) Adenoid cystic carcinoma
(e) Salivary duct carcinoma

Fig. 6.44

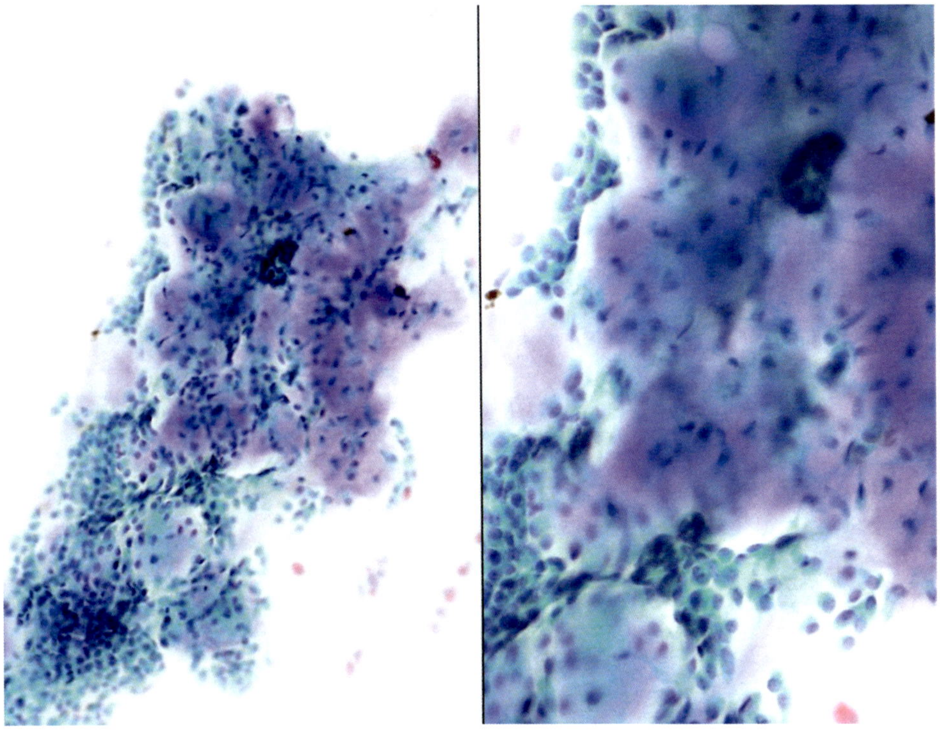

Q-44. A 51-year-old male presented with 2-cm parotid mass. FNA of parotid mass was performed. Representative image is seen below. What is the most likely diagnosis?
(a) Adenoid cystic carcinoma
(b) Acinic cell carcinoma
(c) Warthin tumor
(d) Pleomorphic adenoma (mixed tumor)
(e) Salivary duct carcinoma

Fig. 6.45

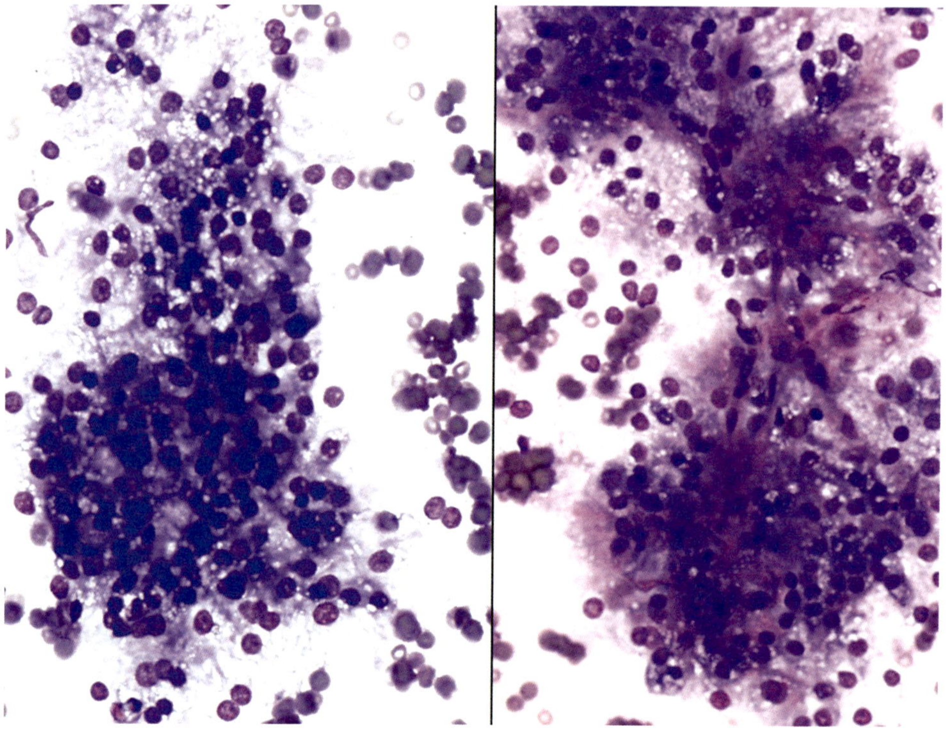

Q-45. A 55-year-old female presented with 3-cm parotid mass and lymphadenopathy. FNA of parotid mass was performed. Representative image is seen below. What is the most likely diagnosis?

(a) Acinic cell carcinoma
(b) Oncocytoma
(c) Basal cell carcinoma
(d) Warthin tumor
(e) Low grade mucoepidermoid carcinoma

6.2 Text-Based Questions 46–65

Q-46. What is the most common benign salivary gland tumor in infants?
(a) Pleomorphic adenoma (mixed tumor)
(b) Low grade mucoepidermoid carcinoma
(c) Hemangioma
(d) Warthin tumor
(e) Oncocytoma

Q-47. Tyrosine rich crystals are likely to be encountered in which of the following lesions?
(a) Warthin tumor
(b) Chronic sialadenitis
(c) Mucoepidermoid carcinoma
(d) Pleomorphic adenoma
(e) Acinic cell carcinoma

Q-48. Which of the following is not a component in benign salivary gland aspirate?
(a) Acinic cells
(b) Duct epithelium
(c) Myoepithelial cells
(d) Fibroadipose cells
(e) Hyaline globules

Q-49. Amylase crystals are mostly seen in which of the following lesions?
(a) Sialadenitis
(b) Mixed tumor
(c) Adenoid cystic carcinoma
(d) Acinic cell carcinoma
(e) Basal cell adenoma/adenocarcinoma

Q-50. Which of the following salivary gland neoplasms is not known to be grossly cystic?
(a) Adenoid cystic carcinoma
(b) Warthin tumor
(c) Low grade mucoepidermoid carcinoma
(d) Mixed tumor
(e) Acinic cell carcinoma

Q-51. Which of the following lesions is more common in HIV infected patients?
(a) Mixed tumors
(b) Acinic cell carcinoma
(c) Warthin tumor
(d) Lymphoepithelial cyst
(e) Adenoid cystic carcinoma

Q-52. Pleomorphic adenoma (mixed tumor) is known to arise from which part of the salivary gland structures?
(a) Acinus
(b) Striated duct
(c) Intercalated duct
(d) Excretory duct
(e) Myoepithelial cells

Q-53. Tumors that arise from which of the following sites are more likely to be malignant?
(a) Parotid gland
(b) Submandibular gland
(c) Sublingual gland
(d) Minor salivary glands
(e) Parotid and submandibular glands

Q-54. Which of the following is true regarding sialometaplasia?
(a) It occurs almost exclusively in the parotid gland.
(b) It is caused by an ischemic necrosis.
(c) The clinical appearance is diagnostic.
(d) Wide surgical excision is the treatment of choice.
(e) Floor of the mouth is a frequent site.

Q-55. Which one of the following salivary gland tumors arises from the striated duct?
(a) Mucoepidermoid carcinoma
(b) Adenoid cystic carcinoma
(c) Pleomorphic adenoma
(d) Warthin tumor
(e) Acinic cell carcinoma

Q-56. Which one of the following salivary neoplasm has no myoepithelial cells component or origin (p63 immunostain is negative)?
(a) Basal cell adenoma
(b) Adenoid cystic carcinoma
(c) Polymorphous low grade adenocarcinoma
(d) Canalicular adenoma
(e) Pleomorphic adenoma

Q-57. Minor salivary gland tumors are most common in which of the following sites?
(a) Nasal cavity
(b) Main bronchi
(c) Esophagus
(d) Maxillary sinus
(e) Palate

Q-58. Which one of the following salivary gland tumors is most common?
(a) Mucoepidermoid carcinoma
(b) Canalicular adenoma
(c) Polymorphous low grade adenocarcinoma
(d) Pleomorphic adenoma
(e) Adenoid cystic carcinoma

Q-59. Perineural invasion is likely present in which of the following salivary gland tumors?
(a) Pleomorphic adenoma
(b) Warthin tumor
(c) Adenoid cystic carcinoma
(d) Canalicular adenoma
(e) Mucoepidermoid carcinoma

Q-60. Numerous lymphocytes are likely to be present in which of the following salivary gland aspirates?
(a) Pleomorphic adenoma
(b) Polymorphous low grade adenocarcinoma
(c) Adenoid cystic carcinoma
(d) Warthin tumor
(e) Canalicular adenoma

Q-61. Which of the following tumors is sometimes bilateral?
(a) Pleomorphic adenoma
(b) Adenoid cystic carcinoma
(c) Salivary duct carcinoma
(d) Warthin tumor
(e) Canalicular adenoma

Q-62. An 80-year-old male presented with a rapidly growing parotid mass associated with facial nerve palsy. Histologic examination of the tumor showed resemblance to comedo duct carcinoma of the breast. This tumor is likely which of the following entities?
(a) Adenoid cystic carcinoma
(b) Recurrent pleomorphic adenoma
(c) Metastatic breast carcinoma
(d) High grade mucoepidermoid carcinoma
(e) Salivary duct carcinoma

Q-63. Which of the following metastatic tumors to salivary gland or intra-parenchymal lymph nodes is most common?
(a) Renal cell carcinoma
(b) Colon adenocarcinoma
(c) Squamous cell carcinoma
(d) Pulmonary small cell carcinoma
(e) Hepatocellular carcinoma

Q-64. Oncocytic cells are not seen in which of the following tumors?
(a) Adenoid cystic carcinoma
(b) Mucoepidermoid carcinoma
(c) Warthin tumor
(d) Pleomorphic adenoma
(e) Acinic cell carcinoma

Q-65. Which of the following statements regarding Warthin tumor is not true?
(a) Almost always occurs in the parotid
(b) Most common benign salivary gland tumor
(c) Associated with cigarette smoking
(d) Always cystic
(e) Most common bilateral salivary gland tumor

6.3 Answers and Discussion of Image-Based Questions 1–45

A-1. **(b) Warthin tumor**
The image displays the classic features of Warthin tumor. There are oncocytes, lymphocytes, and proteinaceous fluid in the background. Oncocytes are characterized by their eosinophilic granular cytoplasm typically present in flat groups. Also, benign lymphocytes are scattered in the background. Warthin tumor is a cystic lesion that often has a doughy feeling on palpation. The aspirate contains a green brown cyst fluid.

A-2. **(d) Acinic cell carcinoma**
The aspirate is cellular with neoplastic acinar cells that are arranged in sheets, crowded clusters, and isolated cells. Cells are large polygonal with indistinct cell borders with vacuolated and abundantly granular cytoplasm. Many naked nuclei are present in the background with or without lymphocytes. Acinic cell carcinoma is the second most common malignant neoplasm of salivary glands accounting for approximately 5 % of all salivary gland neoplasms. It is more common in women, and most of the cases are encountered in the parotid gland. The tumor is bilateral in about 3 % of cases. Rare features of this tumor include clear cell change, psammoma bodies, and cystic changes.

A-3. **(d) Neuroendocrine carcinoma**
The aspirate shows loosely cohesive cells with typical fine and coarse chromatin (neuroendocrine) with nuclear molding and high nuclear-cytoplasmic ratio. Notice the absence of lymphoglandular bodies in the background, which excludes lymphoid elements as a possibility. These cells are often positive for CK20 with the characteristic paranuclear dot pattern. Two metastatic tumors must be excluded since they resemble this tumor to perfection. The first is pulmonary small cell carcinoma, and the second is Merkel cell tumor of the skin.

A-4. **(d) Basal cell adenoma/adenocarcinoma**
There are clusters of basaloid cells with peripheral palisading surrounded by a thin rim of matrix material. Cells are small to intermediate in size. The differential diagnosis of this tumor includes adenoid cystic carcinoma, cellular pleomorphic adenoma, metastatic basal cell carcinoma, and small cell carcinoma. Basal cell adenoma and basal cell adenocarcinoma cannot always be differentiated by cytology, since the designation of carcinoma is based on peripheral invasion of surrounding tissue which can only be appreciated by histology.

A-5. **(c) Mucoepidermoid carcinoma**
The image shows moderate cellularity. Tumor cells are slightly pleomorphic. There is a signet ring cell in addition to few cells with clear cytoplasm. Some cells have epidermoid features. Mucoepidermoid carcinoma is the most common malignant tumor of salivary glands. It is classified into low grade and high grade based on clinical, histologic, and cytologic features. The low grade tumors are commonly cystic whereas high grade tumors are solid, have an infiltrative margin, and require more aggressive treatment.

A-6. **(c) Salivary duct carcinoma**
Image displays overtly malignant cells arranged in sheets and loose clusters. These cells have large irregularly shaped nuclei, prominent nucleoli, and granular and vacuolated cytoplasm. Necrosis is noticed in the background. Salivary duct carcinoma is rare but is an aggressive malignant tumor more common in the parotid gland and in elderly males. It has striking resemblance to breast duct carcinoma. Morphologic differentiation from other high grade malignancies is difficult. Appropriate clinical information is necessary to make the diagnosis.

A-7. **(b) Adenoid cystic carcinoma**
This tumor is composed of basaloid cells arranged in large clusters with three-dimensions. Hyaline matrix globules with sharp circumference are noted and surrounded by basaloid cells. Other loosely cohesive are noted. Adenoid cystic carcinoma is the 3rd most common malignant neoplasm of salivary glands. It occurs more frequently in the submandibular gland. Three variants of this tumor are recognized, tubular, cribriform, and solid, and all three variants could be present in the same tumor. This tumor has a tendency for perineural invasion, and patients may initially present with pain.

A-8. **(d) Epithelial myoepithelial carcinoma**
The aspirate is cellular and has a biphasic cell population, larger myoepithelial cells, and smaller darker cells forming ducts. Acellular matrix material is present, and few naked nuclei are noted in the background. This tumor is low grade and locally aggressive. It represents 1 % of all salivary gland tumors, is more often encountered in the parotid, and is more common in women.

A-9. **(e) Polymorphous low grade adenocarcinoma**
The neoplastic cells are normochromatic and are arranged in acini, tubules, or in a linear arrangement (resembling lobular breast carcinoma). Individual cells have open chromatin (not dark and basaloid as in adenoid cystic carcinoma). Rounded globules of matrix material are noted. The most important differential diagnosis is adenoid cystic carcinoma. This tumor arises almost exclusively in minor salivary glands, and the palate is the most common site. It has a predilection to perineural invasion but the overall prognosis is favorable.

A-10. **(c) Pleomorphic adenoma**
Embedded in a background of fibrillary matrix are groups of myoepithelial cells. The myoepithelial cells are in cohesive groups with variable shapes mostly spindle shaped. Epithelial cells, on the other hand, are recognized by their flat honeycomb arrangement. Pleomorphic adenoma is the most common tumor of all salivary glands. They are most common in the superficial part of the parotid gland toward the tail of the gland near the angle of the mandible. This feature causes elevation of the ear lobule when the tumor is present.

A-11. **(c) Benign acini**
These are normal acini arranged in the typical "clusters of grapes" pattern. Adipose cells are also noted between the acini. Acinar cells are uniform with rounded small nuclei and vacuolated cytoplasm. The small size of the nuclei and the cohesive and intact nature of the cells, in addition to the presence of adipose cells, are important features in differentiating this from acinic cell carcinoma.

A-12. **(a) Benign duct epithelium**
This is a group of benign duct epithelium, characterized by monotonous rounded nuclei and honey comb pattern. Duct epithelium may be seen associated with benign acini as part of normal salivary gland tissue.

A-13. **(e) Sebaceous differentiation**
Sebaceous cells have abundantly vacuolated cytoplasm that contains lipid. They may occur normally in salivary glands or may be associated with lesions such as sebaceous adenoma, sebaceous carcinoma, Warthin tumor, and mucoepidermoid carcinoma.

A-14. **(c) Acute sialadenitis**
This is acute inflammatory exudate with cellular debris. Duct epithelium may occasionally be present. Also, stone fragments may be present in some cases. Occasionally the causative agent (commonly bacteria or fungus) is identified.

A-15. **(b) Pleomorphic adenoma**
Many spindly myoepithelial cells are admixed in the fibrillary matrix material, a diagnostic pattern for pleomorphic adenoma.

A-16. **(c) Chronic sialadenitis**
The image shows a large number of amylase crystalloids with the characteristic elongated polygonal and needle shapes. In addition, there is a reactive group of cells. Nontyrosine crystalloids, like amylase crystalloids, are most often seen in benign non-neoplastic conditions such as chronic sialadenitis. Usually the diagnosis rendered is chronic sialadenitis with crystalloid formation.

A-17. **(d) Pleomorphic adenoma**
The smear shows myoepithelial cells in a cohesive group in a background of chondromyxoid matrix. These features are diagnostic of pleomorphic adenoma. In addition, multiple floret-like crystals are noted which represent tyrosine crystalloids that are commonly encountered in pleomorphic adenoma.

A-18. **(e) Benign intra-parotid lymph node**
The aspirate is composed of reactive lymphocytes with different stages of maturation. In the background are many lymphoglandular bodies that confirm the presence of lymphoid cells. The parotid gland often contains lymph nodes within and around it. This is due to the simultaneous development of the salivary gland and lymphoid tissue in the same location. Many of the lymph nodes may contain salivary remnants from which tumors may arise. Also, these lymph nodes could be the site of metastasis from any primary tumor in the head and neck region.

A-19. **(e) Basaloid neoplasm**
Basaloid neoplasm is one of the most challenging problems in salivary gland fine-needle aspirations. This group includes many lesions such as basal cell adenoma/adenocarcinoma, adenoid cystic carcinoma, chronic sialadenitis, cellular pleomorphic adenoma, metastatic basal cell carcinoma, metastatic basaloid squamous cell carcinoma, and small cell carcinoma. Chronic sialadenitis is a diffuse process rather than a localized mass and often has scant cellularity with inflammatory cells. Absence of mitoses and cellular atypia favors basal cell adenoma. However, absence of mitoses and atypia do not exclude adenoid cystic carcinoma and basal cell adenocarcinoma. Due to the

overlapping features of these lesions it is recommended to report them as basaloid neoplasm and address the specifics in a comment.

A-20. **(d) Low grade mucoepidermoid carcinoma**
Within abundant mucus is group of mucus cells and intermediate cells. There are no squamoid cells which are typically seen in high grade mucoepidermoid carcinoma. Mucus cells are low columnar and cuboidal with mucus in their cytoplasm and no overt malignant features. Mucoepidermoid carcinoma is the most common malignant tumor of salivary glands both in children and adults. It is also the most common malignant neoplasm of major and minor salivary glands.

A-21. **(e) Polymorphous low grade adenocarcinoma**
The tumor is composed of basaloid cells with open chromatin hence they are not hyperchromatic. Tumor cells are arranged in groups forming duct like structures as well as dispersed single cells in the background matrix material. There is no significant atypia, mitoses, or necrosis. The cytologic features and location on the palate confirm the diagnosis.

A-22. **(b) Metastatic spindle cell melanoma**
The aspirate is very cellular. Cells are spindle shaped with slight variation in nuclear size and shape but have no features of high grade malignancy. The differential diagnosis covers a variety of spindle cell tumors that are more frequent in the head and neck region, including spindle cell squamous carcinoma, spindle cell melanoma, myoepithelial carcinoma, schwannoma, and synovial carcinoma. Regarding the choices given in the question, we can easily rule out cellular pleomorphic adenoma based on absence of matrix and epithelial myoepithelial cells. Acinic cell carcinoma is not known to have spindle cell morphology. In salivary duct, carcinoma cells appear more anaplastic in addition to necrosis in the background. Spindle cell squamous carcinoma will have focal squamoid differentiation and a history of irradiation. Spindle cell melanoma is the correct answer based on the history of a malignant skin tumor, the presence of prominent macronucleoli, and the single cell arrangement of cells. Occasionally, melanin can be seen in the cytoplasm of the neoplastic cells or in macrophages. Schwannoma is described in question 29. Myoepithelial carcinoma has plump spindled and plasmacytoid cells with distinct nucleoli and loose stroma described in question 37. Synovial sarcoma is also a consideration in which there is biphasic differentiation. A panel of immunohistochemical stains would be useful to distinguish the entities in this differential diagnosis.

A-23. **(c) Acinic cell carcinoma**
FNA shows a cellular aspirate with cells resembling disorganized serous acini that are irregular. A key feature is the absence of duct epithelium. The cells are large and have granular cytoplasm. Many naked nuclei and cytoplasmic debris are noted in the background. The nuclei are round and uniform. Acinic cell carcinoma is the third most common malignant neoplasm of salivary glands.

A-24. **(c) Warthin tumor**
The smear shows Warthin tumor with squamous metaplasia. There are clusters of oncocytic cells, abundant debris in the background with keratinized squames and lymphocytes. The metaplastic cells are degenerated. Squamous metaplasia and mucinous metaplasia are metaplastic processes that occur in approximately 30 % of Warthin tumors.

A-25. **(e) If untreated, it commonly undergoes sarcomatous changes.**
The image displays one of the characteristic features of pleomorphic adenoma. Groups of spindly myoepithelial cells are admixed with matrix material. Pleomorphic adenoma is the most common salivary gland tumors. It occasionally contains tyrosine crystalloids and can sometimes become cystic. Approximately 30 % of cases undergo squamous or mucinous metaplasia. A sarcomatous change in pleomorphic adenoma is very rare.

A-26. **(a) A Granulomatous sialadenitis**
The image displays the classic features of granulomatous reaction. A crowded group of epithelioid histiocytes is characterized by tapered nuclei. Granulomatous reactions in salivary glands are caused by infections such as fungi, mycobacteria, toxoplasmosis, and cat scratch disease. Other causes include sarcoidosis, lymphoma, and metastatic carcinoma.

A-27. **(e) Lymphoepithelial sialadenitis**
This lesion has been known by several names including: lymphoepithelial lesion, myoepithelial sialadenitis, and Mikulicz disease. The key feature in this lesion is the lymphoepithelial island (formerly, epimyoepithelial island). The aspirate is cellular and contains a mixed population of lymphocytes and plasma cells in addition to the presence of lymphoepithelial islands. This lymphoepithelial island is composed of an aggregate of overlapping ductal cells infiltrated by lymphocytes. The ductal cells display reactive changes and occasionally squamous metaplasia. This lesion is often present in the parotid and

the submandibular gland. It is a disease that frequently affects women, tends to be bilateral in the majority of cases, and is believed to be an autoimmune disease. Almost all patients have Sjogren syndrome.

A-29. (b) **Schwannoma**
The aspirate is moderately cellular. It is composed of spindle-shaped cells in a fibrillary background. The cells have an ill-defined pale cytoplasm, and the nuclei have even chromatin and indistinct nucleoli. The most important differential diagnosis is pleomorphic adenoma and myoepithelioma, which share with schwannoma the abundance of spindle-shaped cells. In contrast to schwannoma that have tapering nuclei to a pointed end, the nuclei of myoepithelial cells have a round end and are less elongated. Another useful feature is the palisading nuclei in schwannoma. Immunostains can be very helpful in this differential. Schwannoma is reactive to s-100 protein, and myoepithelial cells are reactive to p63.

A-30. (b) **Pleomorphic adenoma**
The image shows many discohesive spindly cells with eccentric nuclei (plasmacytoid). The nuclei are round and uniform while the cytoplasm is dense and glassy hence they are called hyaline cells. Hyaline cells are modified myoepithelial cells. The presence of the matrix material in the background supports the diagnosis of pleomorphic adenoma. In the absence of the matrix material, myoepithelioma would be a consideration.

A-31. (b) **Basal cell adenoma/adenocarcinoma**
The image displays thick matrix that lacks fibrillary edges admixed with basaloid cells. The relationship between the matrix and the basaloid cells is disorganized. The matrix lacks the round edge that is typically seen in the classic type of adenoid cystic carcinoma. The findings are characteristic of basal cell adenoma/adenocarcinoma. Warthin tumor with its classic oncocytes, lymphocytes, and cellular debris is clearly not a consideration. There is lack of myoepithelial cells with their spindly shapes, which excludes epithelial myoepithelial carcinoma and pleomorphic adenoma. Polymorphous low grade adenocarcinoma is typically a minor salivary gland tumor and often presents on the palate. In addition, while the latter tumor is composed of basaloid cells, they are usually organized in acinar like structures, and the matrix takes the shape of globules.

A-32. (d) **Mucoepidermoid carcinoma**
The smear is composed of large cells with pleomorphic nuclei with coarse chromatin and thick cytoplasm with occasional mucin vacuoles. Rare necrotic debris is noted in the background. These features are characteristic of high grade mucoepidermoid carcinoma. Pleomorphic adenoma can easily be ruled out based on the absence of epithelial or myoepithelial cells as well as the absence of the characteristic matrix. Basal cell adenoma/adenocarcinoma and adenoid cystic carcinoma are excluded due to absence of basaloid cells and the dense matrix.

A-33. (a) **Metastatic melanoma**
The smear is composed of single cells with large pleomorphic nuclei with prominent macronucleoli. Cells are polyhedral with occasional dirty brown pigment in the cytoplasm suspicious for melanin. So, the discohesive nature, the large macronucleoli, and the pigment in the cytoplasm make metastatic melanoma the most likely diagnosis.

A-34. (b) **Warthin tumor**
The image is diagnostic of Warthin tumor. The three components for the diagnosis, oncocytic cells, lymphocytes, and cyst fluid with cellular debris, are present. Oncocytic mucoepidermoid carcinoma requires the presence of cells with mucin vacuoles and mucin in background. In pleomorphic adenoma, matrix material and epithelial and myoepithelial cells should be present. Oncocytoma requires a predominance of oncocytic cells. Large neoplastic acinic cells in clusters and many bare nuclei and cytoplasmic debris in the background should be seen in acinic cell carcinoma.

A-35. (e) **Cryptococcal sialadenitis**
This is a unique case of cryptoccocal parotid sialadenitis. In a background of reactive and multinucleated macrophages, there are multiple cryptoccocal spores with their characteristic mucin rich capsule. Confirmatory microbiological studies are usually necessary.

A-36. (e) **Warthin tumor with squamous metaplasia**
In this aspirate, cells are mostly degenerated but on closer look one can find features of Warthin tumor such as squamous differentiation and oncocytic cells in a background of debris. The metaplastic squamous cells do not show marked atypia to suspect metastatic squamous cell carcinoma, which is a common pitfall in this lesion. The inflammatory infiltrate is not significant to suspect sialadenitis. Features of pleomorphic adenoma are not seen. In mucoepidermoid carcinoma, a higher grade nuclear atypia is expected in addition to the presence of intracellular and extracellular mucin. In low grade mucoepidermoid

carcinoma, there should be a prevalence of mucinous cells and a background of mucin.

A-37 (c) **Carcinoma expleomorphic adenoma**
In this aspirate, there is a stromal component composed of myxoid matrix in the background and clusters of cells that appear epithelioid and plasmacytoid with high nuclear-to-cytoplasmic ratio and hyperchromatic nuclei and prominent nucleoli. These features are characteristic of myoepithelial carcinoma arising in a background of pleomorphic adenoma. Most cases of myoepithelial carcinoma arise within a preexisting pleomorphic adenoma and more commonly occur in the parotid.

A-38. (b) **Pleomorphic adenoma with tyrosine crystalloids**
The smear shows a myxoid matrix with clusters of epithelial and myoepithelial cells that are characteristic of pleomorphic adenoma. In addition there are multiple floret-like crystalloids, which are known to be most commonly associated with pleomorphic adenoma.

A-39. (e) **Metastatic renal cell carcinoma**
There are large polyhedral cells with clear cytoplasm and large rounded nuclei with prominent magenta red macronucleoli. In addition to these classic features of renal cell carcinoma, the patient history certainly lends more support to the diagnosis. Metastatic tumors to salivary glands are commonly from tumors arising in the head and neck region such as squamous cell carcinoma and melanoma. Renal cell carcinoma is among the more frequent metastasis from outside the head and neck region. Also, it is important to consider primary salivary gland tumors with clear cytoplasm, including epithelial myoepithelial carcinoma, myoepithelioma, oncocytoma, mucoepidermoid carcinoma, and acinic cell carcinoma.

A-40. (e) **Oncocytoma**
This aspirate contains abundant oncocytes with clean cytoplasm (devoid of cellular debris) and lack lymphocytes. The oncocytes have sharply defined cell outlines and granular cytoplasm. The nuclei are small, round, and centrally placed. The nuclei show minimal nuclear variation but no atypia. The differential diagnosis is broad and is based on tumors with oncocytic cells. Many tumors have oncocytic cells such as pleomorphic adenoma (mixed tumor), acinic cell carcinoma, mucoepidermoid carcinoma, oncocytic carcinoma, and Warthin tumor to name a few. The diagnosis is dependent on the other features of the particular tumor.

A-41. (c) **Metastatic rhabdomyosarcoma**
This aspirate is highly cellular and contains abundant of highly atypical pleomorphic spindle cells consistent with sarcoma. Given history of embryonal rhabdomyosarcoma, this aspirate is most consistent with metastatic rhabdomyosarcoma.

Rhabdomyosarcoma (RMS) is a malignant tumor with muscle differentiation that has several subtypes: embryonal, alveolar, and pleomorphic subtypes. Embryonal RMS is the most common variant, which occurs in young children, such as in our case, in the head and neck or urogenital region. It has a better prognosis than alveolar RMS. The embryonal variant may also be subdivided into botryoid, spindle cell, and anaplastic variants). These tumors have complex karyotypes. In alveolar rhabdomyosarcoma (RMS), FISH may detect the FKHR breakpoint and PCR help to identify FKHR-PAX3/PAX7 fusion transcripts. It is of note that the tumor may occasionally stain positive for synaptophysin, chromogranin, and CD 99. The cytomorphology of embryonal RMS overlaps with alveolar RMS. Ancillary studies may show positive immunostains for desmin (cytoplasmic), myogenin (nuclear), MyoD1 (nuclear), and myogenin (nuclear).

A-42. (b) **Acinic cell carcinoma**
The aspirate is cellular and shows relatively small cell type with abundant vacuolated cytoplasm and naked nuclei in the background. There is no matrix material seen. A vague granular background is present. Capillary structures associated with the atypical epithelial cells are also noted. The aspirate shows bland small cells resembling disorganized serous acini that are irregular. A key feature is the absence of duct epithelium. The cells are large and have granular cytoplasm. Many naked nuclei and cytoplasmic debris are noted in the background. The nuclei are round and uniform. These features are consistent with acinic cell carcinoma. Acinic cell carcinoma is the third most common malignant neoplasm of salivary glands.

A-43. (a) **Pleomorphic adenoma**
The aspirate is cellular and shows numerous plasmacytoid myoepithelial cells embedded in extracellular material with a magenta-color fibrillary quality. These features are characteristic of pleomorphic adenoma. The extracellular material in adenoid cystic carcinoma is usually nonfibrillary, homogenous, acellular, and has a sharp border, and the cellular component is basaloid with scant cytoplasm. Warthin tumors are characterized by oncocytic epithelium in a lymphocytic background. Salivary duct carcinoma.

Pleomorphic adenomas are the most common salivary gland neoplasm and account for about 75 % of all neoplasms in major salivary glands. Warthin tumors are the second most common salivary gland tumor. Mucoepidermoid carcinomas are the most common malignant salivary gland tumor. Tyrosinase crystalloids are common in pleomorphic adenomas being seen in up to 30 %. However, tyrosinase crystalloids are not specific for pleomorphic adenoma as they can be seen in adenoid cystic carcinoma, polymorphous low grade adenocarcinoma, and some cysts but less commonly than in pleomorphic adenoma. Amylase crystalloids can also be seen in pleomorphic adenomas but at a lower frequency.

A-44. (**d**) **Pleomorphic adenoma** (**mixed tumor**)
The aspirate is cellular and shows numerous plasmacytoid myoepithelial cells embedded in extracellular materials with a fibrillary quality. These features are characteristic of pleomorphic adenoma. The extracellular material in adenoid cystic carcinoma is usually nonfibrillary, homogenous, acellular, and has a sharp border, and the cellular component is basaloid with scant cytoplasm. Warthin tumors are characterized by oncocytic epithelium in a lymphocytic background. Salivary duct carcinoma.

A-45. (**a**) **Acinic cell carcinoma**
The aspirate is cellular and shows relatively small cell type with abundant vacuolated cytoplasm and naked nuclei in the background. There is no matrix material seen. A vague granular background is present. Capillary structures associated with the atypical epithelial cells are also noted. The aspirate shows bland small cells resembling disorganized serous acini that are irregular. A key feature is the absence of duct epithelium. The cells are large and have granular cytoplasm. Many naked nuclei and cytoplasmic debris are noted in the background. The nuclei are round and uniform. These features are consistent with acinic cell carcinoma. Acinic cell carcinoma is the third most common malignant neoplasm of salivary glands. Oncocytomas do not show cytoplasmic vacuolization.

6.4 Answers and Discussion of Text-Based Questions 46–65

A-46. (c) **Hemangioma**
In children, salivary gland tumors are rare. They account only for less than 3 % of all salivary gland tumors. The most common salivary gland tumors in infants and children are nonepithelial, particularly hemangioma. The most common salivary gland tumor is pleomorphic adenoma (55 %). This is followed by Warthin tumor as the second most common salivary gland tumor. Among all malignant tumors, mucoepidermoid carcinoma is the most common malignant salivary gland neoplasm in both children and adults.

A-47. (d) **Pleomorphic adenoma**
Tyrosine rich crystals are floret shaped and nonbirefringent. Although they are most commonly encountered in pleomorphic adenomas, they are not fully specific for pleomorphic adenoma as they have been reported in adenoid cystic carcinoma and polymorphous low grade adenocarcinoma.

A-48. (e) **Hyaline globules**
Hyaline globules are matrix material present in certain tumors such as pleomorphic adenoma, adenoid cystic carcinoma, and basal cell adenoma/adenocarcinoma. This material is not known to be produced by normal salivary glands.

A-49. (a) **Sialadenitis**
Alpha-amylase crystalloids are known to be associated with chronic sialadenitis.

A-50. (a) **Adenoid cystic carcinoma**
Warthin tumor and low grade mucoepidermoid carcinoma are typically cystic tumors. Both mixed tumor and acinic cell carcinoma have a cystic variant. Adenoid cystic carcinoma is a solid tumor, and the cystic change refers to microscopic appearance.

A-51. (d) **Lymphoepithelial cyst**
In HIV-infected patients, lymphoepithelial cysts are more common and are frequently bilateral. These cysts are lined by squamous epithelium that is surrounded by abundant reactive lymphoid aggregates.

A-52. (c) **Intercalated duct**
Pleomorphic adenomas arise mainly from the intercalated ducts. Acinic cell carcinomas arise from acini, while oncocytoma and Warthin tumor arise from striated ducts. Mucoepidermoid carcinoma and salivary duct carcinoma arise from excretory ducts.

A-53. (d) **Minor salivary glands**
Minor salivary gland tumors are more likely to be malignant compared to tumors from major salivary glands such as parotid, submandibular, or sublingual. Polymorphous low grade adenocarcinoma is almost exclusively a minor salivary gland tumor.

A-54. (b) **Caused by ischemic changes**
Necrotizing sialometaplasia is a rare benign lesion that mimics carcinoma. It is almost exclusively a disease of minor salivary glands and occurs most commonly in the palate. It is caused by ischemic necrosis following trauma or radiation therapy. Clinical history is very useful in making the correct diagnosis.

A-55. (d) **Warthin tumor**
Both Warthin tumor and oncocytoma arise from the striated portion of the salivary duct system. The striated ducts have granular eosinophilic cytoplasm (oncocytic) that resembles the cells in both oncocytoma and Warthin tumor.

A-56. (d) **Canalicular adenoma**
Myoepithelial cells are present in basal cell adenoma, adenoid cystic carcinoma, polymorphous low grade adenocarcinoma, and pleomorphic adenoma as confirmed by positive staining for p63 (a marker for myoepithelial cells). Canalicular adenoma on the other hand is negative for p63, which indicates the absence of myoepithelial cells. Canalicular adenoma is believed to arise from the luminal ductal cells.

A-57. (e) **Palate**
Minor salivary glands are distributed throughout the oral cavity and upper aero-digestive tract. They are composed of a mixture of mucus and serous glands. In reported large series of cases, it was found that the palate is the most common site of tumors of minor salivary glands.

A-58. (d) **Pleomorphic adenoma**
Pleomorphic adenoma is the most common salivary gland neoplasm and accounts for approximately 75 % of all salivary gland tumors.

A-59. (c) **Adenoid cystic carcinoma**
Perineural invasion is more frequently noted in adenoid cystic carcinoma and polymorphous low grade adenocarcinoma. Of the choices given, adenoid cystic carcinoma is the correct response.

A-60. (d) **Warthin tumor**
Of all the choices above, lymphocytes are likely to be present in Warthin tumor. Salivary gland lesions that

contain numerous lymphocytes are intra-parotid lymph node, lymphoma, lymphoepithelial cyst, Warthin tumor, mucoepidermoid carcinoma, acinic cell carcinoma, and lymphoepithelial carcinoma.

A-61. (d) **Warthin tumor**

Tumors that are sometimes bilateral include Warthin tumor, acinic cell carcinoma, lymphoma, lymphoepithelial cyst, amyloidosis, and sialadenitis.

A-62. (e) **Salivary duct carcinoma**

Salivary duct carcinoma is an uncommon tumor of salivary glands. It has a distinctive appearance on cytology and histology. The tumor has striking resemblance to breast comedo duct carcinoma. This tumor has an aggressive clinical course.

A-63. (c) **Squamous cell carcinoma**

Metastatic tumors to the salivary gland or to intraparenchymal lymph nodes are not uncommon. The primary site is often in the head and neck region. Squamous cell carcinoma and melanoma are the most common tumors metastatic to salivary glands.

A-64. (a) **Adenoid cystic carcinoma**

Adenoid cystic carcinoma is composed of basaloid cells and matrix globules. All the remaining tumors may contain oncocytic cells.

A-65. (b) **Most common salivary gland tumor**

Warthin tumor is the second most common salivary gland tumor. Pleomorphic adenoma is the most common salivary gland tumor.

Reading List

Chhieng DC, Cohen J-M, Cangiarella JF. Fine needle aspiration of spindle cell and mesenchymal lesions of the salivary glands. Diagn Cytopathol. 2000;23:253–9.

Flezar M, Pogacnik A. Warthin tumor unusual vs. common morphological findings in fine needle aspiration biopsies. Cytopathology. 2002;13:232–41.

Henry-Stanley MJ, Beneke J, Bardales RH, Stanley MW. Fine-needle aspiration of normal tissue from enlarged salivary glands: Sialosis or missed target? Diagn Cytopathol. 1995;13:300–3.

Kantarcioğlu AS, Gulenc M, Yücel A, Uzun N, Taskin T, Sakiz D, Altas K. Cryptococcal parotid involvement: an uncommon localization of Cryptococcus neoformans. Med Mycol. 2006;44(3):279–83.

Kapila K, Mathur S, Verma K. Schwannoma: a pitfall in the diagnosis of pleomorphic adenomas on fine needle aspiration cytology. Diagn Cytopathol. 2002;27:53–9.

Kawahara A, Harada H, Akiba J, Yokoyama T, Kage M. Fine-needle aspiration cytology of basal cell adenoma of the parotid gland: characteristic cytological features and diagnostic pitfalls. Diagn Cytopathol. 2007;35:85–90.

Khalbuss WE, Monaco SE, Pantanowitz L. Chapter 14. Salivary gland. In: The ASCP Quick Compendium (QC) of cytopathology. Chicago: ASCP Press; 2013. p. 292–312.

Klijanienko J, Lagace R, Servois V, et al. Fine needle sampling of primary neuroendocrine carcinoma of salivary glands: cytohistological correlations and clinical analysis. Diagn Cytopathol. 2001;24:163–6.

Mehta RP, Faquim WC, Deschler DG. Acinic cell carcinoma of the parotid with ductal extension. Arch Otolaryngol Head Neck Surg. 2004;130:792–3.

Nuyens M, Schupbach J, Zbaren P. Metastatic disease to the parotid gland. Otolaryngol Head Neck Surg. 2006;135:844–8.

Pantanowitz L, Goulart R, Cao JK. Salivary glands crystalloids. Diagn Cytopathol. 2006;34:749–50.

Siddiqui NH, Wu SJ. Fine needle aspiration of cystic pleomorphic adenoma with adnexa-like differentiation mimicking mucoepidermoid carcinoma: a case report. Diagn Cytopathol. 2005;32:229–32.

Liver Fine-Needle Aspiration

7

Qing Kay Li and Walid E. Khalbuss

Contents

7.1 **Image-Based Questions 1–38** 412

7.2 **Text-Based Questions 39–75** 450

7.3 **Answers and Discussion of Image-Based Questions 1–38** 454

7.4 **Answers and Discussions of Text-based Questions 39–75** 461

Reading List 467

Q.K. Li, MD, PhD (✉)
Department of Pathology, The Johns Hopkins University School of Medicine, The Johns Hopkins Bayview Medical Center, 4940 Eastern Avenue, AA Building, Room 154B, Baltimore, MD 21224-2780, USA
e-mail: qli23@jhmi.edu

W.E. Khalbuss, MD, PhD, FIAC
Department of Pathology, GE Clarient Diagnostic Services, 31 Columbia, Aliso Viejo, California, 92656, USA
e-mail: Walid.khalbuss@ge.com

W.E. Khalbuss, Q.K. Li (eds.), *Diagnostic Cytopathology Board Review and Self-Assessment*, DOI 10.1007/978-1-4939-1477-7_7, © Springer Science+Business Media New York 2015

Table 7.1 Benign components in liver FNAs

	Descriptions	Differentials
Hepatocytes	Sheets, trabeculae or tissue fragments, and/or dispersed individual cells with centrally located round- to oval-shaped nuclei, small nucleoli, granular chromatin, intranuclear pseudoinclusions, dense cytoplasm, and bile pigment. Binucleation is common	Large oval-shaped cells with granular chromatin, small nucleoli, and dense cytoplasm. Nuclei may show mild atypia, but with smooth nuclear membrane DD: liver cell adenoma, focal nodular hyperplasia, well-differentiated hepatocellular carcinoma, melanoma, and metastatic carcinomas
Bile duct epithelium (bile ductules)	Small clusters or sheets of cuboidal cells, granular chromatin, inconspicuous nucleoli, scant cytoplasm The size of cells is smaller than hepatocytes Nuclear disarray may be present	Bile ductules appear as rows or clusters of epithelial cells with ovoid darkly stained overlapping nuclei and scant cytoplasm DD: cholangiocarcinoma, metastatic adenocarcinoma
Kupffer cells	Intermediate-sized cells with elongated nuclei, vacuolated cytoplasm, and cytoplasmic pigment (hemosiderin)	Resemble macrophages DD: endothelial cells, cholangiocarcinoma, metastatic adenocarcinoma
Histiocytes	Loosely formed two-dimensional clusters or dispersed individual cells, with coffee bean-shape nuclei, fine chromatin, inconspicuous nucleoli, and foamy cytoplasm	Cells have coffee bean-shape nuclei, cytoplasmic vacuoles and pigment, and normal N:C ratio DD: cholangiocarcinoma, hepatocellular carcinoma
Mallory body	Cytoplasmic eosinophilic inclusion, with red color by Papanicolaou stain and blue color by Diff-Quik stain, characteristic twisted-rope appearance Commonly seen in alcohol-related liver disease and hepatocellular carcinoma	It consists of intermediate keratins that have been ubiquinated or bound by other proteins such as heat shock proteins or p62 DD: eosinophilic body in urothelial cell carcinoma
Lipofuscin	Cytoplasmic pigment with golden brown color with Papanicolaou stain, and green-brown color with Diff-Quik stain	Normal findings related to cellular aging and/or degenerative changes DD: melanin pigment
Hemosiderin	Cytoplasmic pigment with yellow-brown color with Papanicolaou stain and blue-brown color with Diff-Quik stain	When present in large quantities, it suggests an abnormal iron metabolism DD: melanin pigment
Bile pigment	Cytoplasmic pigment with dark-green or brown color with Papanicolaou and Diff-Quik stains	It may not be seen in normal hepatocytes by Diff-Quik stain DD: melanin pigment

Table 7.2 Neoplastic lesions in liver FNAs

Conditions	Descriptions	Differentials
Focal nodular hyperplasia	Benign-appearing hepatocytes without atypia Benign bile duct epithelial cells	Absence of nuclear atypia Benign bile duct epithelial cells DD: liver cell adenoma. Regenerating nodule in cirrhosis
Liver cell adenoma	Benign-appearing hepatocytes Absence of bile duct epithelial cells	Scant specimen with mild hepatocyte atypia DD: well-differentiated hepatocellular carcinoma
Bile duct hamartoma	Benign ductal epithelium Benign-appearing hepatocytes Scattered stromal cells	Scant specimen, no malignant features DD: cholangiocarcinoma, metastatic adenocarcinoma
Hepatocellular carcinoma (well differentiated)	Tubules, cords, nests, sheets, or dispersed tumor cells Increased N:C ratio Large round nuclei, granular chromatin, prominent nucleoli Cytoplasmic bile pigment	Tumor cells resemble normal hepatocytes Numerous naked nuclei Endothelial cell surrounding thickened cords of tumor cells DD: regenerating nodule of cirrhosis, liver cell adenoma, focal nodular hyperplasia
Hepatocellular carcinoma (poorly differentiated)	Dyscohesive, dispersed individual tumor cells Markedly pleomorphism Giant tumor cells	Numerous naked nuclei Clear cytoplasm in 10 % of tumors Markedly nuclear atypia DD: metastatic carcinoma, cholangiocarcinoma
Cholangiocarcinoma	Clusters, crowded sheets, and dispersed individual cuboidal cells Large nuclei with variation in size and shape High N:C ratio and scant cytoplasm	Rare or no cytoplasmic bile pigment, no formation of sinusoidal capillaries around tumor cells, no naked nuclei DD: hepatocellular carcinoma Metastatic adenocarcinoma
Metastatic adenocarcinoma	Three-dimensional clusters, papillary and acinar arrangements of columnar cells. Tumor cells have high N/C ratios, prominent nucleoli, coarse chromatin, "lacy" cytoplasm with vacuolization (cytoplasmic mucin)	Columnar cells have high N:C ratio with irregular nuclear membrane, coarse chromatin, prominent nucleoli, and cytoplasmic vacuole (mucin production) DD: cholangiocarcinoma, hepatocellular carcinoma
Metastatic squamous cell carcinoma	Dyscohesive clusters, loosely formed two-dimensional cellular sheets and scattered individual polymorphic cells, with or without keratinization Tumor necrosis	Polygonal, rounded, elongated, or tadpole-shaped cells with large dark nuclei, smudgy chromatin, and dense cytoplasm (cytokeratin formation) DD: poorly differentiated hepatocellular carcinoma
Metastatic small cell carcinoma	Tight clusters of small hyperchromatic cells (2–3 times the size of mature lymphocytes) with nuclear molding and crowding, nuclear stripes (broken nuclear material), inconspicuous nucleoli, scant cytoplasm	Fine chromatin ("salt-pepper" appearance), paranuclear blue bodies, mitosis, necrosis, and apoptotic bodies DD: lymphoma, basaloid squamous cell carcinoma, and poorly differentiated adenocarcinoma
Metastatic melanoma	Scattered individual large cells with prominent nucleoli and cytoplasmic melanin pigment. Binucleation with "mirror" arrangement. Pseudointranuclear inclusions	Large-sized malignant cells with prominent nucleoli, dense cytoplasm DD: poorly differentiated carcinoma, Hodgkin lymphoma, hepatocellular carcinoma
Lymphoma (non-Hodgkin lymphoma)	Dispersed individual atypical lymphoid cells with coarse chromatin and irregular nuclear membrane, prominent nucleoli. High N:C ratio and scant cytoplasm. Increased mitotic activity and the presence of background lymphoglandular bodies	The size of tumor cells ranges from small to large depending on the type of lymphoma. Monomorphic population of lymphocytes is characteristic for SLL/CLL DD: reactive lymphocytes, small cell carcinoma, poorly differentiated carcinoma
Nonepithelial cell neoplasm	Individual or clusters of spindle cells, small round cells, or pleomorphic tumor cells	DD: muscle, nerve tumors, small round cell tumor, and sarcomas

7.1 Image-Based Questions 1–38

Fig. 7.1

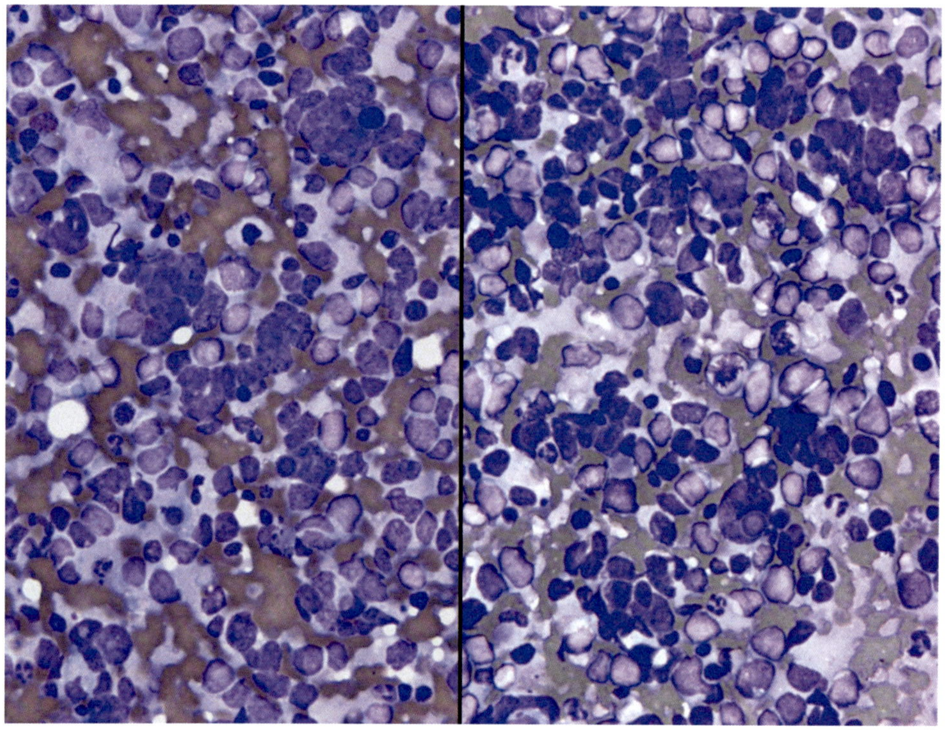

Q-1. A 65-year-old smoker with both lung and liver masses had a CT-guided fine-needle aspiration (FNA) of the liver lesion. What is the diagnosis of the liver FNA?
(a) Lymphoma
(b) Metastatic small cell carcinoma
(c) Poorly differentiated adenocarcinoma
(d) Hepatocellular carcinoma

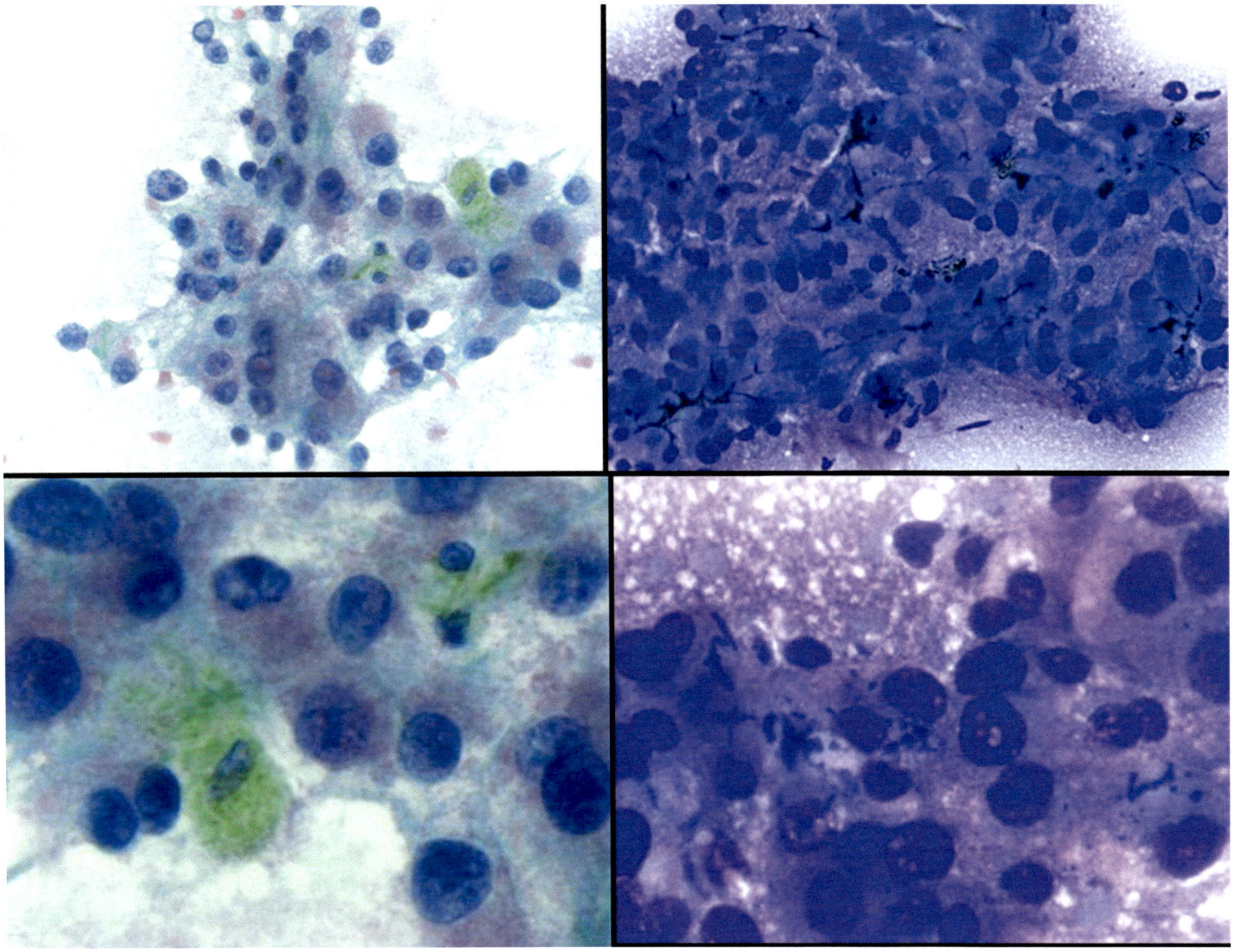

Fig. 7.2

Q-2. All of the following features are seen in a fine-needle aspiration (FNA) of a poorly differentiated hepatocellular carcinoma (HCC), EXCEPT:
(a) Numerous dispersed naked nuclei
(b) Cords and/or individual polygonal cells
(c) Fine and evenly distributed chromatin
(d) Prominent nucleoli

Fig. 7.3

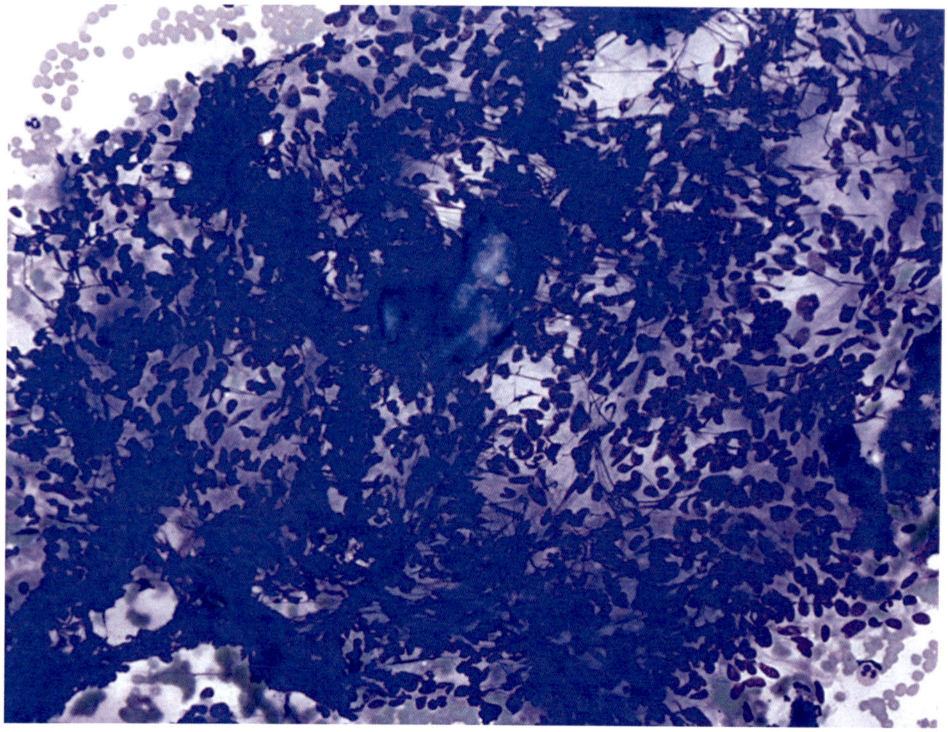

Q-3. A 67-year-old male presented with abdominal pain and discomfort. A CT scan revealed a submucosal mass in the stomach and multiple liver mass. Subsequently, a CT-guided FNA was performed. The differential diagnosis of the lesion includes all of the following, EXCEPT:

(a) Gastrointestinal stromal tumor (GIST)
(b) Sarcomatoid mesothelioma
(c) Angiomyolipoma (AML)
(d) Poorly differentiated adenocarcinoma

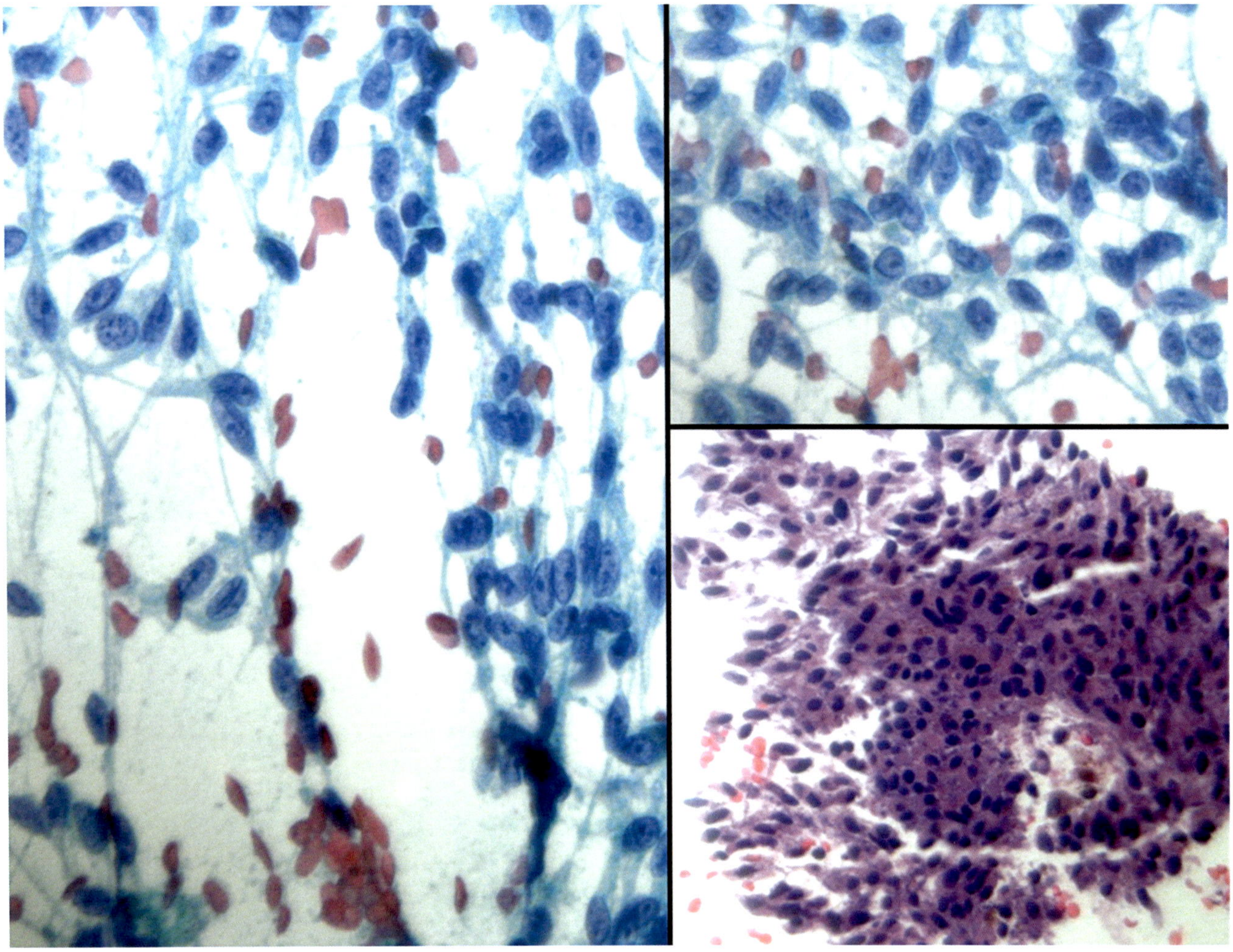

Fig. 7.4

Q-4. A patient who had a history of a "skin tumor" developed multiple liver masses. In FNA smears of the liver mass, scattered "atypical spindle cells" were identified. Which one of the following panels is most useful in confirmation of the diagnosis of this lesion?

(a) S100, HMB45, and Melanin A
(b) C-kit, CD34, and cytokeratin
(c) CK5/6, p63, and p40
(d) CK20, synaptophysin, and chromogranin

Fig. 7.5

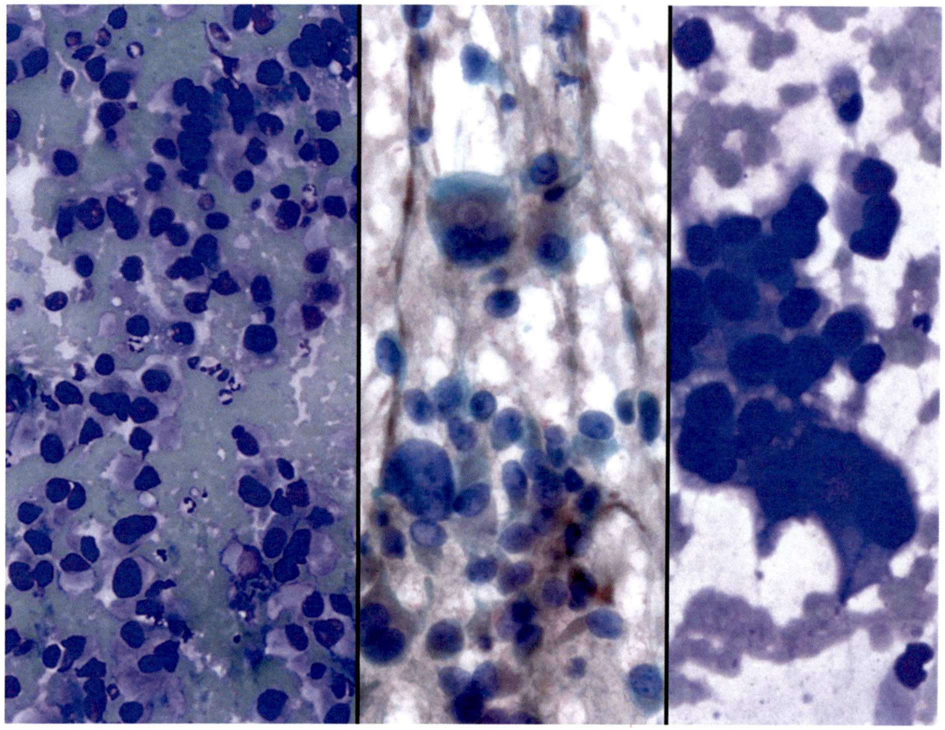

Q-5. An 80-year-old male presented with abdominal pain, jaundice, hematuria, and liver masses. An ultrasound-guided FNA was performed. What is the diagnosis of this liver FNA?

(a) Lymphoma
(b) Metastatic urothelial cell carcinoma
(c) Poorly differentiated adenocarcinoma
(d) Hepatocellular carcinoma

Fig. 7.6

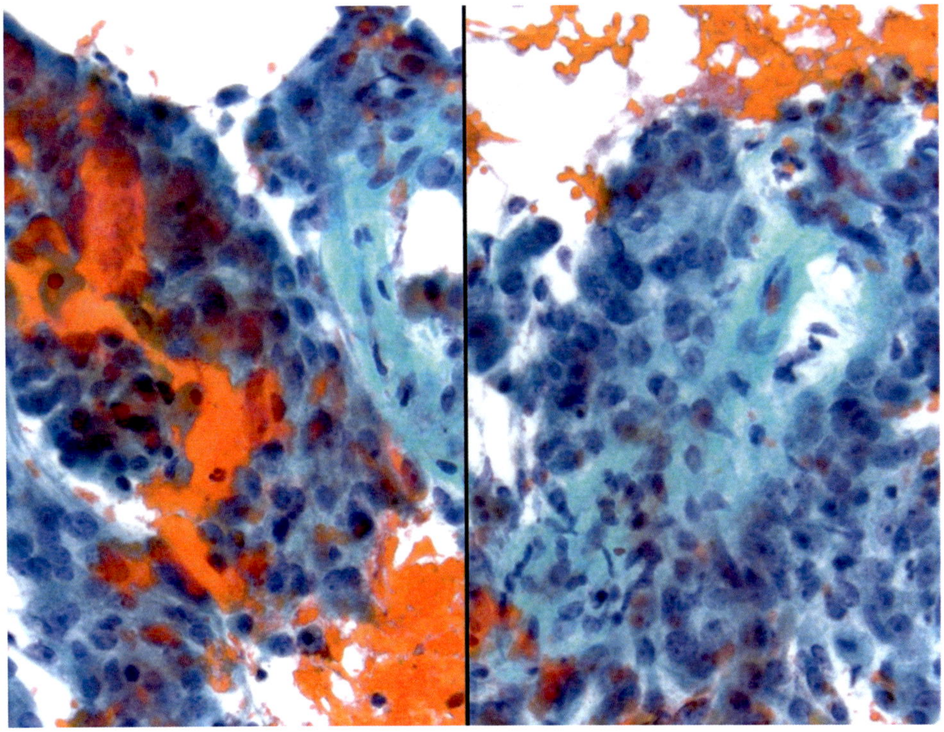

Q-6. A patient with history of kidney cancer developed multiple liver masses and a rapidly enlarging liver. CT-guided FNA of the liver mass was performed. What is the diagnosis of this liver FNA?

(a) Metastatic renal cell carcinoma (RCC)
(b) Metastatic urothelial cell carcinoma
(c) Poorly differentiated adenocarcinoma
(d) Hepatocellular carcinoma

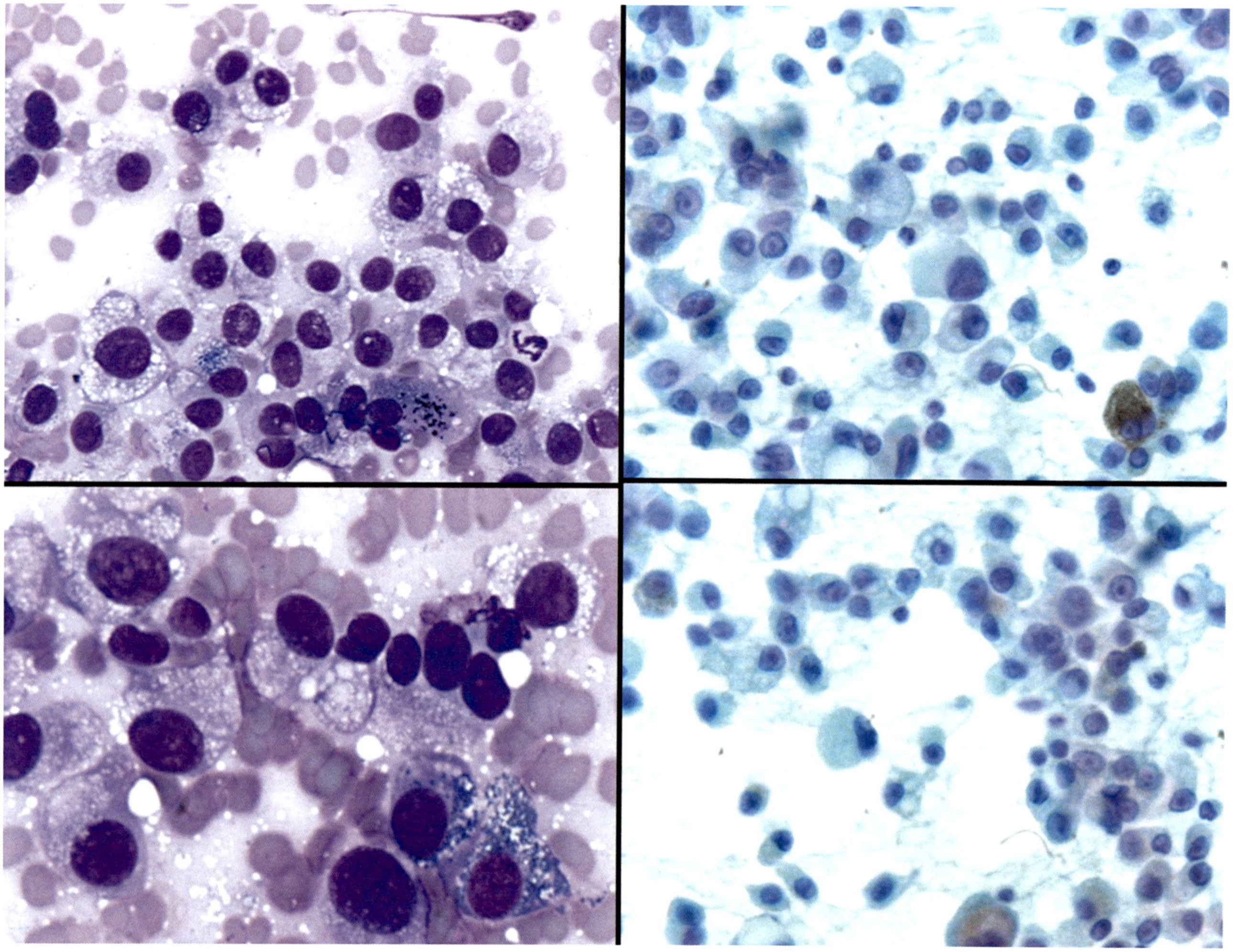

Fig. 7.7

Q-7. A 34-year-old female with a history of "skin cancer" now develops lung and liver masses. What is the diagnosis of this liver FNA?
(a) Metastatic melanoma
(b) Metastatic urothelial cell carcinoma
(c) Poorly differentiated adenocarcinoma
(d) Hepatocellular carcinoma

Fig. 7.8

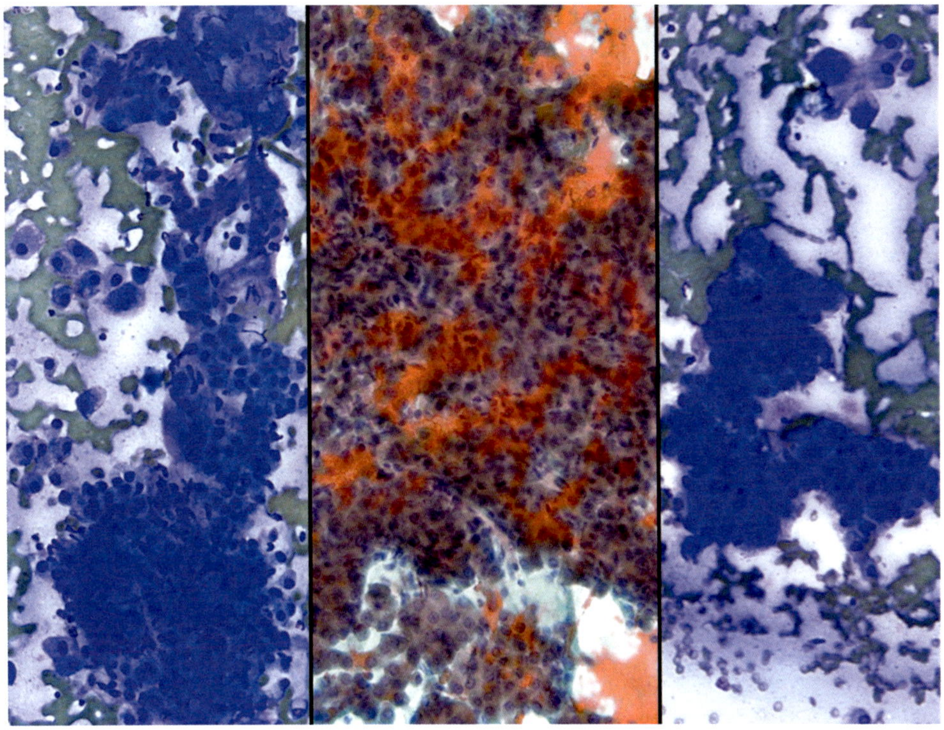

Q-8. A 56-year-old male presented with abdominal pain, jaundice, and liver masses. What is the diagnosis of this liver FNA?
(a) Metastatic poorly differentiated adenocarcinoma
(b) Metastatic melanoma
(c) Hepatocellular carcinoma
(d) Metastatic poorly differentiated squamous cell carcinoma

Fig. 7.9

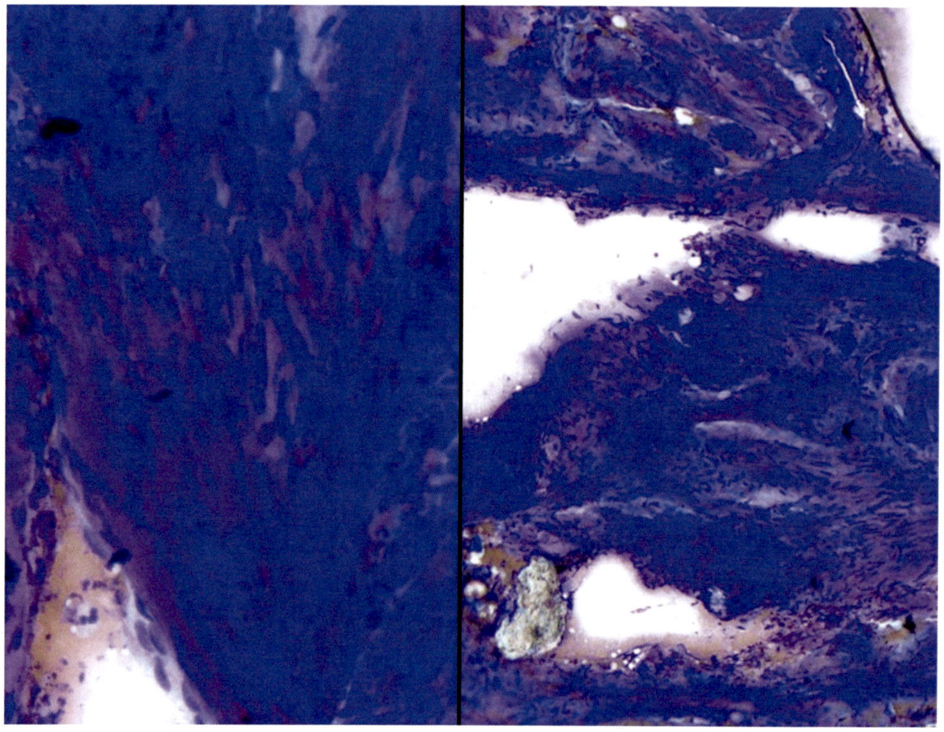

Q-9. A 38-year-old healthy female developed abdominal pain and discomfort. A mass in right liver was found, and a subsequent ultrasound-guided liver mass FNA was performed. What is the diagnosis of this liver FNA?

(a) Granulomatous hepatitis
(b) Leiomyosarcoma
(c) Hepatocellular carcinoma
(d) Hemangioma

Fig. 7.10

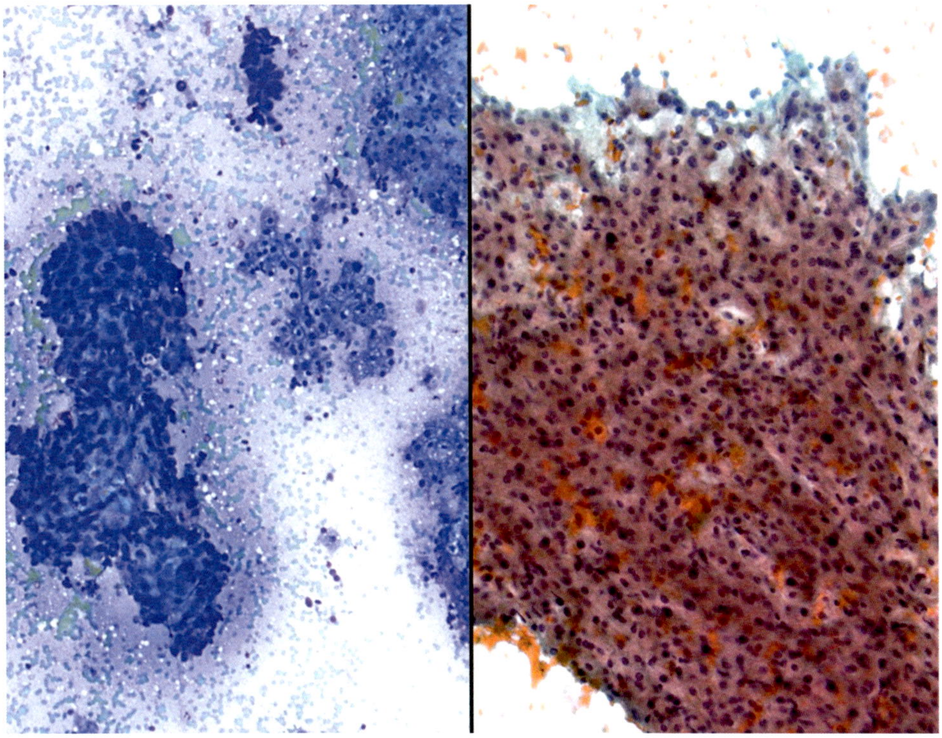

Q-10. A 61-year-old male with clinical presentation of lung and liver masses had an ultrasound-guided FNA of the liver mass. What is the diagnosis of cells seen in this liver FNA?

(a) Metastatic adenocarcinoma of the lung
(b) Hepatocellular carcinoma
(c) Metastatic renal cell carcinoma
(d) Metastatic small cell carcinoma

Fig. 7.11

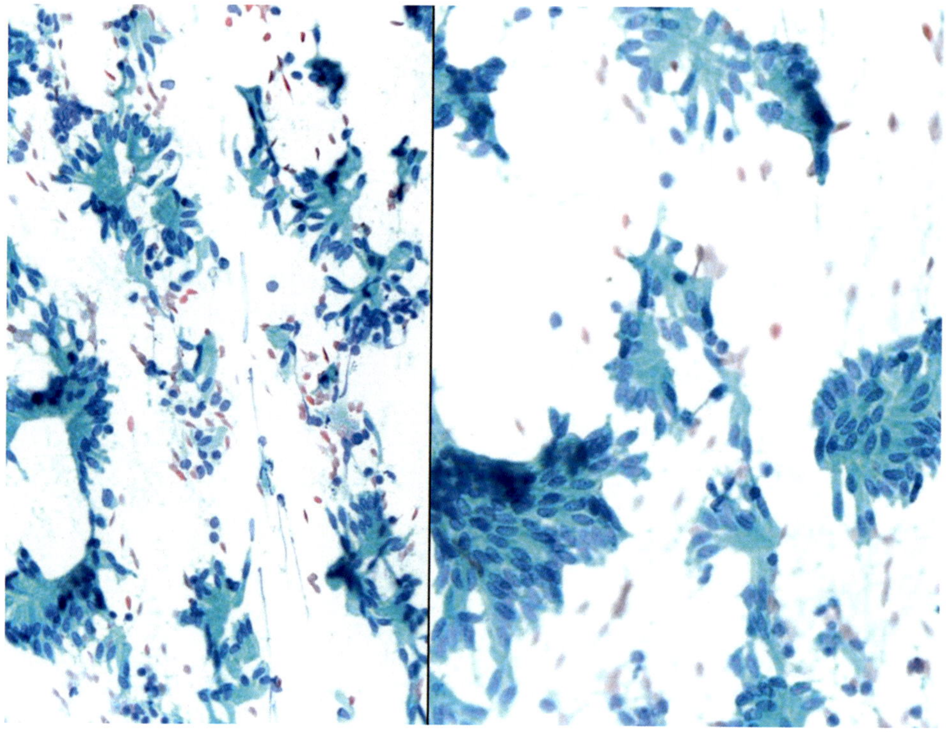

Q-11. A 40-year-old female with bilateral kidney lesions and multiple small liver cystic lesions developed severe abdominal pain and discomfort. Ultrasound-guided liver nodule FNA was performed. What is the diagnosis of this liver FNA?

(a) Metastatic adenocarcinoma
(b) Bile duct hamartoma
(c) Hepatocellular carcinoma
(d) Liver cell adenoma

Fig. 7.12

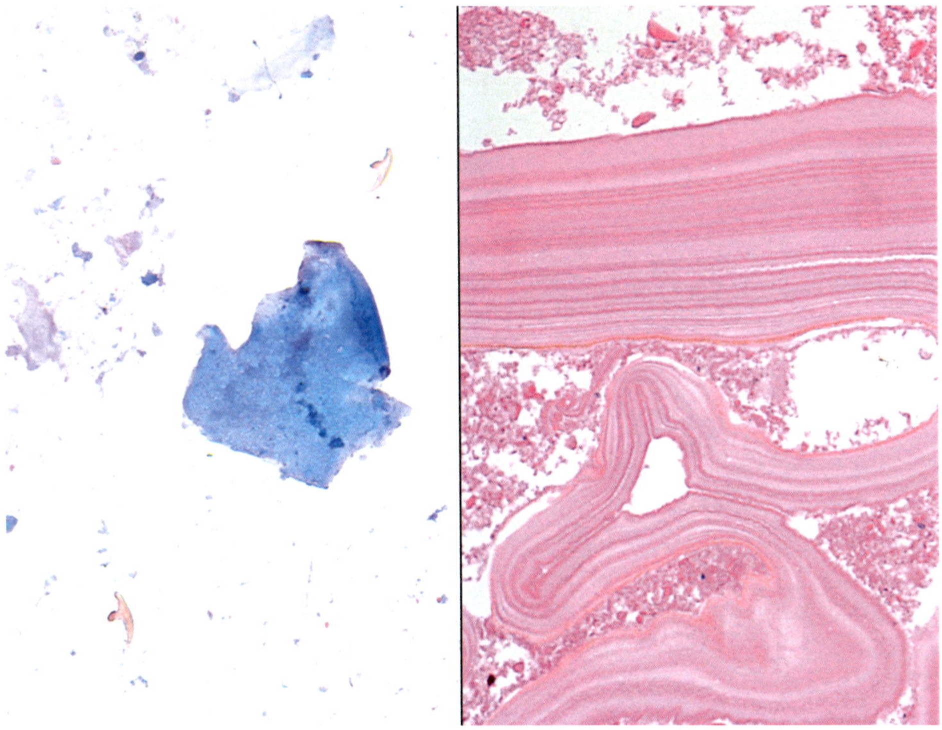

Q-12. A 52-year-old male presented with obstructive jaundice, urticaria, and an enlarged abdomen. A large cystic lesion was found in the liver by ultrasound. If the lesion is aspirated, which one of the following features can be seen, EXCEPT:

(a) Numerous dispersed naked nuclei
(b) Acellular debris
(c) Fragments of the laminated membrane
(d) Scolices and hooklets

Fig. 7.13

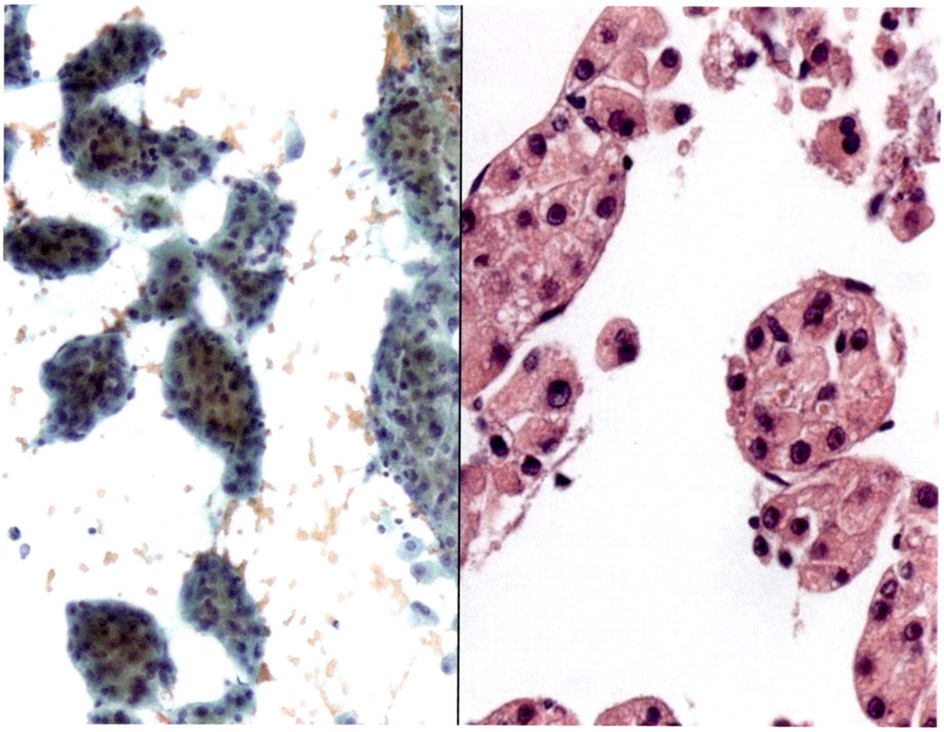

Q-13. A 52-year-old male presented with obstructive jaundice, urticaria, and enlarged abdomen. A large liver mass was found by ultrasound study. What is the diagnosis of this liver FNA?

(a) Metastatic adenocarcinoma
(b) Bile duct hamartoma
(c) Well-differentiated hepatocellular carcinoma
(d) Liver cell adenoma

Fig. 7.14

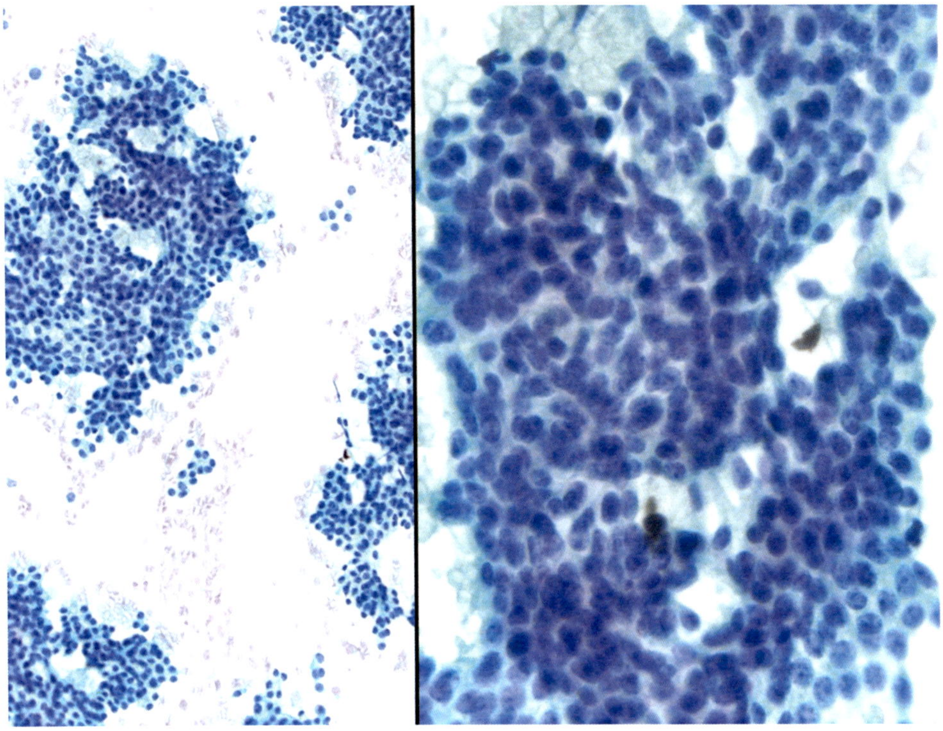

Q-14. A patient presented with diarrhea, abdominal pain, and liver masses. An ultrasound-guided FNA was performed. What is the diagnosis?

(a) Metastatic poorly differentiated adenocarcinoma
(b) Metastatic small cell carcinoma
(c) Hepatocellular carcinoma
(d) Metastatic carcinoid

Fig. 7.15

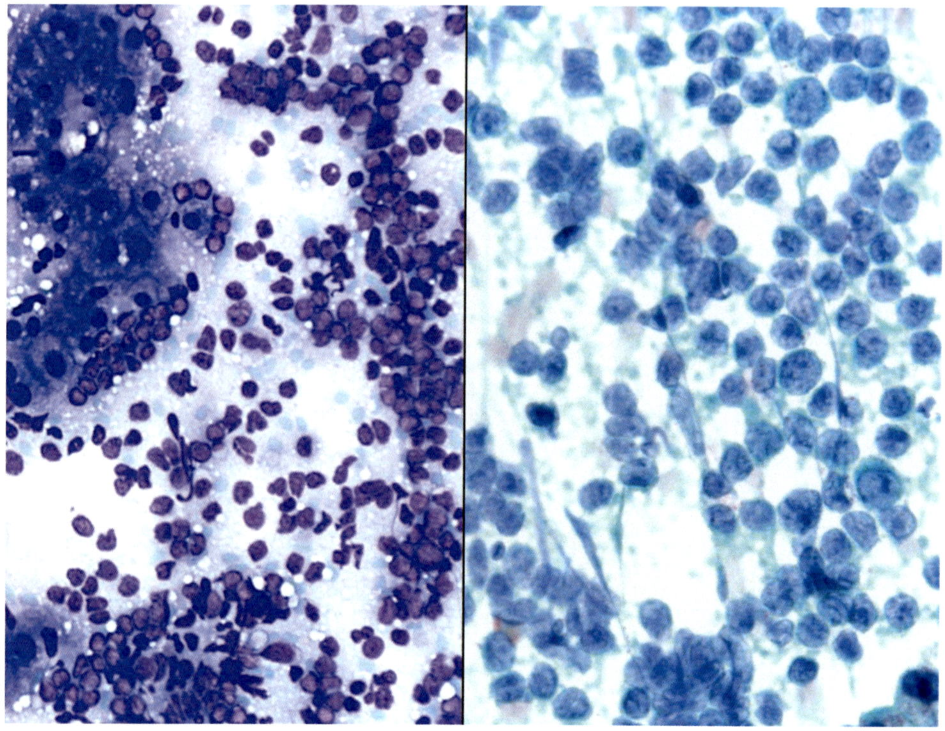

Q-15. A 70-year-old female with a history of breast cancer developed lymphadenopathy, fever, weight loss, and multiple liver masses. What is the diagnosis of this liver FNA?

(a) Metastatic poorly differentiated adenocarcinoma
(b) Metastatic small cell carcinoma
(c) Hepatocellular carcinoma
(d) Diffuse large B-cell lymphoma (DLBCL)

Fig. 7.16

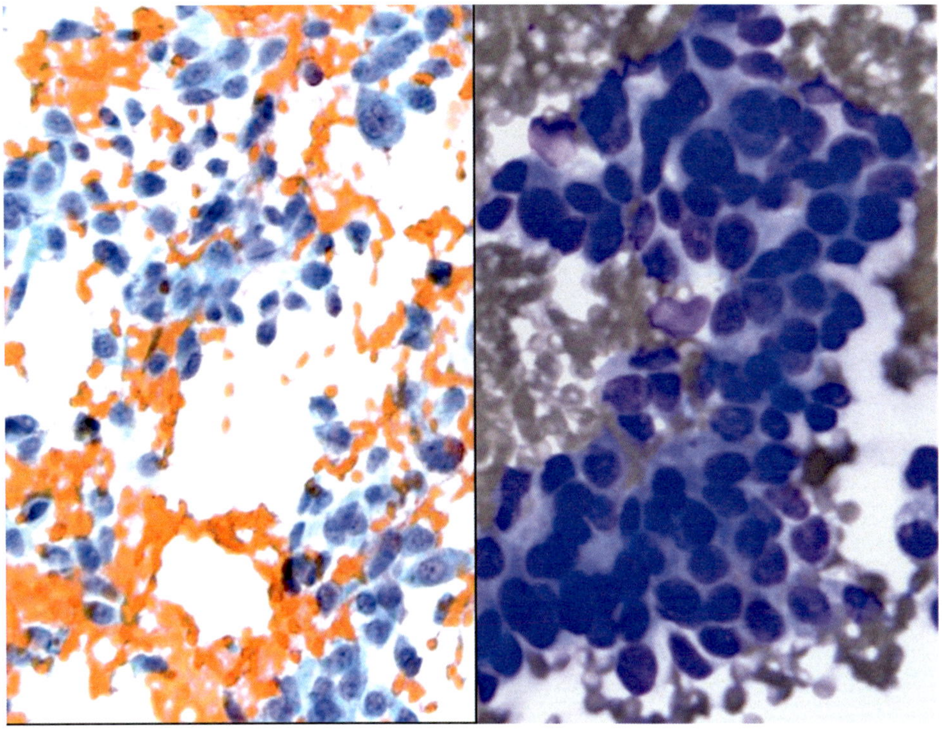

Q-16. A 70-year-old female with a history of primary sclerosing cholangitis developed obstructive jaundice, weight loss, and multiple liver masses. Endoscopic ultrasound-guided FNA (EUS-FNA) was performed. What is the diagnosis of this liver FNA?

(a) Bile duct hamartoma
(b) Metastatic melanoma
(c) Hepatocellular carcinoma
(d) Cholangiocarcinoma

Fig. 7.17

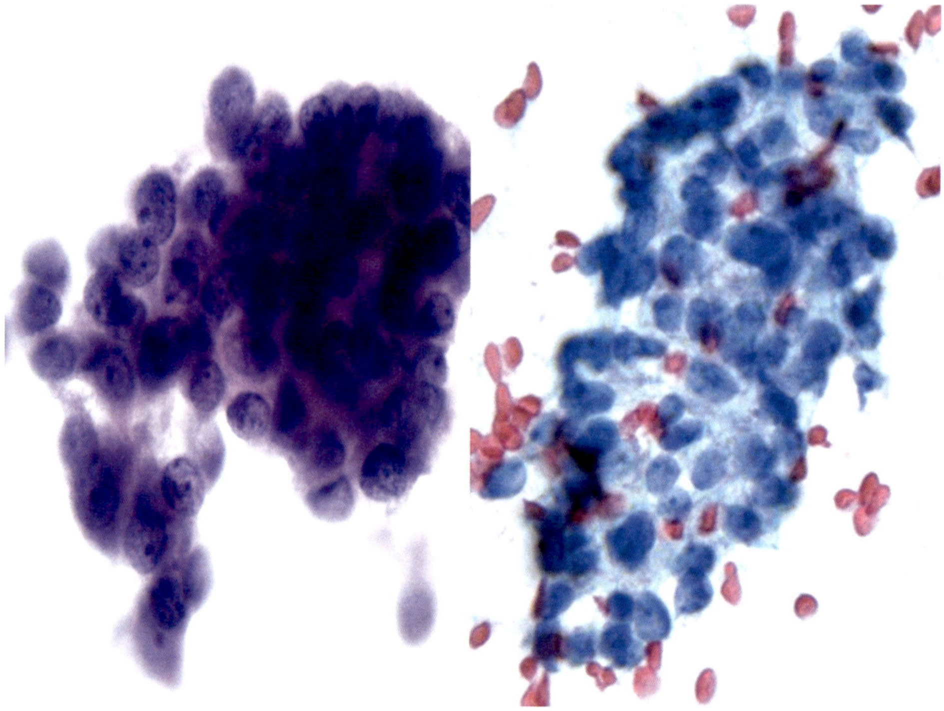

Q-17. A 66-year-old male with malignant history developed multiple liver masses. What is the diagnosis of cells seen in this liver FNA specimen?

(a) Metastatic adenocarcinoma of the lung
(b) Metastatic adenocarcinoma of the prostate
(c) Metastatic adenocarcinoma of the colon
(d) Metastatic small cell carcinoma

Fig. 7.18

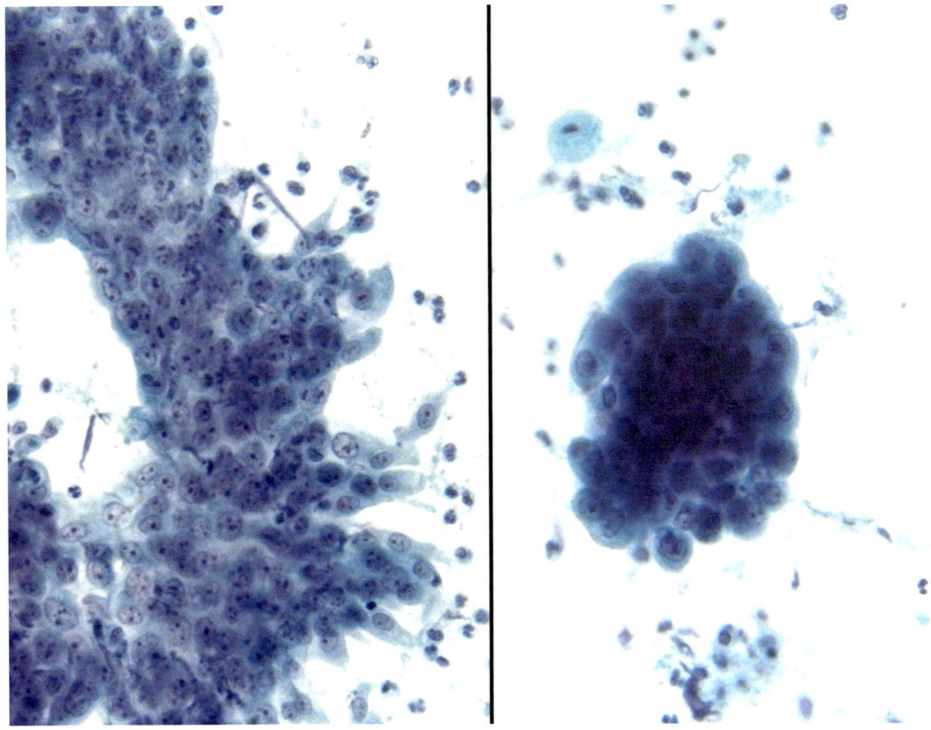

Q-18. A 69-year-old female presented with a right adnexal mass and liver masses. What is the diagnosis of cells seen in this liver FNA?
(a) Metastatic papillary adenocarcinoma of the lung
(b) Metastatic mucinous adenocarcinoma of the ovary
(c) Metastatic adenocarcinoma of the colon
(d) Metastatic small cell carcinoma

Fig. 7.19

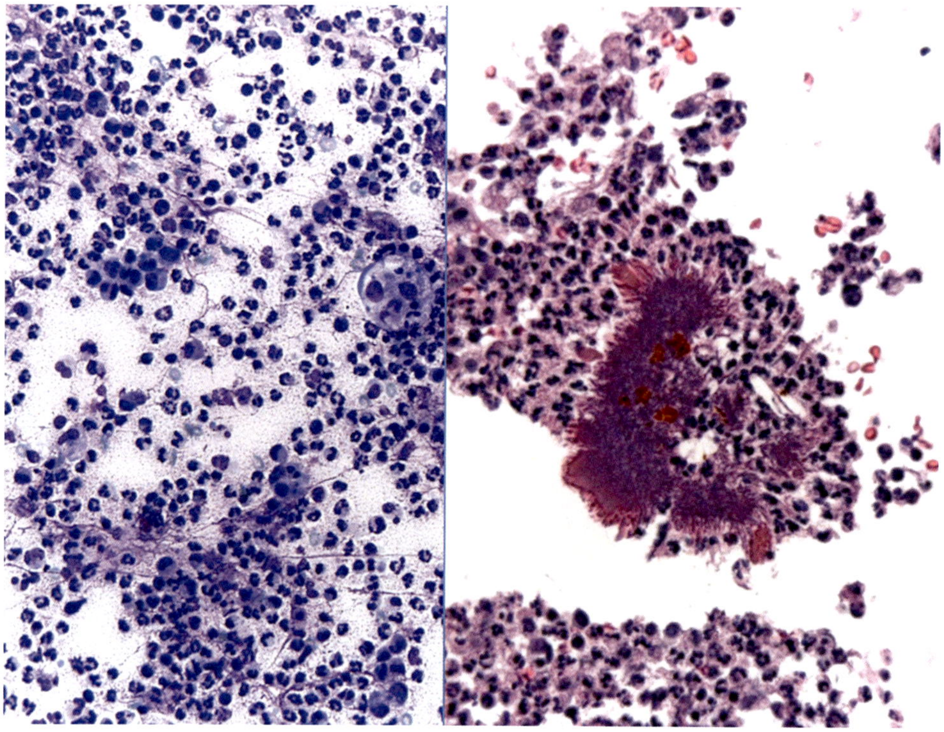

Q-19. An immunocompromised patient develops jaundice, fever, and multiple liver masses. What is the diagnosis of this liver FNA?
(a) Metastatic adenocarcinoma
(b) Lymphoma
(c) Actinomysis
(d) Metastatic small cell carcinoma

Fig. 7.20

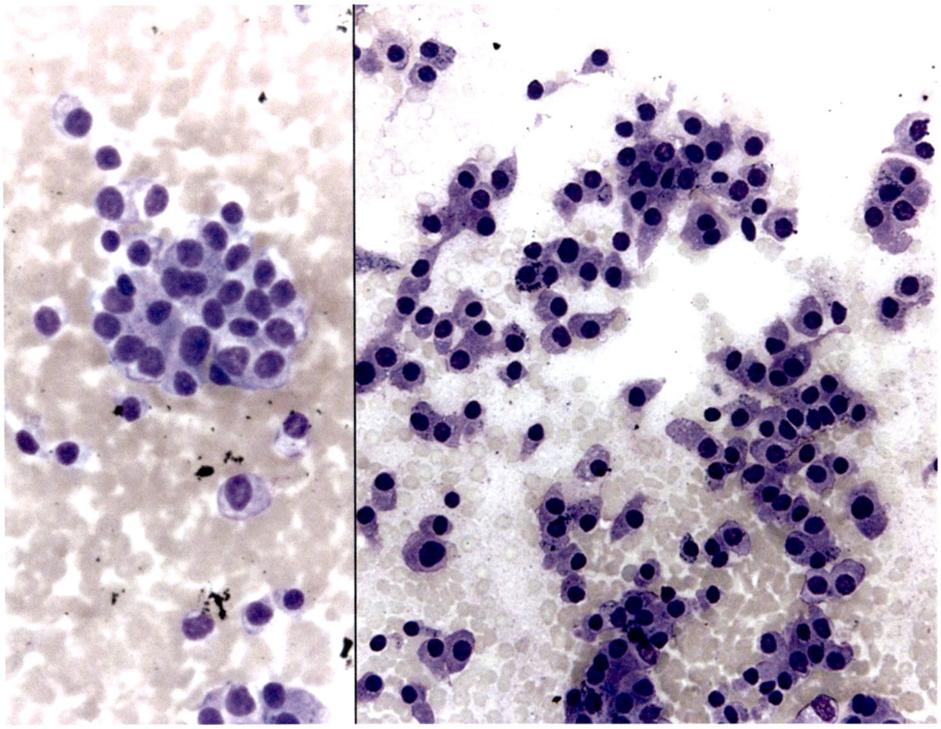

Q-20. What is the diagnosis of this liver mass?
(a) Metastatic small cell carcinoma
(b) Hepatocellular carcinoma
(c) Metastatic carcinoid of the GI tract
(d) Metastatic poorly differentiated adenocarcinoma

Fig. 7.21

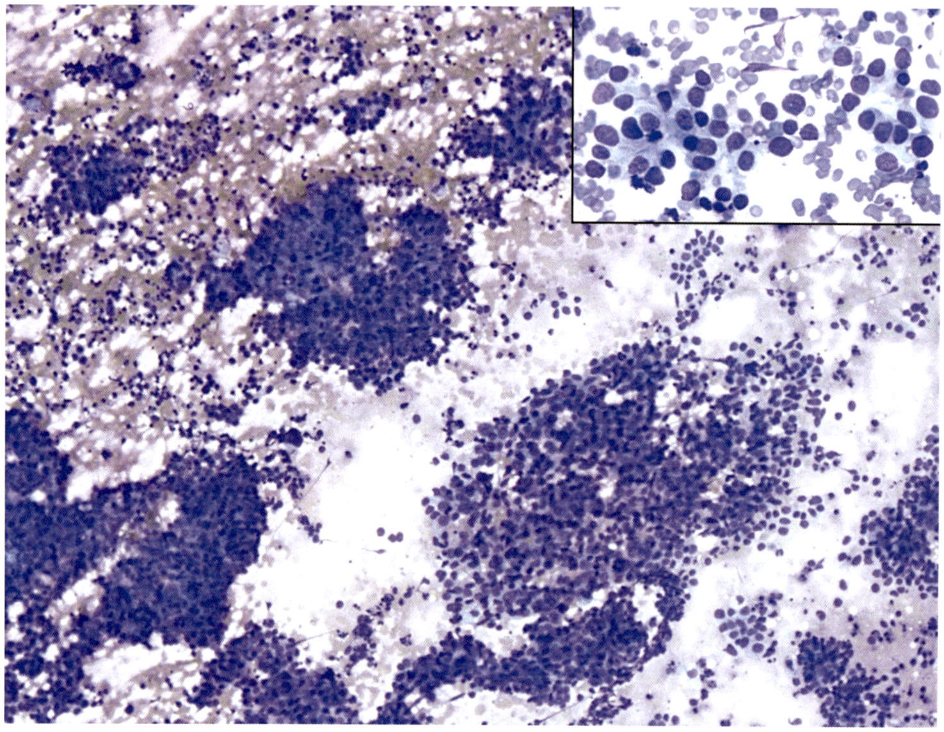

Q-21. What is the diagnosis of this large liver mass from a patient who also has a 1.0 cm mass in the pancreas?
(a) Metastatic small cell carcinoma
(b) Hepatocellular carcinoma
(c) Metastatic endocrine tumor
(d) Metastatic poorly differentiated adenocarcinoma

Fig. 7.22

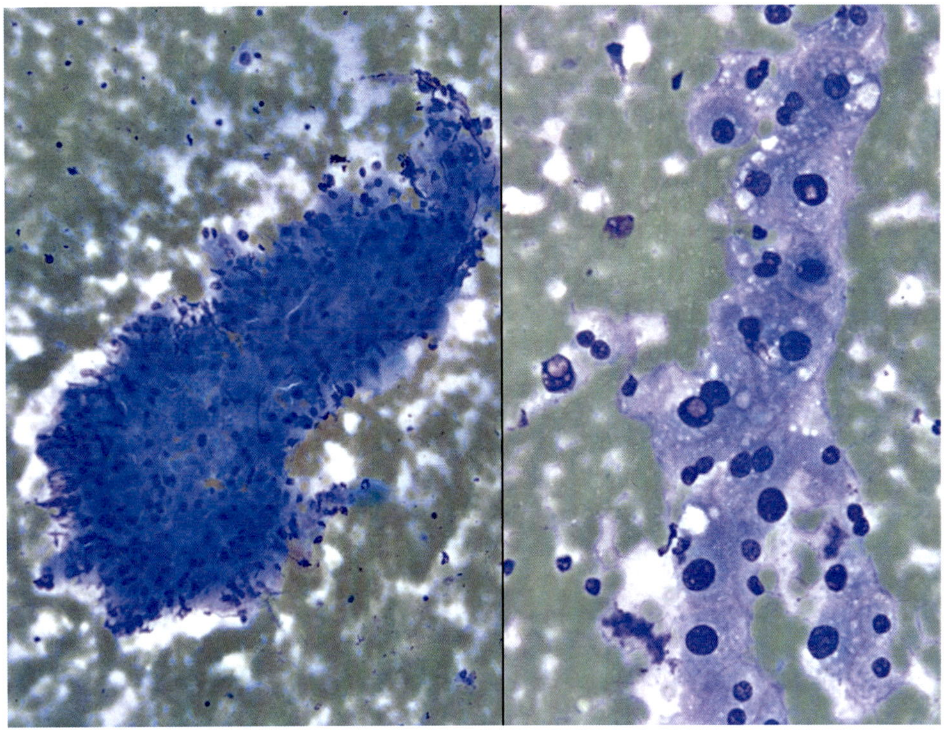

Q-22. What is the diagnosis of this liver FNA?
(a) Metastatic melanoma
(b) Normal liver cells
(c) Poorly differentiated adenocarcinoma
(d) Hepatocellular carcinoma

Fig. 7.23

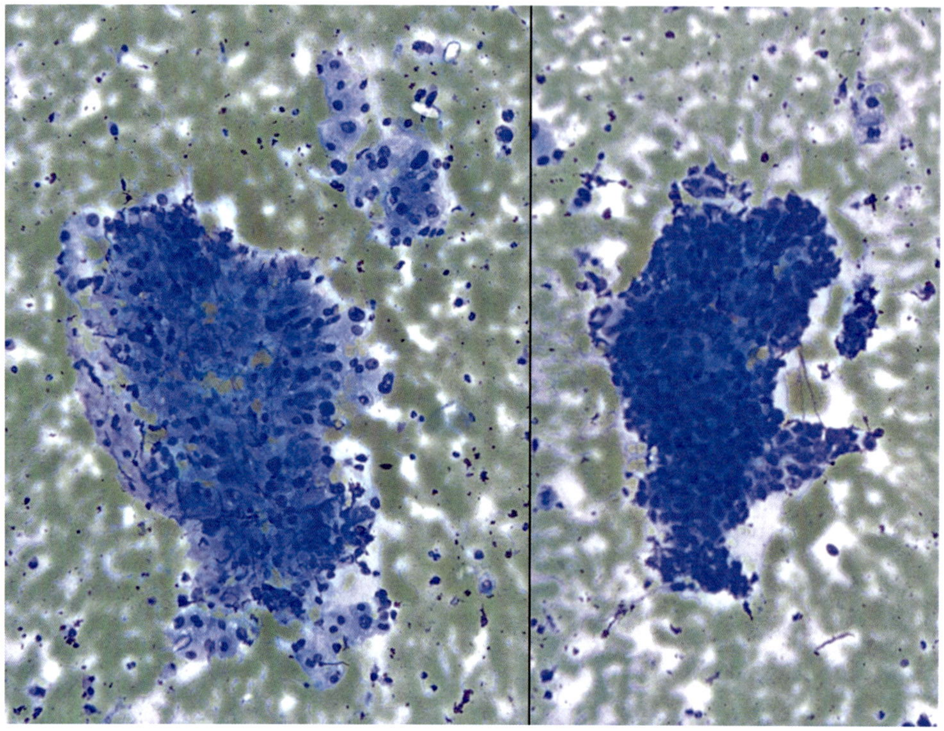

Q-23. A 58-year-old has a history of a stomach tumor and now develops liver masses. What is the diagnosis of this liver FNA?
- (a) Metastatic melanoma
- (b) Normal liver cells
- (c) Metastatic adenocarcinoma
- (d) Hepatocellular carcinoma

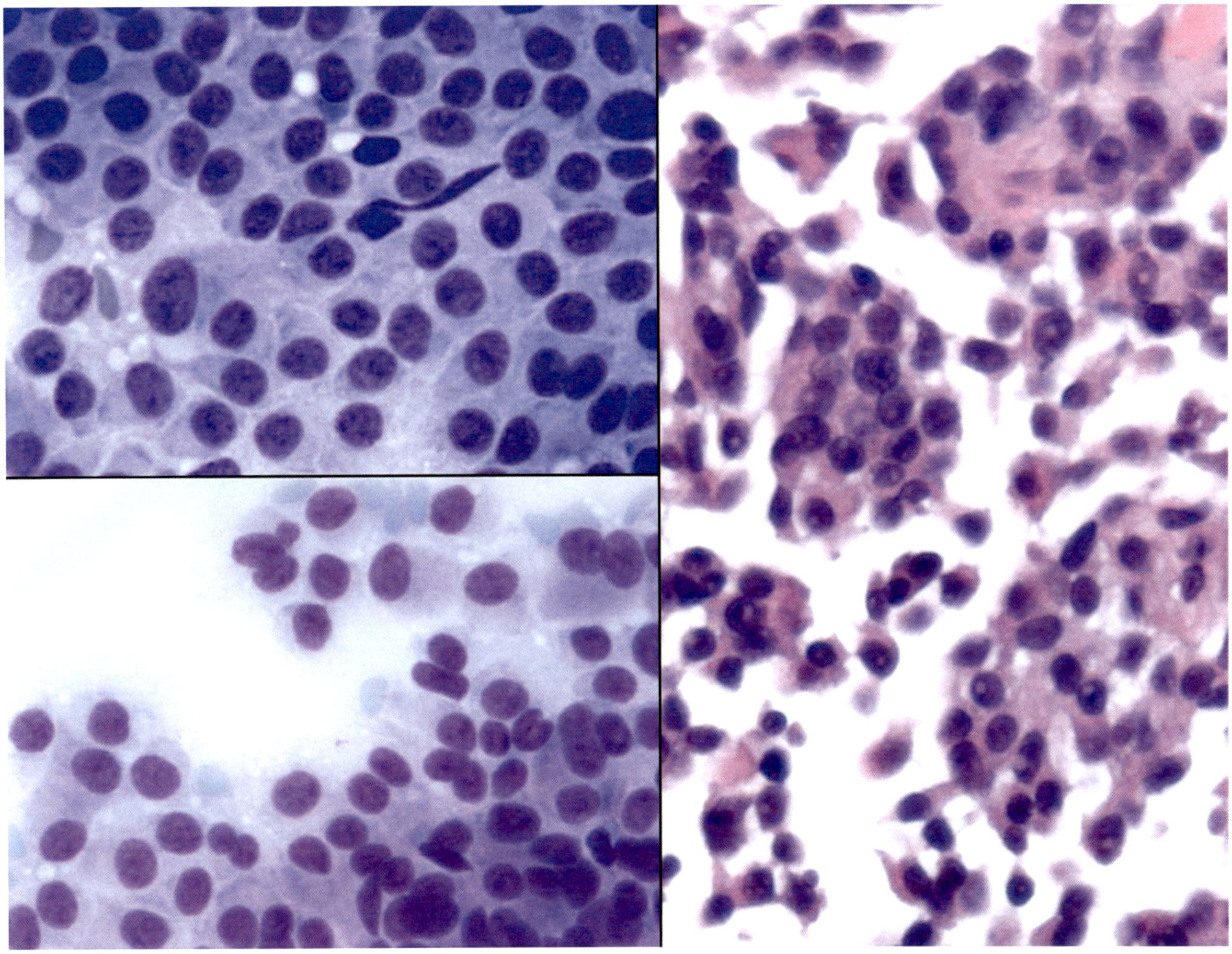

Fig. 7.24

Q-24. What is the diagnosis of this large liver mass?

(a) Normal liver cells
(b) Hepatocellular carcinoma
(c) Endocrine tumor
(d) Metastatic poorly differentiated adenocarcinoma

Fig. 7.25

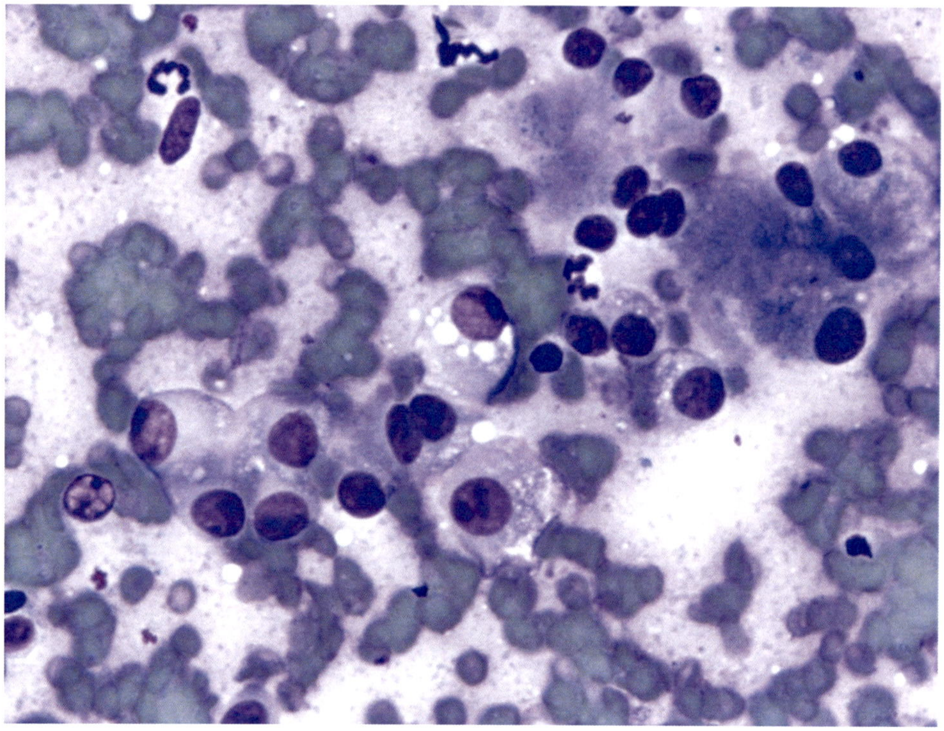

Q-25. A 58-year-old male with a history of "skin cancer" now develops multiple liver masses. What is the diagnosis of this liver FNA?

(a) Metastatic melanoma
(b) Normal liver cells
(c) Poorly differentiated adenocarcinoma
(d) Hepatocellular carcinoma

Fig. 7.26

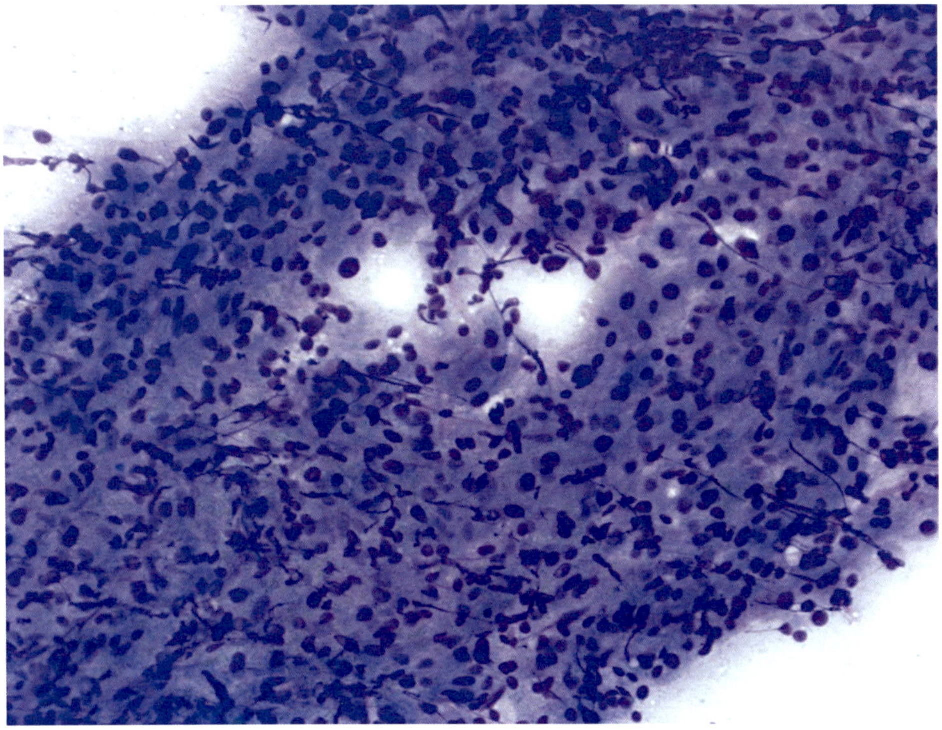

Q-26. A 68-year-old male with a history of alcohol abuse now develops multiple liver masses. What is the diagnosis of this liver FNA?

(a) Metastatic melanoma
(b) Normal liver cells
(c) Poorly differentiated adenocarcinoma
(d) Hepatocellular carcinoma

Fig. 7.27

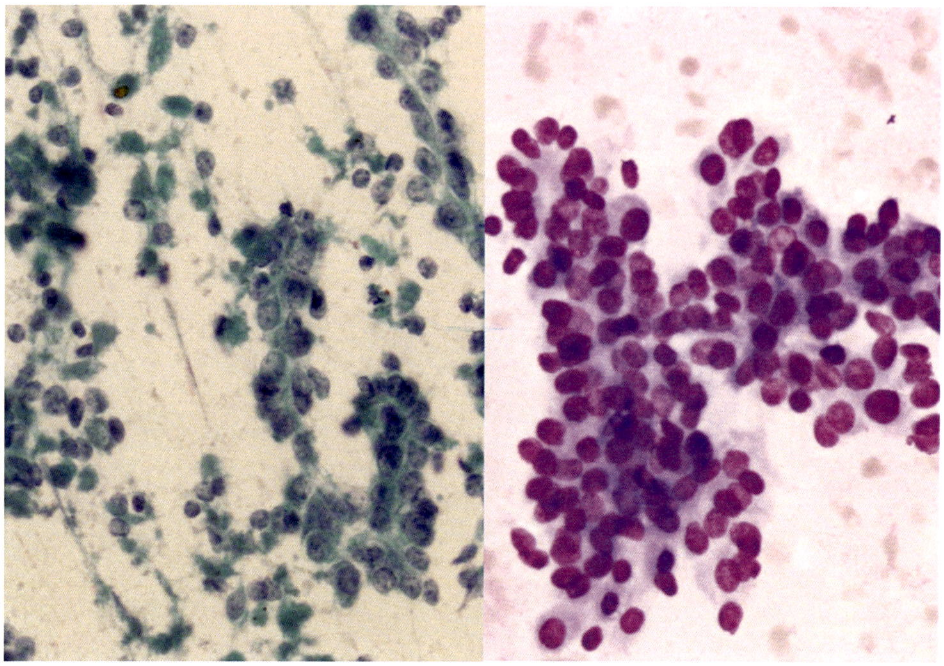

Q-27. A 2-year-old boy with abdominal enlargement is found to have a large liver mass. What is the diagnosis of this liver FNA?

(a) Metastatic small cell carcinoma
(b) Normal liver cells
(c) Hepatoblastoma
(d) Hepatocellular carcinoma

Fig. 7.28

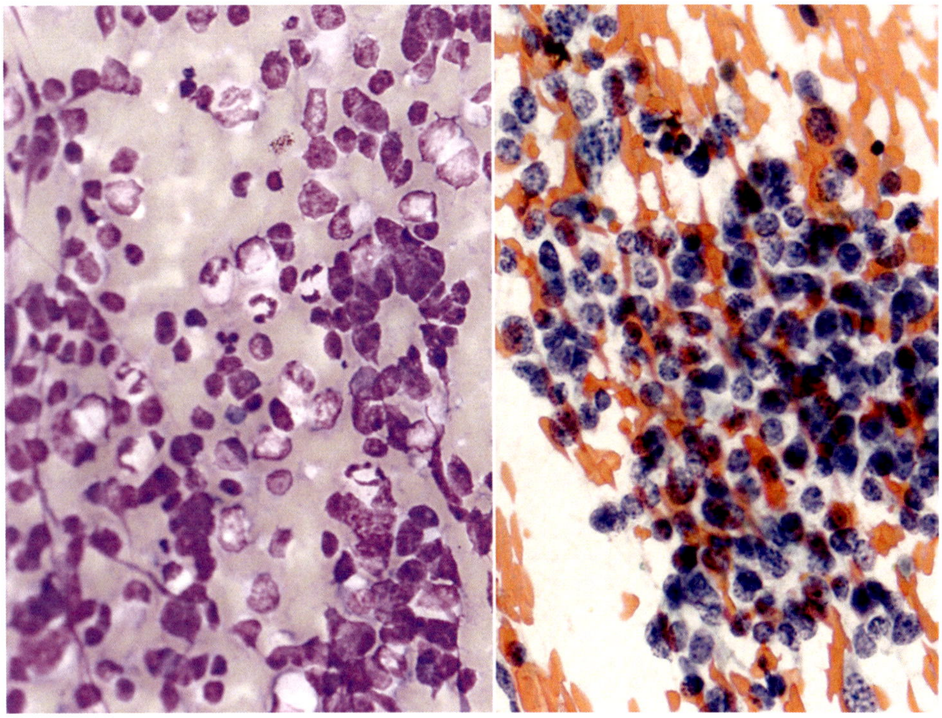

Q-28. A 9-year-old boy with kidney and liver masses had a liver mass FNA. What is the diagnosis of this liver FNA?
(a) Metastatic small cell carcinoma
(b) Normal liver cells
(c) Hepatoblastoma
(d) Metastatic Wilm's tumor

Fig. 7.29

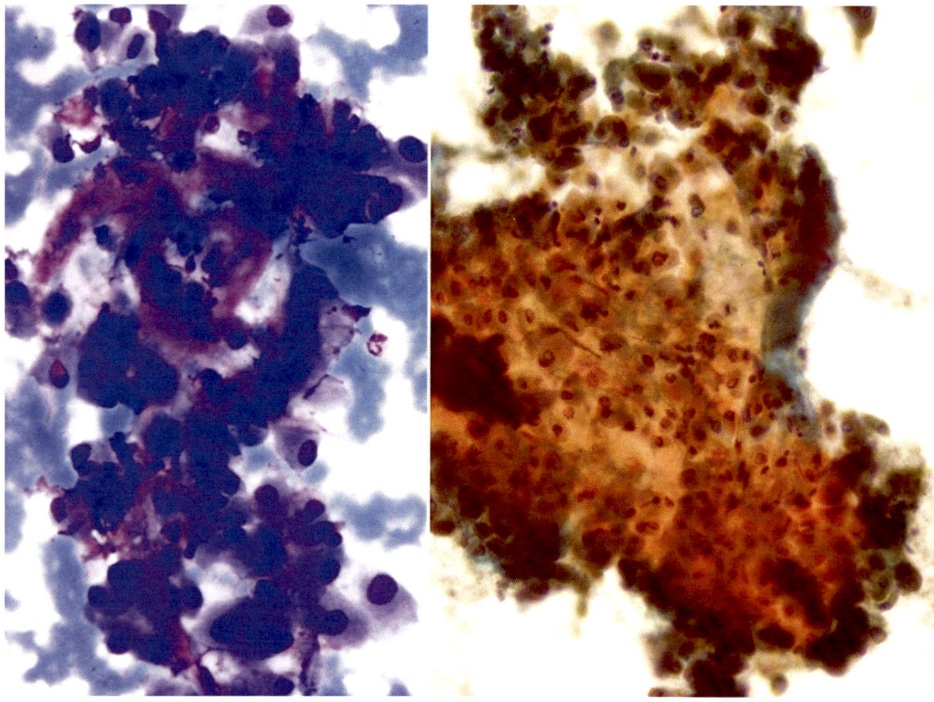

Q-29. A 22-year-old female who has a history of a "uterus tumor" develops a liver mass. What is the diagnosis of this liver FNA?

(a) Fibrolamellar hepatocellular carcinoma
(b) Well-differentiated hepatocellular carcinoma
(c) Cholangiocarcinoma
(d) Metastatic melanoma

Fig. 7.30

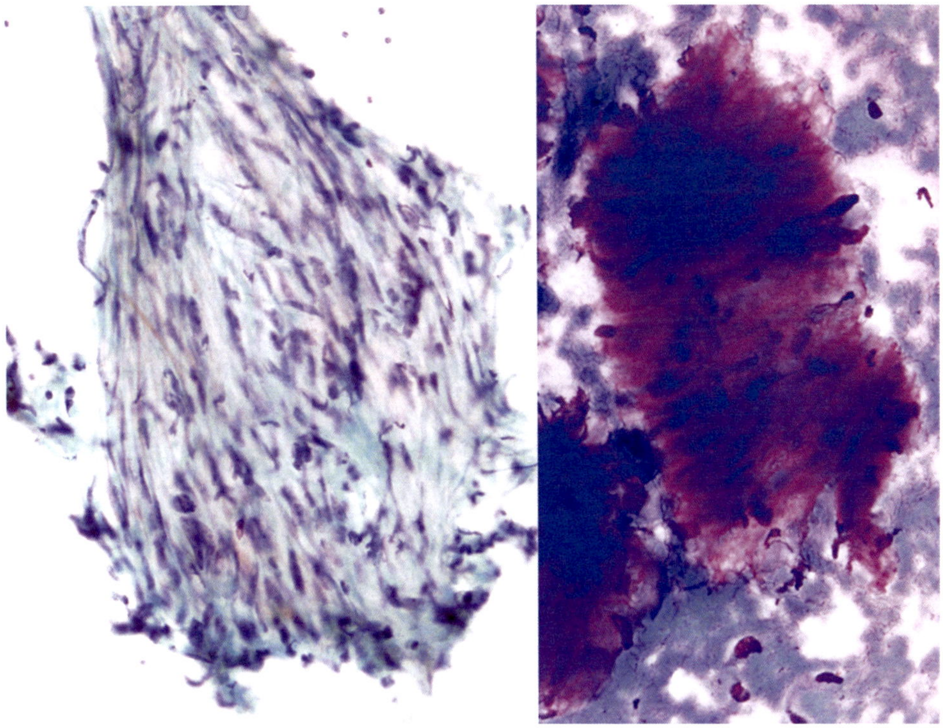

Q-30. A 30-year-old female who has a history of "uterus tumor" develops multiple liver masses. What is the diagnosis of this liver FNA?

(a) Metastatic spindle cell carcinoma
(b) Metastatic spindle cell melanoma
(c) Hemangioma
(d) Metastatic leiomyosarcoma

Fig. 7.31

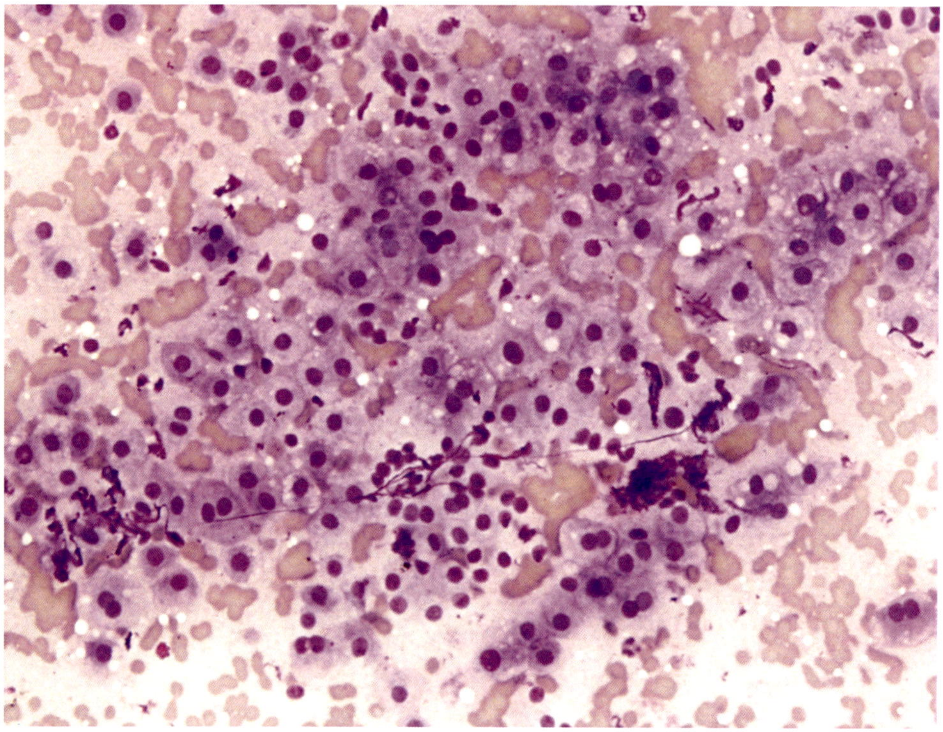

Q-31. What is the diagnosis of this liver FNA?

(a) Metastatic melanoma
(b) Normal liver cells
(c) Poorly differentiated adenocarcinoma
(d) Hepatocellular carcinoma

Fig. 7.32

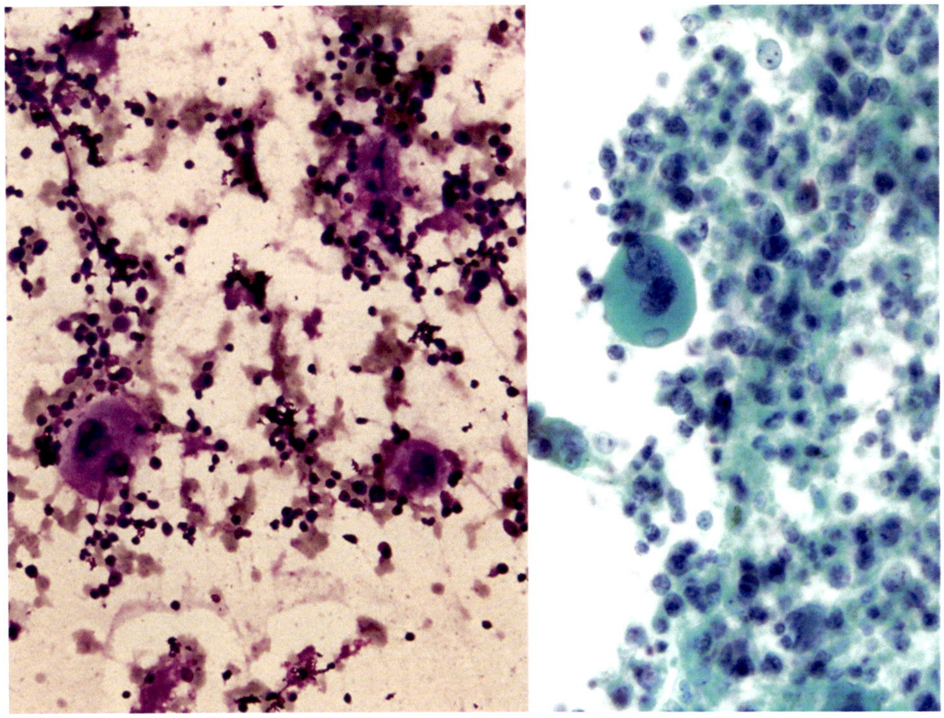

Q-32. A 40-year-old anemic patient develops liver enlargement. What is the diagnosis of this liver FNA?

(a) Reed-Sternberg cells of Hodgkin lymphoma
(b) Normal liver cells
(c) Extramedullary hematopoiesis
(d) Hepatocellular carcinoma

Fig. 7.33

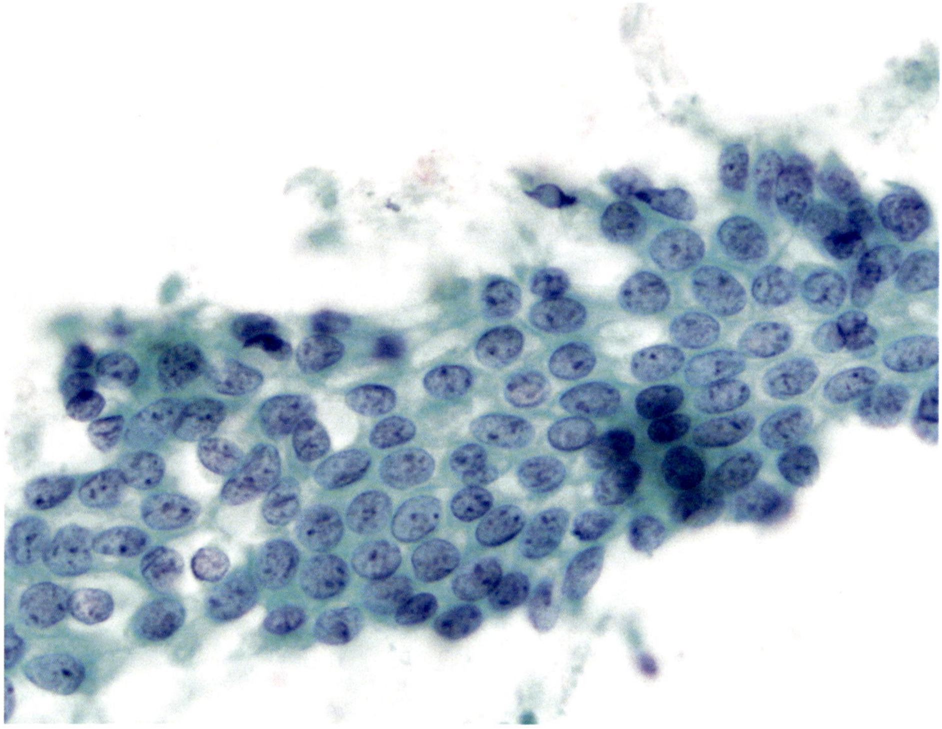

Q-33. What is the diagnosis of this liver FNA?

(a) Carcinoid
(b) Normal liver cells
(c) Benign bile duct epithelial cells
(d) Hepatocellular carcinoma

Fig. 7.34

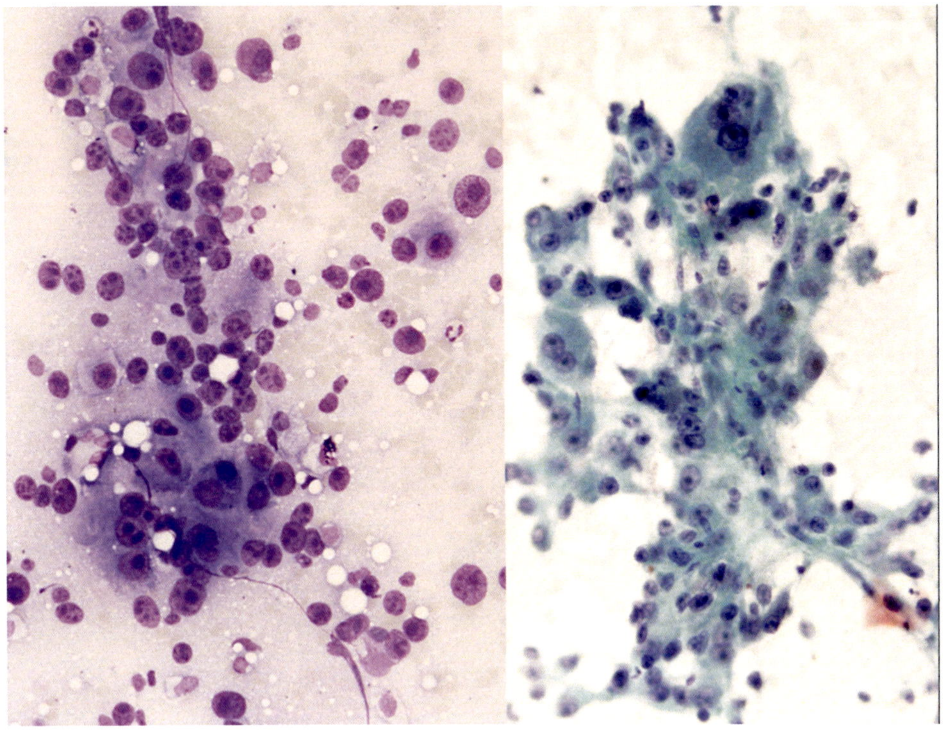

Q-34. What is the diagnosis of this liver FNA?
(a) Carcinoid
(b) Normal liver cells
(c) Poorly differentiated hepatocellular carcinoma
(d) Well-differentiated hepatocellular carcinoma

Fig. 7.35

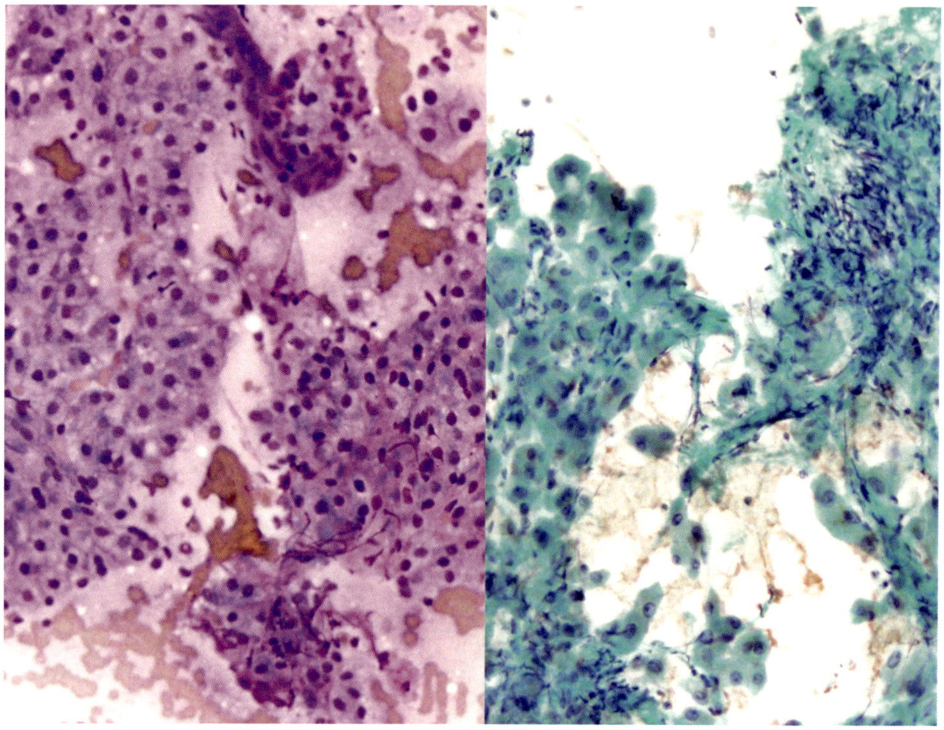

Q-35. What is the diagnosis of this liver FNA from a 42-year-old female?
(a) Liver cell adenoma
(b) Focal nodular hyperplasia
(c) Cholangiocarcinoma
(d) Well-differentiated hepatocellular carcinoma

Fig. 7.36

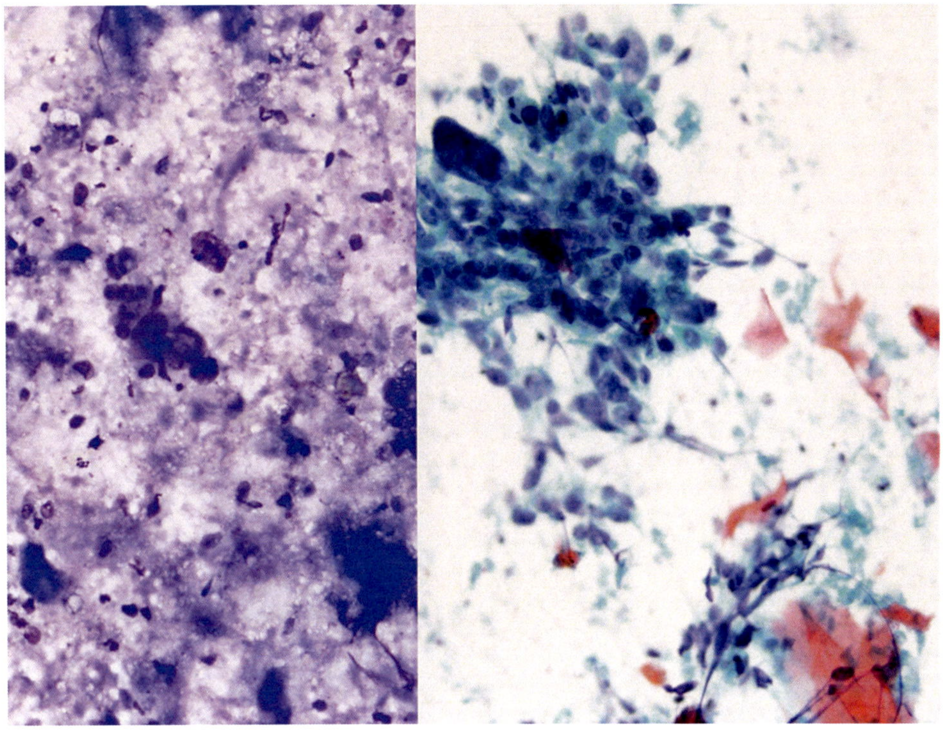

Q-36. An 83-year-old has a history of a skin tumor and develops multiple liver masses. What is the diagnosis of this liver FNA?

(a) Metastatic poorly differentiated adenocarcinoma
(b) Metastatic squamous cell carcinoma
(c) Poorly differentiated hepatocellular carcinoma
(d) Well-differentiated hepatocellular carcinoma

Fig. 7.37

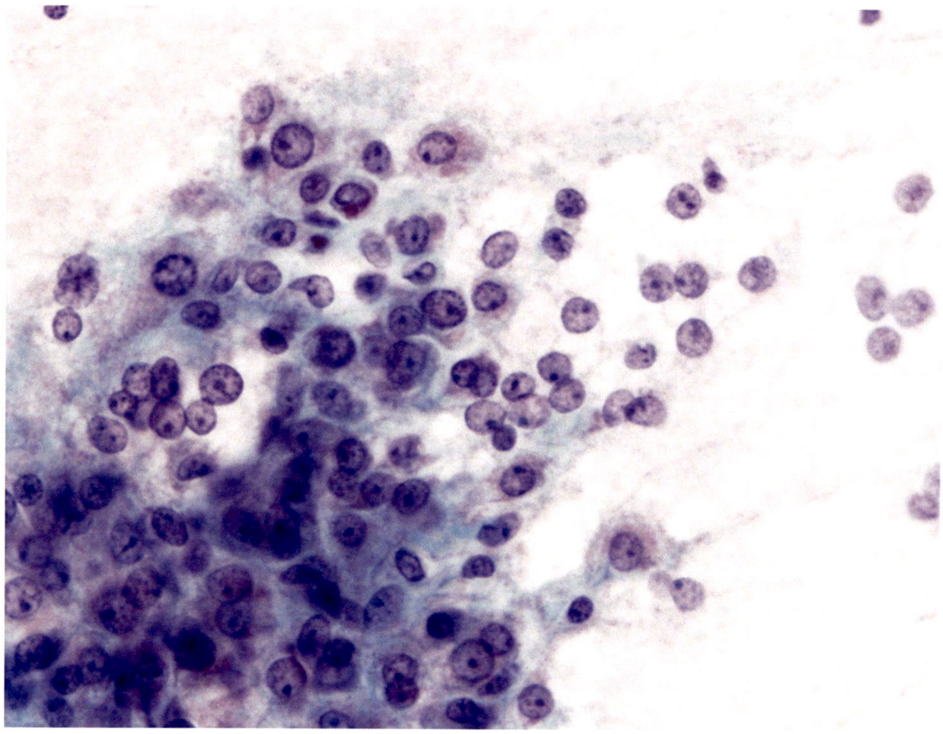

Q-37. What is the diagnosis of this liver FNA?
(a) Carcinoid
(b) Normal liver cells
(c) Cholangiocarcinoma
(d) Hepatocellular carcinoma

Fig. 7.38

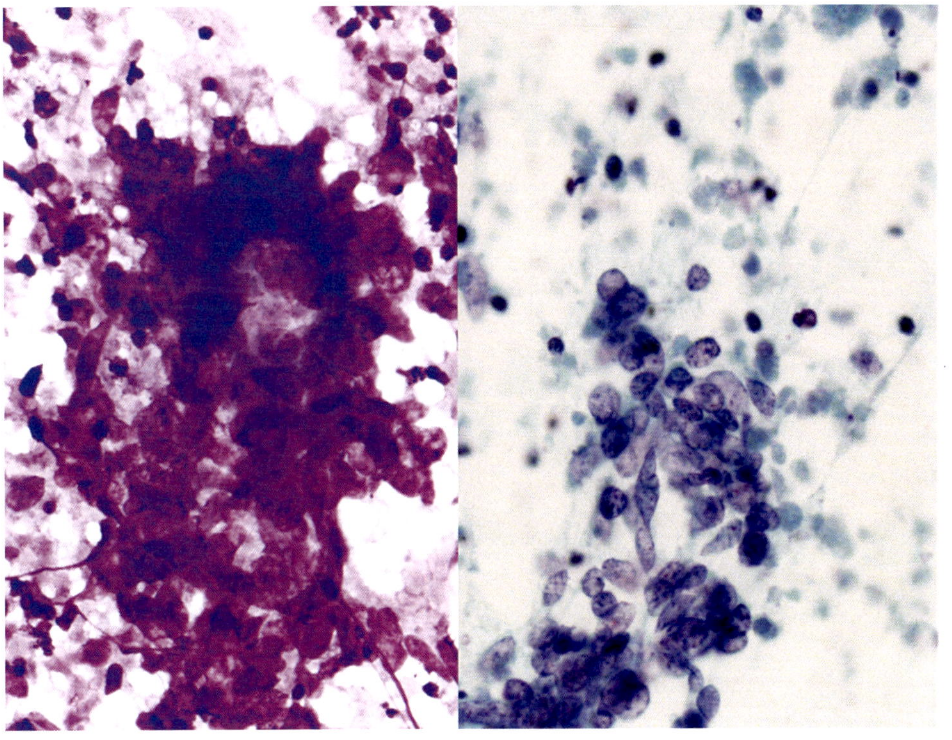

Q-38. A liver FNA was performed on a patient with multiple liver masses. The diagnosis of metastatic adenocarcinoma was made. Which one is the most possible primary site of the tumor?

(a) Breast
(b) Lung
(c) Colon
(d) Renal

7.2 Text-Based Questions 39–75

Q-39. All of the following features are seen in a fine-needle aspiration (FNA) containing benign hepatocytes, EXCEPT:
(a) Numerous dispersed naked nuclei
(b) Sheets of polygonal cells and individual hepatocytes
(c) Centrally placed nuclei with binucleation
(d) Prominent nucleoli

Q-40. Which statement about the liver cell adenoma is correct?
(a) It is a benign tumor and has no risk to progress into malignancy
(b) The tumor reveals clusters of pleomorphic cells and numerous naked nuclei
(c) It commonly occurs in females under the age of 30 and is related to long-term use of oral contraceptives
(d) Tumor necrosis is a common finding

Q-41. All of these cytological features are seen in cholangiocarcinomas, EXCEPT:
(a) Nuclear enlargement and variation in size and shape
(b) Trabeculae, cords, and nested arrangements
(c) Large oval nuclei and coarse chromatin
(d) Numerous naked nuclei

Q-42. Which statement regarding fatty change of the liver is correct?
(a) Fatty change is reported in 40 % of early HCC
(b) Fatty change is only observed in benign hepatocellular lesion
(c) Prevalence of fatty change increases along with increase in tumor size
(d) Fatty change is only observed in benign hepatocellular nodules

Q-43. All of the following cytological features of benign bile duct epithelial cells on a liver FNA specimen are correct, EXCEPT:
(a) The size of bile duct epithelial cells is similar to normal hepatocytes
(b) Bile duct epithelial cells have hyperchromatic nuclei
(c) In benign ductal epithelial cells, nuclear overlapping and disarray are common
(d) Benign bile duct epithelial cells have scant cytoplasm

Q-44. Which cytological feature is most useful in the separation of hepatocellular carcinoma (HCC) from cholangiocarcinoma:
(a) The size of tumor cells, i.e., the tumor cell of HCC is bigger than that of cholangiocarcinoma.
(b) Nuclear enlargement and variation in size and shape
(c) Identification of bile and sinusoidal capillaries
(d) Presence of prominent nucleoli

Q-45. All descriptions of cytological features of hepatic angiomyolipoma (AML) on a liver FNA specimen are correct, EXCEPT:
(a) Presence of extramedullary hematopoiesis
(b) Tumor consists of fat, epithelioid spindle cells (myoid cells), and an increased vascularity
(c) Hepatic AML cannot be diagnosed accurately by FNA
(d) Some of the tumor may have virtually no fat

Q-46. Which immuno panel is most useful in the separation of HCC from a cholangiocarcinoma?
(a) Positive alpha-fetoprotein (AFP), negative CD10
(b) Positive HepPar1, negative CD10
(c) Positive HepPar1 and CD10, negative epithelial membrane antigen (EMA), monoclonal carcinoembryonic antigen (CEA), and CK7
(d) Negative alpha-fetoprotein (AFP), negative CD10

Q-47. For the diagnosis of liver malignancy, ultrasound-and/or CT-guided percutaneous FNA have similar sensitivity and specificity as endoscopic ultrasound-guided FNA (EUS-FNA), true or false?
(a) True
(b) False

Q-48. Which risk factor is NOT significantly associated with cholangiocarcinoma?
(a) Primary sclerosing cholangitis
(b) Cirrhosis
(c) Infection with the parasitic liver flukes *Opisthorchis viverrini* or *Clonorchis sinensis*
(d) Exposure to thorotrast

Q-49. Which cytological feature is NOT seen in liver cell adenoma?
(a) Spindle-shaped endothelial cells
(b) Preserved reticulin scaffold
(c) Prominent bile pigment
(d) Benign bile duct epithelial cells

Q-50. All of the following features can be seen in a well-differentiated HCC, EXCEPT:
(a) Preserved reticulin scaffold pattern
(b) Dense cytoplasm
(c) Prominent nucleoli
(d) Shared cell borders

Q-51. A 65-year-old patient with cirrhosis developed a rapidly enlarged liver mass. On a liver FNA specimen, numerous clusters of liver cells with mild nuclear atypia are identified. Which one of the following tumors is most likely to be diagnosed?
(a) Cholangiocarcinoma
(b) Poorly differentiated hepatocellular carcinoma
(c) Well-differentiated hepatocellular carcinoma
(d) Small cell carcinoma

Q-52. A 60-year-old male patient presents with retroperitoneal lymphadenopathy and diffuse enlargement of the liver. An ultrasound-guided liver FNA was performed. On cytology smear and cell block section, numerous dyscohesive small to intermediate-sized cells with high N:C ratios, hyperchromatic coarse chromatin, and prominent nucleoli are identified. Rare scattered hepatocytes are also present. What is the likely diagnosis of the liver FNA?
(a) Cholangiocarcinoma
(b) Poorly differentiated hepatocellular carcinoma
(c) Lymphoma
(d) Small cell carcinoma

Q-53. A liver FNA was performed on a 60-year-old female smoker who presented with a right liver infiltration and right pleural effusion. On the cytological preparation, large sheets and tight clusters of atypical epithelioid cells are identified; some of them have "signet ring" cell features. What is the diagnosis of the liver FNA?
(a) Metastatic adenocarcinoma of the colon
(b) Metastatic adenocarcinoma of the lung
(c) Cholangiocarcinoma
(d) Well-differentiated hepatocellular carcinoma

Q-54. Immuno marker HepPar1 is positive for hepatocellular carcinoma and negative for cholangiocarcinoma, true or false?
(a) True
(b) False

Q-55. Which of the following cytological feature is most useful in the separation of a metastatic poorly differentiated adenocarcinoma from a metastatic small cell carcinoma in liver FNA specimen?
(a) Prominent nucleoli
(b) Fine or coarse chromatin pattern
(c) Tumor necrosis
(d) Organoid and/or rosettes arrangement of tumor cells

Q-56. A cytological smear of liver FNA reveals a bloody smear with numerous two-dimensional clusters and/or sheets of spindle cells, the differential diagnosis of the lesion includes all of the following, EXCEPT:
(a) Cholangiocarcinoma
(b) Hemangioma
(c) Metastatic melanoma
(d) Angiomyolipoma

Q-57. All of the following cytological features can be seen in metastatic prostate carcinoma, EXCEPT:
(a) Microacini arrangement
(b) Intermediate-sized tumor cells
(c) Paranuclear blue bodies in the cytoplasm
(d) Prominent nucleoli

Q-58. The cytological feature of fibrolamellar hepatocellular carcinoma includes all of them, EXCEPT:
(a) Large polygonal tumor cells with abundant cytoplasm
(b) Intermediate-sized tumor cells
(c) Intracytoplasmic hyaline globules
(d) Prominent nucleoli

Q-59. A liver FNA was performed on a patient with multiple liver masses. On the FNA preparation, it revealed three-dimensional clusters of tall columnar cells with hyperchromatic nuclei, coarse chromatin, prominent nucleoli, irregular nuclear membrane, and feathering cytoplasm. Tumor necrosis is also identified. Which one is the most possible primary site of the tumor?
(a) Breast
(b) Lung
(c) Colon
(d) Kidney

Q-60. A female patient with a breast mass developed liver masses. All of the following features can be seen in a metastatic breast carcinoma. EXCEPT:
(a) Prominent nucleoli
(b) Intracytoplasmic lumina (Magenta body)
(c) Three-dimensional cell clusters
(d) Naked nuclei

Q-61. All of the following features can be seen in a well-differentiated HCC, EXCEPT:
(a) Preserved reticulin scaffold pattern
(b) Dense cytoplasm
(c) Prominent nucleoli
(d) Shared cell borders

Q-62. Cytological features of a metastatic carcinoid tumor may include all of the following, EXCEPT:
(a) Fine chromatin pattern (so-called "salt-and-pepper" pattern)
(b) Inconspicuous or small nucleoli
(c) Scant cytoplasm
(d) Nuclear grooves

Q-63. Which of the following cytological features is helpful in the differential diagnosis of a metastatic carcinoid tumor from cholangiocarcinoma in a liver FNA specimen?
(a) Fine chromatin pattern
(b) Three-dimensional and/or pseudoacinar arrangements of tumor cells
(c) Lacy cytoplasm with vacuolization
(d) Dispersed tumor cells with marked atypia and enlargement

Q-64. A liver FNA specimen characteristic of a metastatic small cell carcinoma includes all of the following, EXCEPT:
(a) Hyperchromatic nuclei and prominent nucleoli
(b) Scant cytoplasm
(c) Three-dimensional cell clusters with nuclear molding
(d) Individual tumor cells with fine chromatin

Q-65. In a FNA specimen, cells reveal "pseudointranuclear inclusions" and mild cytological atypia. All of the following lesions/tumors can have this cytological feature, EXCEPT:
(a) Focal nodular hyperplasia
(b) Liver cell adenoma
(c) Cholangiocarcinoma
(d) Hepatocellular carcinoma

Q-66. In a FNA specimen, atypical cells reveal "clear cytoplasm." All of the following lesions/tumors can have this cytological feature, EXCEPT:
(a) Focal nodular hyperplasia
(b) Renal cell carcinoma
(c) Cholangiocarcinoma
(d) Hepatocellular carcinoma

Q-67. In a FNA specimen, which one of the following features is indicative of a well-differentiated hepatocellular carcinoma (HCC)?
(a) Numerous large clusters of cells
(b) Lacunae spaces on cell block preparation
(c) Presence of a "second population" of cells
(d) Sinusoidal capillaries surrounding the markedly thickened trabeculae of neoplastic cells

Q-68. In a FNA specimen, which one of the following features is best seen in a bile duct hamartoma but not in a metastatic adenocarcinoma?
(a) Sheets or loosely formed clusters of columnar cells
(b) Benign-appearing hepatocytes
(c) Presence of a "second population" of cells
(d) Three-dimensional, dark colored cellular clusters

Q-69. Which of the feature is NOT seen in a metastatic squamous cell carcinoma in a liver FNA specimen?
(a) Large nuclei with smudgy chromatin
(b) Nuclei with variation in size and shape
(c) Pyknotic nuclei
(d) Cytokeratin formation

Q-70. A HIV positive patient developed a diffusely enlarged liver and peripheral lymphadenopathy. Which one of the following lymphomas is associated with c-myc gene rearrangement and shows no evidence of HHV-8 infection?
(a) Burkitt's or Burkitt's-like lymphoma (BL)
(b) Diffuse large B-cell lymphoma (DLBCL)
(c) Peripheral T-cell non-Hodgkin lymphoma (NHL)
(d) Primary effusion lymphoma (PEL)

Q-71. In a FNA specimen, which one of the following features favors the diagnosis of diffuse large B-cell lymphoma (DLBCL) over a metastatic poorly differentiated adenocarcinoma?
(a) Numerous large clusters of cells
(b) Dispersed individual large atypical cells
(c) Presence of a "second population" of cells on the slides
(d) Pseudointranuclear inclusions

Q-72. Which of the following features favors the diagnosis of a metastatic melanoma over the diagnosis of a hepatocellular carcinoma (HCC) in a liver FNA specimen?
(a) Large nuclei with prominent nucleoli

(b) Binucleation with "mirror" image
(c) Variation of nuclear size
(d) Predominantly isolated large cells with "cherry red" nuclei

Q-73. Which statement regarding cholangiocarcinoma is NOT correct?
(a) Cholangiocarcinoma is virtually indistinguishable from a metastatic adenocarcinoma
(b) Cholangiocarcinoma is always seen in a cirrhotic liver
(c) Tumor cells have large oval nuclei and coarse chromatin
(d) Crowded sheets and clusters of tumor cells

Q-74. The most notable features of hepatocellular carcinoma (HCC) include all of the following, EXCEPT:
(a) Polygonal large cells with centrally placed nuclei
(b) Dense cytoplasm and distinct cell border
(c) Large oval nuclei and coarse chromatin
(d) Numerous naked nuclei

Q-75. Which statement regarding the benign hepatocyte is correct?
(a) Numerous dispersed naked nuclei
(b) Clusters of polygonal cells and individual hepatocytes with hyperchromatic nuclei
(c) Centrally placed nuclei with binucleation
(d) Marked variation of size of nuclei

7.3 Answers and Discussion of Image-Based Questions 1–38

A-1. **(b) Metastatic small cell carcinoma**
The diagnosis is metastatic small cell carcinoma of the lung. In small cell carcinomas, tumor cells are relatively small, and they are two- to threefold the size of mature lymphocytes; however, in small cell carcinoma large cell variant, the size of tumor cells can be much larger. Tumor cells show a high N:C ratio, have large nuclei with fine chromatin (salt-and-pepper) pattern, nuclear crowding and molding, and paranuclear blue bodies in the cytoplasm. The prominent nucleolus is not usually seen in a small cell carcinoma. The nucleoli are inconspicuous in small cell carcinomas. In some cases, tumor cells may reveal rare nucleoli, but they are small in size. The background of the smear may also reveal "blue strips" (indicative of breakdown nuclear material). In poorly differentiated adenocarcinomas, tumor cells are larger in size with hyperchromatic nuclei, coarse chromatin, prominent nucleoli, and vacuolated cytoplasm; the tumor also reveals acinar and three-dimensional arrangement. In lymphoma, tumor cells have a high N:C ratio with coarse chromatin and nucleoli, without nuclear molding and crowding. In hepatocellular carcinoma (HCC), tumor cells form cords, tubules, sheets, or isolated individual cells. Tumor cells with hyperchromatic nuclei, coarse chromatin, large prominent nucleoli, intranuclear pseudoinclusion, and cytoplasmic bile/lipofuscin pigments are characteristics seen in HCC. Numerous naked nuclei are also seen in HCC, particularly in poorly differentiated tumor.

A-2. **(c) Fine and evenly distributed chromatin**
In HCC, tumor cells arrange in cords, clusters, tubules, or dispersed individual cells. Tumor cells reveal hyperchromatic nuclei, coarse chromatin, large prominent "cherry-red" nucleoli and intranuclear pseudoinclusions. Dense cytoplasm with cytoplasmic bile/lipofuscin pigments is also characteristic of HCC. Numerous naked nuclei and tumor necrosis are also seen in HCC. In a poorly differentiated HCC, tumor cell pleomorphism and giant tumor cells are also present. Fine and evenly distributed chromatin are features seen in benign hepatocytes rather than HCC. In benign hepatocytes, cells are usually arranged in sheets or isolated cells.

A-3. **(d) Poorly differentiated adenocarcinoma**
The diagnosis of the lesion is a metastatic gastrointestinal stromal tumor (GIST). The cytological features of GIST include sheets or loosely formed clusters of spindle cells with oval or bipolar nuclei, bland chromatin, inconspicuous nucleoli, and vesicular cytoplasm. IHC of tumor cells are positive for c-kit and CD34. The differential diagnosis of a spindle cell lesion in liver FNA cytology is broad, including virtually all tumors with spindle cell morphology such as spindle cell carcinoma, sarcomatoid mesothelioma, melanoma, angiomyolipoma, and others. Therefore, the correlation of cytological features with clinical and image findings is extremely important and may help to narrow down the differential diagnosis. In a poorly differentiated adenocarcinoma, tumor cells form three-dimensional clusters with large hyperchromatic nuclei, coarse chromatin, irregular nuclear membrane, prominent nucleoli, and vacuolated cytoplasm. In AML, cytological features include clusters of epithelioid and spindle cells, fat cells, blood vessels, and extramedullary hematopoiesis. In sarcomatoid mesothelioma, tumor cells have an epithelioid appearance with hyperchromatic oval nuclei, prominent nucleoli, and dense cytoplasm.

A-4. **(a) S100, HMB45, and Melanin A**
The diagnosis is metastatic desmoplastic/spindle melanoma. Tumor cells reveal oval or bizarre nuclei, prominent nucleoli, and no cytoplasmic melanin pigment. Immuno markers S100, HMB45, and MelanA/Mart1 are helpful in the confirmation of the diagnosis. S100 stains the nuclei and cytoplasm with 90 % sensitive but is not specific. HMB45 stains cytoplasm; it is more specific but less sensitive than S100 (only 0–20 % positive in desmoplastic/spindle cell melanoma). MelanA/Mart1 stains cytoplasm and is negative in desmoplastic/spindle cell melanoma. IHC markers of C-kit, CD34, and cytokeratin are for GIST. CK5/6, p63, and p40 are for squamous cell carcinoma. CK20, synaptophysin and chromogranin are for Merkel cell carcinoma.

A-5. **(b) Metastatic urothelial cell carcinoma**
The diagnosis is metastatic urothelial cell carcinoma. The smears reveal clusters and dispersed large malignant epithelial cells with dense cytoplasm. Tumor cells show high N:C ratios, hyperchromatic nuclei with coarse (chunk of charcoal) chromatin, irregular nuclear membrane, and round esosinophilic cytoplasmic inclusions (Melamed-Wolinska body). Melamed-Wolinska bodies are commonly seen in degenerated urothelial cells, particularly in voided urine. The pathogenesis of these bodies is still not fully understood, and they can be found in both benign and malignant conditions. The finding of

Melamed-Wolinska bodies is nonspecific; however, when seen in an extraurinary cytological specimen, the finding may suggest that the lesion is of urothelial origin. The main differential diagnosis of metastatic urothelial cell carcinoma is HCC, since both tumors reveal dense cytoplasm and cytoplasmic material. In HCC, tumor cells have large prominent nucleoli and cytoplasmic bile and/or lipofuscin pigments, which stain golden and brown color with Papanicolaou method. Numerous naked nuclei are also seen in HCC.

A-6. (a) **Metastatic renal cell carcinoma (RCC)**
The diagnosis is metastatic clear cell RCC. In RCC, the most common sites of metastasis are the lung, liver, lymph nodes, and bones. Tumor cells of clear cell RCC arrange in clusters or dispersed individual cells, reveal round to ovoid hyperchromatic nuclei, irregular nuclear membrane, with or without prominent nucleoli, and clear cytoplasm. Focally, tumor cells may also show large, hyperchromatic nuclei with multinucleated giant cells, eosinophilic cytoplasm, and associated areas of necrosis, particularly in Fuhrman Grade III and IV tumors. The background of the smear is bloody with prominent small vessels (hypervascularity).

A-7. (a) **Metastatic melanoma**
In metastatic melanoma, tumor cells are usually arranged in loose clusters or dispersed individual cells. Nuclei of tumor cells are eccentrically located (plasmacytoid appearance) and highly variable in size with finely to coarsely granular chromatin and a single prominent cherry-red nucleoli. The cytoplasm tends to be abundant and may or may not contain melanin pigment. The N/C ratio may not be high. Melanin pigment appears coarsely granular and dark brown on Papanicolaou stain. Other characteristic features include multinucleation, binucleation, and intranuclear inclusions. The main differential diagnosis is hepatocellular carcinoma. In HCC, tumor cells also have large prominent nucleoli and dense cytoplasm which contains cytoplasmic bile and/or lipofuscin pigments, staining golden and brown in color with the Papanicolaou method. Numerous naked nuclei are also seen in HCC.

A-8. (c) **Hepatocellular carcinoma**
The diagnosis is hepatocellular carcinoma. In HCC, tumor cells arrange in cords, clusters, or dispersed individual cells with centrally located nuclei, large prominent nucleoli, and dense cytoplasm containing cytoplasmic bile and/or lipofuscin pigments, and are golden and brown in color with Papanicolaou staining. Numerous naked nuclei are also seen in HCC. In a poorly differentiated tumor, numerous pleomorphic individual cells with hyperchromatic nuclei, prominent nucleoli, and dense granular cytoplasm are characteristic. In adenocarcinomas, tumor cells form three-dimensional clusters with large hyperchromatic nuclei, coarse chromatin, irregular nuclear membrane, prominent nucleoli, and vacuolated cytoplasm.

A-9. (d) **Hemangioma**
The diagnosis is hemangioma. On FNA specimen, several cytological features can be seen, including bloody smear, aggregates of closely packed, thin-walled capillaries with spindle cell clusters, scant benign liver cells, stromal cells, and hemosiderin-laden macrophages. The causes of this liver tumor are not clear. About 30 % of cases have the lesion at the time of birth (indicative of a congenital defect). Studies also show that the development of hemangioma is related to hormonal imbalance, since the usage of steroids and oral contraceptives can exacerbate the growth of the tumor in the liver. The tumor is more commonly seen in the right lobe of the liver than the left. The differential diagnosis includes spindle cell lesions of the liver, such as granulomatous hepatitis, leiomyosarcoma, melanoma, spindle cell carcinoma, and others. Glut1 is an immunohistochemical marker, highly specific for hemangioma, and can be used to differentiate hemangioma from vascular malformations.

A-10. (a) **Metastatic adenocarcinoma of the lung**
The diagnosis is a metastatic adenocarcinoma of the lung. Metastatic adenocarcinoma may have several cytological appearances. In adenocarcinomas, particularly well-differentiated adenocarcinomas, tumor cells form acinar/papillary arrangements or three-dimensional clusters. Tumor cells are intermediate or large in size and reveal hyperchromatic nuclei with coarse chromatin, prominent nucleoli, and vacuolated or clear cytoplasm. Small cell carcinoma has fine (salt-and-pepper) chromatin, nuclear crowding, and molding. Renal cell carcinoma reveals a bloody smear. Tumor cells have hyperchromatic nuclei with coarse chromatin, with or without prominent nucleoli, and clear/eosinophilic cytoplasm. In HCC, tumor cells arrange in cords, clusters, or dispersed individual cells with centrally located nuclei, large prominent nucleoli, and dense cytoplasm containing cytoplasmic bile and/or lipofuscin pigments. Numerous naked nuclei are also seen in HCC.

A-11. (**b**) **Bile duct hamartoma**

The diagnosis is bile duct hamartoma characterized by multiple small nodules dispersed throughout the liver. The FNA reveals bland-appearing columnar cells haphazardly arranged in tubules, sheets and two-dimensional clusters, scattered stromal cells, and benign-appearing hepatocytes. Bile duct hamartoma, also known as von Meyenburg complex, Meyenburg complex, and biliary hamartoma, is a benign tumor-like malformation of the liver and classically associated with polycystic liver disease, may be seen in polycystic kidney disease and Caroli's disease. In adenocarcinomas, tumor cells form three-dimensional clusters with large hyperchromatic nuclei, coarse chromatin, irregular nuclear membrane, prominent nucleoli, and vacuolated cytoplasm. Liver cell adenoma is a benign tumor related to long-term use of oral contraceptives. It is commonly seen in females under the age of 30 and the lesion reveals benign liver cells.

A-12. (**a**) **Numerous dispersed naked nuclei**

The diagnosis is hydatid cyst (echinococcal cyst). The hydatid cyst is caused by infection with the larval stage of the cestode (or tapeworm) *Echinococcus* spp. Transmission is from eggs found in feces of dogs which are accidentally swallowed, usually by children. Larvae develop over many years to form fluid-filled cysts in various organs, particularly the liver. Cysts can grow to considerable size and contain a large amount of fluid and infectious scolices. The cysts have a wall made from both host tissue (pericyst) and larval origin (endocyst). All above cytological features can be seen in the lesion, except numerous dispersed naked nuclei of liver cells, which is the feature seen in HCC.

A-13. (**c**) **Well-differentiated hepatocellular carcinoma**

The diagnosis is a well-differentiated HCC. In HCC, tumor cells arrange in cords, clusters, tubules, or dispersed individual cells. Tumor cells reveal hyperchromatic nuclei, coarse chromatin, large prominent nucleoli, and intranuclear pseudoinclusion. Dense cytoplasm with cytoplasmic bile/lipofuscin pigments is also characteristic of HCC. Numerous naked nuclei and tumor necrosis are also seen in HCC. In a poorly differentiated HCC, tumor cell pleomorphism and giant tumor cells are also present. In bile duct hamartoma, the FNA reveals bland-appearing columnar cells haphazardly arranged in tubules, sheets and two-dimensional clusters, scattered stromal cells, and benign-appearing liver cells. In adenocarcinomas, tumor cells form three-dimensional clusters with large hyperchromatic nuclei, coarse chromatin, irregular nuclear membrane, prominent nucleoli, and vacuolated cytoplasm. Liver cell adenoma reveals benign-appearing liver cells.

A-14. (**d**) **Metastatic carcinoid**

The diagnosis is a metastatic carcinoid of GI tract. Carcinoids are the most common gastrointestinal endocrine tumors and frequently involve the liver. Primary hepatic carcinoids are extremely rare. In FNA specimens, tumor cells reveal acini and/or rosette arrangements and consist of intermediate-sized cells with fine (salt-and-pepper) chromatin with inconspicuous or small nucleoli. Mitoses are rare (low ki67 labeling). In small cell carcinoma, nuclear crowding and molding, and tumor necrosis are characteristic. In HCC, tumor cells reveal hyperchromatic nuclei, coarse chromatin, large prominent nucleoli, and intranuclear pseudoinclusion. Numerous naked nuclei and tumor necrosis are also seen in HCC. In adenocarcinomas, tumor cells form three-dimensional clusters with large hyperchromatic nuclei, coarse chromatin, irregular nuclear membrane, prominent nucleoli, and vacuolated cytoplasm.

A-15. (**d**) **Diffuse large B-cell lymphoma (DLBCL)**

DLBCL is a biological and clinical diverse group of diseases. The FNA reveals a cellular specimen with dyscohesive large atypical lymphoid cells. Three morphological variants are most commonly seen: centroblastic, immunoblastic, and anaplastic variant. Centroblastic variant is the most common subtype and reveals medium-to-large-sized tumor cells with high N:C ratios, oval or round nuclei, fine chromatin, and single or multiple prominent nucleoli. Immunoblasts have a basophilic cytoplasm and a central nucleolus. Most cases are polymorphic, with a mixture of centroblastic and immunoblastic cells. The third morphologic variant, anaplastic variant, consists of large tumor cells with pleomorphic nuclei and may resemble Hodgkin cells or Reed-Sternberg cells. In small cell carcinoma, nuclear crowding and molding, and tumor necrosis are characteristic. In HCC, tumor cells reveal hyperchromatic nuclei, coarse chromatin, large prominent nucleoli, and intranuclear pseudoinclusion. Numerous naked nuclei and tumor necrosis are also seen in HCC. In adenocarcinomas, tumor cells form three-dimensional clusters with large hyperchromatic nuclei, coarse chromatin, irregular nuclear membrane, prominent nucleoli, and vacuolated cytoplasm.

A-16. **(d) Cholangiocarcinoma**
Cholangiocarcinoma can affect any area of the bile ducts, either within or outside the liver. The FNA cytomorphology of the tumor reveals clusters, sheets, or dispersed individual tumor cells with hyperchromatic and variable sized nuclei, coarse chromatin, and prominent nucleoli. The FNA of bile duct hamartoma reveals bland-appearing columnar cells haphazardly arranged in tubules, sheets and two-dimensional clusters, and benign-appearing hepatocytes. In HCC, tumor cells reveal hyperchromatic nuclei, coarse chromatin, large prominent nucleoli, and intranuclear pseudoinclusion. Numerous naked nuclei and tumor necrosis are also seen in HCC. In adenocarcinomas, tumor cells form three-dimensional clusters with large hyperchromatic nuclei, coarse chromatin, irregular nuclear membrane, prominent nucleoli, and vacuolated cytoplasm.

A-17. **(b) Metastatic adenocarcinoma of the prostate**
In metastatic prostate adenocarcinoma, tumor cells form microacinar arrangements or three-dimensional small clusters. Tumor cells are small to intermediate in size, with hyperchromatic nuclei, coarse granular chromatin, prominent nucleoli, and vacuolated or clear cytoplasm. Small cell carcinoma has fine (salt-and-pepper) chromatin, nuclear crowding, and molding. In lung adenocarcinoma, tumor cells have a more pleomorphic appearance with large nuclei, coarse chromatin, prominent nucleoli, and vacuolated cytoplasm. In colonic adenocarcinoma, tumor cells reveal large elongated nuclei (pencil-shaped nuclei), coarse chromatin, prominent nucleoli, and marked tumor necrosis. Immunostains with prostate markers such as PSA (prostate specific antigen), PSAP (prostate specific acid phosphatase), prostate specific membrane antigen, and NKX3 are positive for metastatic tumor cells.

A-18. **(b) Metastatic mucinous adenocarcinoma of the ovary**
Cytological features of mucinous adenocarcinomas include three-dimensional clusters and acinar groups of tumor cells with large round or oval shape nuclei, coarse chromatin, irregular nuclear membrane, and prominent nucleoli. The cytoplasm of tumor cells is vacuolated (indicative of mucin production). Mucinous material can be seen in the background of smears and cell block preparation. In true papillary adenocarcinoma of the lung, numerous papillary structures can be identified. A metastatic colonic adenocarcinoma has hyperchromatic pencil-shaped nuclei and tumor necrosis. Small cell carcinoma has fine (salt-and-pepper) chromatin, nuclear crowding, and molding.

A-19. **(c) Actinomysis**
Actinomysis is caused by systemic dissemination of *Actinomyces israelii* species. The characteristic feature of the smear is the presence of sulfur granules and filamentous bacteria. Sulfur granule forms in the center of purulence surrounded by neutrophils and filamentous bacteria. Sulfur granules look yellow on gross examination and stain blue to purple in color. *Actinomyces* bacteria stain blue with the Papanicolaou method and purple with the Diff-Quik method. They appear as large blue- or purple-colored "cotton balls" on the slide. Clinically, actinomysis is frequently confused with neoplasms due to the formation of mass lesions. However, no malignant features are identified in liver cells.

A-20. **(c) Metastatic carcinoid of the GI tract**
In FNA specimen, the tumor reveals acini and/or rosette arrangements or dispersed individual cells. The tumor consists of intermediate sized cells with fine (salt-and-pepper) chromatin, inconspicuous or small nucleoli. Mitoses are rare (low ki67 labeling). Carcinoids are the most common gastrointestinal endocrine tumors and frequently involve the liver. Primary hepatic carcinoids are extremely rare. In small cell carcinoma, nuclear crowding and molding, and tumor necrosis are characteristic. In HCC, tumor cells reveal hyperchromatic nuclei, coarse chromatin, large prominent nucleoli, and intranuclear pseudoinclusion. Numerous naked nuclei and tumor necrosis are also seen in HCC. In adenocarcinomas, tumor cells form three-dimensional clusters with large hyperchromatic nuclei, coarse chromatin, irregular nuclear membrane, prominent nucleoli, and vacuolated cytoplasm.

A-21. **(c) Metastatic endocrine tumor**
The diagnosis is metastatic endocrine tumor of the pancreas (pancreatic endocrine tumor, PEN). In FNA specimens, the smear is cellular and reveals sheets and clusters of tumor cells with acini and/or rosette arrangements or dispersed individual cells. Tumor cells are small to intermediate in size with round to oval nuclei, fine (salt-and-pepper) chromatin, and inconspicuous nucleoli. PENs occur most commonly in adults. The liver is often involved, even if the primary tumor is only 1–2 cm. The majority of tumors are functional tumors and secrete a variety of hormones, such as insulin, glucagon, somatostatin, vaso-

active intestinal polypeptide (VIP), pancreatic polypeptide, serotonin, adrenocorticotropic hormone (ACTH), or calcitonin. The tumor also stains positive for amyloid.

A-22. (**b**) **Normal liver cells**

This liver FNA reveals normal hepatocytes. A FNA of benign liver may reveal several patterns, including clusters, sheets of cells, or dispersed individual cells. The normal liver cells have centrally placed round- to oval-shaped nuclei, granular chromatin, inconspicuous or small nucleoli, and no hyperchromasia or marked nuclear atypia. Cells also reveal normal N:C ratios. Binucleation is common in cells. Bile and lipofusion pigment can be identified in the cytoplasm. In contrast, in hepatocellular carcinoma (HCC), tumor cells form cords, tubules, sheets, or isolated individual cells. Tumor cells have hyperchromatic nuclei, coarse chromatin, and high N:C ratios. Large prominent nucleoli, marked variation of size of nuclei, and numerous naked nuclei are features seen in HCC.

A-23. (**c**) **Metastatic adenocarcinoma**

The diagnosis is a metastatic adenocarcinoma of the stomach. In metastatic adenocarcinoma, particularly metastasis from stomach, tumor cells form large three-dimensional clusters. Tumor cells are intermediate or large in size and reveal hyperchromatic nuclei with coarse chromatin, prominent nucleoli, and vacuolated cytoplasm. In melanoma, tumor cells are predominantly dispersed as individual cells with large eccentric hyperchromatic nuclei, coarse chromatin, large prominent nucleoli, and cytoplasmic pigment. In HCC, tumor cells arrange in cords, clusters, or dispersed individual cells with centrally located nuclei, large prominent nucleoli, and dense cytoplasm containing cytoplasmic bile and/or lipofuscin pigments. Numerous naked nuclei are also seen in HCC.

A-24. (**c**) **Endocrine tumor**

In FNA specimens, the smear reveals sheets and clusters of tumor cells with acini and/or rosette arrangements or dispersed individual cells. Tumor cells are small to intermediate in size with round to oval nuclei, fine (salt-and-pepper) chromatin, and inconspicuous nucleoli. Almost all endocrine tumors of the liver are metastatic tumors either from the GI tract, pancreas, lung, and other organs. A primary endocrine tumor of the liver is extremely rare.

A-25. (**a**) **Metastatic melanoma**

In metastic melanoma, tumor cells are usually arranged in loose clusters or dispersed individual cells. Nuclei of tumor cells are eccentrically located (plasmacytoid appearance) and highly variable in size with finely to coarsely granular chromatin and a single prominent cherry-red nucleoli. The cytoplasm tends to be abundant and may or may not contain melanin pigment. The N/C ratio may not be high due to abundant cytoplasm. Melanin pigment appears coarsely granular and dark brown on Papanicolaou stain. Other characteristic features include multinucleation, binucleation, and intranuclear inclusions. The main differential diagnosis is hepatocellular carcinoma. In HCC, tumor cells also have large prominent nucleoli and dense cytoplasm which contains cytoplasmic bile and/or lipofuscin pigments, staining golden and brown color with the Papanicolaou method. Numerous naked nuclei are also seen in HCC.

A-26. (**b**) **Normal liver cells**

This liver FNA reveals normal hepatocytes. A FNA of benign liver reveals sheets of cells and dispersed individual cells. The normal liver cells have centrally placed round- to oval-shaped nuclei, granular chromatin, inconspicuous or small nucleoli, and no hyperchromasia or marked nuclear atypia. Cells also reveal normal N:C ratio. Binucleation is common in cells. Bile and lipofusion pigment can be identified in cytoplasm. In contrast, in hepatocellular carcinoma (HCC), tumor cells form cords, tubules, sheets, or isolated individual cells. Tumor cells have hyperchromatic nuclei, coarse chromatin, and high N:C ratios. Large prominent nucleoli, marked variation of size of nuclei, and numerous naked nuclei are features seen in HCC. The finding of benign liver cells may be seen in cirrhosis, liver cell adenomas, focal nodular hyperplasia, nodular regenerative hyperplasia, and others. In this case the FNA findings may be suggestive of cirrhosis and/or nodular regenerative hyperplasia in a cirrhotic liver.

A-27. (**c**) **Hepatoblastoma**

The diagnosis is hepatoblastoma of embryonal cell type. Hepatoblastoma is a rare tumor of infancy and childhood. In FNA specimens, findings vary and depend on the cell type of the tumor. In embryonal variant, the tumor reveals a primitive and undifferentiated appearance with hyperchromatic nuclei and scant cytoplasm, and form rosettes and trabeculae. In anaplastic variant, tumor cells reveal a more pleomorphic appearance. In fetal cell variant, tumor cells resemble normal liver cells. The main differential diagnosis of the tumor is hepatocellular carcinoma and other metastatic small round blue cell tumors.

The positive stain of HePar1 supports the diagnosis of liver primary rather than a nonhepatic origin. Hepatoblastoma is positive for high molecular weight cytokeratin, whereas HCC is negative for high molecular weight cytokeratin. Both tumors are positive for low molecular weight cytokeratin.

A-28. (**d**) **Metastatic Wilm's tumor**
Wilm's tumor is a rare tumor of infancy and childhood. The tumor is bimodal with a mixture of epithelial and mesenchymal component. Occasionally it is triphasic. Generally, in the FNA specimen, numerous dyscohesive small round blue cells are found. Tumor epithelial cells form characteristic tubular-like structure and tight clusters. Tumor cells have hyperchromatic nuclei and scant cytoplasm. The mesenchymal cells are elongated. The main differential diagnosis is rhabdomyosarcoma and PNET. In rhabdomyosarcoma, tumor cells have more eosinophilic cytoplasm. In PNET, tumor cells are more pleomorphic and reveal a tigroid appearance.

A-29. (**a**) **Fibrolamellar hepatocellular carcinoma**
The fibrolamellar variant of hepatocellular carcinoma is usually seen in young patients under the age of 30. It has a favorable prognosis. The cytomorphological features of fibrolamellar hepatocellular carcinoma reveal large polygonal tumor cells separated by fibrous tissue. The size of tumor cells is much larger than well-differentiated HCC. Tumor cells have large nuclei and abundant eosinophilic cytoplasm; therefore, the N:C ratio of tumor cells is normal to slightly increased. Tumor cells also reveal prominent nucleoli and intracytoplasmic hyaline globules. The dense lamellar material is also seen in the slides, separating loosely cohesive tumor cells.

A-30. (**d**) **Metastatic leiomyosarcoma**
The FNA of the lesion reveals clusters of spindle cells with cigar-shaped hyperchromatic nuclei, coarse chromatin, inconspicuous nucleoli, and fibrillar cytoplasm. Tumor necrosis is also present. In desmoplastic/spindle melanoma, tumor cells reveal oval or bizarre nuclei, prominent nucleoli, and do not contain cytoplasmic melanin pigment. In spindle cell carcinoma, tumor cells reveal elongated or bizarre nuclei, prominent nucleoli, and scant cytoplasm. In hemangioma, several cytological features can be seen, including bloody smear, aggregates of closely packed, thin-walled capillaries with spindle cell clusters, scant benign liver cells, and hemosiderin-laden macrophages. Immunostains with muscle markers are helpful in the differential diagnosis of the tumor.

A-31. (**b**) **Normal liver cells**
This liver FNA reveals normal hepatocytes. A FNA of benign liver reveals sheets of cells and dispersed individual cells. The normal liver cells have centrally placed round- to oval-shaped nuclei, granular chromatin, inconspicuous or small nucleoli, and no hyperchromasia or marked nuclear atypia. Cells also reveal normal N:C ratios. Binucleation is common in cells. Bile and lipofusion pigment can be identified in cytoplasm. In contrast, in hepatocellular carcinoma (HCC), tumor cells form cords, tubules, sheets, or isolated individual cells. Tumor cells have hyperchromatic nuclei, coarse chromatin, and high N:C ratio. Large prominent nucleoli, marked variation in the size of nuclei, and numerous naked nuclei are features seen in HCC. The finding of benign liver cells may be seen in cirrhosis, liver cell adenomas, focal nodular hyperplasia, nodular regenerative hyperplasia, and others.

A-32. (**c**) **Extramedullary hematopoiesis**
The diagnosis of this liver FNA is an extramedullary hematopoiesis. It can be caused by myelofibrosis and commonly involves the liver and spleen. The FNA cytology reveals numerous megakaryocytes, nucleated red blood cells, and different stages of nuclear cells. However, no malignant features are seen in the aspirate, excluding the diagnosis of carcinoma. The megakaryocytes are much larger than the Reed-Sternberg cells seen in the Hodgkin's lymphoma and have 3–5 lobes. In addition, other features of Hodgkin's lymphoma are absent in this specimen.

A-33. (**c**) **Benign bile duct epithelial cells**
Benign bile duct epithelium appears as small clusters and/or sheets of cohesive uniform cells. These cells have round to ovoid nuclei, dark granular chromatin, inconspicuous or occasional small nucleoli, and scant cytoplasm. The size of benign bile duct epithelial cells is smaller than that of normal hepatocytes. Nuclear overlapping and nuclear disarray are common findings, mimicking adenocarcinoma. In adenocarcinomas, particularly metastatic adenocarcinomas, tumor cells reveal high N:C ratios, coarse chromatin, prominent nucleoli, and vacuolated cytoplasm.

A-34. (**c**) **Poorly differentiated hepatocellular carcinoma**
The diagnosis is a poorly differentiated hepatocellular carcinoma. In HCC, tumor cells show a wide range of cytomorphology. In poorly differentiated forms, malignant cells are polygonal and dyscohesive with pleomorphic nuclei and giant tumor cells. In well-differentiated forms, tumor cells resemble

normal hepatocytes and form trabeculae, cords, and nests with slightly increased N:C ratios, large round nuclei, prominent nucleoli, naked nuclei, and bile pigment in the cytoplasm. The most notable feature of HCC, particularly in well-differentiated tumors, is the identification of sinusoidal capillaries surrounding markedly thickened trabeculae of neoplastic cells. This feature is not seen in cholangiocarcinoma or other tumors.

A-35. (**b**) **Focal nodular hyperplasia**
The diagnosis is focal nodular hyperplasia. The FNA specimen reveals clusters or dispersed individual benign-appearing hepatocytes with mild nuclear atypia. Cells have abundant granular cytoplasm and normal N:C ratios. Bile ductular epithelial cells are also identified. However, in liver cell adenomas, the bile duct epithelial cells are absent. In a well-differentiated hepatocellular carcinoma, tumor cells resemble normal hepatocytes and form trabeculae, cords, and nests with slightly increased N:C ratios, large round nuclei, prominent nucleoli, naked nuclei, and bile pigment in the cytoplasm. The most notable feature of HCC, particularly in well-differentiated tumors, is the identification of sinusoidal capillaries surrounding markedly thickened trabeculae of neoplastic cells.

A-36. (**b**) **Metastatic squamous cell carcinoma**
The diagnosis is a metastatic squamous cell carcinoma. Metastatic squamous cell carcinoma usually form loose clusters or dispersed individual tumor cells. The cytological features of tumor cells include large nuclei with smudgy chromatin, nuclei with variation in size and shape, and dense cytoplasm (indicative of cytokeratin formation). The dense cytoplasm is blue in color with the Diff-Quik stain and red-pink (eosinophilic) in color with the Papanicolaou stain. Finally, prominent nucleoli can be seen in poorly differentiated squamous cell carcinomas and should not be confused with poorly differentiated adenocarcinomas. Tumor cells of adenocarcinoma have vesicular nuclei, coarse chromatin, and vacuolated cytoplasm.

A-37. (**d**) **Hepatocellular carcinoma**
The diagnosis is hepatocellular carcinoma (moderately differentiated). In HCC, tumor cells show a wide range of cytomorphology. In poorly differentiated forms, malignant cells are polygonal and dyscohesive with pleomorphic nuclei and giant tumor cells. In well-differentiated forms, tumor cells resemble normal hepatocytes and form trabeculae, cords, and nests with slightly increased N:C ratios, large round nuclei, prominent nucleoli, naked nuclei, and bile pigment in the cytoplasm. The most notable feature of HCC, particularly in well-differentiated tumors, is the identification of sinusoidal capillaries surrounding markedly thickened trabeculae of neoplastic cells. This feature is not seen in cholangiocarcinoma or other tumors.

A-38. (**c**) **Colon**
A metastatic colonic adenocarcinoma has unique cytological features. Tumor cells show a tall columnar "picket fence" appearance, hyperchromatic pencil-shaped nuclei, coarse chromatin, and prominent nucleoli. The presence of "dirty" necrosis is also seen. In breast carcinomas, tumor cells form tight three-dimensional "cannon ball" clusters. The size of tumor cells is smaller than that of colon adenocarcinoma. They may have intranuclear inclusion. Renal cell carcinoma usually reveals a centrally located nuclei and clear cytoplasm. Lung adenocarcinoma may have a variety of morphological features. The finding of tall columnar cells favors a colonic primary rather than lung primary. IHC stain of TTF, Napsin A, CK7, CK20, and CDX2 may aid the differential diagnosis in difficult cases. TTF, Napsin A, and CK7 are positive in lung adenocarcinoma, whereas CK20 and CDX2 are positive in colon adenocarcinoma.

7.4 Answers and Discussions of Text-based Questions 39–75

A-39. (**a**) **Numerous dispersed naked nuclei**

A FNA of benign liver reveals sheets of large polygonal and dispersed individual cells. The specimen may also reveal trabeculae arrangements and tissue fragments. Cells have centrally placed round- to oval-shaped nuclei with variation in size, granular chromatin, prominent nucleoli, and normal N:C ratio. Binucleation is common in cells. Bile and lipofusion pigment can be identified in the cytoplasm. Bile stains dark-green by Papanicolaou and Diff-Quik methods, whereas lipofusion stains golden-brown by Papanicolaou and green-brown by Diff-Quik methods. In contrast, in hepatocellular carcinoma (HCC), tumor cells form cords, tubules, sheets, or isolated individual cells. Tumor cells have hyperchromatic nuclei, coarse chromatin, and high N:C ratios. Large prominent nucleoli as well as naked nuclei in the smear are features seen in HCC.

A-40. (**c**) **It commonly occurs in females under the age of 30 and is related to long-term use of oral contraceptives**

The liver cell adenoma is an uncommon benign tumor. It commonly occurs in female under the age of 30 and is related to long-term use of oral contraceptives. Cytologically, the FNA specimen reveals clusters or dispersed individual benign-appearing hepatocytes with mild nuclear atypia. Cells have abundant granular cytoplasm and a normal N:C ratio. No bile duct epithelial cells are present. It is important to distinguish liver cell adenoma from other benign liver tumors, such as hemangiomas (spindle cell lesion, mixed with benign liver cells) and focal nodular hyperplasia (presence of bile duct epithelial cells), because liver cell adenomas have a risk of progressing into a malignancy. When the adenoma grows to a size of more than 6–8 cm, it is considered high risk of developing into an invasive hepatocellular carcinoma. Tumor necrosis, pleomorphic tumor cells, and numerous naked nuclei are features characteristic of hepatocellular carcinoma. The cytological diagnosis of liver cell adenomas can be aided by reticulin stains. In liver cell adenomas, the reticulin scaffold is preserved and hepatocytes do not form layers of more than three cells thick, as is seen in hepatocellular carcinomas.

A-41. (**d**) **Numerous naked nuclei**

Cholangiocarcinoma is known to have the histological and molecular features of adenocarcinoma. Cholangiocarcinoma can affect any area of the bile ducts, either within or outside the liver. The cytomorphology of the tumor includes trabeculae, cords, and nested arrangements, or dispersed individual tumor cells with large oval nuclei and coarse chromatin with scant cytoplasm. The presence of numerous naked nuclei is the feature most commonly seen in HCC. The differential diagnosis of cholangiocarcinoma includes HCC, metastatic adenocarcinomas, and other gastrointestinal tumors.

A-42. (**a**) **Fatty change is reported in 40 % of early HCC**

Fatty change can occur in both benign and malignant liver lesions, as well as all sizes and grades of HCC. It has been reported that fatty change can be identified in 40 % of early HCC. It is also interesting that the prevalence of fatty change decreases along with the increase in tumor size. Fatty change is best appreciated by a Diff-Quik stain as intracytoplasmic vacuoles or as dispersed bubbles in the background of the slide. In a well-differentiated HCC, the finding of tumor cells with prominent fatty change should not be confused as a benign process or benign nodule.

A-43. (**a**) **The size of bile duct epithelial cells is similar to normal hepatocytes**

Benign bile duct epithelium appears as small clusters and/or sheets of cohesive uniform cells. These cells have round to ovoid nuclei, dark granular chromatin, inconspicuous or occasional small nucleoli, and scant cytoplasm. The size of benign bile duct epithelial cells is smaller than that of normal hepatocytes. Nuclear overlapping and nuclear disarray are common findings, mimicking adenocarcinoma. In adenocarcinomas, particular metastatic adenocarcinomas, tumor cells reveal high N:C ratios, coarse chromatin, prominent nucleoli, and vacuolated cytoplasm.

A-44. (**c**) **Identification of bile and sinusoidal capillary**

In HCC, tumor cells show a wide range of cytomorphology. In well-differentiated forms, tumor cells resemble normal hepatocytes and form trabeculae, cords, and nests with a slightly increased N:C ratio, large round nuclei, prominent nucleoli, naked nuclei, and bile pigment in cytoplasm. In poorly differentiated forms, malignant cells are polygonal and dyscohesive with pleomorphic nuclei and giant tumor cells. The most notable feature of HCC, particularly in well-differentiated tumors, is the identification of sinusoidal capillaries surrounding markedly thickened trabeculae of neoplastic cells. This feature is not seen in cholangiocarcinoma. Other features in the question are seen in both HCC and cholangiocarcinoma.

A-45. (c) **Hepatic AML cannot be diagnosed accurately by FNA**

Hepatic AML shares many clinical and cytological features with its renal counterpart. Similar to kidney tumor, it consists of fat, epithelioid spindle cells (myoid cells) with an increased vascularity and frequent extramedullary hematopoiesis. The correct diagnosis depends on the identification of the triad of fat, vessels, and myoid component. The proportions of these components vary considerably from tumor to tumor. Some tumors are composed predominantly of fat, whereas others have virtually no fat and are almost exclusively myoid cells (smooth muscle). In difficult cases, immunohistochemical (IHC) staining with HMB45 is helpful and positive for the neoplastic cells.

A-46. (c) **Positive HepPar1 and CD10, negative epithelial membrane antigen (EMA), monoclonal carcinoembryonic antigen (CEA), and CK7**

For HCC, the panel should include Hep Par 1, CD10, and CAM5.2 or CK8/18. For cholangiocarcinoma, the panel should include poly- or monoclonal carcinoembryonic antigen (CEA), CK7, and CD15. pCEA (and CD10) demonstrate a canalicular staining pattern in HCC but a cytoplasmic pattern in cholangiocarcinoma. The demonstration of AFP positivity points toward a malignant tumor of hepatocellular origin, however, it is also positive in nonseminomatous germ cell tumors and extrahepatic AFP-producing carcinomas. Cautious use of Hep Par1 antibody in a panel with other positive (alpha-fetoprotein, CD10, polyclonal carcinoembryonic antigen) and negative (epithelial membrane antigen, monoclonal carcinoembryonic antigen, CD15) markers of hepatocellular differentiation may aid in the accurate diagnosis of HCC.

A-47. (a) **True**

The sensitivity and specificity of percutaneous FNA biopsy for detection of liver malignancy have been reported to be around 90 % (range, 67–100 %) and 100 %, respectively. A variety of factors may affect the sensitivity, such as the size and location of the lesion, number of FNA passes, operator's skill and experience, quality of smears, and cytopathologist's expertise. The positive and negative predictive values and overall accuracy of percutaneous FNA biopsy for liver malignancy were reported in one large study to be 100, 59.1, and 92.4 %. Endoscopic ultrasound-guided FNA (EUS-FNA) is the latest diagnostic and staging tool with a sensitivity of 82–94 % and specificity of 90–100 %. The procedure is safe and accurate, but highly operator dependent. Furthermore, EUS-FNA can access the left lobe of liver, hilum, proximal right lobe, gallbladder, extrahepatic biliary system, and perihilar lymph nodes. It is especially useful for small and deep-seated left lobe lesions, which cannot be easily accessed by percutaneous FNA.

A-48. (b) **Cirrhosis**

Known risk factors for cholangiocarcinoma include primary sclerosing cholangitis, congenital liver malformations, infection with the parasitic liver flukes *Opisthorchis viverrini* or *Clonorchis sinensis*, and exposure to thorotrast (thorium dioxide), a chemical formerly used in medical imaging. However, most patients with cholangiocarcinoma have no identifiable specific risk factors. Cirrhosis has not been found to associate with cholangiocarcinoma, although it is a significant risk factor for HCC.

A-49. (d) **Benign bile duct epithelial cells**

In liver cell adenomas, the FNA specimen reveals clusters or dispersed individual benign-appearing hepatocytes with mild nuclear atypia. Cells have abundant granular cytoplasm and normal N:C ratio. However, bile ductular epithelial cells are not identified. The cytological diagnosis of liver cell adenomas can be aided by reticulin stains. In liver cell adenomas, the reticulin scaffold is preserved and hepatocytes do not form layers of more than three cells thick, as is seen in hepatocellular carcinoma. It is important to distinguish liver cell adenomas from other benign liver tumors, such as hemangiomas (spindle cell lesion, mixed with benign liver cells) and focal nodular hyperplasia (presence of bile duct epithelial cells), because liver cell adenomas have a risk of progressing into a malignancy.

A-50. (a) **Preserved reticulin scaffold pattern**

In a well-differentiated HCC, tumor cells resemble normal hepatocytes and form trabeculae, cords, and nests with a slightly increased N:C ratio, have large round nuclei with prominent nucleoli, and may contain prominent bile pigment in cytoplasm. Naked nuclei can also be present. In poorly differentiated tumors, malignant cells are polygonal and dyscohesive with pleomorphic nuclei and giant tumor cells. The most notable feature in HCC, particularly in well-differentiated tumors, is the loss of reticulin scaffold pattern and the presence of sinusoidal capillaries surrounding the markedly thickened trabeculae of neoplastic cells. This feature is best seen on cell block preparations.

A-51. (c) **Well-differentiated hepatocellular carcinoma**
Cirrhotic liver is a well-known risk factor for the development of HCC. In this liver FNA, the most important differential diagnosis is a well-differentiated HCC. In HCC, tumor cells show a wide range of cytomorphology. In well-differentiated forms, tumor cells resemble normal hepatocytes and form trabeculae, cords, and nests and have an increased N:C ratio, large round nuclei, prominent nucleoli, naked nuclei, and bile pigment in cytoplasm. In poorly differentiated forms, malignant cells are markedly polygonal and dyscohesive with pleomorphic nuclei and giant tumor cells. The most notable feature of HCC, particularly in well-differentiated tumors, is the identification of sinusoidal capillaries surrounding the markedly thickened trabeculae of neoplastic cells. This feature is not seen in cholangiocarcinoma. In addition, mild nuclear atypia of hepatocytes can be seen in nodular regenerative hyperplasia of cirrhosis; however, the patient's clinical presentation of "rapidly enlarged liver mass" precludes the diagnosis.

A-52. (c) **Lymphoma**
The most likely diagnosis of this liver FNA is lymphoma. The cytological features of numerous dyscohesive small- to intermediate-sized cells with high N:C ratios and hyperchromatic coarse chromatin are characteristic of lymphoma. The monomorphic appearance of the lesion represents a monoclonal proliferation of lymphoma cells. Other cytological features of lymphoma include hyperchromatic nuclei with clumped (soccer-ball-like) chromatin, irregular nuclear membrane, and scant basophilic cytoplasm. Lymphoglandular bodies can also be seen in the background. In cholangiocarcinoma, tumor cells form clusters with large nuclei, hyperchromatic nuclei, and prominent nucleoli. In HCC, tumor cells are large with centrally located nuclei and large nucleoli, dense cytoplasm, and numerous naked nuclei. In small cell carcinomas, tumor cells reveal fine (salt-and-pepper) chromatin with nuclear crowding and molding.

A-53. (b) **Metastatic Adenocarcinoma of the lung**
The differential diagnosis of carcinoma with "signet ring" cells features is broad, including breast, lung, stomach, and other carcinomas. In metastatic adenocarcinomas of the lung, tumor cells form three-dimensional clusters with hyperchromatic nuclei, prominent nucleoli, and vacuolated cytoplasm. In metastatic adenocarcinoma of colon, tumor cell reveals elongated nuclei and prominent tumor necrosis. Cholangiocarcinoma has many overlapping cytological features with metastatic adenocarcinomas, and it is difficult to separate the tumor from metastatic adenocarcinoma based on morphology alone. The immunostains of TTF1 and Napsin A may help in the differential diagnosis of lung adenocarcinoma from other carcinomas. In a metastatic lung adenocarcinoma, TTF1 and Napsin A are usually positive.

A-54. (b) **False**
Hep Par 1 (hepatocyte Paraffin 1) antibody (clone OCH1E5.2.10) was developed in 1993 by Wennerberg et al. and it stains normal and neoplastic hepatocytes. Several studies have reported this antibody to be a sensitive marker for HCC (80–90 %). However, recent studies also found that it also frequently stains gastric carcinomas (30–47 %). It is not, however, entirely specific, showing frequent staining in gastric carcinomas. Several other tumors also stain occasionally, including yolk sac tumors as well as carcinomas of the adrenal cortex, lung, colon, and ovary. It also stains cholangiocarcinoma (50 %). In addition, poorly differentiated HCCs are more likely to be negative for Hep Par 1 than are better differentiated cases.

A-55. (a) **Prominent nucleoli**
The presence of prominent nucleoli is not a feature seen in small cell carcinoma. All other features can be seen in both adenocarcinoma and small cell carcinoma. In adenocarcinomas, tumor cells form acini and/or three-dimensional clusters and reveal hyperchromatic nuclei, vesicular or coarse chromatin, prominent nucleoli, and vacuolated cytoplasm (indication of mucin production). In small cell carcinoma, tumor cells reveal acini/rosettes arrangements with hyperchromatic nuclei, fine (salt-and-pepper) chromatin, inconspicuous nucleoli, and scant cytoplasm. In addition, in small cell carcinoma, nuclear crowding and molding are common features. Tumor necrosis can be seen in both adenocarcinoma and small cells carcinoma.

A-56. (a) **Cholangiocarcinoma**
The differential diagnosis of spindle cells lesion is broad, including all of tumors in the question except cholangiocarcinoma. In hemangiomas, several cytological features can be seen, including bloody smear, aggregates of closely packed, thin-walled capillaries with spindle cell clusters, scant benign liver cells, and hemosiderin-laden macrophages. In cholangiocarcinomas, tumor cells resemble adenocarcinoma and form clusters with large nuclei, hyperchromatic nuclei, and prominent nucleoli. In angiomyolipoma, the tumor reveals fat, spindle myoid cells, blood vessels, and extramedullary hematopoiesis. Glut1 is an

immunohistochemical marker, highly specific for hemangioma and can be used to differentiate hemangioma from vascular malformations.

A-57. (c) **Paranuclear blue bodies in the cytoplasm**
In metastatic prostate carcinoma, tumor cells are intermediate in size and reveal microacini arrangement or small three-dimensional clusters. Tumor cells show high N:C ratios, large nuclei with fine chromatin, small prominent nucleoli, and vesicular cytoplasm. Paranuclear blue bodies in the cytoplasm are features seen in small cell carcinoma. Some prostate carcinomas may have neuroendocrine differentiation and reveal salt-and-pepper chromatin pattern. Immunostains of prostate markers such as PSA (prostate specific antigen), PSAP (prostate specific acid phosphatase), prostate specific membrane antigen, and NKX3 are positive for metastatic tumor cells.

A-58. (b) **Intermediate-sized tumor cells**
The cytomorphological features of fibrolamellar hepatocellular carcinoma reveal large polygonal tumor cells separated by fibrous tissue. The size of tumor cells is much larger than well-differentiated HCC. Tumor cells have large nuclei and abundant eosinophilic cytoplasm; therefore, the N:C ratio of tumor cells is normal to slightly increased. Tumor cells also reveal prominent nucleoli and intracytoplasmic hyaline globules. The fibrolamellar variant of hepatocellular carcinoma is usually seen in young patient under the age of 30. It has a favorable prognosis.

A-59. (c) **Colon**
A metastatic colonic adenocarcinoma has these classic cytological features. Tumor cells show a tall columnar "picket fence" appearance, hyperchromatic pencil-shaped nuclei, coarse chromatin, and prominent nucleoli. The presence of "dirty" necrosis is usually not as apparent as seen in histological sections. In breast carcinomas, tumor cells form tight three-dimensional "cannon ball" clusters. The size of tumor cells is smaller than that of colon adenocarcinoma; they may have intranuclear inclusions. Renal cell carcinoma usually reveals a centrally located nuclei and clear cytoplasm. Lung adenocarcinoma may have a variety of morphological features. The finding of tall columnar cells favors a colonic primary rather than the lung primary. IHC stain of TTF, Napsin A, CK7, CK20, and CDX2 may aid to the differential diagnosis in difficult cases. TTF, Napsin A, and CK7 are positive in lung adenocarcinoma, whereas CK20 and CDX2 are positive in colon adenocarcinomas.

A-60. (d) **Naked nuclei**
The presence of naked nuclei is not a feature seen in metastatic breast carcinoma. In a metastatic breast carcinoma, tumor cells form tight three-dimensional clusters. The size of tumor cells is relatively smaller than that of metastatic adenocarcinoma from the lung and/or GI tract. The presence of intracytoplasmic lumina, so-called Magenta body, is also one of the characteristics of metastatic breast carcinoma. Magenta bodies are variably sized red-to-purple perinuclear inclusions seen by Diff-Quik stains. The prominent nucleoli are a common cytological feature seen in a variety of adenocarcinomas. Naked nuclei can be seen in metastatic melanoma and hepatocellular carcinoma.

A-61. (a) **Preserved reticulin scaffold pattern**
In a well-differentiated HCC, tumor cells resemble normal hepatocytes and form trabeculae, cords, and nests with a slightly increased N:C ratio and have large round nuclei with prominent nucleoli, naked nuclei, and may contain prominent bile pigment in the cytoplasm. In poorly differentiated tumors, malignant cells are polygonal and dyscohesive with pleomorphic nuclei and giant tumor cells. The most notable feature in HCC, particularly in well-differentiated tumors, is the loss of reticulin scaffold pattern and the presence of sinusoidal capillaries surrounding the markedly thickened trabeculae of neoplastic cells. This feature is best seen on cell block preparations.

A-62. (d) **Nuclear grooves**
Metastatic carcinoids in the liver most often come from a primary tumor in the intestine, pancreas, or the lungs. Carcinoids, despite differing embryological origin, have common phenotypic characteristics. The cytological features of carcinoids are characterized by acini arrangements, small clusters, and dispersed individual tumor cells. Tumor cells reveal a fine chromatin (salt-and-pepper chromatin) pattern, inconspicuous or small nucleoli, and scant cytoplasm. Mitoses are extremely rare. Nuclear grooves are not features seen in carcinoid. In addition, the cellular proliferative rate (Ki67 labeling) should be performed in tumors, since it has been considered as a useful marker for the classification of the tumor. An increased labeling pattern may indicate an adverse prognosis.

A-63. **(d) Dispersed tumor cells with marked atypia and enlargement**
As discussed in A-24, the cytological features of carcinoid are characterized by small acini/pseudorosette arrangements, small clusters, and/or dispersed individual tumor cells. Tumor cells reveal a fine chromatin (salt-and-pepper chromatin) pattern, inconspicuous or small nucleoli, and scant cytoplasm; mitoses are extremely rare. Whereas, cholangiocarcinoma form two- or three-dimensional clusters, crowded sheets, or dispersed large typical cells. Tumor cells have coarse granular rather than fine chromatin, and lacy or vacuolated cytoplasm. In difficult cases, diagnosis of carcinoid versus a cholangiocarcinoma depends on IHC staining with neuroendocrine markers. Carcinoid tumors are positive for synaptophysin, chromogranin, and CD56.

A-64. **(a) Hyperchromatic nuclei and prominent nucleoli**
The presence of prominent nucleoli is not a feature seen in small cell carcinomas. All other features can be seen in small cell carcinoma. In small cell carcinoma, tumor cells form three-dimensional clusters or dispersed individual cells, reveal hyperchromatic nuclei with fine (salt-and-pepper) chromatin, and scant cytoplasm. In addition, nuclear crowding, molding, apoptotic bodies, and mitotic figures are common features. The background of the smear may also reveal "blue strips" (indicative of breakdown nuclear material). Tumor necrosis is also a feature commonly seen in metastatic small cell carcinomas.

A-65. **(c) Cholangiocarcinoma**
"Pseudointranuclear inclusions" have been found in normal hepatocyte, benign and malignant liver lesions. A mild cytological atypia can also be found in both benign and malignant liver lesions. Pseudointranuclear inclusions and mild cytological atypia are not features seen in cholangiocarcinoma. In cholangiocarcinoma, tumor cells form two- or three-dimensional clusters, crowded sheets, or dispersed large typical cells. They have large hyperchromatic nuclei with coarse chromatin, prominent nucleoli, scant cytoplasm, high N:C ratios, and lacy or vacuolated cytoplasm.

A-66. **(c) Cholangiocarcinoma**
The cytological finding of clear cytoplasm can be seen in a variety of tumors, such as mucin producing adenocarcinoma, renal cell carcinoma, hepatocellular carcinoma, and steroid/lipid producing tumors. This feature is not seen in cholangiocarcinoma. The cytological features of renal cell carcinoma (clear cell renal cell carcinoma) include loosely cohesive clusters and/or scattered individual tumor cells. They have slightly enlarged round nuclei with or without nucleoli depending on the Fuhrman grade of the tumor. The background of smears can be bloody with vascular structures, best seen on cell block preparations. In hepatocellular carcinoma, particularly in poorly differentiated forms, 10 % of tumors may have prominent clear cytoplasm.

A-67. **(d) Sinusoidal capillaries surrounding the markedly thickened trabeculae of neoplastic cells**.
In HCC, tumor cells show a wide range of cytomorphology. In well-differentiated forms, tumor cells resemble normal hepatocytes and form trabeculae, cords, and nests and have a slightly increased N:C ratio, large round nuclei, prominent nucleoli, naked nuclei, and bile pigment in the cytoplasm. In poorly differentiated forms, malignant cells are markedly polygonal and dyscohesive with pleomorphic nuclei and giant tumor cells. The most notable feature of HCC, particularly in well-differentiated tumors, is the identification of sinusoidal capillaries surrounding the markedly thickened trabeculae of neoplastic cells. This feature is not seen in benign liver lesions or cholangiocarcinoma. The presence of lacunae spaces on a cell block preparation is the feature seen in adenocarcinomas.

A-68. **(a) Sheets or loosely formed clusters of columnar cells**
Bile duct hamartoma (also known as von Meyenburg complex, Meyenburg complex, and biliary hamartoma) is a benign tumor-like malformation of the liver. It is classically associated with polycystic liver disease and may be seen in polycystic kidney disease and Caroli's disease. The bile duct hamartoma is characterized by multiple small nodules dispersed throughout the liver. The FNA reveals bland-appearing columnar cells haphazardly arranged in tubules, sheets and two-dimensional clusters, scattered stromal cells, and benign-appearing hepatocytes. In adenocarcinomas, tumor cells form three-dimensional clusters with large hyperchromatic nuclei, coarse chromatin, irregular nuclear membrane, prominent nucleoli, and vacuolated cytoplasm.

A-69. **(c) Pyknotic nuclei**
Metastatic squamous cell carcinomas usually form loose clusters and dispersed individual tumor cells. The cytological features of tumor cells include large

nuclei with smudgy chromatin, nuclei with variation in size and shape, dense cytoplasm (indicative of cytokeratin formation). The dense cytoplasm is blue in color with a Diff-Quik stain and red-pink (eosinophilic) color with Papanicolaou stain. Pyknotic nuclei are usually seen in reactive and/or benign squamous cells. Finally, prominent nucleoli can be seen in poorly differentiated squamous cell carcinomas and should not be confused with poorly differentiated adenocarcinomas. Tumor cells of adenocarcinoma have vesicular nuclei, coarse chromatin, and vacuolated cytoplasm.

A-70. (**a**) **Burkitt's or Burkitt's-like lymphoma (BL)**
The most common types of AIDS-related non-Hodgkin lymphoma (ARL) include Burkitt's or Burkitt's-like lymphoma (BL), diffuse large B-cell lymphoma (DLBCL) (including the subtypes of immunoblastic and centroblastic lymphoma), plasmablastic lymphoma (including oral cavity involved and multicentric Castleman's disease [MCD] associated), and primary effusion lymphoma (PEL). Among them, BL tumor cells are positive for the characteristic c-myc gene rearrangement and show no evidence of HHV-8 infection. Peripheral T-cell NHLs can usually be distinguished by routine immunohistochemistry for T-cell markers or T-cell receptor (TCR) gene rearrangement studies. Both DLBCL and PEL can have similar cytomorphology. In DLBCL, tumor cells are positive for Epstein-Barr virus, but negative for HHV-8. In PEL, tumor cells are negative for Epstein-Barr virus, but positive for HHV-8.

A-71. (**b**) **Dispersed individual large atypical cells**
DLBLC is a good mimic of carcinoma. In DLBCL, the FNA reveals a cellular specimen with dyscohesive large atypical lymphoid cells. Tree morphological variants are most commonly seen: centroblastic, immunoblastic, and anaplastic variant. Centroblastic variant is the most common subtype and reveals medium-to-large-sized tumor cells with high N:C ratios, oval or round nuclei, fine chromatin, and single or multiple prominent nucleoli. Immunoblasts have a basophilic cytoplasm and a central nucleolus. Most cases are polymorphic, with a mixture of centroblastic and immunoblastic cells. The third morphologic variant, anaplastic variant, consists of large tumor cells with pleomorphic nuclei, and may resemble Hodgkin cells or Reed-Sternberg cells. In a poorly differentiated adenocarcinoma, tumor cells can be dyscohesive and presented as dispersed individual cells or form three-dimensional clusters with large hyperchromatic nuclei, coarse chromatin, irregular nuclear membrane, prominent nucleoli, and vacuolated cytoplasm. In difficult cases, IHC stains for lymphoma and adenocarcinoma markers are necessary for an accurate diagnosis.

A-72. (**d**) **Predominantly isolated large cells with "cherry red" nuclei**
The cytological differential diagnosis of a metastatic melanoma and HCC can be difficult. The cytological features of a metastatic melanoma include: individual large cells with prominent large nucleoli, intranuclear inclusion, cytoplasmic melanin pigment, binucleation, and the presence of plasmacytoid cells. In HCC, tumor cells form loose clusters or dispersed individual cells and reveal hyperchromatic nuclei, coarse chromatin, large prominent nucleoli, and intranuclear pseudoinclusion. Numerous naked nuclei and tumor necrosis are also seen in HCC. The predominant dyscohesive arrangement of tumor cells favors the diagnosis of a metastatic melanoma. In difficult cases, IHC stains of HMB45 and Melanin A may help.

A-73. (**b**) **Cholangiocarcinoma is always seen in a cirrhotic liver**
Cholangiocarcinoma is known to have the histological and molecular features of adenocarcinoma. Cirrhotic liver is not a significant risk factor for developing cholangiocarcinoma. The cytomorphology of the tumor includes trabeculae, cords, crowded sheets and nests arrangements, or dispersed individual tumor cells with large oval nuclei and coarse chromatin, and scant cytoplasm. The differential diagnosis of cholangiocarcinoma includes HCC, metastatic adenocarcinoma, and other gastrointestinal tumors.

A-74. (**b**) **Dense cytoplasm and distinct cell border**
In hepatocellular carcinoma, tumor cells form cords, tubules, sheets, or isolated individual cells. Tumor cells have hyperchromatic nuclei, coarse chromatin, and high N:C ratio. Large prominent nucleoli, marked variation of size of nuclei, and numerous naked nuclei are also features seen in HCC. However, the cytoplasm of HCC is vesicular, granular, and/or clear. The dense cytoplasm and distinct cell border are not seen in HCC.

A-75. (**c**) **Centrally placed nuclei with binucleation**
A FNA of benign liver reveals sheets of large polygonal and dispersed individual cells. The specimen may also reveal trabecular arrangements and tissue fragments. Cells have centrally placed round- to oval-shaped nuclei with mild variation in size, granular chromatin, prominent nucleoli, no hyperchromasia,

and a normal N:C ratio. Binucleation is common in cells. Bile and lipofusion pigment can be identified in the cytoplasm. In contrast, in hepatocellular carcinoma (HCC), tumor cells form cords, tubules, sheets, or isolated individual cells. Tumor cells have hyperchromatic nuclei, coarse chromatin, and high N:C ratios. Large prominent nucleoli, marked variation of size of nuclei, and numerous naked nuclei are features seen in HCC.

Reading List

Balani S, Malik R, Malik R, Kapoor N. Cytomorphological variables of hepatic malignancies in fine needle aspiration smears with special reference to grading of hepatocellular carcinoma. J Cytol. 2013;30:116–20.

Bibbo M, Wood MD, Fitzpatrick BT. Peritoneal washings and ovary. In: Bibbo M, Wilbur D, editors. Comprehensive cytopathology. 3rd ed. Philadelphia: Saunders/Elsevier; 2008.

Cibas ES. Peritoneal washings. In: Cibas ES, Ducatman BS, editors. Cytology: diagnostic principles and clinical correlates. Philadelphia: Saunders/Elsevier; 2009.

DeMay RM. Chapter 6. Cerebrospinal fluid. In: The art and science of cytopathology, exfoliative cytology, vol. 1. 2nd ed. Chicago: ASCP Press; 2012. p. 490–525.

Geramizadeh B, Asadi N, Tabei SZ. Cytologic comparison between malignant and regenerative nodules in the background of cirrhosis. Hepat Mon. 2012;12:448–52.

Khalbuss WE, Monaco SE, Pantanowitz L. Chapter 16. Liver. In: The ASCP Quick Compendium (QC) of cytopathology. Chicago: ASCP Press; 2013. p. 340–65.

VandenBussche C, Gocke CD, Li QK. Fine needle aspiration of metastatic papillary thyroid carcinoma found in the liver. Diagn Cytopathol. 2013;41:418–24.

Wee A. Fine needle aspiration biopsy of hepatocellular carcinoma and hepatocellular nodular lesions: role, controversies and approach to diagnosis. Cytopathology. 2011;22:287–305.

Pancreatic Fine-Needle Aspiration

8

Abdelmonem Elhosseiny and Walid E. Khalbuss

Contents

8.1 **Image-Based Questions 1–40** 472
8.2 **Text-Based Questions 41–68** 512
8.3 **Answers and Discussion of Image-Based Questions 1–40** 514
8.4 **Answers and Discussion of Text-Based Questions 41–62** 517
Reading List 518

Table 8.1 Pancreatic FNA: indications, contraindication, accuracy, and complication

Indication	Evaluation of suspicious pancreatic solid or cystic masses
Accuracy	*Sensitivity*: 80–95 % and *specificity* approaches 100 % *Causes of false negative cases*: Sampling errors (small lesions, difficult anatomic target, and extensive fibrosis or bleeding) Interoperation errors, well-differentiated adenocarcinoma (as benign duct cells) *Causes of false positive cases*: Over-interpretation of atypia in cases of chronic pancreatitis can lead to false positive diagnosis
Contraindications	Bleeding diathesis, upper GI obstruction, and difficult anatomic sites
Complications	Rare; acute pancreatitis and extensive bleeding

Table 8.2 Normal pancreatic FNA

Acini/acinar cells	Acini are the predominant component Cohesive clusters, single cells, and rarely bare nuclei The nuclei are round, regular, and central, with evenly distributed fine chromatin and prominent nucleoli The cytoplasm is abundant and granular with occasional vacuoles The architecture of the acinar cells in smears is often described as that of clusters of grapes
Ducts/ducal cells	Sheets of flat cohesive glandular epithelium Cells are round, uniform, evenly spaced nuclei (classic honey comb pattern)
Endocrine cells	Endocrine cells are rarely seen in normal pancreatic FNA Small cells with granular cytoplasm and eccentric small nuclei

A. Elhosseiny, MD (✉)
Fletcher Allen Health Care, University of Vermont,
111 Colchester Avenue, Burlington, VT 05405, USA
e-mail: abdel.elhosseiny@vtmednet.org

W.E. Khalbuss, MD, PhD, FIAC
Department of Pathology, GE Clarient Diagnostic Services,
31 Columbia, Aliso Viejo, California, 92656, USA
e-mail: Walid.khalbuss@ge.com

W.E. Khalbuss, Q.K. Li (eds.), *Diagnostic Cytopathology Board Review and Self-Assessment*,
DOI 10.1007/978-1-4939-1477-7_8, © Springer Science+Business Media New York 2015

Table 8.3 Pancreatic duct adenocarcinoma

Clinical:
More in the head of the pancreas (80–90 %)
The most common tumor of the pancreas (90 %)
The fourth leading cause of cancer death in the USA
Most cases occur between the ages of 60 and 80 years
Cigarette smoking has been identified as a risk factor for pancreatic cancer
More in men than in women; ages of 60–80 years and 10 % are familial
Poor prognosis (5-year survival rate is <5 %)
Cytological features:
Cellular aspirate
Cells are arranged in 3D groups, single cells, or small clusters
The tumor cells have enlarged nuclei with nuclear size up to 4 times the nuclear size of acinar cells. Cells within the groups are overlapping with irregular nuclear contour. Mitotic activity is significant. Clusters with cribriform pattern are also seen. The background may show: cell necrosis, mucin, and ghost tumor cells
In well-differentiated adenocarcinoma the nuclear enlargement is less than the above and the cell crowding is more subtle. Loss of polarity is an important feature. The spaces between the neoplastic cells are wide and uneven which leads to focal overlapping of the nuclei. The nuclear contour irregularity is less obvious. The cytoplasm is often mucinous
Immunostain:
Duct adenocarcinoma: p53 (positive), SMAD4 (negative), and CDx2 (weak or focal reactivity)
Chronic pancreatitis and GI contaminants: p53 (negative), SMAD4 (positive), and CDx2 (positive)
Variants of pancreatic adenocarcinoma
Adenosquamous carcinoma (3 %)
Poorly differentiated (anaplastic) adenocarcinoma

Table 8.4 Acinic Cell Carcinoma (ACC)

Clinical:
Rare (2 %); occurs in patients age 60 or older (rare in children and adolescents)
This tumor resembles pancreatic acini and produces pancreatic enzymes
Survival rate is as poor as pancreatic duct adenocarcinoma
Cytologic features:
Cellular aspirate
Cells are arranged single cells and in small groups
Background of bare nuclei is common
Many cell groups are arranged in small acini and loosely cohesive groups
The nuclei are large relative to normal acini with even chromatin and prominent nucleoli
The nuclear contour is mildly irregular
The cytoplasm varies from granular to foamy
The cytoplasm is positive for PAS/dPAS
Differential diagnosis:
Pancreatic endocrine tumor (PEN), solid pseudopapillary tumor and normal acini
Immunostain:
Positive for trypsin, chymotrypsin, alpha-1-chymotrypsin, and CK

Table 8.5 Pancreatic Endocrine Neoplasm (PEN)

Clinical:
Low grade well differentiated neoplasms
Represent 3–5 % of all pancreatic tumors
The mean age for these tumors is 40–60 years
These tumors may be functioning in 50 % of cases causing hypoglycemia, GI ulcers, or diarrhea with dehydration
Cytologic features:
Cellular aspirates
Uniform population of cells of small- to medium-sized polygonal cells
Eccentric nuclei (plasmacytoid appearance)
The nuclei have the neuroendocrine chromatin pattern and nucleoli are inconspicuous
Rare variant of this tumor has oncocytic cytoplasm
Poorly differentiated variant (small cell carcinoma and large cell endocrine carcinoma)
Differential diagnosis:
Acinic cell tumor, solid pseudopapillary tumor, and normal acini (pitfall)
Immunostain:
Reactive for CAM 5.2, AE1/AE3, chromogranin, synaptophysin, and NSE

Table 8.6 Solid Pseudopapillary Neoplasm (SPN)

Clinical:
Uncommon 2–3 %, more in females (9:1), age 7–79 years
A low grade malignant neoplasm
Solid or with secondary cystic degeneration
Excellent prognosis (only 15 % recurrence or metastatic disease)
Complete surgical resection in a node negative patient is considered curative
Cytological features:
Highly cellular smears
Monotonous cuboidal cells in single and loosely cohesive groups
Single or multiple cells around vascular structures
The vascular structures have a myxoid or hyalinized stroma (Figs. 8.26 and 8.27)
Differential diagnosis:
PENs and ACC
Immunostain:
Negative for keratins and synaptophysin but usually reactive to B-catenin

Table 8.7 Pancreatic cystic lesions

General	Pancreatic cysts are uncommon (10 %) Analysis of the enzyme and tumor markers in cyst fluid is helpful Pseudocysts display the highest amylase and lipase activity Tumor markers such as CEA are elevated in mucinous cysts
Pancreatic pseudocyst	Most common cyst of the pancreas, 5–10 cm Occurs in the setting of acute pancreatitis (auto digestion) Cyst filled with fluid secondary to inflammation, necrosis, or hemorrhage More adjacent to the tail of the pancreas and has no lining cells Chemical analysis of cyst fluid yields high amylase, normal CEA, and low viscosity
Cytologic features	Cloudy, turbid, or dark fluid with cellular debris Hemosiderin laden macrophages and normal components of pancreatic tissue
Lymphoepithelial cyst	Benign cysts lined by squamous epithelium and reactive lymphoid nodules Rare (0.05 % of all pancreatic cysts) More in men and in older patients (mean age of 56 years)
Cytologic features	Nucleated and anucleated squamous cells Debris; cholesterol clefts, histiocytes, and lymphocytes
Serous cystadenoma	Benign, rare (2 % of all pancreatic cysts) and often microcystic More in female (mean age is 65 years) Small cuboidal cells with high glycogen content and secrete clear serous fluid There is an association with von Hippel–Lindau syndrome
Cytologic features	The cyst contents are sparsely cellular Clear or granular background Fat sheets of cuboidal cells with clear or granular cytoplasm The nuclei are central, round, fine chromatin and inconspicuous nucleoli Rare bare nuclei are sometimes noted Cyst fluid: low amylase and CEA (rules out pseudocyst)
Mucinous cystic neoplasms (MCN)	5 % of pancreatic neoplasms, more in the tail and body of the pancreas Cysts are lined by mucinous epithelium and not communicating with the pancreatic duct. Specialized stroma of the ovarian type is located beneath the epithelium This stroma expresses receptors for estrogen and progesterone
Intraductal papillary mucinous neoplasms (IPMN)	4 % of all pancreatic neoplasms, more in men and more in the head of the pancreas Connect to the main pancreatic duct May have a spectrum of dysplastic changes (benign, borderline to invasive carcinoma)
Cytologic features	MCN and IPMC have same cytological characteristics Both MCN and IPMN yield scant cellular samples with thick mucus and columnar epithelium arranged in single cells or arranged in papillae or sheets The sensitivity of cytology in these lesions is close to 50 %

Table 8.8 Metastatic neoplasms to the pancreas

Most common : renal cell carcinoma and melanoma
Others: lung, breast, lymphomas, ovary, colon, gallbladder, stomach, prostate, and sarcoma
Thorough clinical history, review of prior material and immunostains can be useful

8.1 Image-Based Questions 1–40

Fig. 8.1

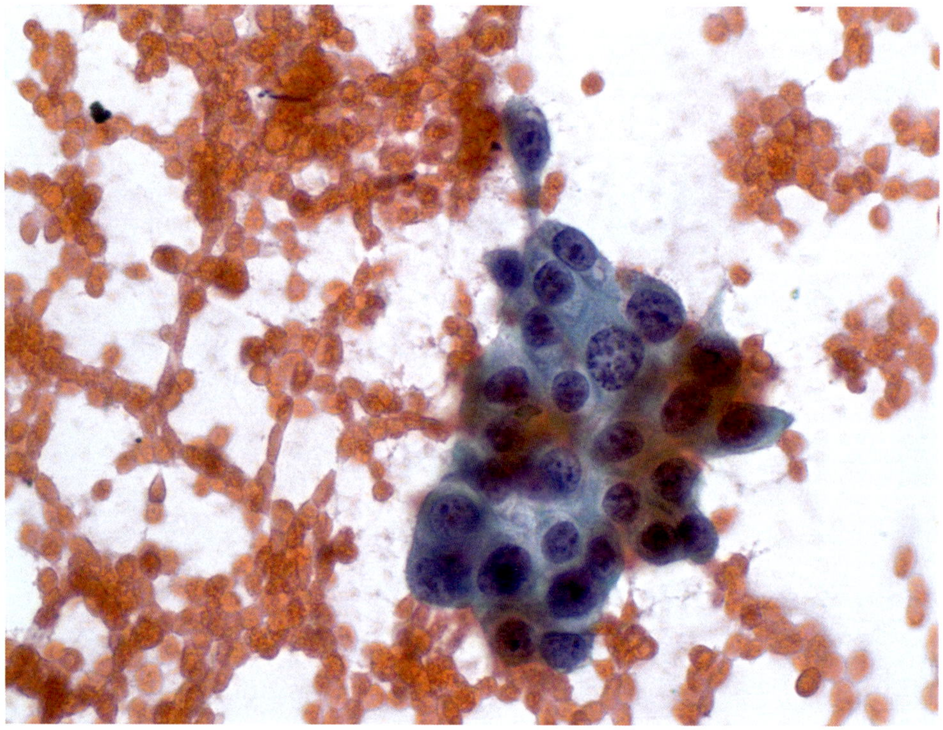

Q-1. A 68-year old male was found to have a 4-cm mass in the head of the pancreas. AN EUS-guided FNA of this mass is shown. What is your diagnosis?

(a) Moderately differentiated adenocarcinoma
(b) Acinic cell carcinoma
(c) Intraductal papillary mucinous tumor
(d) Gastric contaminant
(e) Pancreatic endocrine tumor

Fig. 8.2

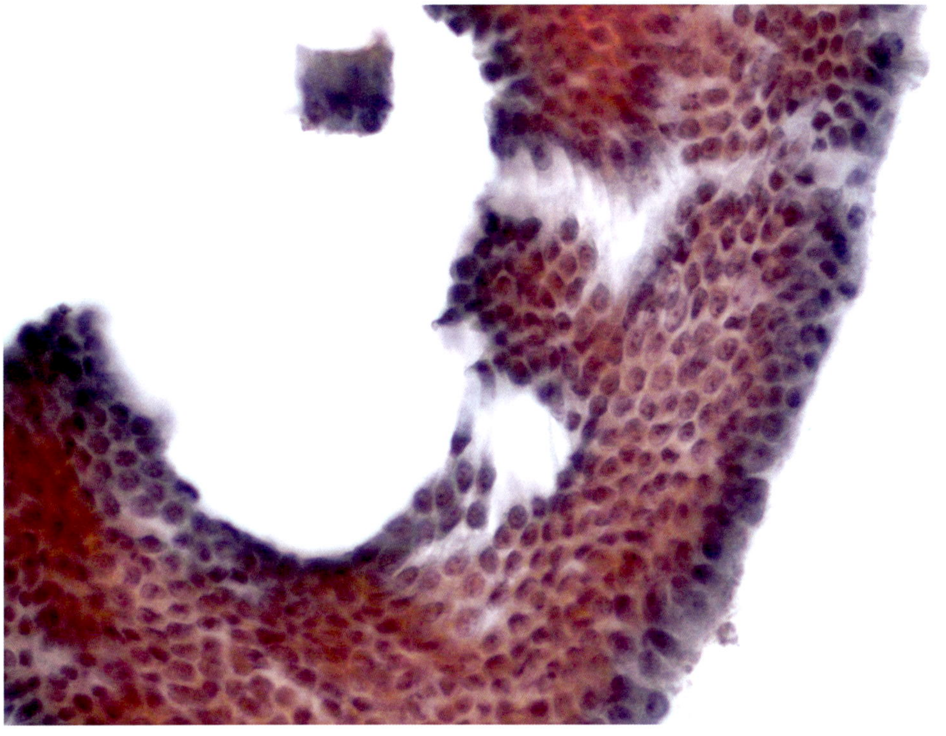

Q-2. EUS-guided FNA of a cystic mass in the tail of the pancreas in a 65-year old female. What is the most likely diagnosis?

(a) Well-differentiated adenocarcinoma
(b) Mucinous cystic neoplasm
(c) Intraductal papillary mucinous tumor
(d) Gastric contaminant
(e) Serous cyst adenoma

Fig. 8.3

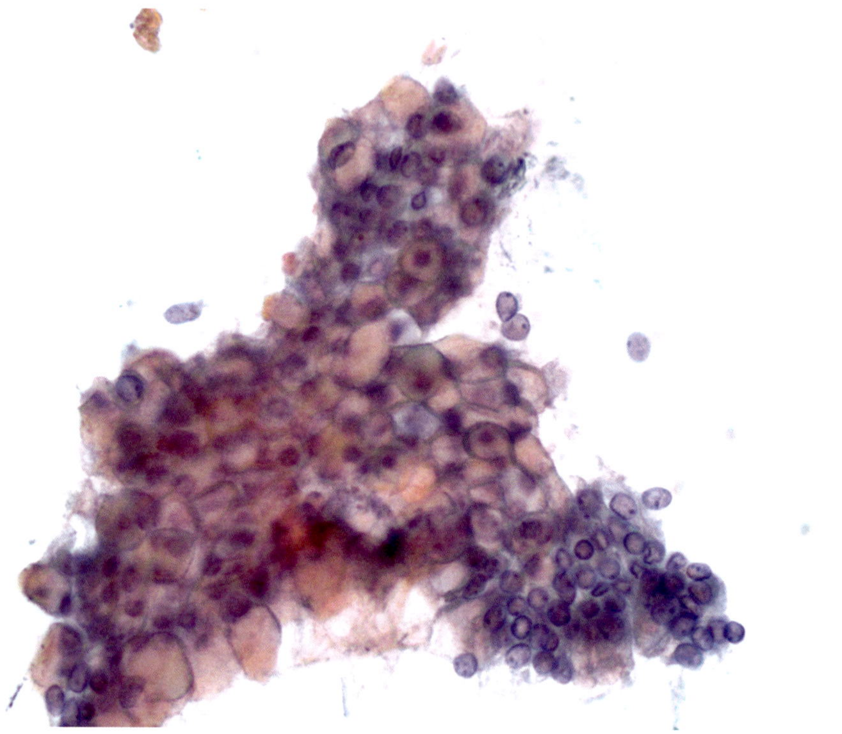

Q-3. EUS-guided FNA of a solid pancreatic head mass from a 59-year old female. What is your diagnosis?
(a) Mucinous cyst adenoma
(b) Intraductal papillary mucinous tumor
(c) Mucinous adenocarcinoma
(d) Gastric contaminant
(e) Reactive duct epithelium

Fig. 8.4

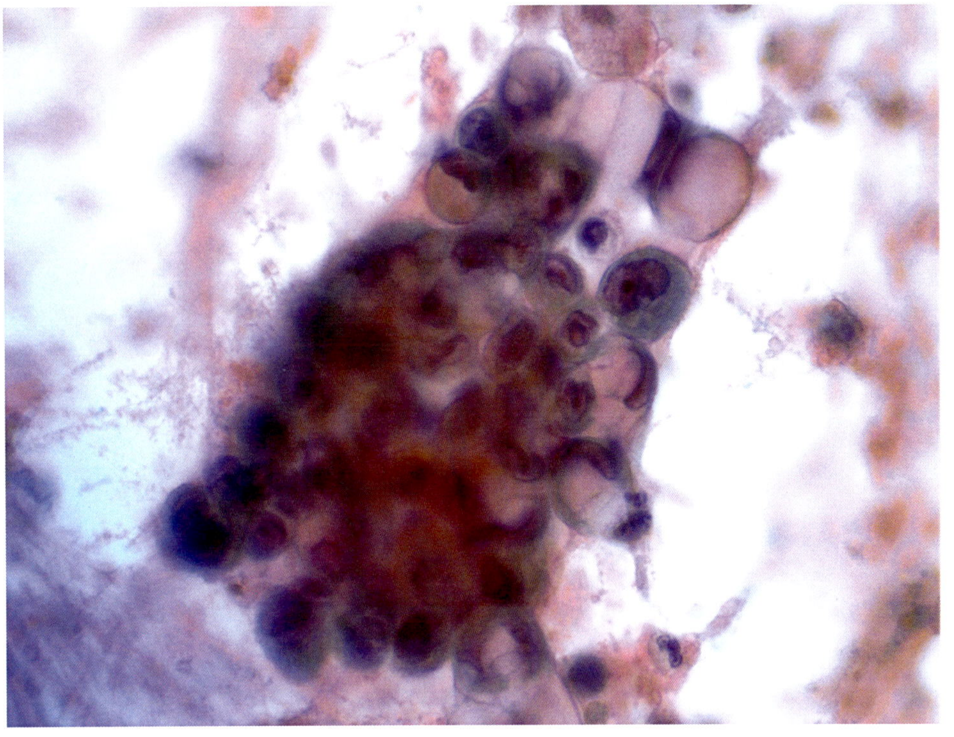

Q-4. EUS-guided FNA of a 3-cm solid mass in the head of the pancreas from a 59-year-old male. Tumor as immunoreactive to CK19. What is your best diagnosis?
(a) Mucinous cystadenoma
(b) Acinic cell carcinoma
(c) Mucinous adenocarcinoma with signet ring cells
(d) Adenosquamous carcinoma
(e) Solid pseudopapillary tumor

Fig. 8.5

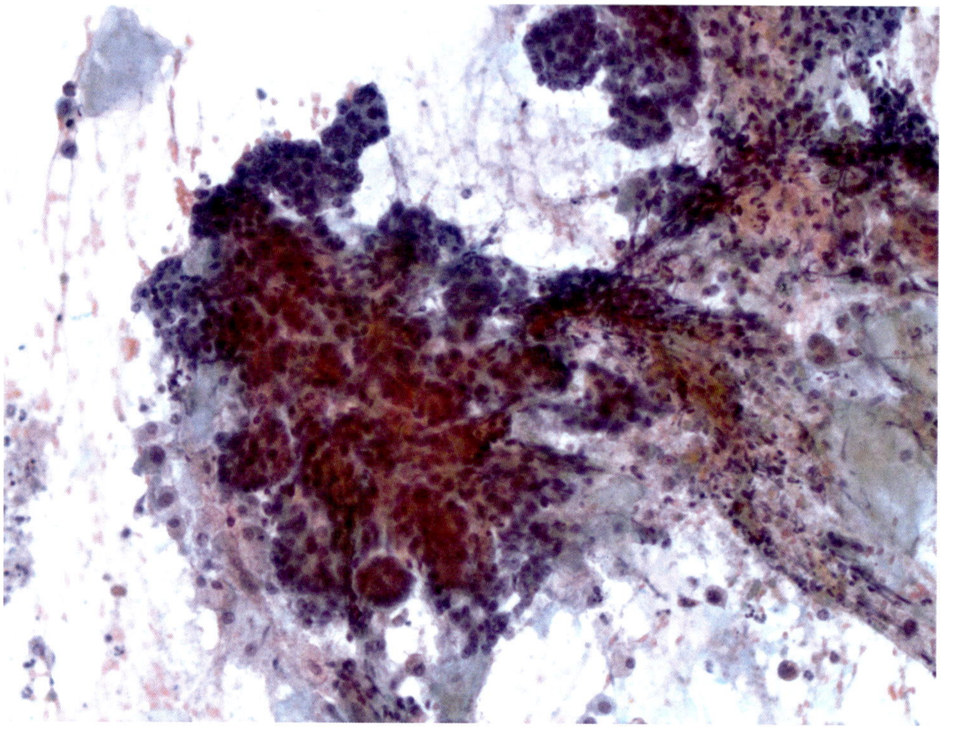

Q-5. EUS FNA of a mass in the head of the pancreas in a 68-year-old male. What is your best diagnosis?
(a) Acinic cell carcinoma
(b) Well-differentiated adenocarcinoma
(c) Serous cystadenoma
(d) Chronic pancreatitis
(e) Normal pancreas

Fig. 8.6

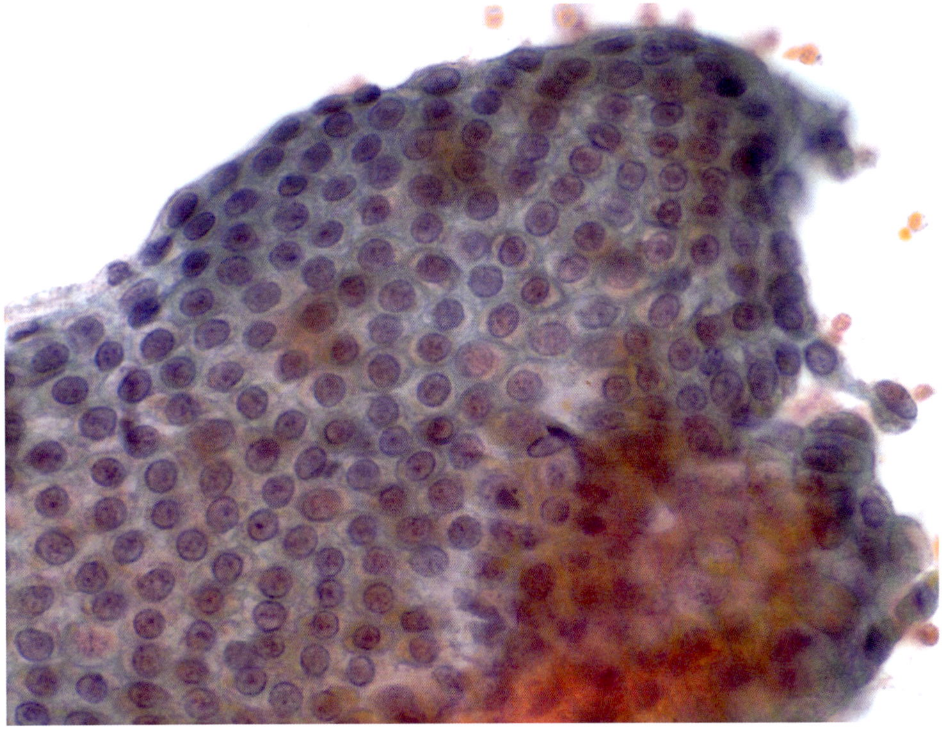

Q-6. A 67-year-old woman underwent EUS-guided FNA of a cystic mass in the body of the pancreas. What is your diagnosis?
(a) Mucinous cystadenoma
(b) Well-differentiated pancreatic adenocarcinoma
(c) Serous cystadenoma
(d) Duodenal contaminant
(e) Gastric contaminant

Fig. 8.7

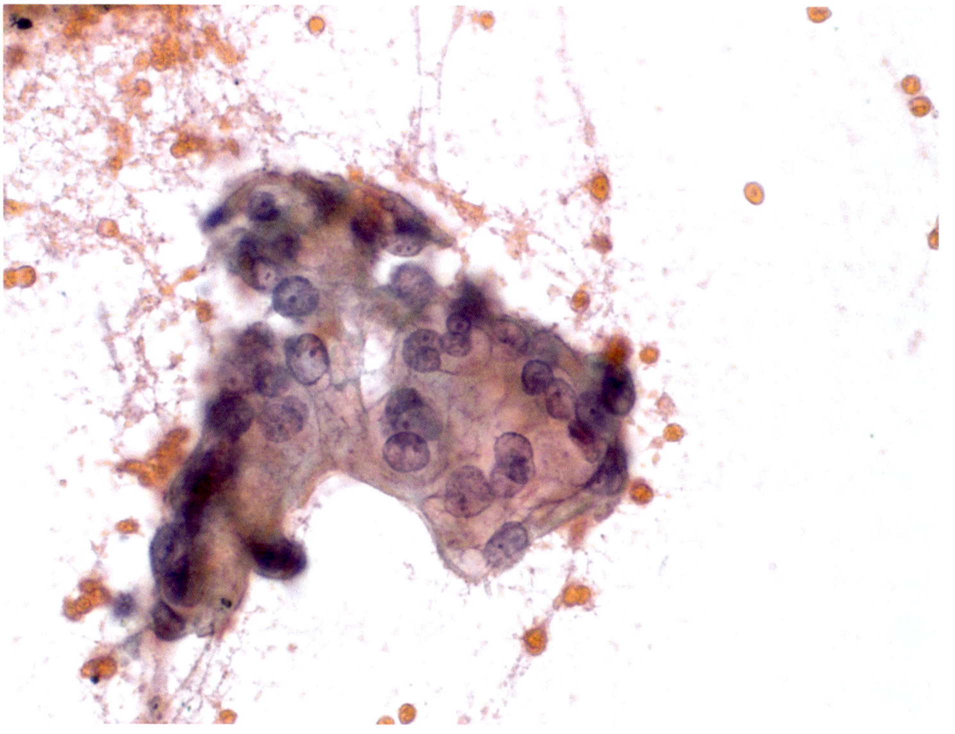

Q-7. FNA of a 3-cm pancreatic body mass in a 65-year-old female. What is your best diagnosis?
(a) Gastric contamination
(b) Granular adenocarcinoma
(c) Mucinous cyst adenoma
(d) Acinic cell carcinoma
(e) Serous cyst adenoma

Fig. 8.8

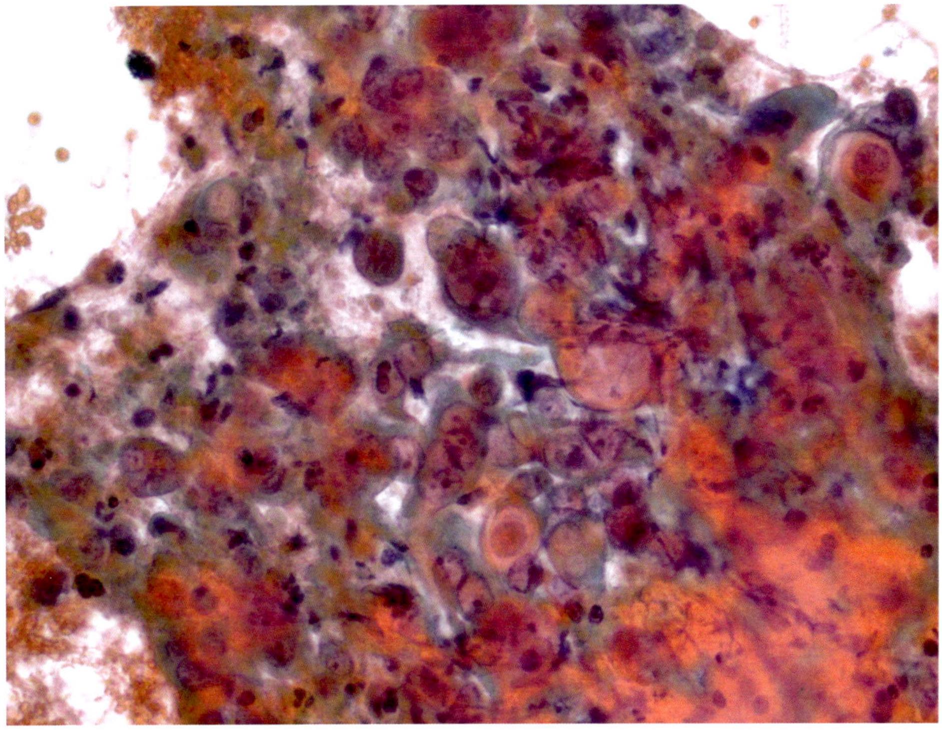

Q-8. EUS-guided FNA of a 5.5 cm mass in the head of the pancreas from a 78-year-old male. The pancreatic duct is dilated and patient is jaundiced. What is the most likely diagnosis?

(a) Pancreatoblastoma
(b) Adenocarcinoma, poorly differentiated
(c) Adenosquamous carcinoma
(d) Metastatic squamous carcinoma
(e) Anaplastic carcinoma with giant cells

Fig. 8.9

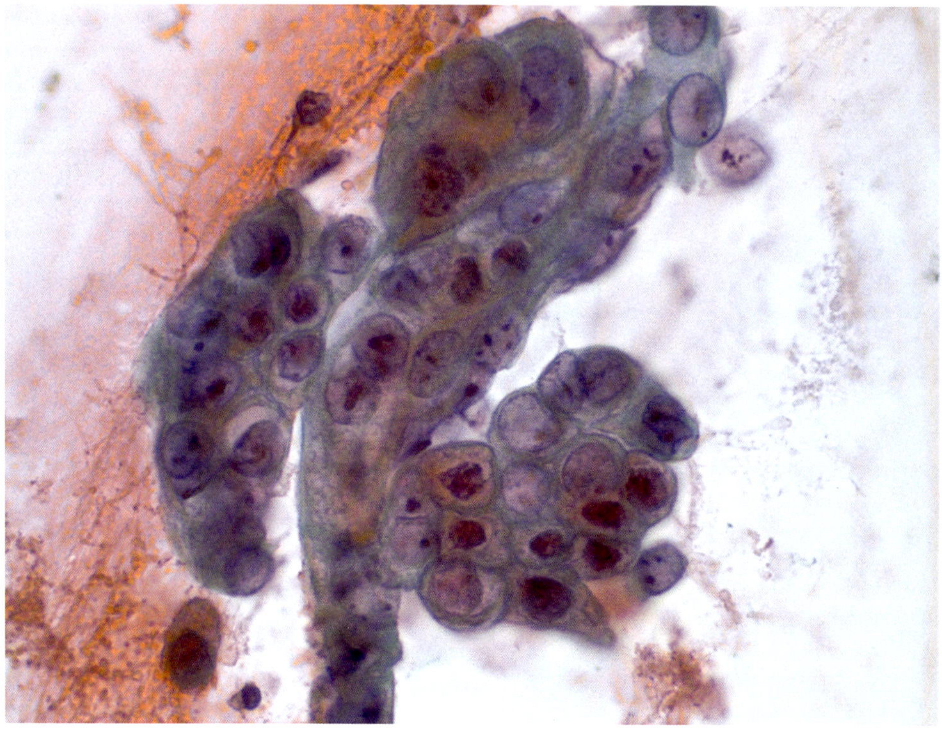

Q-9. A 78-year-old woman was found to have a 3-cm pancreatic mass in the region of the head. The depicted image is from an aspirate of this mass. The best diagnosis is:
- (a) Pancreatic endocrine tumor
- (b) High grade lymphoma
- (c) Pancreatic adenocarcinoma, moderately differentiated
- (d) Acinic cell carcinoma
- (e) Solid pseudopapillary tumor

Fig. 8.10

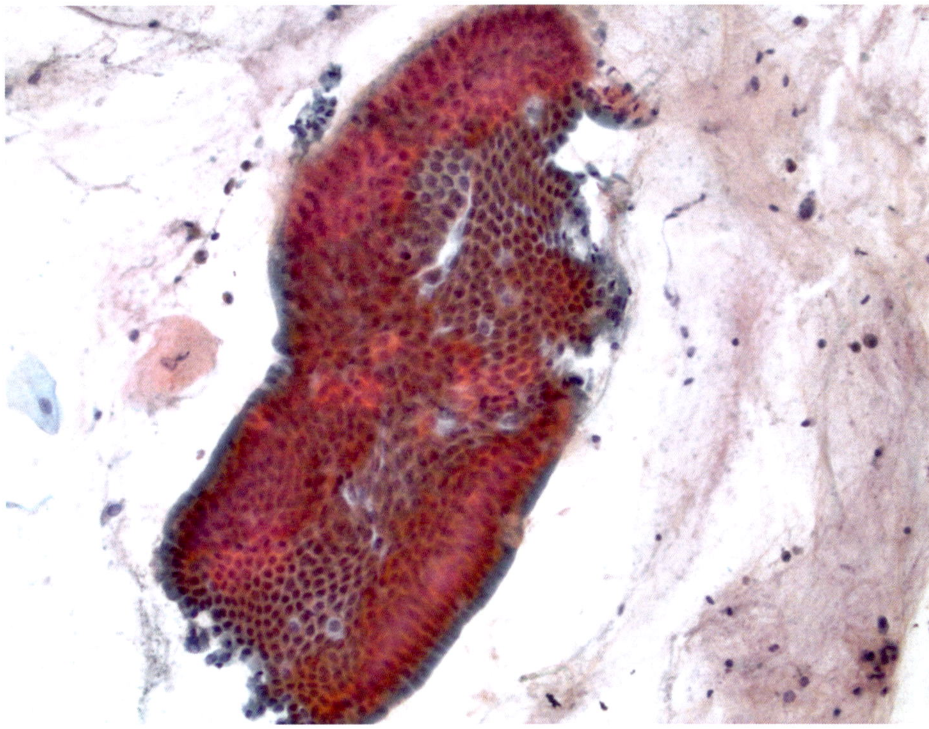

Q-10. FNA of a 4.5 cystic mass in the head of the pancreas in a 59-year-old male. What is your best diagnosis?
(a) Mucinous cyst adenoma
(b) Intraductal papillary mucinous tumor
(c) Adenocarcinoma, well differentiated
(d) Gastric contaminant
(e) Duodenal contaminant

Fig. 8.11

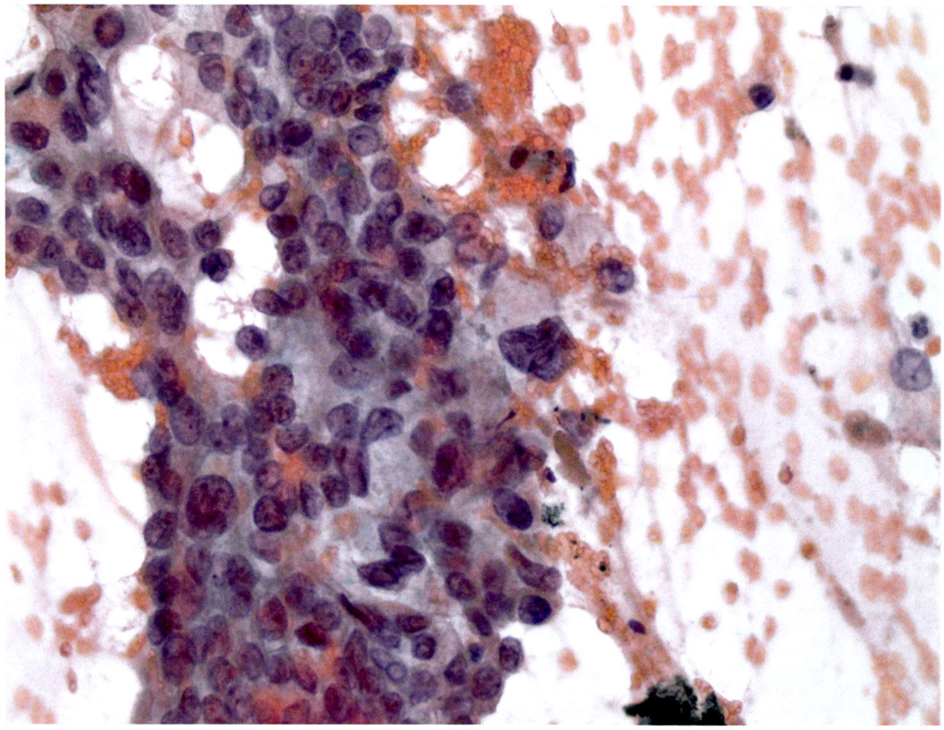

Q-11. EUS-guided FNA of a 4-cm mass from a 70-year-old male. What is your best diagnosis?

(a) Adenocarcinoma, moderately differentiated
(b) Pancreaticoblastoma
(c) Adenosquamous carcinoma
(d) Acinic cell carcinoma
(e) Pancreatic endocrine tumor

Fig. 8.12

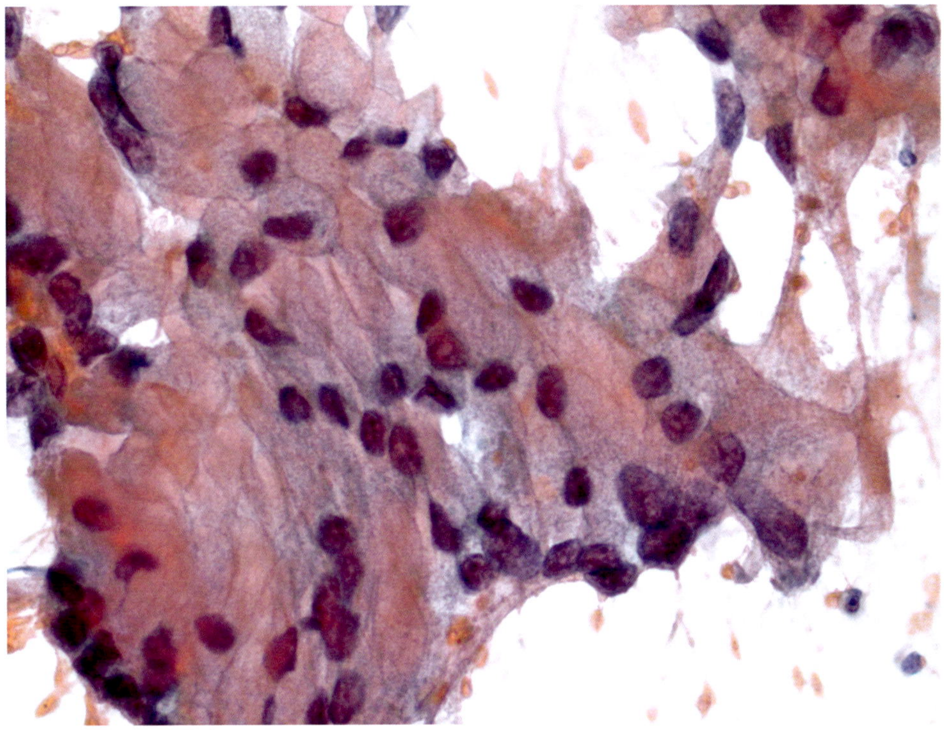

Q-12. FNA of a solid mass of pancreas from a 59-year-old woman. What is the best diagnosis?
(a) Atypia due to chronic pancreatitis
(b) Acinic cell carcinoma
(c) Pancreatic endocrine tumor
(d) Solid pseudopapillary tumor
(e) Mucinous adenocarcinoma

Fig. 8.13

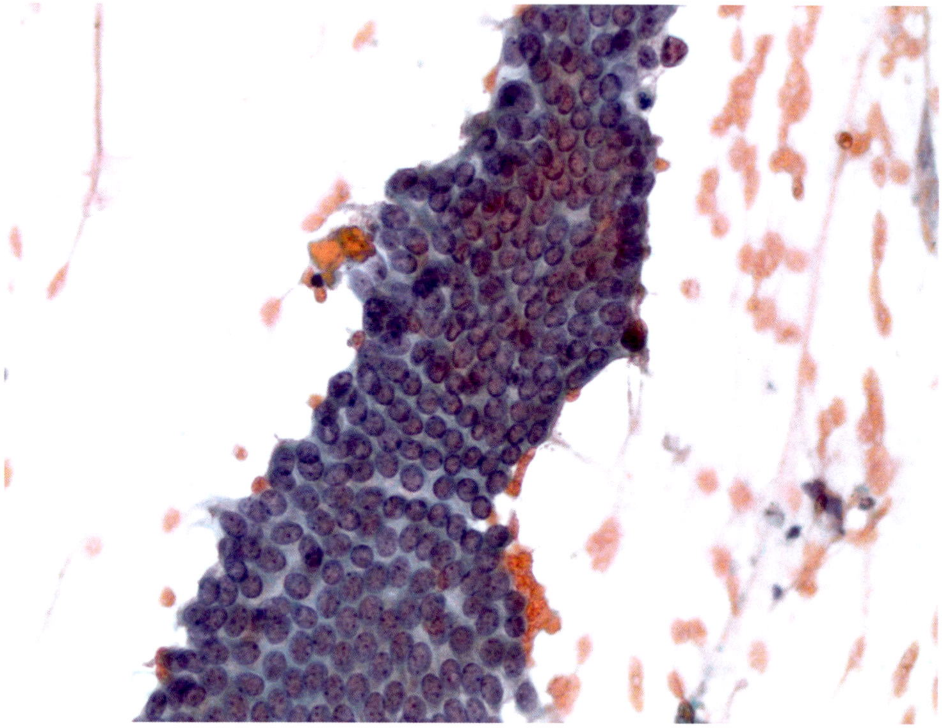

Q-13. EUS-guided FNA of a mass in the head of the pancreas from a 75-year-old male. The diagnosis is?
(a) Well-differentiated adenocarcinoma
(b) Atypia due to chronic pancreatitis
(c) Acinic cell carcinoma
(d) Benign pancreatic duct epithelium
(e) Serous cystadenoma

Fig. 8.14

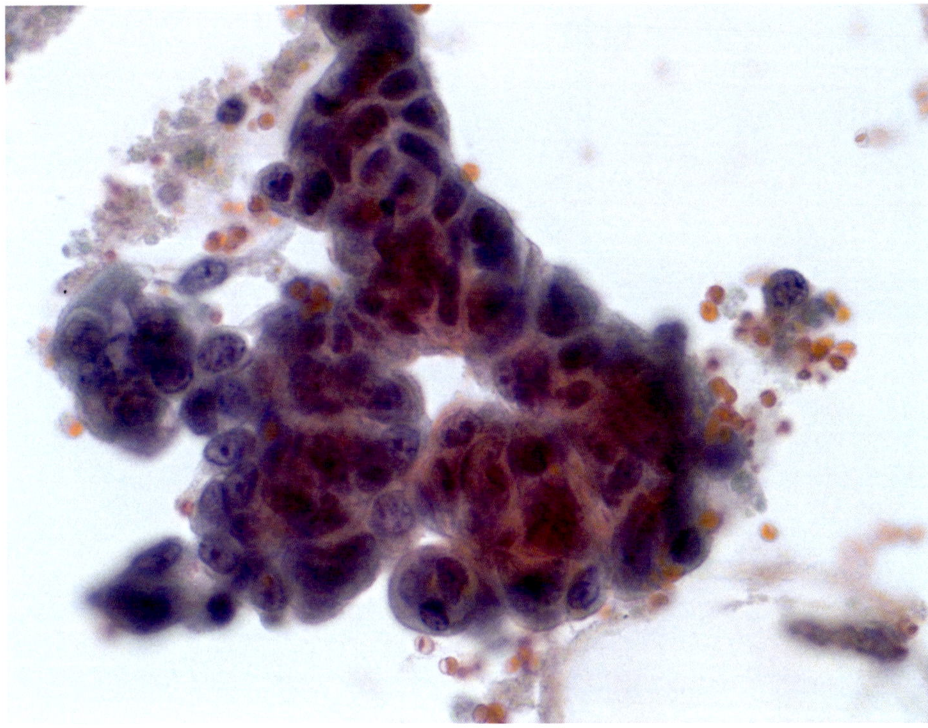

Q-14. This is an aspirate from a pancreatic mass from an 80-year-old woman who was jaundiced and had a dilated common bile duct. The best diagnosis is:
(a) Pancreaticoblastoma
(b) Adenocarcinoma poorly differentiated
(c) Acinic cell carcinoma
(d) Solid pseudopapillary tumor
(e) Pancreatic endocrine tumor

Fig. 8.15

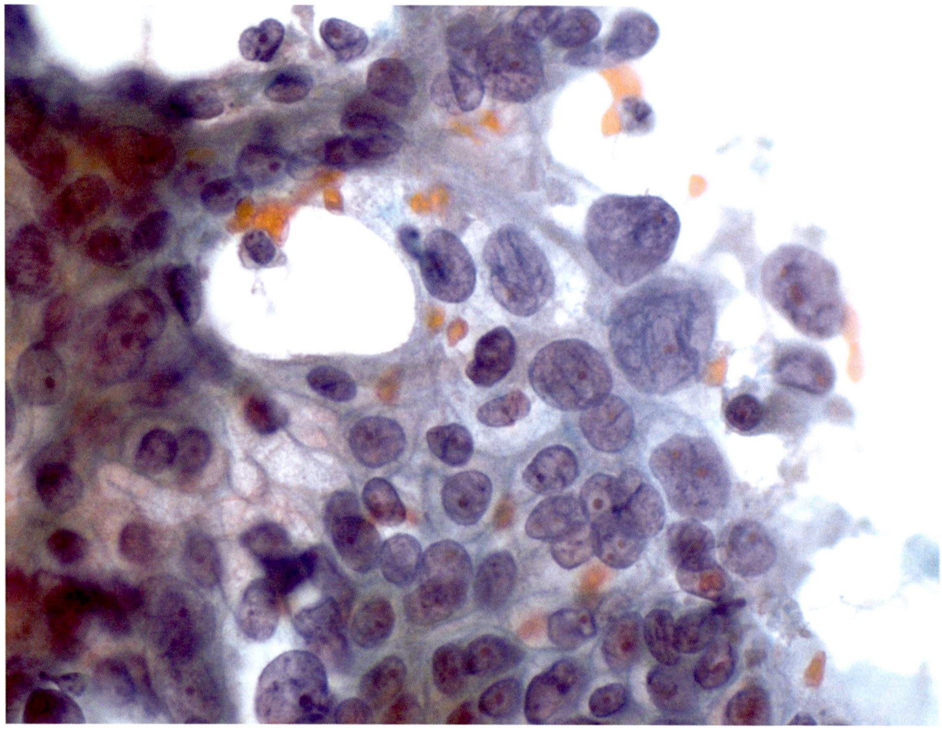

Q-15. EUS-guided FNA of a pancreatic mass from a 68-year-old male. Upper endoscopy is negative. Tumor cells were reactive to CK 19. What is the best diagnosis?

(a) Pancreatic duct adenocarcinoma, moderately differentiated
(b) Clear cell adenocarcinoma
(c) Acinic cell carcinoma
(d) Metastatic gastric carcinoma
(e) Pancreaticoblastoma

Fig. 8.16

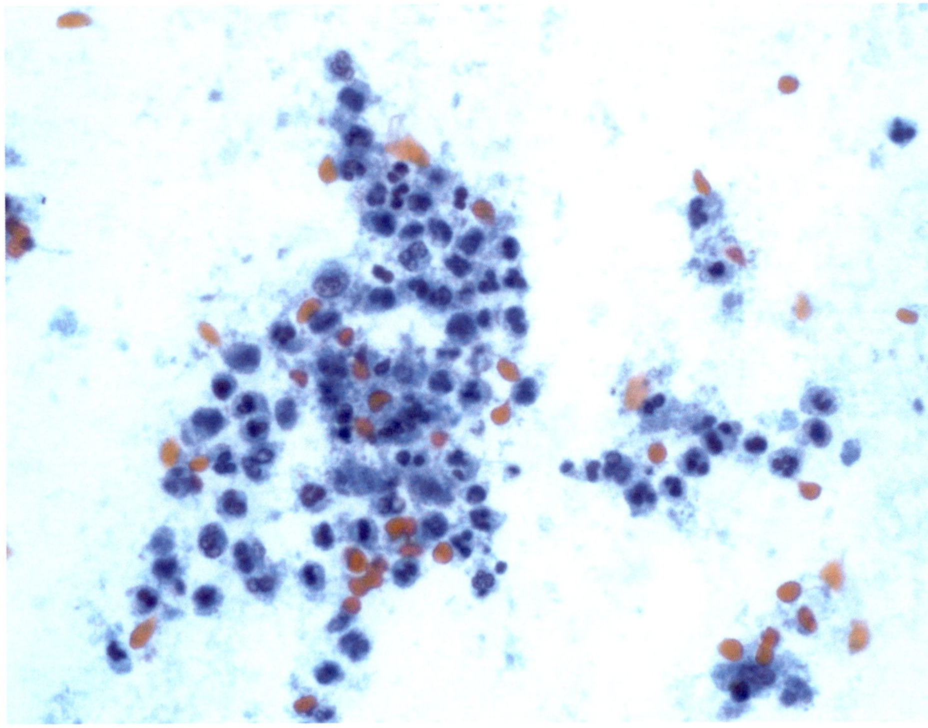

Q-16. A 59-year-old male who had history of alcohol abuse developed a 8-cm parapancreatic cyst. All of the following regarding this lesion are correct except:

(a) This cyst has no true epithelial lining
(b) This is the most common cyst of the pancreas
(c) CEA is elevated in the cyst contents
(d) Amylase is commonly elevated in cyst contents
(e) This cyst has no malignant potential

Fig. 8.17

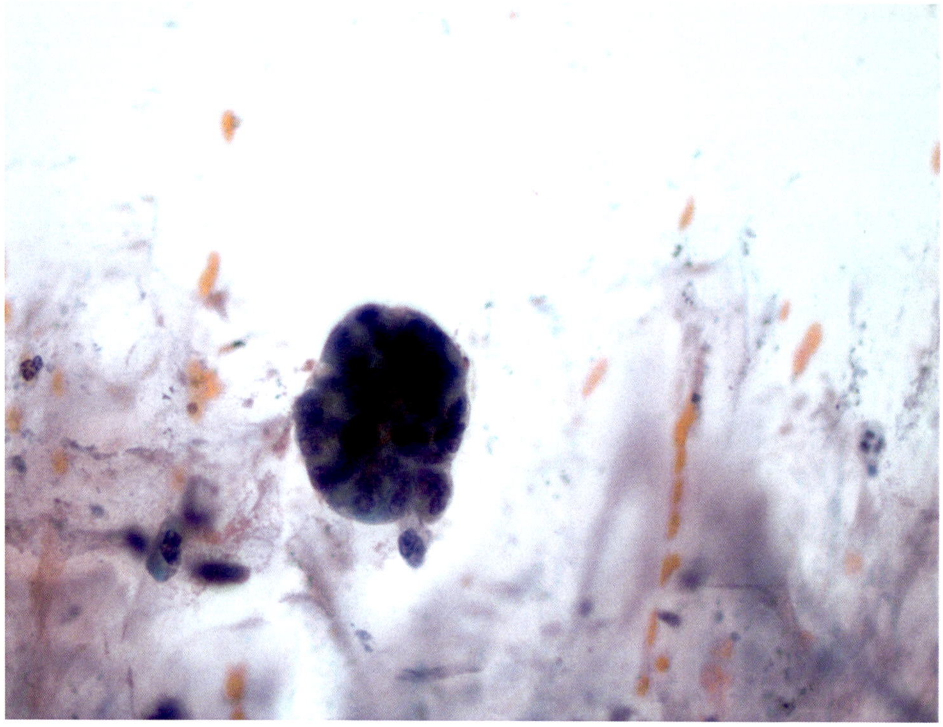

Q-17. A 65-year-old female was found to have a 3.5 cm cystic mass in the body of the pancreas. She underwent EUS-guided FNA. What is your best diagnosis?
(a) Pancreatic duct adenocarcinoma
(b) Mucinous cystadenoma
(c) Intraductal papillary mucinous adenoma
(d) Gastric contaminant
(e) Mucinous cystadenocarcinoma

Fig. 8.18

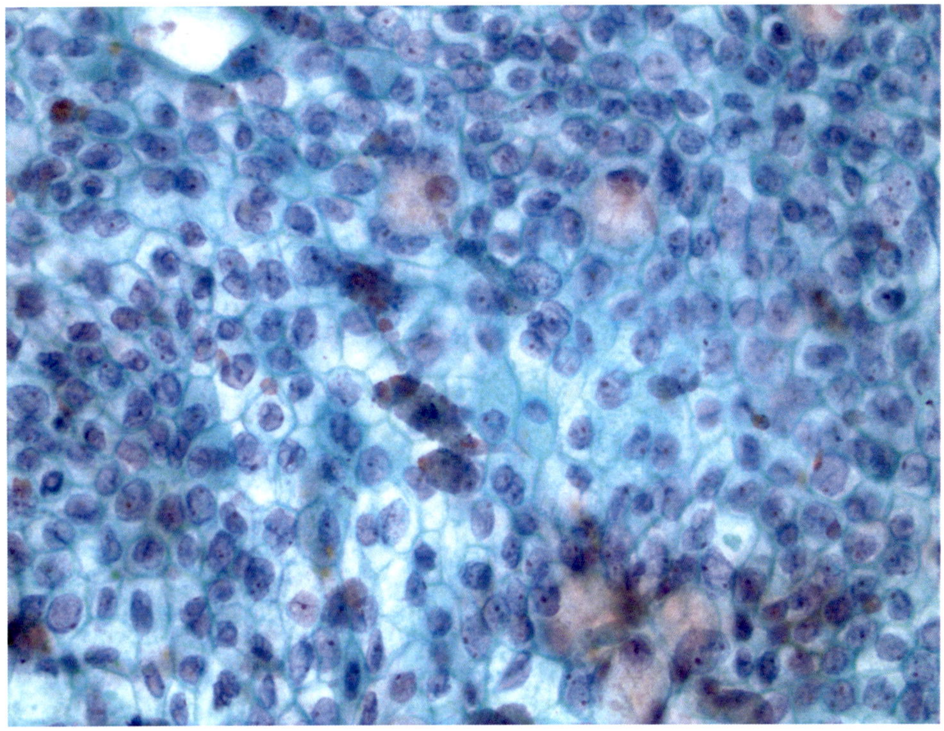

Q-18. This is an EUS-guided FNA of a 3-cm mass in the head of the pancreas from a 68-year-old male with history of ethanol abuse. What is the diagnosis?

(a) Chronic pancreatitis
(b) Adenocarcinoma, well differentiated
(c) Reactive pancreatic duct epithelium
(d) Acinic cell carcinoma
(e) Serous cystadenoma

Fig. 8.19

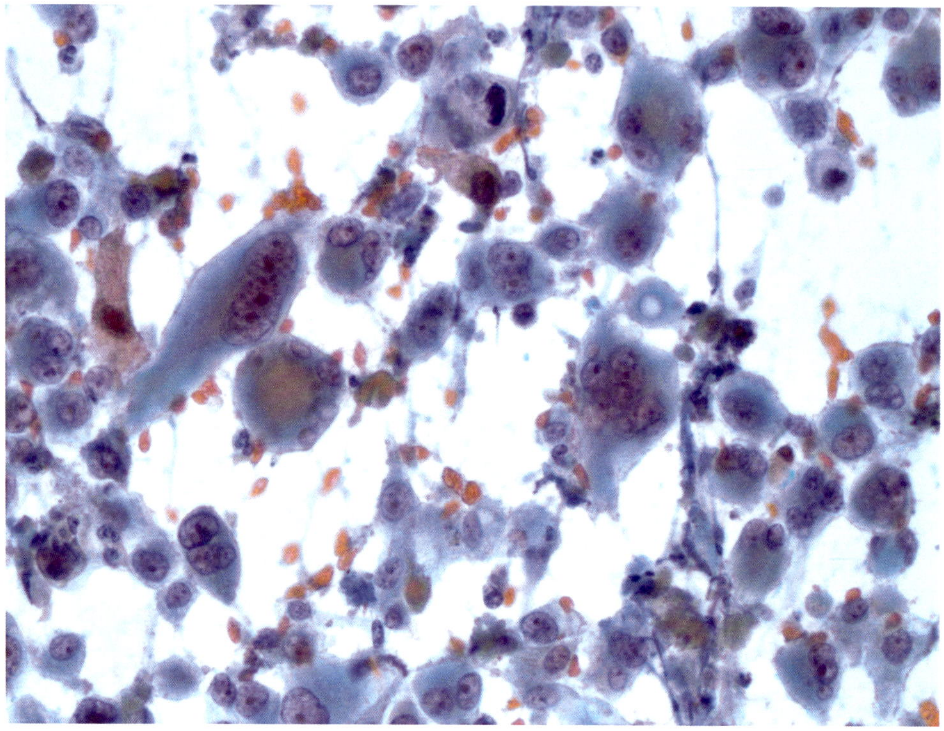

Q-19. EUS-guided FNA of a 4.5-cm mass in body of the pancreas of a 70-year-old female. What is your best diagnosis?
(a) Inflammatory granulomatous reaction
(b) Metastatic giant cell tumor of bone
(c) Undifferentiated adenocarcinoma with giant cells
(d) Pancreatic endocrine tumor
(e) Solid pseudopapillary tumor

Fig. 8.20

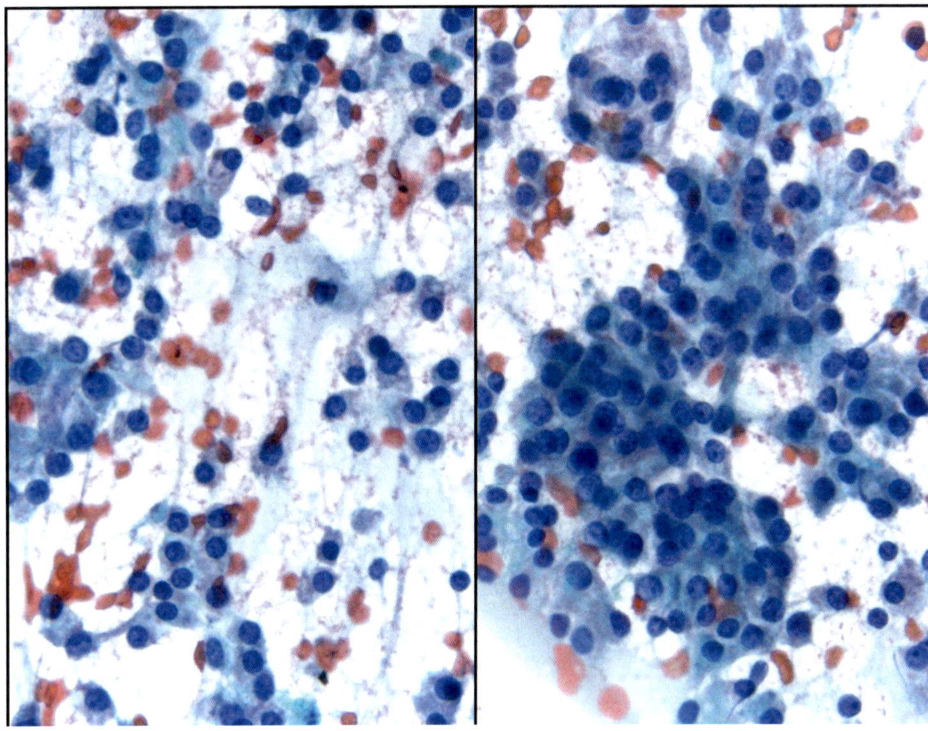

Q-20. A 67-year-old male underwent EUS-guided FNA of a 4-cm partially cystic pancreatic body mass. What is your best diagnosis?

(a) Well-differentiated adenocarcinoma
(b) Pancreatic endocrine tumor
(c) Acinic cell carcinoma
(d) Serous cystadenoma
(e) Pancreaticoblastoma

Fig. 8.21

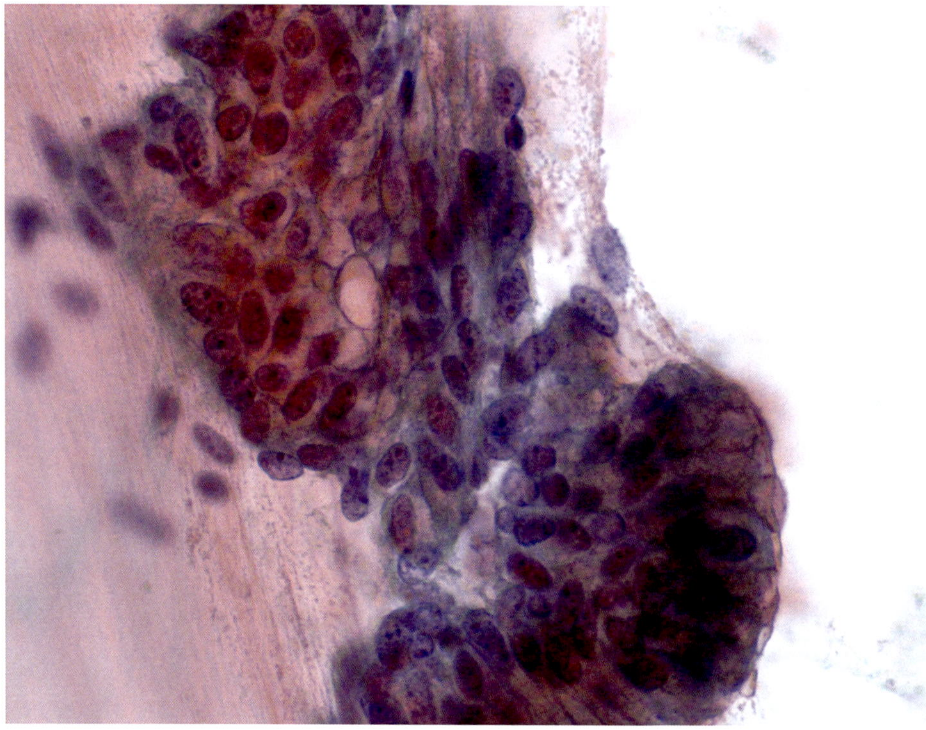

Q-21. A 62-year-old woman was found to have a 4-cm cystic lesion in the body of the pancreas. The lesion was detected during CT scan of the abdomen and pelvis to evaluate an ovarian mass. She underwent EUS-guided FNA of the cyst. What is your best diagnosis?

(a) Unsatisfactory for evaluation
(b) Mucinous cystic neoplasm adenoma
(c) Pseudocyst
(d) Contaminant gastric mucin
(e) Borderline mucinous lesion

Fig. 8.22

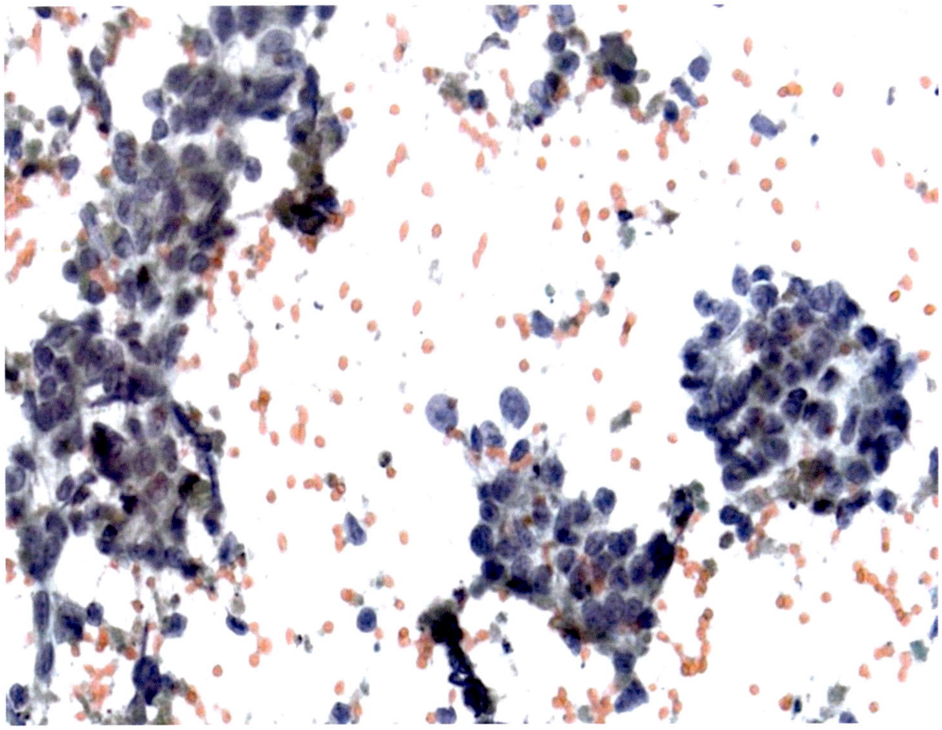

Q-22. A 74-year-old male was found to have a mass in the head of the pancreas. Patient had history of prostatic adenocarcinoma (Gleason 8) a year ago. Patient underwent EUS-guided FNA of the pancreatic lesion. Which of the following antibodies will be most helpful?

(a) CK 19
(b) B catenin
(c) A1 antitrypsin
(d) TTF1
(e) PSA

Fig. 8.23

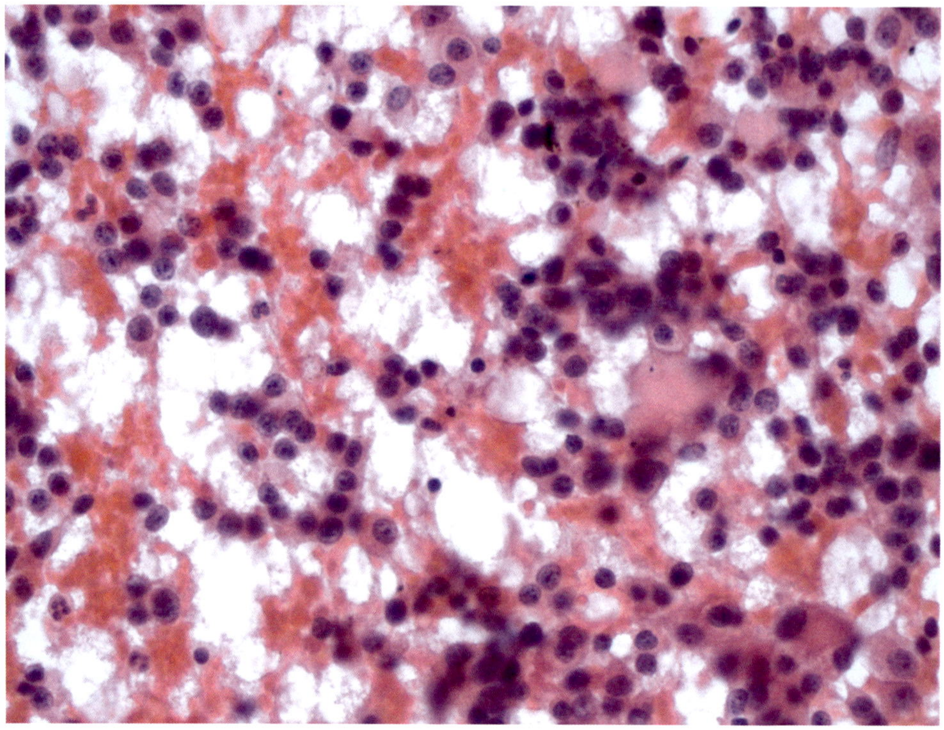

Q-23. Pancreatic mass aspirate from a 57-year-old female. Which of the following immunostains is helpful?
(a) B catenin
(b) CK-19
(c) Synaptophysin
(d) Trypsin
(e) Vimentin

Fig. 8.24

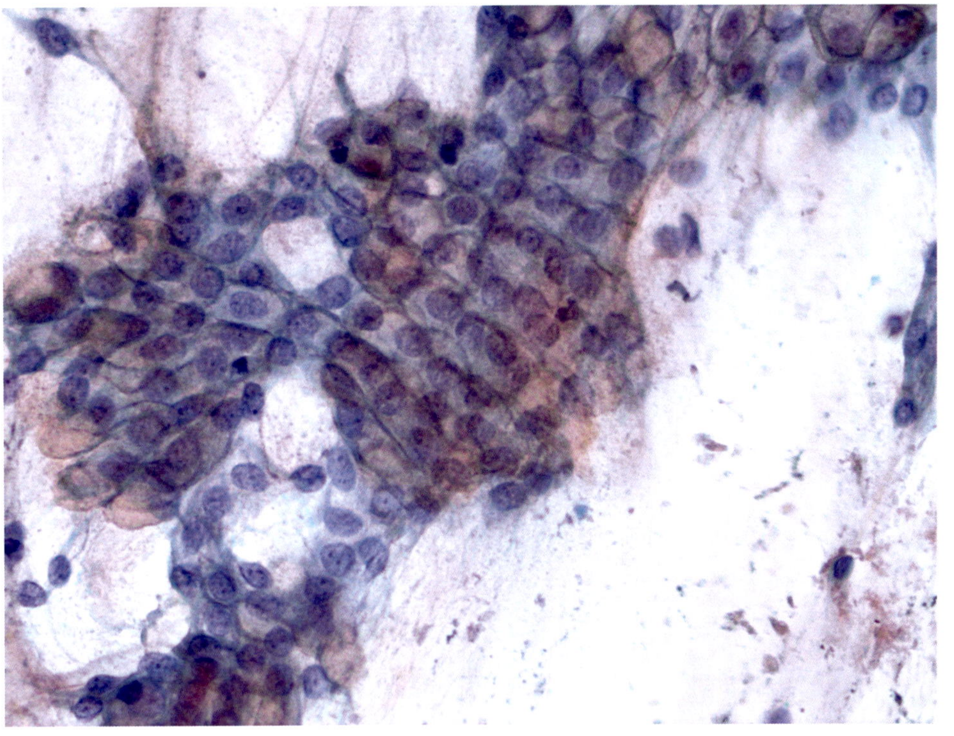

Q-24. This is an aspirate from a 79-year-old female who has a 3-cm mass in the body of the pancreas. What is your best diagnosis?
(a) Unsatisfactory, gastric contaminant
(b) Mucinous neoplasm-adenoma
(c) Solid pseudopapillary tumor
(d) Pancreatic endocrine neoplasm
(e) Lymphoma, low grade

Fig. 8.25

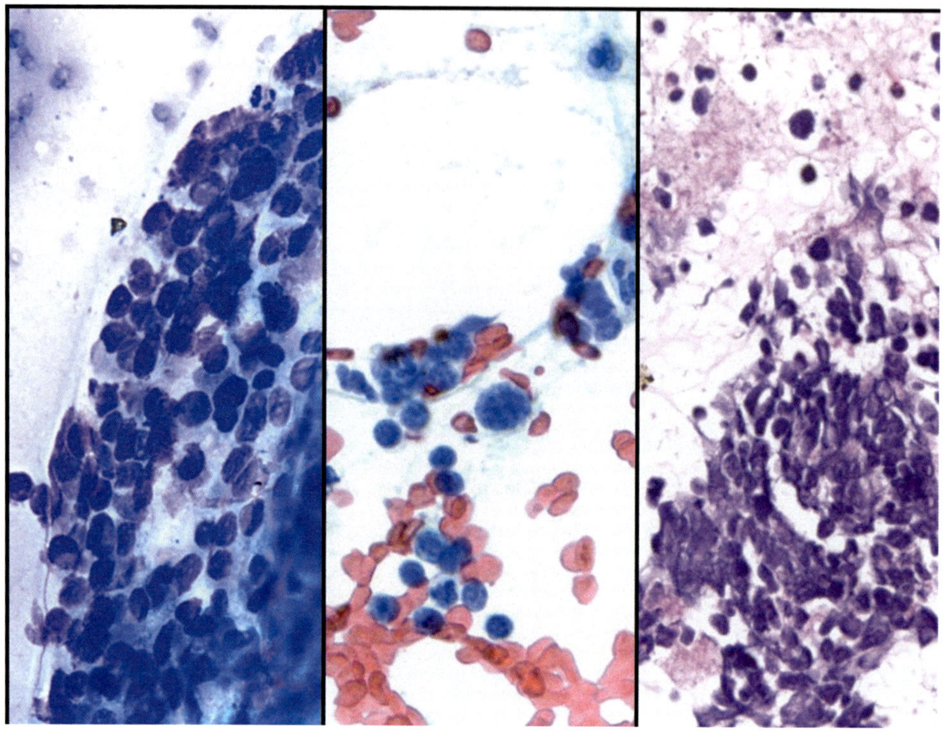

Q-25. A 78-year-old male who had lung carcinoma 6 months ago. A pancreatic mass was detected during a follow-up CT scan. What is your best diagnosis?

(a) Metastatic small cell carcinoma
(b) Pancreatic endocrine tumor
(c) Lymphoma small cell
(d) Adenocarcinoma, poorly differentiated
(e) Acinic cell carcinoma

Fig. 8.26

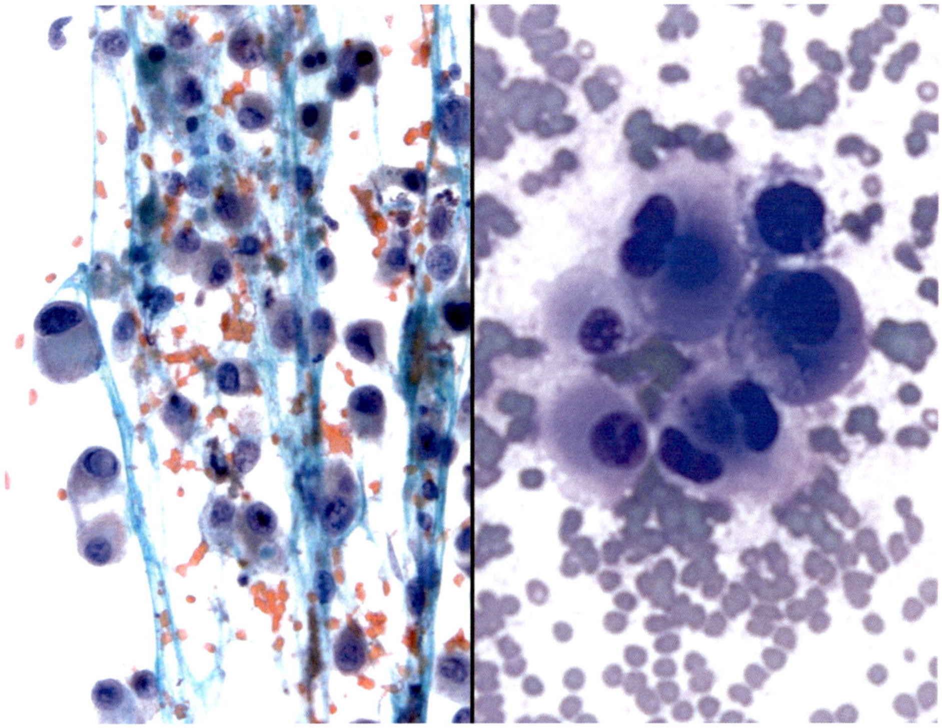

Q-26. Pancreatic aspirate from a 75-year-old male. Patient had history of excision of a malignant skin lesion 9 years ago. Which of the following immunostains is helpful?

(a) CK7, CK20
(b) B catenin, CD10
(c) Synaptophysin
(d) S100, HMB 45
(e) Trypsin, chymotrypsin

Fig. 8.27

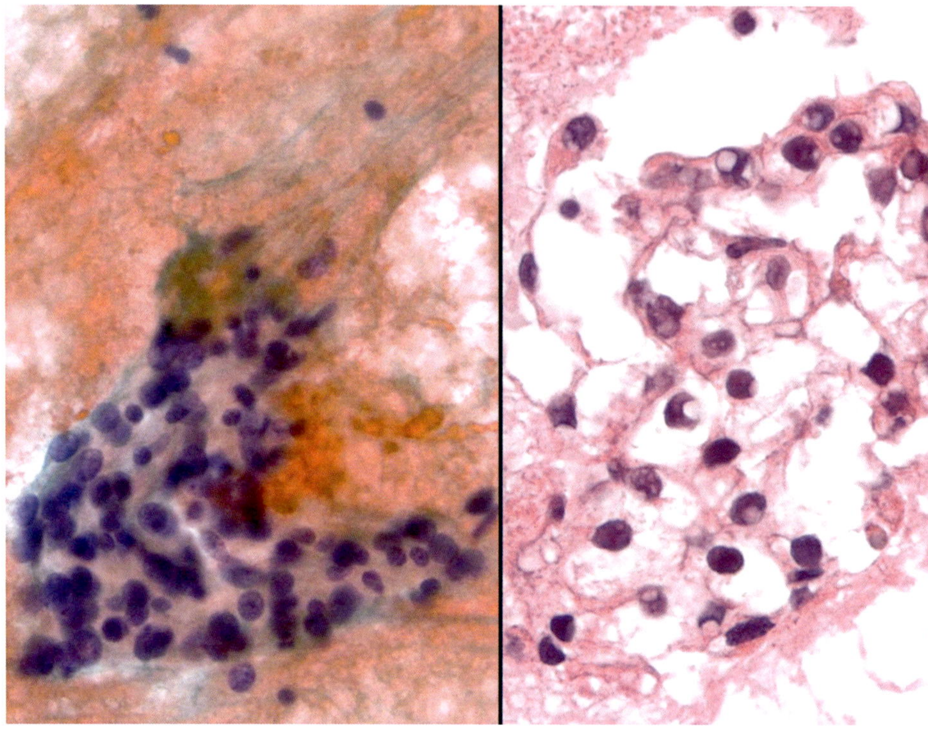

Q-27. A pancreatic aspirate from a 77-year-old male. Patient had history of left nephrectomy for carcinoma. What is the most likely diagnosis?
(a) Clear cell pancreatic carcinoma
(b) Acinic cell carcinoma
(c) Pancreatic endocrine tumor
(d) Mucinous neoplasm
(e) Metastatic renal cell carcinoma

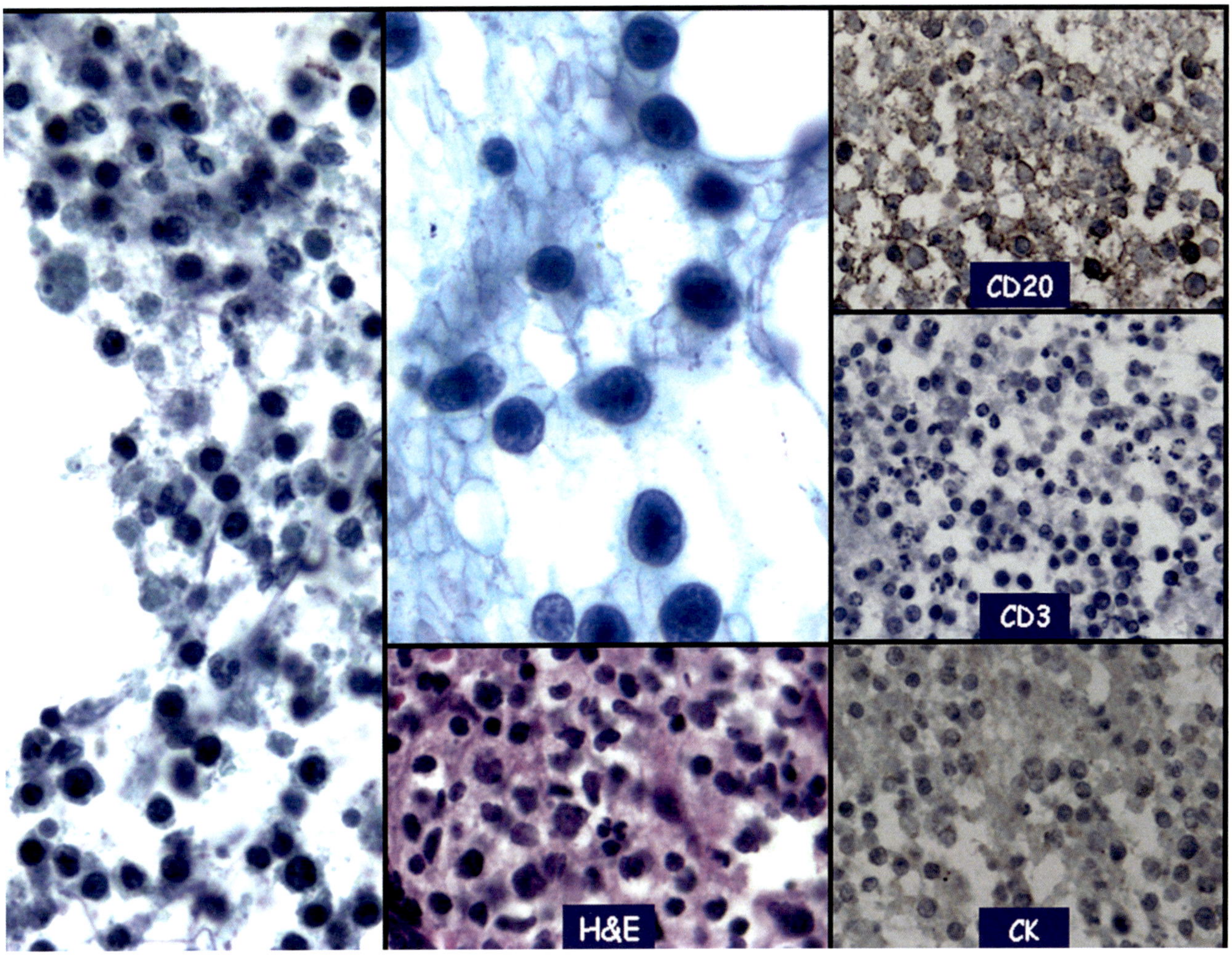

Fig. 8.28

Q-28. An HIV Positive 43-year-old male presented to his family physician with lymphadenopathy and neck and pancreatic masses. What is your diagnosis?
(a) Lymphoma
(b) Pancreatic endocrine neoplasm
(c) Acinic cell carcinoma
(d) Chronic pancreatitis
(e) Adenocarcinoma

Fig. 8.29

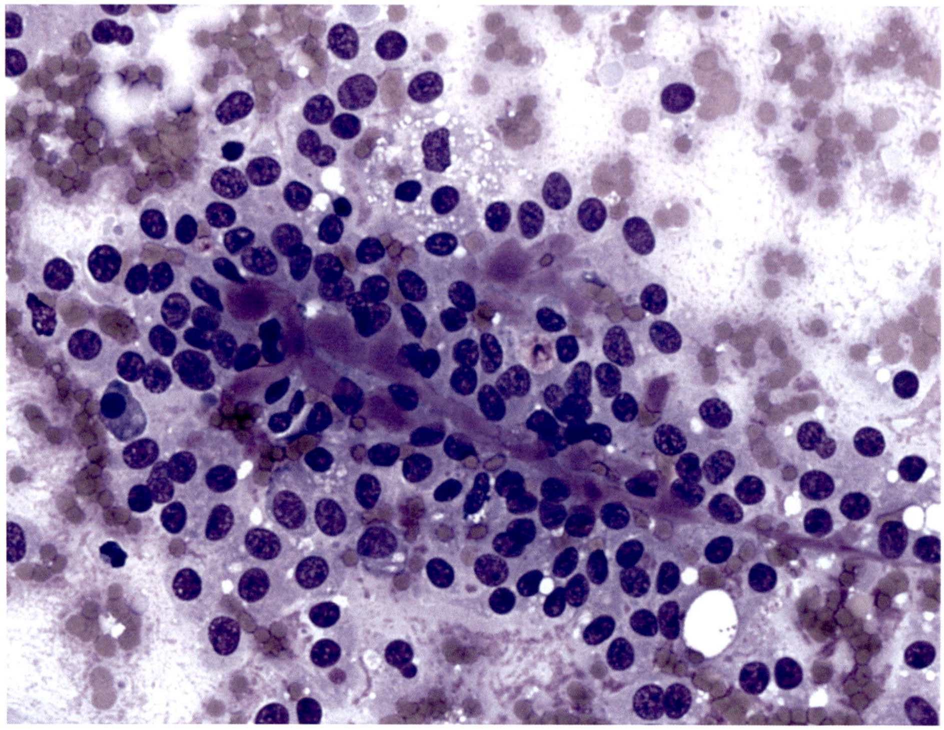

Q-29. EUS-guided aspiration of a pancreatic mass from a 37-year-old female. What is the best diagnosis?

(a) Pancreatic endocrine tumor
(b) Acinic cell carcinoma
(c) Adenocarcinoma well differentiated
(d) Solid pseudopapillary tumor
(e) Pancreaticoblastoma

Fig. 8.30

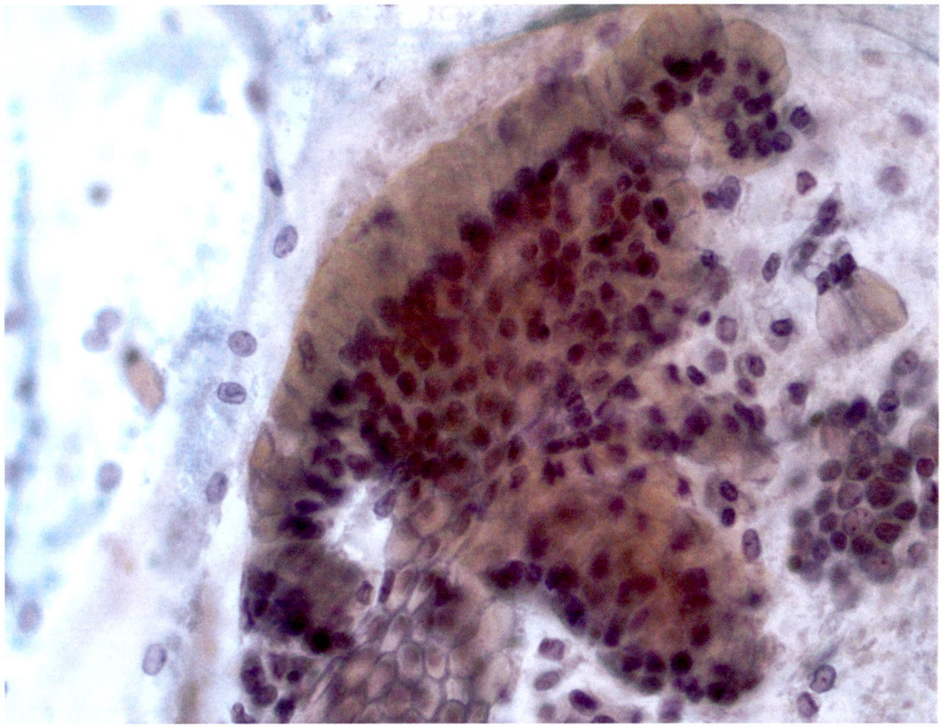

Q-30. Aspirate from a solid pancreatic body lesion from a 57-year-old female. What is your best diagnosis?
(a) Pseudocyst
(b) Serous cystadenoma
(c) Mucinous noncystic neoplasm-adenoma
(d) Cystic endocrine tumor
(e) Cystic acinic cell carcinoma

Fig. 8.31

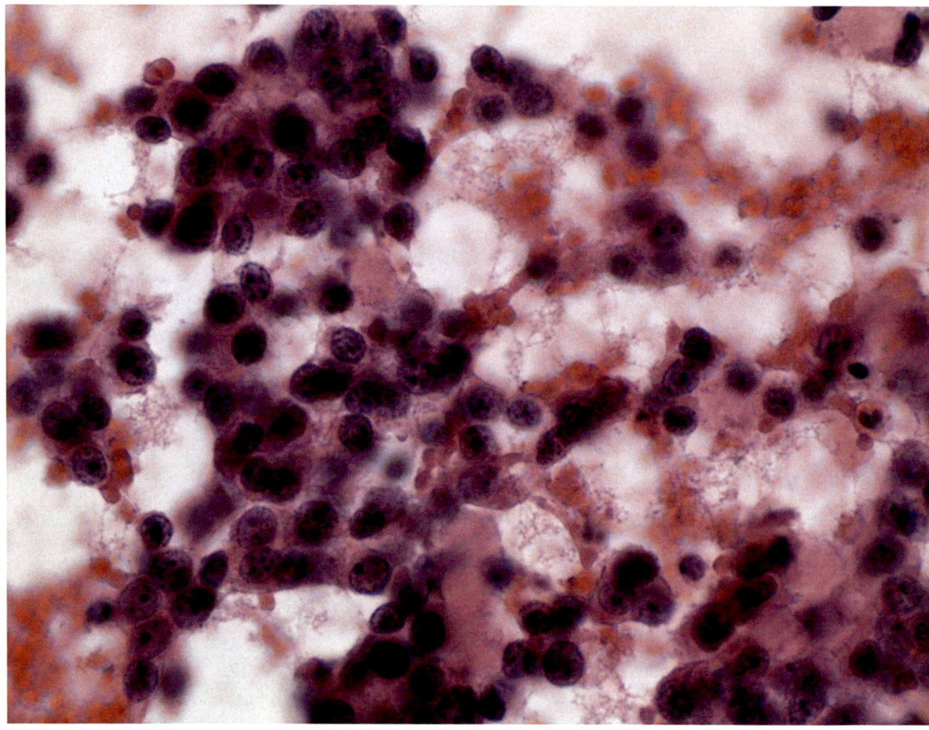

Q-31. Aspirate from a pancreatic tail mass from a 68-year-old female. What is the most likely diagnosis?
(a) Pancreatic adenocarcinoma
(b) Pancreatic endocrine neoplasm
(c) Lymphoma
(d) Acinic cell carcinoma
(e) Small cell carcinoma

Fig. 8.32

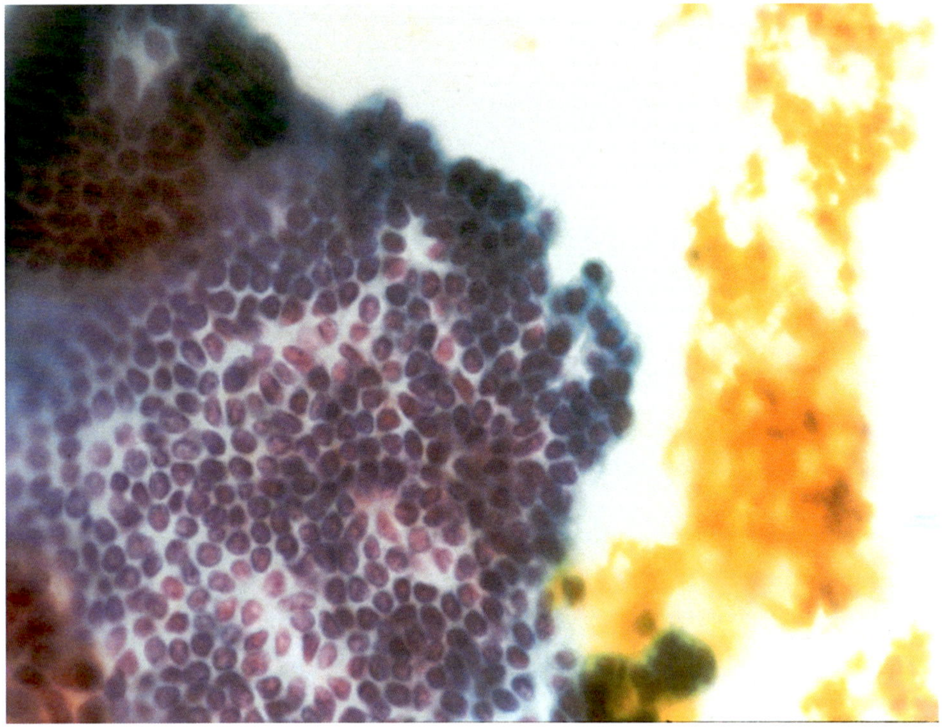

Q-32. Biliary brushing from a 67-year-old male who was found to have a stricture. The best diagnosis is:
(a) Well-differentiated adenocarcinoma
(b) Atypia of biliary epithelium
(c) Benign biliary epithelium
(d) Moderately differentiated adenocarcinoma
(e) Suspicious for adenocarcinoma

Fig. 8.33

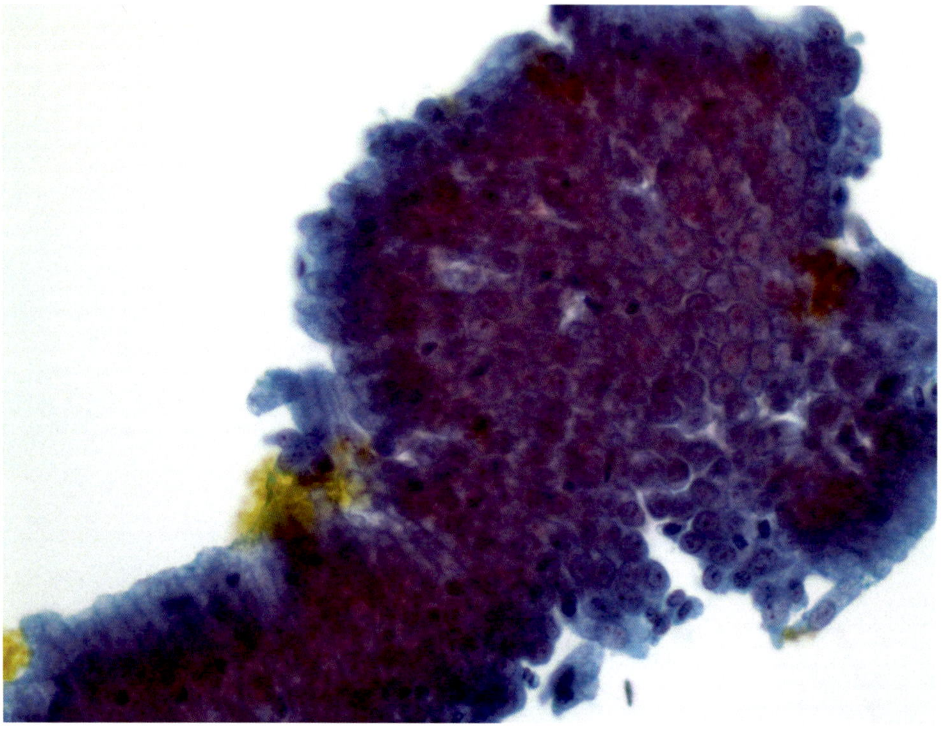

Q-33. Biliary brushing from a 55-year-old male with history of ulcerative colitis. A stent was placed a month ago. What is the best interpretation?
(a) Well-differentiated adenocarcinoma
(b) Atypia of biliary epithelium
(c) Benign biliary epithelium
(d) Moderately differentiated adenocarcinoma
(e) Suspicious for adenocarcinoma

Fig. 8.34

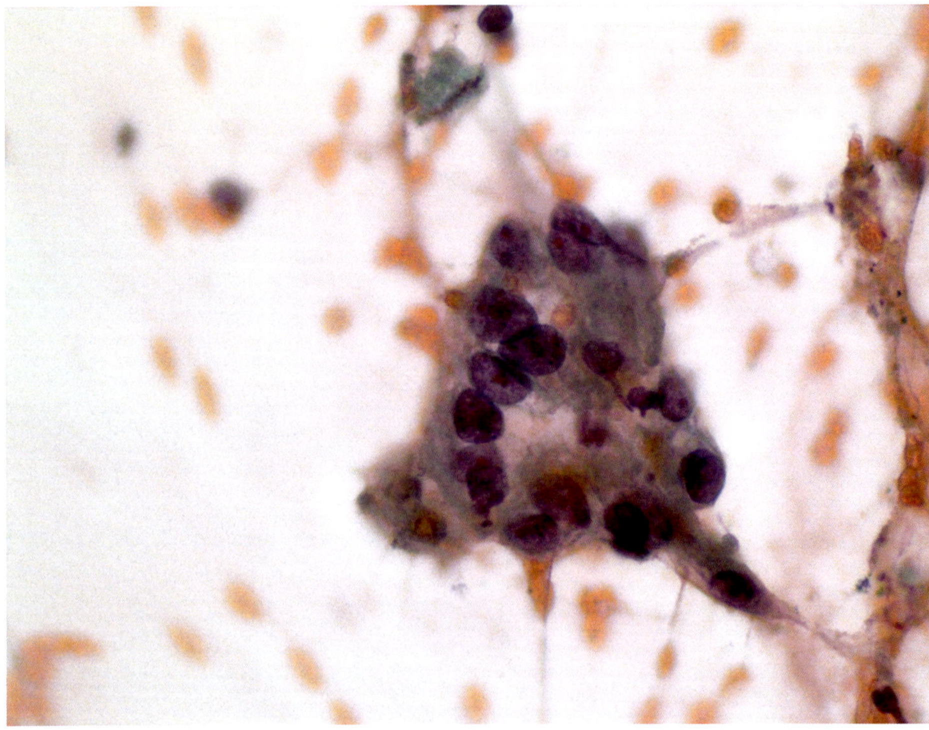

Q-34. Biliary brushing from a 59-year-old male with a stricture. What is the best interpretation?
(a) Well-differentiated adenocarcinoma
(b) Atypia of biliary epithelium
(c) Benign biliary epithelium
(d) Moderately differentiated adenocarcinoma
(e) Suspicious for adenocarcinoma

Fig. 8.35

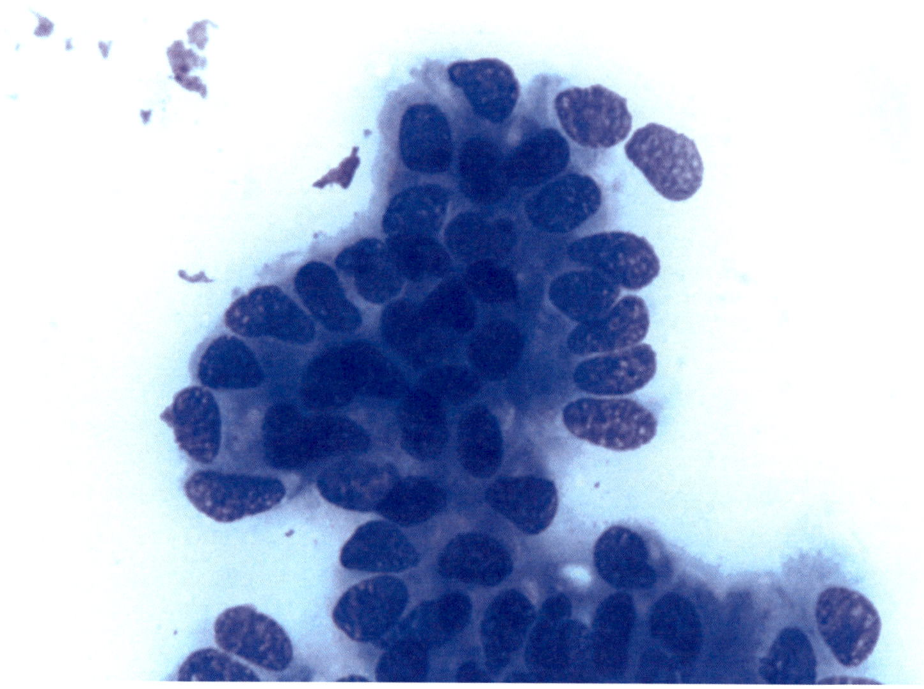

Q-35. Biliary brushing from a 67-year-old male with long history of ulcerative colitis. What is the best interpretation?

(a) Well-differentiated adenocarcinoma
(b) Atypia of biliary epithelium
(c) Benign biliary epithelium
(d) Moderately differentiated adenocarcinoma
(e) Suspicious for adenocarcinoma

Fig. 8.36

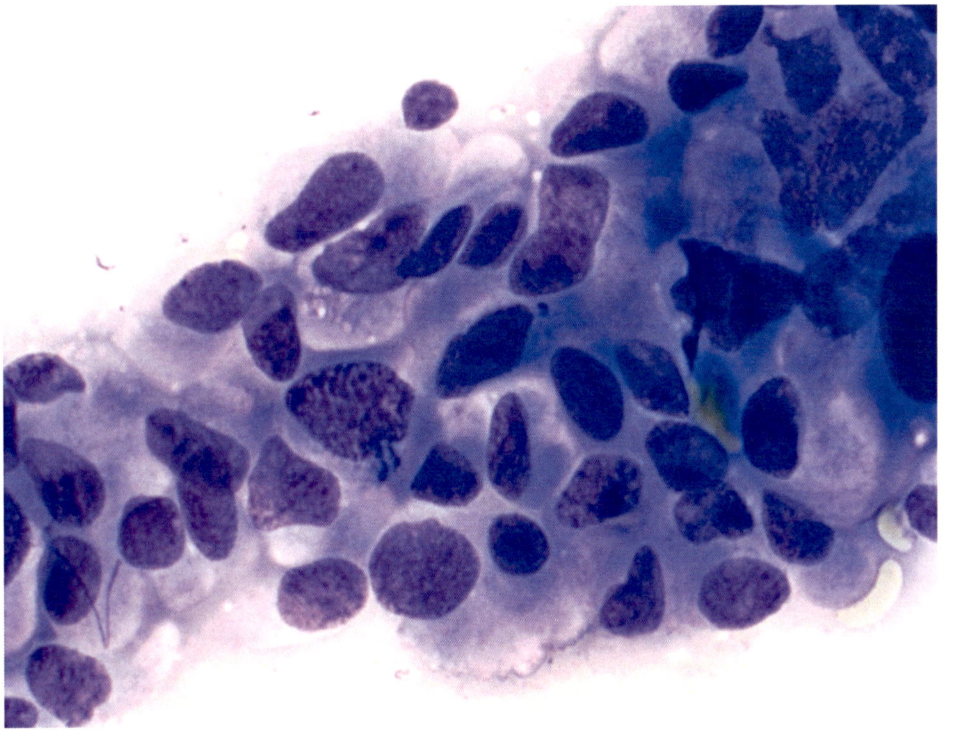

Q-36. A 65-year-old female underwent biliary brushing and a stent insertion because of a obstructive mass and jaundice. What is the best interpretation?
(a) Well-differentiated adenocarcinoma
(b) Atypia of biliary epithelium
(c) Benign biliary epithelium
(d) Poorly differentiated adenocarcinoma
(e) Suspicious for adenocarcinoma

Fig. 8.37

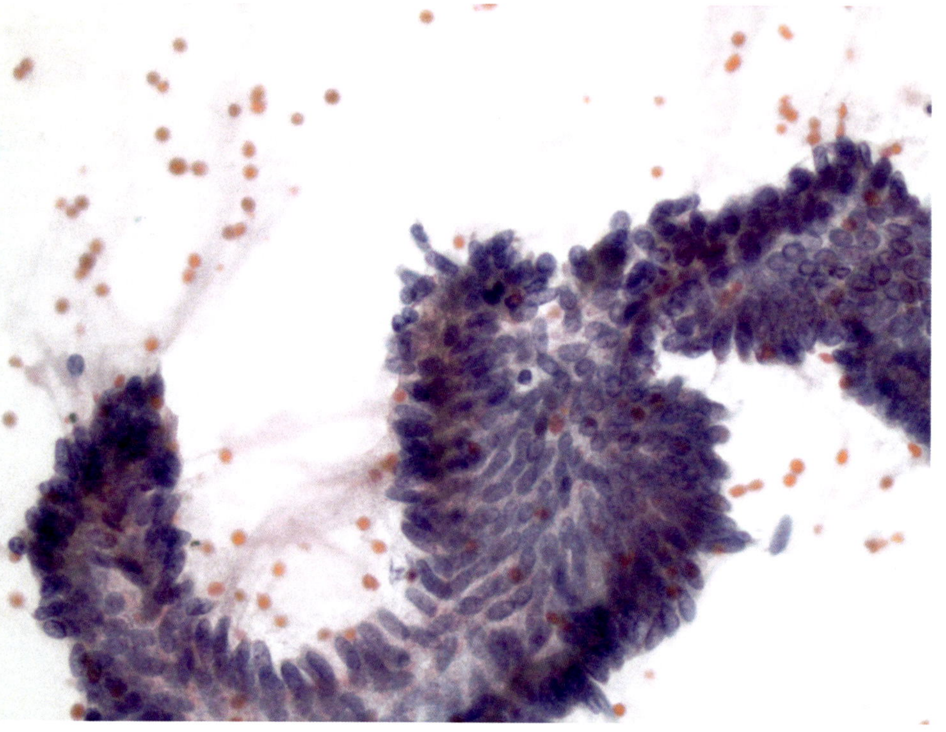

Q-37. Biliary brushing from a 59-year-old female because of a mass lesion. What is the best interpretation?

(a) Well-differentiated adenocarcinoma
(b) Atypia of biliary epithelium
(c) Benign biliary epithelium
(d) Moderately differentiated adenocarcinoma
(e) Suspicious for adenocarcinoma

Fig. 8.38

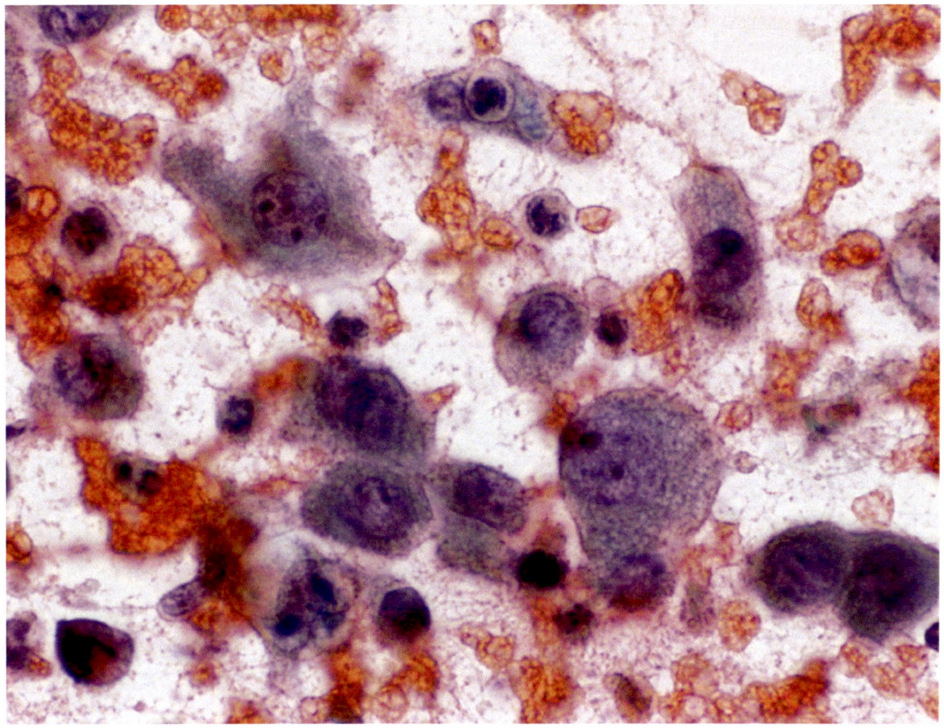

Q-38. EUS-guided FNA of a pancreatic mass from a 65-year-old female. Tumor cells are reactive to hepar-1 and CK 19. What is the best diagnosis?
(a) Normal hepatocytes
(b) Hepatocellular carcinoma, metastatic
(c) Pancreatic adenocarcinoma, hepatoid type
(d) Giant cell carcinoma
(e) Metastatic melanoma

Fig. 8.39

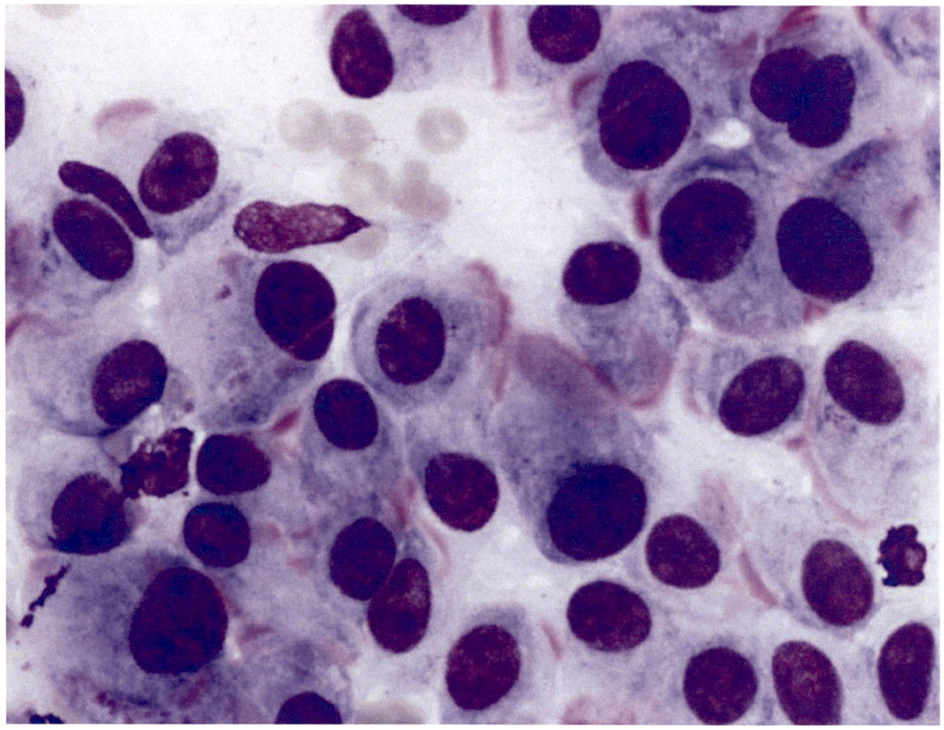

Q-39. A 57-year-old female was found to have a mass in the body of the pancreas on CT scan as part of work up for persistent back pain. Which of the following antibodies is likely to be reactive?

(a) Trypsin
(b) TTF1
(c) Synaptophysin
(d) CD 45
(e) Vimentin

Fig. 8.40

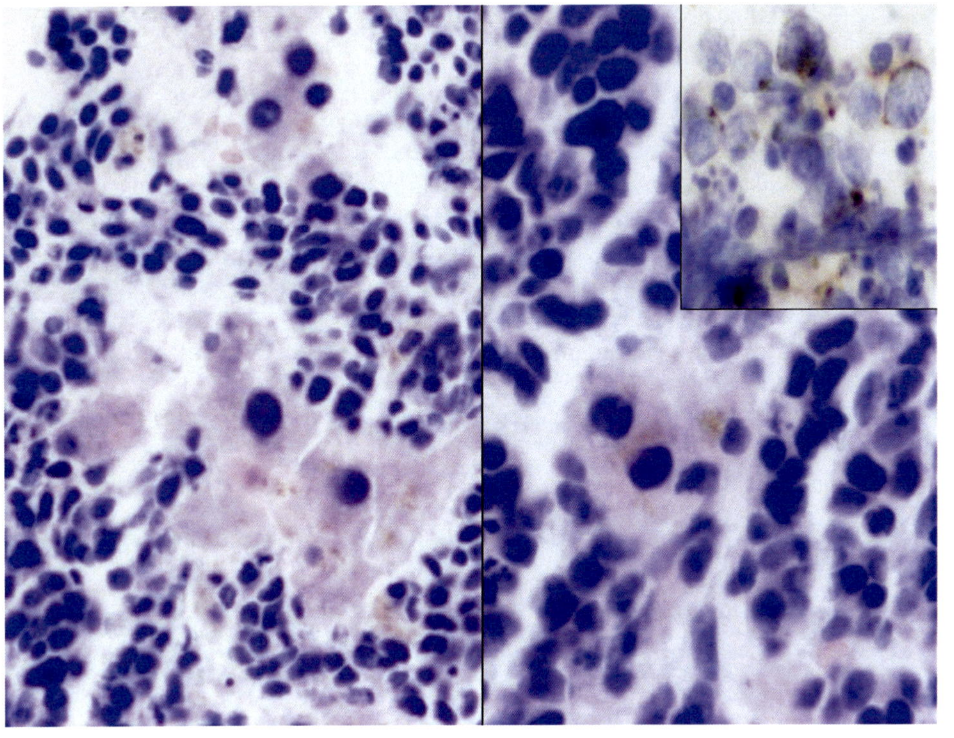

Q-40. EUS-guided FNA of a 3.5 cm pancreatic mass in the head region of a 78-year-old male. Patient is jaundiced and lost 20 lbs. Patient had history of lung cancer few months earlier. What is the best diagnosis?

(a) Pancreatic duct adenocarcinoma
(b) Pancreatic endocrine tumor
(c) Lymphoma
(d) Small cell carcinoma
(e) Acinic cell carcinoma

8.2 Text-Based Questions 41–68

Q-41. A 63-year-old male with jaundice underwent US-guided FNA of a 2 cm solid mass in the head of the pancreas. The aspirate revealed cells arranged in flat sheets with loss of polarity and single cells. Many cells have slightly enlarged nuclei and clear cytoplasm. No acinar arrangement is noted. The best diagnosis is:
(a) Well-differentiated adenocarcinoma
(b) Duodenal contaminant
(c) Reactive duct epithelium
(d) Pancreatic endocrine tumor
(e) Mucinous intraductal neoplasm

Q-42. An US-guided FNA of a pancreatic mass in a 43-year-old man revealed abundant single cells with eccentric nuclei. The cells are monotonous, small, and with no significant anisocytosis. The best diagnosis is:
(a) Acinic cell tumor
(b) Adenocarcinoma
(c) Pancreatic endocrine tumor
(d) Solid pseudopapillary tumor
(e) Lymphoma

Q-43. Contaminants commonly encountered in endoscopic FNA of pancreatic tail lesions are frequently from:
(a) Spleen
(b) Colon
(c) Duodenum
(d) Stomach
(e) Esophagus

Q-44. What is the most common solid malignant neoplasm of the pancreas in a 55-year-old female?
(a) Duct adenocarcinoma
(b) Acinic cell carcinoma
(c) Pancreatic endocrine neoplasm
(d) Solid pseudopapillary tumor
(e) Pancreaticoblastoma

Q-45. The most common cyst of the pancreas is:
(a) Pancreatic mucinous cystic neoplasm
(b) Intraductal papillary mucinous neoplasm
(c) Lymphoepithelial cyst
(d) Cystic acinic tumor
(e) Pancreatic pseudocyst

Q-46. Acinic cell carcinoma can be distinguished cytologically from normal pancreas by:
(a) Cell arrangement
(b) Cell size
(c) Granularity of the cytoplasm
(d) The presence of prominent nucleoli
(e) The presence of a mucin vacuole

Q-47. Which of the following is the most useful histologic feature in distinguishing intraductal papillary mucinous neoplasm from mucinous neoplasm?
(a) Papillary cyst lining
(b) Presence of oncocytic metaplasia
(c) Ovarian stroma
(d) Grade of dysplasia
(e) Gastric foveolar lining epithelium

Q-48. Which of the following cysts is likely if amylase is elevated?
(a) Mucinous cystic neoplasm
(b) Serous cystadenoma
(c) Lymphoepithelial cyst
(d) Cystic acinic cell carcinoma
(e) Intraductal papillary mucinous cyst

Q-49. Which of the following is most challenging in diagnosing pancreatic lesions by EUS-guided FNA?
(a) Cell debris
(b) Mucin
(c) Clinical correlation
(d) G.I. contaminants
(e) Identifying neoplastic cells

Q-50. A 27-year-old female has an incidentally discovered 3.5 cm complex pancreatic mass. EUS-guided FNA revealed small monotonous cells which were negative for synaptophysin and trypsin but positive for B catenin and CD10. What is the most likely diagnosis?
(a) Pancreatic endocrine tumor
(b) Lymphoepithelial cyst
(c) Acinic cell carcinoma
(d) Solid pseudopapillary tumor
(e) Mucinous cyst

Q-51. Which of the following is not a risk factor for pancreatic duct carcinoma?
(a) Age
(b) Smoking
(c) Familial
(d) Peutz–Jeghers Syndrome
(e) Drinking coffee

Q-52. Which of the following is the most commonly utilized method in sampling pancreatic lesions?
(a) US-guided transabdominal FNA
(b) CT-guided transabdominal FNA
(c) Biliary brushing

(d) Endoscopic US-guided FNA
(e) ERCP and pancreatic duct sampling

Q-53. Which one of the following pancreatic tumors is the most common?
(a) Acinic cell carcinoma
(b) Pancreatic endocrine tumor
(c) Mucinous cystadenoma
(d) Intraductal papillary mucinous
(e) Duct adenocarcinoma

Q-54. Which of the following neoplasms is most common in children?
(a) Solid pseudopapillary tumor
(b) Acinic cell carcinoma
(c) Serous cyst adenoma
(d) Pancreatic endocrine tumor
(e) Pancreaticoblastoma

Q-55. An aspirate from a mass in the head of the pancreas in an 82-year-old male yielded a mixed population of adenocarcinoma and squamous cell carcinoma. What is the most likely diagnosis?
(a) Pancreaticoblastoma
(b) Metastatic carcinoma
(c) Primary adenosquamous carcinoma
(d) Adenocarcinoma and metastatic squamous carcinoma
(e) Adenocarcinoma and squamous metaplasia

Q-56. The differential diagnosis of pancreaticoblastoma includes which of the following?
(a) Solid pseudopapillary tumor
(b) Acinic cell carcinoma
(c) Serous cyst adenoma
(d) Pancreatic endocrine tumor
(e) Pancreatic adenocarcinoma

Q-57. A 60-year-old woman was found to have a cystic lesion in the pancreas. An FNA yielded scant clusters of monotonous cuboidal cells with central rounded nuclei and vacuolated cytoplasm. The background is clean. These cells are mostly reactive with CK 19. All of the following statements about this lesion are correct *except*:
(a) Malignant transformation is rare
(b) May be associated with VHL-gene abnormalities
(c) The cytoplasm is positive for PAS stain
(d) The cyst contents show high CEA levels
(e) Commonly multicystic

Q-58. A 50-year-old man who had an episode of acute pancreatitis few months ago was found to have an 18-cm unilocular peripancreatic cystic lesion on CT scan. All of the following about this lesion are correct *except*:
(a) It is the most common cyst of the pancreas
(b) It has focal mucinous lining
(c) It occurs in the postnecrotic resorption of fat
(d) The contents yield high amylase
(e) The aspirate contains degenerated and inflammatory cells

Q-59. Which of the following is not characteristic of acinic cell carcinoma?
(a) Abundant stripped naked nuclei
(b) Granular cytoplasm
(c) Immunoreactive to trypsin
(d) CAM 5.2 is nonreactive
(e) Tumor cells form small acinar structure

Q-60. Which set of immunohistochemical stains is useful in differentiating pancreatic endocrine tumor (PEN) from acinic cell carcinoma (ACC).
(a) Cam 5.2 and CK7
(b) Amylase and CEA
(c) PAS-D
(d) Synaptophysin and trypsin
(e) B-catenin and AE1/AE3

Q-61. Which of the following is not typical of solid pseudopapillary tumor of the pancreas?
(a) Cystic changes
(b) Keratin and synaptophysin reactivity
(c) Hyaline globules
(d) Vimentin and B-Catenin expression
(e) Zone of foamy macrophages

Q-62. Tumor cells derived from pancreatic duct adenocarcinoma are likely to be diffusely positive for which one of the following markers?
(a) Chromogranin
(b) Cytokeratin 7
(c) Trypsin
(d) Cytokeratin 20
(e) Beta-Catenin

In question 63–68 match the following entities on the left with the most appropriate related response on the right. Each response on the right may be used once, more than once, or not at all.

Q-63. Pancreaticoblastoma	(a) Von Hippel–Lindau Syndrome
Q-64. Pancreatic pseudocysts	(b) Peutz–Jeghers Syndrome
Q-65. Serous cystadenomas	(c) Beckwith–Wiedmann Syndrome
Q-66. Solid pseudopapillary tumors	(d) Most common non-neoplastic cyst
Q-67. Mucinous cystadenomas	(e) Ovarian stroma
Q-68. Pancreatic duct adenocarcinomas	(f) Female to male ratio 9:1

8.3 Answers and Discussion of Image-Based Questions 1–40

A-1. (**a**) **Moderately differentiated adenocarcinoma**.
The image displays a flat sheet with cells showing anisocytosis; notice the variation in nuclear size. The chromatin is coarse and the n/c ratio is high. Ductal carcinoma of the pancreas frequently involves the head of the pancreas (80–90 %). It is the most common tumor of the pancreas comprising approximately 90 % of all pancreatic tumors. It is more common in men than in women (male to female ratio, 1.30–1.0). Generally aspirates are cellular. Cells are arranged in three-dimensional groups and single cells or small clusters. The tumor cells have enlarged nuclei with nuclear size up to four times the nuclear size of acinar cells. Cells within the groups are overlapping with irregular nuclear contour. Mitotic activity is significant. Clusters with cribriform pattern are also seen. In the background there are cell necrosis, mucin, and ghost tumor cells.

A-2. (**b**) **Mucinous cystic neoplasm** (**MCN**) displays bland epithelium, honeycomb pattern and shows diffuse cytoplasmic mucin with columnar nuclei. MCN contribute about 5 % of pancreatic neoplasm. They are most common in women with a mean age of 50 years. They are commonly located in the body and tail of pancreas. Cysts are lined by mucinous epithelium and usually do not communicate with the pancreatic duct. Specialized stroma of the ovarian type is located beneath the epithelium which defines this neoplasm. This stroma expresses receptors for estrogen and progesterone. Histologically, MCN may have a spectrum of dysplastic changes that varies from benign to frankly invasive carcinoma. The lining of a single cyst could display the entire spectrum.

A-3. (**c**) **Mucinous noncystic adenocarcinoma**.
Tumor cells are arranged in a three-dimensional pattern with individual cells have vacuolated cytoplasm with occasional signet ring cells.

A-4. (**c**) **Mucinous adenocarcinoma with signet ring cells**.
This tumor is recognized by the prominence of signet ring cells and the cytoplasmic vacuoles. The cytoplasmic vacuoles compress the nuclei and push them to the periphery of the cell.

A-5. (**e**) **Normal pancreatic tissue**.
The cells display the normal cellular architecture of the pancreas; cells are monotonous and form cohesive grape-like structures. Occasional stripped nuclei are noted. The nuclear size is within normal limits with no variation. A small group of benign duct epithelium is noted adjacent to the cell groups.

A-6. (**e**) **Gastric contaminant**.
Cells are noted in flat sheet, evenly spaced with monotonous nuclei and no evidence of atypia or nuclear overlapping.

A-7. (**b**) **Granular adenocarcinoma** is a rare variant of duct adenocarcinoma that is characterized by neoplastic cells with granular cytoplasm and enlarged nuclei with prominent nucleoli and fine chromatin.

A-8. (**c**) **Adenosquamous carcinoma** is characterized by a mixture of glandular and a squamous component. The squamous component shows infiltrating sheets of polygonal cells with varying degrees of cytoplasmic keratinization in addition to the usual cells of adenocarcinoma.

A-9. (**c**) **Moderately differentiated adenocarcinoma**.
The cells are slightly crowded with enlarged nuclei. The nuclei show marked variation in size. The chromatin is fine and varies from hyperchromatic to hypochromasia. Large prominent nuclei are noticed.

A-10. (**e**) **Duodenal contaminant**.
The duodenal epithelium is characterized by its sheet-like arrangement with many goblet cells seeded with the epithelium. The luminal edge displays a brush border which is another characteristic feature. The nuclei are small, uniform, and evenly spaced.

A-11. (**a**) **Moderately differentiated adenocarcinoma**.
This is another example of pancreatic adenocarcinoma which displays a crowded group of neoplastic cells with remarkable nuclear size variation. Within the same group some nuclei are four times bigger than other nuclei (an important feature in pancreatic adenocarcinoma). In addition, high N/C ratio, fine chromatin, and prominent nucleoli are evident.

A-12. (**e**) **Mucinous adenocarcinoma**.
A crowded group of large polyhedral cells are characterized by abundant cytoplasm rich in mucin with nuclei showing variable sizes. Mucin is also noted in the background.

A-13. (**d**) **Pancreatic duct epithelium**.
There is a flat sheet of cells with small rounded, evenly spaced uniform nuclei. This is the typical honey comb pattern of benign pancreatic duct epithelium.

A-14. (b) **Poorly differentiated adenocarcinoma**.
There is a crowded three-dimensional group of cells that display nuclear density and pleomorphism. The nuclei are hyperchromatic with irregular nuclear membrane and occasional prominent nucleoli. A rare single cell and necrosis is noted in background.

A-15. (a) **Moderately differentiated adenocarcinoma**.
This group of neoplastic cells displays the remarkable variation in nuclear size with some cells being four times as big compared to other cells in the same group. In addition, there are nuclear membrane irregularities. The fine chromatin and the prominent nucleoli are other features.

A-16. (c) **CEA is elevated in cyst contents**.
The history and the image support the diagnosis of a pseudocyst of the pancreas. The photograph displays acute inflammatory cells and cellular debris in the background, a feature characteristic of this type of cyst. Pancreatic pseudocyst is the most common non-neoplastic cyst of the pancreas. By definition this type of cyst lacks epithelial lining and it is not known to have malignant potential.

A-17. (e) **Mucinous cystadenocarcinoma**.
There is a crowded three-dimensional group containing cells with hyperchromasia, irregular nuclear contour, and nucleoli. The background shows abundant mucin.

A-18. (b) **Well-differentiated adenocarcinoma**.
This well-differentiated adenocarcinoma is characterized by subtlety crowded neoplastic nuclei with chromatin clearing and peripheral clumping. Notice the nuclear crowding and the enhanced cell walls.

A-19. (c) **Undifferentiated adenocarcinoma with giant cells**.
This tumor is characterized by the formation of large, bizarre, anaplastic and pleomorphic mononuclear and multinucleated giant tumor cells.

A-20. (c) **Acinic cell carcinoma**.
This tumor is characterized by small glandular structures and single cells. Many stripped nuclei in the background. Cells are bland with almost uniform nuclei that have coarse chromatin. Granular material is present in the background.

A-21. (b) **Mucinous cystic neoplasm**.
There is colloid like mucin in the background. The cell group noted has a uniform honeycomb pattern. The cells in the group are columnar with abundant intracellular mucin. Cells are uniform and have no atypical features.

A-22. (a) **The aspirate reveals neoplastic cells in small glandular formation**.
Individual tumor cells have high n/c ratio and prominent nuclei. There is striking resemblance between tumor cells and prostatic adenocarcinoma; PSA would be the most likely stain to use to rule out metastatic prostatic adenocarcinoma.

A-23. (c) **Synaptophysin**.
The aspirate is composed of dyshesive and single cell arrangement. Cells are uniform with monotonous nuclei which have an eccentric position. The chromatin is coarse (salt and pepper) with prominent nucleoli. Cytoplasm is eosinophilic and granular (oncocytic).

A-24. (b) **Mucinous neoplasm**.
There is abundant mucin in the background. The epithelium is arranged in a honey comb pattern. Individual cells are columnar with abundant cytoplasmic mucin and uniform nuclei.

A-25. (a) **Metastatic small cell carcinoma**.
In view of this patient history of lung carcinoma, the present tumor displays the characteristic features of small cell carcinoma making it the most likely diagnosis.

A-26. (d) **S100 and HMB45**.
The aspirate reveals single malignant cells with large nuclei and prominent nucleoli. In view of patient history of excision of a malignant skin tumor and the morphologic appearance of the aspirate does also resemble melanoma, consideration should be given to rule out melanoma.

A-27. (e) **Metastatic renal cell carcinoma**.
The aspirate shows many large polyhedral cells with clear cytoplasm and central nuclei and prominent nucleoli. In view of the patient history of nephrectomy for carcinoma and the morphology, consideration should be given to renal cell carcinoma as the likely diagnosis.

A-28. (a) **Lymphoma**.
The aspirate displays a monotonous population of single cells with the morphologic appearance of lymphocytes. The staining pattern clearly defined these lymphocytes as B cells.

A-29. (**d**) **Solid pseudo papillary tumor**.
The aspirate is cellular and shows small uniform cells in a cohesive pattern intermixed with single cells. The nuclei of these single cells are finely granular and the nucleoli are inconspicuous. No atypia noted. Hyaline material is noted between the cells.

A-30. (**c**) **Mucinous noncystic neoplasm-adenoma**.
The aspirate shows abundant mucin in the background and a sheet of uniform cells with columnar nuclei. The cytoplasm is rich in mucin. Nuclei don't show atypical features and have a honeycomb pattern.

A-31. (**b**) **Pancreatic endocrine tumor**.
The aspirate yields a single cell population with eccentric monotonous nuclei, endocrine chromatin (salt and pepper), and granular eosinophilic cytoplasm. These features are characteristic of pancreatic endocrine tumor.

A-32. (**c**) **Benign biliary epithelium**.
This cohesive, flat, round, uniform, evenly spaced nuclei with a honey comb pattern. Bile is noted adjacent to the cells. These are the features of benign biliary epithelium.

A-33. (**b**) **Reactive biliary epithelium**.
While the polarity of the cells in a honey comb pattern is essentially maintained, there is slight enlargement of the nuclei with prominence of the nucleoli. Cells display occasional chromatin clumping. Features are characteristic of reactive biliary epithelium.

A-34. (**a**) **Well-differentiated adenocarcinoma**.
The gland forming cells in the aspirate have variable nuclear size, fine chromatin, and prominent nucleoli. The n/c ratio is high. Features are diagnostic of adenocarcinoma.

A-35. (**d**) **Moderately differentiated adenocarcinoma**.
The displayed cells have pleomorphic, hyperchromatic nuclei, and prominent nucleoli. The cell group maintains a community border. Features are consistent with moderately differentiated adenocarcinoma.

A-36. (**d**) **Poorly differentiated adenocarcinoma**.
This three-dimensional group of pleomorphic cells shows remarkable variation in nuclear size, shape, and color. Occasional large prominent nucleoli are noted. The cellular features are diagnostic of poorly differentiated adenocarcinoma.

A-37. (**c**) **Benign biliary epithelium**.
This group of columnar epithelial cells has an intact polarity. The cells are organized and do not display any significant cellular crowding or atypia. These cells are characteristic of benign biliary epithelium.

A-38. (**c**) **Pancreatic adenocarcinoma**, **hepatoid type**.
These bizarre cells are clearly neoplastic. The cells have a granular oncocytic cytoplasm. The staining reactive is very informative. Most of hepatoid neoplasms, regardless of their origin, react with hepar-1but the CK19 in this context is helpful in supporting a diagnosis of adenocarcinoma.

A-39. (**c**) **Synaptophysin**.
The displayed cells show rounded nuclei with endocrine chromatin (salt and pepper) and eccentric nuclei. These features are characteristic of pancreatic endocrine neoplasm.

A-40. (**d**) **Small cell carcinoma**.
The cells display the characteristic features of small cell carcinoma in the form of their hyperchromatic appearance, molding, neuroendocrine chromatin, and the characteristic parachromatin staining of the nuclei with keratin AE1/AE3.

8.4 Answers and Discussion of Text-Based Questions 41–62

A-41. (a) **Well-differentiated adenocarcinoma**.
Cells of ductal adenocarcinoma are larger than their normal counterpart. Loss of polarity is typical of ductal adenocarcinoma cells and is manifested by crowding and uneven spacing of neoplastic cells. A disordered honeycomb-like arrangement is known as Drunken honeycomb is characterized by anisocytosis is often one of the clues to well-differentiated ductal adenocarcinoma.

A-42. (c) **Pancreatic endocrine tumor**
Pancreatic endocrine tumor in its well-differentiated form is characterized by increased cellularity with the majority of cells isolated with bare nuclei. Intact cells reveal eccentric nuclei. Chromatin is typically "salt and pepper."

A-43. (d) **Stomach**
Endoscopic ultrasound fine needle aspiration of pancreatic lesions are done through the duodenum for lesions in the head of the pancreas and are done through the stomach for lesions in the body and tail of the pancreas.

A-44. (a) **Duct adenocarcinoma**
Duct adenocarcinoma is the 4th leading cause of death due to cancer in men and women in U.S. It the 8th leading cause of cancer death worldwide. Ductal adenocarcinoma is the most common cancer of the pancreas.

A-45. (e) **Pancreatic pseudocyst**
Pancreatic pseudocyst is the most common non-neoplastic cyst in the pancreas. They occur as a result of damage to the pancreatic parenchyma which results in hemorrhage and necrosis as well as autodigestion of pancreatic tissue due to the release of pancreatic enzymes. Alcohol abuse is the most common etiology. Approximately 10 % of patients with acute pancreatitis will develop a pseudocyst.

A-46. (a) **Cell arrangement**
Fine needle aspiration of acinic cell carcinoma gives rise to loose clusters, crowded acinar-like cells, and isolated cells with coarsely granular cytoplasm. The nuclei are larger than those of normal acinar cells. The nuclei have smooth nuclear contour, mixed fine and coarse chromatin with a single prominent nucleolus.

A-47. (c) **Ovarian stroma**
The distinction between mucinous neoplasms MCN and intraductal papillary mucinous neoplasms IPMN is not possible by cytology. The distinction requires clinical and imaging correlations. MCN occur mostly in women and commonly located in the body or tail areas. MCNs are lined by mucinous epithelium that form closed cyst without communication with the pancreatic duct. A defining feature is the presence of ovarian stroma beneath the mucinous epithelium.

A-48. (e) **Intraductal papillary mucinous cyst**
IPMN is distinguished from duct carcinoma and MCN because it is connected to and grows into the pancreatic duct system. IPMN are more common in men and are often located in the pancreatic head. Amylase is elevated in the cyst fluid of IPMN.

A-49. (d) **G.I. contaminants**
The recognition of gastric and duodenal epithelial contamination is critical for accurate interpretation of endoscopic ultrasound guided FNA. Duodenal epithelium is recognized by its sheet-like arrangement and the presence of goblet cells. Gastric epithelium also occurs in sheets and unlike duodenal mucosa lack goblet cells and brush borders. Gastric epithelium is commonly nonmucinous.

A-50. (d) **Solid pseudopapillary tumor**
Solid pseudopapillary neoplasm is a neoplasm of low grade malignancy, mostly solid with secondary cystic changes. The tumor cells are small and lack significant atypia and are of uncertain origin. The tumor occurs almost exclusively in women with a female-to-male ratio of 9:1. The cells are usually positive for a1 antitrypsin, CD10, B catenin, NSE, CD56. Tumor cells are negative for CK7 and CK19.

A-51. (e) **Drinking coffee**
Although a well-publicized study suggested a link between coffee consumption and pancreatic cancer, further subsequent studies have shown no link between coffee consumption and pancreatic cancer.

A-52. (d) **Endoscopic US-guided FNA**
Currently endoscopic ultrasound-guided FNA is the procedure of choice in sampling pancreatic lesions.

A-53. (e) **Duct adenocarcinoma**
Duct adenocarcinoma is the 4th leading cause of death due to cancer in men and women in U.S. It the

8th leading cause of cancer death worldwide. Ductal adenocarcinoma is the most common cancer of the pancreas.

A-54. (e) **Pancreaticoblastoma**
Pancreaticoblastoma is a malignant neoplasm with multiple lines of epithelial differentiation, most commonly acinar differentiation. It often contains squamous nests and a mesenchymal component. It is an extremely rare tumor with approximately two thirds occurring in children, representing approximately 25 % of all pancreatic neoplasm in the pediatric population.

A-55. (c) **Primary adenosquamous carcinoma**
Adenosquamous carcinoma is an extremely aggressive variant of ductal adenocarcinoma in which both glandular and squamous differentiations are present. The cytologic diagnosis depends on recognizing the two components on smears.

A-56. (b) **Acinic cell carcinoma**
In contrast to pancreaticoblastoma, acinic cell carcinoma will not display squamous nests.

A-57. (d) **The cyst contents show high CEA levels**
This is the classic cytomorphologic features of serous cystadenoma. It is a benign tumor that is typically microcystic. The cysts are lined by cells rich in cytoplasmic glycogen which produce the serous cyst fluid. There is association with von Hippel–Lindau syndrome. Cells are typically PAS-positive and d-PAS negative which confirms cytoplasmic glycogen. The cyst fluid is low in amylase and CEA.

A-58. (b) **It has focal mucinous lining**
Pancreatic pseudocyst is the most common non-neoplastic cyst in the pancreas. They occur as a result of damage to the pancreatic parenchyma which results in hemorrhage and necrosis as well as autodigestion of pancreatic tissue due to the release of pancreatic enzymes. The cyst characteristically has no epithelial lining. Alcohol abuse is the most common etiology. Aspiration of this cyst often yields degenerated cells and inflammatory cells. Approximately 10 % of patients with acute pancreatitis will develop a pseudocyst.

A-59. (d) **CAM 5.2 is nonreactive**
Aspirates from acinic cell carcinoma are usually moderately cellular and display a clean background which may contain cytoplasmic granules. The nuclei resemble lymphocytes. Many striped nuclei are characteristic. Tumor cells form sheets, irregular clusters, as well as small acinar formation. Tumor cells are positive for trypsin, chymotrypsin, CAM 5.2, AE1/AE3 but negative for CK 7, CK 19, and CK 20.

A-60. (d) **Synaptophysin and trypsin**
Synaptophysin is typically positive in pancreatic endocrine tumor while trypsin is usually positive in acinic cell carcinoma.

A-61. (b) **Keratin and synaptophysin reactivity**
Solid pseudopapillary tumor of the pancreas has the following staining characteristics: Usually positive for a1 antitrypsin, CD10, B catenin, vimentin, and cytokeratin AE1/AE3 and CAM 5.2.

A-62. (b) **Cytokeratin 7**
Pancreatic adenocarcinoma is reactive to CytokeratinsCk8, AE1/AE3, CAM 5.2, CK7, CK13, CK18, and CK19. Chromogranin is mostly reactive in pancreatic endocrine tumors. Cytokeratin 20 is negative in pancreatic carcinoma. Trypsin is reactive in acinic cell carcinoma while B-catenin is reactive in pancreatic solid pseudopapillary tumors.

A-63 (**c**, **Beckwith-Wiedmann Syndrome**), A-64 (**d**, **Most common non-neoplastic cyst**), A-65 (**a**, **Von Hippel–Lindau Syndrome**), A-66 (**f**, **Female-to-Male ratio 9:1**), A-67 (**e**, **Ovarian stroma**), A-68 (**b**, **Peutz–Jeghers Syndrome**).
Syndromes that are associated with pancreatic tumors are Peutz–Jeghers with pancreatic adenocarcinoma, Von Hippel–Landau with serous cystadenoma, and Beckwith–Wiedmann with pancreaticoblastoma.

Mucinous cystadenomas have the characteristic ovarian stroma. Pseudocyst of the pancreas is considered the most common non-neoplastic cyst of the pancreas; its incidence is approximately 10 % in patients with alcoholic pancreatitis. Solid pseudopapillary tumor of the pancreas is almost exclusively in women with a female-to-male ratio of 9:1.

Reading List

Adsay NV, Hasteh F, Cheng JD, et al. Lymphoepithelial cysts of the pancreas: a report of 12 cases and a review of the literature. Mod Pathol. 2002;15(5):492–501.

Al-Haddad M, Schmidt CM, Sandrasegaran K, Dewitt J. Cystic pancreatic tumors: state of the art review. Clin Gastroenterol Hepatol. 2011. Available at: http://www.ncbi.nlm.nih.gov/pubmed/21397725. Accessed 27 Apr 2011.

Brugge WR. Role of endoscopic ultrasound in the diagnosis of cystic lesions of the pancreas. Pancreatology. 2001;1(6):637–40.

Chang F, Chandra A, Culora G, et al. Cytologic diagnosis of pancreatic endocrine tumors by endoscopic ultrasound-guided fine-needle aspiration: a review. Diagn Cytopathol. 2006;34(9):649–58.

Deshpande V, Mino-Kenudson M, Brugge WR, et al. Endoscopic ultrasound guided fine needle aspiration biopsy of autoimmune pancreatitis: diagnostic criteria and pitfalls. Am J Surg Pathol. 2005;29(11):1464–71.

Eloubeidi MA, Chen VK, Jhala NC, et al. Endoscopic ultrasound-guided fine needle aspiration biopsy of suspected cholangiocarcinoma. Clin Gastroenterol Hepatol. 2004;2(3):209–13.

Khalbuss WE, Monaco SE, Pantanowitz L. Chapter 17. Pancreas. In: The ASCP Quick Compendium (QC) of cytopathology. Chicago: ASCP Press; 2013. p. 366–85.

Klimstra DS, Pitman MB, Hruban RH. An algorithmic approach to the diagnosis of pancreatic neoplasms. Arch Pathol Lab Med. 2009; 133(3):454–64.

Layfield LJ, Cramer H. Fine-needle aspiration cytology of intraductal papillary-mucinous tumors: a retrospective analysis. Diagn Cytopathol. 2005;32(1):16–20.

Maire F, Couvelard A, Hammel P, et al. Intraductal papillary mucinous tumors of the pancreas: the preoperative value of cytologic and histopathologic diagnosis. Gastrointest Endosc. 2003;58(5):701–6.

Michaels PJ, Brachtel EF, Bounds BC, Brugge WR, Pitman MB. Intraductal papillary mucinous neoplasm of the pancreas: cytologic features predict histologic grade. Cancer. 2006;108(3): 163–73.

Solé M, Iglesias C, Fernández-Esparrach G, et al. Fine-needle aspiration cytology of intraductal papillary mucinous tumors of the pancreas. Cancer. 2005;105(5):298–303.

Gastrointestinal and Bile Duct Brushing Cytology

9

Qing Kay Li and Walid E. Khalbuss

Contents

9.1 **Image-Based Questions 1–31** 524

9.2 **Text-Based Questions 32–61** 555

9.3 **Answers and Discussion of Image-Based Questions 1–31** 558

9.4 **Answers and Discussion of Text-Based Questions 32–61** 565

Reading List 571

Q.K. Li, MD, PhD (✉)
Department of Pathology, The Johns Hopkins University
School of Medicine, The Johns Hopkins Bayview Medical Center,
4940 Eastern Avenue, AA Building, Room 154B,
Baltimore, MD 21224-2780, USA
e-mail: qli23@jhmi.edu

W.E. Khalbuss, MD, PhD, FIAC
Department of Pathology, GE Clarient Diagnostic Services,
31 Columbia, Aliso Viejo, California, 92656, USA
e-mail: Walid.khalbuss@ge.com

W.E. Khalbuss, Q.K. Li (eds.), *Diagnostic Cytopathology Board Review and Self-Assessment*,
DOI 10.1007/978-1-4939-1477-7_9, © Springer Science+Business Media New York 2015

Table 9.1 Benign components and conditions in G.I. and bile duct cytology

	Descriptions	Differentials
Squamous cells	Sheets or scattered individual cells with small (pyknotic) nuclei and dense cytoplasm with cytokeratin formation (purple color on Diff-Quik stain and orangeophilic color on Papanicolaou stain)	Cells have an oval- or spindle-shaped, low N/C ratio, and benign nuclear features DD: squamous cell carcinoma
Reactive squamous cells	Sheets of cells with streaming pattern and scattered individual cells with small nuclei and dense cytoplasm	Cells have mild nuclear atypia, normal N/C ratio, and benign nuclear features DD: squamous cell carcinoma
Benign glandular cells	Clusters of columnar cells with picket fence arrangement, oval nuclei, vesicular chromatin, inconspicuous or small nucleoli, abundant cytoplasm with vacuoles	No nuclear overlapping, no nuclear atypia DD: adenocarcinoma
Smooth muscle cells	Sheets of spindle-shaped cells with blunt-ended nuclei and abundant fibrillar cytoplasm	No markedly nuclear variations, no nuclear atypia DD: sarcomas, GIST
Goblet cells	Single or clusters of cells with abundant mucin-filled cytoplasm and eccentrically located nuclei, "signet ring" appearance	Cells are without nuclear atypia DD: mucinous adenocarcinoma, signet ring cell carcinoma
Chief cells	Polygonal cells with small round nuclei, fine chromatin, inconspicuous nucleoli, and cytoplasmic basophilic zymogen granules	Similar to acinar cells of the pancreas DD: parietal cells
Parietal cells	Pyramidal or flask-shaped cells with coarse chromatin, inconspicuous or small nucleoli, cytoplasmic eosinophilic granules	The size of cells is larger than chief cells DD: chief cells
Bile ductal glandular cells	Sheets or small clusters of cuboidal cells, round nuclei with evenly distributed chromatin, regular nuclear membrane, and inconspicuous nucleoli	Preserved N:C ratio, no overlapping nuclei, no large prominent nucleoli DD: adenocarcinoma
Histiocytes	Loosely formed two-dimensional clusters or dispersed individual cells, with coffee bean-shaped nuclei, fine chromatin, inconspicuous nucleoli, and foamy cytoplasm	Cells have coffee bean-shaped nuclei, cytoplasmic vacuoles and pigment, and normal N:C ratio DD: adenocarcinoma, signet ring cell carcinoma
Candidiasis	Budding yeast with pseudohyphae	Pseudohyphae are 2–10 μm in diameter and branch at a 90° angle
Herpes simplex virus (HSV)	Multinucleated large cells with ground-glass chromatin, Cowdry A bodies, and nuclear molding	Multinucleation, ground-glass chromatin, and intranuclear inclusion DD:CMV infection
Cytomegalovirus (CMV)	Large cells with single enlarged nuclei, single large basophilic intranuclear inclusion, perinuclear halo, and cytoplasmic CMV inclusions	Mononucleation, single intranuclear inclusion DD: HSV infection

Table 9.2 Malignant conditions in G.I. and bile duct cytology

Conditions	Descriptions	Differentials
Adenocarcinoma	Three-dimensional clusters and acinar arrangements of columnar cells. Tumor cells have hyperchromasia, high N:C ratio, prominent nucleoli, coarse chromatin, "lacy" cytoplasm with vacuolization (cytoplasmic mucin)	Columnar cells have high N:C ratio with irregular nuclear membrane, coarse chromatin, prominent nucleoli, and cytoplasmic vacuole (mucin production) DD: reactive atypia, poorly differentiated squamous cell carcinoma
Squamous cell carcinoma	Dyscohesive clusters, loosely formed two-dimensional cellular sheets and scattered individual polymorphic cells, hyperchromatic nuclei, irregular nuclear membrane, with or without keratinization Tumor necrosis	Polygonal, rounded, elongated, or tadpole-shaped cells with large dark nuclei, smudgy chromatin, and dense cytoplasm (cytokeratin formation) DD: poorly differentiated adenocarcinoma
Carcinoid	Loosely cohesive clusters and scattered individual cells arranged in rosette-like architectures. Tumor cells are relatively uniform with fine (salt-and-pepper) chromatin. No mitoses or necrosis	Uniform tumor cells form rosettes, with inconspicuous or occasional small nucleoli. Branching capillaries in the background DD: small cell carcinoma, poorly differentiated adenocarcinoma, lymphoma
Small cell carcinoma	Tight clusters of small hyperchromatic cells (two to three times of the size of mature lymphocytes) with nuclear molding and crowding, nuclear stripes (broken nuclear material), inconspicuous nuclei, scant cytoplasm	Fine (salt-and-pepper) chromatin, nuclear molding and crowding, paranuclear blue bodies, mitosis, necrosis, and apoptotic body DD: lymphoma, basaloid squamous cell carcinoma, and poorly differentiated adenocarcinoma
Gastrointestinal stromal tumor (GIST)	Clusters of spindle cells or epithelioid cells with oval nuclei, granular chromatin, inconspicuous nucleoli, wispy cytoplasm and long extension	Lack of markedly nuclear atypia DD: leiomyosarcoma
Metastatic melanoma	Scattered individual large cells with prominent nucleoli and cytoplasmic melanin pigment. Binucleation, multinucleation with prominent nucleoli in "mirror" arrangement. Pseudointranuclear inclusions	Large-sized malignant cells with prominent nucleoli, dense cytoplasm DD: poorly differentiated carcinoma, Hodgkin lymphoma, hepatocellular carcinoma
Lymphoma (non-Hodgkin lymphoma)	Dispersed individual atypical lymphoid cells with coarse chromatin and irregular nuclear membrane, prominent nucleoli. High N:C ratio and scant cytoplasm. Increased mitotic activity and the presence of background lymphoglandular bodies	The size of tumor cells ranges from small to large depending on the type of lymphoma. Monomorphic population of lymphocytes is characteristic for SLL/CLL DD: reactive lymphocytes, small cell carcinoma, poorly differentiated carcinoma
Non-epithelial cell neoplasm	Individual or clusters of spindle cells, small round cells, or pleomorphic tumor cells	DD: muscle, nerve tumors, small round cell tumor, and sarcomas

9.1 Image-Based Questions 1–31

Fig. 9.1

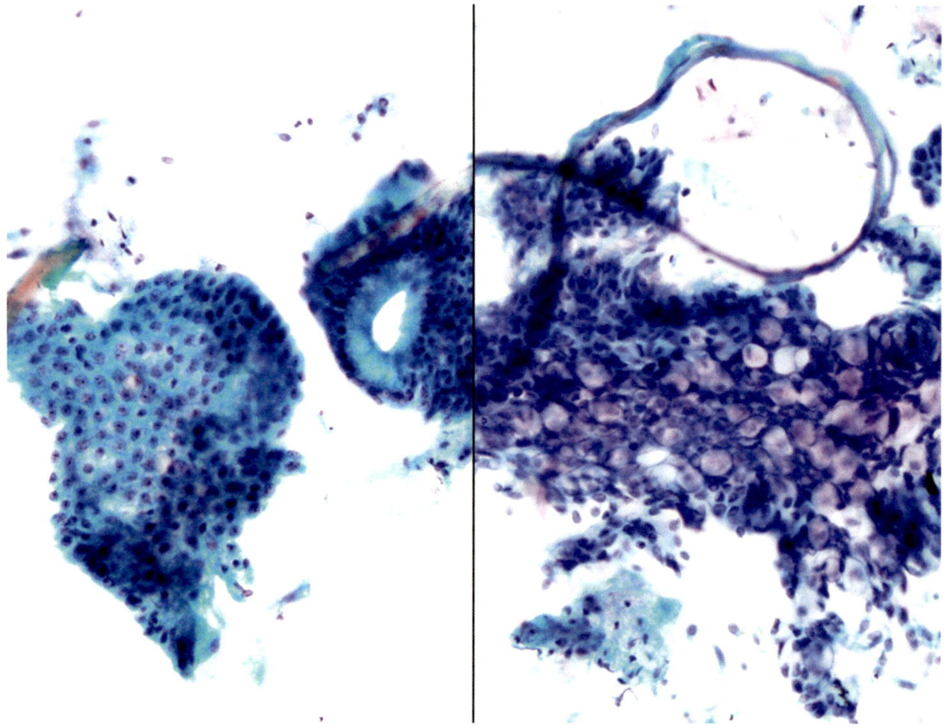

Q-1. A 58-year-old male with reflex symptoms had an endoscopic esophageal brushing. What is the diagnosis of this cytological specimen?
(a) Well-differentiated adenocarcinoma
(b) Barrett esophagus
(c) Poorly differentiated adenocarcinoma
(d) Reactive/regenerative glandular atypia

Fig. 9.2

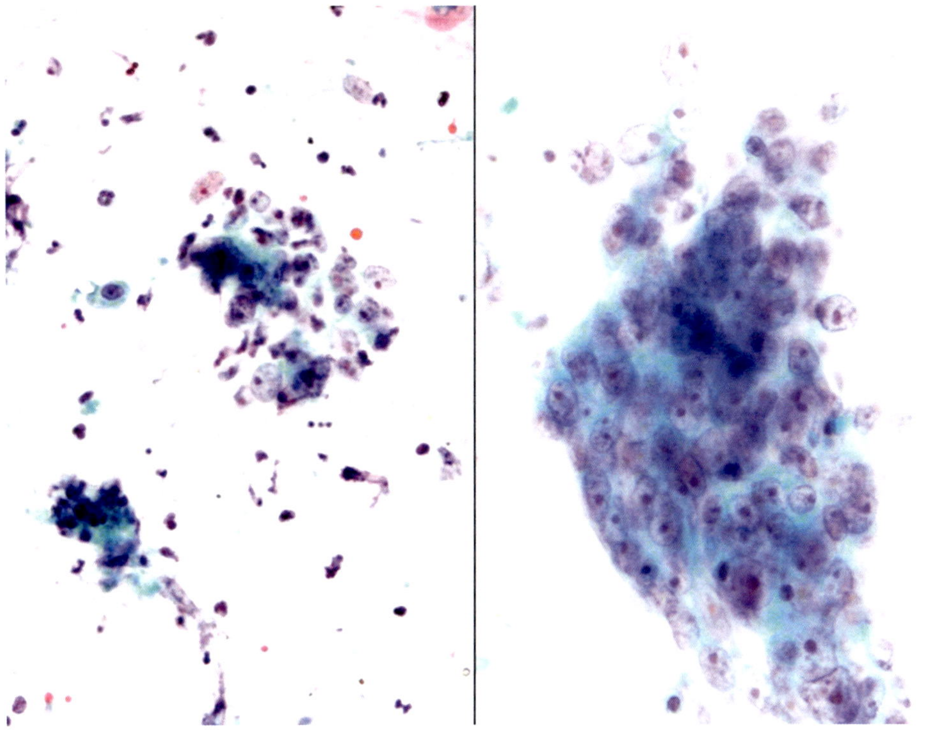

Q-2. A 59-year-old male with abdominal pain and weight loss had an endoscopic esophageal brushing. What is the diagnosis of this cytological specimen?
(a) Adenocarcinoma
(b) Barrett esophagus
(c) Poorly differentiated squamous cell carcinoma
(d) Reactive/regenerative glandular atypia

Fig. 9.3

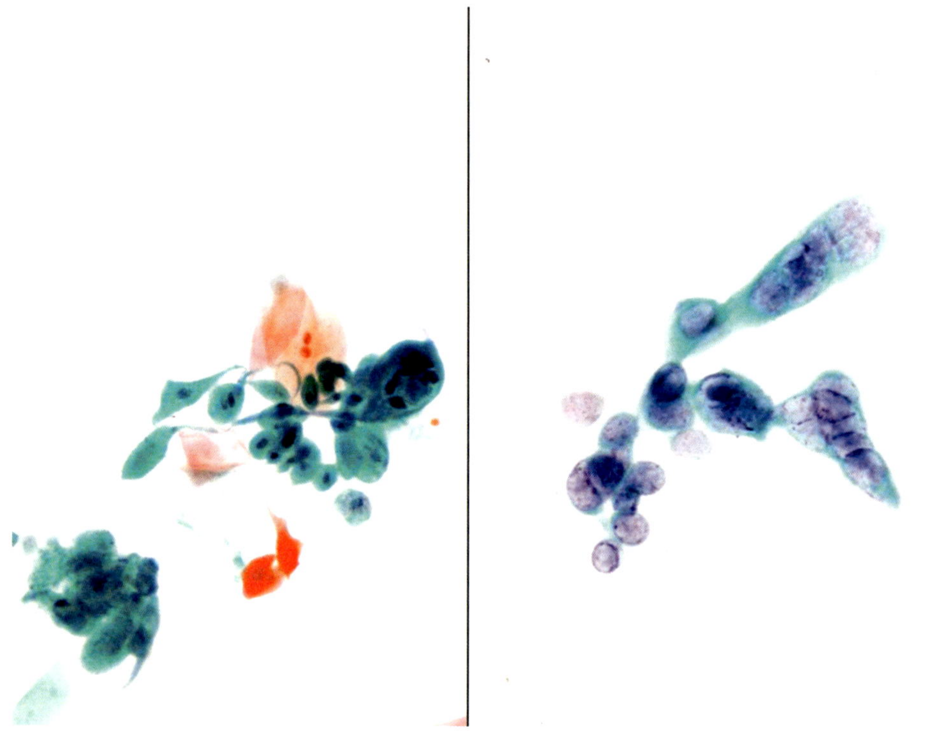

Q-3. A 25-year-old HIV-positive patient presented with severe heart burn and weight loss, who underwent an endoscopic esophageal brushing. What is the diagnosis of this cytological specimen?

(a) Adenocarcinoma
(b) Barrett esophagus
(c) Poorly differentiated squamous cell carcinoma
(d) Herpes simplex virus (HSV) infection

Fig. 9.4

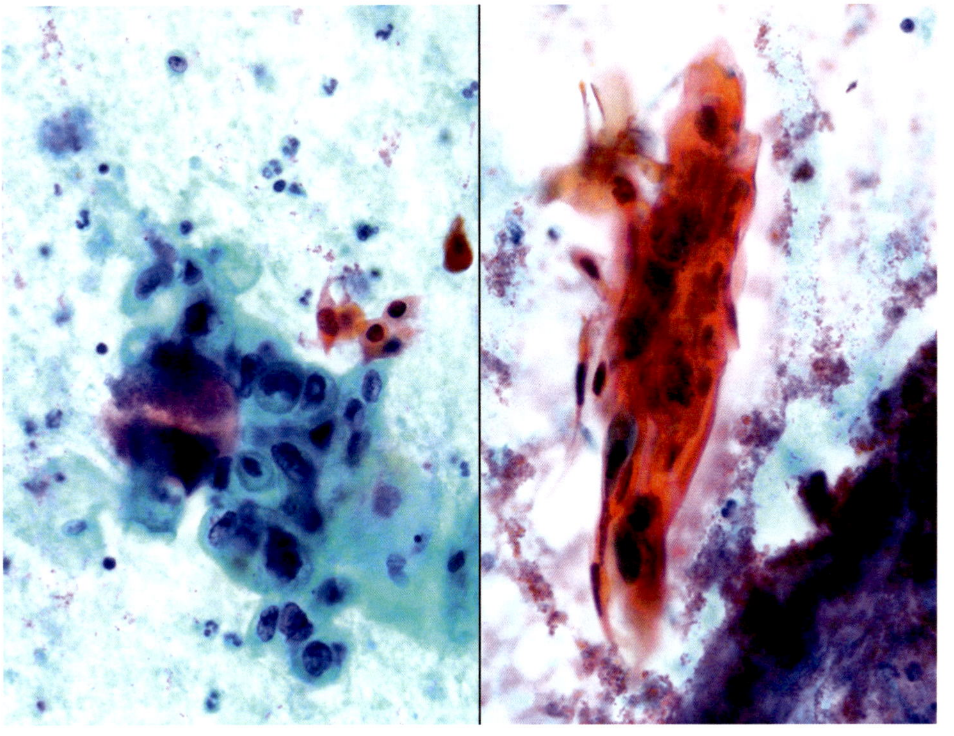

Q-4. A 68-year-old female with abdominal pain and weight loss had an endoscopic esophageal brushing. What is the diagnosis of this cytological specimen?
(a) Adenocarcinoma
(b) Barrett esophagus
(c) Squamous cell carcinoma
(d) Reactive/regenerative atypia

Fig. 9.5

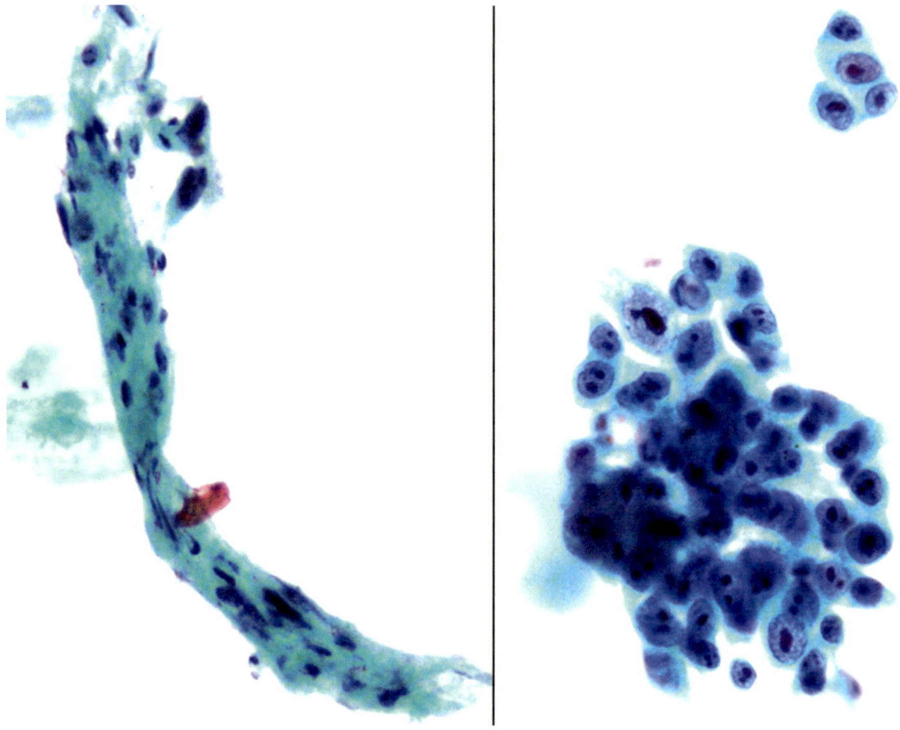

Q-5. A 70-year-old male with abdominal pain and weight loss had an endoscopic esophageal brushing. What is the diagnosis of this cytological specimen?
(a) Adenocarcinoma
(b) Barrett esophagus
(c) Poorly differentiated squamous cell carcinoma
(d) Reactive/regenerative atypia

Fig. 9.6

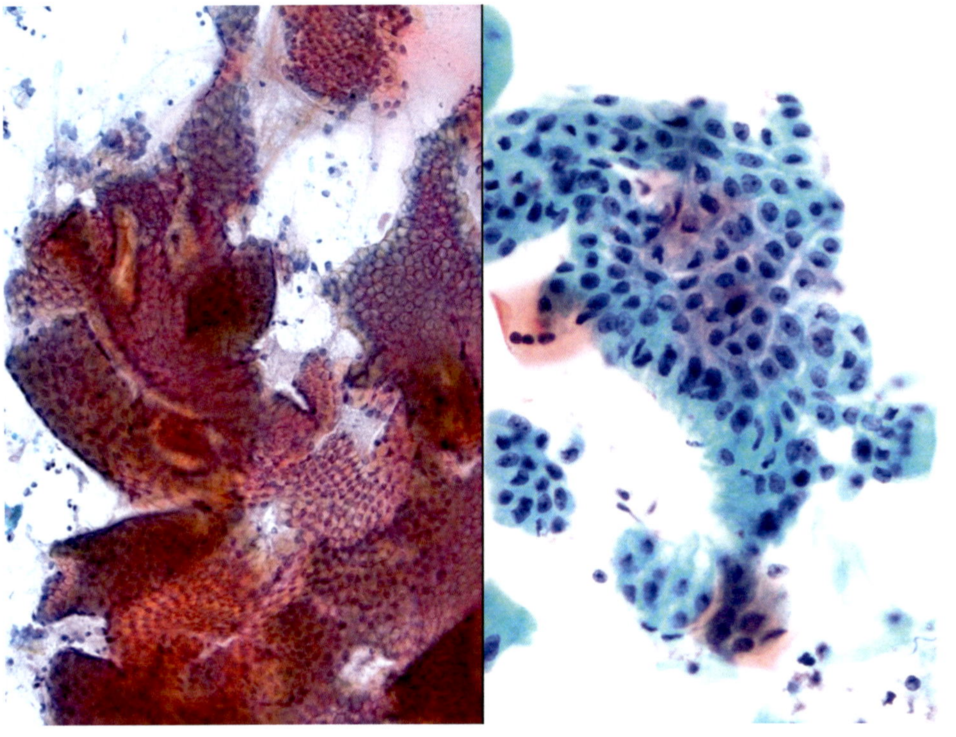

Q-6. A 67-year-old male with abdominal pain and weight loss had an endoscopic procedure. In his stomach, edematous gastric mucosa was revealed, and a gastric brushing was performed. What is the diagnosis of this cytological specimen?
(a) Adenocarcinoma
(b) Barrett esophagus
(c) Benign-appearing gastric mucosa
(d) Reactive/regenerative atypia

Fig. 9.7

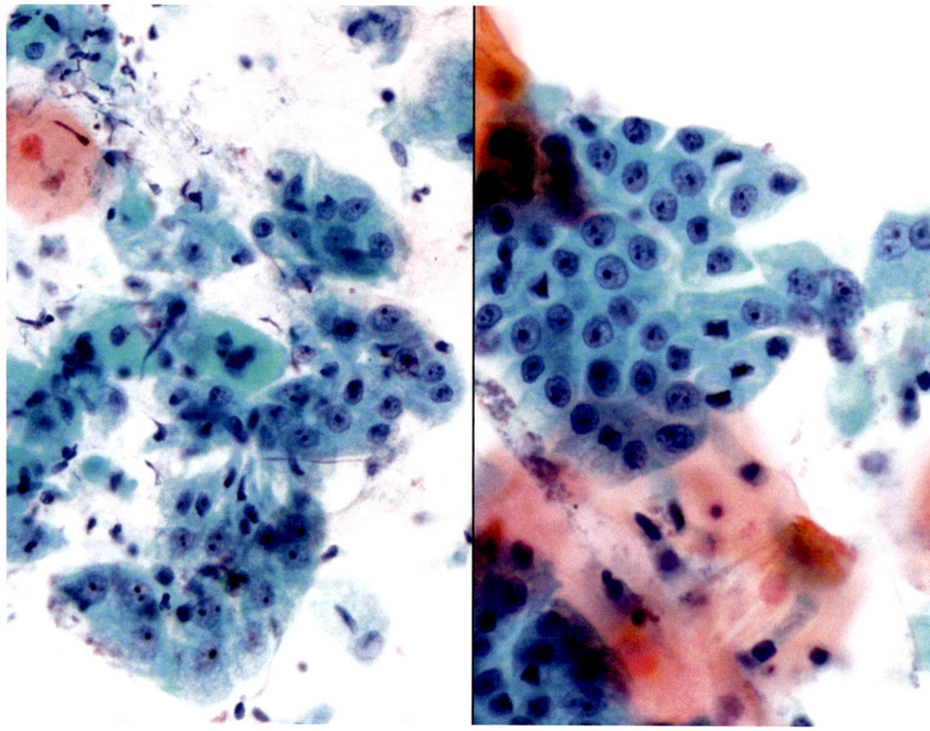

Q-7. A 37-year-old male with abdominal pain had a gastric brushing. What is the diagnosis of this cytological specimen?
(a) Adenocarcinoma
(b) Barrett esophagus
(c) Benign-appearing gastric mucosa
(d) Gastric mucosa with reactive changes

Fig. 9.8

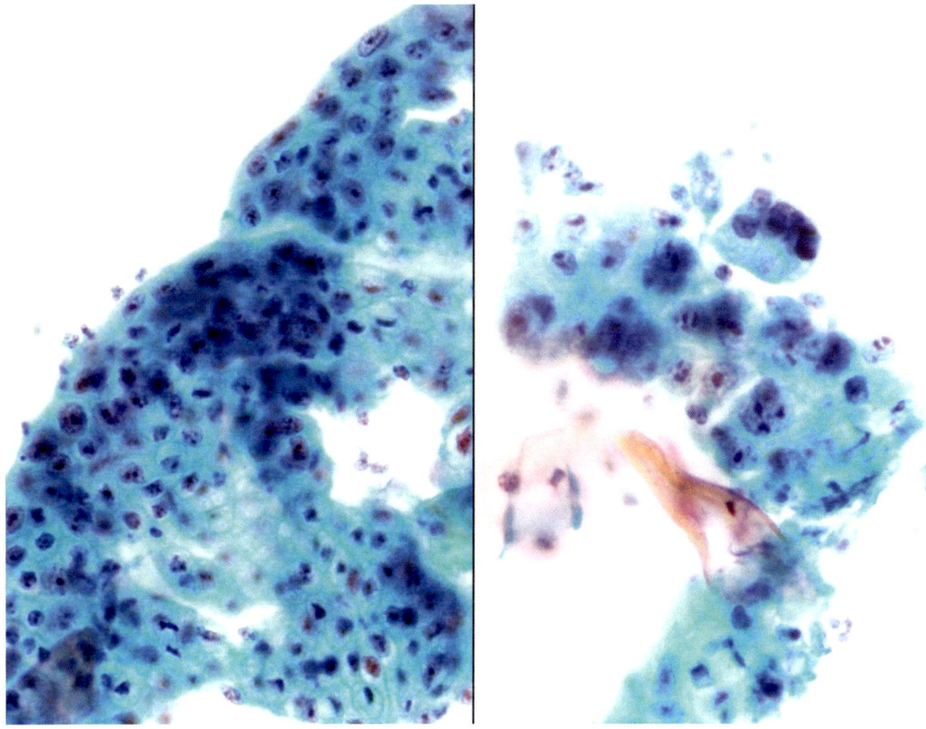

Q-8. A 56-year-old male with abdominal pain had an endoscopic procedure. A 1.0 cm gastric ulcer was found; and a gastric brushing was performed. What is the diagnosis of this cytological specimen?

(a) Adenocarcinoma
(b) Poorly differentiated squamous cell carcinoma
(c) Benign-appearing gastric mucosa
(d) Gastric mucosa with reactive changes consistent with a benign gastric ulcer

Fig. 9.9

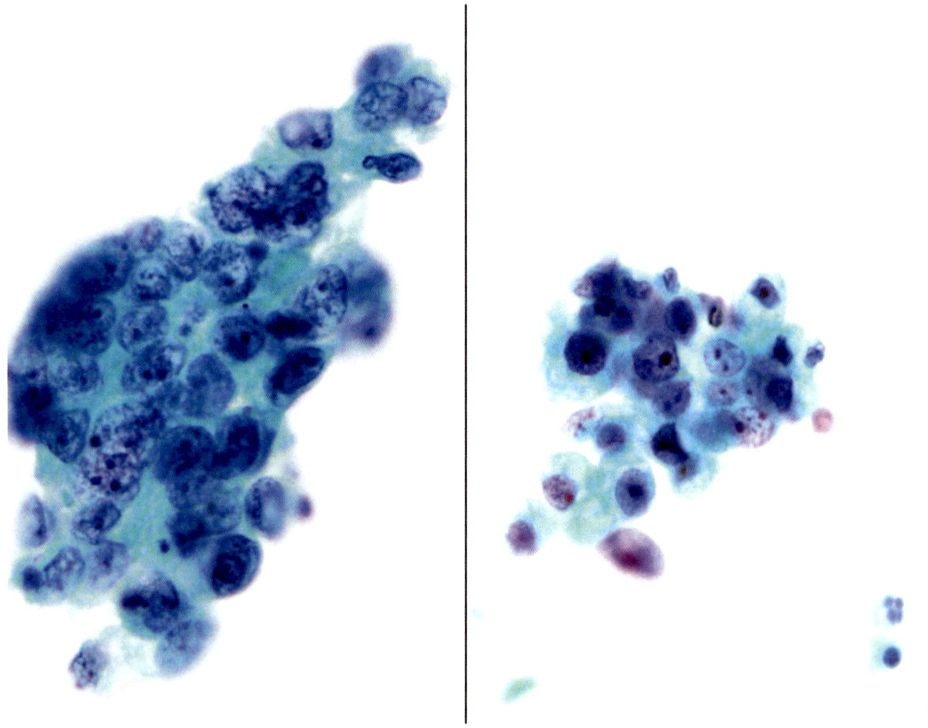

Q-9. A 78-year-old female presented with abdominal pain and weight loss. An upper GI endoscopy revealed a 2.0 cm gastric ulcer. A gastric brushing was performed. What is the diagnosis of this cytological specimen?

(a) Adenocarcinoma
(b) Poorly differentiated squamous cell carcinoma
(c) Benign-appearing gastric mucosa
(d) Gastric mucosa with reactive changes consistent with a benign gastric ulcer

Fig. 9.10

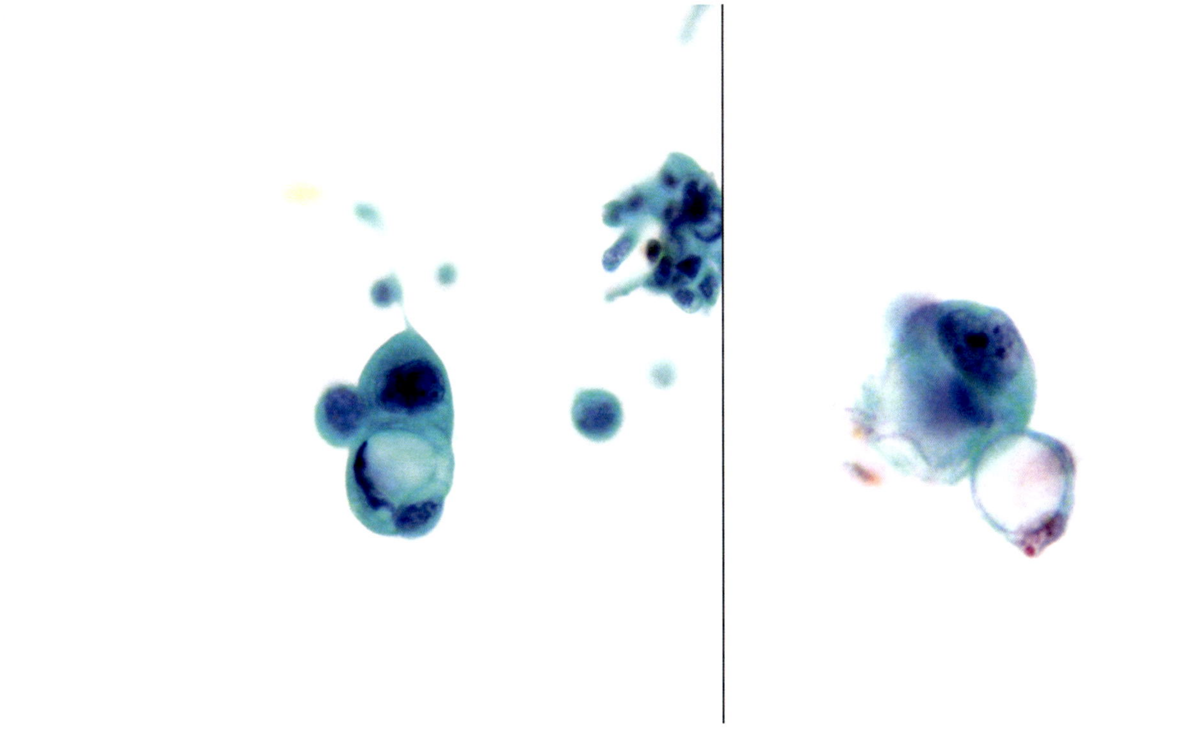

Q-10. An upper GI endoscopic ultrasound-guided procedure was performed on a 74-year-old female smoker who presented with abdominal pain, weight loss, and right pleural effusion. On the cytological brushing specimen, tight clusters and dispersed individual atypical epithelioid cells were identified. What is the diagnosis of the EUS brushing?

(a) Metastatic adenocarcinoma of the breast
(b) Metastatic adenocarcinoma of the lung
(c) Signet ring cell carcinoma of the stomach
(d) Reactive histiocytes

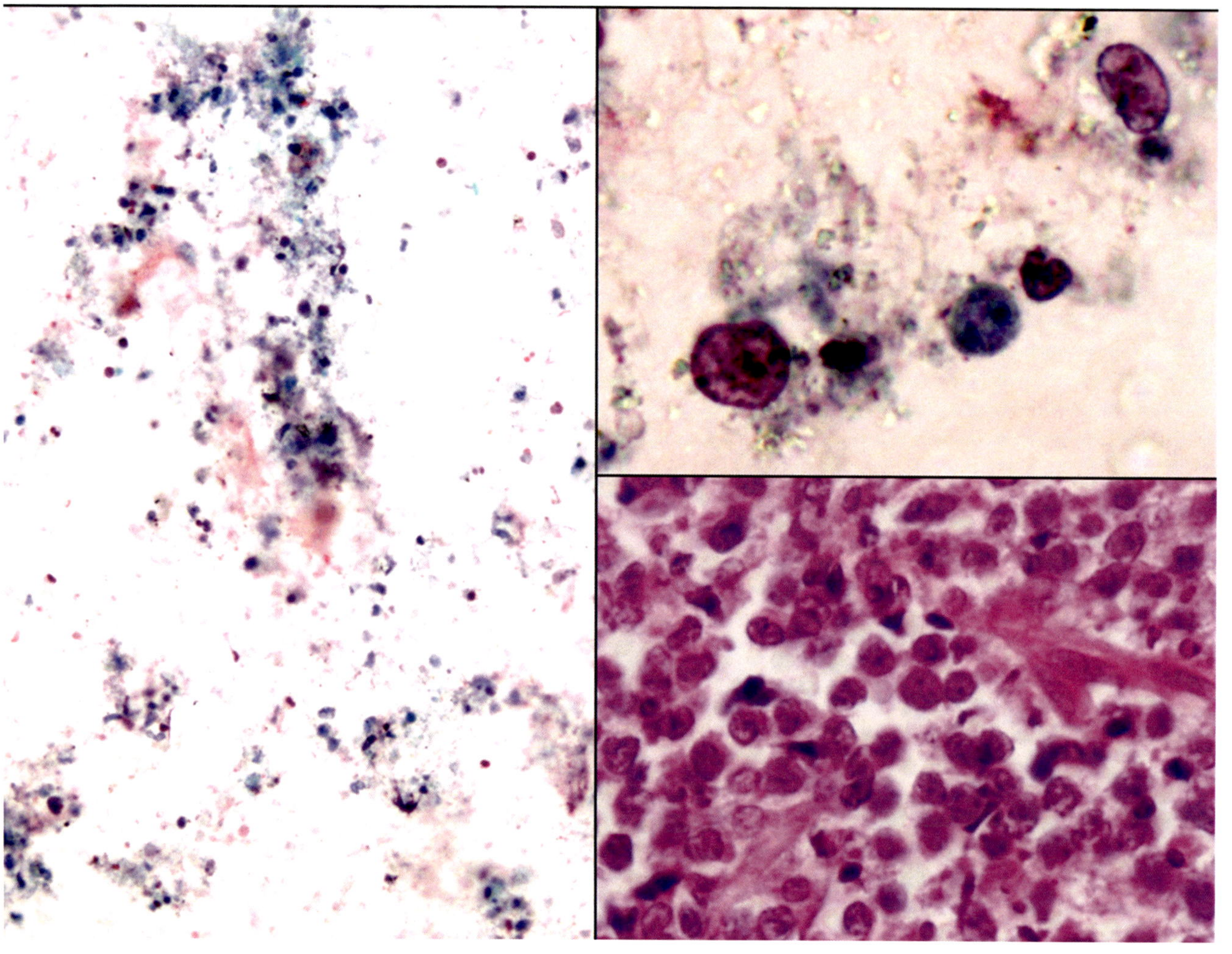

Fig. 9.11

Q-11. An upper GI endoscopic ultrasound-guided (EUS) procedure was performed on a 75-year-old female who presented with stomach bleeding, fever, lymphadenopathy, and weight loss. On the cytological brushing specimen, numerous dispersed individual atypical cells were identified. What is the diagnosis of the EUS brushing?

(a) Poorly differentiated adenocarcinoma
(b) Poorly differentiated squamous cell carcinoma
(c) Benign-appearing gastric mucosa
(d) Diffuse large B cell lymphoma (DLBCL)

Fig. 9.12

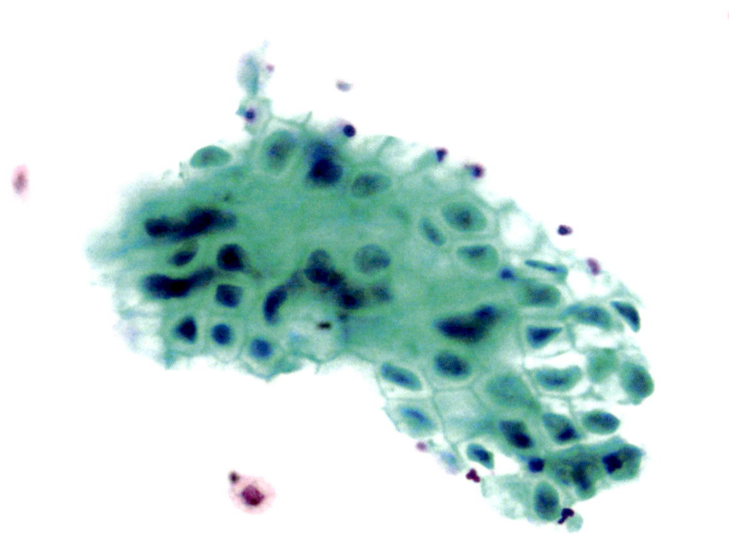

Q-12. A gastric brushing was performed on a patient with a gastric ulcer. What is the diagnosis of this cytological specimen?
(a) Adenocarcinoma
(b) Poorly differentiated squamous cell carcinoma
(c) Reactive gastric glandular cells
(d) Vegetable cells

Fig. 9.13

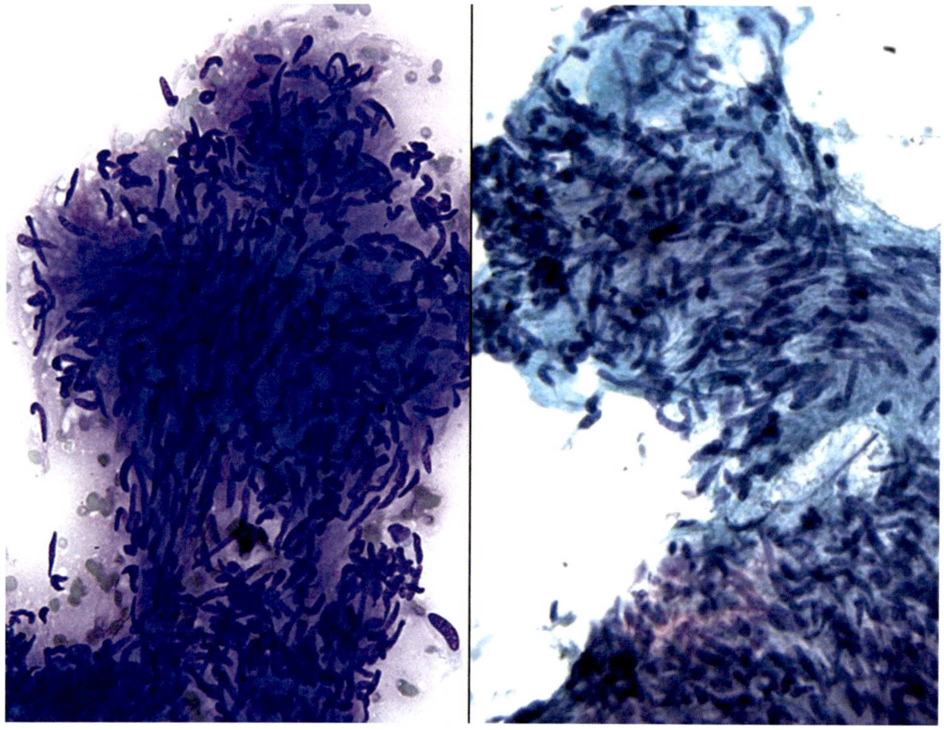

Q-13. A 73-year-old female with a history of breast carcinoma presented with stomach pain and abdominal discomfort. CT scan revealed a 1.0 cm submucosal mass in the stomach. Subsequently, endoscopic ultrasound-guided FNA was performed. What is the diagnosis of this cytological specimen?

(a) Adenocarcinoma
(b) Poorly differentiated carcinoma
(c) Reactive gastric glandular cells
(d) Gastrointestinal stromal tumor (GIST)

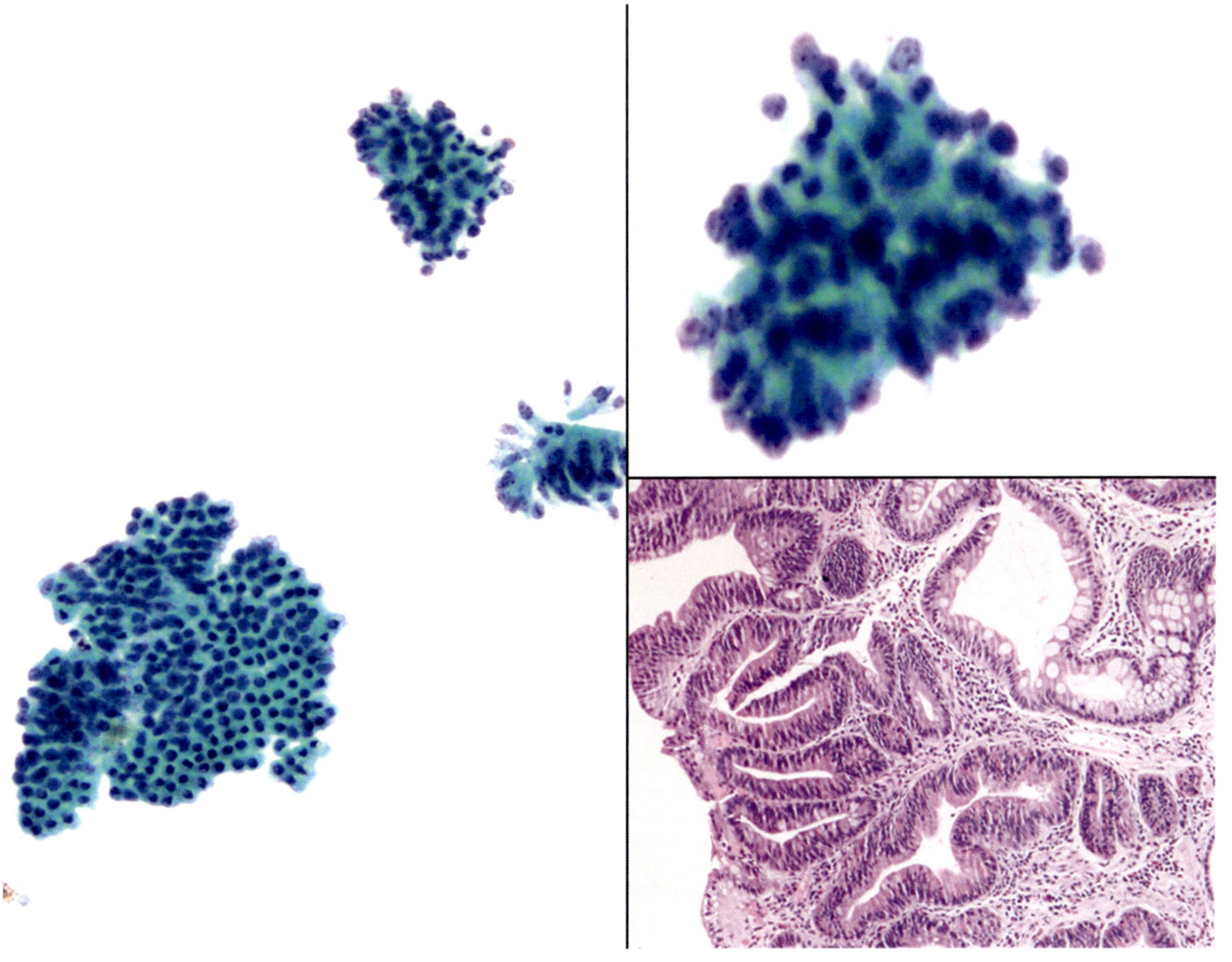

Fig. 9.14

Q-14. A 36-year-old female with abdominal pain had an endoscopic ultrasound-guided FNA. During the procedure, a small polypoid lesion was seen in the duodenum. What is the diagnosis of this brushing specimen from the duodenum?

(a) Adenocarcinoma
(b) Poorly differentiated carcinoma
(c) Adenoma
(d) Carcinoid

Fig. 9.15

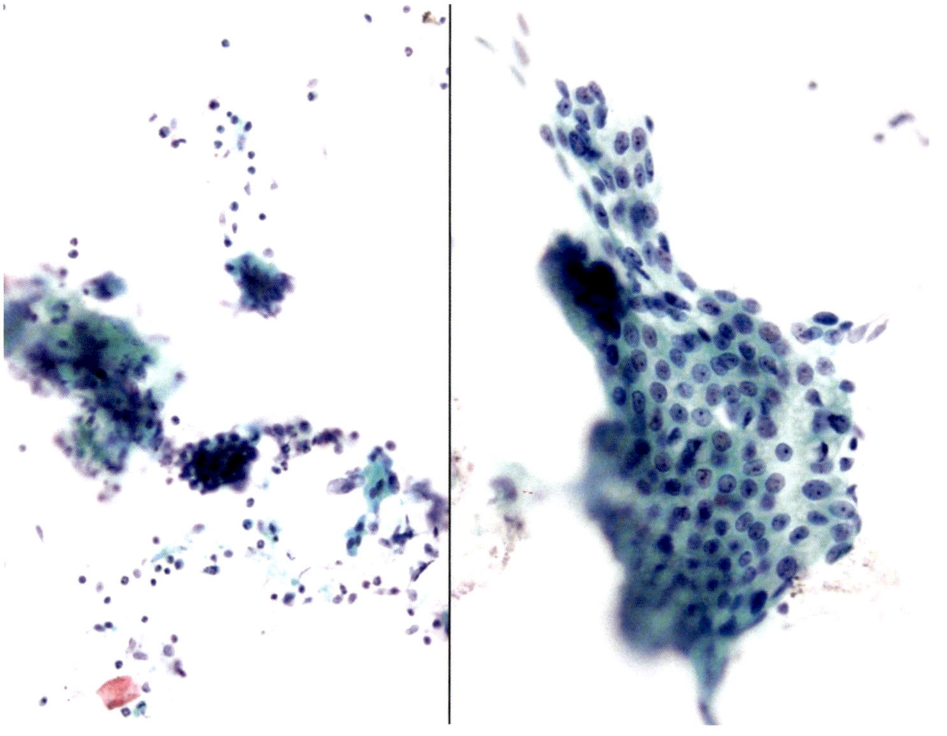

Q-15. A 64-year-old female with abdominal pain and enlarged liver had an endoscopic ultrasound-guided FNA. A biliary tree brushing was performed. What is the diagnosis of this brushing specimen?
(a) Adenocarcinoma
(b) Poorly differentiated carcinoma
(c) Reactive glandular cells
(d) Carcinoid

Fig. 9.16

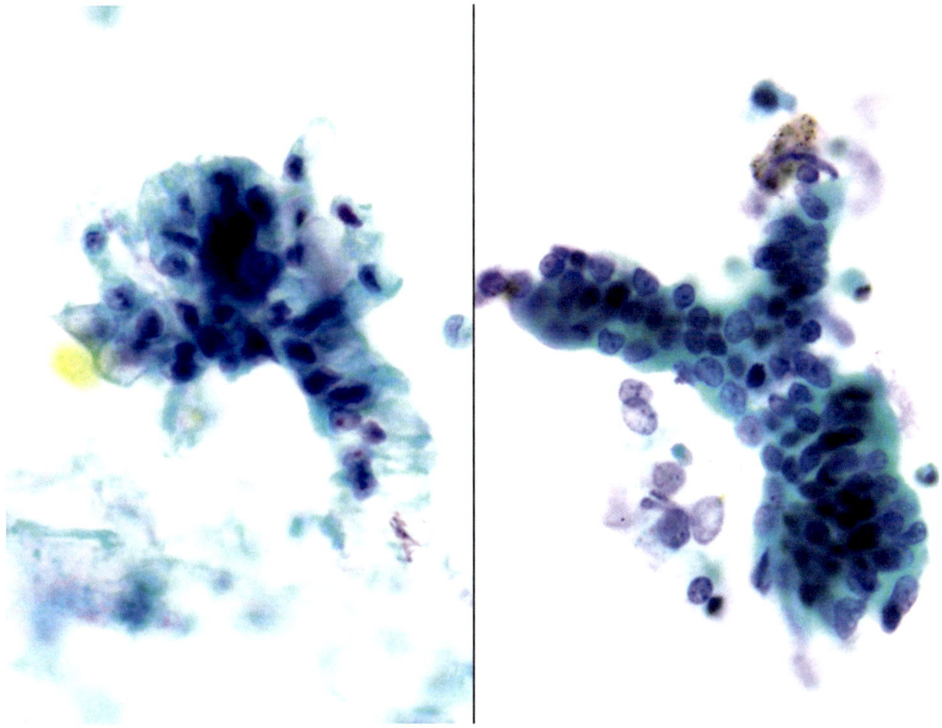

Q-16. A 64-year-old female had a history of biliary tree tumor with a biliary tree stent placement, now presented with jaundice. An endoscopic ultrasound-guided FNA was performed. A biliary tree brushing was done. What is the diagnosis of this brushing specimen?
(a) Adenocarcinoma
(b) Poorly differentiated carcinoma
(c) Reactive glandular cells
(d) Carcinoid

Fig. 9.17

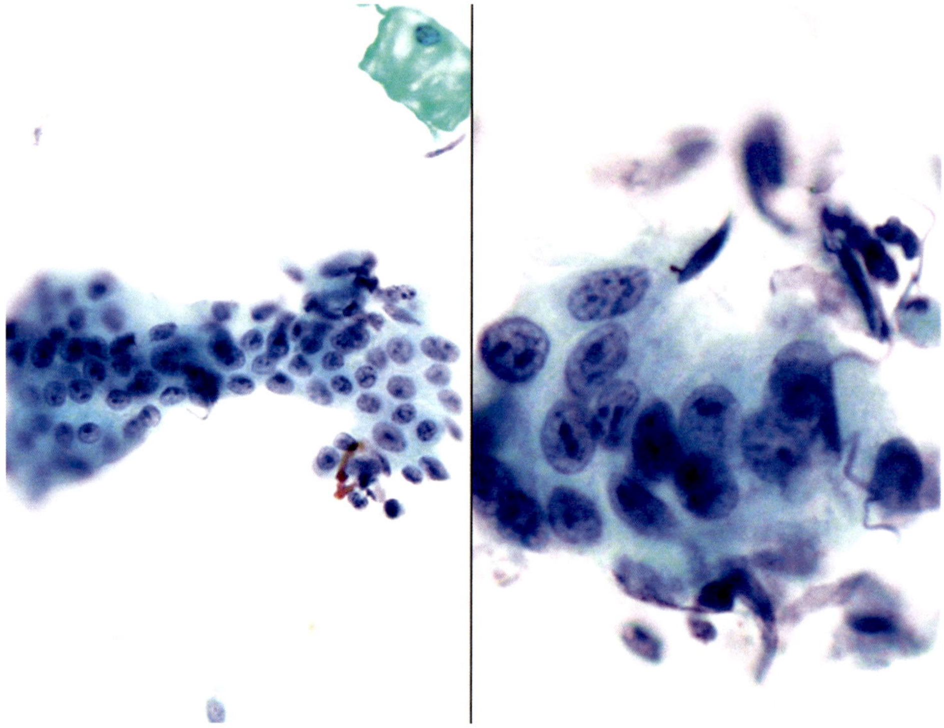

Q-17. A 70-year-old female had a history of biliary tree adenocarcinoma with chemo- and radiation therapy, now presented with jaundice. A biliary tree brushing was performed. What is the diagnosis of this brushing specimen?
(a) Adenocarcinoma
(b) Poorly differentiated carcinoma
(c) Reactive glandular cells
(d) Carcinoid

Fig. 9.18

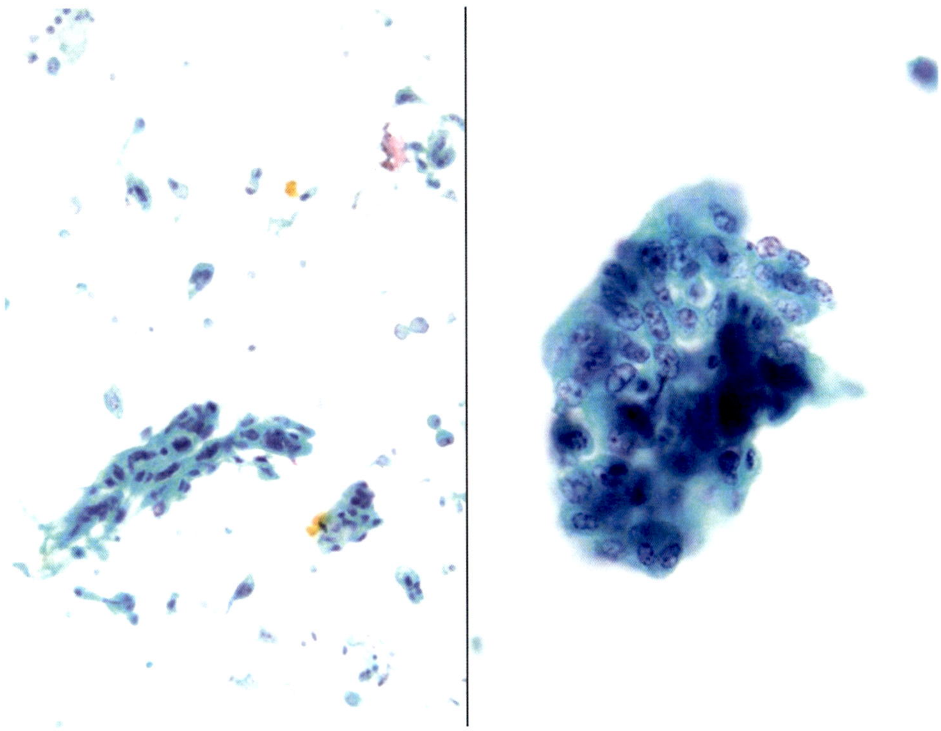

Q-18. A biliary tree brushing was performed on a patient with jaundice. What is the diagnosis of this brushing specimen?
(a) Adenocarcinoma
(b) Poorly differentiated squamous cell carcinoma
(c) Reactive glandular cells
(d) Carcinoid

Fig. 9.19

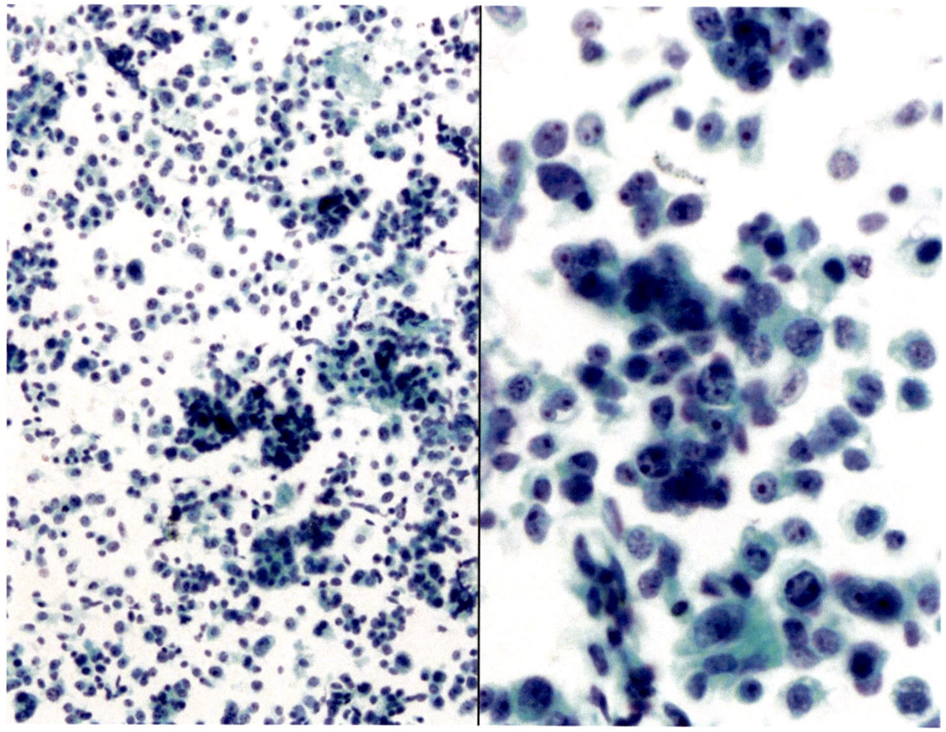

Q-19. An 81-year-old female presented with jaundice and abdominal pain. A biliary tree brushing was performed. What is the diagnosis of this brushing specimen?
(a) Carcinoid
(b) Lymphoma
(c) Melanoma
(d) Adenocarcinoma

Fig. 9.20

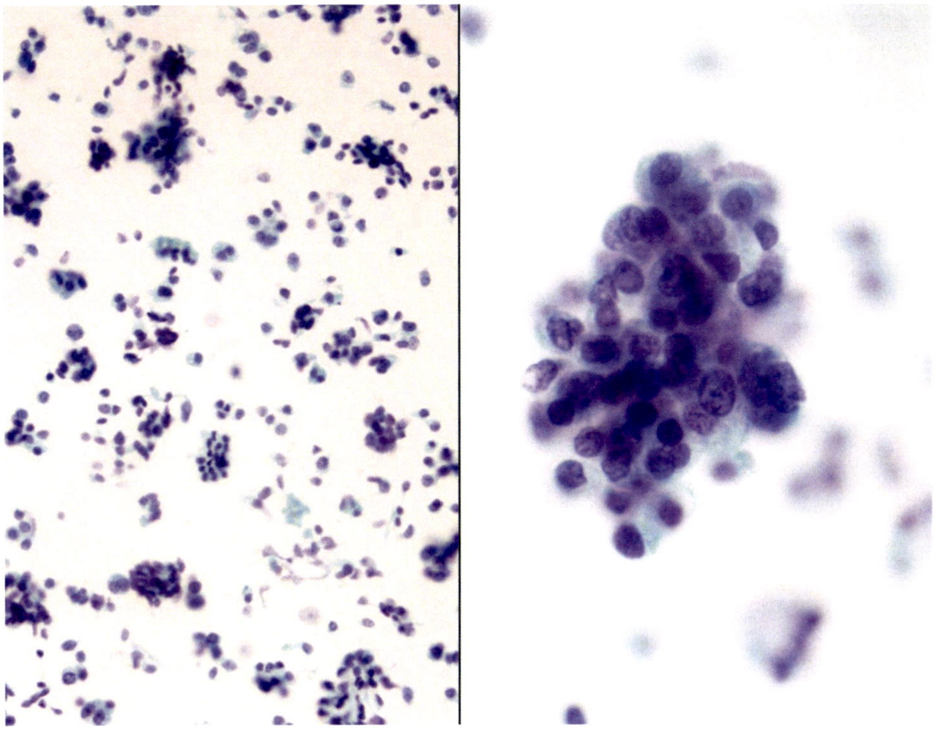

Q-20. A biliary tree brushing was performed on a patient with abdominal pain. What is the diagnosis of this brushing specimen?

(a) Adenocarcinoma
(b) Poorly differentiated squamous cell carcinoma
(c) Reactive glandular cells
(d) Carcinoid

Fig. 9.21

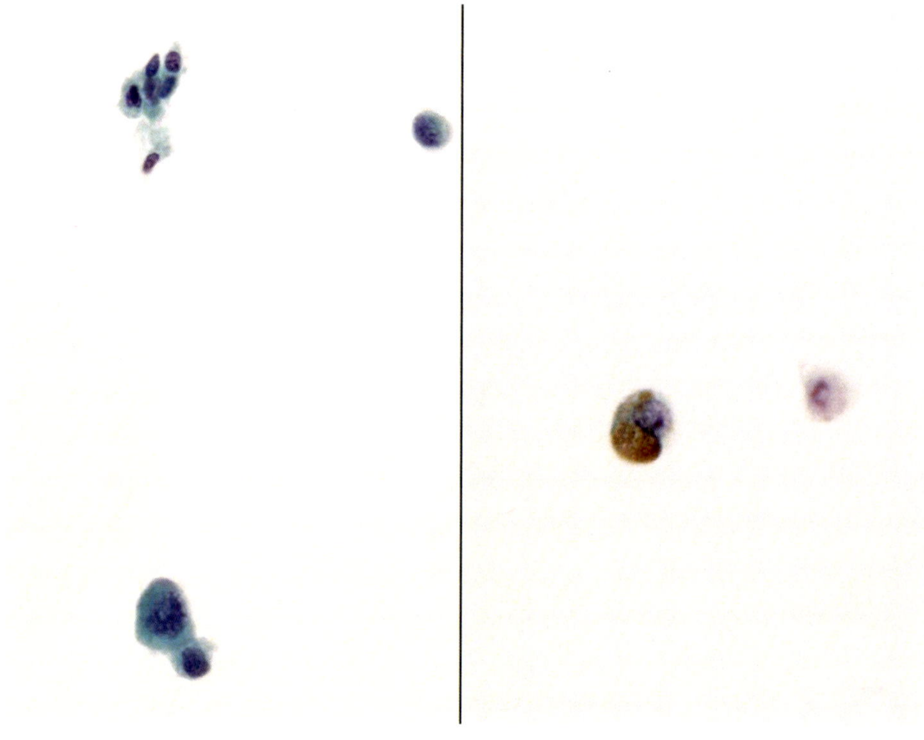

Q-21. A 54-year-old female presented with jaundice and abdominal pain. A biliary tree brushing was performed. What is the diagnosis of this brushing specimen?

(a) Carcinoid
(b) Lymphoma
(c) Melanoma
(d) Adenocarcinoma

Fig. 9.22

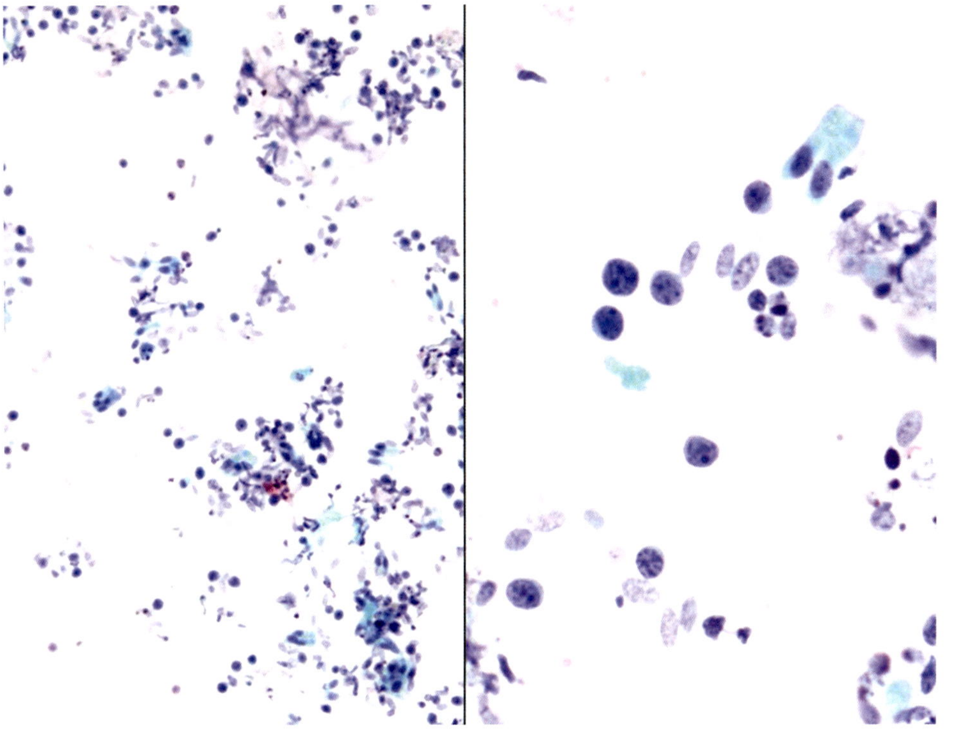

Q-22. A 60-year-old male patient presented with abdominal pain, jaundice, and retroperitoneal lymphadenopathy. An endoscopic ultrasound-guided biliary tree brushing was performed. What is the diagnosis of this brushing specimen?

(a) Adenocarcinoma
(b) Poorly differentiated hepatocellular carcinoma
(c) Lymphoma
(d) Small cell carcinoma

Fig. 9.23

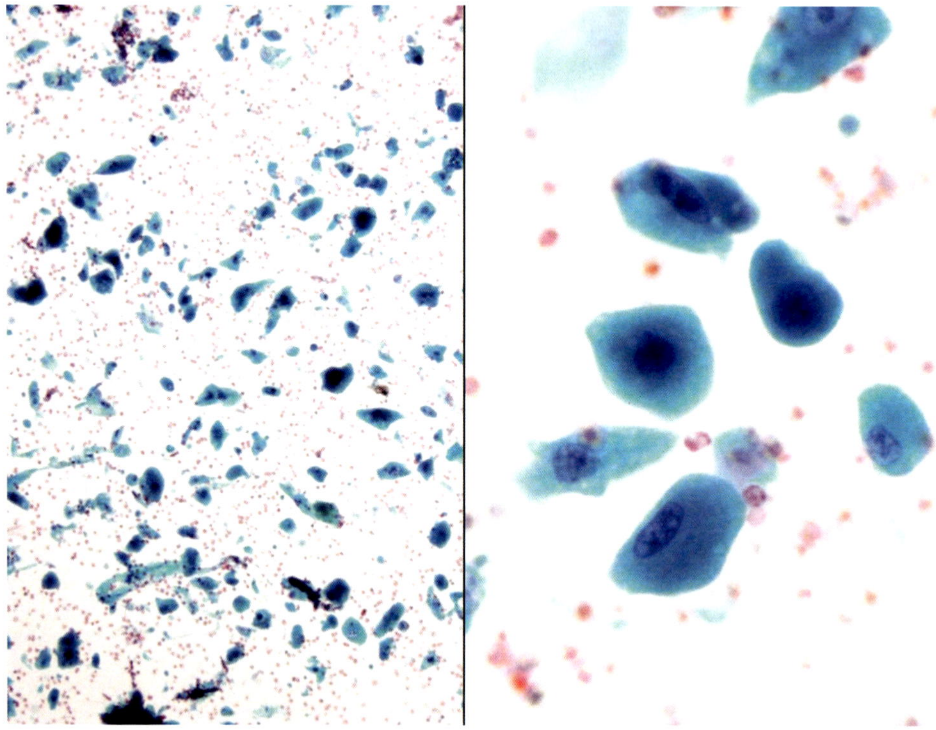

Q-23. A 78-year-old male patient presented with abdominal pain and jaundice. An endoscopic ultrasound-guided biliary tree brushing was performed. What is the diagnosis of this brushing specimen?

(a) Adenocarcinoma
(b) Hepatocellular carcinoma (HCC)
(c) Diffuse large B cell lymphoma (DLBCL)
(d) Melanoma

Fig. 9.24

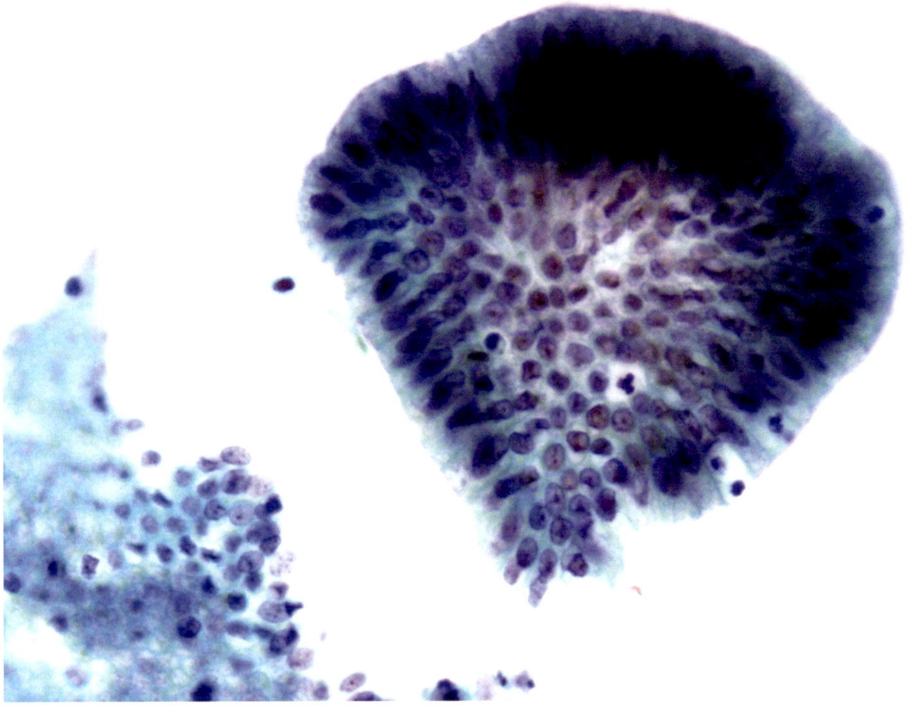

Q-24. A 64-year-old female with abdominal pain and diarrhea had a colon brushing. What is the diagnosis of this brushing specimen?

(a) Adenocarcinoma
(b) Poorly differentiated carcinoma
(c) Benign glandular cells
(d) Carcinoid

Fig. 9.25

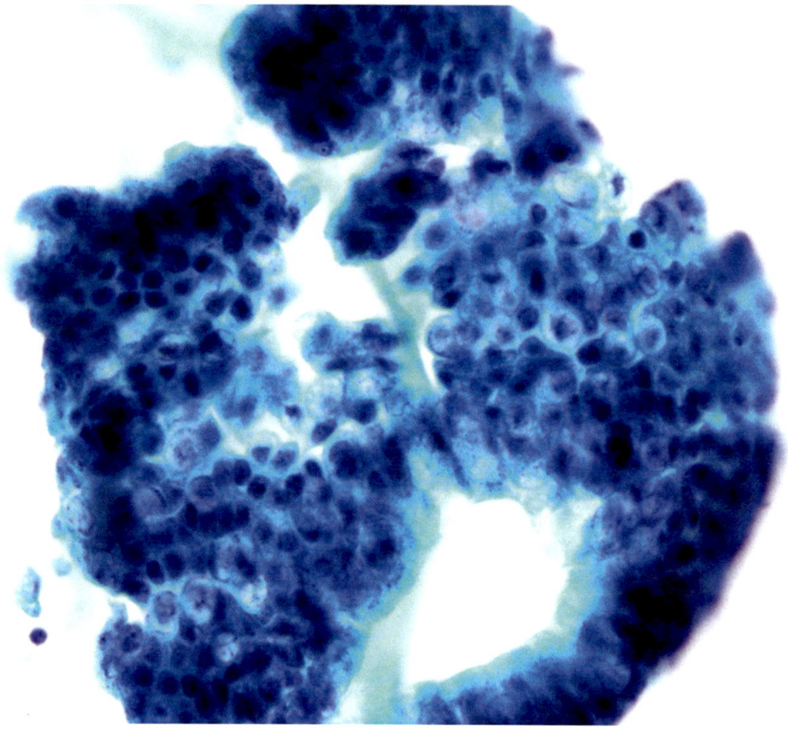

Q-25. A 72-year-old patient with a history of colonic adenocarcinoma and surgical resection of the tumor now presented with diarrhea. A colon brushing was performed. What is the diagnosis of this brushing specimen?

(a) Adenocarcinoma
(b) Small cell carcinoma
(c) Reactive glandular cells
(d) Carcinoid

Fig. 9.26

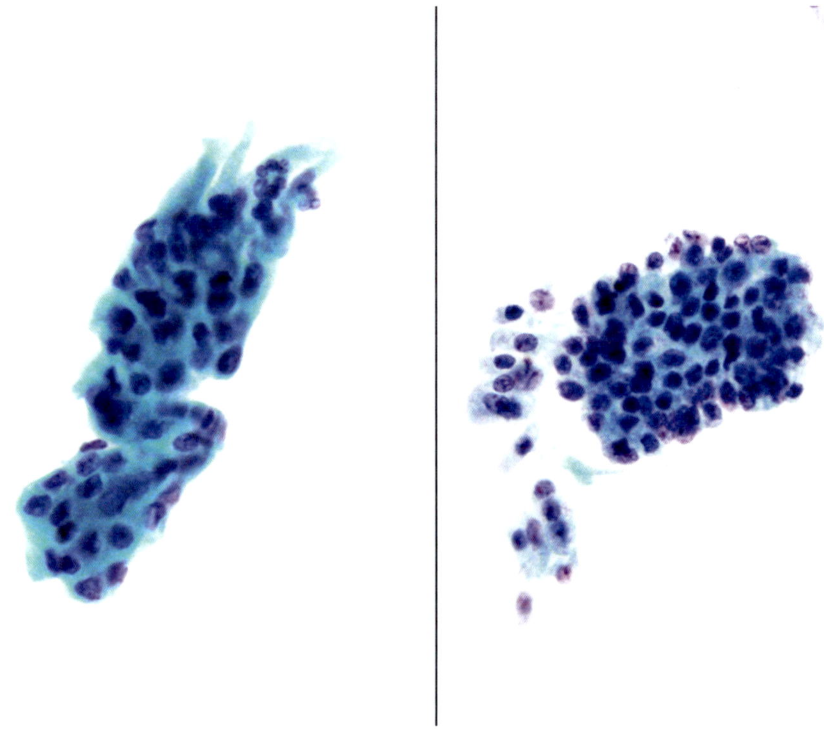

Q-26. A 42-year-old patient had a history of chronic diarrhea, and a colon brushing was performed. What is the diagnosis of this brushing specimen?

(a) Adenocarcinoma
(b) Small cell carcinoma
(c) Reactive glandular cells
(d) Carcinoid

Fig. 9.27

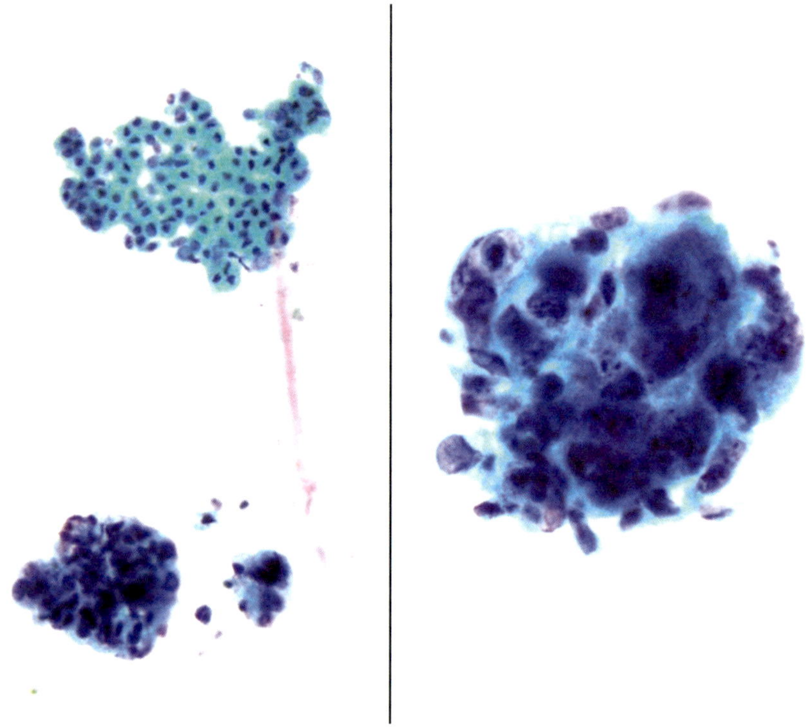

Q-27. A colon brushing was performed on a patient with a history of ulcerative colitis, now developed multiple liver nodules. What is the diagnosis of this colon brushing?

(a) Adenoma
(b) Adenocarcinoma
(c) Reactive glandular cells
(d) Ulcerative colitis

Fig. 9.28

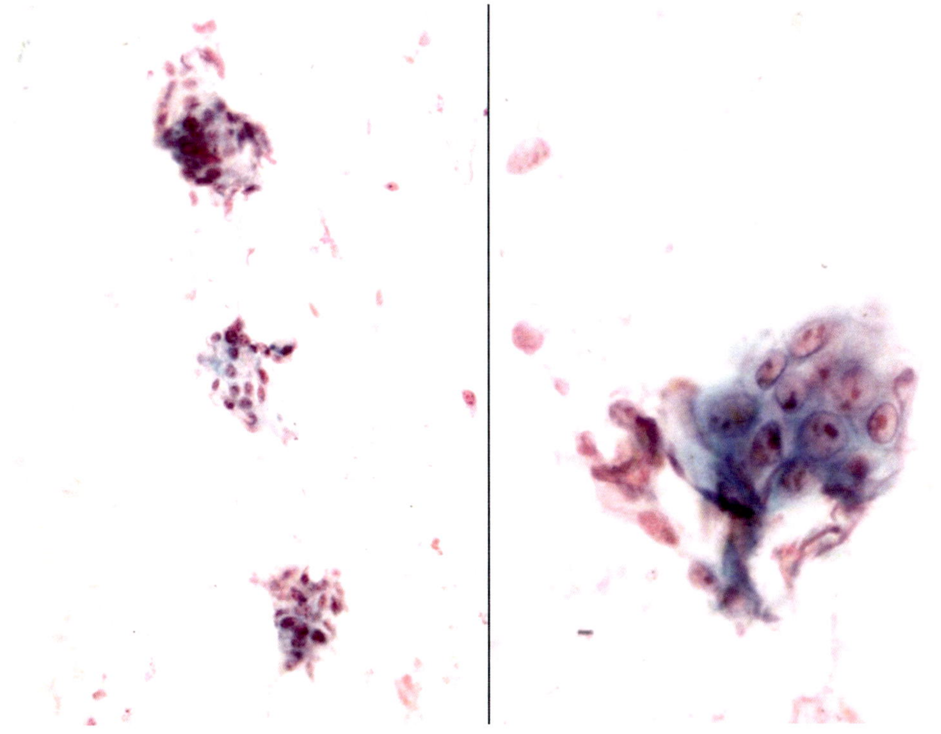

Q-28. A colon brushing was performed on a patient with a history of diarrhea. What is the diagnosis of this colon brushing?

(a) Adenoma
(b) Adenocarcinoma
(c) Reactive glandular cells
(d) Ulcerative colitis

Fig. 9.29

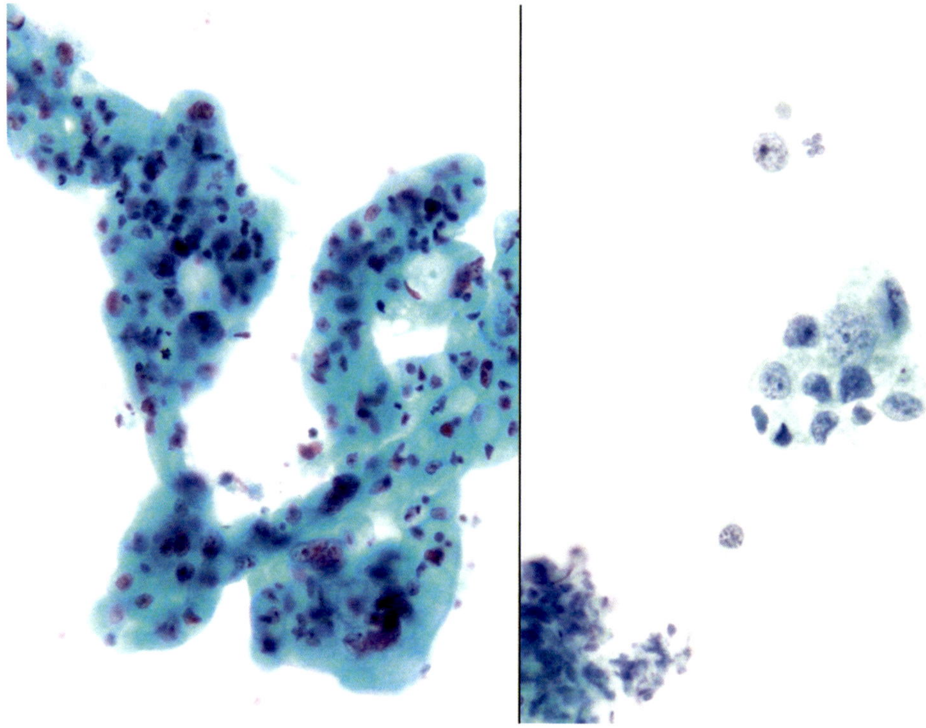

Q-29. A 57-year-old patient presented with stomach pain and bleeding; an upper GI endoscopy revealed a gastric ulcer. A gastric brushing was performed. What is the diagnosis of this cytological specimen?
(a) Adenocarcinoma
(b) Poorly differentiated squamous cell carcinoma
(c) Reactive gastric mucosa
(d) Gastric mucosa with reactive changes consistent with a benign gastric ulcer

Fig. 9.30

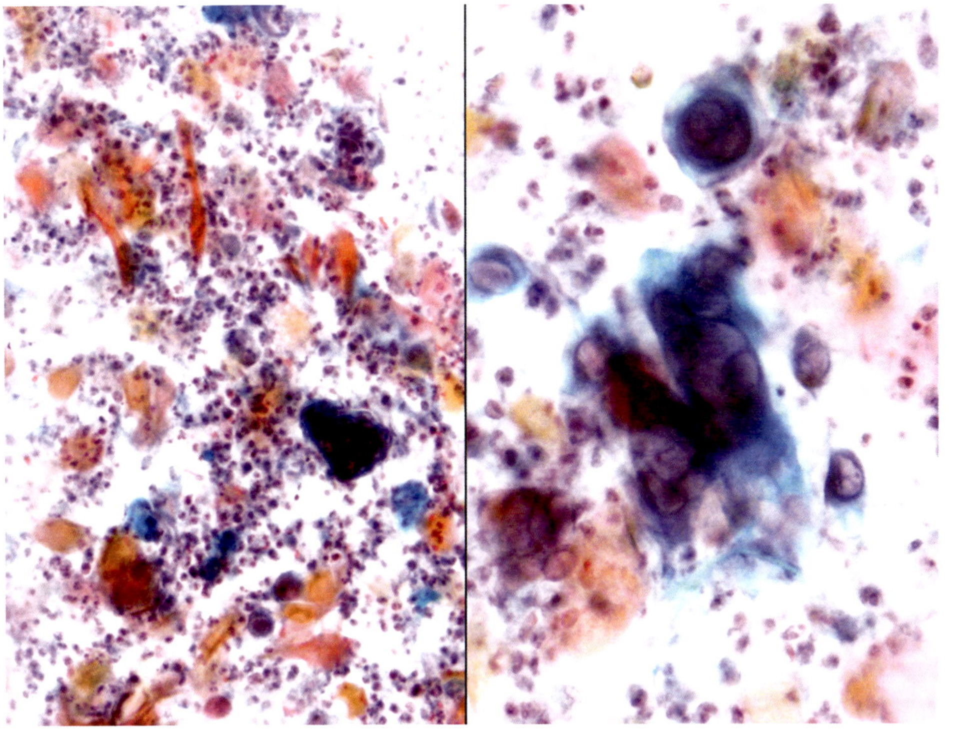

Q-30. A 30-year-old female presented with severe rectal pain and bleeding, who underwent a rectal brushing. What is the diagnosis of this cytological specimen?
(a) Adenocarcinoma
(b) Squamous cell carcinoma
(c) Cytomegalovirus (CMV) infection
(d) Herpes simplex virus (HSV) infection

Fig. 9.31

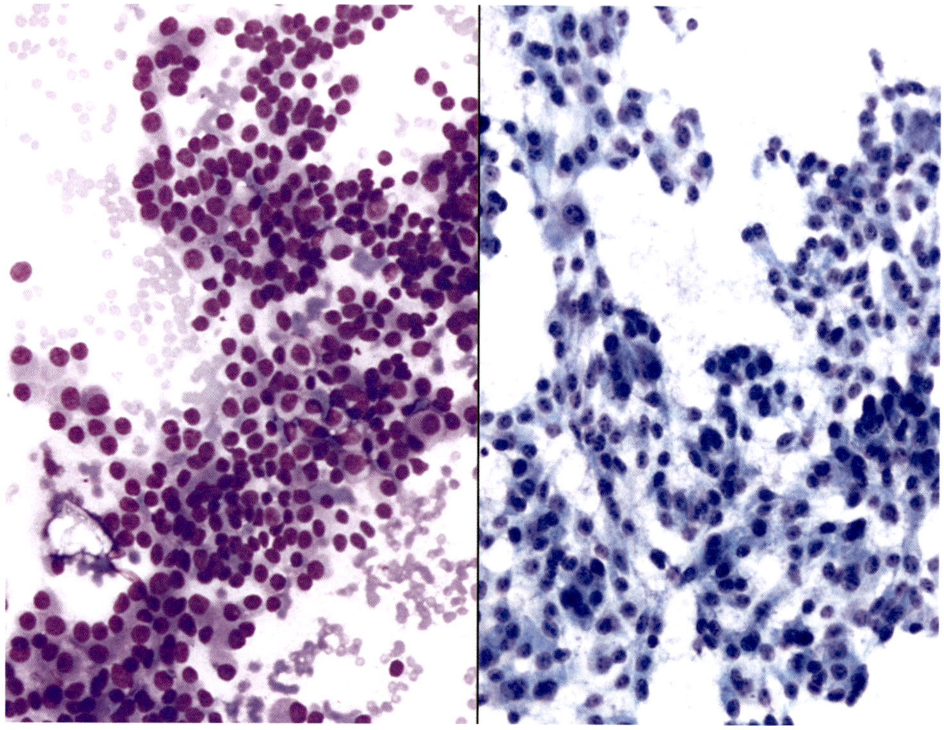

Q-31. A 52-year-old female presented with severe rectal pain and underwent a rectal brushing. What is the diagnosis of this cytological specimen?
(a) Adenocarcinoma
(b) Squamous cell carcinoma
(c) Carcinoid
(d) Small cell carcinoma

9.2 Text-Based Questions 32–61

Q-32. All features are seen in reactive/reparative squamous cells on an esophageal brushing EXCEPT:
(a) Irregular nuclear membrane and coarse chromatin
(b) Small centrally located nucleoli
(c) Streaming pattern of cellular arrangement
(d) Mild enlargement of nuclei

Q-33. All features are seen in benign gastric mucous glandular cells on an endoscopic gastric brushing specimen EXCEPT:
(a) Granular chromatin and inconspicuous nucleoli
(b) Sheets or two-dimensional cluster of glandular cells
(c) Tight three-dimensional cluster of glandular cells with dark nuclei
(d) Abundant cytoplasm with vacuolization

Q-34. On an endoscopic ultrasound-guided esophagus-gastric fine-needle aspiration (FNA) specimen, which feature is best seen in an adenocarcinoma of the esophagus-gastric junction rather than in a reactive glandular atypia?
(a) Enlarged nuclei and prominent nucleoli
(b) Sheets or two-dimensional cluster of glandular cells
(c) Hyperchromatic nuclei with irregular nuclear membrane
(d) Abundant cytoplasm with vacuolization

Q-35. Which feature is not seen in radiation- and chemotherapy-induced glandular cell changes?
(a) Prominent nucleoli
(b) Multinucleation and a vesicular chromatin pattern
(c) Hyperchromatic nuclei and clumped chromatin
(d) Cytomegaly with proportional nuclear enlargement

Q-36. A 49-year-old male had a routine lower gastrointestinal endoscopy; and a small sessile submucosal mass was found in the rectum; an endoscopic ultrasound-guided FNA of the mass was performed. Tumor cells revealed plasmacytoid appearances and were arranged in cords and nests, with relatively uniform nuclei, fine chromatin, and inconspicuous nucleoli. Neither mitosis nor tumor necrosis was identified. Which panel of IHC markers will help you to confirm the diagnosis?
(a) CK7, CK20, and mucin stain
(b) Synaptophysin, chromogranin, and CD56
(c) C-kit and CD34
(d) P63, P40, and CK5/CK6

Q-37. Cytological features of a carcinoid include all of following EXCEPT:
(a) Cords, nests, and rosette of intermediate-sized tumor cells
(b) Fine chromatin and small or inconspicuous nucleoli
(c) Coarse chromatin and large prominent nucleoli
(d) Uniform cells and occasional pleomorphic cells

Q-38. A 67-year-old male presented with stomach pain and abdominal discomfort. CT scan revealed a submucosal mass in the stomach. Subsequently, ultrasound-guided endoscopic FNA was performed. The diagnosis of gastrointestinal stromal tumor (GIST) was made. Which statement regarding GIST is TRUE?
(a) Most GISTs are benign tumors.
(b) Spindle-shaped or epithelioid tumor cells with bland nuclei.
(c) The presence of spindle cells and fat with or without prominent vessels are characteristics of the tumor.
(d) CD117 is the only marker for GIST.

Q-39. Which one of the following tumor is most easily confused with a GIST?
(a) Metastatic spindle cell carcinoma
(b) Metastatic melanoma
(c) Leiomyosarcoma
(d) Spindle cell carcinoid

Q-40. Which statement regarding herpes simplex virus (HSV) infection is CORRECT?
(a) Intranuclear Cowdry B body
(b) Large single basophilic intranuclear inclusion
(c) Multinucleation
(d) Perinuclear halo

Q-41. All of following features are seen in a bile duct brushing specimen from the patient with a biliary stent EXCEPT:
(a) Prominent nucleoli and a vesicular chromatin pattern
(b) Cohesive sheets of cells with streaming pattern
(c) Hyperchromatic nuclei, clumped chromatin, and irregular nuclear membrane
(d) Coarse chromatin and large prominent nucleoli

Q-42. Which statement regarding endoscopic ultrasound-guided fine-needle aspiration (EUS-FNA) is NOT correct?
(a) EUS-FNA can be used for the evaluation of intra-abdominal and intrathoracic lesions.

(b) EUS-FNA can be used for staging of lung cancer.
(c) EUS-FNA is particularly helpful in identifying the origin of the lesion.
(d) EUS-FNA biopsy has similar accuracy as endoscopic mucosal forceps biopsy for submucosal lesions.

Q-43. A 59-year-old male presented with abdominal pain and weight loss. A gastric endoscopy revealed thickened gastric folds. FNA was performed and showed monomorphic population of small- to intermediate-sized lymphocytes. Which statement is INCORRECT?
(a) The mucosa-associated lymphoid tissue (MALT) lymphoma is also called extranodal marginal zone B cell lymphoma.
(b) MALT lymphoma (MALToma) reveals monomorphic population of small- to intermediate-sized lymphocytes.
(c) The presence of plasma cells is a helpful feature for MALT.
(d) The lymphoma is caused by the clonal expansion of subpopulations of T cells.

Q-44. In an FNA specimen, which one of the following features favors the diagnosis of a MALT lymphoma rather than a carcinoid?
(a) Numerous clusters of cells
(b) Monomorphic population of cells
(c) Lymphoglandular bodies
(d) Fine (salt-and-pepper) chromatin and inconspicuous nucleoli

Q-45. In an FNA specimen, which one of the following features favors the diagnosis of a poorly differentiated adenocarcinoma over a diffuse large B cell lymphoma (DLBCL)?
(a) Three-dimensional clusters of atypical cells.
(b) Dispersed individual large atypical cells.
(c) Large cells have round or markedly atypical nuclei with multiple nucleoli and scant cytoplasm.
(d) Large cells have bizarre or pleomorphic nuclei with multinucleation and prominent nucleoli.

Q-46. All cytological features of benign bile ductal epithelial cells on a brushing specimen are correct EXCEPT:
(a) Vesicular chromatin and smooth nuclear membrane
(b) Hyperchromatic nuclei and irregular nuclear membrane
(c) Honeycomb arrangement of glandular cells
(d) Small or inconspicuous nucleoli

Q-47. In addition to chemo- and radiation therapy, which one of the following is the most common cause of bile ductal reactive atypia?
(a) HSV infection
(b) Biliary stent
(c) Tuberculosis
(d) CMV infection

Q-48. An upper GI EUS-FNA was performed on a 72-year-old male smoker who presented with abdominal pain, weight loss, and right pleural effusion. On the cytological preparation, tight clusters and dispersed individual atypical epithelioid cells are identified and reveal "signet ring" cell features. What is the diagnosis of the EUS-FNA?
(a) Metastatic adenocarcinoma of the colon
(b) Metastatic adenocarcinoma of the lung
(c) Signet ring cell carcinoma
(d) Reactive histiocytes

Q-49. Which of the following cytological feature is most useful in the separation of a metastatic poorly differentiated adenocarcinoma from a metastatic small cell carcinoma in esophageal FNA specimen?
(a) Prominent nucleoli
(b) Fine or coarse chromatin pattern
(c) Tumor necrosis
(d) Organoid and/or rosette arrangement of tumor cells

Q-50. A colon brushing was performed on a patient with a history of ulcerative colitis, who now developed multiple liver nodules. On the cytological preparation, it revealed three-dimensional clusters of tall columnar cells with hyperchromatic nuclei, coarse chromatin, prominent nucleoli, irregular nuclear membrane and feathering cytoplasm, and a background of necrotic debris. What is the most likely diagnosis of this lesion?
(a) Adenoma
(b) Adenocarcinoma
(c) Reactive glandular cells
(d) Ulcerative colitis

Q-51. Cytological features of a carcinoid tumor may include all of following EXCEPT:
(a) Fine (so-called "salt-and-pepper") chromatin pattern
(b) Nuclear molding and crowding
(c) Moderate to scant cytoplasm
(d) Inconspicuous or small nucleoli

Q-52. Which of the features is NOT seen in an esophageal well-differentiated squamous cell carcinoma on a brushing specimen?
(a) Large nuclei with smudgy chromatin
(b) Nuclei with variation in size and shape
(c) Large prominent nucleoli
(d) Cytokeratin formation

Q-53. A 60-year-old male presented with a diffuse thickening of stomach wall and retroperitoneal lymphadenopathy. An ultrasound-guided FNA of the stomach was performed. On cytology smear and cell block section, numerous dyscohesive small- to intermediate-sized cells with coarse chromatin and scant cytoplasm are identified. What is the likely diagnosis of the FNA?
(a) Carcinoid
(b) Poorly differentiated carcinoma
(c) Lymphoma
(d) Small cell carcinoma

Q-54. Which of the features is NOT seen in an esophageal poorly differentiated squamous cell carcinoma on an FNA specimen?
(a) Large nuclei with smudgy chromatin
(b) Nuclei with variation in size and shape
(c) Pyknotic nuclei
(d) Large prominent nucleoli

Q-55. All features are seen in Barrett with low-grade dysplasia EXCEPT:
(a) Elongated nuclei with vesicular chromatin
(b) Nuclei with mild variation in size and shape
(c) Crowed clusters of glandular cells with stratification
(d) Hyperchromatic nuclei, prominent nucleoli, and coarse chromatin

Q-56. A gastric brushing from a 2.0 cm ulcer reveals a cellular specimen with loosely cohesive glandular cells and a markedly inflamed background. In addition, scattered clusters and dispersed individual large cells with enlarged hyperchromatic nuclei, coarse chromatin, and irregular nuclear membrane are identified. What is the likely diagnosis?
(a) Suspicious for an adenocarcinoma
(b) Melanoma
(c) Gastritis
(d) Reactive atypia

Q-57. The most useful feature to separate Barrett with low-grade dysplasia from a high-grade dysplasia is
(a) Elongated nuclei with vesicular chromatin
(b) Nuclei with mild variation in size and shape
(c) Crowded clusters of glandular cells with stratification
(d) Hyperchromatic nuclei, prominent nucleoli, and coarse chromatin

Q-58. In a patient with Barrett's esophagus, the brushing specimen reveals loosely cohesive and occasional single glandular cells with markedly enlarged hyperchromatic nuclei, coarse chromatin, prominent nucleoli, and irregular nuclear membrane. What is the most likely diagnosis?
(a) Barrett with low-grade dysplasia
(b) Barrett without dysplasia
(c) Lymphoma
(d) Barrett with a high-grade dysplasia, suspicious for adenocarcinoma

Q-59. A HIV-positive patient had an esophageal ulcer. Esophageal brushing was performed. On cytological preparations, scattered epithelial cells with large single basophilic intranuclear inclusions are identified. What is the most likely diagnosis?
(a) Melanoma
(b) Poorly differentiated carcinoma
(c) Cytomegalovirus (CMV) infection
(d) Herpes simplex virus (HSV) infection

Q-60. A patient has an esophageal ulcer. On an esophageal brushing specimen, all features are seen in reactive epithelial atypia EXCEPT:
(a) Elongated nuclei with vesicular chromatin
(b) Hyperchromatic nuclei, coarse chromatin, and irregular nuclear membrane
(c) Nuclei with mild variation in size and shape
(d) Crowded clusters of cells with streaming pattern

Q-61. In a biliary brush specimen, which one of the following features is the most useful one in the separation of a hepatocellular carcinoma from an adenocarcinoma?
(a) Numerous large clusters of cells
(b) Lacunae spaces on cell block preparation
(c) Presence of "second population" cells
(d) Dispersed large polygonal cells with large nuclei, hyperchromatic chromatin, prominent nucleoli, and dense granular cytoplasm

9.3 Answers and Discussion of Image-Based Questions 1–31

A-1. **(b) Barrett esophagus**
In Barrett esophagus, the specimen reveals sheets and clusters of well-organized glandular cells with dispersed goblet cells. The presence of many goblet cells gives rise to a Swiss appearance on the honeycomb sheet of glandular cells. Goblet cells are characterized by a single large cytoplasmic vacuole and peripherally located nuclei. The cytoplasmic mucin reveals blue to clear color with Papanicolaou stain. There is no dysplasia identified in this specimen. In reactive/reparative changes, glandular cells reveal slightly enlarged nuclei with vesicular chromatin and prominent nucleoli; and cells are arranged in sheets with "streaming" pattern and occasional single cells. There are no goblet cells identified. In reactive/regenerative cells, nuclei is slightly enlarged, but the N:C ratio is preserved. Nuclei show evenly distributed chromatin, regular nuclear membrane, and small nucleoli. In contrast, in adenocarcinomas, tumor cells are arranged in three-dimensional clusters and dispersed individual cells with hyperchromatic large nuclei, coarse chromatin, and irregular nuclear membrane. In a poorly differentiated adenocarcinoma, tumor cells are arranged predominately in single cells.

A-2. **(a) Adenocarcinoma**
In adenocarcinomas, tumor cells form three-dimensional clusters, acinar arrangements, and dispersed individual cells with high N:C ratio, hyperchromatic or vesicular nuclei, coarse chromatin, irregular nuclear membrane, and prominent nucleoli. Nuclear overlapping and variation in size are prominent. Tumor necrosis may be also seen on the slide. In reactive glandular atypia, cells are arranged in sheets and/or two-dimensional clusters with streaming pattern; cells reveal slightly enlarged nuclei, finely granular chromatin, regular and smooth nuclear membrane, and small prominent nucleoli. Although the nuclei is bigger, the normal N:C ratio is maintained. Reactive glandular cells may lose the polarity, but no markedly nuclear overlapping and pleomorphism are seen. Cytoplasmic vacuoles are seen in both adenocarcinoma and reactive glandular cells. Tumor cells of squamous cell carcinomas have hyperchromatic nuclei, smudgy chromatin, dense cytoplasm, and cytokeratin formation.

A-3. **(d) Herpes simplex virus (HSV) infection**
In HSV infection, cells reveal multinucleation, nuclear molding, ground-glass chromatin, and margination of chromatin in nuclei. Cowdry A bodies may also be present, which are eosinophilic nuclear inclusions composed of nucleic acid and protein seen in cells infected with HSV. The differential diagnosis is cytomegalovirus (CMV) infection. In CMV infection, large single basophilic intranuclear inclusions and perinuclear halos are characteristics of CMV infected cells.

A-4. **(c) Squamous cell carcinoma**
The diagnosis is squamous cell carcinoma. Tumor cells of squamous cell carcinomas form loosely clusters or dispersed individual cells with hyperchromatic nuclei, smudgy chromatin, dense cytoplasm, and cytokeratin formation. In a well-differentiated tumor, numerous spindle-shaped malignant cells with prominent cytoplasmic keratin are identified. Cytokeratin stains purple to blue color with Diff-Quik method and orangeophilic with Papanicolaou method. In reactive/reparative changes, squamous cells reveal slightly enlarged nuclei with vesicular chromatin and small nucleoli; and cells are arranged in sheets with "streaming" pattern; the normal N:C ratio is maintained. In adenocarcinomas, tumor cells are arranged in tight three-dimensional clusters. Tumor cells of adenocarcinomas have hyperchromatic nuclei, coarse chromatin, prominent nucleoli, and vacuolated cytoplasm (indicative of mucin production). In Barrett, both glandular cells and goblet cells are identified, and cells have normal N:C ratio and have no significant nuclear atypia.

A-5. **(c) Squamous cell carcinoma**
In squamous cell carcinomas, tumor cells form loosely clusters or dispersed individual cells with hyperchromatic nuclei, smudgy chromatin, dense cytoplasm, and cytokeratin formation. In a well-differentiated tumor, numerous spindle-shaped malignant cells with prominent cytoplasmic cytokeratin are identified. However, in a poorly differentiated squamous cell carcinoma, tumor cells may be arranged in clusters and round up with prominent nucleoli and less or no cytokeratin formation. These features of a poorly differentiated squamous cell carcinoma can be confused with adenocarcinoma. In adenocarcinomas, tumor cells are arranged in tight three-dimensional clusters and have hyperchromatic nuclei, coarse chromatin, prominent nucleoli, and vacuolated cytoplasm (indicative of mucin production). In reactive/reparative changes, squamous cells reveal slightly enlarged nuclei with vesicular chromatin and small nucleoli; cells are arranged in sheets with "streaming" pattern; the normal N:C ratio is maintained.

In Barrett, both glandular cells and goblet cells are identified, and cells reveal normal N:C ratio and have no significant nuclear atypia.

A-6. (c) **Benign-appearing gastric mucosa**
The diagnosis is benign-appearing gastric mucosa. A gastric brushing specimen usually contains numerous gastric glandular cells. The benign gastric glandular cells are arranged in honeycomb sheets or two-dimensional clusters with bland basal nuclei and abundant apical mucin characteristic of a polarized appearance. Polarized glandular cells are best seen at peripheral area of cellular arrangements. Cells reveal oval nuclei, smooth nuclear membrane, inconspicuous nucleoli, normal N:C ratio, and absence of nuclear overlapping. Occasionally, goblet cells may be identified in cellular arrangements, indicative of either intestinal metaplasia or duodenal mucosa. In adenocarcinomas, tumor cells are arranged in tight three-dimensional clusters and have hyperchromatic nuclei, coarse chromatin, prominent nucleoli, vacuolated cytoplasm (indicative of mucin production), and a high N:C ratio. In reactive/reparative atypia, cells reveal slightly enlarged nuclei with vesicular chromatin and small nucleoli; cells are arranged in sheets with "streaming" pattern; the normal N:C ratio is maintained.

A-7. (d) **Gastric mucosa with reactive changes**
The diagnosis is gastric mucosa with reactive changes. In reactive cellular changes, cells reveal a mild to moderate atypia. Cytological features include sheets and/or loose cluster of epithelial cells with elongated/enlarged nuclei, single or multiple small nucleoli, and mild nuclear atypia; cells are still arranged in an orderly fashion with a streaming appearance. No significant nuclear atypia is seen. N:C ratio is normal in reactive cells. In contrast, in adenocarcinomas, tumor cells form acini and/or three-dimensional clusters or many dyscohesive individual tumor cells with large hyperchromatic nuclei, coarse chromatin, irregular nuclear membrane, prominent nucleoli, overlapping nuclei, and high N:C ratio. Therefore, careful evaluation of nuclear features is crucial in the differential diagnosis of reactive atypia from adenocarcinomas.

A-8. (d) **Gastric mucosa with reactive changes consistent with a benign gastric ulcer**
The diagnosis is a benign gastric ulcer. The brushing cytology reveals a cellular specimen with sheets and/or loose clusters of glandular cells with enlarged nuclei, single or multiple small nucleoli, finely granular chromatin, and smooth nuclear membrane. Cells are still arranged in an orderly fashion with a streaming appearance. No significant nuclear atypia is seen. Normal N:C ratio is still maintained in cells. In the background of the slides, mixed inflammatory cells and necrotic debris are present. The inflammatory cells are also admixed with sheets of glandular cells. Taken together, all features are consistent with gastric mucosa with reactive changes characteristic of a benign ulcer. In adenocarcinomas, tumor cells form acini and/or three-dimensional clusters or many dyscohesive individual tumor cells with large hyperchromatic nuclei, coarse chromatin, irregular nuclear membrane, prominent nucleoli, overlapping nuclei, and high N:C ratio.

A-9. (a) **Adenocarcinoma**
The diagnosis is adenocarcinoma of the stomach. The slide reveals hyperchromatic clusters of cells with enlarged nuclei. In adenocarcinomas, tumor cells are arranged in three-dimensional clusters, acini and glandular structures, or many dyscohesive individual cells. Tumor cells have large hyperchromatic overlapping nuclei, coarse chromatin, irregular nuclear membrane, prominent nucleoli, vacuolated cytoplasm, and high N:C ratio. In reactive cellular changes, cell reveals sheets and/or loose clusters of glandular cells with mild to moderate enlarged nuclei, single or multiple small nucleoli, finely granular chromatin, and smooth nuclear membrane. Cells are still arranged in an orderly fashion with a streaming appearance. No significant nuclear atypia is seen. Normal N:C ratio is still maintained in cells. In squamous cell carcinomas, tumor cells form loosely clusters or dispersed individual cells with hyperchromatic nuclei, smudgy chromatin, dense cytoplasm, and cytokeratin formation.

A-10. (c) **Signet ring cell carcinoma of the stomach**
In signet ring cell carcinoma of the stomach, tumor cells are arranged in small clusters or dispersed individual cells with large cytoplasmic vacuoles (mucin) that push the nuclei to eccentric location (signet ring appearance). The nuclei are large with hyperchromasia, coarse chromatin, and irregular nuclear membrane. Histiocytes and macrophages may reveal signet ring cell features; however, no nuclear atypia is identified in these cells. Several other carcinomas may reveal "signet ring" cell morphology, such as some variants of breast and lung carcinomas, due to the production of cytoplasmic mucin. In adenocarcinomas of the lung, tumor cells form large three-dimensional clusters and reveal a variety of cytomorphologies; tumor cells have hyperchromatic

nuclei, prominent nucleoli, and vacuolated cytoplasm. In breast carcinomas, the size of tumor cells is smaller than that of GI carcinomas; tumor cells are arranged in tight three-dimensional clusters or acini with coarse chromatin, prominent nucleoli, and scant cytoplasm. In difficult cases, IHC stains of lung markers (TTF1 and napsin A) and breast markers (ER, PR, and GATA3) may help for the differential diagnosis.

A-11. (d) **Diffuse large B cell lymphoma** (**DLBCL**)
In DLBCL, the cytological specimen, including brushing, reveals dyscohesive large atypical lymphoid cells. Within atypical lymphoid cells, three variants are most commonly seen: centroblastic, immunoblastic, and anaplastic variant. Centroblastic variant is the most common subtype and reveals medium- to large-sized tumor cells with high N:C ratio, oval or round nuclei, fine chromatin, and single or multiple prominent nucleoli. Immunoblasts have a basophilic cytoplasm and a central nucleolus. The third morphologic variant, anaplastic variant, consists of large tumor cells with pleomorphic nuclei and may resemble Hodgkin cells (Reed-Sternberg cells). Most cases of DLBCL are polymorphic, with a mixture of centroblastic and immunoblastic cells. DLBLC is a good mimic of a poorly differentiated adenocarcinoma. In poorly differentiated adenocarcinomas, tumor cells can be dyscohesive and presented as dispersed individual cells or form three-dimensional clusters with large hyperchromatic nuclei, coarse chromatin, irregular nuclear membrane, prominent nucleoli, and vacuolated cytoplasm. Careful examination of the cytomorphology of tumor cells helps with the differential diagnosis. In difficult cases, IHC stains of epithelial markers (AE1/AE3, CAM5.2, and others) and lymphoid markers (CD45, CD20, BCL2, BCL6, and others) can help with the differential diagnosis.

A-12. (d) **Vegetable cells**
The slide reveals sheets of rectangular-shaped, uniform cells with cellulose wall. These cells have large nuclei, resembling tumor cells of squamous cell carcinomas. In squamous cell carcinomas, tumor cells form loosely clusters or dispersed individual cells with hyperchromatic nuclei, smudgy chromatin, dense cytoplasm, and cytokeratin formation. Cytokeratin stains purple to blue color with Diff-Quik method and orangeophilic with Papanicolaou method. In adenocarcinomas, tumor cells are arranged in tight three-dimensional clusters or dispersed individual cells with hyperchromatic nuclei, coarse chromatin, prominent nucleoli, irregular nuclear membrane, and vacuolated cytoplasm (indicative of mucin production). The N:C ratio of cells is high. In reactive cellular changes, it reveals sheets and/or loose clusters of glandular cells with enlarged nuclei, single or multiple small nucleoli, finely granular chromatin, and smooth nuclear membrane. Cells are still arranged in an orderly fashion with a streaming appearance. No significant nuclear atypia is seen. Normal N:C ratio is still maintained in cells.

A-13. (d) **Gastrointestinal stromal tumor** (**GIST**)
The diagnosis is GIST. GIST is the most common mesenchymal tumor of the gastrointestinal tract, representing 1–3 % of all gastrointestinal malignancies. The majority of GISTs present at ages 50–70 years. The cytological features of GIST reveal sheets or loosely formed clusters of spindle or epithelioid cells with oval or bipolar nuclei, granular chromatin, inconspicuous nucleoli, wispy cytoplasm, and long extension. Most GISTs (70–80 %) have spindle cell appearance; and the rest of them have either epithelioid appearance or a combined appearance. IHC of tumor cells are positive for CD117 and CD34. If the CD117 stain is negative in a GIST, the newer antibody DOG-1 (discovered on GIST-1) can be used. Also sequencing of *Kit* and *PDGFRA* gene may be used to prove the diagnosis. The differential diagnosis of a spindle cell lesion in FNA cytology is broad, including spindle cell carcinoma, leiomyoma, leiomyosarcoma, melanoma, nerve tumors, fibrous tumors, and others. The leiomyosarcoma is easily confused with a GIST. In a leiomyosarcoma, tumor cells have "cigar-shaped" nuclei and finely granular cytoplasm. Naked nuclei and increased mitosis are also commonly seen in the tumor. IHC stains of tumor cells are positive for desmin and myogenin. In spindle cell carcinomas, tumor cells form clusters with large hyperchromatic nuclei, coarse chromatin, irregular nuclear membrane, prominent nucleoli, and scant cytoplasm. Stains of cytokeratin are positive for tumor cells.

A-14. (c) **Adenoma**
The slides reveal sheets and two-dimensional clusters of glandular cells with slightly enlarged nuclei, single small nucleoli, evenly distributed chromatin, and smooth nuclear membrane. Cells are arranged in an orderly fashion and have normal N:C ratio. These features in conjunction with the clinical finding of a polypoid lesion are consistent with an adenoma. In adenocarcinomas, tumor cells are arranged in tight three-dimensional clusters or dispersed individual cells with large hyperchromatic nuclei, coarse chromatin, prominent nucleoli, irregular nuclear

membrane, vacuolated cytoplasm (indicative of mucin production), and high N:C ratio. Cytological features of a carcinoid tumor reveal a cellular specimen forming cords, nests, and rosette-like structures. Tumor cells are intermediate in size with relatively uniform nuclei, fine (salt-and-pepper) chromatin, and small or inconspicuous nucleoli.

A-15. (c) **Reactive glandular cells**

The slide reveals small clusters and/or honeycomb sheets of cohesive uniform cells with round to ovoid nuclei, dark granular chromatin, inconspicuous or occasional small nucleoli, and scant cytoplasm. In some of the cellular arrangements, they reveal slightly enlarged nuclei with vesicular chromatin, small nucleoli, smoother nuclear membrane, and normal N:C ratio. Although nuclear overlapping and mild nuclear disarray are common findings (mimicking adenocarcinoma), cells are still in an orderly arrangements. In adenocarcinomas and poorly differentiated carcinomas, tumor cells are arranged in three-dimensional clusters or dispersed individual cells with large hyperchromatic nuclei, high N:C ratio, coarse chromatin, prominent nucleoli, and vacuolated cytoplasm. In carcinoids, tumor cells are intermediate in size and form cords, nests, and rosette-like structures with relatively uniform nuclei, fine (salt-and-pepper) chromatin, and small or inconspicuous nucleoli.

A-16. (c) **Reactive glandular cells**

The diagnosis is reactive glandular cells. The biliary stricture and the placement of biliary tree stent are the common causes of bile ductal reactive atypia on a brushing specimen. The slide reveals cohesive groups of glandular cells with slightly enlarged nuclei and nuclear angulations and small or inconspicuous nucleoli. Other features include small clusters and/or sheets of two-dimensional columnar cells with round to ovoid nuclei, dark granular chromatin, inconspicuous or occasional small nucleoli, and scant cytoplasm. Mild nuclear overlapping and nuclear disarray are common findings, mimicking adenocarcinoma. However, the nuclear membrane is smooth and N:C ratio is still in the normal range. The most important differential diagnosis of bile duct brushing from a biliary stent specimen is an adenocarcinoma, particularly a well-differentiated adenocarcinoma. In adenocarcinomas, tumor cells reveal markedly nuclear atypia, hyperchromasia, coarse chromatin, irregular nuclear membrane, prominent nucleoli, and high N:C ratio. Tumor cells are also arranged in tight three-dimensional clusters or dispersed individual tumor cells. Nuclear disorganization and crowding are commonly seen. Dispersed individual tumor cells may be also identified. An increased mitotic activity and necrotic debris (tumor diathesis) in the background may be also suggestive of the diagnosis of adenocarcinoma. In carcinoids, tumor cells are intermediate in size and form cords, nests, and rosette-like structures with relatively uniform nuclei, fine (salt-and-pepper) chromatin, and small or inconspicuous nucleoli.

A-17. (c) **Reactive glandular cells**

Cytological features of radiation- and chemotherapy-induced glandular cell changes include sheets and two-dimensional clusters of cells with cytomegaly; but the nuclei to cytoplasmic ratio is still in a normal range (proportional enlargement of nuclei and cytoplasm). Multinucleation and prominent nucleoli are common. The most important differential diagnosis of radiation- and chemotherapy-induced glandular cell changes is the residual and/or recurrent adenocarcinoma. In adenocarcinomas, tumor cells reveal markedly nuclear atypia, hyperchromasia, coarse chromatin, prominent nucleoli, and high N:C ratio. Tumor cells are also arranged in tight three-dimensional clusters or dispersed individual tumor cells. Hyperchromatic nuclei, clumped chromatin, irregular nuclear membrane, and high N:C ratio are not features seen in reactive atypia, and they are features characteristic of adenocarcinomas. In carcinoids, tumor cells are intermediate in size and form cords, nests, and rosette-like structures with relatively uniform nuclei, fine (salt-and-pepper) chromatin, and small or inconspicuous nucleoli.

A-18. (a) **Adenocarcinoma**

The slide reveals tight clusters and dispersed individual hyperchromatic cells. In adenocarcinomas, tumor cells are arranged in tight three-dimensional clusters or dispersed individual tumor cells with hyperchromatic nuclei, coarse chromatin, prominent nucleoli, irregular nuclear membrane, and high N:C ratio. Markedly nuclear disarray and disorganization are also characteristics of adenocarcinomas. An increased mitotic activity, particularly abnormal mitotic figures, and necrotic debris (tumor diathesis) in the background may be also suggestive of the diagnosis of an adenocarcinoma. Cytological features of reactive glandular cell changes include sheets and two-dimensional clusters of cells with slightly enlarged nuclei, small nucleoli, smooth nuclear membrane, and normal N:C ratio. In carcinoids, tumor cells are intermediate in size and form cords, nests, and rosette-like structures with relatively uniform nuclei, fine (salt-and-pepper) chromatin, and small or inconspicuous nucleoli.

A-19. **(d) Adenocarcinoma**
The slide reveals predominately dispersed individual hyperchromatic cells and loosely formed clusters. In adenocarcinomas, particularly in a poorly differentiated adenocarcinomas, tumor cells are arranged in dispersed individual tumor cells and loose clusters with hyperchromatic nuclei, coarse chromatin, prominent nucleoli, irregular nuclear membrane, vacuolated cytoplasm, and high N:C ratio. Markedly nuclear disarray and disorganization are also characteristic of adenocarcinoma. An increased mitotic activity, particularly abnormal mitotic figures, and necrotic debris (tumor diathesis) in the background may be also suggestive of the diagnosis of an adenocarcinoma. In lymphomas, tumors consist of atypical lymphoid cells with hyperchromatic nuclei, coarse chromatin, irregular nuclear membrane, and scant basophilic cytoplasm. The identification of lymphoglandular bodies in the slide is characteristic for lymphoma. In melanomas, tumor cells reveal plasmacytoid appearance with binucleation and single large nucleoli. Cytoplasmic melanin pigments may be seen.

A-20. **(a) Adenocarcinoma**
The slide reveals tight clusters and dispersed individual hyperchromatic cells. In adenocarcinomas and poorly differentiated carcinomas, tumor cells are arranged in tight three-dimensional clusters or dispersed individual tumor cells with hyperchromatic nuclei, coarse chromatin, prominent nucleoli, irregular nuclear membrane, and high N:C ratio. Markedly nuclear disarray and disorganization are also commonly seen in adenocarcinomas. An increased mitotic activity, particularly abnormal mitotic figures, and necrotic debris (tumor diathesis) in the background may be also suggestive of the diagnosis of adenocarcinoma. Cytological features of reactive glandular cell changes include sheets and two-dimensional clusters of cells with slightly enlarged nuclei, small nucleoli, smooth nuclear membrane, and normal N:C ratio. In carcinoids, tumor cells are intermediate in size and form cords, nests, and rosette-like structures with relatively uniform nuclei, fine (salt-and-pepper) chromatin, and small or inconspicuous nucleoli.

A-21. **(c) Melanoma**
The diagnosis is melanoma. The slide reveals predominately dispersed individual hyperchromatic cells and loosely formed clusters. In melanomas, tumor cells are dyscohesive and form small clusters or dispersed individual cells. Tumor cells are large in size and with a plasmacytoid appearance. Binucleation and multinucleation are common features. Tumor cells also reveal large nuclei with single large nucleoli and cytoplasmic melanin pigment. In adenocarcinomas, tumor cells are arranged in three-dimensional clusters and dispersed individual tumor cells with hyperchromatic nuclei, coarse chromatin, prominent nucleoli, irregular nuclear membrane, vacuolated cytoplasm, and high N:C ratio. In carcinoids, tumor cells are intermediate in size and form cords, nests, and rosette-like structures with relatively uniform nuclei, fine (salt-and-pepper) chromatin, and small or inconspicuous nucleoli. In lymphomas, tumors consist of atypical lymphoid cells with hyperchromatic nuclei, coarse chromatin, irregular nuclear membrane, and scant basophilic cytoplasm. The identification of lymphoglandular bodies in the slide is characteristic for lymphoma.

A-22. **(c) Lymphoma**
The diagnosis is lymphoma. The slides reveal numerous dyscohesive small- to intermediate-sized cells with high N:C ratio, hyperchromatic nuclei, and scant basophilic cytoplasm. The monomorphic appearance of the lesion represents a monoclonal proliferation of lymphoma cells. Other cytological features of lymphoma include hyperchromatic nuclei with clumped (soccer ball-like) chromatin, irregular nuclear membrane, and scant basophilic cytoplasm. Lymphoglandular bodies can also be seen in the background. In adenocarcinomas and poorly differentiated carcinomas, tumor cells are bigger in size and arranged in three-dimensional clusters and dispersed individual tumor cells with hyperchromatic nuclei, coarse chromatin, prominent nucleoli, irregular nuclear membrane, vacuolated cytoplasm, and high N:C ratio. In HCC, it reveals dispersed large polygonal cells with a centrally located large nucleus, hyperchromatic chromatin, prominent nucleoli, dense granular cytoplasm, and numerous naked nuclei. In small cell carcinomas, tumor cells reveal fine (salt-and-pepper) chromatin with nuclear crowding and molding.

A-23. **(b) Hepatocellular carcinoma (HCC)**
The diagnosis is HCC. The slide reveals numerous dispersed large polygonal cells with a centrally located large nucleus, hyperchromatic chromatin, prominent nucleoli, and dense granular cytoplasm. In HCC, tumor cells show a wide range of cytomorphology. In well-differentiated tumors, cells resemble normal hepatocytes; form clusters, trabeculae, cords, and nest; and have a slightly increased N:C ratio, large round nuclei, prominent nucleoli, naked nuclei, and bile pigment in the cytoplasm. In poorly differentiated tumors,

cells are markedly polygonal and dyscohesive with pleomorphic nuclei and giant tumor cells. Tumor cells reveal large nuclei, hyperchromatic chromatin, prominent nucleoli, and dense granular cytoplasm. In adenocarcinomas, tumor cells form three-dimensional clusters with hyperchromatic nuclei, vesicular or coarse chromatin, irregular nuclear membrane, prominent nucleoli, and vacuolated cytoplasm. In DLBCLs, tumors consist of atypical lymphoid cells with hyperchromatic nuclei, coarse chromatin, irregular nuclear membrane, prominent nucleoli, and scant basophilic cytoplasm. In melanomas, tumor cells reveal plasmacytoid appearance with binucleation and single large nucleoli. Cytoplasmic melanin pigment may be seen.

A-24. (c) **Benign glandular cells**
The diagnosis is benign glandular cells. Benign glandular cells appear as small clusters and/or honeycomb sheets of cohesive uniform cells with round to ovoid nuclei, evenly distributed chromatin, inconspicuous or occasional small nucleoli, and abundant cytoplasm. In reactive cells, it reveals elongated nuclei with vesicular chromatin, small nucleoli, smoother nuclear membrane, and normal N:C ratio; and cells are still arranged in an orderly fashion. In adenocarcinomas and poorly differentiated carcinomas, tumor cells form three-dimensional clusters and dispersed individual cells with hyperchromatic nuclei, vesicular or coarse chromatin, irregular nuclear membrane, prominent nucleoli, vacuolated cytoplasm, and high N:C ratio. Tumor necrosis is also present. In carcinoids, tumor cells are intermediate in size and form cords, nests, and rosette-like structures with relatively uniform nuclei, fine (salt-and-pepper) chromatin, and small or inconspicuous nucleoli.

A-25. (c) **Reactive glandular cells**
The diagnosis is reactive glandular cells. Cytological features of reactive glandular cell changes include sheets and two-dimensional clusters of cells with elongated nuclei; but the nucleus to cytoplasmic ratio is still in a normal range. Multinucleation and prominent small nucleoli are common features. The elongated nuclei reveal vesicular chromatin and smoother nuclear membrane; and cells are still arranged in an orderly fashion. In adenocarcinomas, tumor cells reveal tall columnar "picket fence" appearance and are arranged in three-dimensional clusters with markedly nuclear atypia; they have hyperchromatic pencil-shaped nuclei, coarse chromatin, irregular nuclear membrane, and prominent nucleoli. The presence of "dirty" necrosis is usually seen. In carcinoids, tumor cells are intermediate in size and form cords, nests, and rosette-like structures with relatively uniform nuclei, fine (salt-and-pepper) chromatin, and small or inconspicuous nucleoli. In small cell carcinomas, tumor cells reveal fine (salt-and-pepper) chromatin with nuclear crowding and molding.

A-26. (c) **Reactive glandular cells**
The diagnosis is reactive glandular cells. Cytological features of reactive glandular cell changes include sheets and two-dimensional clusters of cells with elongated nuclei; but the nucleus to cytoplasmic ratio is still in a normal range. Multinucleation and prominent small nucleoli are common features. The elongated nuclei reveal vesicular chromatin and smoother nuclear membrane; and cells are still arranged in an orderly fashion. In adenocarcinomas, tumor cells reveal tall columnar "picket fence" appearance and are arranged in three-dimensional clusters with markedly nuclear atypia; they have hyperchromatic pencil-shaped nuclei, coarse chromatin, irregular nuclear membrane, and prominent nucleoli. The presence of "dirty" necrosis is usually seen. In carcinoids, tumor cells are intermediate in size and form cords, nests, and rosette-like structures with relatively uniform nuclei, fine (salt-and-pepper) chromatin, and small or inconspicuous nucleoli. In small cell carcinomas, tumor cell reveals fine (salt-and-pepper) chromatin with nuclear crowding and molding.

A-27. (b) **Adenocarcinoma**
The brushing cytology showed cytological features of a colonic adenocarcinoma, characteristic by three-dimensional clusters of hyperchromatic malignant cells. In patients with inflammatory bowel disease such as ulcerative colitis, long-term surveillance is needed. The distinction between reactive/reparative glandular cells and adenocarcinoma on cytological preparation can be confusing and difficult. In reactive glandular cells, cohesive clusters of stratified glandular cells are seen; cells are arranged in an orderly fashion with slightly enlarged nuclei and mild nuclear atypia. In adenocarcinomas, tumor cells reveal tall columnar "picket fence" appearance and are arranged in three-dimensional clusters with markedly nuclear atypia; they have hyperchromatic pencil-shaped nuclei, coarse chromatin, irregular nuclear membrane, and prominent nucleoli. The presence of "dirty" necrosis is usually seen. However, cytological examination of colonic adenomas cannot be relied on to exclude the possibility of adenocarcinoma/invasive carcinoma, since spectrum of nuclear atypia can be seen in colonic adenomas ranging from moderate to marked, overlapping with adenocarcinomas. Thus, brushing cytology has its limitation in the differential diagnosis of colon adenomas from adenocarcinomas.

A-28. (a) **Adenoma**

The diagnosis is a colonic adenoma. The slide reveals sheets and two-dimensional clusters of glandular cells with spectrum of nuclear atypia ranging from moderate to marked. The nuclei are enlarged with prominent nucleoli and vesicular chromatin. The most important differential diagnosis of adenomas is the adenocarcinoma. In adenocarcinomas, tumor cells reveal tall columnar "picket fence" appearance and are arranged in three-dimensional clusters with markedly nuclear atypia; they have hyperchromatic pencil-shaped nuclei, coarse chromatin, irregular nuclear membrane, and prominent nucleoli. The presence of "dirty" necrosis is usually seen. However, cytological examination of colonic adenomas cannot be relied on to exclude the possibility of an adenocarcinoma/invasive carcinoma, since spectrum of nuclear atypia can be seen in colonic adenomas ranging from moderate to marked, overlapping with adenocarcinoma. Thus, brushing cytology has its limitation in the differential diagnosis of colon adenomas from adenocarcinomas.

A-29. (a) **Adenocarcinoma**

The diagnosis is adenocarcinoma of the stomach. The slide reveals hyperchromatic clusters of cells. In adenocarcinomas, tumor cells are arranged in three-dimensional clusters, acini and glandular structures, or many dyscohesive individual cells. Tumor cells have large hyperchromatic nuclei, coarse chromatin, irregular nuclear membrane, prominent nucleoli, overlapping nuclei, vacuolated cytoplasm, and high N:C ratio. In squamous cell carcinomas, tumor cells form loosely clusters or dispersed individual cells with hyperchromatic nuclei, smudgy chromatin, dense cytoplasm, and cytokeratin formation. In reactive cellular changes, cells reveal sheets and/or loose clusters of glandular cells with enlarged nuclei, single or multiple small nucleoli, finely granular chromatin, and smooth nuclear membrane. Cells are still arranged in an orderly fashion with a streaming appearance. No significant nuclear atypia is seen. Normal N:C ratio is still maintained in cells. In benign gastric ulcers, it reveals reactive cellular changes without malignant nuclear features, inflammatory cells, and necrotic debris.

A-30. (d) **Herpes simplex virus (HSV) infection**

The diagnosis is HSV infection. In HSV infection, cells reveal enlarged nuclei with multinucleation, nuclear molding, ground-glass chromatin, and margination of chromatin in nuclei. Cowdry A bodies may also present in the nuclei, which are eosinophilic nuclear inclusions composed of nucleic acid and protein. In CMV infection, nuclei reveal large single basophilic intranuclear inclusions and perinuclear halos. In adenocarcinomas, tumor cells reveal tall columnar "picket fence" appearance and are arranged in three-dimensional clusters with markedly nuclear atypia; they have hyperchromatic pencil-shaped nuclei, coarse chromatin, irregular nuclear membranes, and prominent nucleoli. The presence of "dirty" necrosis is usually seen. In squamous cell carcinomas, tumor cells form loosely clusters or dispersed individual cells with hyperchromatic nuclei, smudgy chromatin, dense cytoplasm, and cytokeratin formation.

A-31. (c) **Carcinoid**

The diagnosis is a carcinoid. Cytological features of a carcinoid tumor reveal a cellular specimen forming cords, nests, and rosette-like structures. Tumor cells are intermediate in size with relatively uniform nuclei, fine (salt-and-pepper) chromatin, and small or inconspicuous nucleoli. The cytoplasm is abundant. Plasmacytoid cells and occasional pleomorphic cells are commonly seen. No mitosis or tumor necrosis is identified. The important differentiation of a carcinoid is adenocarcinoma. In adenocarcinomas, particularly in a well-differentiated adenocarcinoma, tumor cells are arranged predominantly in three-dimensional clusters and dispersed individual cells with large hyperchromatic nuclei, coarse chromatin, and irregular nuclear membranes. The cytoplasm is scant and contains cytoplasmic vacuoles. In squamous cell carcinomas, tumor cells form loosely clusters or dispersed individual cells with hyperchromatic nuclei, smudgy chromatin, dense cytoplasm, and cytokeratin formation. In small cell carcinomas, tumor cells reveal fine (salt-and-pepper) chromatin with nuclear crowding and molding.

9.4 Answers and Discussion of Text-Based Questions 32–61

A-32. (a) **Irregular nuclear membrane and coarse chromatin**

In reactive/reparative squamous cells, cytological specimen from esophageal brushings shows sheets of cells with "streaming" pattern and occasional single cells. In these cells, nuclei is slightly enlarged, but the N:C ratio is preserved. Nuclei show evenly distributed chromatin, regular nuclear membrane, and small nucleoli. Degenerating squamous cells may show cytoplasmic cyanophilia and vacuolization. In contrast, in squamous cell carcinomas, tumor cells are dyscohesive and arranged predominantly in dispersed individual cell pattern with hyperchromatic large nuclei, smudgy chromatin, and irregular nuclear membrane. In a poorly differentiated tumor, the presence of prominent nucleoli is commonly seen.

A-33. (c) **Tight three-dimensional cluster of glandular cells with dark nuclei**

A brushing specimen usually contains numerous gastric mucous/glandular cells. The benign gastric glandular cells are arranged in honeycomb sheets or two-dimensional clusters with bland basal nuclei and abundant apical mucin characteristic of a polarized appearance. Polarized glandular cells are best seen at peripheral area of cellular arrangements. Cells reveal oval nuclei, smooth nuclear membrane, inconspicuous nucleoli, normal N:C ratio, and without nuclear overlapping. Occasionally, goblet cells may be identified in cellular arrangements, indicative of either intestinal metaplasia or duodenal mucosa. Tight three-dimensional clusters of glandular cells with hyperchromatic nuclei are features usually seen in adenocarcinomas.

A-34. (c) **Hyperchromatic nuclei with irregular nuclear membrane**

In an adenocarcinoma of the esophagus-gastric junction, tumor cells form three-dimensional clusters, acinar arrangements, and dispersed individual cells with high N:C ratio, hyperchromatic nuclei, coarse chromatin, irregular nuclear membrane, and prominent nucleoli. Nuclear overlapping and variation in size are prominent. Tumor necrosis may also be seen on the slide. In reactive glandular atypia, cells are arranged in sheets and/or two-dimensional clusters with streaming pattern; cells reveal slightly enlarged nuclei, finely granular chromatin, regular/smooth nuclear membrane, and small prominent nucleoli. Although the nuclei are bigger, the normal N:C ratio is maintained. Reactive glandular cells may lose the polarity, but no markedly nuclear overlapping and pleomorphism are seen. Cytoplasmic vacuoles are seen in both adenocarcinoma and reactive glandular cells.

A-35. (c) **Hyperchromatic nuclei and clumped chromatin**

The most important differential diagnosis of radiation- and chemotherapy-induced glandular cell changes is the residual and/or recurrent adenocarcinoma, since the patient has the history of adenocarcinoma and chemo- and/or radiation therapy. Cytological features of radiation- and chemotherapy-induced glandular cell changes include sheets and two-dimensional clusters of cells with cytomegaly; but the nuclei to cytoplasmic ratio is still in a normal range (proportional enlargement of nuclei and cytoplasm). Multinucleation and prominent nucleoli are common. However, hyperchromatic nuclei, clumped chromatin, and irregular nuclear membrane are not features seen in reactive atypia. The finding of these features is diagnostic for adenocarcinoma.

A-36. (b) **Synaptophysin, chromogranin, and CD56**

The diagnosis of the lesion is a carcinoid. Rectal carcinoids are typically diagnosed during routine lower gastrointestinal endoscopy as small, sessile masses or thickened submucosal areas. African-American males had the highest incidence in some published series (2.12 per 100,000 population per year). Clinical symptoms, only presented in half of patients, include abdominal discomfort, change in bowel habits, constipation, and bleeding. The overall 5-year survival rate ranges from 88.3 to 98.3 %. The size of rectal carcinoids correlates closely with the likelihood of metastases. Tumors smaller than 1 cm are rarely metastatic; however, tumors larger than 2 cm may be metastatic in 70 % of patients. The panel of synaptophysin, chromogranin, and CD56 will confirm the diagnosis. Immunostain of Ki67 is necessary for an accurate diagnosis and classification of neuroendocrine tumors. CK7, CK20, and mucin stains are markers for adenocarcinomas. C-kit and CD34 are markers for GIST. P63, P40, and CK5/CK6 are markers for squamous cell carcinoma.

A-37. (c) **Coarse chromatin and large prominent nucleoli**

Cytological features of a carcinoid tumor reveal a cellular specimen forming cords, nests, and rosette-like structures. Tumor cells are intermediate in size with relatively uniform nuclei, fine (salt-and-pepper) chromatin, and small or inconspicuous nucleoli. The cytoplasm is abundant. Plasmacytoid cells and occasional pleomorphic cells are commonly seen. Neither mitosis nor tumor necrosis is identified. The important differentiation of carcinoid is adenocarcinoma. In adenocarcinomas, particularly in a well-differentiated adenocarcinoma, tumor cells are arranged predominantly in three-dimensional clusters and dispersed individual cells with large hyperchromatic nuclei, coarse chromatin, and irregular nuclear membrane. The cytoplasm is scant and contains cytoplasmic vacuoles. In a poorly differentiated adenocarcinoma, tumor cells also reveal prominent nuclear pleomorphism.

A-38. (**b**) **Spindle-shaped or epithelioid tumor cells with bland nuclei**

Gastrointestinal stromal tumor (GIST) is the most common mesenchymal tumor of the gastrointestinal tract, representing 1–3 % of all gastrointestinal malignancies. All GIST tumors are now considered to have malignant potential, and no GIST tumor can be definitively classified as "benign." The majority of GISTs present at ages 50–70 years. The estimated incidence of GIST in the United States is approximately 5,000 cases annually. The cytological features of GIST reveal sheets or loosely formed clusters of spindle or epithelioid cells with oval or bipolar nuclei, granular chromatin, inconspicuous nucleoli, wispy cytoplasm, and long extension. Most GISTs (70–80 %) have spindle cell appearance, and the rest of them have either epithelioid appearance or a combined appearance. The behavior of GIST is driven by mutations in the *kit* gene or platelet-derived growth factor receptor alpha (*PDGFR-alpha*) gene. Approximately 85 % GISTs are associated with an abnormal expression of C-kit pathway (CD117). IHC of tumor cells are positive for CD117 and CD34. If the CD117 stain is negative in a GIST, the newer antibody DOG-1 (discovered on GIST-1) can be used. Also sequencing of *Kit* and *PDGFRA* gene may be used to prove the diagnosis. The presence of spindle cells and fat with or without prominent vessels is a characteristic of angiomyolipoma.

A-39. (**c**) **Leiomyosarcoma**

The differential diagnosis of a spindle cell lesion in FNA cytology is broad, including spindle cell carcinoma, leiomyoma, leiomyosarcoma, melanoma, nerve tumors, fibrous tumors, and others. The leiomyosarcoma is easily confused with a GIST. In a leiomyosarcoma, tumor cells have "cigar-shaped" nuclei and finely granular cytoplasm. Naked nuclei and increased mitosis are also common in the tumor. IHC stains of tumor cells are positive for desmin and myogenin. The cytological features of GIST reveal sheets or loosely formed clusters of spindle or epithelioid cells with oval or bipolar nuclei, granular chromatin, inconspicuous nucleoli, wispy cytoplasm, and long extension. IHC stains of tumor cells are positive for CD117 and CD34. In spindle cell carcinoma, tumor cells form clusters with large hyperchromatic nuclei, coarse chromatin, irregular nuclear membrane, prominent nucleoli, and scant cytoplasm. In spindle cell carcinoid, tumor cells reveal neuroendocrine cell features with uniform oval nuclei, fine chromatin, inconspicuous nucleoli, and abundant cytoplasm.

A-40. (**c**) **Multinucleation**

In HSV infection, cells reveal multinucleation, nuclear molding, ground-glass chromatin, and margination of chromatin in nuclei. Cowdry bodies are eosinophilic nuclear inclusions composed of nucleic acid and protein seen in cells infected with HSV, varicella-zoster virus, and cytomegalovirus (CMV). There are two variants: type A is seen in HSV infection and type B (antiquated and perhaps illusory type) is seen in poliovirus infections. Large single basophilic intranuclear inclusion and perinuclear halo are characteristics of CMV infection.

A-41. (**c**) **Hyperchromatic nuclei, clumped chromatin, and irregular nuclear membrane**

Cytological features of bile duct brushing from a patient with bile duct stent may reveal markedly reactive cellular atypia. On the slide, the specimen is cellular and consists of sheets and two-dimensional clusters of columnar cells with streaming patterns. Cells may have enlarged nuclei, dense chromatin, and small nucleoli. Sometimes, coarse chromatin and large prominent nucleoli may also be present. However, the nuclear membrane is smooth and N:C ratio is normal or slightly increased. The most important differential diagnosis of bile duct brushing from a biliary stent specimen is an adenocarcinoma, particularly a well-differentiated adenocarcinoma. In adenocarcinomas, tumor cells form three-dimensional clusters with hyperchromatic nuclei, clumped chromatin, and irregular nuclear membrane. Nuclear disorganization and crowding are commonly seen. Dispersed individual tumor cells may also be identified. An increased mitotic activity and necrotic debris (tumor diathesis) in the background may also be suggestive of the diagnosis of adenocarcinomas.

A-42. (**d**) **EUS-FNA biopsy has similar accuracy as endoscopic mucosal forceps biopsy for submucosal lesions**.

Endoscopic ultrasound-guided fine-needle aspiration (EUS-FNA) has been increasingly used in recent years for the diagnosis and staging of intra-abdominal and certain intrathoracic lesions. For GI tract lesions, EUS procedure is particularly helpful for identifying the origin/location of the lesion, i.e., whether the lesion arises in the wall, submucosal, or mucosal area. EUS can also identify which layer of the GI wall is involved by the lesion. The procedure can be used to evaluate the extent and the border of the lesion. EUS-FNA can also be used for staging of lung cancer regarding the mediastinum involvement. However, the definitive diagnosis between benign and malignant lesions cannot be made by EUS imaging alone. Therefore, FNA and tissue biopsy is required to establish a conclusive diagnosis. The diagnostic accuracy of endoscopic FNA is approximately 94 % and significantly higher than that of endoscopic mucosal forceps biopsy (87 %); this is particularly true in the case of submucosal lesions and infiltrative malignancies.

A-43. (**d**) **The lymphoma is caused by the clonal expansion of subpopulations of T cells**.

The vast majority of GI MALT lymphomas are thought to be related to H. pylori infection. The chronic antigenic stimulation of the infection leads to malignant transformation and the clonal expansion of subpopulations of B cells. Although it frequently involves the stomach, virtually any mucosal site can be affected. Gastric MALT lymphoma is frequently associated with chronic *Helicobacter pylori* infection in 70–90 % of patients. The cure of *H. pylori* infection is associated with complete remission in approximately 80 % of patients with low-grade MALT lymphoma in an early stage of the disease. The FNA of the lesion reveals a cellular specimen with monomorphic population of lymphocytes. Lymphoma cells are dyscohesive and have round or irregular nuclei, coarse granular chromatin, inconspicuous nucleoli, and scant cytoplasm. Numerous lymphoglandular bodies and scattered plasma cells may be seen in the background. No specific IHC marker is available, CD20 stain is diffusely positive for tumor cells, and aberrant coexpression of CD43 by neoplastic B cells is found in up to 50 % of cases. The t(11;18)(q21;q21) is the most common translocation. It involves the *API2/MALT1* (the fusion of the N-terminus of *API2* (apoptosis inhibitor-2) on chromosome 11 and the C-terminus of *MALT1* (MALT lymphoma-associated translocation 1) on chromosome 18). The translocation can be found in 25 % of gastric and 40–60 % of small intestinal MALT lymphomas, respectively.

A-44. (**c**) **Lymphoglandular bodies**

Both MALT lymphoma and carcinoid involve the wall of GI tract. Both of them consist of relatively uniform population of tumor cells with fine granular chromatin pattern. The FNA of a MALT lymphoma reveals a dyscohesive monomorphic population of lymphocytes. Lymphoma cells have round or irregular nuclei, coarse granular chromatin, inconspicuous nucleoli, and scant cytoplasm. The identification lymphoglandular bodies on the slide is consistent with a lymphoid lesion. In carcinoids, tumor cells have uniform appearance but reveal acini and/or rosette arrangements; they are intermediate in size (larger than that of lymphoma cells) with fine salt-and-pepper chromatin, inconspicuous or small nucleoli, and fair amount of cytoplasm. IHC stains of neuroendocrine markers (synaptophysin, chromogranin, and CD56) are positive for tumor cells.

A-45. (**a**) **Three-dimensional clusters of atypical cells**

DLBLC is a good mimic of a poorly differentiated adenocarcinoma. In a poorly differentiated adenocarcinoma, tumor cells can be dyscohesive and presented as dispersed individual cells or form three-dimensional clusters with large hyperchromatic nuclei, coarse chromatin, irregular nuclear membrane, prominent nucleoli, and vacuolated cytoplasm. In DLBCLs, the FNA reveals a cellular specimen with dyscohesive large atypical lymphoid cells. Within cellular morphology, three variants are most commonly seen: centroblastic, immunoblastic, and anaplastic variant. Centroblastic variant is the most common subtype and reveals medium- to large-sized tumor cells with high N:C ratio, oval or round nuclei, fine chromatin, and single or multiple prominent nucleoli. Immunoblasts have a basophilic cytoplasm and a central nucleolus. The third morphologic variant, anaplastic variant, consists of large tumor cells with pleomorphic nuclei and may resemble Hodgkin cells (Reed-Sternberg cells). Most cases of DLBCL are polymorphic, with a mixture of centroblastic and immunoblastic cells.

A-46. (**b**) **Hyperchromatic nuclei and irregular nuclear membrane**

Benign bile ductal epithelium is arranged in small clusters and/or sheets of cohesive uniform cells with honeycomb appearances. These cells have round to ovoid nuclei, granular chromatin, inconspicuous or occasional small nucleoli, and scant cytoplasm.

In reactive bile ductal epithelial cells, specimen reveals cohesive groups of glandular cells with slightly enlarged nuclei, nuclear angulations, and small or inconspicuous nucleoli. Mild nuclear overlapping and nuclear disarray are also commonly seen. In benign and reactive bile ductal epithelium, the N:C ratio of cells is normal. In adenocarcinomas, tumor cells form tight three-dimensional clusters and reveal large nuclei with coarse chromatin, prominent nucleoli, irregular nuclear membrane, and vacuolated cytoplasm. The N:C ratio is high.

A-47. (**b**) **Biliary stent**
The biliary stricture and the placement of biliary stent are common causes of bile ductal reactive atypia found on a brushing specimen. The brushing specimen from biliary stent patient reveals cohesive groups of glandular cells with slightly enlarged nuclei, nuclear angulations, and small or inconspicuous nucleoli. Other features include small clusters and/or sheets of cohesive columnar cells with round to ovoid nuclei, dark granular chromatin, inconspicuous or occasional small nucleoli, and scant cytoplasm. Mild nuclear overlapping and nuclear disarray are common findings, mimicking adenocarcinomas. In adenocarcinomas, tumor cells reveal markedly nuclear atypia, hyperchromasia, coarse chromatin, prominent nucleoli, and high N:C ratio. Tumor cells are also arranged in tight three-dimensional clusters or dispersed individual tumor cells. An increased mitotic activity and necrotic debris (tumor diathesis) in the background may also be suggestive of the diagnosis of adenocarcinoma.

A-48. (**c**) **Signet ring cell carcinoma**
The diagnosis is a signet ring cell carcinoma of the stomach. In signet ring cell carcinoma of the stomach, tumor cells are arranged in clusters or dispersed individual cells with large cytoplasmic vacuoles (mucin) that push the nuclei to eccentric location (signet ring appearance). The nucleus is large with hyperchromasia, coarse chromatin, and irregular nuclear membrane. Although histiocytes and macrophages may reveal signet ring cell features, no nuclear atypia is identified in them. Therefore, careful evaluation of nuclear morphology is critical for separating benign from malignant cells. In addition, other carcinomas may reveal "signet ring" features, such as certain carcinomas of breast and lung, due to the production of cytoplasmic mucin. In adenocarcinomas of the lung, tumor cells form large three-dimensional clusters and reveal variable appearances; they have hyperchromatic nuclei, prominent nucleoli, and vacuolated cytoplasm. In breast carcinoma, the size of tumor cells is smaller than that of GI carcinoma; tumor cells are arranged in tight three-dimensional clusters or acini with coarse chromatin, prominent nucleoli, and scant cytoplasm. In adenocarcinomas of colon, tumor cell reveals elongated nuclei and prominent tumor necrosis.

A-49. (**a**) **Prominent nucleoli**
The presence of prominent nucleoli is the feature of adenocarcinomas and is not usually seen in small cell carcinomas. All other features can be seen in both adenocarcinomas and small cell carcinomas. In adenocarcinomas, tumor cells form acini and/or three-dimensional clusters and can be confused with rosettes in a suboptimally prepared slides; tumor cells reveal hyperchromatic nuclei, vesicular or coarse chromatin, prominent nucleoli, and vacuolated cytoplasm (indicative of mucin production). In small cell carcinomas, the size of tumor cells is smaller than that of adenocarcinoma; tumor cells reveal acini/rosettes arrangements with hyperchromatic nuclei, fine granular (salt-and-pepper) chromatin, inconspicuous nucleoli, and scant cytoplasm. In addition, in small cell carcinomas, nuclear crowding and molding are characteristic features. The background of the smear may also reveal "blue strips" (indicative of breakdown of nuclear material). Tumor necrosis can be seen in both adenocarcinomas and small cell carcinomas.

A-50. (**b**) **Adenocarcinoma**
The brushing cytology showed cytological features of a colonic adenocarcinoma. In ulcerative colitis patients, long-term surveillance is needed to identify the presence of adenocarcinomas. In patients with inflammatory bowel disease, the distinction among reactive/repair, adenoma, and adenocarcinoma on cytological preparation is very difficult. In adenocarcinomas, tumor cells reveal tall columnar "picket fence" appearance and are arranged in three-dimensional clusters with markedly nuclear atypia; they have hyperchromatic pencil-shaped nuclei, coarse chromatin, and prominent nucleoli. The presence of "dirty" necrosis is usually seen. In reactive glandular cells, a cohesive cluster of stratified glandular cells is seen; cells are arranged in an orderly fashion with slightly enlarged nuclei and mild nuclear atypia. Cytological examination of colonic adenomas cannot be relied on to exclude the possibility of an invasive carcinoma, since spectrum of nuclear atypia can be seen in adenomas ranging from moderate to marked. Thus, brushing cytology has its limitation in the diagnosis of colon lesions.

A-51. (b) **Nuclear molding and crowding**
Carcinoid tumors comprise 1–2 % of all gastrointestinal malignancies. The most common sites of primary disease are the appendix (35 %), small intestine (25 %), and rectum (12 %). The cytological features of carcinoids are characterized by acini arrangements, small clusters, and dispersed individual tumor cells. Tumor cells reveal fine granular chromatin (salt-and-pepper chromatin) pattern, inconspicuous or small nucleoli, and moderate to scant cytoplasm. Mitosis is extremely rare. Nuclear molding and crowding are not features seen in carcinoids. In addition, cellular proliferative rate (Ki67 labeling) should be performed in all tumors, since it has been considered a marker for the classification of the tumor and related to the clinical behavior of the tumor.

A-52. (c) **Large prominent nucleoli**
In a well-differentiated squamous cell carcinoma, tumor cells are arranged in loose clusters and/or dispersed individual tumor cells. The cytological features of tumor cells include large nuclei with variation in size and shape, smudgy chromatin, irregular nuclear membrane, and dense cytoplasm (indicative of cytokeratin formation). The cytokeratin is purple color with Diff-Quik stain and red-pink (eosinophilic) to blue color with Papanicolaou stain. Spindle-shaped keratinizing malignant cells are also seen. Degenerated cells with pyknotic nuclei may be identified in the background. Necrotic debris and inflammatory cells are usually present. Finally, the presence of prominent nucleoli is not the feature of a well-differentiated squamous cell carcinoma and can be seen in poorly differentiated squamous cell carcinomas and should not be confused with poorly differentiated adenocarcinomas. Tumor cells of adenocarcinoma reveal vesicular nuclei, coarse chromatin, and vacuolated cytoplasm.

A-53. (c) **Lymphoma**
The most likely diagnosis of this FNA is a lymphoma. The cytological features of numerous dyscohesive small- to intermediate-sized cells with high N:C ratio and hyperchromatic coarse chromatin are characteristics of lymphoma. The monomorphic appearance of the lesion represents a monoclonal proliferation of lymphoma cells. Other cytological features of lymphomas include hyperchromatic nuclei with clumped (soccer ball-like) chromatin, irregular nuclear membrane, and scant basophilic cytoplasm. Lymphoglandular bodies can also be seen in the background. In poorly differentiated carcinomas, tumor cells are large in size and form clusters; they reveal large nuclei, hyperchromatic nuclei, and prominent nucleoli. In carcinoids, tumor cells have uniform appearance but reveal acini and/or rosette arrangements; they are intermediate in size (larger than that of lymphoma cells) with fine salt-and-pepper chromatin, inconspicuous or small nucleoli, and a fair amount of cytoplasm. In small cell carcinomas, tumor cells reveal salt-and-pepper chromatin, nuclear molding and crowding, and numerous apoptotic bodies and mitotic figures.

A-54. (c) **Pyknotic nuclei**
In a poorly differentiated squamous cell carcinoma, tumor cells reveal less cytokeratin formation and are predominately arranged in clusters and/or dispersed as individual tumor cells. Tumor cells have large nuclei with coarse chromatin, prominent nucleoli, and indistinct cell borders. Pyknotic nuclei are usually not seen. The presence of prominent nucleoli should not be confused with poorly differentiated adenocarcinomas. Tumor cells of adenocarcinomas have vesicular nuclei, coarse chromatin, and vacuolated cytoplasm.

A-55. (d) **Hyperchromatic nuclei, prominent nucleoli, and coarse chromatin**
In a low-grade Barrett mucosa, cytological features include sheets and/or loose cluster of glandular cells with stratification and elongated nuclei with mild nuclear atypia; cells are arranged in an orderly fashion. No significant nuclear atypia is identified. In adenocarcinomas, tumor cells form acini and/or three-dimensional clusters and many dyscohesive individual tumor cells with large hyperchromatic nuclei, coarse chromatin, irregular nuclear membrane, prominent nucleoli, and vacuolated cytoplasm (indicative of mucin production). Therefore, features of hyperchromatic nuclei, prominent nucleoli, and coarse chromatin are characteristics of adenocarcinomas.

A-56. (a) **Suspicious for adenocarcinoma**
The most likely diagnosis of this FNA is suspicious for adenocarcinoma. In adenocarcinomas, tumor cells form acini and/or three-dimensional clusters and many dyscohesive individual tumor cells with large hyperchromatic nuclei, coarse chromatin, irregular nuclear membrane, prominent nucleoli, and vacuolated cytoplasm. Therefore, features of hyperchromatic nuclei, prominent nucleoli, and coarse chromatin are characteristics of adenocarcinomas. In reactive glandular cells and gastritis, glandular cells are arranged in cohesive clusters with a streaming

pattern or in an orderly fashion; reactive glandular cells reveal slightly enlarged nuclei with mild nuclear atypia and small or inconspicuous nucleoli. In melanomas, tumor cells are dyscohesive, large in size, and with a plasmacytoid appearance. Multinucleation and large prominent nucleoli are commonly seen in melanomas.

A-57. **(d) Hyperchromatic nuclei, prominent nucleoli, and coarse chromatin**
Currently, there are no well-accepted criteria for separating Barrett low-grade dysplasia from a high-grade dysplasia. In low-grade Barrett mucosa, cytological features include sheets and/or loose cluster of glandular cells with stratification and elongated nuclei with mild nuclear atypia; cells are arranged in an orderly fashion. No significant nuclear atypia is identified. In a Barrett with high-grade dysplasia, cytological features significantly overlap with adenocarcinoma; the distinction of these two lesions is extremely difficult with brushing cytology. Therefore, they are best considered a group of disease. In general, in this group, cells form acini and/or three-dimensional clusters and many dyscohesive individual atypical cells with large hyperchromatic nuclei, coarse chromatin, irregular nuclear membrane, prominent nucleoli, and vacuolated cytoplasm. Therefore, features of hyperchromatic nuclei, prominent nucleoli, and coarse chromatin are characteristics of high-grade dysplasia/adenocarcinoms.

A-58. **(d) Barrett with a high-grade dysplasia, suspicious for adenocarcinoma**
Currently, there are no well-accepted criteria for separating Barrett high-grade dysplasia from an adenocarcinoma. In a Barrett with high-grade dysplasia, cytological features significantly overlap with adenocarcinoma; the distinction of these two lesions is extremely difficult with brushing cytology. Therefore, they are best considered a group of disease. In general, in this group, cells form acini and/or three-dimensional clusters and many dyscohesive individual atypical cells with large hyperchromatic nuclei, coarse chromatin, irregular nuclear membrane, prominent nucleoli, and vacuolated cytoplasm. Therefore, features of hyperchromatic nuclei, prominent nucleoli, and coarse chromatin are characteristics of high-grade dysplasia/adenocarcinoms.

A-59. **(c) Cytomegalovirus (CMV) infection**
The diagnosis of this esophageal brushing is CMV infection. Large single basophilic intranuclear inclusions and perinuclear halos are characteristics of CMV infection. In HSV infection, cells reveal multinucleation, nuclear molding, ground-glass chromatin, and margination of chromatin in nuclei. Cowdry type A bodies are also seen in cells infected with HSV. The large intranuclear inclusions of viral infection can be confused with malignant lesions. In a poorly differentiated carcinoma, cells form three-dimensional clusters or dyscohesive individual tumor cells with large hyperchromatic nuclei, coarse chromatin, irregular nuclear membrane, prominent nucleoli, and vacuolated cytoplasm. In melanoma, tumor cells reveal large "cherry-red" intranuclear inclusions and other malignant nuclear features and melanin pigment in the cytoplasm.

A-60. **(b) Hyperchromatic nuclei, coarse chromatin, and irregular nuclear membrane**
In reactive atypia, cytological features include sheets and/or loose cluster of epithelial cells with elongated nuclei and mild nuclear atypia; cells are arranged in an orderly fashion with a streaming appearance. No significant nuclear atypia is seen. In contrast, in carcinoma, tumor cells form acini and/or three-dimensional clusters or many dyscohesive individual tumor cells with large hyperchromatic nuclei, coarse chromatin, and irregular nuclear membrane. Therefore, features of hyperchromatic nuclei, coarse chromatin, and irregular nuclear membrane are not seen in reactive epithelial atypia.

A-61. **(d) Dispersed large polygonal cells with large nuclei, hyperchromatic chromatin, prominent nucleoli, and dense granular cytoplasm**
In HCC, tumor cells show a wide range of cytomorphology. In well-differentiated tumors, cells resemble normal hepatocytes and form clusters, trabeculae, cords, and nests and have a slightly increased N:C ratio, large round nuclei, prominent nucleoli, naked nuclei, and bile pigment in cytoplasm. In poorly differentiated tumors, cells are markedly polygonal and dyscohesive with pleomorphic nuclei and giant tumor cells. The useful feature of HCC is the identification of dispersed large polygonal cells with large nuclei, hyperchromatic chromatin, prominent nucleoli, and dense granular cytoplasm. In adenocarcinomas, tumor cells form three-dimensional clusters with hyperchromatic nuclei, vesicular or coarse chromatin, irregular nuclear membrane, prominent nucleoli, and vacuolated cytoplasm. The presence of lacunae spaces on a cell block preparation is the feature seen in adenocarcinomas.

Reading List

Bibbo M, Wood MD, Fitzpatrick BT. Peritoneal washings and ovary. In: Bibbo M, Wilbur D, editors. Comprehensive cytopathology. 3rd ed. Philadelphia: Saunders/Elsevier; 2008.

Capelli P, Fassan M, Scarpa A. Pathology – grading and staging of GEP-NETs. Best Pract Res Clin Gastroenterol. 2012;26:705–17.

Cibas ES. Peritoneal washings. In: Cibas ES, Ducatman BS, editors. Cytology: diagnostic principles and clinical correlates. Philadelphia: Saunders/Elsevier; 2009.

DeMay RM. The art and science of cytopathology, exfoliative cytology, vol. 1. 2nd ed. Chicago: ASCP Press; 2012.

Engstrand L, Lindberg M. Helicobacter pylori and the gastric microbiota. Best Pract Res Clin Gastroenterol. 2013;27:39–45.

Khalbuss WE, Monaco SE, Pantanowitz L. Chapter 21. Gastrointestinal tract & bile ducts. In: The ASCP Quick Compendium (QC) of cytopathology. Chicago: ASCP Press; 2013. p. 484–507.

Khalbuss WE, Yang H, Lian Q, Elhosseiny A, Pantanowitz L, Monaco SE. The cytomorphologic spectrum of small-cell carcinoma and large-cell neuroendocrine carcinoma in body cavity effusions: a study of 68 cases. Cytojournal. 2011;8:18.

Kiśluk J, Gryko M, Guzińska-Ustymowicz K, Kemona A, Kędra B. Immunohistochemical diagnosis of gastrointestinal stromal tumors – an analysis of 80 cases from 2004 to 2010. Adv Clin Exp Med. 2013;22:33–9.

Maleki Z, Erozan Y, Geddes S, Li QK. Endorectal ultrasound-guided fine needle aspiration: a useful diagnostic tool for peri-rectal and intraluminal lesions. Acta Cytol. 2013;57:9–18.

Wheeler YR, Burroughs F, Li QK. Fine needle aspiration of a well-differentiated papillary mesothelioma in the hernia sac: case report and review of literature. Diagn Cytopathol. 2009;37: 748–54.

Renal and Adrenal Fine-Needle Aspiration

10

Qing Kay Li and Walid E. Khalbuss

Contents

10.1 **Image-Based Questions 1–25** 576

10.2 **Text-Based Questions 26–50** 601

10.3 **Answers and Discussions of Image-Based Questions 1–25** 604

10.4 **Answers and Discussions of Text-Based Questions 26–50** 611

Reading List 615

Q.K. Li, MD, PhD (✉)
Department of Pathology, The Johns Hopkins Bayview Medical Center, The Johns Hopkins University School of Medicine, 4940 Eastern Avenue, AA Building, Room 154B, Baltimore, MD 21224-2780, USA
e-mail: qli23@jhmi.edu

W.E. Khalbuss, MD, PhD, FIAC
Department of Pathology, GE Clarient Diagnostic Services, 31 Columbia, Aliso Viejo, California, 92656, USA
e-mail: Walid.khalbuss@ge.com

W.E. Khalbuss, Q.K. Li (eds.), *Diagnostic Cytopathology Board Review and Self-Assessment*, DOI 10.1007/978-1-4939-1477-7_10, © Springer Science+Business Media New York 2015

Table 10.1 Benign components in renal and adrenal FNAs

	Descriptions	Differentials
Glomeruli	Large globular and/or clusters of cells with scalloped border and scattered red blood cells	Oval- and spindle-shaped cells with low N:C ratios, dense nuclei, and benign nuclear features DD: low-grade clear cell and papillary renal cell carcinoma
Tubular cells	Loosely formed sheets and dispersed individual cells with round nuclei, fine chromatin, small nucleoli, granular cytoplasm, and indistinct cytoplasmic border	Cells with uniform appearances, minimal nuclear variations, normal N:C ratios, and benign nuclear features DD: low-grade clear cell and papillary renal cell carcinoma
Benign renal cysts	Scattered macrophages with oval nuclei, vesicular chromatin, inconspicuous or small nucleoli, abundant foamy cytoplasm with vacuoles. Amorphous debris in the background	Nuclei without variations, no nuclear atypia DD: cystic renal cell carcinoma
Liesegang rings	Laminated ringlike structures with double-layer outer walls, radial cross striations, and an amorphous central nidus. It consists of organic substances and stains blue in color with the hematoxylin-eosin (H&E) and the Papanicolaou methods	Most commonly seen in a benign cystic fluid DD: parasites, parasitic eggs, algae, calcifications, and psammoma bodies

Table 10.2 Neoplastic conditions in renal and FNAs

Conditions	Descriptions	Differentials
Oncocytoma	Dispersed individual cells and small flat cluster of cells with round nuclei, fine chromatin, inconspicuous or small nucleoli, abundant dense granular cytoplasm, and distinct cytoplasmic borders	Cells with abundant dense granular cytoplasm and mild nuclear atypia DD: low-grade clear cell and papillary renal cell carcinoma, chromophobe renal cell carcinoma, and hepatocytes
Angiomyolipoma	Clusters of spindle cells, fat cells (fat vacuoles), and blood vessels	Spindle cells may have a mild nuclear atypia. Thick-walled blood vessels are rarely seen on smears DD: renal cell carcinoma
Metanephric adenoma	Cohesive sheets and clusters of cells with round- and oval-shaped nuclei and scant cytoplasm	Cells look similar to renal tubular cells but have uniform nuclei, dense chromatin, inconspicuous or small nucleoli, and scant cytoplasm DD: Wilms' tumor and papillary renal cell carcinoma
Clear cell renal cell carcinoma (RCC)	Cohesive two-dimensional clusters and scattered individual cells with large eccentrically placed nuclei, vesicular chromatin, and granular or vacuolated cytoplasm	Intercellular pink color strand-like material (basement membrane material) may be seen by the Diff-Quik stain. Nucleoli vary in size depending on the Fuhrman grade DD: benign renal tubular cells, hepatocytes, and papillary renal cell carcinoma
Cystic renal cell carcinoma	Rare small groups and scattered individual cells with large eccentrically placed nuclei, vesicular chromatin, and granular or vacuolated cytoplasm	Scant specimen with rare tumor cells. Difficult to make the diagnosis DD: benign renal cysts
Sarcomatoid renal cell carcinoma	Clusters of oval- and spindle-shaped cells with high N:C ratio, large nuclei, coarse chromatin, irregular nuclear membrane, prominent nucleoli, and elongated cytoplasm	Tumor cells are arranged haphazardly and with marked nuclear atypia DD: angiomyolipoma and sarcoma
Translocation-associated renal cell carcinoma (Xp11 TRCC)	Mixed papillary and clusters of cuboidal cells with granular or clear cytoplasm	Tumor cells are positive for TFE3 and involves *TFE3* gene on chromosome X (Xp11) DD: clear cell renal cell carcinoma, and papillary renal cell carcinoma
Papillary renal cell carcinoma	Papillary and spherule clusters of cells with dense nuclei and scant-to-moderate granular cytoplasm. Foamy macrophages in the background	True fibrovascular cores. Nucleoli vary in size. Type 1 variant with mild nuclear atypia. Type 2 variant with marked nuclear atypia DD: glomeruli, metanephric adenoma, and clear cell renal cell carcinoma (RCC)
Chromophobe renal cell carcinoma	Sheets of cells with small nuclei, hyperchromatic chromatin, inconspicuous nucleoli, abundant vacuolated cytoplasm, and distinct cell borders	Tumor cells have small dense nuclei, cytoplasm with a moth-eaten appearance, and well-defined cell borders DD: clear cell renal cell carcinoma and oncocytoma

(continued)

Table 10.2 (continued)

Conditions	Descriptions	Differentials
Collecting duct carcinoma (Bellini tumor)	Acinar and trabecular arrangement of cuboidal cells with hyperchromatic nuclei, coarse chromatin, irregular nuclear membrane, prominent nucleoli, and scant cytoplasm	Tumor cells resembles metastatic adenocarcinomas DD: metastatic adenocarcinomas, papillary renal cell carcinoma, and medullary carcinoma
Renal urothelial cell carcinoma	Cohesive two-dimensional clusters and dispersed individual cells with large hyperchromatic nuclei, dense chromatin, inconspicuous nucleoli, and dense cytoplasm	Tumor cells with elongated cytoplasm and cercariform cells DD: renal cell carcinoma and metastatic squamous cell carcinoma
Wilms' tumor	Mixture of clusters and dispersed individual cells with hyperchromatic nuclei and scant cytoplasm and spindle cells	Bimodal population of cells with small blue cells (epithelial cells) and spindle cells (mesenchymal cells) DD: lymphoma, Ewing's/PNET, and small cell carcinomas
Benign adrenal cortical cells	Small sheets and dispersed individual cells with round nuclei, granular chromatin and small nucleoli, clear and/or granular cytoplasm, and indistinct cell borders	Round nuclei without nuclear atypia DD: adrenal cortical carcinoma
Adrenal cortical adenoma	Dispersed individual cells and small sheets of cells with round nuclei, granular chromatin and small nucleoli, and granular cytoplasm and indistinct cell borders	Round nuclei with mild nuclear atypia. Naked nuclei float in a sea of frothy cytoplasmic remnants DD: adrenal cortical carcinoma
Adrenal cortical carcinoma	Sheets and dispersed individual cells with large round nuclei, granular chromatin and prominent nucleoli, and scant granular cytoplasm	Large tumor cells with marked nuclear variations and atypia and increased mitoses DD: adrenal cortical adenoma, and renal cell carcinoma
Pheochromocytoma	Dispersed individual cells and small sheets of cells with pleomorphic nuclei, granular chromatin and prominent nucleoli, granular cytoplasm, and distinct cell borders	Pleomorphic large tumor cells with marked nuclear atypia and dense granular cytoplasm. Bizarre giant tumor cells DD: adrenal cortical carcinoma
Metastatic adenocarcinoma	Three-dimensional clusters and acinar arrangements of columnar cells. Tumor cells have hyperchromasia, high N:C ratio, prominent nucleoli, coarse chromatin, "lacy" cytoplasm with vacuolization (cytoplasmic mucin)	Columnar cells have high N:C ratio with irregular nuclear membrane, coarse chromatin, prominent nucleoli, and cytoplasmic vacuole (mucin production) DD: glomeruli and papillary renal cell carcinoma
Metastatic squamous cell carcinoma	Discohesive clusters, loosely formed two-dimensional cellular sheets and scattered individual polymorphic cells, hyperchromatic nuclei, irregular nuclear membrane, with or without keratinization Tumor necrosis	Polygonal, rounded, elongated, or tadpole-shaped cells with large dark nuclei, smudgy chromatin, and dense cytoplasm (cytokeratin formation) DD: urothelial cell carcinoma
Metastatic small cell carcinoma	Tight clusters of small hyperchromatic cells (two to three times the size of mature lymphocytes) with nuclear molding and crowding, nuclear stripes (broken nuclear material), inconspicuous nuclei, scant cytoplasm	Fine (salt-and-pepper) chromatin, nuclear molding and crowding, paranuclear blue bodies, mitosis, necrosis and apoptotic body DD: lymphoma, and poorly differentiated adenocarcinoma
Metastatic melanoma	Scattered individual large cells with prominent nucleoli and cytoplasmic melanin pigment. Binucleation, multinucleation with prominent nucleoli in "mirror" arrangement. Pseudointranuclear inclusions	Large-sized malignant cells with prominent nucleoli, dense cytoplasm DD: poorly differentiated carcinoma, Hodgkin lymphoma, and pheochromocytoma
Lymphoma (non-Hodgkin lymphoma)	Dispersed individual atypical lymphoid cells with coarse chromatin and irregular nuclear membrane, prominent nucleoli. High N:C ratio and scant cytoplasm. Increased mitotic activity and the presence of background lymphoglandular bodies	The size of tumor cells ranges from small to large depending on the type of lymphoma. Monomorphous population of lymphocytes is characteristic for SLL/CLL DD: reactive lymphocytes and metastatic small cell carcinoma
Non-epithelial cell neoplasm	Individual or clusters of spindle cells, small round cells, or pleomorphic tumor cells	DD: muscle, nerve tumors, small round cell tumor, and sarcomas

10.1 Image-Based Questions 1–25

Fig. 10.1

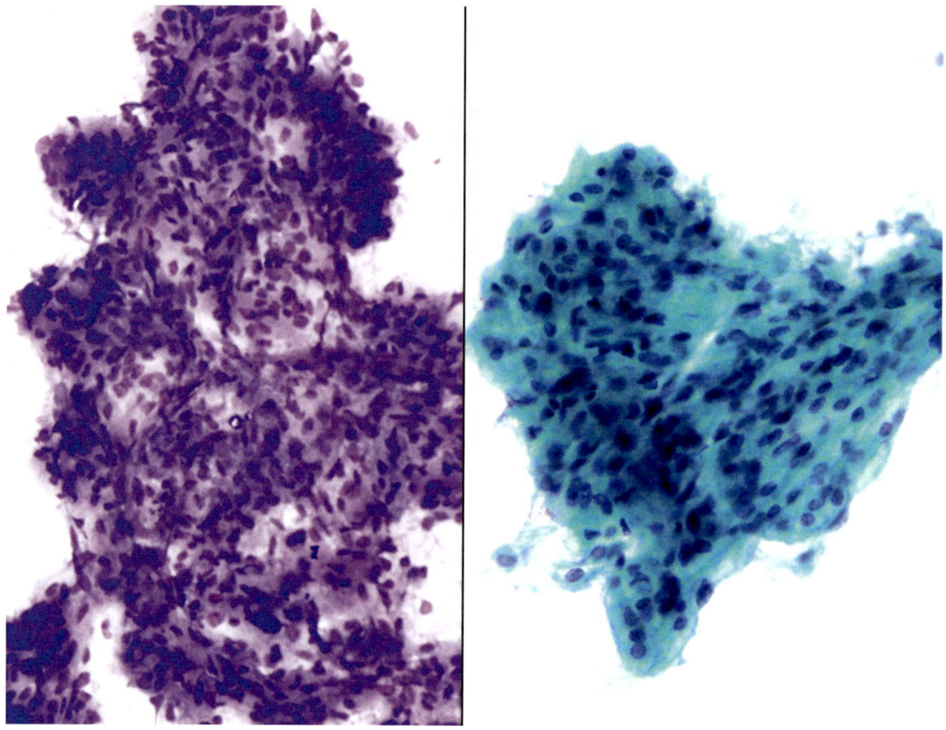

Q-1. What is the diagnosis of the image?
(a) Metastatic adenocarcinoma
(b) Clear cell renal cell carcinoma (RCC)
(c) Glomerulus
(d) Papillary renal cell carcinoma (RCC)

Fig. 10.2

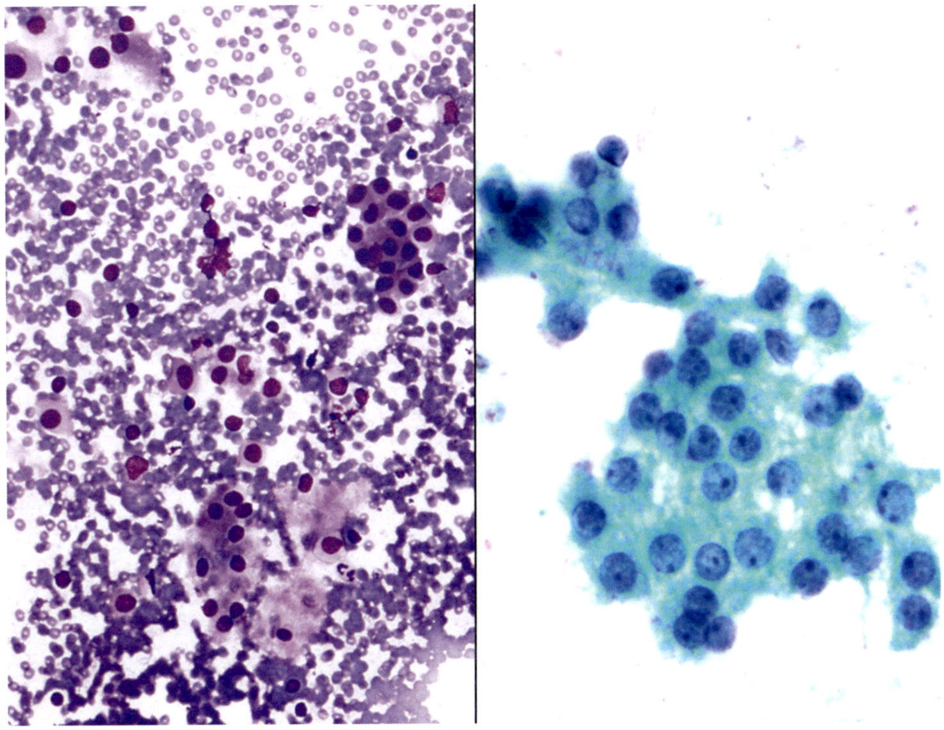

Q-2. A 65-year-old female had a right renal mass. A CT-guided FNA was performed. What is the diagnosis of the image?

(a) Metastatic adenocarcinoma
(b) Clear cell renal cell carcinoma (RCC)
(c) Benign renal tubular cells
(d) Papillary renal cell carcinoma (RCC)

Fig. 10.3

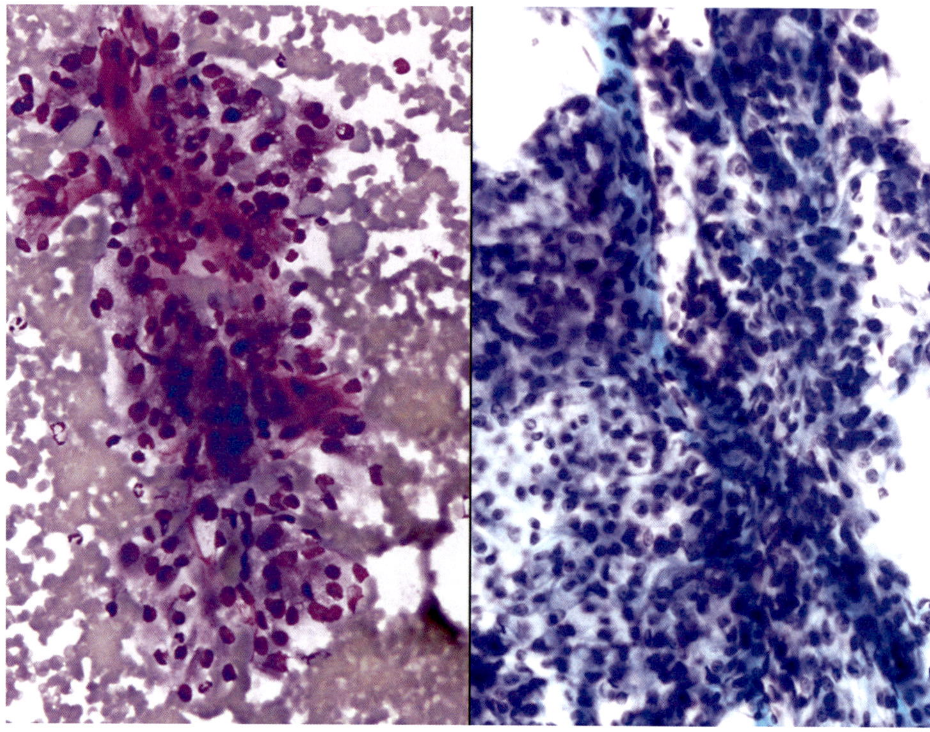

Q-3. A 64-year-old male had a right renal mass. A CT-guided FNA was performed. What is the diagnosis of the image?
(a) Metastatic adenocarcinoma
(b) Clear cell renal cell carcinoma (RCC)
(c) Benign renal tubular cells
(d) Papillary renal cell carcinoma (RCC)

Fig. 10.4

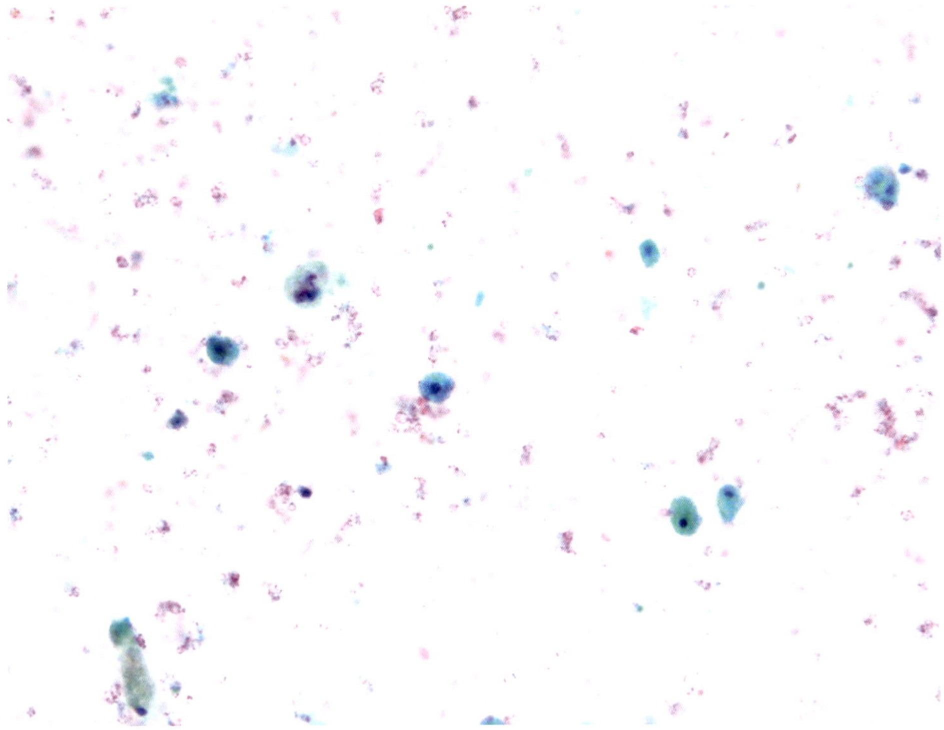

Q-4. A 50-year-old male had a large right cyst. An ultrasound-guided FNA was performed. What is the diagnosis of the image?
(a) Benign renal cyst
(b) Cystic renal cell carcinoma (RCC)
(c) Benign renal tubular cells
(d) Papillary renal cell carcinoma (RCC)

Fig. 10.5

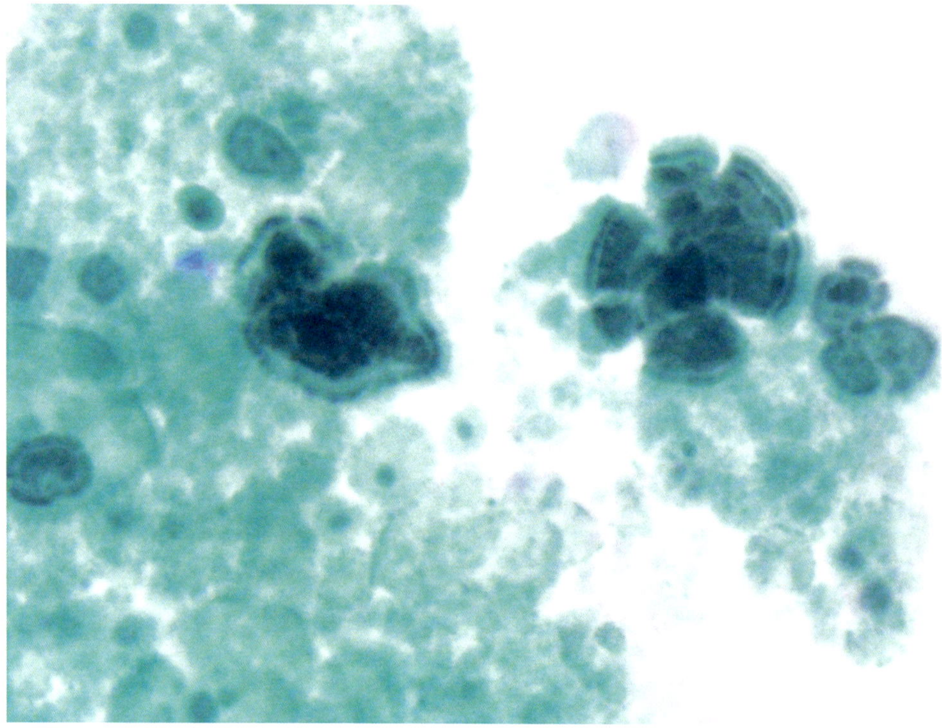

Q-5. What is the diagnosis of the image?
- (a) Psammoma bodies
- (b) Liesegang rings
- (c) Charcot-Leyden crystals
- (d) Michaelis-Gutmann bodies

Fig. 10.6

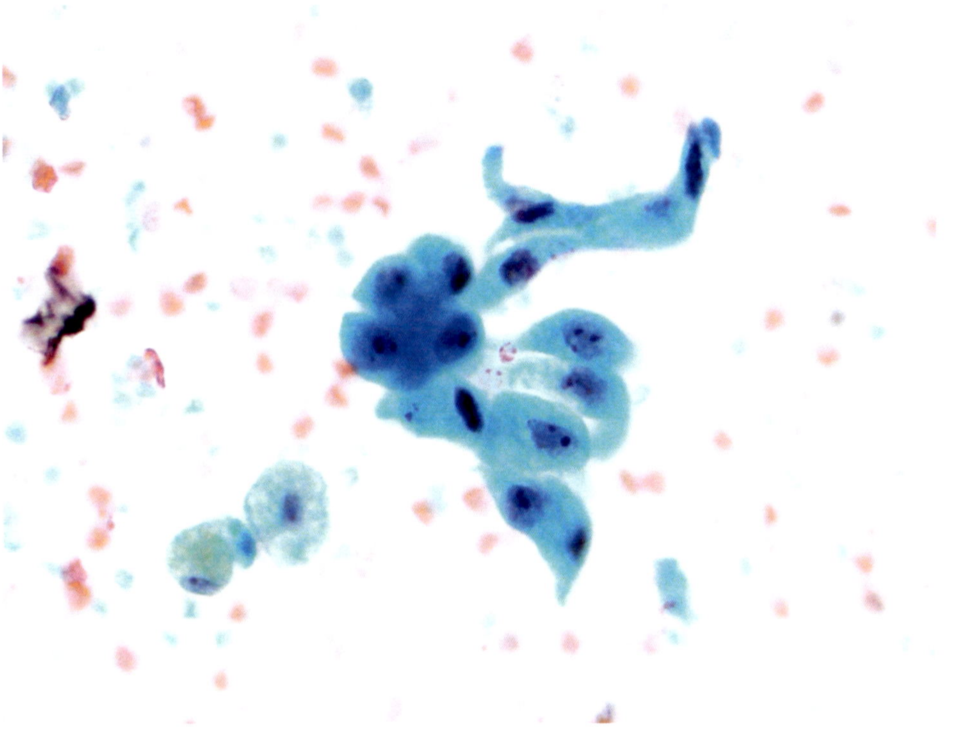

Q-6. A 70-year-old male had a left renal cyst. An ultrasound-guided FNA was performed. What is the diagnosis of the image?
(a) Metastatic adenocarcinoma
(b) Papillary renal cell carcinoma (RCC)
(c) Benign renal tubular cells
(d) Cystic renal cell carcinoma (RCC)

Fig. 10.7

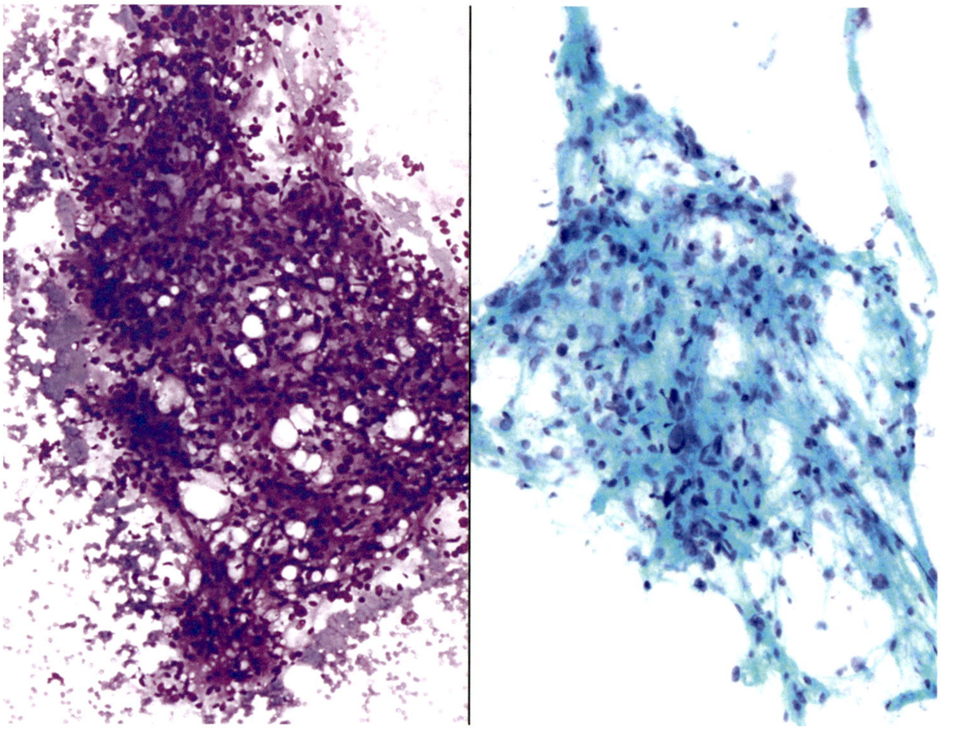

Q-7. A 23-year-old male had a left renal mass. An ultrasound-guided FNA was performed. What is the diagnosis of the image?

(a) Metastatic adenocarcinoma
(b) Clear cell renal cell carcinoma (RCC)
(c) Angiomyolipoma (AML)
(d) Papillary renal cell carcinoma (RCC)

Fig. 10.8

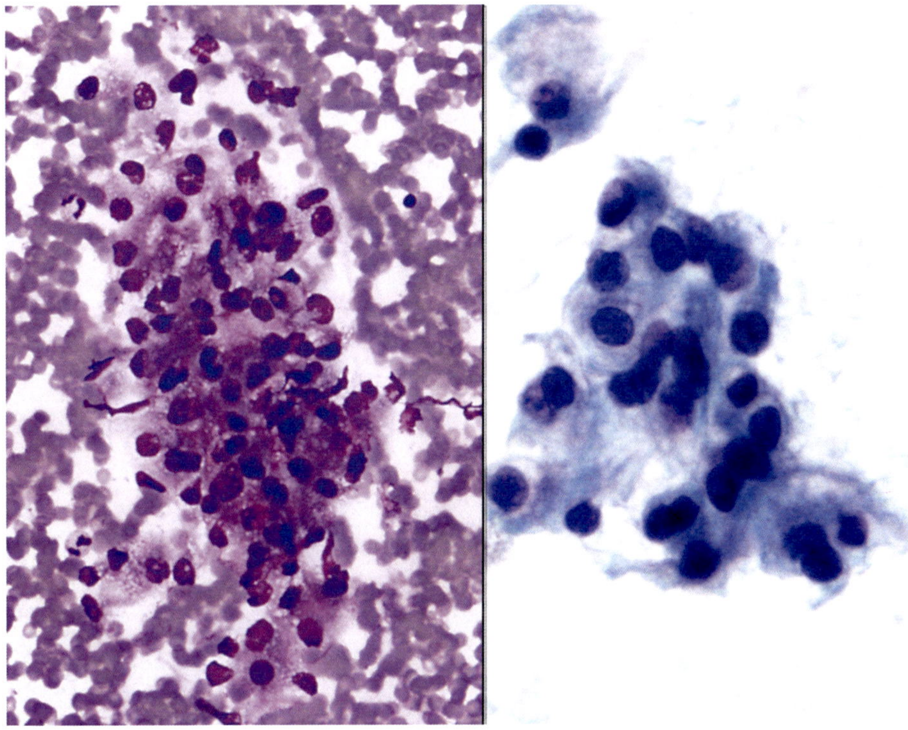

Q-8. A 58-year-old male had a right renal mass. A CT-guided FNA was performed. What is the diagnosis of the FNA?
(a) Metastatic adenocarcinoma
(b) Papillary renal cell carcinoma (RCC)
(c) Benign renal tubular cells
(d) Clear cell renal cell carcinoma (RCC)

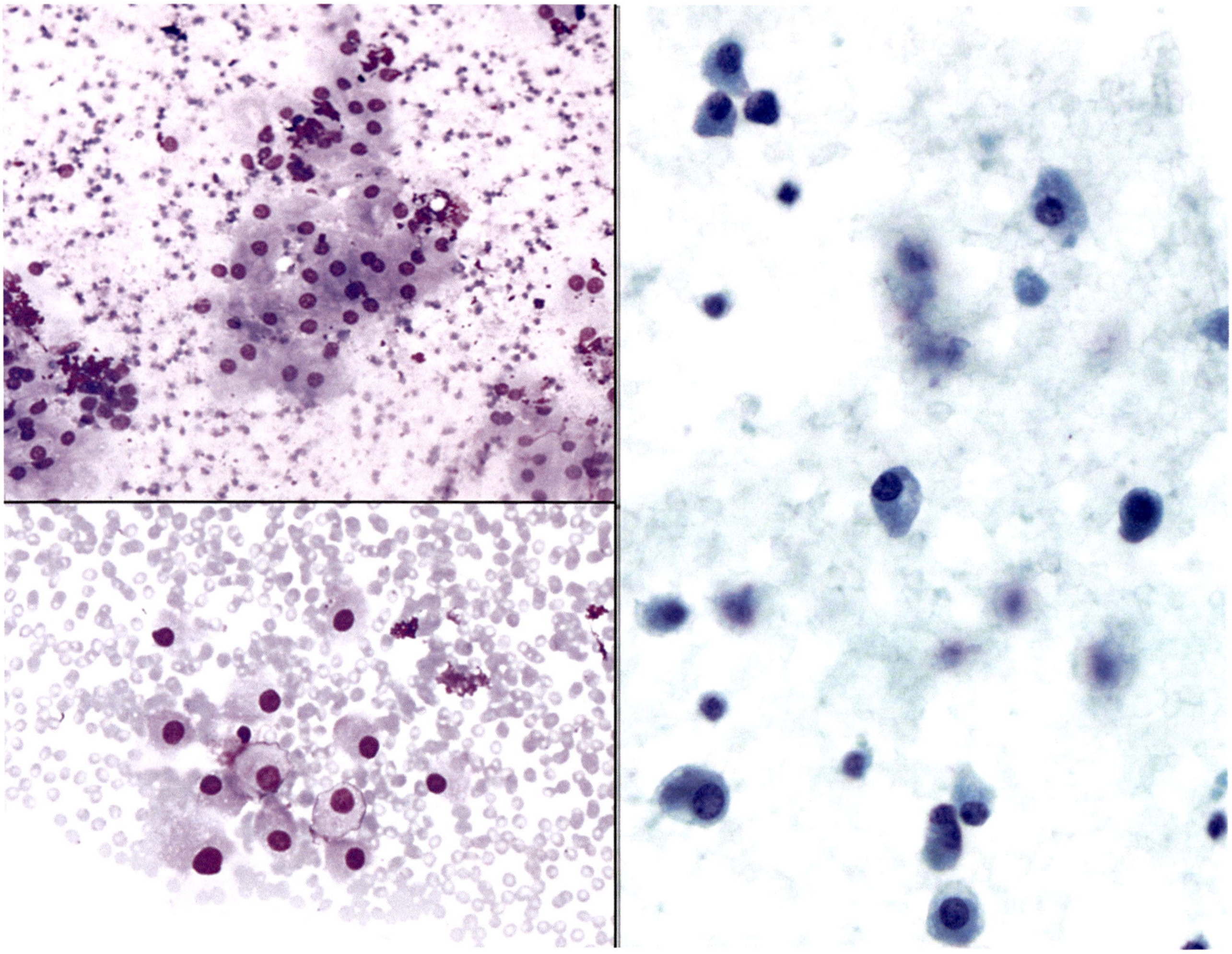

Fig. 10.9

Q-9. A 77-year-old female had a right renal mass. A CT-guided FNA was performed. What is the diagnosis of the FNA?

(a) Papillary renal cell carcinoma (RCC)
(b) Oncocytoma
(c) Benign renal tubular cells
(d) Cystic renal cell carcinoma (RCC)

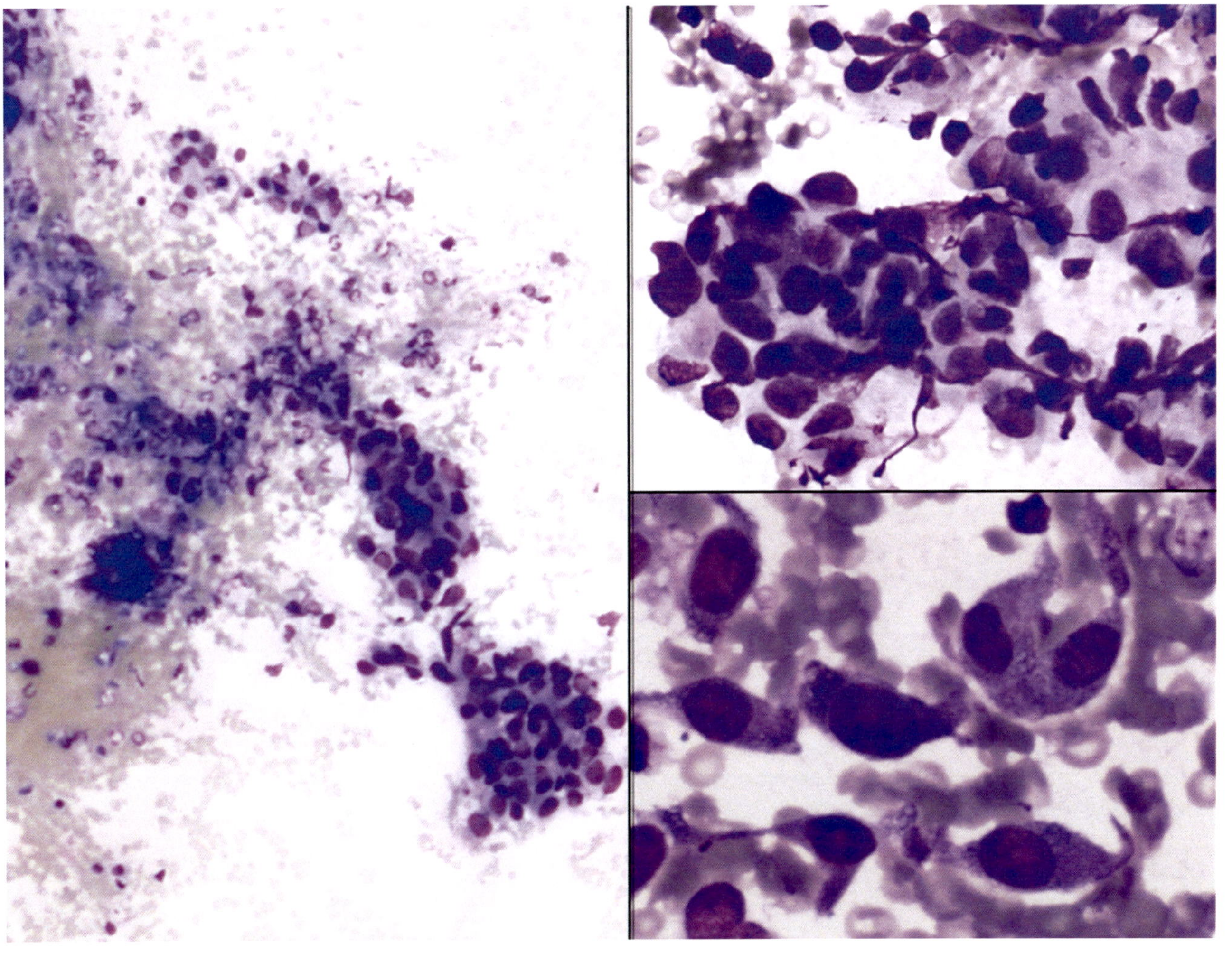

Fig. 10.10

Q-10. A 58-year-old male had a left renal mass. An ultrasound-guided FNA was performed. What is the diagnosis of the image?

(a) Metastatic adenocarcinoma
(b) Oncocytoma
(c) Benign renal tubular cells
(d) Urothelial cell carcinoma

Fig. 10.11

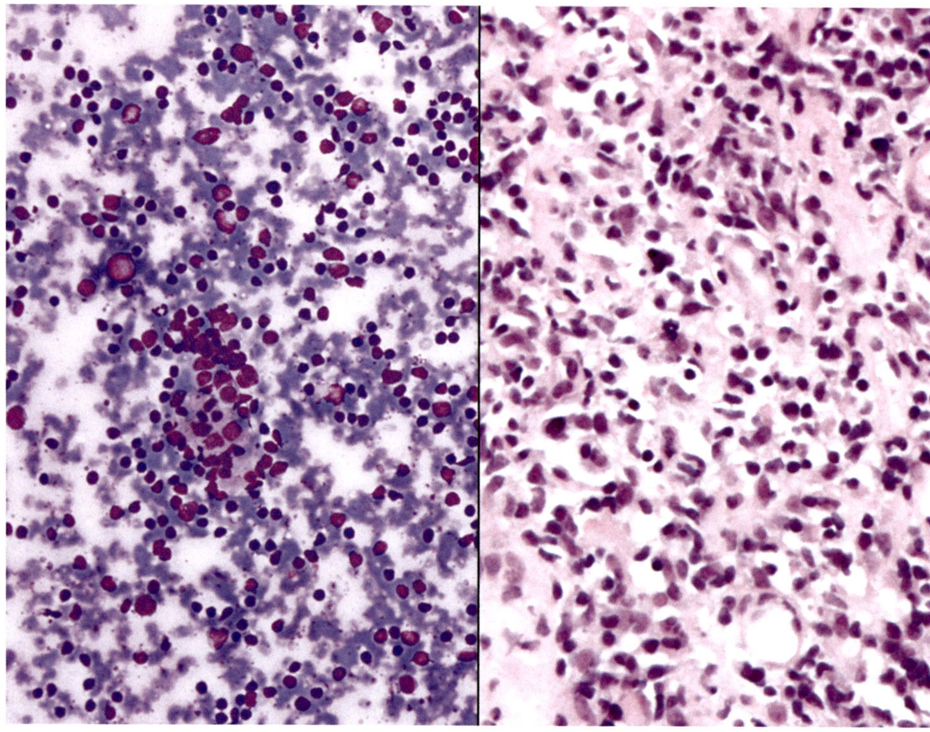

Q-11. A 60-year-old male had a right renal mass. An ultrasound-guided FNA was performed. What is the diagnosis of the FNA?

(a) Reactive lymphocyte hyperplasia
(b) Oncocytoma
(c) Benign renal tubular cells
(d) Diffuse large B cell lymphoma (DLBCL)

Fig. 10.12

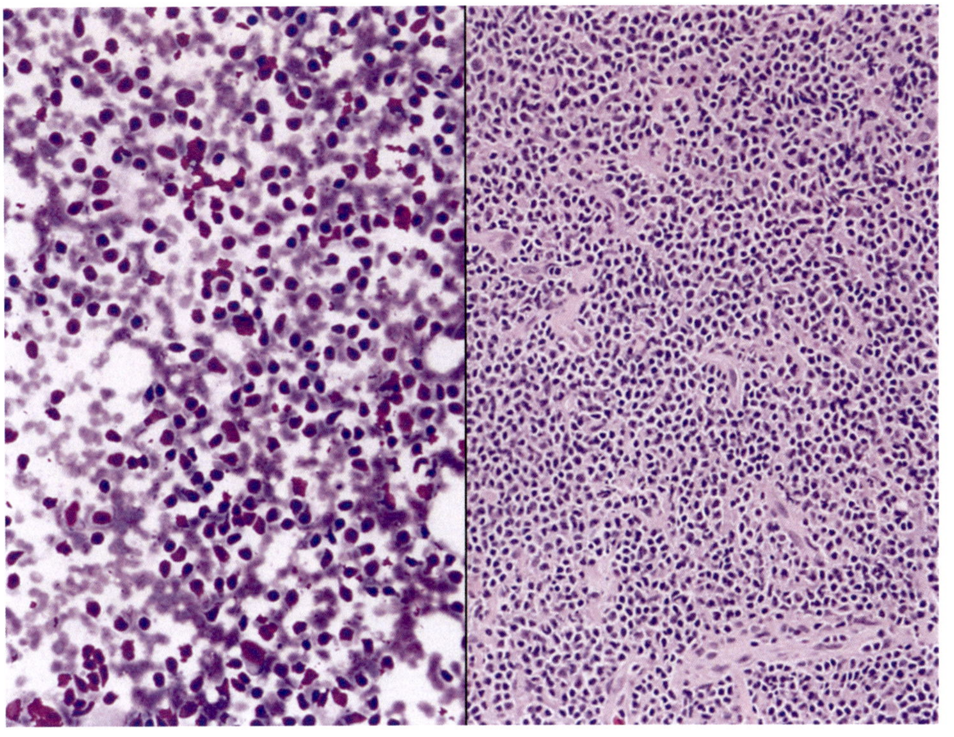

Q-12. A 63-year-old male had a left renal mass. An ultrasound-guided FNA was performed. What is the diagnosis of the FNA?

(a) Low-grade B cell lymphoma
(b) Oncocytoma
(c) Benign renal tubular cells
(d) Reactive lymphocyte hyperplasia

Fig. 10.13

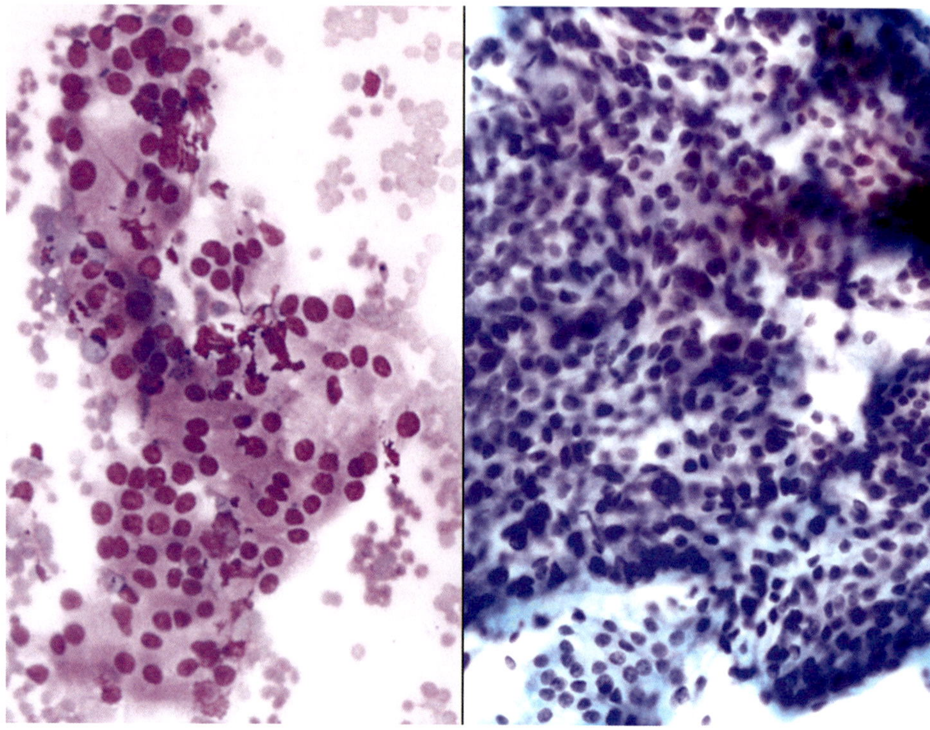

Q-13. A 65-year-old female had a left renal mass. A CT-guided FNA was performed. What is the diagnosis of the FNA?
(a) Benign renal tubular cells
(b) Papillary renal cell carcinoma (RCC)
(c) Differentiated, epithelial-predominant Wilms' tumor
(d) Metanephric adenoma (MA)

Fig. 10.14

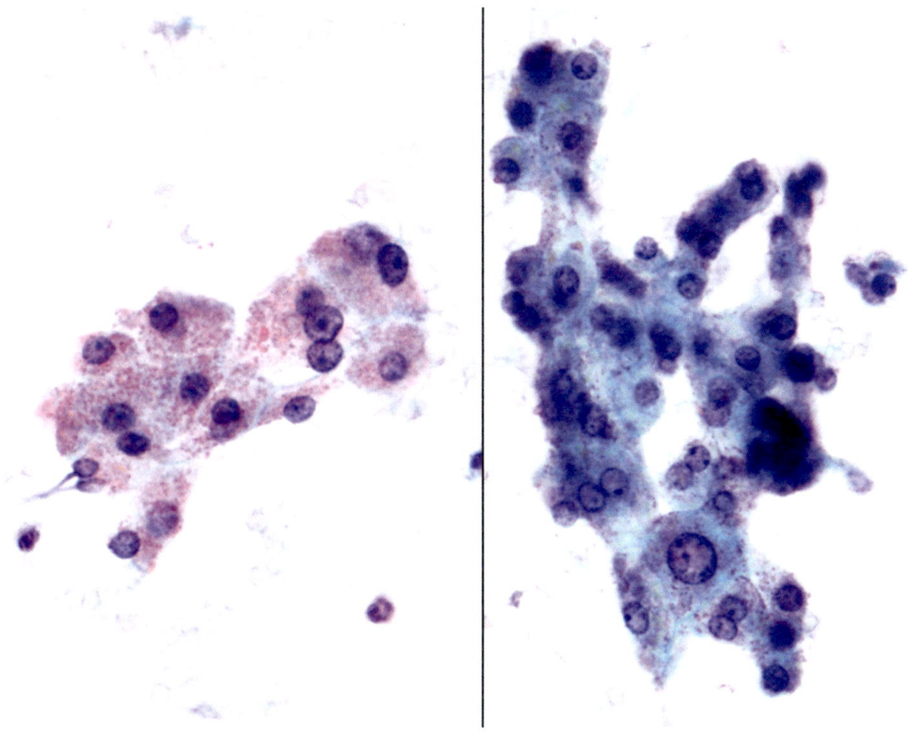

Q-14. A 52-year-old male had a left adrenal mass. A CT-guided FNA was performed. What is the diagnosis of the image?

(a) Normal adrenal cortical cells
(b) Oncocytoma
(c) Clear cell renal cell carcinoma (RCC)
(d) Adrenal cortical carcinoma

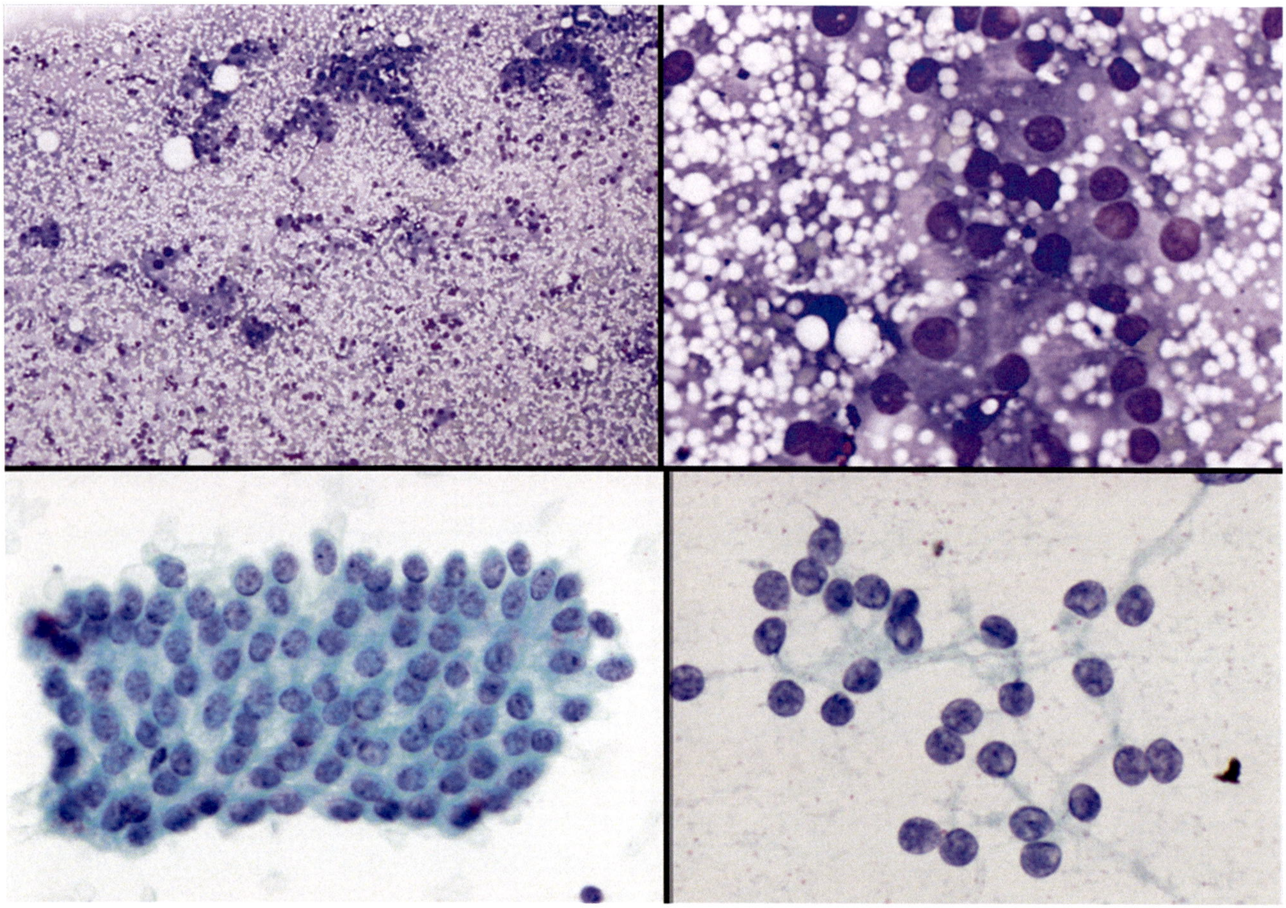

Fig. 10.15

Q-15. A 48-year-old female had a right adrenal mass. A CT-guided FNA was performed. What is the diagnosis of the image?
(a) Adrenal cortical adenoma
(b) Oncocytoma
(c) Clear cell renal cell carcinoma (RCC)
(d) Adrenal cortical carcinoma

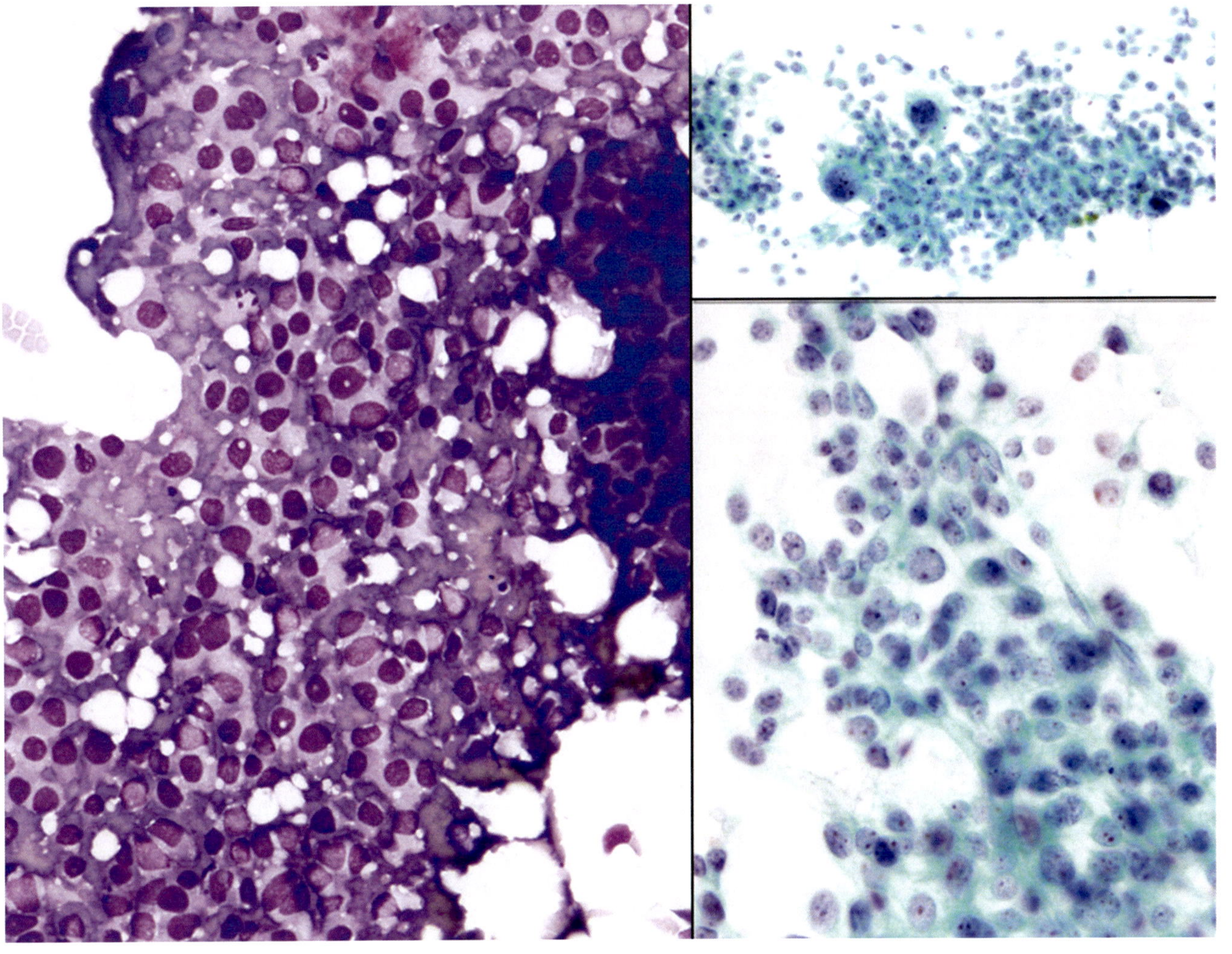

Fig. 10.16

Q-16. A 53-year-old female had a left adrenal mass. A CT-guided FNA was performed. What is the diagnosis of the FNA?

(a) Adrenal cortical adenoma
(b) Oncocytoma
(c) Adrenal cortical carcinoma
(d) Clear cell renal cell carcinoma (RCC)

Fig. 10.17

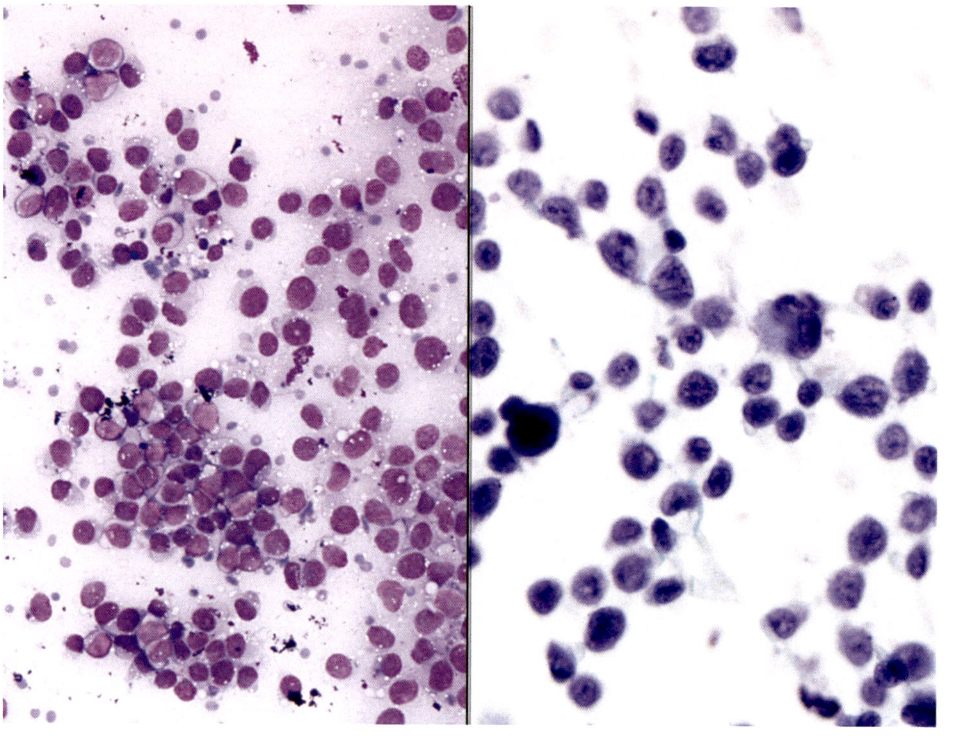

Q-17. A 70-year-old male had a left renal cyst. A CT-guided FNA was performed. What is the diagnosis of the FNA?

(a) Lymphoma
(b) Metastatic melanoma
(c) Adrenal cortical carcinoma
(d) Clear cell renal cell carcinoma (RCC)

Fig. 10.18

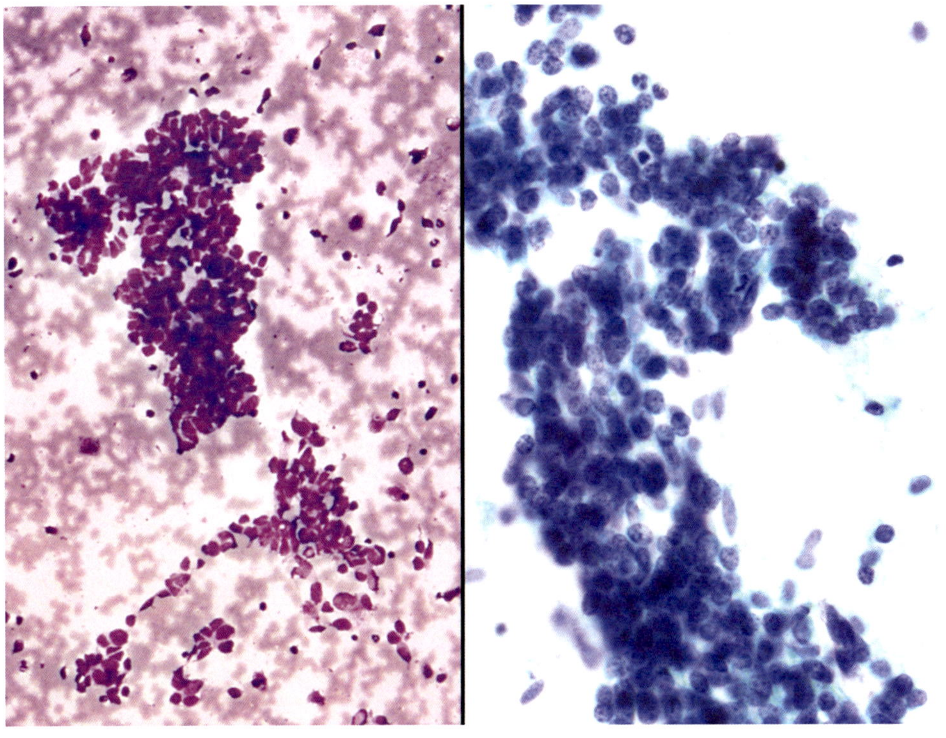

Q-18. An 83-year-old male has a lung mass and bilateral adrenal masses. A CT-guided FNA was performed. What is the diagnosis of the FNA?

(a) Lymphoma
(b) Metastatic small cell carcinoma
(c) Metastatic adenocarcinoma
(d) Clear cell renal cell carcinoma (RCC)

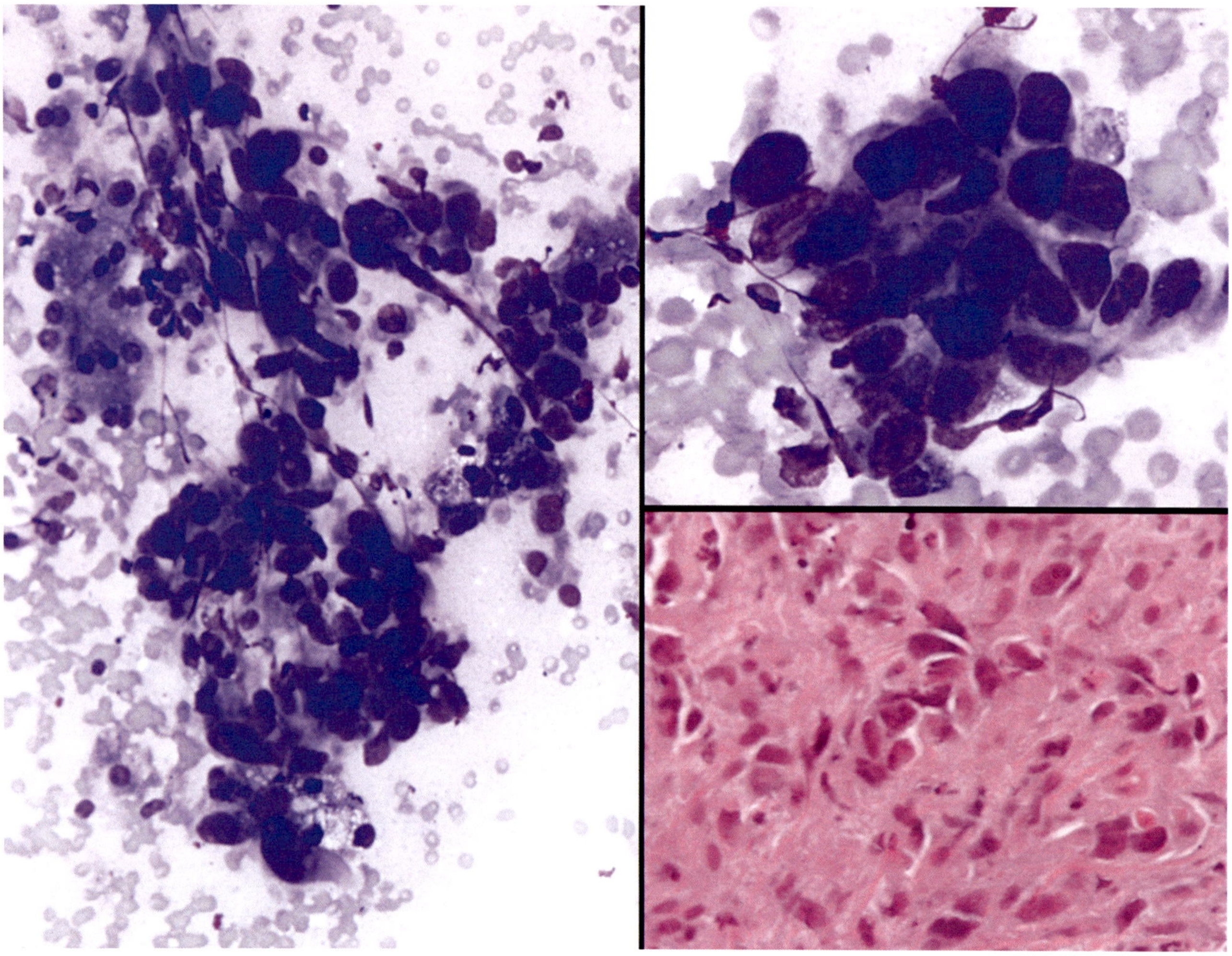

Fig. 10.19

Q-19. A 47-year-old male has a bladder mass and left renal cyst. A CT-guided FNA was performed. What is the diagnosis of the image?

(a) Metastatic melanoma
(b) Metastatic hepatocellular carcinoma (HCC)
(c) Metastatic renal cell carcinoma (RCC)
(d) Metastatic urothelial cell carcinoma

Fig. 10.20

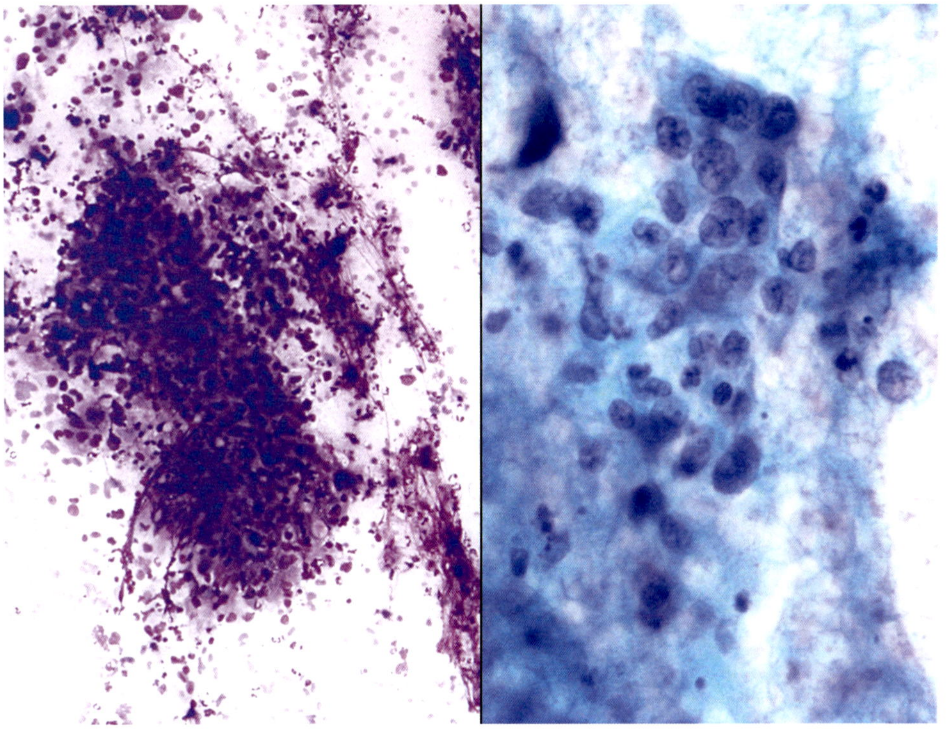

Q-20. A 65-year-old female has a uterine mass and a right adrenal mass. A CT-guided FNA was performed. What is the diagnosis of the image?

(a) Metastatic endometrial carcinoma
(b) Metastatic small cell carcinoma
(c) Metastatic melanoma
(d) Metastatic urothelial cell carcinoma

Fig. 10.21

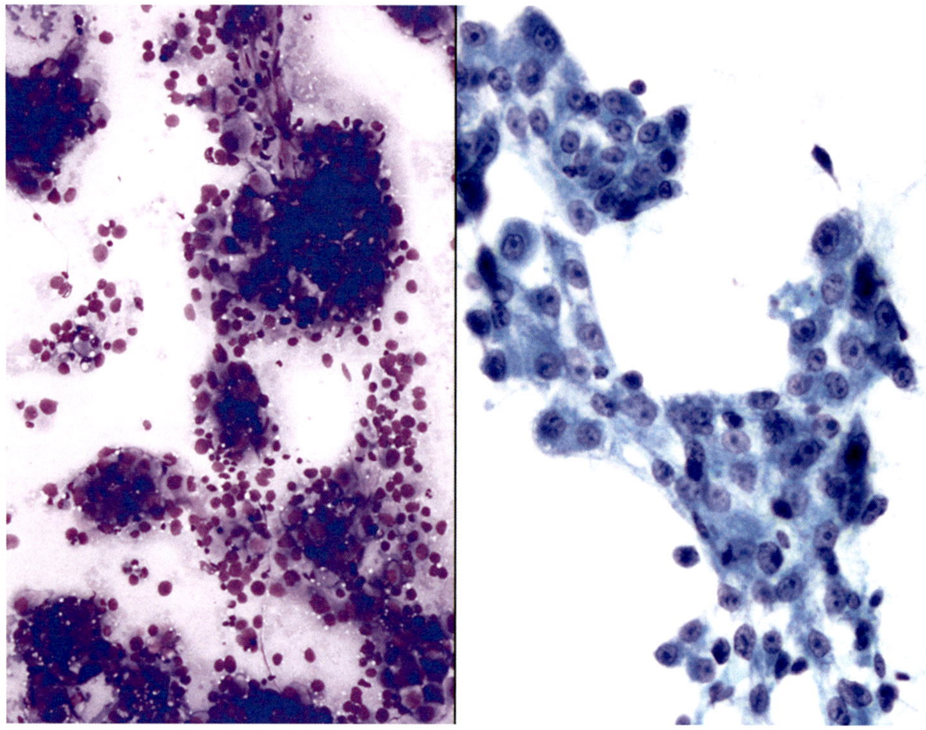

Q-21. A 63-year-old male has a liver mass and a right adrenal mass. A CT-guided FNA was performed. What is the diagnosis of the FNA?

(a) Metastatic adenocarcinoma
(b) Metastatic hepatocellular carcinoma (HCC)
(c) Metastatic melanoma
(d) Metastatic urothelial cell carcinoma

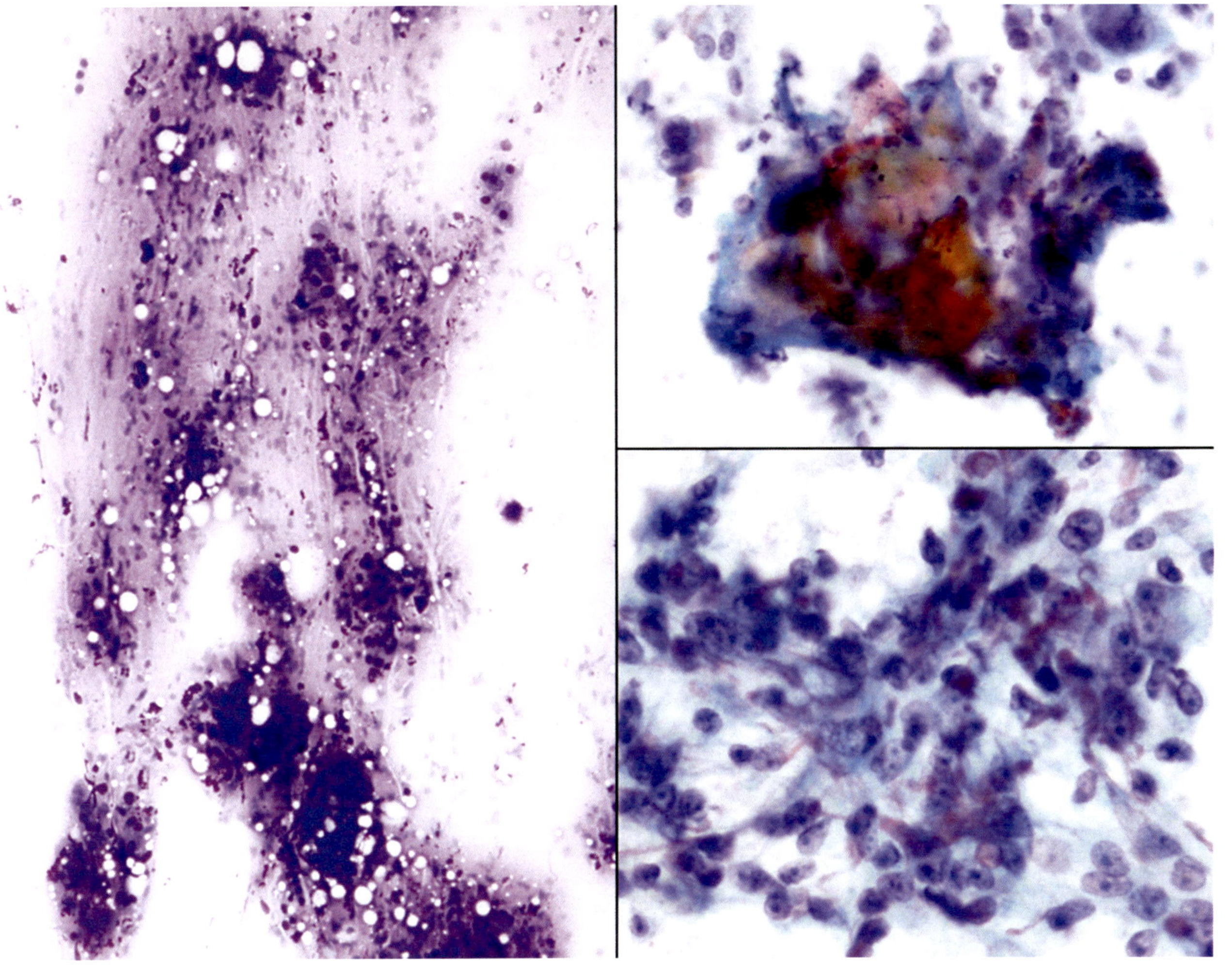

Fig. 10.22

Q-22. A 78-year-old male has a lung mass and a left adrenal mass. A CT-guided FNA was performed. What is the diagnosis of the FNA?

(a) Metastatic adenocarcinoma
(b) Metastatic urothelial cell carcinoma
(c) Metastatic squamous cell carcinoma
(d) Metastatic melanoma

Fig. 10.23

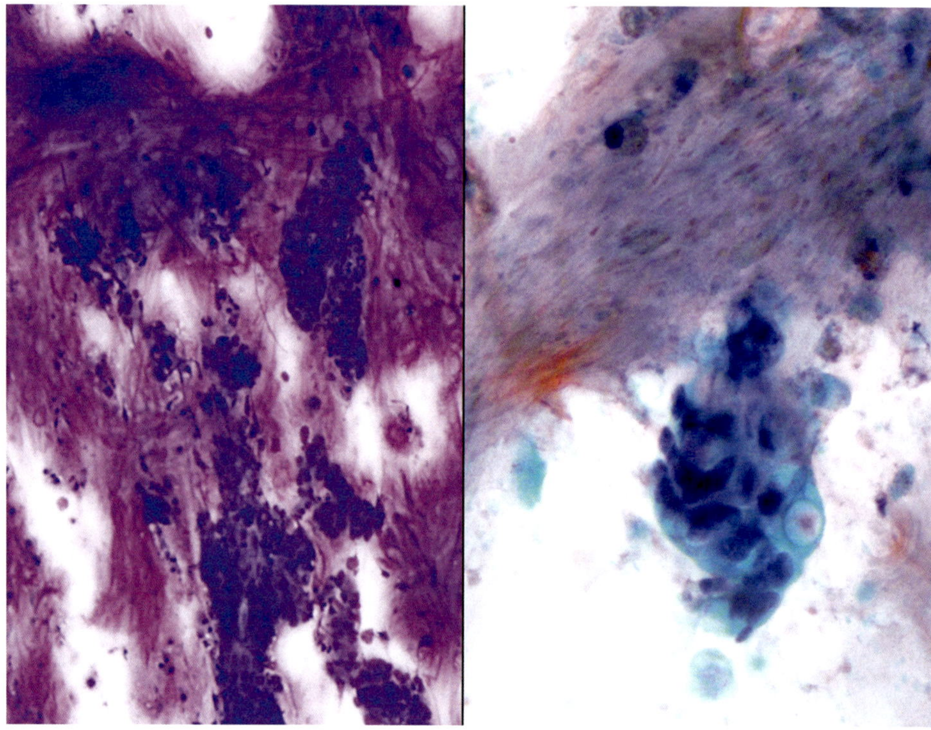

Q-23. A 69-year-old male has a small bowel mass and a left renal mass. A CT-guided FNA was performed. What is the diagnosis of the FNA?
(a) Metastatic mucinous adenocarcinoma
(b) Metastatic hepatocellular carcinoma (HCC)
(c) Metastatic squamous cell carcinoma
(d) Metastatic urothelial cell carcinoma

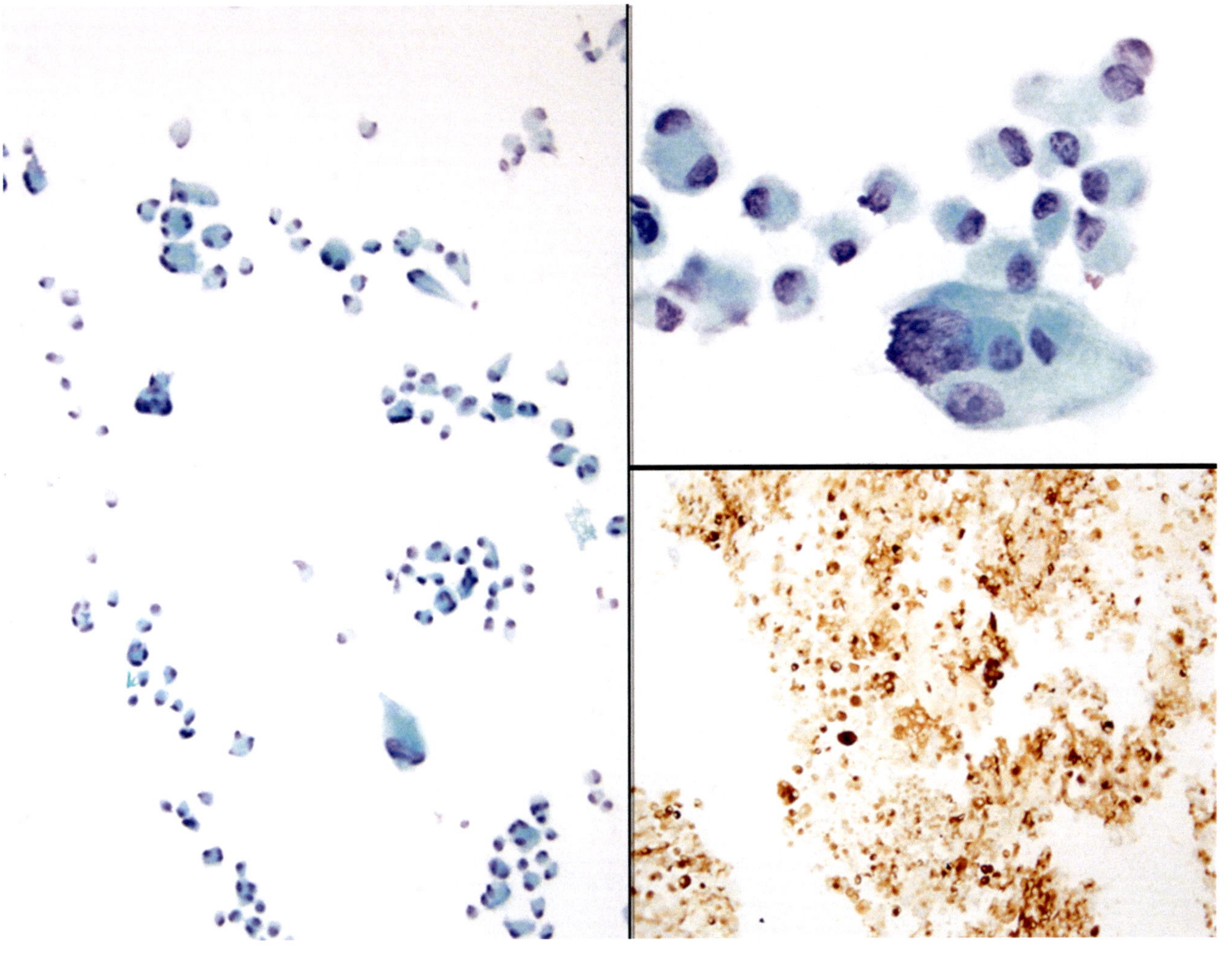

Fig. 10.24

Q-24. A 46-year-old male had a left adrenal mass. A CT-guided FNA was performed. What is the diagnosis of the FNA?
(a) Metastatic melanoma
(b) Metastatic hepatocellular carcinoma (HCC)
(c) Pheochromocytoma
(d) Metastatic squamous cell carcinoma

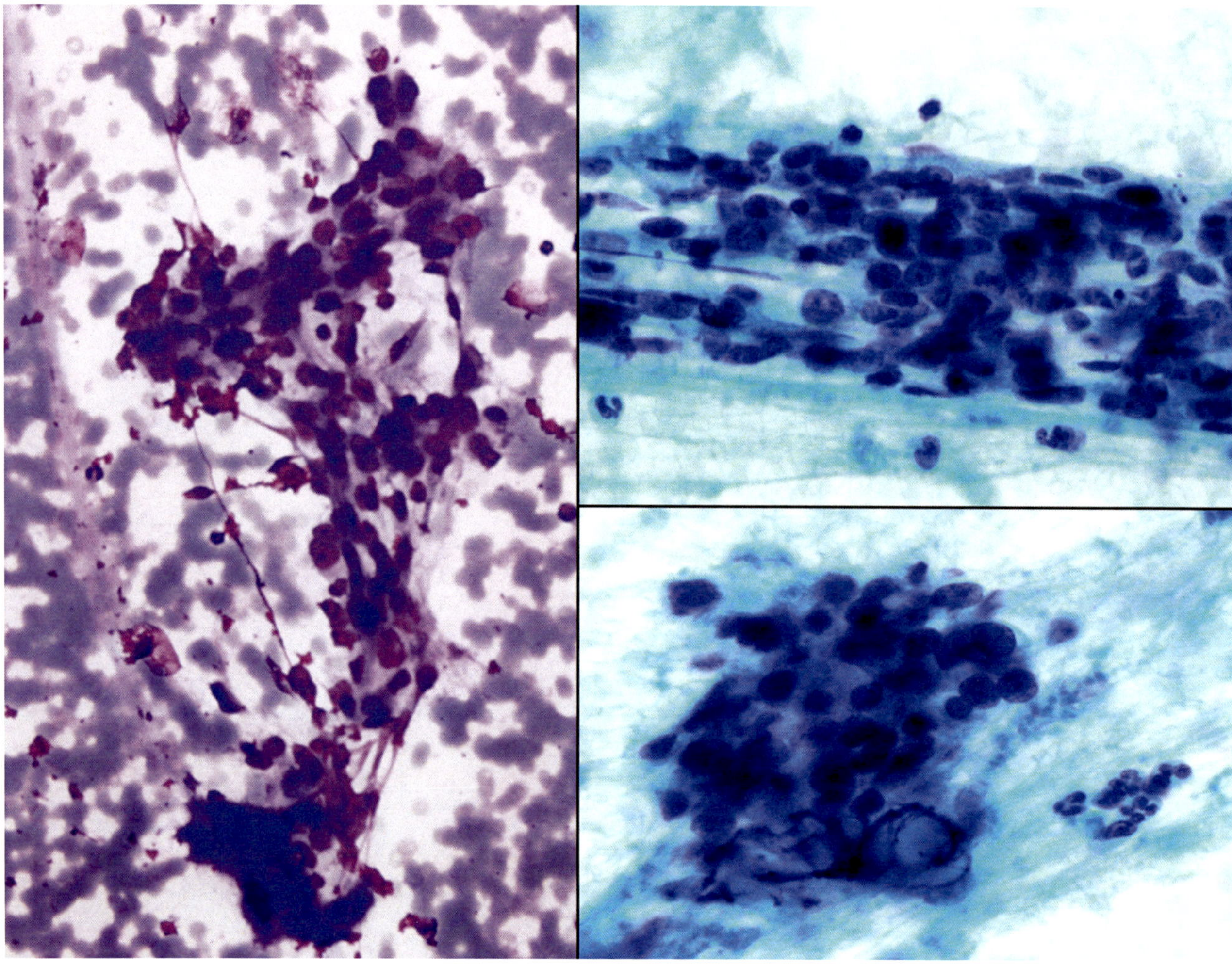

Fig. 10.25

Q-25. A 66-year-old male had a left renal cyst. An ultrasound-guided FNA was performed. What is the diagnosis of the image?
(a) Metastatic small cell carcinoma
(b) Metastatic prostate carcinoma
(c) Metastatic squamous cell carcinoma
(d) Metastatic urothelial cell carcinoma

10.2 Text-Based Questions 26–50

Q-26. All of the following cytological features are seen in clear cell renal cell carcinomas (RCCs), except:
(a) Abundant clear and/or granular cytoplasm
(b) Cohesive clusters and dispersed individual cells
(c) Eccentrically placed large round nuclei
(d) Numerous naked nuclei

Q-27. All of the following cytological features are seen in benign renal tubular cells, except:
(a) Nuclear enlargement and variation in size and shape
(b) Abundant granular cytoplasm
(c) Round nuclei and small nucleoli
(d) Small sheets and scattered individual cells

Q-28. Which statement about cystic renal cell carcinoma (RCC) is more accurate?
(a) Scant specimen with rare scattered tumor cells
(b) Trabecular, cord, and nest arrangement of tumor cells
(c) Large nuclei, scant cytoplasm, and high N:C ratios of tumor cells
(d) Numerous naked nuclei

Q-29. All of the following features are seen in a fine-needle aspiration (FNA) specimen containing benign renal tubular cells, except:
(a) Granular cytoplasm and indistinct cell borders
(b) Sheets and dispersed polygonal cells
(c) Uniform cells with centrically placed round nuclei
(d) Granular chromatin and small nucleoli

Q-30. Which statement about adrenal cortical adenoma is correct?
(a) The tumor involves bilateral adrenals.
(b) Clusters of uniform cells and numerous naked nuclei.
(c) Most of tumors are functioning and secret hormones.
(d) Tumor necrosis is a common finding.

Q-31. All of the following cytological features are seen in adrenal cortical carcinomas, except:
(a) Nuclear enlargement and variation in size and shape
(b) Clusters, sheets, and dispersed individual cells
(c) Large oval nuclei and coarse chromatin
(d) Numerous naked nuclei

Q-32. All descriptions of cytological features of angiomyolipoma (AML) in a renal FNA are correct, except:
(a) Thick-walled blood vessels are a common finding on the slide.
(b) Tumor consists of fat, myoid cells, and blood vessels.
(c) AML can be diagnosed by FNA.
(d) Some of the tumor may have virtually no fat component.

Q-33. A 68-year-old male presents with a right kidney mass and retroperitoneal lymphadenopathy. An ultrasound-guided FNA of the kidney mass was performed. On cytology smear and cell block section, numerous discohesive small- to intermediate-sized cells with high N:C ratio, hyperchromatic nuclei, and scant cytoplasm are identified. What is the most likely diagnosis of the FNA?
(a) Benign renal tubular cells
(b) Clear cell renal cell carcinoma (RCC)
(c) Lymphoma
(d) Small cell carcinoma

Q-34. Which statement regarding the angiomyolipoma (AML) is not correct?
(a) The tumors are commonly seen in elderly male patients.
(b) The tumor derives from perivascular epithelial cells.
(c) Tumor cells are positive for HMB45 and MART-1.
(d) Epithelioid cell variant of AMLs has metastatic potentials.

Q-35. Which statement about cystic renal cell carcinomas (RCCs) is correct?
(a) Adequate sampling of a cystic RCC is difficult.
(b) Cystic RCCs are difficult to distinguish from benign cysts.
(c) The diagnostic rate of cystic RCCs is low.
(d) All of the above.

Q-36. Which statement about adrenal cortical carcinomas is correct?
(a) The tumor involves bilateral adrenals.
(b) Clusters of uniform cells and numerous naked nuclei.
(c) Tumor cells have marked nuclear variations and atypia.
(d) Tumor necrosis is a rare finding.

Q-37. Which statement about translocation-associated renal cell carcinomas (Xp11 TRCCs) is correct?
(a) Tumors only involve children.
(b) Xp11 TRCCs have better prognosis than clear cell RCCs.
(c) The tumor has a distinct histomorphology and without clear cell morphology.
(d) Translocations on chromosome X involves the transcription factor E3 (*TFE3*) gene.

Q-38. Which statement about cytological features of glomeruli is correct?
(a) Glomerulus can only be found in the FNA of a benign lesion.
(b) It may be confused with papillary RCCs.
(c) Marked nuclear variations and atypia are characteristics.
(d) It contains flat sheets of cells.

Q-39. All of the following cytological features of oncocytomas in a renal FNA are correct, except:
(a) Tumor cells with bland nuclei and abundant granular cytoplasm.
(b) Tumor cells are arranged in small flat sheets and dispersed individual cells.
(c) No mitosis or tumor necrosis.
(d) Tumor cells with marked nuclear variations and atypia.

Q-40. On a cell block preparation, which of following cytological findings is the most useful feature in the differential diagnosis of an oncocytoma from a chromophobe renal cell carcinoma (RCC)?
(a) Tumor cells with bland nuclei, abundant granular cytoplasm, and distinct cell borders.
(b) Tumor cells are arranged in round circumscribed nests.
(c) Positive Hale's colloidal iron stains.
(d) Tumor cells with distinct cell borders.

Q-41. In a renal FNA specimen, cercariform cells are identified. What is the most likely diagnosis?
(a) Metastatic squamous cell carcinoma
(b) Metastatic melanoma
(c) Benign renal tubular cells
(d) Urothelial cell carcinoma

Q-42. In the FNA specimen of a kidney mass, which one of following features favors the diagnosis of a lymphoma?
(a) Numerous clusters of cells
(b) Monomorphous population of cells
(c) Lymphoglandular bodies
(d) Vesicular chromatin and inconspicuous nucleoli

Q-43. All of the following cytological features of Wilms' tumors in a renal FNA are correct, except:
(a) Bland nuclei and abundant granular cytoplasm
(b) Numerous discohesive small blue cells
(c) Mitoses and tumor necrosis
(d) Marked nuclear atypia

Q-44. Which statement about clear cell renal cell carcinomas (RCCs) is correct?
(a) Focally, tumor cells may show large hyperchromatic nuclei, multinucleation, and eosinophilic cytoplasm.
(b) The tumor may be composed of clear cells or granular cells or both. Sarcomatoid and other variants also occur.
(c) The smear reveals prominent small vessels (hypervascularity).
(d) All of the above.

Q-45. In an FNA specimen, which one of following features favors the diagnosis of a diffuse large B cell lymphoma (DLBCL)?
(a) Three-dimensional clusters of atypical large cells
(b) Discohesive and/or dispersed individual large atypical cells
(c) Clusters of large cells have markedly atypical nuclei and abundant cytoplasm
(d) Acini/papillary groups of large cells with pleomorphic nuclei and abundant cytoplasm

Q-46. All of the following cytological features of urothelial cell carcinomas in a renal FNA are correct, except:
(a) Tumor cells with bland nuclei and abundant granular cytoplasm
(b) Large tumor cells with hyperchromatic nuclei and inconspicuous nucleoli
(c) Dense cytoplasm
(d) Tumor cells with marked nuclear variations and atypia

Q-47. Which statement about adrenal cortical neoplasms is correct?
(a) Focally, tumor cells of carcinomas can be bland, whereas adenoma can be atypical.
(b) The tumor may be composed of clear cells or granular cells or both.
(c) Normal adrenal cortex and adenomas can be difficult to distinguish by cytology alone.
(d) All of the above.

Q-48. All of the following cytological features of pheochromocytoma in a renal FNA are correct, except:
(a) Three-dimensional clusters of cells with bland nuclei and abundant granular cytoplasm

(b) Large tumor cells with hyperchromatic nuclei and inconspicuous nucleoli
(c) Dense cytoplasm
(d) Tumor cells with marked nuclear variations and atypia

Q-49. Which of the features is not seen in a metastatic squamous cell carcinoma in an FNA specimen?
(a) Large nuclei with smudgy chromatin
(b) Nuclei with variation in size and shape
(c) Small pyknotic nuclei
(d) Large prominent nucleoli

Q-50. In an FNA specimen of a kidney mass, epithelioid cells with "clear cytoplasm" are identified. All of the following tumors can have this cytological feature, except:
(a) Oncocytoma
(b) Clear cell renal cell carcinoma (RCC)
(c) Papillary renal cell carcinoma (RCC)
(d) Benign renal tubular cells

10.3 Answers and Discussions of Image-Based Questions 1–25

A-1. **(c) Glomerulus**

In a renal FNA, glomeruli are large globular and/or lobulated structures with scalloped borders and contain spindled endothelial cells, oval-shaped mesangial cells, and capillary loops. Cells of glomeruli reveal normal N:C ratios, dense chromatin, and moderate cytoplasm. In clear cell RCCs, tumor cells form cohesive two-dimensional clusters and have large eccentrically placed nuclei, vesicular chromatin, and granular or vacuolated cytoplasm. Intercellular pink color strand-like material (basement membrane material) may be seen by the Diff-Quik stain. Nucleoli vary in size depending on the Fuhrman grade. In papillary RCCs, tumor cells form papillae with true fibrovascular cores and reveal dense nuclei and scant-to-moderate granular cytoplasm. Type 1 variant of papillary RCC reveals mild nuclear atypia, and type 2 variant reveals marked nuclear atypia. Foamy macrophages may also be identified in the background. In metastatic adenocarcinomas, tumor cells form acini and/or three-dimensional clusters and reveal hyperchromatic nuclei, coarse chromatin, prominent nucleoli, and vacuolated cytoplasm (indicative of mucin production).

A-2. **(c) Benign renal tubular cells**

Benign renal tubular cells, particularly proximal tubular cells, are arranged in loosely formed sheets and dispersed individual cells; they have a uniform appearance with round nuclei, fine granular chromatin, small nucleoli, abundant granular cytoplasm, and indistinct cytoplasmic border. Cells also reveal minimal nuclear variations and normal N:C ratios. In clear cell RCCs, tumor cells form cohesive two-dimensional clusters and have large eccentrically placed nuclei, vesicular chromatin, and granular or clear cytoplasm. Intercellular pink color strand-like material (basement membrane material) may be seen by the Diff-Quik stain. Nucleoli vary in size depending on the Fuhrman grade. In papillary RCCs, tumor cells form papillae with true fibrovascular cores and reveal dense nuclei and scant-to-moderate granular or clear cytoplasm. Type 1 variant of papillary RCC reveals mild nuclear atypia, and type 2 variant reveals marked nuclear atypia. Foamy macrophages may also be identified in the background. In metastatic adenocarcinomas, tumor cells form acini and/or three-dimensional clusters and reveal hyperchromatic nuclei, coarse chromatin, prominent nucleoli, and vacuolated cytoplasm (indicative of mucin production).

A-3. **(b) Clear cell renal cell carcinoma (RCC)**

The clear cell RCC variant (conventional renal cell carcinomas) is the most common histologic subtype of malignant renal tumors and accounts for 70 % of renal cell carcinomas. The "clear cell" appearances of tumor cells are due to the cytoplasmic glycogen and lipid that are dissolved during tissue processing. In RCCs, particularly in clear cell RCCs, tumor cells are arranged in clusters or dispersed individual cells and have round- to oval-shaped hyperchromatic nuclei; granular chromatin, with or without prominent nucleoli (depending on the Fuhrman grade); and clear or granular cytoplasm. Intercellular pink color strand-like material (basement membrane material) may be seen by the Diff-Quik stain. Focally, tumor cells may also show large hyperchromatic nuclei, multinucleation, and eosinophilic cytoplasm. Tumor necrosis may be seen, particularly in the Fuhrman grade III and IV tumors. The background of smear is bloody and with prominent small vessels (hypervascularity). In papillary RCCs, tumor cells form papillae with true fibrovascular cores and reveal dense nuclei and scant-to-moderate granular cytoplasm. Type 1 variant of papillary RCC reveals mild nuclear atypia, and type 2 variant reveals marked nuclear atypia. Foamy macrophages may also be identified in the background. In metastatic adenocarcinomas, tumor cells form acini and/or three-dimensional clusters and reveal hyperchromatic nuclei, coarse chromatin, prominent nucleoli, and vacuolated cytoplasm (indicative of mucin production). In benign renal tubular cells, particularly proximal tubular cells, they are arranged in loosely formed sheets and have round nuclei, fine chromatin, small nucleoli, abundant granular cytoplasm, and indistinct cytoplasmic border. Cells also reveal minimal nuclear variations and normal N:C ratios.

A-4. **(a) Benign renal cyst**

An FNA of a benign renal cyst reveals scant cellularity with scattered foamy macrophages and amorphous material in the background. The main differential diagnosis of benign renal cysts is cystic RCCs. In cystic RCCs, tumor cells are scant and reveal dispersed individual cells with round- to oval-shaped hyperchromatic nuclei; granular chromatin, with or without prominent nucleoli (depending on the Fuhrman grade); and clear or granular cytoplasm. In papillary RCCs, tumor cells form papillae with true fibrovascular cores and reveal dense nuclei and scant-to-moderate granular cytoplasm. Type 1 variant of papillary RCC reveals mild nuclear atypia, and type 2 variant reveals marked nuclear atypia. Foamy macrophages may also be identified in the background. In benign renal tubular cells, particularly proximal tubular cells, they are arranged in loosely formed sheets and have round nuclei, fine chromatin, small nucleoli, abundant granular cytoplasm, and indistinct cytoplasmic border. Cells also reveal minimal nuclear variations and normal N:C ratios.

A-5. (**b**) **Liesegang rings**
Liesegang rings are large laminated ringlike structures with double-layer outer walls, radial cross striations, and an amorphous central nidus. They are most commonly seen in a benign cystic fluid such as in renal and breast cysts and are composed of organic substances most likely formed by the precipitation from the cystic fluid. They stain blue in color with the hematoxylin-eosin (H&E) and the Papanicolaou methods. The differential diagnoses include parasites, parasitic eggs, algae, calcifications, and psammoma bodies. Awareness of the Liesegang phenomenon within cystic lesions will decrease the possibility of erroneous misdiagnosis as another type of pathologic process. The Charcot-Leyden crystals are a needle-shaped, orangeophilic structure derived from degenerated eosinophils; they may be found in a variety of lung diseases associated with increased eosinophils. Psammoma bodies are structures with concentrically laminated calcifications and a circumferential thin layer of epithelial cells; it is commonly seen in both carcinomas and benign conditions. The Michaelis-Gutmann bodies are small intracytoplasmic basophilic inclusions and measure 2–10 μm in diameter. They are composed of iron and calcium and associated with malakoplakia.

A-6. (**d**) **Cystic renal cell carcinoma** (**RCC**)
The main differential diagnosis of renal cysts is cystic RCCs. In cystic RCCs, tumor cells are scant and reveal dispersed individual cells with round- to oval-shaped hyperchromatic nuclei; granular chromatin, with or without prominent nucleoli (depending on the Fuhrman grade); and clear or granular cytoplasm. In papillary RCCs, tumor cells form papillae with true fibrovascular cores and reveal dense nuclei and scant-to-moderate granular cytoplasm. Type 1 variant of papillary RCC reveals mild nuclear atypia, and type 2 variant reveals marked nuclear atypia. Foamy macrophages may also be identified in the background. In benign renal tubular cells, particularly proximal tubular cells, they are arranged in loosely formed sheets and have round nuclei, fine chromatin, small nucleoli, abundant granular cytoplasm, and indistinct cytoplasmic border. Cells also reveal minimal nuclear variations and normal N:C ratios. In metastatic adenocarcinomas, tumor cells form acini and/or three-dimensional clusters and reveal hyperchromatic nuclei, coarse chromatin, prominent nucleoli, and vacuolated cytoplasm (indicative of mucin production).

A-7. (**c**) **Angiomyolipoma** (**AML**)
AML is a rare benign mesenchymal tumor and composed of mature fat cells, epithelioid spindle cells (smooth muscle cells), and blood vessels. The diagnosis depends on the identification of the triad. However, proportions of these components vary considerably from tumor to tumor. Some tumors are composed predominantly of fat, whereas others have virtually no fat and almost exclusive myoid cells (smooth muscle). In difficult cases, the immunohistochemical (IHC) stain of HMB45 is helpful and positive for the neoplastic cells. In RCCs, particularly in clear cell RCCs, tumor cells are arranged in clusters or dispersed individual cells and have round- to oval-shaped hyperchromatic nuclei; granular chromatin, with or without prominent nucleoli (depending on the Fuhrman grade); and clear or granular cytoplasm. Intercellular pink color strand-like material (basement membrane material) may be seen by the Diff-Quik stain. Focally, tumor cells may also show large hyperchromatic nuclei, multinucleation, and eosinophilic cytoplasm. Tumor necrosis may be seen, particularly in the Fuhrman grade III and IV tumors. The background of smear is bloody and with prominent small vessels (hypervascularity). In papillary RCCs, tumor cells form papillae with true fibrovascular cores and reveal dense nuclei and scant-to-moderate granular cytoplasm. Type 1 variant of papillary RCC reveals mild nuclear atypia, and type 2 variant reveals marked nuclear atypia. Foamy macrophages may also be identified in the background. In metastatic adenocarcinomas, tumor cells form acini and/or three-dimensional clusters and reveal hyperchromatic nuclei, coarse chromatin, prominent nucleoli, and vacuolated cytoplasm (indicative of mucin production).

A-8. (**d**) **Clear cell renal cell carcinoma** (**RCC**)
In clear cell RCC, tumor cells are arranged in clusters or dispersed individual cells and have round- to oval-shaped hyperchromatic nuclei; granular chromatin, with or without prominent nucleoli (depending on the Fuhrman grade); and clear or granular cytoplasm. Intercellular pink color strand-like material (basement membrane material) may be seen by the Diff-Quik stain. Focally, tumor cells may also show large

hyperchromatic nuclei, multinucleation, and eosinophilic cytoplasm. Tumor necrosis may be seen, particularly in the Fuhrman grade III and IV tumors. The background of smear is bloody and with prominent small vessels (hypervascularity). In papillary RCCs, tumor cells form papillae with true fibrovascular cores and reveal dense nuclei and scant-to-moderate granular cytoplasm. Type 1 variant of papillary RCC reveals mild nuclear atypia, and type 2 variant reveals marked nuclear atypia. Foamy macrophages may also be identified in the background. In benign renal tubular cells, particularly proximal tubular cells, they are arranged in loosely formed sheets and have round nuclei, fine chromatin, small nucleoli, abundant granular cytoplasm, and indistinct cytoplasmic border. Cells also reveal minimal nuclear variations and normal N:C ratios. In metastatic adenocarcinomas, tumor cells form acini and/or three-dimensional clusters and reveal hyperchromatic nuclei, coarse chromatin, prominent nucleoli, and vacuolated cytoplasm (indicative of mucin production).

A-9. (**b**) **Oncocytoma**

Oncocytoma is a benign tumor and comprises less than 5 % of all renal tumors. The FNA reveals a cellular specimen. Tumor cells are arranged in small flat clusters and dispersed individual cells and reveal bland nuclei and abundant granular cytoplasm. Nuclei are round in shape with fine chromatin, inconspicuous or small nucleoli, abundant dense granular cytoplasm, and distinct cytoplasmic borders. In cystic RCCs, tumor cells are scant and reveal dispersed individual cells with round- to oval-shaped hyperchromatic nuclei; granular chromatin, with or without prominent nucleoli (depending on the Fuhrman grade); and clear or granular cytoplasm. In papillary RCCs, tumor cells form papillae with true fibrovascular cores and reveal dense nuclei and scant-to-moderate granular cytoplasm. Type 1 variant of papillary RCC reveals mild nuclear atypia, and type 2 variant reveals marked nuclear atypia. Foamy macrophages may also be identified in the background. In benign renal tubular cells, particularly proximal tubular cells, they are arranged in loosely formed sheets and have round nuclei, fine chromatin, small nucleoli, abundant granular cytoplasm, and indistinct cytoplasmic border. Cells also reveal minimal nuclear variations and normal N:C ratios.

A-10. (**d**) **Urothelial cell carcinoma**

Urothelial cell carcinomas arise in the renal pelvis. Tumor cells are large in size and arranged in cohesive two-dimensional clusters and dispersed individual cells with large hyperchromatic nuclei, dense chromatin, inconspicuous nucleoli, and dense cytoplasm. Some of the tumor cells with elongated cytoplasm and flared cytoplasmic ends form the so-called cercariform cells, characteristics of urothelial cell neoplasm. The cercariform appearance is the result of pseudostratification of urothelial cells. In metastatic adenocarcinomas, tumor cells form acini and/or three-dimensional clusters and reveal hyperchromatic nuclei, coarse chromatin, prominent nucleoli, and vacuolated cytoplasm (indicative of mucin production). In oncocytomas, tumor cells are arranged in small flat clusters and dispersed individual cells and reveal bland nuclei and abundant granular cytoplasm. Nuclei are round in shape with fine chromatin, inconspicuous or small nucleoli, abundant dense granular cytoplasm, and distinct cytoplasmic borders. In benign renal tubular cells, particularly proximal tubular cells, they are arranged in loosely formed sheets and have round nuclei, fine chromatin, small nucleoli, abundant granular cytoplasm, and indistinct cytoplasmic border. Cells also reveal minimal nuclear variations and normal N:C ratios.

A-11. (**d**) **Diffuse large B cell lymphoma (DLBCL)**

DLBCL is a biological and clinical diverse group of diseases. The FNA reveals a cellular specimen with discohesive large atypical lymphoid cells. Three morphological variants are most commonly seen: centroblastic, immunoblastic, and anaplastic variant. Centroblastic variant is the most common subtype and reveals medium- to large-sized tumor cells with high N:C ratios, oval or round nuclei, fine chromatin, and single or multiple prominent nucleoli. Immunoblasts have a basophilic cytoplasm and a central nucleolus. The third morphologic variant, anaplastic variant, consists of large tumor cells with pleomorphic nuclei and may resemble the Hodgkin cells or Reed-Stemberg cells. Most cases of DLBCL are polymorphic, with a mixture of centroblastic and immunoblastic cells. Reactive lymphoid hyperplasia contains a heterogeneous mixture of lymphocytes, including small lymphocytes, centrocytes/centroblasts, immunoblasts, tingible body macrophages, and other cells. There is a great variation of cellular sizes and appearances, characteristic of polymorphous population of cells. In oncocytomas, tumor cells are arranged in small flat clusters and dispersed individual cells and reveal bland nuclei and abundant granular cytoplasm. Nuclei are round in shape with fine chromatin, inconspicuous or small nucleoli, abundant dense granular cytoplasm, and distinct cytoplasmic borders. In benign renal tubular cells, particularly proximal tubular cells, they are arranged in loosely formed sheets and have round nuclei, fine chromatin, small nucleoli, abundant granular cytoplasm, and indistinct cytoplasmic border. Cells also reveal minimal nuclear variations and normal N:C ratios.

A-12. (a) **Low-grade B cell lymphoma**
The FNA of a lymphoma reveals a cellular specimen with monomorphous population of lymphocytes, particularly in low-grade B cell lymphoma and/or small lymphocytic lymphomas/chronic lymphocytic leukemia (SLL/CLL). It represents a monoclonal proliferation of lymphoma cells. Other cytological features of a low-grade B cell lymphoma include discohesive tumor cells with hyperchromatic nuclei, clumped (soccer-ball-like) chromatin, irregular nuclear membranes, inconspicuous nucleoli and scant cytoplasm, and rare or absence of tingible body macrophages. Reactive lymphoid hyperplasia contains a heterogeneous mixture of lymphocytes, including small lymphocytes, centrocytes/centroblasts, immunoblasts, tingible body macrophages, and other cells. There is a great variation of cellular sizes and appearances, characteristic of polymorphous population of cells.

A-13. (d) **Metanephric adenoma** (MA)
MA is a rare benign tumor and most commonly occurs in females in the fifth decade. Histologically, MA is composed of closely packed acinar or tubular structures lined by bland cells with scanty interposed stroma. On cytological preparations, cells are arranged in tight clusters and loose sheets and have small round nuclei, inconspicuous or small nucleoli, and scant cytoplasm. Mitoses are conspicuously absent. Cells of MA are also positive for WT1 stain. The main differential diagnoses of MA are papillary RCC and differentiated, epithelial-predominant Wilms' tumor. In papillary RCCs, tumor cells form papillae with true fibrovascular cores and reveal dense nuclei and scant-to-moderate granular cytoplasm. Type 1 variant of papillary RCC reveals mild nuclear atypia, and type 2 variant reveals marked nuclear atypia. Foamy macrophages may also be identified in the background. Wilms' tumors involve infants and young children and are triphasic neoplasms, which contain blastemal components (closely packed small blue cells), mesenchymal components (spindle cells), and epithelial components (packed tubular structures). Therefore, MA can be difficult to distinguish from differentiated, epithelial-predominant Wilms' tumor. In differentiated, epithelial-predominant Wilms' tumor, cells are more hyperchromatic and with abundant mitoses.

A-14. (a) **Normal adrenal cortical cells**
Normal adrenal cortical cells are arranged in small sheets and dispersed individual cells with small round nuclei, granular chromatin, small centrically located nucleoli, and abundant clear and/or granular cytoplasm. In adrenal cortical carcinomas, tumor cells have marked nuclear variations and atypia, abundant mitoses, and necrotic debris. In oncocytomas, tumor cells are arranged in small flat clusters and dispersed individual cells and reveal bland nuclei and abundant granular cytoplasm. Nuclei are round in shape with fine chromatin, inconspicuous or small nucleoli, abundant dense granular cytoplasm, and distinct cytoplasmic borders. In clear cell RCC, tumor cells are arranged in clusters or dispersed individual cells and have round- to oval-shaped hyperchromatic nuclei; granular chromatin, with or without prominent nucleoli (depending on the Fuhrman grade); and clear or granular cytoplasm. Intercellular pink color strand-like material (basement membrane material) may be seen by the Diff-Quik stain. Focally, tumor cells may also show large hyperchromatic nuclei, multinucleation, and eosinophilic cytoplasm. Tumor necrosis may be seen, particularly in the Fuhrman grade III and IV tumors. The background of smear is bloody and with prominent small vessels (hypervascularity).

A-15. (a) **Adrenal cortical adenoma**
Adrenal cortical adenomas contain normal-appearing adrenal cortical cells, which are arranged in small sheets and dispersed individual cells. Tumor cells have small round nuclei, granular chromatin, small centrically located nucleoli, and abundant clear and/or granular cytoplasm. No mitosis is identified. Numerous naked nuclei floating in a frothy granular background is also a characteristic. Tumor necrosis is not a common finding in adrenal cortical adenomas. In adrenal cortical carcinomas, tumor cells have marked nuclear variations and atypia, abundant mitoses, and necrotic debris. In oncocytomas, tumor cells are arranged in small flat clusters and dispersed individual cells and reveal bland nuclei and abundant granular cytoplasm. Nuclei are round in shape with fine chromatin, inconspicuous or small nucleoli, abundant dense granular cytoplasm, and distinct cytoplasmic borders. In clear cell RCC, tumor cells are arranged in clusters or dispersed individual cells and have round- to oval-shaped hyperchromatic nuclei; granular chromatin, with or without prominent nucleoli (depending on the Fuhrman grade); and clear or granular cytoplasm.

A-16. (**c**) **Adrenal cortical carcinoma**

Histologically, the diagnosis of adrenal cortical carcinomas requires to follow strict criteria, such as nuclear grade, necrosis, capsular invasion, mitotic rate, and atypical mitoses. These features are difficult to evaluate on a cytological specimen. Nevertheless, most of the adrenal masses can be correctly classified as benign or malignant by FNAs. In adrenal cortical carcinomas, FNA reveals a cellular specimen. Tumor cells are arranged in loose clusters, sheets, and dispersed individual cells and have marked nuclear variations and atypia, abundant mitoses, and necrotic debris. Adrenal cortical adenomas contain normal-appearing adrenal cortical cells, which are arranged in small sheets and dispersed individual cells with small round nuclei, granular chromatin, small centrically located nucleoli, and abundant clear and/or granular cytoplasm. No mitosis or necrosis is identified. Numerous naked nuclei floating in a frothy granular background is also a characteristic. In oncocytomas, tumor cells are arranged in small flat clusters and dispersed individual cells and reveal bland nuclei and abundant granular cytoplasm. Nuclei are round in shape with fine chromatin, inconspicuous or small nucleoli, abundant dense granular cytoplasm, and distinct cytoplasmic borders. In clear cell RCC, tumor cells are arranged in clusters or dispersed individual cells and have round- to oval-shaped hyperchromatic nuclei; granular chromatin, with or without prominent nucleoli (depending on the Fuhrman grade); and clear or granular cytoplasm.

A-17. (**b**) **Metastatic melanoma**

In metastatic melanoma, tumor cells are usually arranged in loose clusters or dispersed individual cells. The nuclei of tumor cells are eccentrically located (plasmacytoid appearance) and highly variable in size with finely to coarsely granular chromatin and a single prominent cherry-red nucleoli. The cytoplasm tends to be abundant and may or may not contain melanin pigment. The N:C ratio may not be high. Melanin pigment appears coarsely granular and dark brown on the Papanicolaou stain. Other characteristic features include multinucleation, binucleation, and intranuclear inclusions. In lymphomas, tumor cells reveal a monomorphous appearance and lymphoglandular bodies. In adrenal cortical carcinomas, FNA reveals a cellular specimen. Tumor cells are arranged in loose clusters and dispersed individual cells and have marked nuclear variations and atypia, abundant mitoses, and necrotic debris. In clear cell RCC, tumor cells are arranged in clusters or dispersed individual cells and have round- to oval-shaped hyperchromatic nuclei; granular chromatin, with or without prominent nucleoli (depending on the Fuhrman grade); and clear or granular cytoplasm. In difficult cases, immunomarkers S100, HMB45, and MelanA/Mart1 are helpful in the differential diagnosis of melanomas.

A-18. (**b**) **Metastatic small cell carcinoma**

In small cell carcinomas, the size of tumor cells is smaller. Tumor cells reveal acini and/or pseudorosette arrangements, with hyperchromatic nuclei, fine (salt-and-pepper) chromatin, inconspicuous nucleoli, and scant cytoplasm. Nuclear crowding and molding are characteristic features. The background of the smear may also reveal "blue strips" (indicative of breakdown of nuclear material), abundant mitoses, and tumor necrosis. In adenocarcinoma, tumor cells form acini and/or three-dimensional clusters and can be confused with rosettes in a suboptimal prepared slides; tumor cells reveal hyperchromatic nuclei, vesicular or coarse chromatin, prominent nucleoli, and vacuolated cytoplasm (indicative of mucin production). In lymphoma, tumor cells are discohesive with clump chromatin and scant cytoplasm. Lymphoglandular bodies may be identified in the background of the smear. Metastatic melanoma reveals large discohesive tumor cells with prominent nucleoli and cytoplasmic pigment. In clear cell RCC, tumor cells are arranged in clusters or dispersed individual cells and have round- to oval-shaped hyperchromatic nuclei; granular chromatin, with or without prominent nucleoli (depending on the Fuhrman grade); and clear or granular cytoplasm.

A-19. (**d**) **Metastatic urothelial cell carcinoma**

The smears reveal a cellular specimen. Tumor cells are large in size and arranged in cohesive two-dimensional clusters and dispersed individual cells with large hyperchromatic nuclei, dense chromatin, inconspicuous nucleoli, and dense cytoplasm. Some of the tumor cells with elongated cytoplasm form the so-called cercariform cells, characteristics of urothelial cell neoplasm. In HCCs, tumor cells have large prominent nucleoli and cytoplasmic bile and/or lipofuscin pigments, which stain golden and brown color with the Papanicolaou method. Numerous naked nuclei are also seen in HCCs. Metastatic melanoma reveals large discohesive tumor cells with prominent nucleoli and cytoplasmic pigment. In clear cell RCC, tumor cells are arranged in clusters or dispersed individual cells and have round- to oval-shaped hyperchromatic nuclei; granular chromatin, with or without prominent nucleoli (depending on the Fuhrman grade); and clear or granular cytoplasm.

A-20. **(a) Metastatic endometrial carcinoma**
The smears reveal cohesive two-dimensional clusters, acini, and dispersed individual cells with high N:C ratios. Tumor cells have large hyperchromatic nuclei, coarse chromatin, conspicuous nucleoli, irregular nuclear membranes, and vesicular cytoplasm. These findings are consistent with a metastatic adenocarcinoma of the uterus primary. In metastatic urothelial cell carcinomas, tumor cells are large in size and arranged in cohesive two-dimensional clusters and dispersed individual cells with large hyperchromatic nuclei, dense chromatin, inconspicuous nucleoli, and dense cytoplasm. Some of the tumor cells with elongated cytoplasm form the so-called cercariform cells, characteristics of urothelial cell neoplasm. Metastatic melanoma reveals large discohesive tumor cells with prominent nucleoli and cytoplasmic pigment. In small cell carcinomas, the size of tumor cells is smaller. Tumor cells reveal acini and/or pseudorosette arrangements, with hyperchromatic nuclei, fine (salt-and-pepper) chromatin, inconspicuous nucleoli, and scant cytoplasm. Nuclear crowding and molding are characteristic features. The background of the smear may also reveal "blue strips" (indicative of breakdown nuclear material), abundant mitoses, and tumor necrosis.

A-21. **(b) Metastatic hepatocellular carcinoma (HCC)**
In metastatic HCCs, tumor cells show a wide range of cytomorphology. In poorly differentiated forms, malignant cells are polygonal and discohesive with pleomorphic nuclei and giant tumor cells. In well-differentiated forms, tumor cells resemble normal hepatocytes and form trabeculae, cords, and nests with slightly increased N:C ratios, large round nuclei, prominent nucleoli, naked nuclei, and bile pigment in the cytoplasm. The most notable features of HCCs are large polygonal cells with prominent nucleoli, dense cytoplasm which contains cytoplasmic bile and/or lipofuscin pigments, and numerous naked nuclei. In metastatic urothelial cell carcinomas, tumor cells are large in size and arranged in cohesive two-dimensional clusters and dispersed individual cells with large hyperchromatic nuclei, dense chromatin, inconspicuous nucleoli, and dense cytoplasm. Some of the tumor cells with elongated cytoplasm form the so-called cercariform cells, characteristics of urothelial cell neoplasm. Metastatic melanoma reveals large discohesive tumor cells with prominent nucleoli and cytoplasmic pigment. In metastatic adenocarcinomas, tumor cells form acini and/or three-dimensional clusters and reveal hyperchromatic nuclei, coarse chromatin, prominent nucleoli, and vacuolated cytoplasm (indicative of mucin production).

A-22. **(c) Metastatic squamous cell carcinoma**
Metastatic squamous cell carcinoma usually forms loose clusters or dispersed individual tumor cells. The cytological features of tumor cells include large nuclei with smudgy chromatin, nuclei with variation in size and shape, and dense cytoplasm (indicative of cytokeratin formation). The dense cytoplasm is blue in color with the Diff-Quik stain and red pink (eosinophilic) in color with the Papanicolaou stain. Prominent nucleoli can be seen in poorly differentiated squamous cell carcinomas and should not be confused with poorly differentiated adenocarcinomas. In metastatic adenocarcinomas, tumor cells form acini and/or three-dimensional clusters and reveal hyperchromatic nuclei, coarse chromatin, prominent nucleoli, and vacuolated cytoplasm (indicative of mucin production). In metastatic urothelial cell carcinomas, tumor cells are large in size and arranged in cohesive two-dimensional clusters and dispersed individual cells with large hyperchromatic nuclei, dense chromatin, inconspicuous nucleoli, and dense cytoplasm. Some of tumor cells with elongated cytoplasm form the so-called cercariform cells, characteristics of urothelial cell neoplasm. Metastatic melanoma reveals large discohesive tumor cells with prominent nucleoli and cytoplasmic pigment.

A-23. **(a) Metastatic mucinous adenocarcinoma**
The smears reveal abundant mucinous material and cohesive three-dimensional clusters of tumor cells with high N:C ratios. Tumor cells have large hyperchromatic nuclei, coarse chromatin, conspicuous nucleoli, irregular nuclear membranes, and cytoplasmic mucin. These findings are consistent with a metastatic mucinous adenocarcinoma of the intestinal primary. In metastatic urothelial cell carcinomas, tumor cells are large in size and arranged in cohesive two-dimensional clusters and dispersed individual cells with large hyperchromatic nuclei, dense chromatin, inconspicuous nucleoli, and dense cytoplasm. Some of the tumor cells with elongated cytoplasm form the so-called cercariform cells, characteristics of urothelial cell neoplasm. Metastatic melanoma reveals large discohesive tumor cells with prominent nucleoli and cytoplasmic pigment. In metastatic squamous cell carcinomas, cytological features of tumor cells include large nuclei with smudgy chromatin, nuclei with variation in size and shape, and dense cytoplasm (indicative of cytokeratin formation). In metastatic HCCs, the most notable features are large polygonal cells with prominent nucleoli, dense cytoplasm which contains cytoplasmic bile and/or lipofuscin pigments, and numerous naked nuclei.

A-24. (**c**) **Pheochromocytoma**

Pheochromocytoma is rarely aspirated due to the risk of hypertensive crisis. However, about 10 % of tumors are nonfunctional and may be aspirated. The FNA specimen reveals dispersed pleomorphic tumor cells with large hyperchromatic nuclei, granular chromatin, prominent nucleoli, and dense cytoplasm. Giant tumor cells with multinucleation and bizarre tumor cells are also common findings. Numerous mitoses may be present. Tumor cells are positive for chromogranin and synaptophysin. In metastatic squamous cell carcinomas, cytological features of tumor cells include large nuclei with smudgy chromatin, nuclei with variation in size and shape, and dense cytoplasm (indicative of cytokeratin formation). In metastatic HCCs, the most notable features are large polygonal cells with prominent nucleoli, dense cytoplasm which contains cytoplasmic bile and/or lipofuscin pigments, and numerous naked nuclei. Metastatic melanoma reveals large discohesive tumor cells with prominent nucleoli and cytoplasmic pigment. Finally, pheochromocytomas can behave in a benign or malignant fashion; morphology is not always predictive of clinical behaviors.

A-25. (**b**) **Metastatic prostate carcinoma**

The smears reveal three-dimensional clusters of hyperchromatic cells with acinar arrangements and high N:C ratios. In metastatic prostate carcinomas, tumor cells are intermediate in size with hyperchromatic nuclei, coarse chromatin, irregular nuclear membrane, prominent nucleoli, and vacuolated cytoplasm. In metastatic small cell carcinomas, tumor cells are small with fine (salt-and-pepper) chromatin and scant cytoplasm. Nuclear crowding and molding and tumor necrosis are also characteristics of a small cell carcinoma. In metastatic squamous cell carcinomas, cytological features of tumor cells include large nuclei with smudgy chromatin, nuclei with variation in size and shape, and dense cytoplasm (indicative of cytokeratin formation). In metastatic urothelial cell carcinomas, tumor cells are large in size and arranged in cohesive two-dimensional clusters and dispersed individual cells with large hyperchromatic nuclei, dense chromatin, inconspicuous nucleoli, and dense cytoplasm. Some of the tumor cells with elongated cytoplasm form the so-called cercariform cells, characteristics of urothelial cell neoplasm.

10.4 Answers and Discussions of Text-Based Questions 26–50

A-26. **(d) Numerous naked nuclei**
The clear cell RCC variant (conventional renal cell carcinomas) is the most common histologic subtype of malignant renal tumors and accounts for 70 % of renal cell carcinomas. The "clear cell" appearances of tumor cells are due to the cytoplasmic glycogen and lipids that are dissolved during tissue processing. In clear cell RCCs, tumor cells are arranged in clusters or dispersed individual cells and have round- to oval-shaped hyperchromatic nuclei; granular chromatin, with or without prominent nucleoli (depending on the Fuhrman grade); and clear or granular cytoplasm. Intercellular pink color strand-like material (basement membrane material) may be seen by the Diff-Quik stain. Focally, tumor cells may also show large hyperchromatic nuclei, multinucleation, and eosinophilic cytoplasm. Tumor necrosis may be seen, particularly in the Fuhrman grade III and IV tumors. The background of smear is bloody and with prominent small vessels (hypervascularity). Numerous naked nuclei are the feature seen in adrenal cortical adenomas; it is not the feature seen in clear cell RCCs.

A-27. **(a) Nuclear enlargement and variation in size and shape**
Benign renal tubular cells, particularly proximal tubular cells, are arranged in loosely formed sheets and dispersed individual cells; they have a uniform appearance with round nuclei, fine granular chromatin, small nucleoli, abundant granular cytoplasm, and indistinct cytoplasmic borders. Cells also reveal minimal nuclear variations and normal N:C ratios. Nuclear enlargement and variation in size and shape are not features seen in benign renal tubular cells.

A-28. **(a) Scant specimen with rare scattered tumor cells**
In cystic renal lesions, the main differential diagnosis is cystic RCC. In cystic RCCs, tumor cells are scant and have low N:C ratios; therefore, it is difficult to make the diagnosis. Tumor cells of cystic RCCs have similar cytological features as seen in clear cell RCCs, including dispersed individual cells with round- to oval-shaped hyperchromatic nuclei; granular chromatin, with or without prominent nucleoli (depending on the Fuhrman grade); and clear or granular cytoplasm. Trabecular, cord, and nest arrangements of tumor cells with large nuclei, scant cytoplasm, high N:C ratios, and numerous naked nuclei are not features seen in cystic RCCs. Finally, the diagnosis of cystic RCCs should be correlated with radiographic findings.

A-29. **(b) Sheets and dispersed polygonal cells**
Benign renal tubular cells, particularly proximal tubular cells, are arranged in loosely formed sheets and dispersed individual cells; they have a uniform appearance with round nuclei, fine granular chromatin, small nucleoli, abundant granular cytoplasm, and indistinct cytoplasmic border. Cells also reveal minimal nuclear variations and normal N:C ratios. Sheets and dispersed polygonal cells are not features seen in benign renal tubular cells.

A-30. **(b) Clusters of uniform cells and numerous naked nuclei**
Adrenal cortical adenomas are quite common and involve approximately 5 % of adults. In contrast to adrenal cortical carcinomas, more than 85 % of adenomas are nonfunctioning. The tumor usually occurs unilaterally. The adrenal cortical adenomas contain normal-appearing adrenal cortical cells, which are arranged in small sheets and dispersed individual cells. Tumor cells have small round nuclei, granular chromatin, small centrically located nucleoli, and abundant clear and/or granular cytoplasm. No mitosis is identified. Numerous naked nuclei floating in a frothy granular background are also characteristics. Tumor necrosis is not a common finding in adrenal cortical adenomas.

A-31. **(d) Numerous naked nuclei**
In adrenal cortical carcinomas, FNA reveals a cellular specimen. Tumor cells are arranged in loose clusters, sheets, and dispersed individual cells and have marked nuclear variations and atypia, abundant mitoses, and necrotic debris. Histologically, the diagnosis of adrenal cortical carcinomas requires to follow strict criteria, such as nuclear grade, tumor necrosis, capsular invasion, mitotic rate, and atypical mitoses. These features are difficult to evaluate in a cytological specimen. Nevertheless, most of the adrenal masses can be correctly classified as benign or malignant by FNAs. Numerous naked nuclei floating in a frothy granular background are characteristics of adrenal cortical adenomas.

A-32. **(a) Thick-walled blood vessels are a common finding on the slide**
The diagnosis of AML depends on the identification of the triad of mature fat, spindle ells (smooth muscle cells), and blood vessels. However, proportions of three components vary considerably from tumor to tumor. Some tumors are composed predominantly of fat, whereas others have virtually no fat and almost exclusively myoid cells (smooth muscle cells).

In general, tumor reveals cohesive clusters of spindle-shaped smooth muscle cells, fat cells, and vessels. Occasionally, thick-walled blood vessels are seen on FNA slides. But it is not a common finding. In difficult cases, the immunohistochemical (IHC) stain of HMB45 is helpful and positive for the neoplastic cells.

A-33. **(c) Lymphoma**

The most likely diagnosis of this FNA is a lymphoma. The cytological features of numerous discohesive small- to intermediate-sized cells with high N:C ratio, hyperchromatic nuclei, and scant cytoplasm are characteristics of lymphomas. The monomorphous appearance of the lesion represents a monoclonal proliferation of lymphoma cells. Other cytological features of lymphoma include hyperchromatic clumped (soccer-ball-like) chromatin, irregular nuclear membrane, and scant basophilic cytoplasm. Lymphoglandular bodies can also be seen in the background. In small cell carcinomas, tumor cells reveal salt-and-pepper chromatin, nuclear molding and crowding, numerous apoptotic bodies, and mitotic figures. Benign renal tubular cells, particularly proximal tubular cells, are arranged in loosely formed sheets and dispersed individual cells; they have a uniform appearance with round nuclei, fine granular chromatin, small nucleoli, abundant granular cytoplasm; and indistinct cytoplasmic borders. Cells also reveal minimal nuclear variations and normal N:C ratios. In clear cell RCCs, tumor cells form cohesive two-dimensional clusters and have large eccentrically placed nuclei, vesicular chromatin, and granular or vacuolated cytoplasm. Intercellular pink color strand-like material (basement membrane material) may be seen by the Diff-Quik stain.

A-34. **(a) The tumors are commonly seen in elderly male patients**

AML is a rare benign mesenchymal tumor and occurs in two distinct clinical settings: in young adults with tuberous sclerosis (TS) and/or in young and middle-aged females without clinical syndrome. The diagnosis of the tumor depends on the identification of the triad of mature fat, spindle cells (smooth muscle cells), and blood vessels. However, proportions of the three components vary considerably from tumor to tumor. Some tumors are composed predominantly of fat, whereas others have virtually no fat and almost exclusive myoid cells (smooth muscle). In difficult cases, the immunohistochemical (IHC) stain of HMB45 is helpful and positive for the neoplastic cells. Although AML is considered as a benign tumor, the epithelioid cell variant has a potential risk for metastasis.

A-35. **(d) All of the above**

In cystic renal lesions, the main differential diagnosis is cystic RCC. In cystic RCCs, tumor cells are scant and have low N:C ratios; therefore, it is difficult to make the diagnosis. Tumor cells of cystic RCCs have similar cytological features as seen in clear cell RCCs, including dispersed individual cells with round- to oval-shaped hyperchromatic nuclei; granular chromatin, with or without prominent nucleoli (depending on the Fuhrman grade); and clear or granular cytoplasm. Adequate sampling of a cystic RCC is difficult. The cytological diagnostic rate of cystic RCCs is low. Finally, the diagnosis of cystic RCCs should be correlated with radiographic findings.

A-36. **(c) Tumor cells have marked nuclear variation and atypia**

In adrenal cortical carcinomas, FNA reveals a cellular specimen. Tumor cells are arranged in loose clusters, sheets, and dispersed individual cells and have marked nuclear variations and atypia, abundant mitoses, and necrotic debris. Histologically, the diagnosis of adrenal cortical carcinomas requires to follow strict criteria, such as nuclear grade, tumor necrosis, capsular invasion, mitotic rate, and atypical mitoses. These features are difficult to evaluate on a cytological specimen. Nevertheless, most of the adrenal masses can be correctly classified as benign or malignant by FNAs. Clusters of uniform cells and numerous naked nuclei floating in a frothy granular background are characteristics of adrenal cortical adenoma.

A-37. **(d) Translocations on chromosome X involves the transcription factor E3 (*TFE3*) gene**

Xp11 TRCC is a rare variant of RCCs and may be found in both pediatric and adult population. Tumors usually present at an advanced stage with metastases and universally have an aggressive clinical course and poor prognosis. The gross pathologic feature of Xp11 TRCCs reveals a well-circumscribed tumor without areas of hemorrhage or necrosis. Histological examination of the tumor reveals nests, loosely formed clusters, and papillary arrangements of cells with granular and/or clear cytoplasm. These features are often confused with papillary RCCs and/or clear cell RCCs. The most common genetic abnormality of Xp11 TRCCs is the Xp11 mutations, which result in gene fusion products between the helix-loop-helix leucine zipper transcription factor (*TFE3*) and the alveolar soft part sarcoma locus (*ASPL*). A strong clinical suspicion and a positive immunostain of TEF3 are necessary to distinguish Xp11 TRCCs from papillary and clear cell RCCs.

A-38. (**b**) **It may be confused with papillary RCCs**
Normal elements are frequently encountered on renal FNAs, particularly when a small lesion is sampled. Therefore, glomeruli can be found on slides from both benign and malignant lesions. In a renal FNA, glomeruli are large globular and/or lobulated structures with scalloped borders and contain spindled endothelial cells, oval-shaped mesangial cells, and capillary loops. Cells of glomeruli reveal normal N:C ratios, dense chromatin, and moderate cytoplasm. Marked nuclear variations and atypia are not seen in glomerulus. Glomerulus may be confused with papillary RCCs. In papillary RCCs, tumor cells form papillae with true fibrovascular cores and reveal dense nuclei and scant-to-moderate granular cytoplasm. Type 1 variant of papillary RCC reveals mild nuclear atypia, and type 2 variant reveals marked nuclear atypia. Foamy macrophages may also be identified in the background.

A-39. (**d**) **Tumor cells with marked nuclear variations and atypia**
Oncocytoma is a benign tumor and comprises less than 5 % of all renal tumors. The FNA reveals a cellular specimen. Tumor cells are arranged in small flat clusters and dispersed individual cells and reveal bland nuclei and abundant granular cytoplasm. Nuclei are round in shape with fine chromatin, inconspicuous or small nucleoli, abundant dense granular cytoplasm, and distinct cytoplasmic borders. No mitosis or tumor necrosis is present. Tumor cells with marked nuclear variations and atypia are not features seen in oncocytomas.

A-40. (**b**) **Tumor cells are arranged in round circumscribed nests**
The distinction between oncocytomas and chromophobe RCCs can be difficult due to overlapping cytological features between the two tumors. In oncocytomas, tumor cells reveal bland nuclei and abundant granular cytoplasm. Nuclei are round in shape with fine chromatin, inconspicuous or small nucleoli, abundant dense granular cytoplasm, and distinct cytoplasmic borders. In chromophobe RCCs, tumor cells reveal similar cytological features, such as bland nuclei, abundant granular cytoplasm, and distinct cell borders. Furthermore, both tumors can be positive for Hale's colloidal iron stain, although oncocytoma is focally positive and chromophobe RCC is diffusely positive. Therefore, the most useful cytological feature for the differential diagnosis of oncocytomas is the cellular arrangement on cell block preparations. Tumor cells of oncocytomas are arranged in round circumscribed nests, whereas tumor cells of chromophobe RCCs are arranged in "endless sheets."

A-41. (**d**) **Urothelial cell carcinoma**
Cercariform cells are urothelial cells with elongated cytoplasm and flared cytoplasmic ends. They are tadpole-like cells and a characteristic of urothelial cell carcinomas. Other cytological findings of urothelial cell carcinomas include large tumor cells with hyperchromatic nuclei, dense chromatin, inconspicuous nucleoli, and dense cytoplasm. In metastatic melanoma, tumor cells are usually arranged in loose clusters or dispersed individual cells. The nuclei of tumor cells are eccentrically located (plasmacytoid appearance), highly variable in size with finely to coarsely granular chromatin, and a single prominent cherry-red nucleoli. Cytoplasmic melanin pigments may also be present. In benign renal tubular cells, particularly proximal tubular cells, they are arranged in loosely formed sheets and have round nuclei, fine chromatin, small nucleoli, abundant granular cytoplasm, and indistinct cytoplasmic border. Cells also reveal minimal nuclear variations and normal N:C ratios. In metastatic squamous cell carcinomas, polygonal tumor cells have large nuclei, smudgy chromatin, and dense cytoplasmic keratin formation.

A-42. (**b**) **Monomorphous population of cells**
The FNA of a lymphoma reveals a cellular specimen with monomorphous population of lymphocytes, particularly in low-grade B cell lymphoma, and/or small lymphocytic lymphomas/chronic lymphocytic leukemia (SLL/CLL). It represents a monoclonal proliferation of lymphoma cells. Other cytological features of a lymphoma include discohesive tumor cells with hyperchromatic nuclei, clumped (soccer-ball-like) chromatin, irregular nuclear membranes, inconspicuous nucleoli, scant cytoplasm, and rare or absent tingible body macrophages. Reactive lymphoid hyperplasia contains a heterogeneous mixture of lymphocytes, including small lymphocytes, centrocytes/centroblasts, immunoblasts, tingible body macrophages, and other cells. There is a great variation of cellular sizes and appearances, characteristic of polymorphous population of cells. Lymphoglandular bodies can be seen in both lymphomas and reactive lymphocytes.

A-43. **(a) Bland nuclei and abundant granular cytoplasm**
Wilms' tumor is a rare tumor of infancy and childhood. Histologically, the tumor contains blastemal component (closely packed small blue cells) and mesenchymal component (spindle cells). Therefore, it may be confused with the other so-called small blue round cell tumors, such as Ewing/PNETs, rhabdomyosarcomas, and small cell carcinomas. In the FNA specimen of Wilms' tumor, numerous discohesive small round blue cells are found and arranged in tubular-like structure and dispersed individual cells. Tumor cells have hyperchromatic nuclei and scant cytoplasm. The mesenchymal cells are elongated spindle-shaped cells. In rhabdomyosarcoma, tumor cells have more eosinophilic cytoplasm. In Ewing/PNET, tumor cells are more pleomorphic and reveal a tigroid appearance. In small cell carcinomas, tumor cells reveal acinar/rosette arrangements with hyperchromatic nuclei, fine (salt-and-pepper) chromatin, inconspicuous nucleoli, scant cytoplasm, nuclear crowding, and molding.

A-44. **(d) All of the above**
The clear cell RCC variant (conventional renal cell carcinomas) is the most common histologic subtype of malignant renal tumors and accounts for 70 % of renal cell carcinomas. The "clear cell" appearances of tumor cells are due to the cytoplasmic glycogen and lipid that are dissolved during tissue processing. In RCCs, particularly in clear cell RCCs, tumor cells are arranged in clusters or dispersed individual cells and have round- to oval-shaped hyperchromatic nuclei; granular chromatin, with or without prominent nucleoli (depending on the Fuhrman grade); and clear or granular cytoplasm. Intercellular pink color strand-like material (basement membrane material) may be seen by the Diff-Quik stain. Focally, tumor cells may also show large hyperchromatic nuclei, multinucleation, and eosinophilic cytoplasm. Tumor necrosis may be seen, particularly in the Fuhrman grade III and IV tumors. The background of smear is bloody and with prominent small vessels (hypervascularity).

A-45. **(b) Discohesive and/or dispersed individual large atypical cells**
In DLBCL, the FNA reveals a cellular specimen with discohesive large atypical lymphoid cells. Three morphological variants are most commonly seen: the centroblastic, immunoblastic, and anaplastic variant. Centroblastic variant is the most common subtype and reveals medium- to large-sized tumor cells with high N:C ratio, oval or round nuclei, fine chromatin, and single or multiple prominent nucleoli. Immunoblasts have basophilic cytoplasm and a central nucleolus. The third morphologic variant, anaplastic variant, consists of large tumor cells with pleomorphic nuclei and may resemble the Hodgkin cells (Reed-Stemberg cells). Most cases are mixtures of centroblastic and immunoblastic cells.

A-46. **(a) Tumor cells with bland nuclei and abundant granular cytoplasm**
In urothelial cell carcinomas, tumor cells are large in size and arranged in two-dimensional clusters and dispersed individual cells with large hyperchromatic nuclei, dense chromatin, inconspicuous nucleoli, and dense cytoplasm. Some of the tumor cells with elongated cytoplasm and flared cytoplasmic ends form the so-called cercariform cells, characteristics of urothelial cell neoplasm. The cercariform appearance is the result of pseudostratification of urothelial cells.

A-47. **(d) All of the above**
There is some morphological overlapping between adrenal cortical adenomas and carcinomas. Adrenal cortical adenomas contain normal-appearing adrenal cortical cells, which are arranged in small sheets and dispersed individual cells. Tumor cells have small round nuclei, granular chromatin, small centrically located nucleoli, and abundant clear and/or granular cytoplasm. No mitosis is identified. Numerous naked nuclei floating in a frothy granular background are also characteristics. Tumor necrosis is not a common finding in adrenal cortical adenomas. Histologically, the diagnosis of adrenal cortical carcinomas requires to follow strict criteria, such as nuclear grade, necrosis, capsular invasion, mitotic rate, and atypical mitoses. These features are difficult to evaluate on a cytological specimen. Nevertheless, most of the adrenal masses can be correctly classified as benign or malignant by FNAs. In adrenal cortical carcinomas, FNA reveals a cellular specimen. Tumor cells are arranged in loose clusters, sheets, and dispersed individual cells and have marked nuclear variations and atypia, abundant mitoses, and necrotic debris.

A-48. **(a) Three-dimensional clusters of cells with bland nuclei and abundant granular cytoplasm**
Pheochromocytoma is rarely aspirated due to the risk of hypertensive crisis. However, about 10 % of tumors are nonfunctional and may be aspirated. The FNA specimen reveals dispersed pleomorphic tumor cells with large hyperchromatic nuclei, granular chroma-

tin, prominent nucleoli, and dense cytoplasm. Giant tumor cells with multinucleation and bizarre tumor cells are also common findings. Numerous mitoses may be present. Tumor cells are positive for chromogranin and synaptophysin. Pheochromocytomas can behave in a benign or malignant fashion; morphology is not always predictive of clinical behaviors.

A-49. **(c) Small pyknotic nuclei**
In metastatic squamous cell carcinomas, tumor cells are predominately arranged in clusters and/or dispersed as individual tumor cells. Tumor cells have large nuclei with smudgy or coarse chromatin, prominent nucleoli, and dense cytoplasm with cytokeratins. Pyknotic nuclei are features seen in benign squamous cells and usually not seen in squamous cell carcinomas. The presence of prominent nucleoli should not be confused with poorly differentiated adenocarcinomas. Tumor cells of adenocarcinomas have vesicular nuclei, coarse chromatin, and vacuolated cytoplasm.

A-50. **(a) Oncocytoma**
In oncocytomas, tumor cells reveal bland round nuclei with fine chromatin, inconspicuous or small nucleoli, abundant dense granular cytoplasm, and distinct cytoplasmic borders. Benign renal tubular cells, particularly proximal tubular cells, have a uniform appearance with round nuclei, fine granular chromatin, small nucleoli, abundant granular or clear cytoplasm, and indistinct cytoplasmic borders. Cells also reveal minimal nuclear variations and normal N:C ratios. In clear cell RCCs, tumor cells form cohesive two-dimensional clusters and have large eccentrically placed nuclei, vesicular chromatin, and clear cytoplasm. Intercellular pink color strand-like material (basement membrane material) may be seen by the Diff-Quik stain. Nucleoli vary in size depending on the Fuhrman grade. In papillary RCCs, tumor cells form papillae with true fibrovascular cores and reveal dense nuclei and scant-to-moderate granular or clear cytoplasm. Type 1 variant of papillary RCC reveals mild nuclear atypia, and type 2 variant reveals marked nuclear atypia. Foamy macrophages may also be identified in the background.

Reading List

Argani P, Lal P, Hutchinson B, et al. Aberrant nuclear immunoreactivity for TFE3 in neoplasms with TFE3 gene fusions: a sensitive and specific immunohistochemical assay. Am J Surg Pathol. 2003; 27:750–61.

Bibbo M, Wood MD, Fitzpatrick BT. Peritoneal washings and ovary. In: Bibbo M, Wilbur D, editors. Comprehensive cytopathology. 3rd ed. Philadelphia: Saunders/Elsevier; 2008.

Cibas ES. Peritoneal washings. In: Cibas ES, Ducatman BS, editors. Cytology: diagnostic principles and clinical correlates. Philadelphia: Saunders/Elsevier; 2009.

DeMay RM. The art and science of cytopathology, exfoliative cytology, vol. 1. 2nd ed. Chicago: ASCP Press; 2012.

Dusenbery D, Dekker A. Needle biopsy of the adrenal gland: retrospective review of 54 cases. Diagn Cytopathol. 1996;14:126–34.

Jhala NC, Darshana J, Eloubeidi MA, Chhieng DC, Ralph Crowe D, Janie R, Isam E. Endoscopic ultrasound-guided fine-needle aspiration biopsy of the adrenal glands. Cancer Cytopathol. 2004;102:308–14.

Khalbuss WE, Monaco SE, Pantanowitz L. Chapter 20. Renal, adrenal & retroperitoneum. In: The ASCP Quick Compendium (QC) of cytopathology. Chicago: ASCP Press; 2013. p. 448–83.

Lam KY, Lo CY. Metastatic tumors of the adrenal glands: a 30-year experience in a teaching hospital. Clin Endocrinol (Oxf). 2002; 56:95–101.

Powers CN, Elbadawi A. "Cercariform" cells: a clue to the cytodiagnosis of transitional cell origin of metastatic neoplasms? Diagn Cytopathol. 1995;13:15–21.

Raso DS, Greene WB, Finley JL, Silverman JF. Morphology and pathogenesis of Liesegang rings in cyst aspirates: report of two cases with ancillary studies. Diagn Cytopathol. 1998;19:116–9.

Subhawong AP, Subhawong TK, Li QK. Fine needle aspiration of a metastatic prostate carcinoma simulating a primary adrenal cortical neoplasm: A case report and review of literature. Diagn Cytopathol. 2010;38:147–53.

Urine Cytopathology

11

Ehab A. ElGabry and Walid E. Khalbuss

Contents

11.1 **Image-Based Questions 1–36** 619
11.2 **Text-Based Questions 37–61** 655
11.3 **Answers and Discussion of Image-Based Questions 1–36** 658
11.4 **Answers and Discussion of Text-Based Questions 37–61** 665
Reading List 668

Table 11.1 Advantages of urine cytology testing

Simple, cost-effective and noninvasive for detection of bladder cancers
Diagnosis of primary and metastatic bladder cancers in symptomatic patients
Follow-up for recurrence of urothelial carcinoma
Screening high-risk populations for developing bladder cancer (industrial exposure to arylamines, heavy smokers, endemic *Schistosoma haematobium*)
Evaluation tool for patients with hematuria
High sensitivity and specificity for high-grade neoplasms (high-grade urothelial carcinoma and secondary malignancies)

Table 11.2 Bladder malignancy subtyping

Primary tumors: 90 %
Urothelial carcinoma, low grade
Urothelial carcinoma, high grade
Squamous cell carcinoma
Adenocarcinoma
Small cell carcinoma
Carcinosarcoma
Secondary tumors : 10 %
Direct involvement: 70 %: prostatic/GYN malignancies and colorectal carcinomas
Distant metastases: 30 %: melanoma, GI malignancies, breast carcinomas, renal cell carcinoma, and lung carcinomas

E.A. ElGabry, MD (✉)
Department of Pathology, University of Pittsburgh Medical Center (UPMC)-Shadyside, 5150 Centre Avenue; POB2, Suite 201, Pittsburgh, PA 15232, USA
e-mail: drgabry2013@gmail.com

W.E. Khalbuss, MD, PhD, FIAC
Department of Pathology, GE Clarient Diagnostic Services, 31 Columbia, Aliso Viejo, California, 92656, USA
e-mail: Walid.khalbuss@ge.com

W.E. Khalbuss, Q.K. Li (eds.), *Diagnostic Cytopathology Board Review and Self-Assessment*,
DOI 10.1007/978-1-4939-1477-7_11,

Table 11.3 Malignancy criteria in urothelial carcinomas

Low-grade urothelial carcinomas:
Architecture atypia
Papillary fragments
Cell cluster with irregular borders and loss of polarity (mild)
Cytological and nuclear features
Nuclear enlargement
Mild pleomorphism
Irregular nuclear contour
Fine, evenly distributed chromatin
Homogeneous cytoplasm
High-grade urothelial carcinomas:
Architecture atypia
Papillary fragments or single cells or both
Cell cluster with irregular borders and loss of polarity (marked)
Cytological and nuclear features
Nuclear enlargement and high N/C ratio
Marked cellular pleomorphism
Marked nuclear hyperchromasia
Coarsely granular chromatin
Irregular nuclear contour
Necrosis
Squamous, glandular, or neuroendocrine differentiation

11.1 Image-Based Questions 1–36

Fig. 11.1

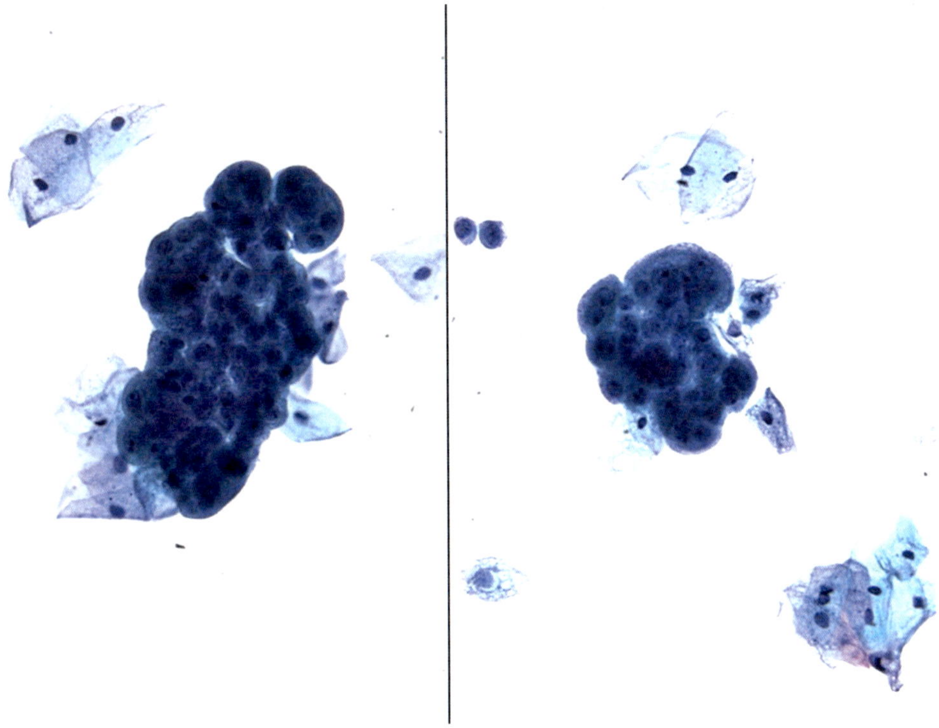

Q-1. The image shown is from a catheterized urine specimen of 73-year-old man with microscopic hematuria. What is the most likely diagnosis?
(a) Squamous cell carcinoma
(b) Reactive urothelial cells
(c) Urolithiasis
(d) Urothelial carcinoma, low grade
(e) Urothelial carcinoma, high grade

Fig. 11.2

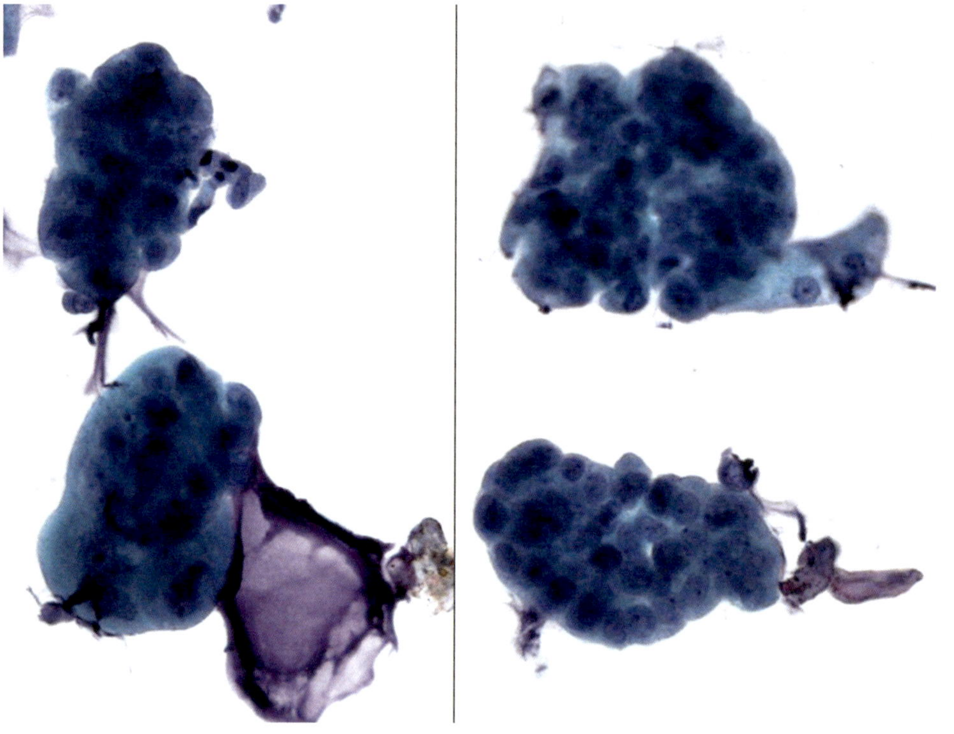

Q-2. These images represent a urine specimen of a 68-year-old man with painless gross hematuria. The specimen shows (see images) numerous clusters with mild cytological atypia and no obvious umbrella cells. The most likely diagnosis is:
(a) Reactive urothelial cells
(b) Urothelial carcinoma, high grade
(c) Urothelial carcinoma, low grade
(d) Urolithiasis
(e) Instrumentation atypia

Fig. 11.3

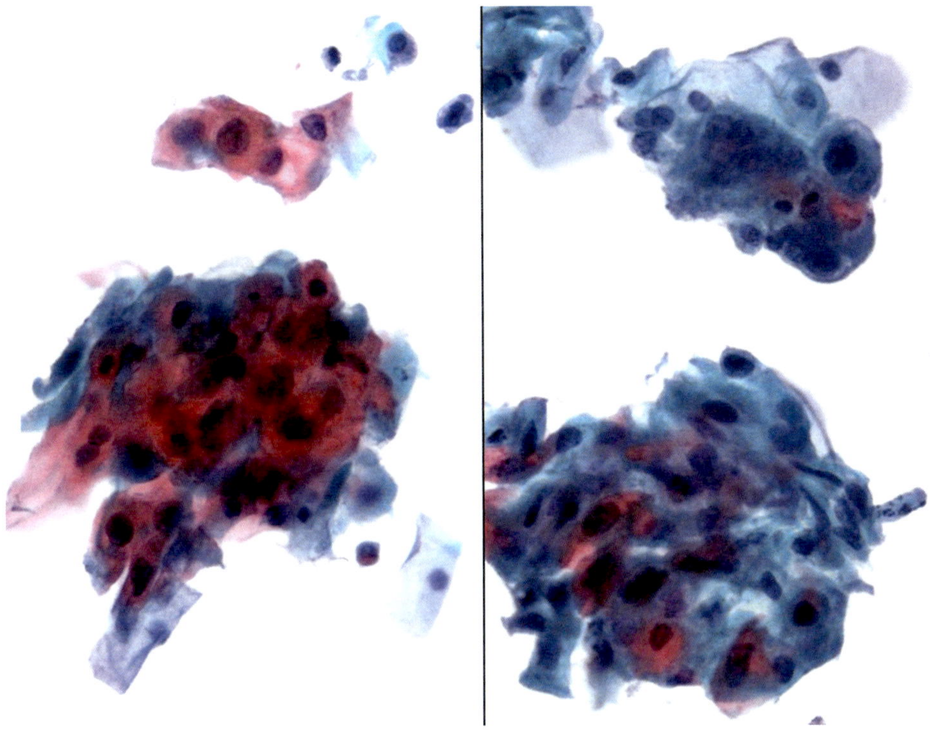

Q-3. These images are from the voided urine specimen of a 68-year-old woman with painless gross hematuria. The most likely diagnosis is:

(a) Reactive urothelial and squamous cells
(b) Urothelial carcinoma, low grade with squamous differentiation
(c) Urothelial carcinoma, high grade with squamous differentiation
(d) Schistosoma haematobium infection
(e) Urolithiasis

Fig. 11.4

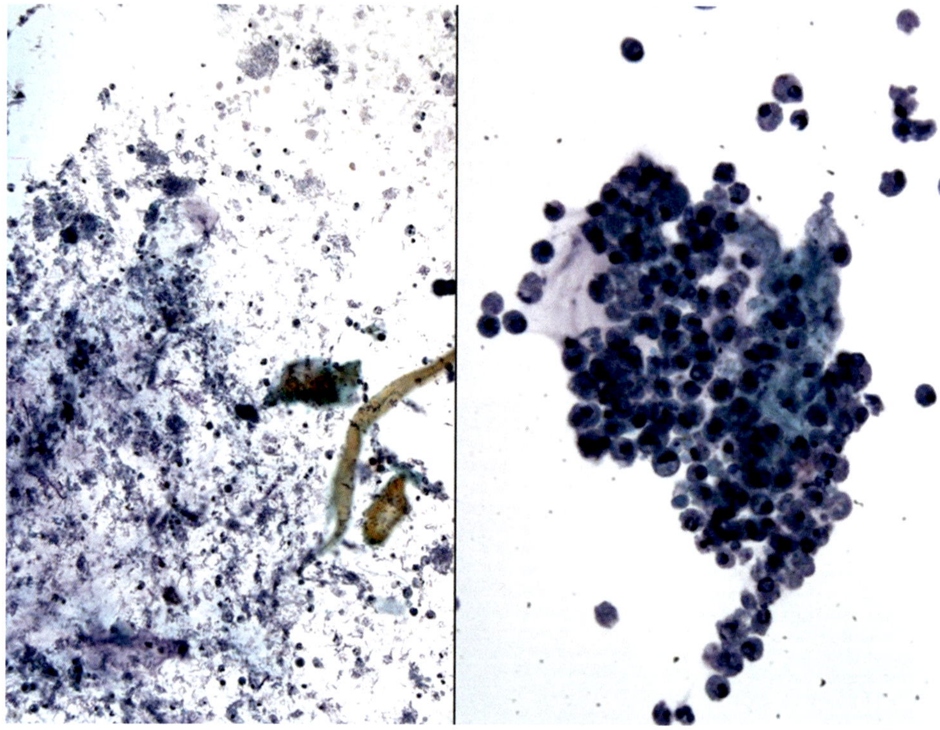

Q-4. These images are from urine specimen of a 69-year-old male who underwent surgery for bladder cancer 2 years ago. The most likely diagnosis is:
(a) Small cell carcinoma
(b) Adenocarcinoma
(c) Urothelial carcinoma, low grade
(d) Urothelial carcinoma, high grade, recurrence
(e) Benign, negative for malignancy

Fig. 11.5

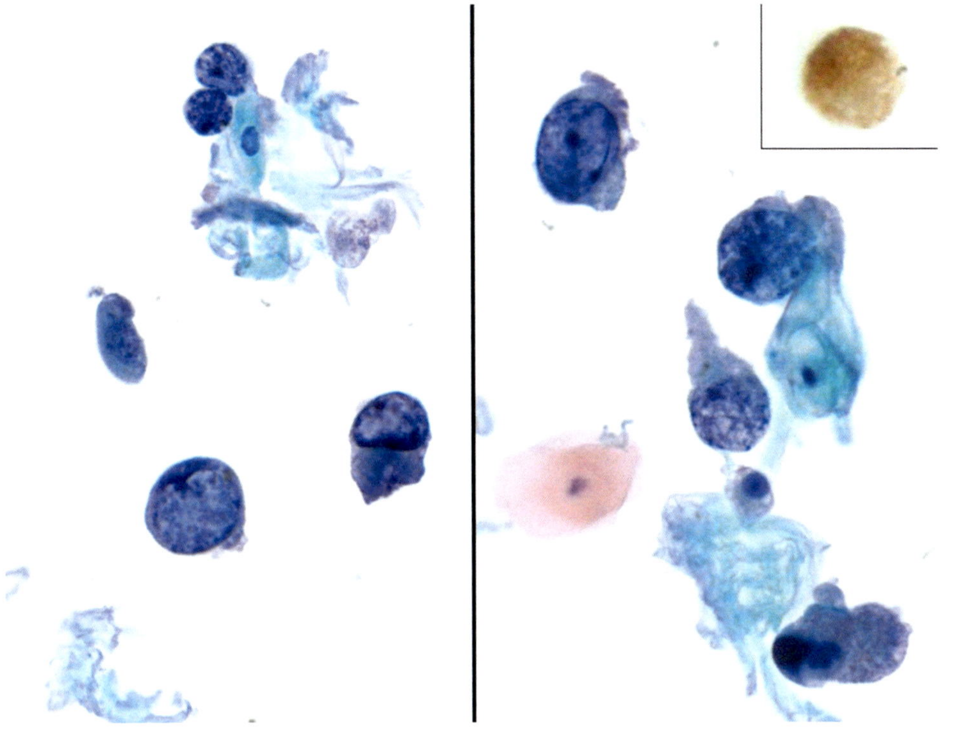

Q-5. This image is from a voided urine specimen from a 45-year-old man with a history of renal transplant. The insert image is most likely showing a positive stain for:

(a) P53 (positive in urothelial carcinoma)
(b) P63 (positive in squamous or urothelial cells/carcinoma)
(c) Polyomavirus immunostain (SV40)
(d) TTF-1 (positive in lung and thyroid carcinoma)
(e) Ki67 (proliferate index marker)

Fig. 11.6

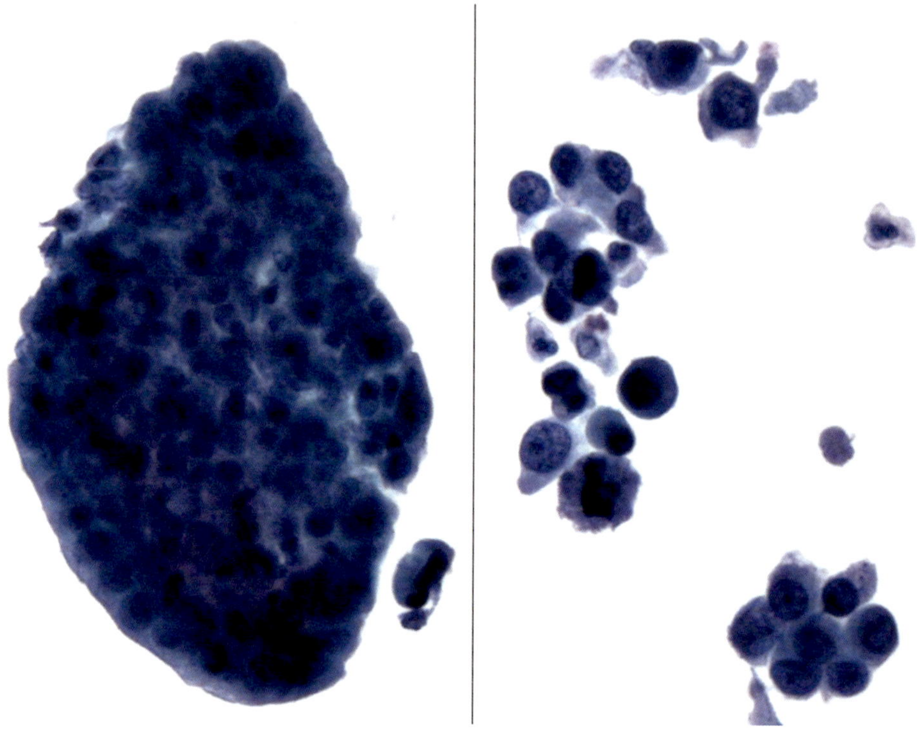

Q-6. These images are from the voided urine specimen of a 53-year-old female with painless gross hematuria. The most likely diagnosis is:
(a) Reactive urothelial and squamous cells and Candida infection
(b) Polyomavirus infection
(c) High-grade urothelial carcinoma or carcinoma in situ (CIS)
(d) Small cell carcinoma
(e) Vaginal contaminant: endometrial cell and Candida microorganisms

Fig. 11.7

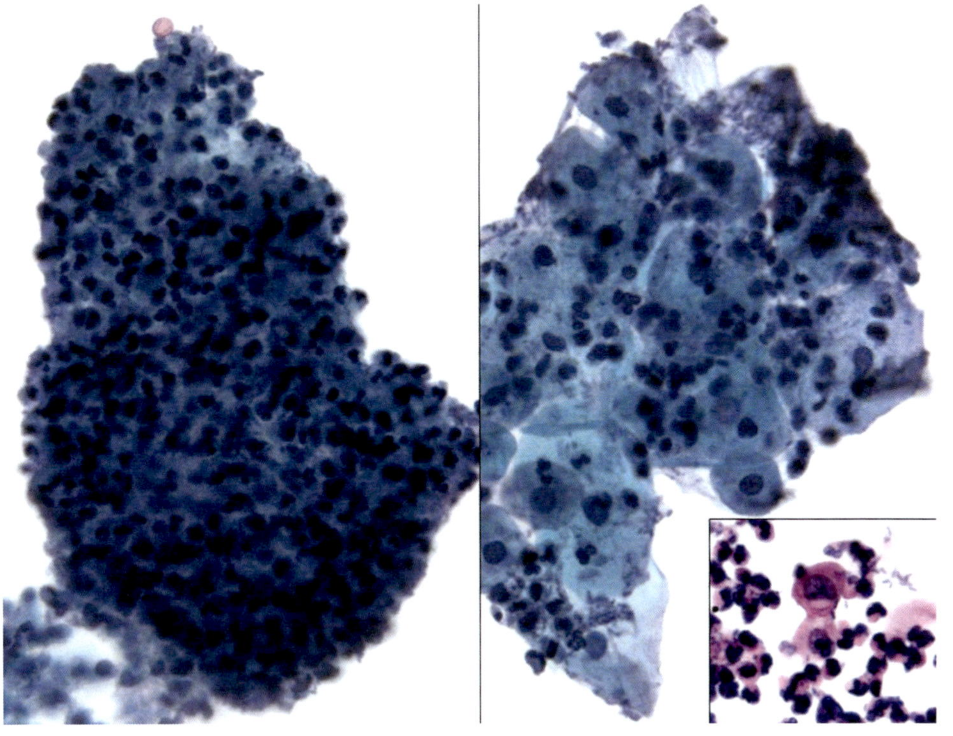

Q-7. The images are from the urine of a 54-year-old woman. Which of the following is the most likely diagnosis?

(a) Urothelial carcinoma favor low grade
(b) Urothelial carcinoma favor high grade
(c) Squamous cell Ca
(d) Acute cystitis
(e) Unsatisfactory for evaluation, suggest resampling

Fig. 11.8

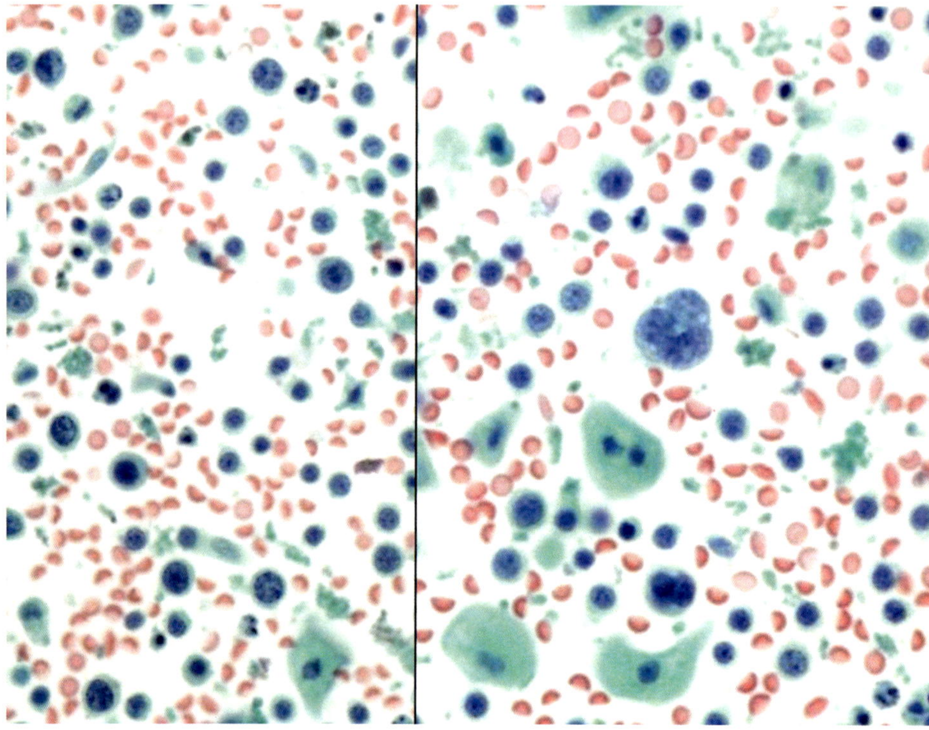

Q-8. 48-year-old woman, S/P chemotherapy for malignancy, presented with hematuria. A voided urine sample was submitted for cytological examination. The most likely diagnosis of this case is:

(a) Negative for malignancy, follicular cystitis
(b) Suspicious for small cell carcinoma
(c) Suspicious for malignant lymphoma
(d) Negative for malignancy, acute cystitis
(e) Negative for malignancy, granulomatous cystitis

Fig. 11.9

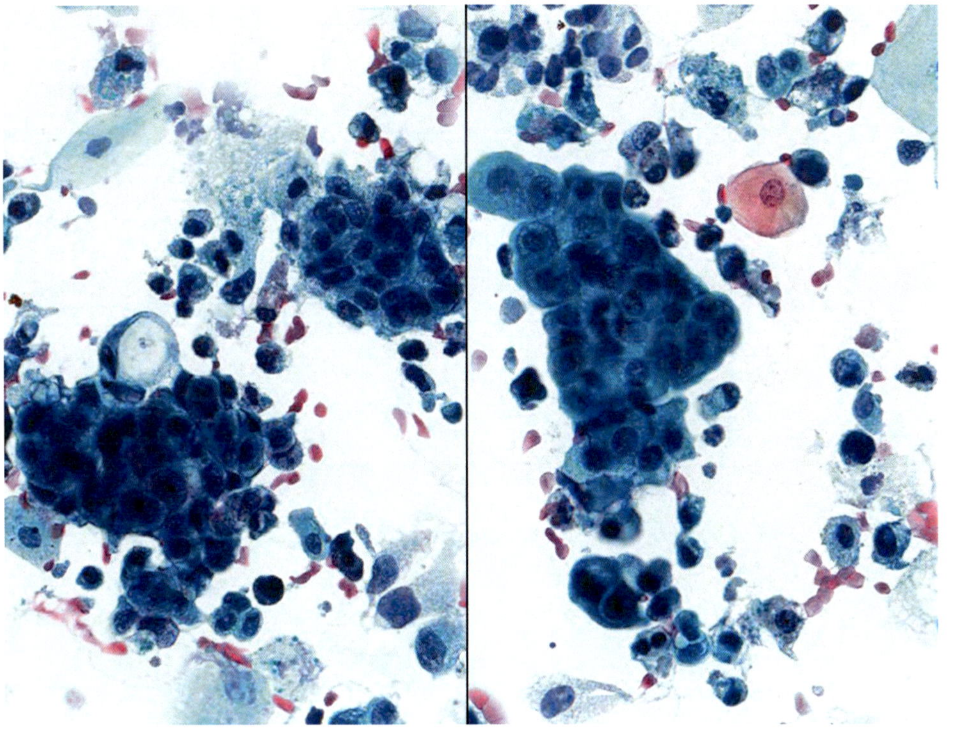

Q-9. These images are from the voided urine specimen of a 68-year-old man with hematuria. The positivity of CK 20 would favor which diagnosis:
(a) Reactive urothelial cells
(b) Urothelial carcinoma, low grade
(c) Instrumentation atypia
(d) Urolithiasis
(e) Infectious atypia

Fig. 11.10

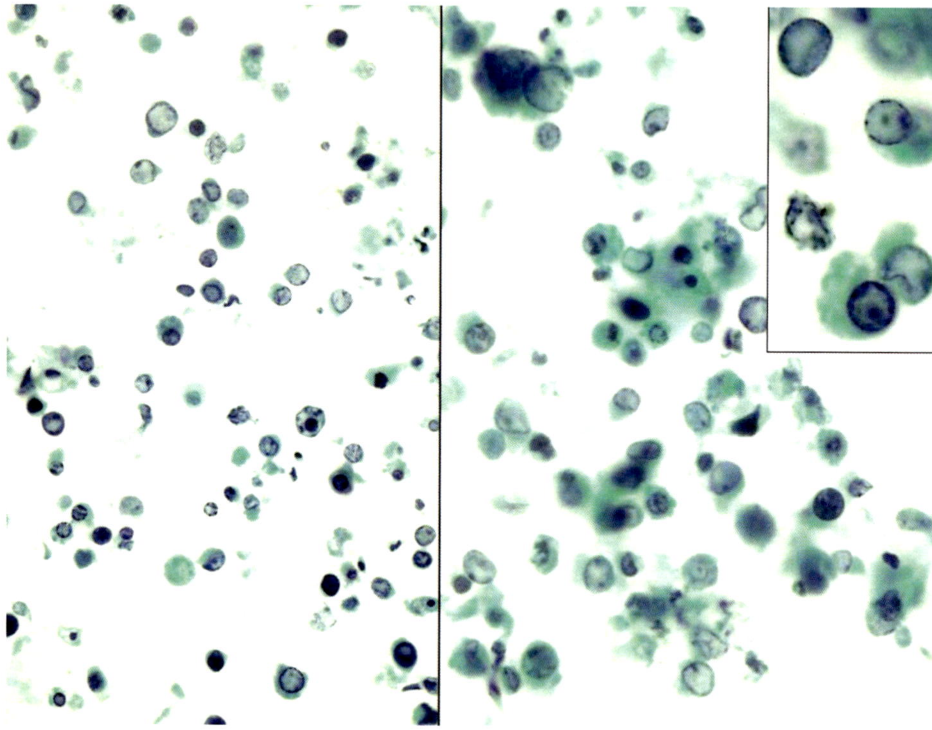

Q-10. These images are from the voided urine specimen from a 46-year-old female. The most likely diagnosis is:
(a) Polyomavirus infection
(b) Urothelial carcinoma, low grade
(c) Urothelial carcinoma in situ
(d) Urothelial carcinoma, high grade, invasive
(e) Lymphoma

Fig. 11.11

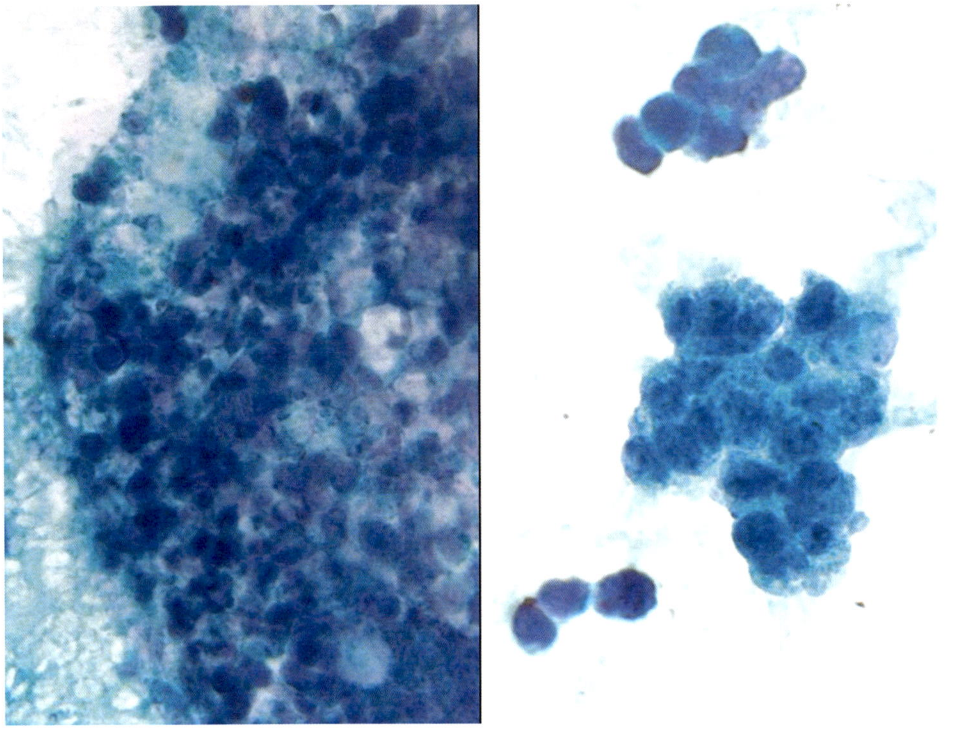

Q-11. These images are from the voided urine specimen of a 63-year-old man with a hematuria. The most likely diagnosis is:

(a) Reactive urothelial atypia with lymphocytosis
(b) Urothelial carcinoma, low grade
(c) Urothelial carcinoma in situ
(d) High-grade urothelial carcinoma with small cell features
(e) Urolithiasis

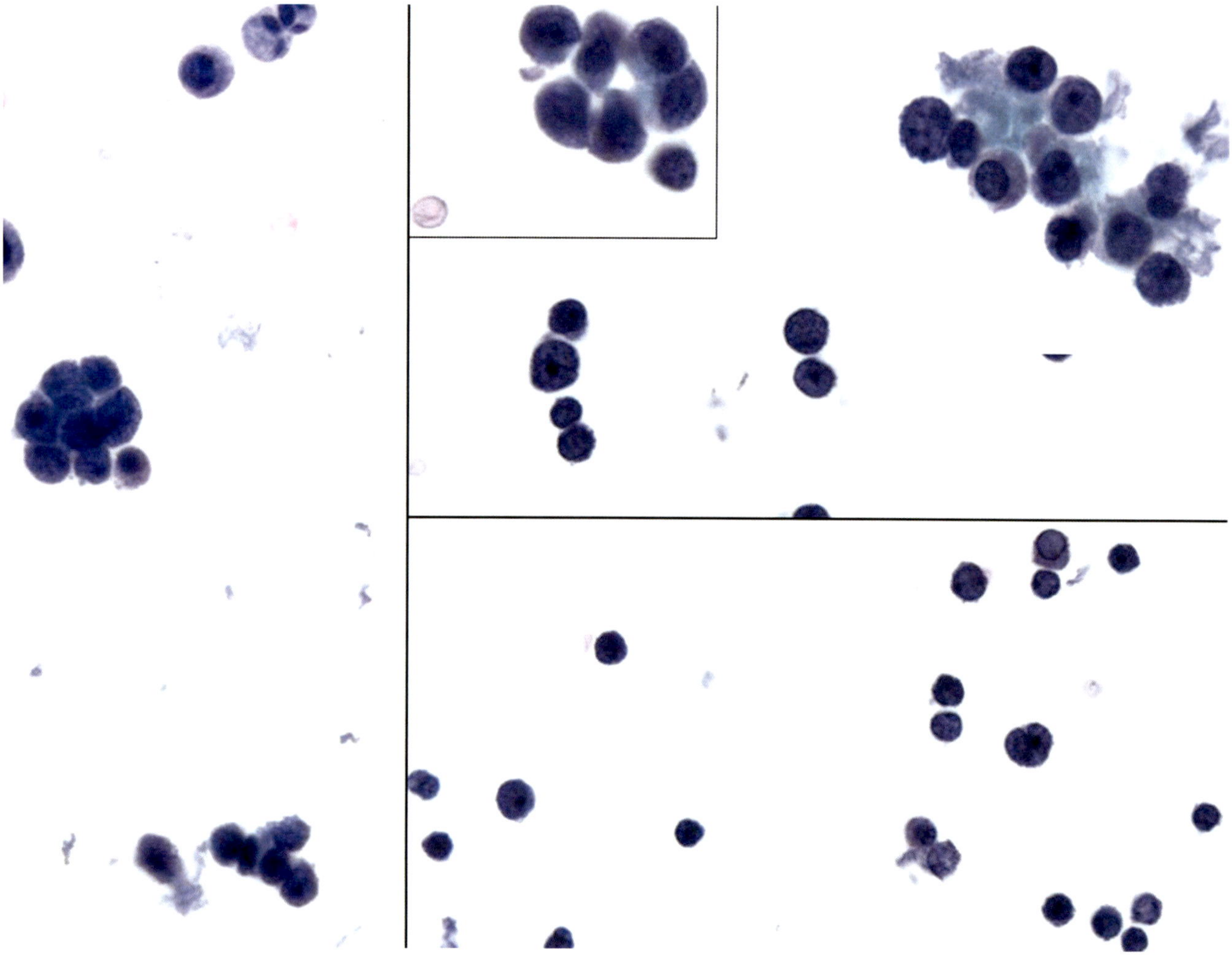

Fig. 11.12

Q-12. The images are from the voided urine of a 65-year-old woman with painless gross hematuria. Which of the following is the most likely diagnosis?
(a) Instrumentation artifact
(b) Urothelial carcinoma, high grade
(c) Reactive urothelial cells
(d) Squamous cell Ca
(e) Urothelial carcinoma, low grade

Fig. 11.13

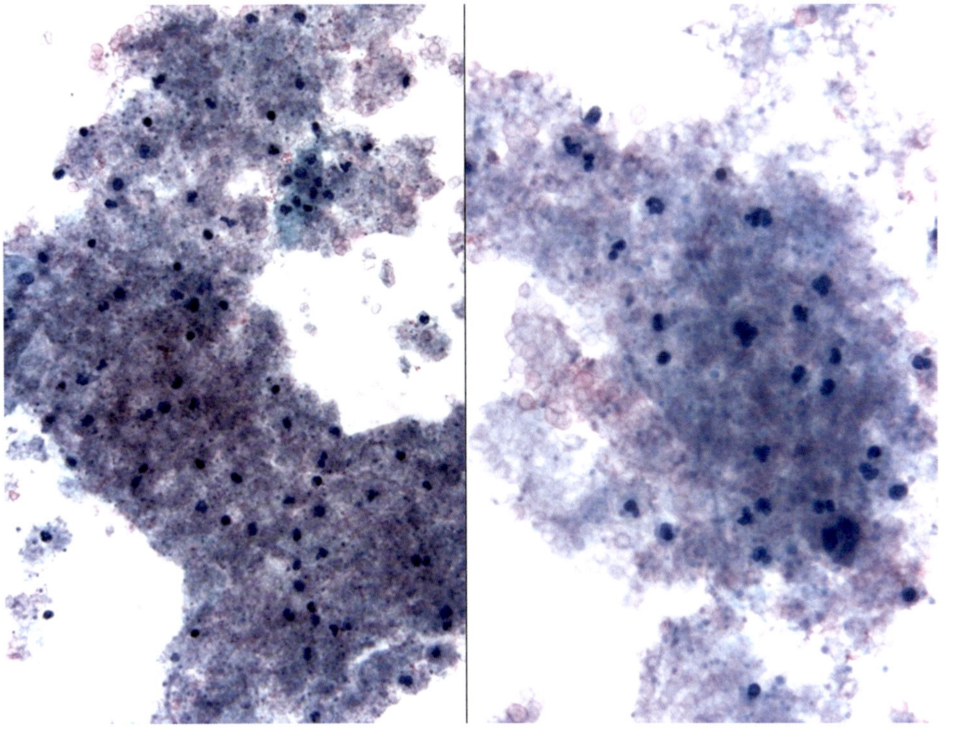

Q-13. The images are from the urine of a 46-year-old woman with history of smoking who presented with hematuria. Which of the following is the most likely diagnosis?
(a) Urothelial carcinoma favor low grade
(b) Urothelial carcinoma favor high grade
(c) Squamous cell Ca
(d) Acute cystitis
(e) Unsatisfactory for evaluation, suggest resampling

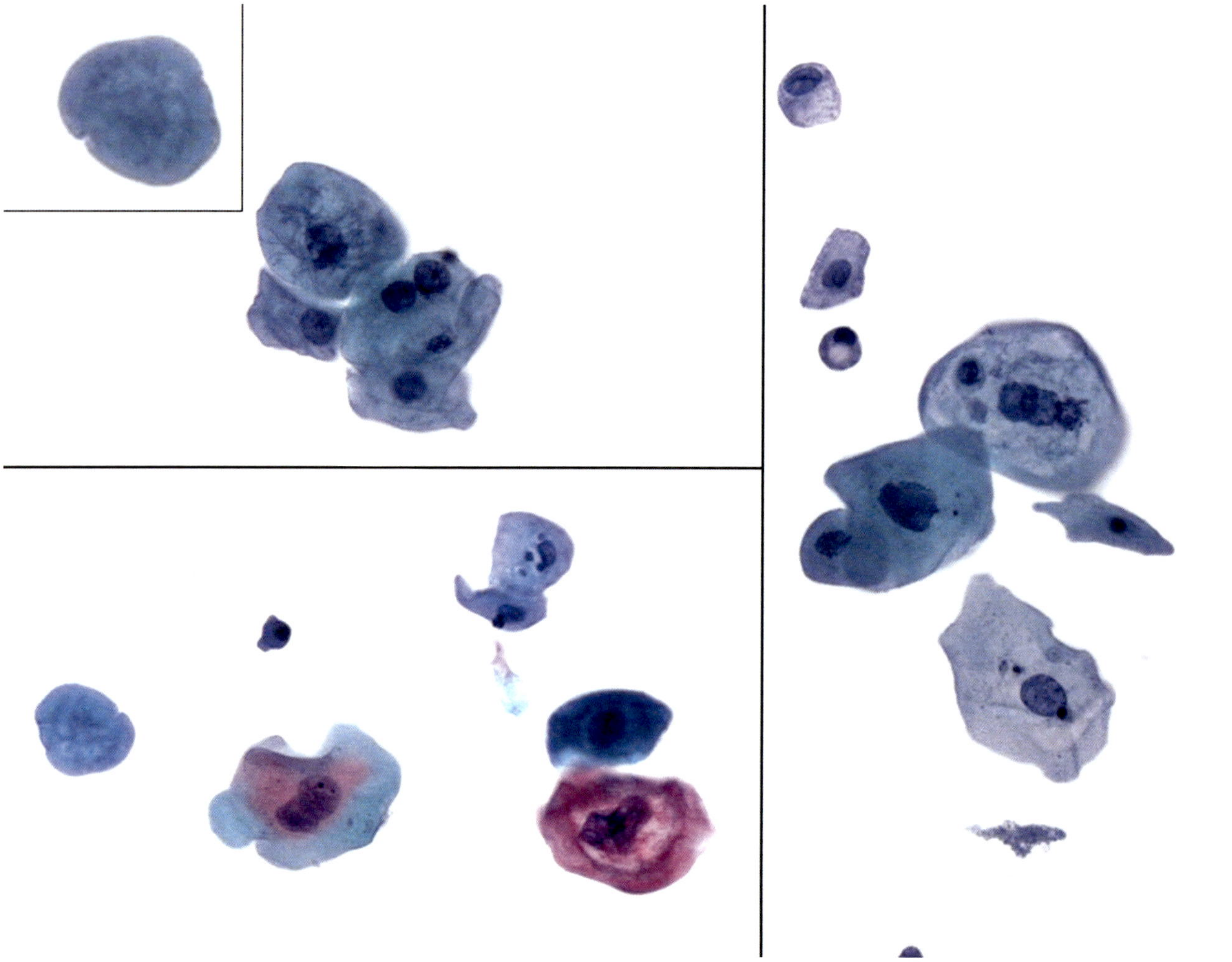

Fig. 11.14

Q-14. These images are from voided urine specimen from patient with hematuria. The most likely diagnosis is:
- (a) Reactive urothelial cells
- (b) Urothelial carcinoma, low grade
- (c) Urothelial carcinoma in situ
- (d) Squamous intraepithelial lesion, low grade (CIN-1)
- (e) Squamous cell carcinoma

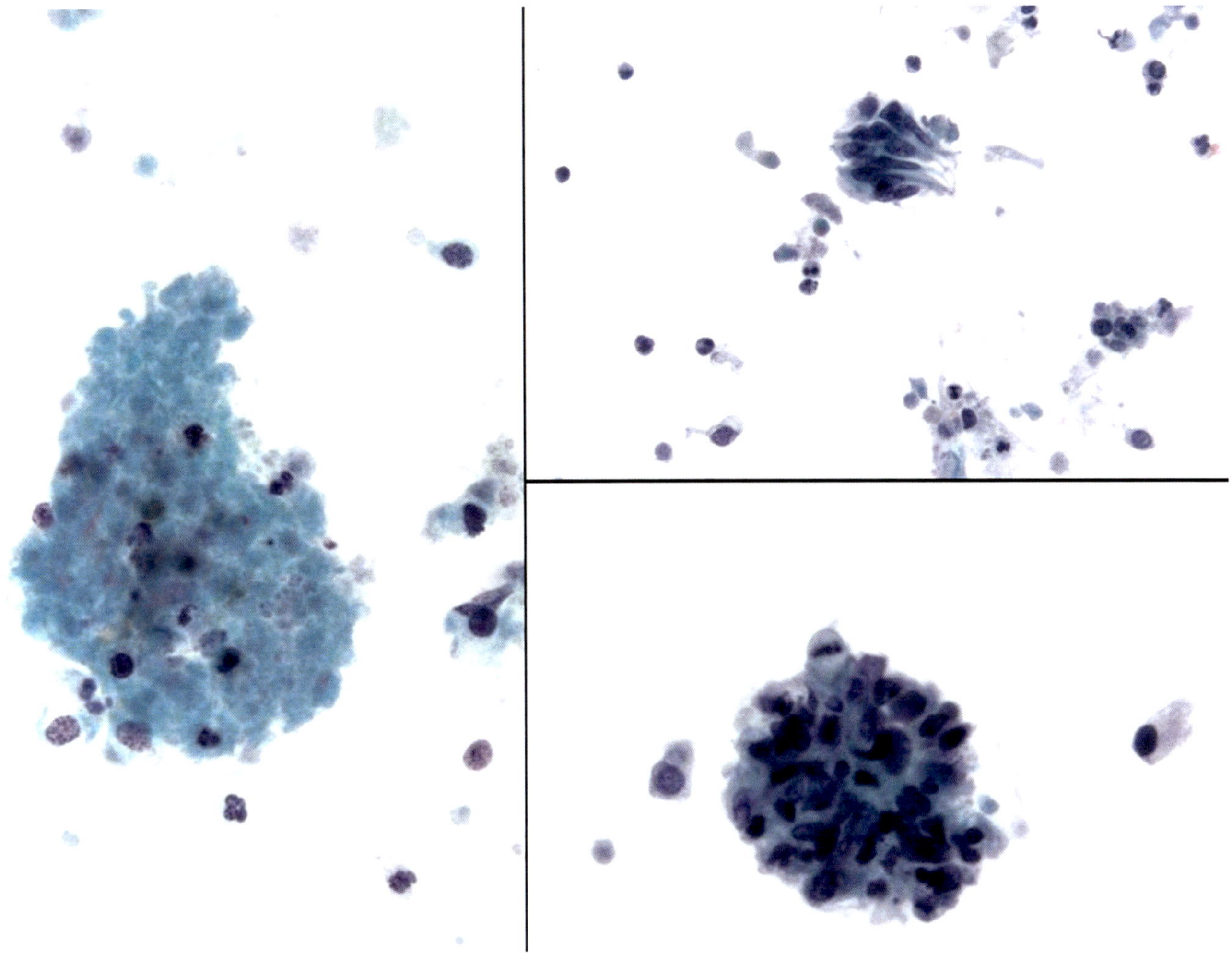

Fig. 11.15

Q-15. The images are from the urine of a 68-year-old man. Immunostain study on cell block showed: CK20+, CK7−, CEA+, and CDx2+. Which of the following is the most likely diagnosis?

(a) Metastatic colonic adenocarcinoma
(b) Urothelial carcinoma, low grade
(c) Reactive urothelial cells
(d) Cystitis cystica or glandularis
(e) Squamous cell carcinoma

Fig. 11.16

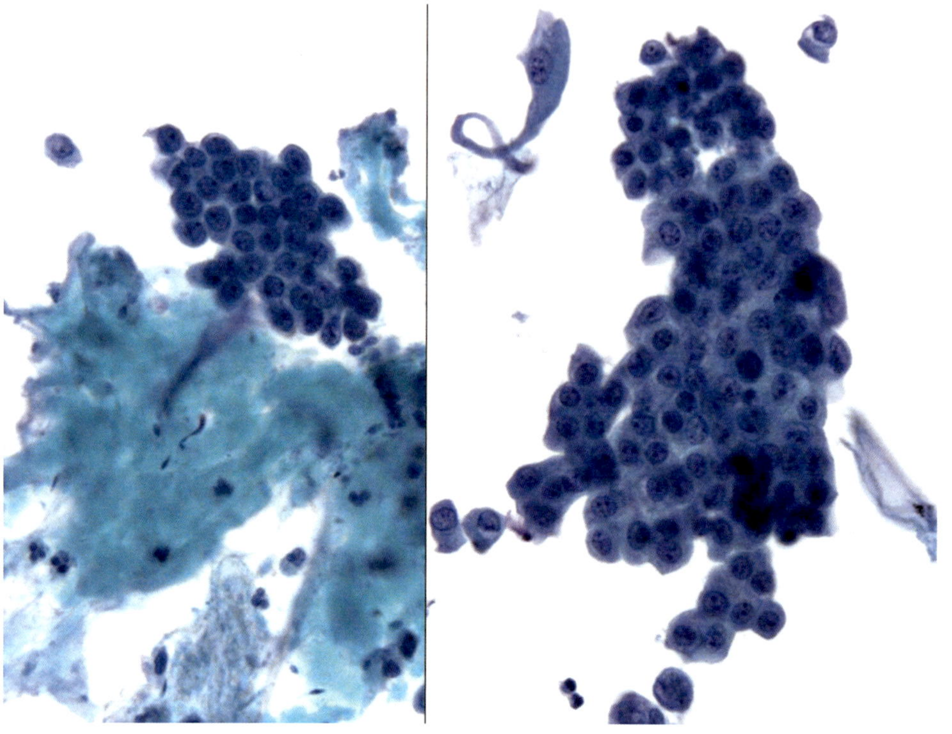

Q-16. These images are from a catheterized urine specimen of a patient with hematuria. The most likely diagnosis is:
(a) Reactive urothelial cells
(b) Urothelial carcinoma, low grade
(c) Urothelial carcinoma in situ
(d) Granulomatous cystitis
(e) Urolithiasis

Fig. 11.17

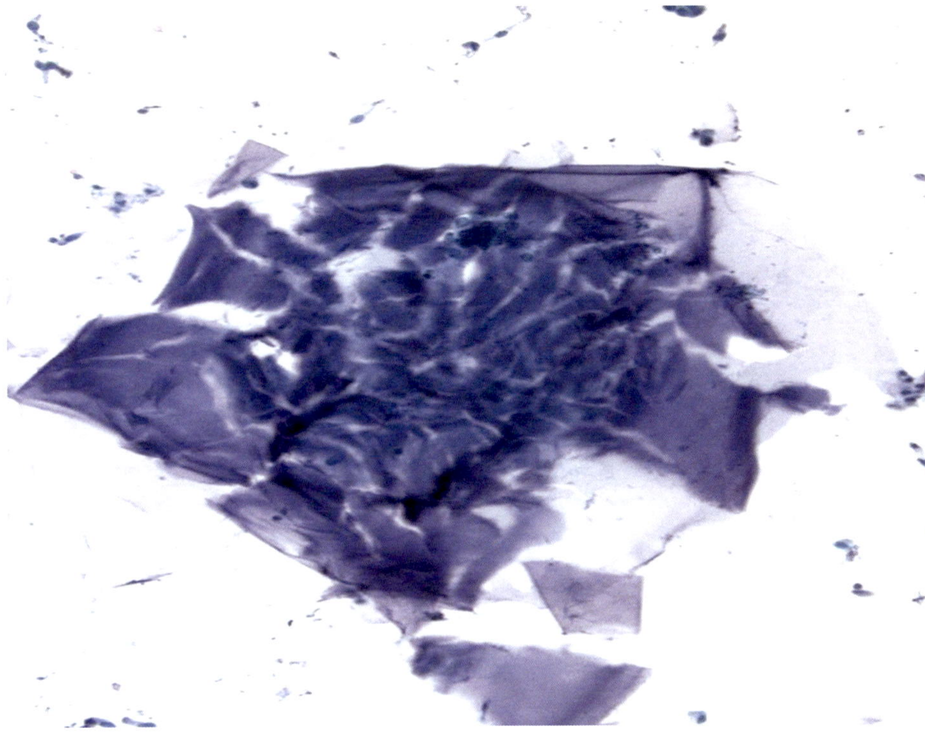

Q-17. The images are from catheterized urine specimen of a 58-year-old man with history of high-grade urothelial carcinoma. The most likely diagnosis of this case is:

(a) Urothelial carcinoma, low grade
(b) Mucinous adenocarcinoma
(c) Unsatisfactory, obscuring lubricant.
(d) Cystitis cystica or glandularis
(e) Polyomavirus infection

Fig. 11.18

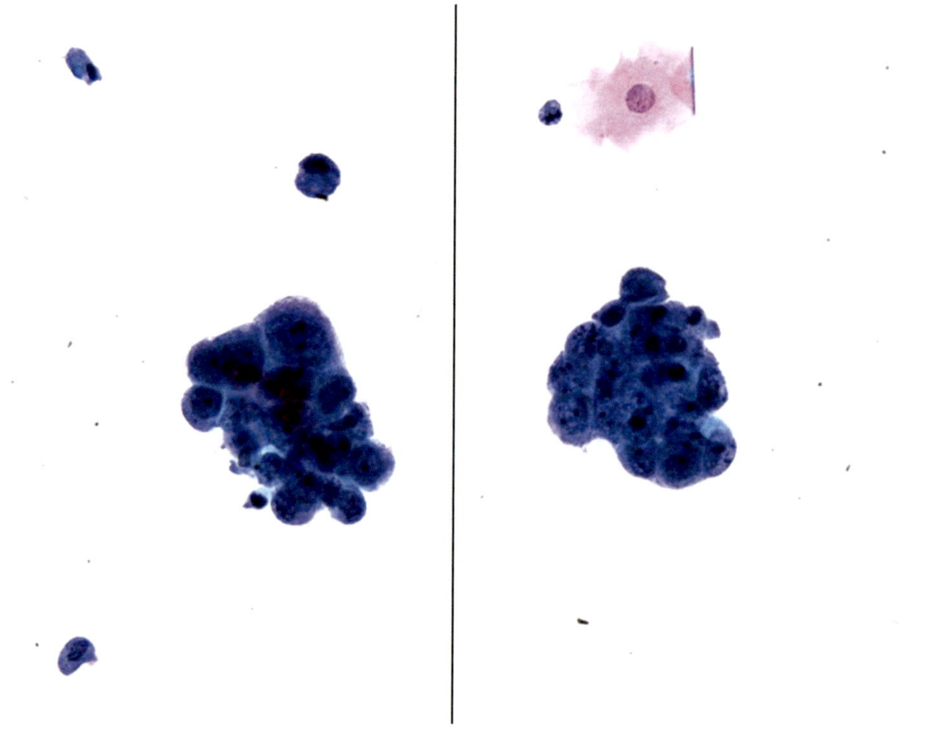

Q-18. The images are from the urine of a 72-year-old woman with hematuria. Which of the following is the most likely diagnosis?

(a) Urothelial carcinoma, favor low grade
(b) Urothelial carcinoma, favor high grade
(c) Reactive urothelial cells
(d) Squamous cell Ca
(e) Degenerative changes, suggest resampling

Fig. 11.19

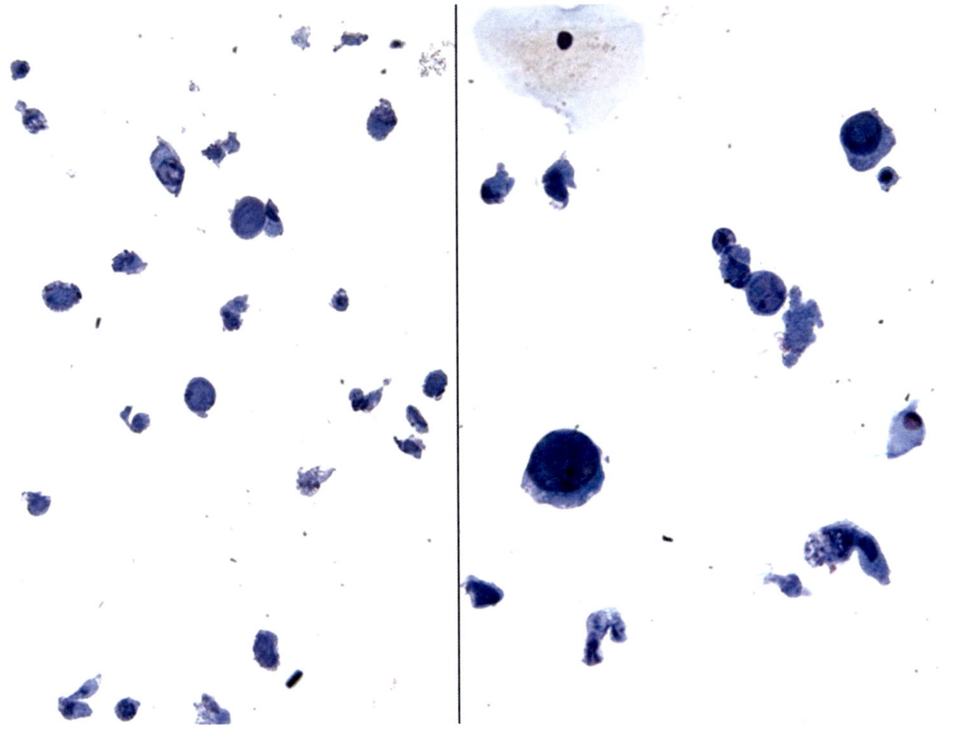

Q-19. The images are from the voided urine of a 69-year-old diabetic man who was thought to have high-grade urothelial carcinoma. All of the following are TRUE of this entity, EXCEPT:

(a) This virus belongs to the Papovaviridae family and is related to HPV.
(b) Infection by this virus is acquired late in life.
(c) There are two strains of this virus: JC (associated with PML in the brain) and BK (associated with urinary tract, renal transplant).
(d) Infection by this virus can be confirmed with an immunohistochemical stain to SV40 virus, which shares antigenic properties with polyomavirus.
(e) Infection by this virus is acquired in childhood and is nearly universal.

Fig. 11.20

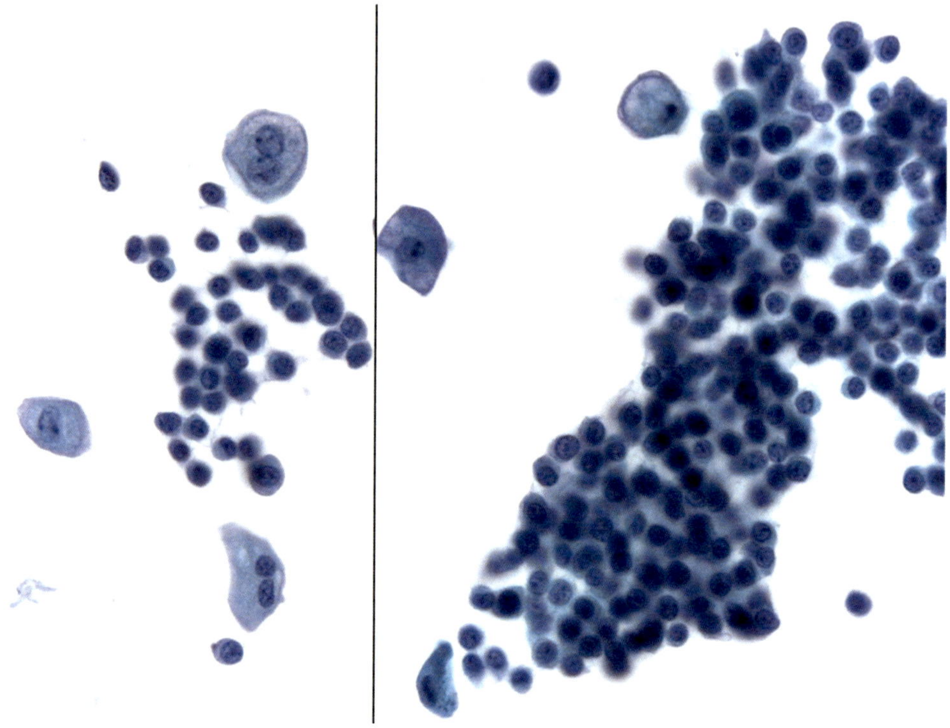

Q-20. These images are from catheterized urine specimen of a 49-year-old woman with a hematuria. The most likely diagnosis is:
(a) Granulomatous inflammation
(b) Urolithiasis
(c) Reactive urothelial cells
(d) Urothelial carcinoma, low grade
(e) Urothelial Carcinoma, high grade

Fig. 11.21

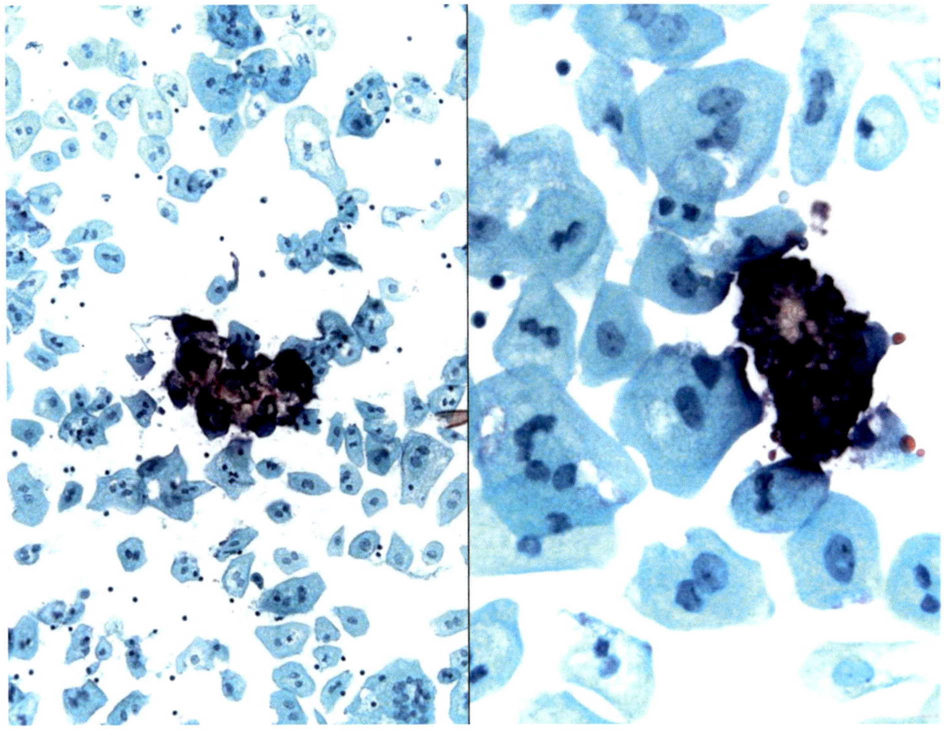

Q-21. These images are from catheterized urine specimen from a 34-year-old man with painful gross hematuria. The most likely diagnosis is:
(a) Squamous cell carcinoma
(b) Reactive urothelial cells
(c) Urolithiasis
(d) Urothelial carcinoma, low grade
(e) Urothelial carcinoma, high grade

Fig. 11.22

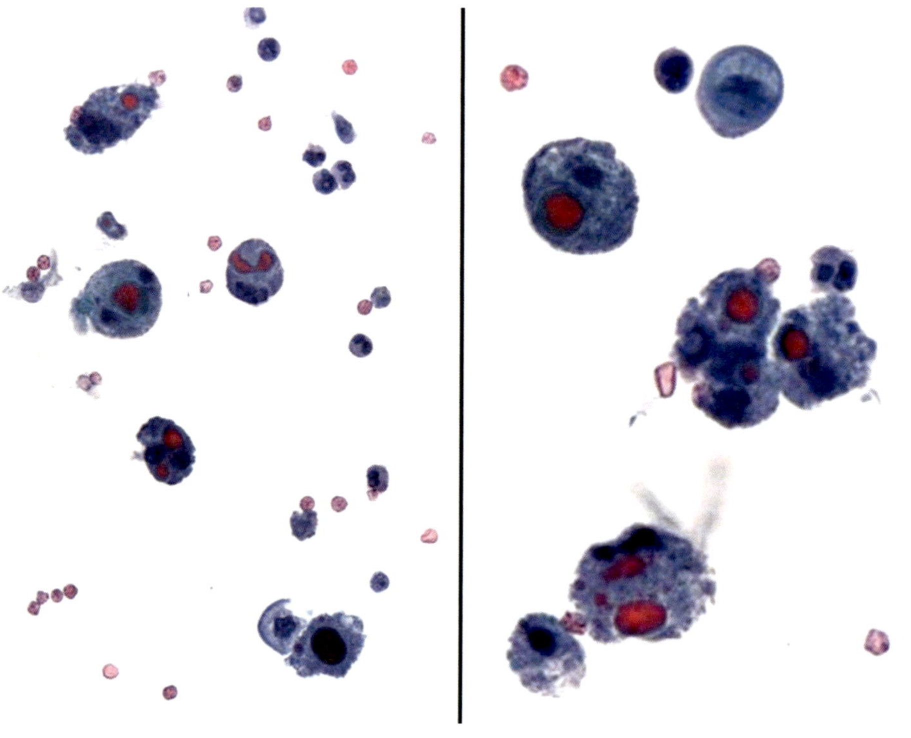

Q-22. The urine cytology images provided show:
(a) Polyomavirus-infected cells
(b) CMV-infected cells
(c) Malakoplakia
(d) Herpes-infected cells
(e) Melamed-Wolinska bodies

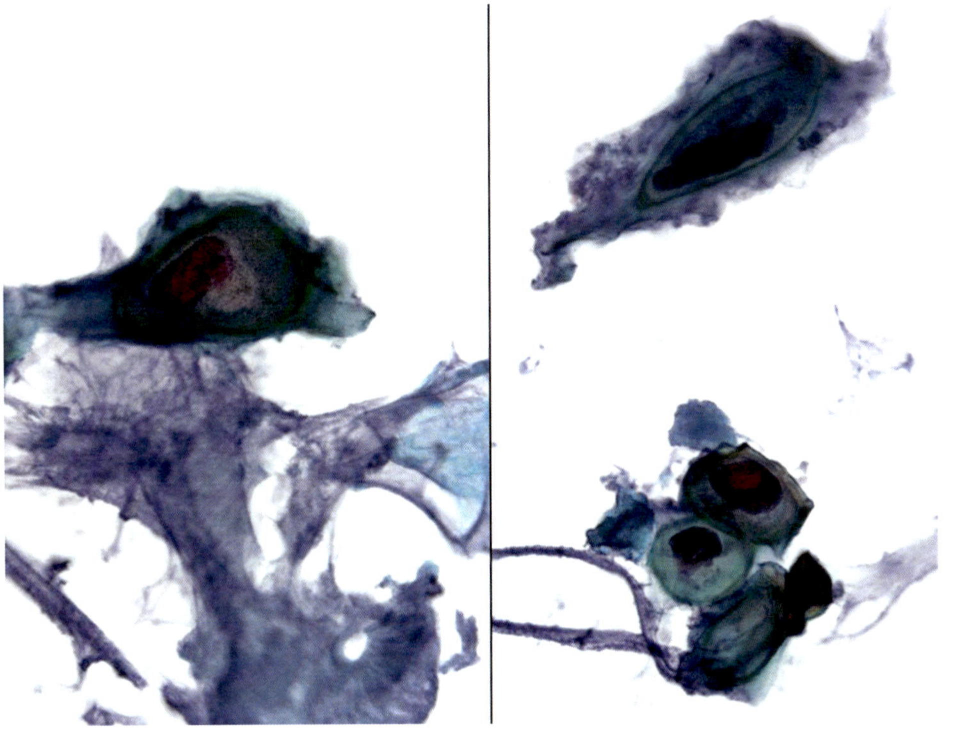

Fig. 11.23

Q-23. The urine cytology images provided which are from a 68-year-old man with urinary diversion (ileal conduit specimen) show:
(a) Gel lubricant
(b) Corpora amylacea
(c) Vegetable cell
(d) A and C
(e) None of the above

Fig. 11.24

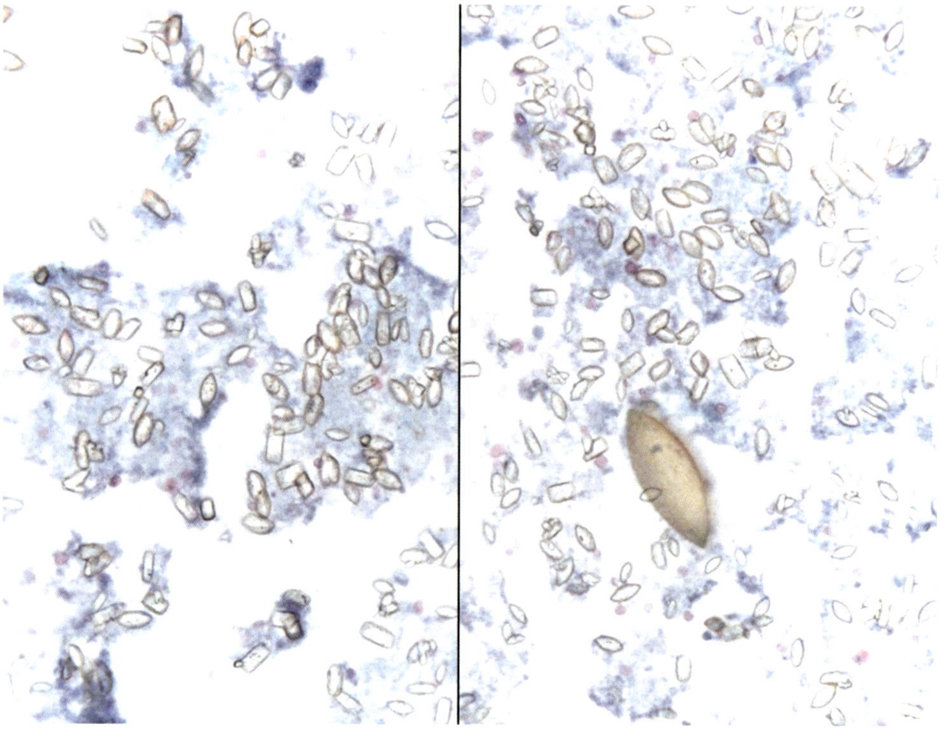

Q-24. The images are from the urine specimen of a 34-year-old woman with hematuria. Which of the following is the most likely diagnosis?
(a) Urothelial carcinoma favor low grade
(b) Urothelial carcinoma favor high grade
(c) Squamous cell Ca
(d) Unsatisfactory for evaluation, suggest resampling
(e) Urolithiases

Fig. 11.25

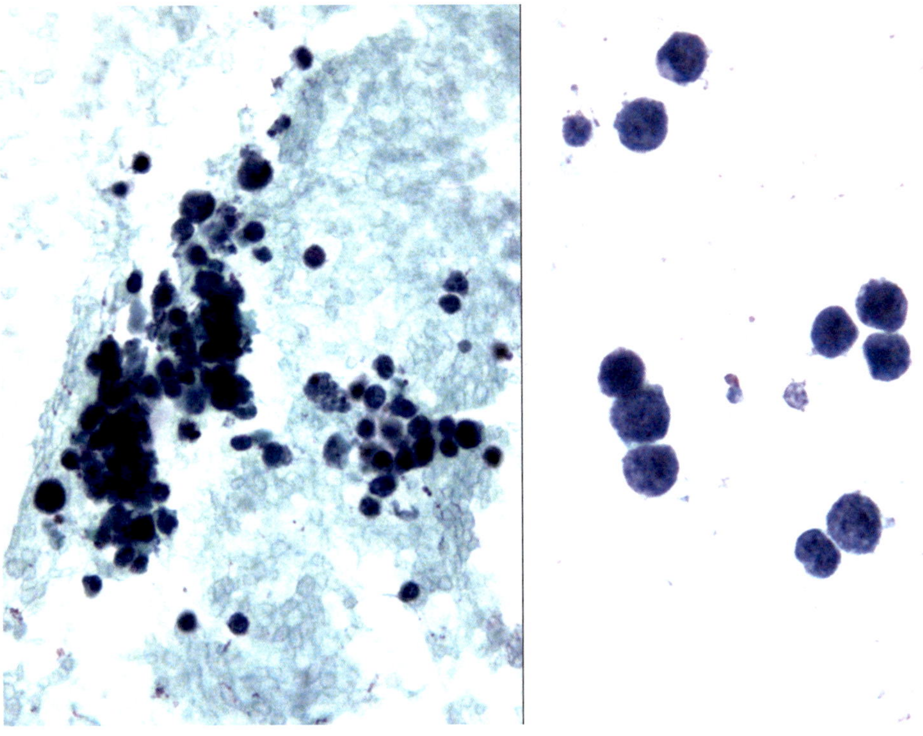

Q-25. The images are from the urine of a 68-year-old man with hematuria and previous history of lung carcinoma. Immunostain of the block showed shows positive staining for chromogranin (neuroendocrine marker) and TTF-1, CK7+, and CK20 – which of the following is the most likely diagnosis?

(a) Metastatic lung non-small carcinoma/squamous cell carcinoma
(b) Metastatic lung non-small cell carcinoma/large cell carcinoma
(c) Metastatic lung non-small cell carcinoma/adenocarcinoma
(d) Metastatic lung small cell carcinoma
(e) Urothelial carcinoma in situ (CIS)

Fig. 11.26

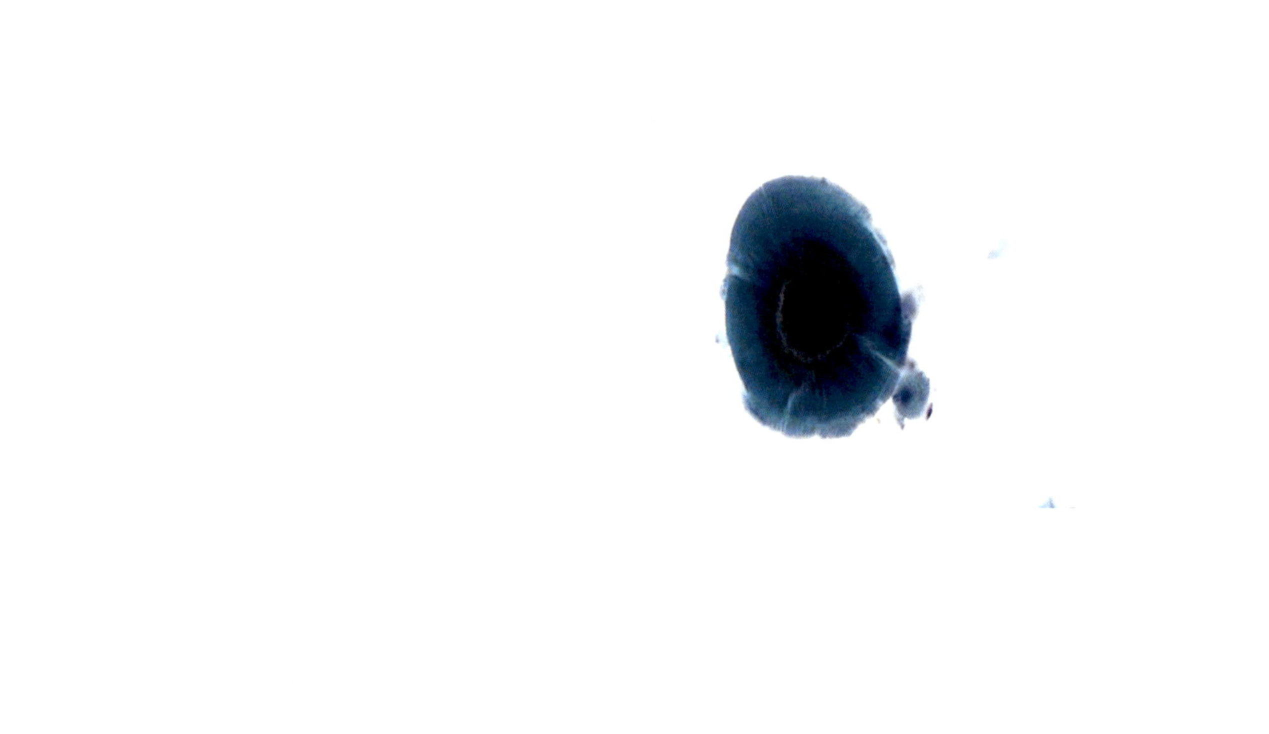

Q-26. This urine cytology specimen is showing the image of:

(a) Vegetable cell
(b) Umbrella cell
(c) Decoy cell
(d) Corpora amylacea
(e) Non of the above

Fig. 11.27

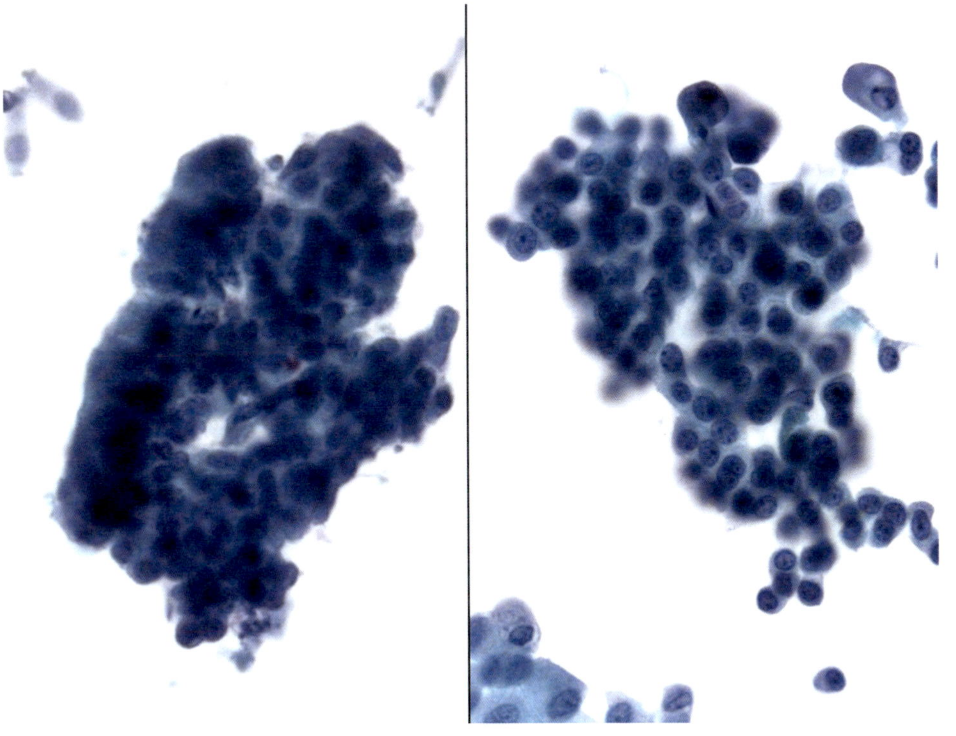

Q-27. The image shown is of a catheterized urine cytology specimen of a 68-year-old man. What are these cells?

(a) Columnar cells
(b) Urothelial cells, basal
(c) Urothelial cells, umbrella cells
(d) A and B
(e) Non of the above

Fig. 11.28

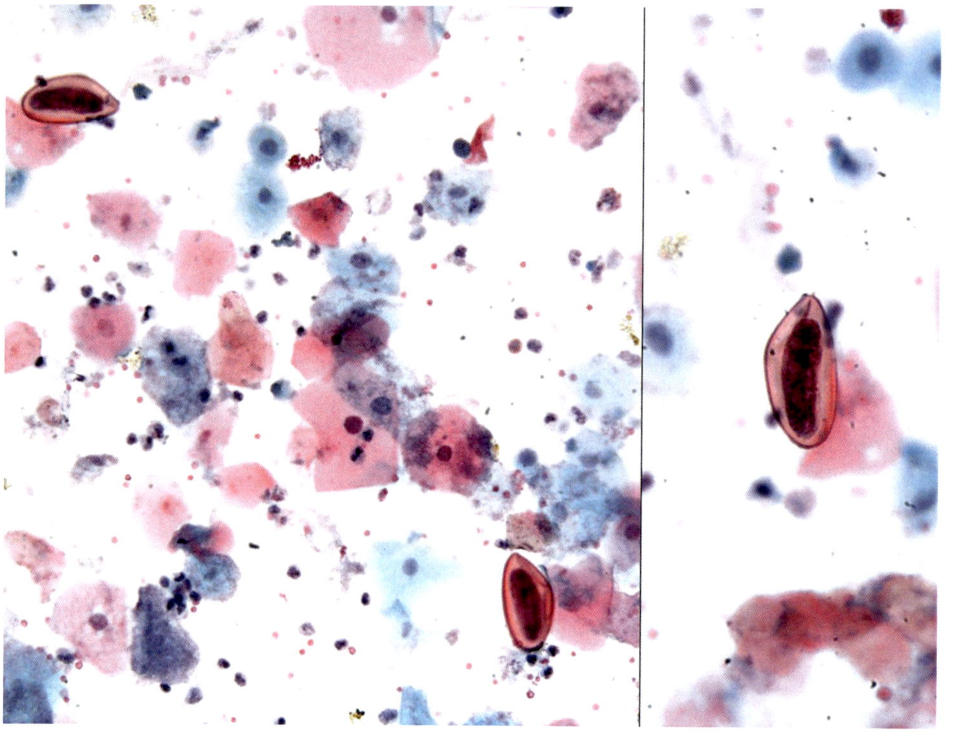

Q-28. The image shown is a urine cytology of a young female. What is the most likely diagnosis?

(a) *Schistosoma haematobium*
(b) *Ent*erobius vermicularis
(c) Herpes simplex type 1
(d) Herpes simplex type 2
(e) CMV

Fig. 11.29

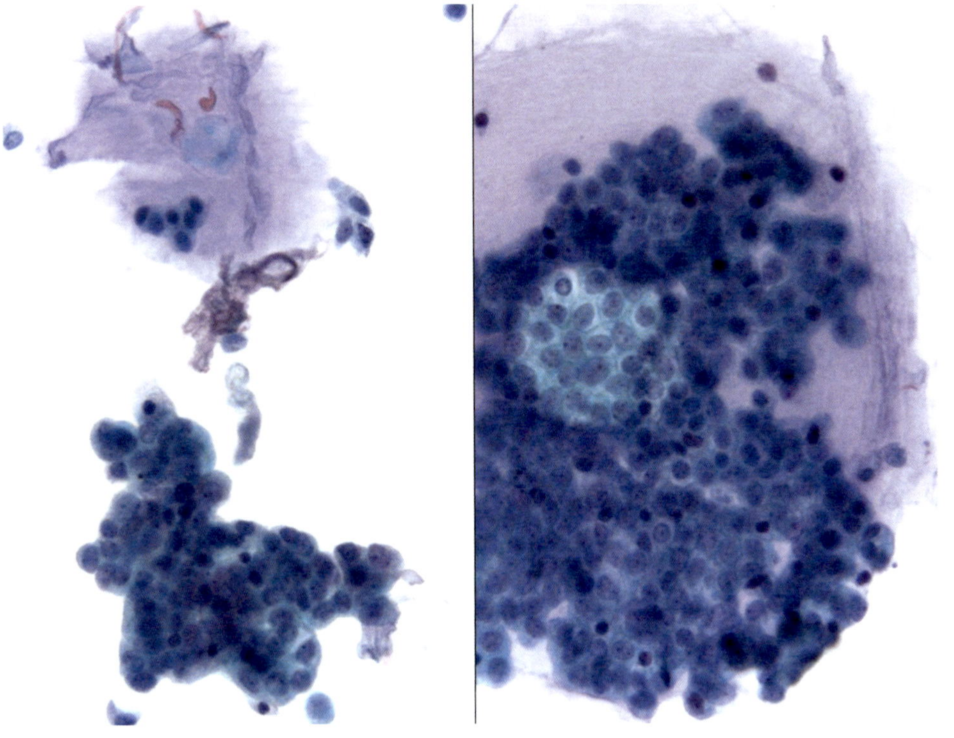

Q-29. These images are from a catheterized urine specimen of a 81 year-old man with hematuria. The most likely diagnosis is:

(a) Reactive urothelial cells
(b) Urothelial carcinoma, low grade
(c) Urothelial carcinoma in situ
(d) Small cell carcinoma
(e) Urolithiasis

Fig. 11.30

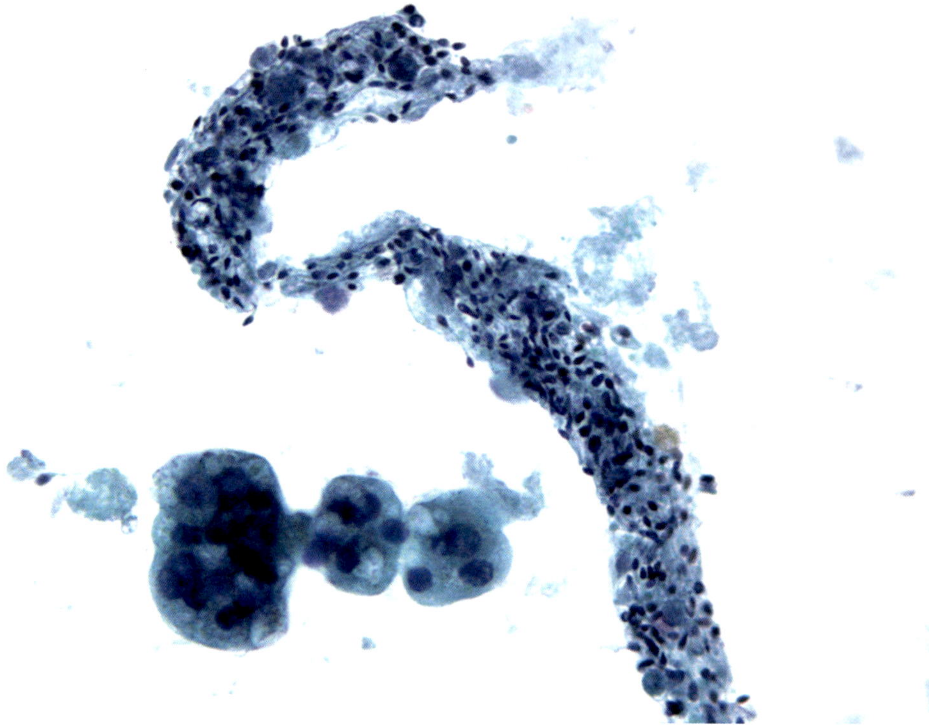

Q-30. These images are from a voided urine specimen of a patient with hematuria. The most likely diagnosis is:
(a) Reactive urothelial cells
(b) Adenocarcinoma
(c) Melanoma
(d) Granulomatous cystitis
(e) Unsatisfactory, non-urothelial elements.

Fig. 11.31

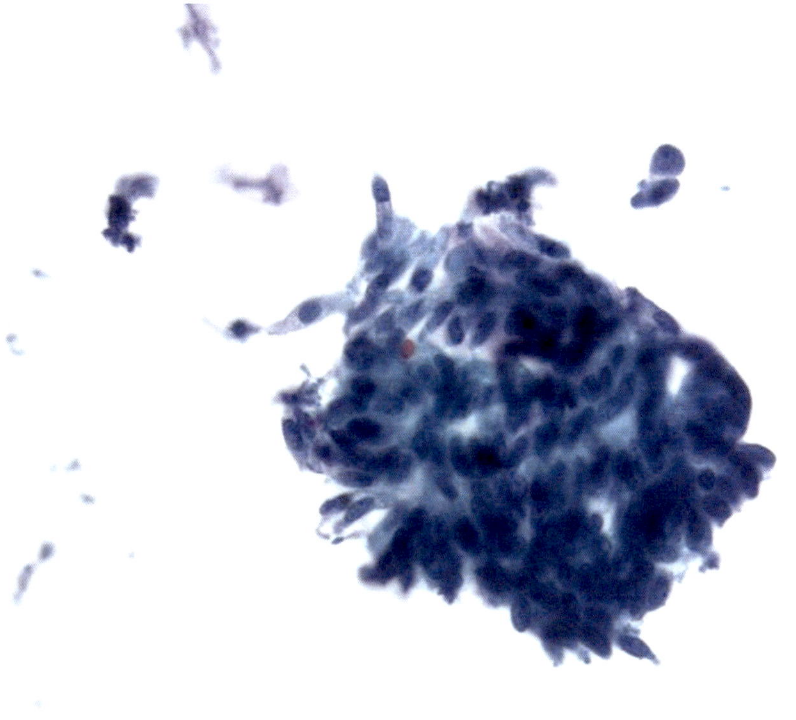

Q-31. The images are from the catheterized urine of a patient with previous history of high-grade urothelial carcinoma. The most likely diagnosis is:

(a) Positive, favor UC, low grade
(b) Positive, favor urothelial carcinoma, high grade (recurrence)
(c) Positive, well-differentiated adenocarcinoma
(d) Negative, degenerative changes
(e) Negative, benign columnar cells suggestive of cystitis glandularis or cystitis cystica

Fig. 11.32

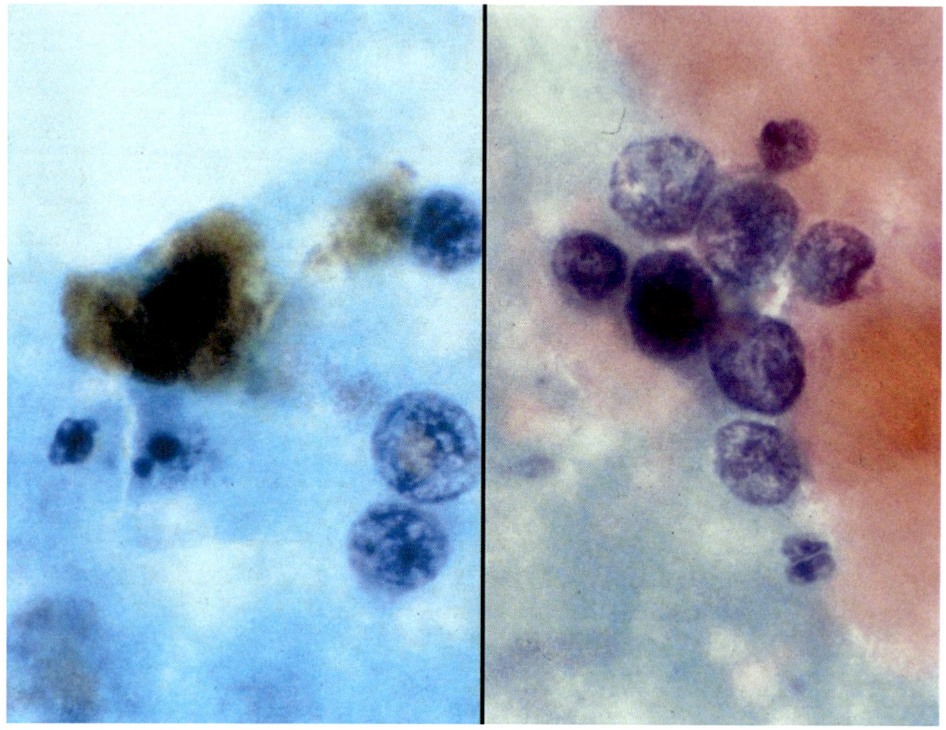

Q-32. This urine sample was collected from a 62-year-old woman with hematuria. The cytological features are consistent with:

(a) Urothelial carcinoma
(b) Atypia suggestive of chemotherapy
(c) Polyomavirus infection
(d) Benign cells from seminal vesicle
(e) Melanoma

Fig. 11.33

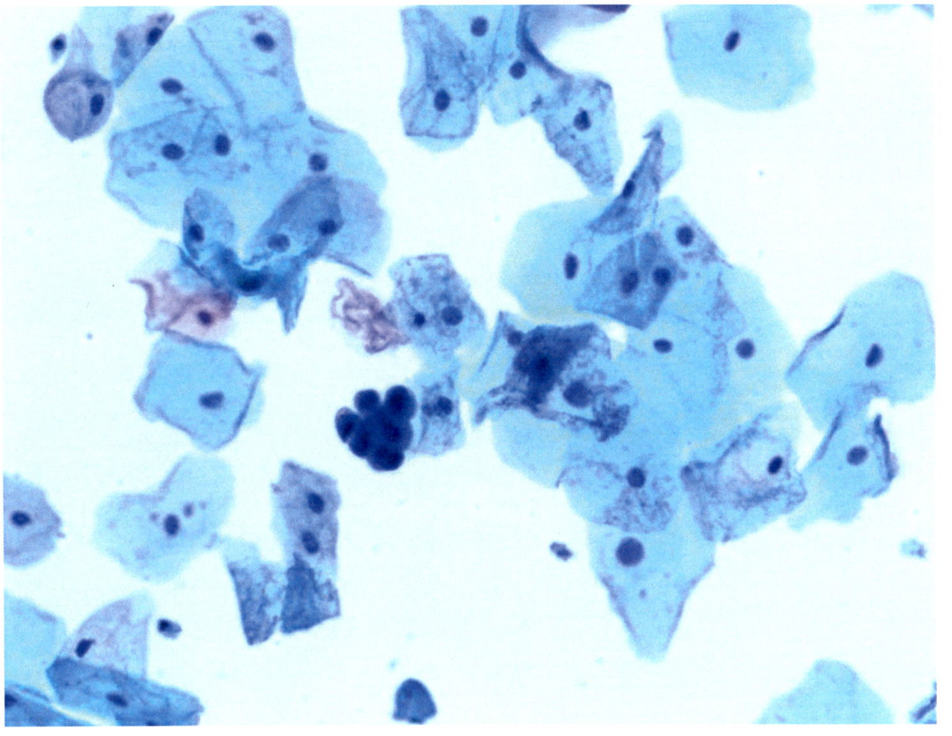

Q-33. Voided urine from a 48-year-old woman. History of hematuria. Cystoscopy and bladder washings were negative. The most likely diagnosis is:
(a) High-grade urothelial carcinoma
(b) Benign, decoy cells
(c) Adenocarcinoma
(d) Reactive urothelial cells
(e) Benign, endometrial cells

Fig. 11.34

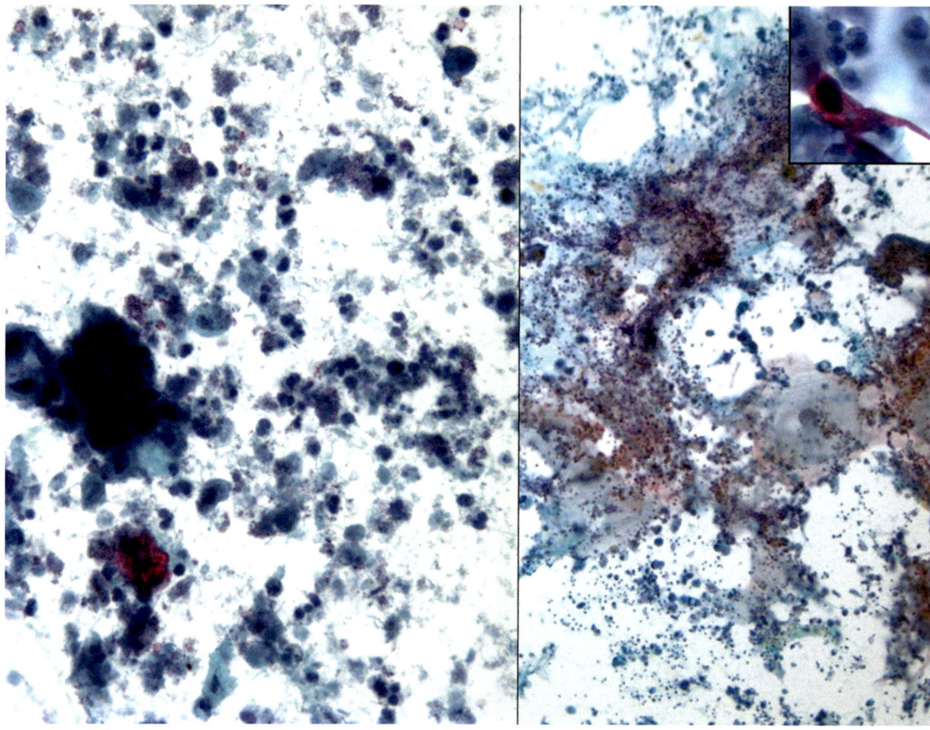

Q-34. The images are from voided urine of a 63-year-old woman with hematuria and status post chemotherapy for rectal cancer. Which of the following is true about these images?

(a) There is inflammatory/infectious necrosis due to chemotherapy effect.
(b) Tumor necrosis is present, the diagnosis is at least suspicious for malignancy.
(c) There is ischemic necrosis due to therapy effect.
(d) The morphology is consistent with acute cystitis.
(e) The morphology is consistent with chronic cystitis.

Fig. 11.35

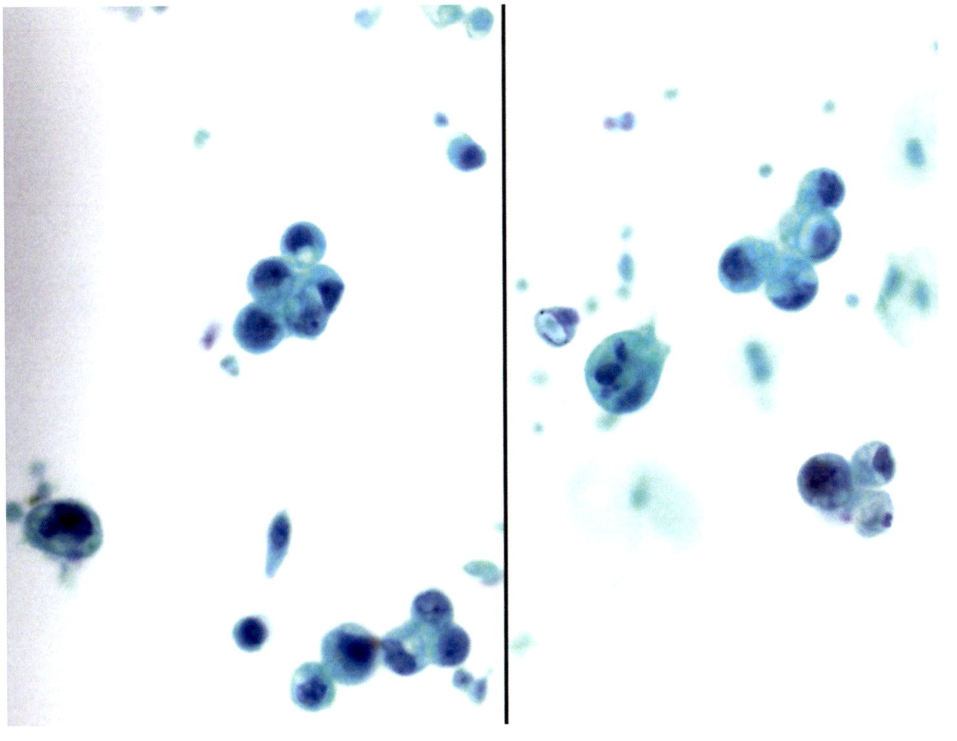

Q-35. The images are from ThinPrep preparation of urine specimen of a 73-year-old woman, who has a history of endometrial adenocarcinoma with positive lymph nodes. Which of the following is the most likely diagnosis?

(a) Urothelial carcinoma, high grade
(b) Reactive urothelial cells
(c) Cystitis cystica or glandularis
(d) Metastatic endometrial adenocarcinoma
(e) Squamous cell carcinoma

Fig. 11.36

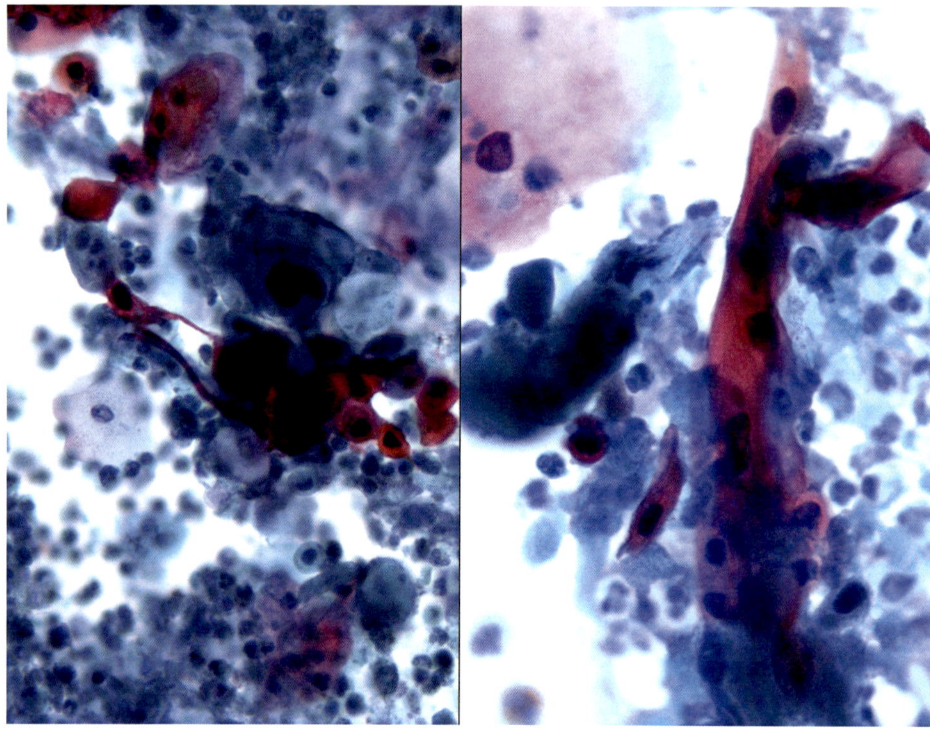

Q-36. These images are from the catheterized urine specimen of a 59-year-old man with painless gross hematuria. The most likely diagnosis is:
(a) Reactive urothelial and squamous cells
(b) Urothelial carcinoma, high grade
(c) Squamous intraepithelial lesion, low grade (CIN 1)
(d) Squamous intraepithelial lesion, high grade (CIS)
(e) Urothelial carcinoma, high grade with squamous differentiation

11.2 Text-Based Questions 37–61

Q-37. All the following criteria for diagnosing low-grade urothelial carcinoma in cytological specimens are correct except:
(a) Nuclear enlargement and high nuclear to cytoplasmic ratio
(b) Necrosis
(c) Papillary fragments with fibrovascular cores
(d) Cell clusters without cores
(e) Irregular cell clusters

Q-38. Urothelial cells with large nuclear basophilic inclusions and perinuclear haloes are most likely infected with which virus:
(a) HIV virus
(b) Herpes simplex type 1 virus
(c) Cytomegalovirus
(d) Herpes simplex type 2 virus
(e) Human polyomavirus

Q-39. A 58-year-old man with smoking history presents with painless gross hematuria. Urothelial carcinoma is suspected and FISH is ordered on urine specimen. Which is the earliest genetic alteration in urothelial carcinoma that may be revealed by FISH?
(a) EGFR overexpression
(b) P53 gene alteration
(c) Chromosome 9 alteration
(d) A and C
(e) None of the above

Q-40. All the following statements regarding "Immunocyt" test are correct *except*:
(a) The Immunocyt test combines cytology with an immunofluorescence assay of three fluorescent monoclonal antibodies.
(b) The Immunocyt test combines cytology with an immunofluorescence assay of two fluorescent monoclonal antibodies.
(c) The technique requires 20–40 ml of urine that is fixed immediately in 50 % ethanol
(d) This technique has approximately 77 % sensitivity in diagnosing urothelial carcinoma
(e) None of the above

Q-41. Which initial cystoscopic surveillance protocol is mostly applied for newly diagnosed patients with bladder cancer that did not invade the muscularis propria?
(a) 0–3 months for 2 years
(b) 3–6 months for 2 years
(c) 6–9 months for 5 years
(d) 9–12 months for 5 years
(e) 1–2 years for 10 years

Q-42. Which of the following collection methods is the least to yield benign urothelial clusters in urine cytology?
(a) Bladder washings
(b) Voided urine
(c) Bladder brushings
(d) Catheterized urine
(e) Urolithiasis

Q-43. Decoy cells are associated with:
(a) An unknown etiology
(b) Prostatic adenocarcinoma
(c) Catheterized urine
(d) Urothelial carcinoma
(e) Viral infection

Q-44. Which immunohistochemical stain results would support diagnosis of B-cell lymphoma?
(a) Predominant of CD20+ cells
(b) Predominant of ALK+ cells
(c) Predominant of LCA+ cells
(d) Predominant of CD30+ cells
(e) Predominant of CD3+ cells

Q-45. Which preservative is used for urine specimens when immediate cytopreparation is not possible?
(a) Buffered formalin
(b) 40 % ethyl alcohol
(c) 50 % ethyl alcohol
(d) Normal saline
(e) Xylene

Q-46. Which is the most common fungus seen in urine?
(a) *Aspergillus*
(b) *Candida albicans*
(c) *Torulopsis*
(d) *Histoplasmosis*
(e) *Coccidiomycosis*

Q-47. The marked urothelial cellular changes in status post chemotherapy include :
(a) Increased cellularity
(b) Cellular degeneration
(c) High N/C ratio
(d) Nuclear membrane irregularities
(e) All of the above

Q-48. Bacillus Calmette-Guerin (BCG) therapy for superficial bladder cancer would most likely result in:
(a) Non-necrotizing granulomatous inflammation
(b) Necrotizing granulomatous inflammation
(c) Urothelial carcinoma
(d) A and C
(e) None of the above

Q-49. All the following statements are true regarding Melamed-Wolinska bodies except:
(a) They are diagnostic of herpes virus infection
(b) They can be seen in almost 50 % of urine specimens
(c) They can suggest a urothelial origin
(d) They are round eosinophilic cytoplasmic inclusions of varying sizes
(e) None of the above

Q-50. Examination of urine cytology specimen of a 24-year-old woman showed urothelial cells with nuclear molding, chromatin margination, and multinucleation. These features are most consistent with:
(a) Herpes simplex virus (HSV)
(b) Human papillomavirus (HPV)
(c) Cytomegalovirus (CMV)
(d) Polyomavirus
(e) Human immunodeficiency virus (HIV)

Q-51. Cyclophosphamide therapy may cause all of the following changes *except* :
(a) Hematuria
(b) Squamous carcinoma of the bladder
(c) Urothelial atypia mimicking viral cytopathic effect
(d) Radiation-like-induced changes
(e) Urothelial carcinoma

Q-52. Intranuclear inclusions are caused by all of the following *except:*
(a) Lead poisoning
(b) Cytomegalovirus infection
(c) Herpes virus infection
(d) Polyomavirus infection
(e) Malakoplakia

Q-53. Malakoplakia of the bladder is associated with:
(a) Schistosomiasis
(b) Keratinized mucosal plaque(s)
(c) Increased risk for squamous carcinoma
(d) Granulomatous inflammation
(e) Viral etiology

Q-54. The presence of cancer cells in bladder washings in the absence of cystoscopically visible tumor is likely to indicate:
(a) Renal pelvis urothelial carcinoma
(b) Renal cell carcinoma
(c) Instrumentation atypia
(d) Viral infection
(e) Flat carcinoma in situ

Q-55. Squamous carcinoma may be associated with all of the following *except*:
(a) Schistosomiasis
(b) Metastatic carcinoma from cervix uteri
(c) Diverticular disease of the bladder
(d) Patent urachus
(e) Chronic bladder irritation

Q-56. What is the best time of the day to collect voided urine specimen?
(a) Early morning, first void
(b) Midmorning
(c) Noon
(d) 2 p.m.
(e) Time of day does not matter

Q-57. What percent of bladder neoplasms are diagnosed on the first-voided urine specimen?
(a) 100 %
(b) 80 %
(c) 20 %
(d) 5 %
(e) 1 %

Q-58. Which is true regarding the sensitivity of urine cytology?
(a) More sensitive for high-grade lesions.
(b) More sensitive for low-grade lesions.
(c) Equally sensitive for high- and low-grade lesions.
(d) Washings of the ureter and pelvis are more sensitive than urine cytology.

Q-59. Which of the following may mimic carcinoma in urine cytology and can contribute to false positives?
(a) Urolithiasis
(b) Chemotherapy
(c) Human polyomavirus
(d) Seminal vesicle cells
(e) All of the above

Q-60. In urine cytology specimens, all of the following are true about superficial (umbrella) cells except:
(a) Umbrella cells are a common component of ALL urine specimens regardless of the type of sample or collection technique.
(b) Umbrella cells are the largest of the urothelial cells and may have single, double, or multiple nuclei.
(c) The cytoplasm of umbrella cells is abundant and is usually eosinophilic, finely granular, and sometimes vacuolated, with a cell membrane that is sharply demarcated and often slightly rolled.

(d) The nuclei of umbrella cells may vary in size but they are spherical or slightly ovoid with finely textured chromatin and a well-defined nuclear membrane.
(e) Umbrella cells are more common in voided urine.

Q-61. All of the following are true about UroVysion FISH Testing except:
(a) This test is FDA approved.
(b) Start-up costs are very high, since a quality immunofluorescence microscope with four filters connected to a computer with a digital camera are required in addition to dark-field space and technical personnel licensed for complex procedures.
(c) UroVysion FISH test is basically a cytogenetics test that searches for abnormalities in chromosomes 3 (polysomy), 7 (polysomy), 9 (deletion of 9p21),and 17 (polysomy).
(d) A positive UroVysion FISH result indicates the presence of a urothelial neoplasm.
(e) According to the protocol, at least 25 nuclei must be recordable before a specimen can be considered informative.

11.3 Answers and Discussion of Image-Based Questions 1–36

A-1. **(b) Reactive urothelial cells**
The images show the cytomorphologic features of reactive urothelial cells in catheterized urine. In comparison to voided urine, catheterized specimens may yield larger number of umbrella cells and groups of urothelial cells and may show superficial, intermediate, and deep basal cell. The key is to compare the nucleus and the chromatin with other obvious benign intermediate cells. Reactive or inflammatory processes may have prominent nucleoli. In general, cells are mostly rounded, but elongated or columnar cells may be seen. Squamous cells in male patients may be present normally in urine specimens, and if abundant, they may signify squamous metaplasia. Contamination from the skin usually shows numerous nonnucleated squamous cells. Low-grade urothelial carcinoma cellular features are homogenous cytoplasm, definitive increase in N/C ratio, slight contour irregularity, mild loss of polarity, cellular and nuclear enlargement, and large clustering with irregular clustering border. In high-grade urothelial carcinoma, there are more single cells and marked cytological atypia (nuclear enlargement, irregular nuclear contour; loss of polarity) and the chromatin is usually coarsely clumped. In urolithiasis, benign reactive urothelial clusters may be abundance and crystals may be seen.

A-2. **(c) Urothelial carcinoma, low grade**
The image provided depicts the cytomorphologic features of low-grade urothelial carcinoma: homogenous cytoplasm with absence of vacuoles, definitive increase in N/C ratio, slightly irregular contours, mild loss of polarity with haphazard growth pattern, cellular enlargement, large clusters with irregular borders, nuclear enlargement, eccentric nucleus, uniform granular chromatin, and no obvious umbrella cells. In comparison to high-grade lesions, this case has predominance of clustering with no significant single cell present and no necrosis in the background. Clinical and endoscopic correlation may help in difficult cases.

A-3. **(c) Urothelial carcinoma, high grade with squamous differentiation**
The images show features of high-grade urothelial carcinoma with squamous differentiation which include marked irregular nuclear contour, variable increase in N/C ratio, single cells, coarse chromatin, and no umbrella cells. Necrotic background may be seen. In bladder squamous cell carcinoma, the squamous carcinoma component has to be predominant, and this is challenging to ascertain in cytology. Accordingly, cytology cases should be designated as high-grade urothelial carcinoma with squamous differentiation. Low-grade urothelial carcinoma does not show squamous differentiation, glandular differentiation, or small cell/neuroendocrine differentiation. The differential diagnosis of urothelial carcinoma with squamous cell differentiation includes: squamous cell carcinoma (primary or metastatic), intraepithelial squamous dysplastic lesion (low or high grade), or benign squamous cells with reactive atypia. *Schistosoma haematobium* is endemic in Egypt and may cause bladder squamous cell carcinoma, but, outside the endemic areas, the ova are rarely found.

A-4. **(e) Benign, negative for malignant, consistent with urinary diversion specimen**
The images show the cytomorphologic features of urine diversion urine specimen, which can be obtained from patients who underwent cystectomy. The specimen usually shows markedly degenerated, round/cuboidal intestinal cells with pyknotic eccentric nuclei, granular cytoplasm, and indistinct cytoplasmic borders. RBCs and inflammation are usually absent. Benign columnar cells of the bowel mucosa are a normal component of ileal urine and should not be confused for adenocarcinoma. The conduit urine is examined for possible detection of concurrent carcinoma of the upper urinary tract. In high-grade urothelial carcinoma the cells show nuclear enlargements, high N/C ratio, marked irregular nuclear contour, coarse chromatin, and a background of necrosis and no umbrella cells.

A-5. **(c) Polyomavirus immunostain (SV40)**
Human polyomaviruses are small, non-enveloped, double-stranded DNA viruses classified into two main strains: BK and JC, where BK strain affects the kidney and can be detected in the urine. The image display polyomavirus-infected single cells showing cellular enlargement, very high N/C ratios, and ground glass nuclei with homogenous basophilic intranuclear inclusions that fill the nuclear area. The nuclear membrane contour shows no irregularity. Clustering is not a feature of polyomavirus infection. Polyomavirus nephropathy is becoming a common infection after kidney transplant. The infected cells show nuclear positivity when stained with (SV40).

A-6. **(c) Urothelial carcinoma in situ (CIS)**
The images show features of urothelial carcinoma in situ (CIS) which are similar to features of high-grade

urothelial carcinoma without a necrotic background. The cells are classically single and enlarged (about x4 lymphocyte). In addition, they display very high N/C ratio, coarsely clumped chromatin, irregular nuclear contour, and loss of polarity (when are clustered) and may have prominent nucleoli. Due to the non-cohesive and actively proliferating nature of the disease, they exfoliate in disproportionately large numbers. Small cell carcinoma will show significant necrosis, pleomorphism, salt and pepper chromatin, and almost no cytoplasm and the cells are of a smaller size (2–3 lymphocyte size). Polyomavirus infection does not cause clustering or irregular nuclear membrane irregularities.

A-7. **(d) Acute cystitis**
The image displays acute inflammatory cells, lysed blood, and extensive degeneration. Reactive urothelial cells with nuclear enlargement, hypochromasia, and round regular nuclear contour are present. These reactive cells exhibit low N/C ratios. Unsatisfactory diagnosis should be used when no well-visualized epithelial cells are present to be evaluated or due to obscuring factors such as lubricant, blood, and marked inflammation. If cellular atypia is present, then the diagnosis should be at least atypical with mentioning of the scant cellularity or obscuring factors as a quality indicator. For urothelial carcinoma (low and high grade), cytological atypia must be present, which is not seen in this case.

A-8. **(c)Suspicious for malignant lymphoma**
The specimen shows a fairly monotonous population of dyshesive single cells. Cells are small to intermediate with high nuclear/cytoplasmic ratio. Cells have irregular distributed chromatin with visible nucleoli. The background is unremarkable with no atypical urothelial cells seen. The absence of true tissue aggregates is very useful key. These features are highly suspicious for malignant lymphoma involving urinary bladder and flow cytometric study is indicated for confirming the diagnosis.

The differential diagnosis of bladder lymphoma includes follicular cystitis, granulomatous cystitis, small cell carcinoma, and high-grade urothelial carcinoma. The key for diagnosis is the presence of monotonous population of lymphoma-like cells. In follicular cystitis, lymphocytes vary in maturation but are mostly small mature lymphocytes accompanied by immature follicular center lymphocytes and tingible-body macrophages. Immunostain of both CD20 and CD3 confirms a reactive process (more CD3 cells than CD20 cells).

Chronic cystitis should yield multipopulation of inflammatory cells including lymphocytes and plasma cells. The absence of a significant histiocytes and giant cells precludes the diagnosis of granulomatous cystitis.

A-9. **(b) Urothelial carcinoma, low grade**
The specimen shows clusters and isolated urothelial cells showing mild nuclear enlargement, mild loss of polarity, mild high N/C ratio, and mild irregular nuclear contour. The differential diagnosis includes reactive atypia vs. low-grade urothelial carcinoma. The positivity of CK20 (in non-umbrella cells) is suggestive of urothelial carcinoma. It has been shown that normal urothelial cells express cytokeratin 19 (CK19) and cytokeratin 8 (CK8). However, cytokeratin 20 (CK20) has shown to be selectively expressed in malignant urothelial cells. In addition to immunohistochemistry, reverse transcriptase polymerase chain reaction (RT-PCR) technique can be used to detect CK20 gene expression. The overall sensitivity of CK20 is 91 % (87–94 %), and overall specificity is 78 % (67–97 %).

A-10. **(a) Polyomavirus infection**
The image show features of polyomavirus infections: cellular enlargement, very high N/C ratios, and ground glass nuclei with homogenous basophilic intranuclear inclusions entirely filling the nuclear area. A zone of clearing surrounding the inclusion caused by degeneration of the viral particles is seen in addition to chromatin margination. Nuclear membrane contours are regular and no clustering is seen. Polyomavirus-infected cells may mimic high-grade urothelial carcinoma; however, the lack of irregular contour and clustering favors polyomavirus infection. Polyomavirus-infected cells are sometimes referred to as "BK cells" or "decoy cells." Activation of polyomavirus is most commonly observed in immune deficient or suppressed patients following organ transplants or chemotherapy.

A-11. **(d) High-grade urothelial carcinoma with small cell features**
The images show small cells arranged singly and in clusters in a necrotic hemorrhagic background displaying marked pleomorphism, hyperchromatic nuclei with karyorrhectic/apoptotic nuclei, nuclear molding, and salt and pepper chromatin. These features are consistent with small cell carcinoma. These cases are better diagnosed as high-grade urothelial carcinoma with small cell features. Ancillary studies including neuroendocrine markers should be done to

further confirm the diagnosis. Exclusion of a metastasis from other sites should be done before diagnosing a primary small cell carcinoma of the bladder.

A-12. **(b) Urothelial carcinoma, high grade**
The images show large single cells with marked cytological atypia, nuclear enlargement, irregular nuclear contour, and coarsely clumped chromatin. The cytoplasm is homogenous with no vacuoles. These features are consistent with high-grade tumors which are commonly composed of markedly disorganized hyperplastic urothelium with enlarged, irregular, and hyperchromatic nuclei. Classically, the nuclear configuration would be angular with coarse chromatin and mitotic figures. Nucleoli are not a prominent feature. Due to the actively proliferating, discohesive, and exfoliative nature of the disease, cytology can be an excellent adjunctive diagnostic tool.

In low-grade urothelial carcinoma, the cells are large with homogenous cytoplasm that shows no visible vacuoles, definitive increase in N/C ratio, slight contour irregularity, mild loss of polarity, and no obvious umbrella cells.

A-13. **(e) Unsatisfactory for evaluation, suggest resampling**
Guidelines for urine specimen adequacy have not been established with some authors suggesting at least 15 well-visualized basal and intermediate cells per slide as a perquisite for adequacy. This case is a "blood only specimen" composed of lysed blood and inflammatory cells. No diagnosis could be rendered; accordingly, it should be designated as unsatisfactory (non-diagnostic) specimen. In general, unsatisfactory diagnosis should be reserved for extremely hypocellular specimen with no well-visualized epithelial cells for evaluation. Also, the presence of obscuring factors such as lubricant, blood, and marked inflammation can render the specimen non-diagnostic. If cytological atypia is present, an atypical diagnosis should be generated with a comment mentioning the scant cellularity or obscuring factors as a quality indicator. Please, note that any specimen with clearly abnormal cells is satisfactory for evaluation.

A-14. **(d) Squamous intraepithelial lesion, low grade (CIN-1)**
Human papillomavirus infection (HPV) has been reported in the squamous mucosa of the bladder and distal urethra. The image shows squamous cells with cytomorphologic features of mild dysplasia (CIN-1) displaying the characteristic cytopathic changes (koilocytes).

Bladder condyloma affects more women than men and usually develops in the setting of immunosuppression. Human papillomavirus has been found in bladder condyloma. The cells show a wrinkled, hyperchromatic nucleus, a perinuclear cavity with thick outlines, binucleation, and dense cytoplasm.

In squamous cell carcinoma, the cells show marked irregular nuclear contour, variable increase in N/C ratio, numerous single cells, coarse chromatin, and background of necrosis. Squamous cell carcinoma also shows squamous differentiation with bright cytoplasmic keratinization and hyperchromatic nucleoli.

A-15. **(a) Metastatic colonic adenocarcinoma**
Adenocarcinoma is a rare finding in urine cytology and can be primary or secondary, with the primary tumors accounting for less than 3 % and mostly associated with the urachal remnant at the bladder dome. In metastatic colonic adenocarcinoma, the cells are columnar shape with variable necrosis in the background. Poorly differentiated adenocarcinoma may mimic urothelial carcinoma; thus, clinical correlation and/or ancillary studies are important to make this distinction. The most frequent primary sites for metastatic adenocarcinoma are gastrointestinal (colonic and rectal), breast, kidney, and prostate. Tumors of colonic origin may show CK20+, CK7, CEA+, and CDx2+.

A-16. **(a) Reactive urothelial cells**
The image shows a tight cluster of basal cells with low N/C ratios. Although hyperchromasia (degeneration) is seen, there is no irregular nuclear contours. These cells are more common in catheterized specimens than voided urine. There is no significant increase in nuclear size.

The groups of cells in this setting should not misdiagnosed as papillary tumor. A useful clue to their reactive nature is that the nuclei maintain a relatively smooth contour.

A-17. **(c) Unsatisfactory, obscuring lubricants**
This case shows almost no urothelial cells with abundance of lubricants/gel. Lubricants appears as a well-delineated, flat, opaque, amorphous fragment. It is usually has a grayish-blue color and frayed or speculated borders. The identification of lubricant in a urine specimen indicates the use of an instrument for obtaining the urine sample. Therefore, urothelial cellular changes related to instrumentation must be considered in the differential diagnosis of a low-grade urothelial carcinoma. Distinguishing of lubricant from a mucinous background of mucinous adenocarcinoma may be challenging and requires search of atypical or

malignant glandular cells. The mucinous background is diffuse and abundant and not well delineated and localized.

A-18. (**b**) **Urothelial carcinoma, high grade**
The images show the cytomorphologic features of high-grade urothelial carcinoma which include large loosely cohesive clusters of highly atypical cells showing marked cytological atypia (nuclear enlargement, irregular nuclear contour, loss of polarity) and the chromatin is coarsely clumped. The cytoplasm is homogenous (absence of vacuoles) and the cluster borders are irregular. The clusters are markedly disorganized with enlarged, irregular, and hyperchromatic nuclei. Nuclear configuration is angular and chromatin is coarse. In low-grade urothelial carcinoma, there is a homogenous cytoplasm (absence of vacuoles), definitive increase in N/C ratio, slight contour irregularity, mild loss of polarity (haphazard growth pattern), cellular enlargement, large clustering with irregular clustering border, nuclear enlargement, eccentric nucleus, uniform granular chromatin, and no obvious umbrella cells.

A-19. (**b**) **Infection by this virus is acquired late in life.**
There is almost universal infection by human polyomavirus in childhood, thus the cytological manifestations reflect reactivation or super infection with the virus. Polyomaviruses have a smaller genome and are differently organized than the papillomaviruses, but they are part of same family and EM looks similar. The image shows cells infected with polyomavirus showing very high N/C ratios and ground glass nuclei with homogenous basophilic intranuclear inclusions that fill the nuclear area entirely. Few cells show zone of clearing due to degeneration of the viral particles and also causing some margination of chromatin. There is no irregularity in the nuclear membrane contour. Clustering also is not seen in polyomavirus infection. Polyomavirus infection is common after cancer treatment or among transplanted patents. Immunostain of polyomavirus (SV40) can be used on smear or cell block to confirm the diagnosis in difficult cases. It should be nuclear positivity.

A-20. (**c**) **Reactive urothelial cells**
The specimen contains some umbrella cells and basal urothelial cells. Instrumented urine such as catheterized specimen in this case will show superficial, intermediate, and deep cells. The umbrella cells are a common component of the urine sediment regardless of the type of sample or collection technique, and they can be numerous in bladder washing specimens. They are the largest of the urothelial cells and may have single, double, or multiple nuclei. Their abundant cytoplasm is usually eosinophilic, finely granular, and sometimes vacuolated, with a cell membrane that is sharply demarcated and often slightly rolled. Nuclei may vary in size but they are spherical or slightly ovoid with finely textured chromatin and a well-defined nuclear membrane. The mechanism of formation of these giant cells is not clear but appears to be an artifact. The basal cells shown have abundant and vacuolated cytoplasm and display round shape nucleus with slightly dark/hyperchromatic chromatin; however, the nuclear contours are uniform and the chromatin is powdery which argues against neoplastic nature.

In low-grade urothelial carcinoma, the cells usually show homogenous cytoplasm, definitive increase in N/C ratio, slight irregular contour irregularity, mild loss of polarity, cellular and nuclear enlargement, and large clustering with irregular clustering border. In high-grade urothelial carcinoma, there is more single cells and marked cytological atypia (nuclear enlargement, irregular nuclear contour, loss of polarity) and the chromatin is usually coarsely clumped.

A-21. (**c**) **Urolithiasis**
Irregular basophilic noncellular material representing stone fragments is seen. The abrasive effect of stone produces exfoliation of urothelial cells and cause reactive atypia. The cytomorphologic features of the urothelial cells (mostly umbrella cells) shown in the image display mild atypia mainly in the form of nuclear enlargement; however, the chromatin is powdery and similar in color and texture to neighboring nonreactive benign urothelial cells. Urolithiasis may mimic malignancy causing false-positive diagnosis particularly low-grade urothelial carcinoma. In low-grade urothelial carcinoma, the cells have homogenous cytoplasm with no vacuoles, definitive increase in N/C ratio, contour irregularity and nuclear enlargement (nucleus > 3 RBCs size), and no obvious umbrella cells. In high-grade urothelial carcinoma, there are more single cells and marked cytological atypia (nuclear enlargement, irregular nuclear contour; loss of polarity) and the chromatin is usually coarsely clumped. The background is granular with lysed RBCs present.

A-22. (**e**) **Melamed-Wolinska bodies**
The image show degenerated urothelial cells with Melamed-Wolinska bodies (eosinophilic cytoplasmic inclusions). These bodies are seen in almost 50 % of urine specimens. Although they have no diagnostic value, they are helpful in suggesting a urothelial origin when dealing with a metastatic carcinoma of

unkown primary. Sometimes they can be seen in human polyomavirus infection and ileal conduit intestinal cells.

A-23. (e) **None of the above**
The image display of thick-walled cells contained dense, smudged cores and pericentral clearing in a grayish-blue background of amorphous fragment with frayed borders consistent with lubricant material. The board rigid-like contours and thick uniform wall help identify them as vegetable cells. On rare occasions, vegetable cell-like structures are identified in urinary diversion specimens, possibly as a contaminant from stoma care material. Recognitions of their peculiar morphology will help in distinguishing theme from pathologic conditions involving parasitic ova or koilocytes.

A-24. (**d**) **Unsatisfactory for evaluation, suggest repeat sampling**.
The images show numerous crystals with no urothelial cells seen. Therefore, the diagnosis should be unsatisfactory (non-diagnostic) specimen. Unsatisfactory diagnosis should be used for very hypocellular specimen (no well-visualized epithelial cells to be evaluated) or due to presence of obscuring factors such as lubricant, blood, and marked inflammation unless there is evidence of cytological atypia. Then, the diagnosis should be at least atypical with mentioning of the scant cellularity or obscuring factors as a quality indicator.

Specific guidelines for determining the adequacy of urine specimens have not been established. Some authors have suggested that a slide should contain at least 15 well-visualized basal and intermediate cells to be classified as adequate. Any other quality factors should be described immediately after the satisfactory and unsatisfactory terms (i.e., low cellularity, poor preservation, obscuring blood, or inflammation). Crystals may be present in urolithiases, but it is not adequate for such diagnosis. The abrasive effect of stone produces exfoliation of single urothelial cells and cell clusters. Ancillary studies and clinical and radiological correlation may help in difficult cases.

A-25. (c) **Metastatic lung small cell carcinoma**
The images show the cytomorphologic features of small cell carcinoma which include small cells arranged singly and in clusters, marked pleomorphism, hyperchromatic nuclei with karyorrhectic nuclei/apoptotic nuclei, nuclear molding, salt and pepper chromatin, and necrotic hemorrhagic background. The smears are highly cellular and show small, round to oval, pleomorphic hyperchromatic nuclei with very scant cytoplasm. The cells arranged singly and in clusters of variable cohesiveness and often display nuclear molding. Karyorrhectic nuclei, blood, acute inflammation, and necrotic debris are common. Ancillary studies performed on cell block material show positive staining for chromogranin (neuroendocrine marker) and TTF-1 (lung and thyroid malignancy marker), CK7+, and CK20 – which confirm the presence of small cell carcinoma of lung origin. Primary small cell carcinoma of the bladder is very rare entity. Therefore, a diagnosis of primary small cell carcinoma of the bladder should only be made after exclusion of a metastasis from other sites such as lung and prostate in male and lung and cervix in female.

A-26. (**d**) **Corpora amylacea**
The image shows large acellular spherical structures with fine radial striations and concentric laminations suggestive of *Corpora amylacea*. They are more commonly seen in older individuals, and in urine cytology they are mostly from a prostate origin. They carry no known clinical significance.

A-27. (**d**) **A and B**
The images show display columnar cells and basal urothelial cells. The columnar cells are characterized by their elongated cytoplasm and polar nuclei. Benign features include: oval, uniform, bland nuclei with a finely granular chromatin pattern. Benign columnar cells in urine are a normal finding and should not be misdiagnosed for adenocarcinoma. They may represent metaplastic or glandular epithelium, from the urethra. In males, they may also represent exfoliation of prostatic columnar cells or seminal vesicles cells. Most columnar cells are non-ciliated; however, ciliated columnar cells may be from vasa deferentia or epididymis origin. Basal cells are also a normal component of urine cytology, mostly seen in instrumented urine and rarely seen in voided specimens. They are predominantly oval, with basophilic, dense cytoplasm and single nuclei. Their relative contour smoothness and low N/C ratio should help differentiating them from neoplastic cells.

A-28. (**b**) ***Enterobius vermicularis***
Enterobius vermicularis "pinworm" is a small, thin, white roundworm that most commonly occurs among children, institutionalized persons, and household members of persons with pinworm infection and has a high rate of reinfection. The image shown display *Enterobius vermicularis eggs* which have double

walled and smooth shell with an embryo inside. The eggs usually measure 50–60 μm by 20–25 μm. The alimentary tract is the most common site for infection; however, the eggs can show in urine as a contaminant or as a result of urinary infection especially among women with poor personal hygiene.

A-29. (a) **Reactive urothelial cells**
The image shows a large cluster of reactive urothelial cells and gel materials. The reactive urothelial cells show uniform, relatively small nuclei with smooth nuclear contours indicating benign nature. Neoplastic cells tend to display nuclear enlargements and marked size difference/pleomorphism. The cells are very viable and abundance due to the specimen being instrumented in urine specimen. Degenerative changes are common in voided urine and frequently show dark and smudgy chromatin with frayed-like cytoplasmic changes; however, the cells should maintain small nuclei.

A-30. (e) **Unsatisfactory, non-urothelial elements**
The image shows non-urothelial elements: sperms and seminal vesicle cells. There is no urothelial or epithelial cells present; therefore, the specimen is unsatisfactory for evaluation.

A-31. (e) **Negative, suggestive of cystitis glandularis or cystitis cystica**
There specimen shows reactive benign epithelial cells with columnar differentiation suggestive of cystitis glandularis. When columnar cells are predominant in urine specimen, it is most likely arising from areas of cystitis glandularis or cystitis cystica in the bladder. However, in men they may originate also from the prostate or seminal vesicles. In both men and women, columnar cells can rarely arise from the glandular epithelium of paraurethral glands, which extend from the ducts to the urethral surface mucosa. Cystitis cystica and cystitis glandularis are lesions related to Von Brunn's nests. Cystitis cystica is present in approximately 60 % of bladders. It is most common in adults but also occurs in children. The cysts are formed by degeneration of urothelium in the central portion of Brunn's nests, leaving a peripheral lining of one or several layers of urothelium or metaplastic cuboidal epithelium. The central cystic space is filled with eosinophilic fluid and sometimes a few inflammatory cells. In cystitis glandularis, the epithelium lining the cysts of cystitis cystica is transformed by metaplasia into mucus-secreting glandular epithelium of intestinal type. Cystitis glandularis is almost as common as cystitis cystica and is also present mostly in the trigone.

A-32. (e) **Melanoma**
The images show the cytomorphologic features of malignant melanoma which include variable amount of intracellular melanin pigment or melanophages, large dissociated cells with marked nuclear atypia. The cytoplasm is dense and cyanophilic and contains a fine dusty to coarse granular brown-black melanin pigments. The differential diagnosis includes melanosis of the kidney (melanin-pigmented renal tubular cells that can be seen in the urine). Ancillary studies can be performed on cytospin or cell block material to confirm the diagnosis. Melanoma usually positive for S100, Melan-A, and HMB45 and negative for cytokeratin. Urothelial carcinoma is usually positive for pan cytokeratin, CK7, CK20, p63, p53, and p16 and negative for S100, Melan-A, and HMB45. Most malignant melanoma in the bladder are metastasis from know primary. However, primary bladder melanoma does occur, but very rare, and requires strict criteria to be met (see references).

A-33. (e) **Endometrial cells**
Vaginal contamination is common in voided urine specimen from female patients. This includes squamous cells from vaginal origin and glandular epithelium including cervical and endometrial. The presence of abundance squamous cells with lactobacilli is indicative of vaginal contamination. Endometrial epithelium may also seen in urine sample such is this case. The size of nuclei similar to squamous intermediate cells is one clue (about ×1 RBC). The endometrial cells have high N/C ratio and smudgy, dark, pyknotic, and crowded nuclei.

Small cell carcinoma shows cellular specimen with single and small cluster of viable pleomorphic small cells, larger than normal endometrial nuclei (2–3 RBC) with necrotic background.

A-34. (b) **There is a tumor necrosis; the diagnosis is at least suspicious for malignancy**.
The images show the cytomorphologic features of tumor necrosis. Tumor necrosis characterizes by presence of cellular debris that include nuclear debris and atypical cells. Viable atypical cells are occasionally very rare, and therefore, suspicious diagnosis is rendered in such specimens. The necrotic debris may clumped in liquid-based cytology preparation giving clinging necrosis appearances. Inflammatory necrosis

does not have atypical cells. Instead, there is marked acute inflammatory cells present. Ischemic necrosis is extremely rare in exfoliative cytology. The specimen will show numerous ghost of single and clusters of cells with no cytological atypia seen.

A-35. **(d) Metastatic endometrial adenocarcinoma**
Adenocarcinoma is a rare finding in urine cytology and can be primary or secondary. Bladder primary adenocarcinoma accounts for less than 3 % and mostly associated with the urachal remnant at the bladder dome. In metastatic adenocarcinoma the cells are glandular, with cytoplasmic vacuolization and nuclear enlargements and irregularities. Necrosis may be seen and marked in colonic origin adenocarcinoma. Poorly differentiated adenocarcinoma may mimic urothelial carcinoma; thus, clinical correlation and/or ancillary studies are important to make this distinction. The most frequent primary sites for metastatic adenocarcinoma are gastrointestinal (colonic and rectal), gynecological malignancies, breast, kidney, and prostate. Tumors of endometrial origin may show vimentin+, ER+, PR+, and WT1.

A-36. **(e) Urothelial carcinoma, high grade with squamous differentiation**
The images show features of high-grade urothelial carcinoma with squamous differentiation which include marked pleomorphic cells (cell and nuclear pleomorphism), irregular nuclear contour, and coarse chromatin in necrotic background. In bladder squamous cell carcinoma, the squamous carcinoma component has to be predominant, and this is challenging to ascertain in cytology. Accordingly, cytology cases should be designated as high-grade urothelial carcinoma with squamous differentiation. Low-grade urothelial carcinoma does not show squamous differentiation, glandular differentiation, or small cell/neuroendocrine differentiation. The differential diagnosis of urothelial carcinoma with squamous cell differentiation includes squamous cell carcinoma (primary or metastatic), intraepithelial squamous dysplastic lesion (low or high grade), or benign squamous cells with reactive atypia. *Schistosoma haematobium* is endemic in Egypt and may cause bladder squamous cell carcinoma but is rare in the USA.

11.4 Answers and Discussion of Text-Based Questions 37–61

A-37. (**b**) **Necrosis**
Diagnostic criteria for low-grade urothelial carcinoma can be divided into architectural atypia and cytological atypia. Architectural findings include the presence of papillary fragments or single cells with nuclear enlargements, homogenous cytoplasm, and plasmacytoid morphology. The cytological criteria include a high nuclear to cytoplasmic ratio, homegenious cytoplasm, and mild irregular nuclear membranes and no necrosis. Necrosis is indicative of high-grade urothelial carcinoma.

A-38. (**c**) **Cytomegalovirus**
Cytomegalovirus (CMV) can infect urothelial cells; however, it most frequently affects renal tubular epithelial cells. Morphologically infected cells are enlarged with a single large nucleus and the characteristic of perinuclear halo/large intranuclear basophilic inclusions. Smaller cytoplasmic inclusion may also be seen. Both herpes and polyomaviruses show nuclear inclusions. In addition, herpes usually display multinucleation, molding and chromatin margination (3 Ms). Degenerated CMV-infected cells should not be misdiagnosed for high-grade urothelial carcinoma.

A-39. (**c**) **Chromosome 9 alteration**
The earliest genetic alteration of urothelial carcinoma is p16 gene deletion at chromosome 9p21 which can be detected by FISH. P53 and Rb alterations have been implicated in the progression of superficial urothelial carcinoma into muscle invasive urothelial carcinoma. In general, FISH assay appears to enhance the sensitivity of routine urine cytology analysis.

A-40. (**b**) **The Immunocyt test combines cytology with an immunofluorescence assay of two fluorescent monoclonal antibodies**.
The Immunocyt test combines cytology with an immunofluorescence assay of three fluorescent monoclonal antibodies M344 and LDQ10 (green fluorescence) and 19A21 (red fluorescence). It requires 20–40 ml of urine that is fixed immediately in 50 % ethanol and a special fixative solution; then, the cells are collected by filtration and are processed for immunocytochemical assessment before fluorescent microscope examination. This technique is helpful in diagnosing urothelial carcinoma, with 77 % sensitivity and 76 % specificity.

A-41. (**b**) **3–6 months for 2 years**
Although cystoscopic surveillance protocols for newly diagnosed patients with superficial bladder cancer (no invasion of the muscularis propria) may vary per different institutional protocols, most authorities would agree on initial cystoscopic surveillance with urine cytology every 3–6 months for the first 2 years. Afterword and according to surveillance findings, this protocol can be modified to accommodate less frequent testing in later years.

A-42. (**b**) **Voided urine**
The finding of urothelial clusters in voiding urine is very rare. Due to the vigorous nature of the bladder washings, brushings, and catheterization, they are more likely to yield urothelial clusters.

A-43. (**e**) **Viral infection**
Polyomavirus infection is widespread, usually acquired during childhood or young adult life. The cellular expression of viral changes in urothelial cells is considered a reactivation process. Infected cells are sometimes referred to as "BK cells" for the initials of the patient in whom this disease was first described. They are also called "decoy cells," a name given by Andrew Ricci, a cytotechnologist at Memorial Hospital, because they were often misinterpreted as malignant cells by newcomers to the laboratory. Activation of polyomavirus is most commonly observed in immune deficient or suppressed patients, for example, those receiving organ transplant and patients on chemotherapy.

A-44. (**a**) **Predominant of CD20+ cells**
The morphologic hallmark for lymphoma is a discohesive monotonous population of large atypical cells. Identification of this morphology mandates ordering flow cytometry and immunohistochemical panels to further diagnose the case. Primary lymphoma of the urinary bladder is rare and correlation with clinical history is crucial; hence, a history of high-grade lymphoma or human immunodeficiency virus (HIV) is usually present. CD19, CD20, CD22, CD79a, CD79b, and PAX-5 are markers for pan-B and pan-pre-B cells. CD2, CD3, CD4, CD5, CD8, and CD1a are T-cell markers.

A-45. (**c**) **50 % ethyl alcohol**
Normal urine is not isotonic; it has a low pH and high content of urea and other organic compounds, making it a hostile medium for desquamated cells and an excellent medium for growth of microorganisms.

Thus, when immediate cytopreparation of a urine specimen is not possible, the addition of a preservative is recommended, for example, 50 % ethyl alcohol added to an approximately equal volume of urine.

A-46. (**b**) ***Candida albicans***
In general, *Candida albicans* is the common fungus in urine and more commonly found in immunocompromised patients or as a diabetic complication. In women, especially with a background composed of many squamous cells, bacteria, and few neutrophils, it may represent vaginal contamination. Rarely *Torulopsis* or *Aspergillus* is detected in urine.

A-47. (**b**) **Cellular degeneration**
Chemotherapy effect can mimic high-grade urothelial carcinoma. The cytomorphologic features of chemotherapy include increased cellularity, cellular degeneration, high N/C ratio, and nuclear membrane irregularities. A helpful clue is the nuclear chromatin which tends to be homogenously dark status post-treatment but more textured in high-grade urothelial carcinoma. Correlation with clinical history is required.

A-48. (**b**) **Necrotizing granulomatous inflammation**
In a select group of patients with superficial bladder cancer (no muscularis propria invasion), bacillus Calmette-Guerin (BCG) can be used as a topical immunotherapy. This therapy usually leads to a necrotizing granulomatous inflammatory response in both the bladder and prostrate associated with dysuria. Microscopically, it would show as collections of epithelioid cells, giant cells, and a necrotic background.

A-49. (**a**) **They are diagnostic of herpes virus infection**.
Melamed-Wolinska bodies are eosinophilic cytoplasmic inclusions of urothelial cells seen in almost 50 % of urine specimens. Although they have no diagnostic value, they are helpful in suggesting a urothelial origin when dealing with a metastatic carcinoma of unknown primary. Sometimes they can be seen in human polyomavirus infection and ileal conduit intestinal cells.

A-50. (**a**) **Herpes simplex virus** (**HSV**)
The viral cytopathic changes of herpes simplex virus (HSV) infection include multinucleation, ground glass chromatin, nuclear molding, and peripheral condensation of chromatin.

A-51. (**c**) **Urothelial atypia mimicking viral cytopathic effect**
Cyclophosphamide is an alkylating agent used for the treatment of malignant tumors and is known to induce changes in the urothelium that may be difficult to differentiate from carcinoma. It also may cause severe hemorrhagic cystitis, squamous metaplasia, and squamous or urothelial carcinoma.

A-52. (**e**) **Malakoplakia**
Malakoplakia is a chronic granulomatous inflammation that can affect any part of the urinary tract, but the bladder is the most common site. The disease is characterized by multiple soft umbilicated yellow plaques and is caused by an impaired cellular response to invading bacteria, most commonly *Escherichia coli*. The bacteria are incorporated into the lysosomes of phagocytic macrophages but not properly digested and later became the nidus for calcification, resulting in the formation of Michaelis-Gutmann bodies. Michaelis-Gutmann bodies are eosinophilic; granular cytoplasmic inclusions may present mineralized fragments of bacteria due to impaired autophagolysosomal activity of the cell to kill phagotized bacteria. They are PAS, calcium, and iron positive.

A-53. (**d**) **Granulomatous inflammation**
Malakoplakia is a chronic granulomatous inflammation of unknown etiology that can affect any part of the urinary tract, but the bladder is the most common site. The disease is characterized by multiple soft umbilicated yellow plaques and is caused by an impaired cellular response to invading bacteria, most commonly *Escherichia coli*. The bacteria are incorporated into the lysosomes of phagocytic macrophages but not properly digested and later became the nidus for calcification, resulting in the formation of Michaelis-Gutmann bodies. Michaelis-Gutmann bodies are eosinophilic; granular cytoplasmic inclusions may present mineralized fragments of bacteria due to impaired autophagolysosomal activity of the cell to kill phagotized bacteria. They are PAS, calcium, and iron positive.

A-54. (**e**) **Flat carcinoma in situ** (**CIS**)
In carcinoma in situ, cells are usually shed singly and show the nuclear changes of carcinoma without cellular enlargement or pleomorphism. Occasional red cells are present in almost all cases but the background is otherwise "clean." Invasive carcinoma is marked by much greater viability in nuclear and

cellular size and shape. These cancers typically shed cells with large and often bizarre nuclei and often with squamous differentiation. There is much inflammation in the background, with degenerated cellular debris and a variable number of red blood cells.

This is the most important high-grade neoplastic lesion of the urothelium and is composed of cytologically malignant urothelial cells in a non-papillary flat mucosa. The normal urothelium is totally replaced by cancer cells that have not invaded through the basement membrane. Flat carcinoma in situ is often found in association with papillary tumors and is believed to be the source of invasive carcinoma in many of those patients with perhaps only 20 % of invasive carcinomas arising from (high-grade) papillary carcinoma. CIS is most common in men above the age of 50 years. Symptoms include dysuria, frequency, and microscopic hematuria. Gross hematuria is not common, unlike invasive carcinoma. A substantial number of patients with CIS may be asymptomatic. Most CIS cases are multifocal, appearing cystoscopically as one or several red, velvety patches. However, in some cases the mucosa may appear normal to the cystoscopist. Cytology is extremely useful in detection of CIS. The cells derived from this lesion are typically non-cohesive and actively proliferating, and they exfoliate in disproportionately large numbers. The tumor cells may be only slightly enlarged but they have relatively large hyperchromatic nuclei, irregular nuclear contours, and coarse chromatin. Nucleoli are absent or inconspicuous. Cytoplasm is usually scant.

A-55. (**d**) **Patent urachus**

Bladder urachus may cause primary adenocarcinoma. Primary bladder adenocarcinoma accounts for less than 2–3 % of malignant bladder tumors. It is divided into two principal categories: arising from the urachus and those arising in the bladder proper. Urachal carcinomas must invade into the dome of the bladder before they exfoliate tumor cells. Non-urachal carcinoma accounts for 60–80 % of primary adenocarcinomas of the bladder and is believed to arise in cystitis glandularis. They have the potential for earlier detection than urachal carcinoma because they arise from the mucosal epithelium. Nevertheless, adenocarcinoma in 40 % of patients is already advanced at the time of presentation. Hematuria is the most common presenting symptom.

A-56. (**b**) **Midmorning**

Explanation: The first-voided specimen in the morning is usually cellular, but the cells are mostly degenerated. The second- or later-voided sample provides generally better preserved cells. Thus, specimen from morning's second voiding is best (3–4 h after last urination). It is recommended to collect three samples on three consecutive days which are diagnostically optimal. The midstream clean-catch urine is best.

A-57. (**b**) **80** %

Of the neoplasms diagnosed with voided urine → 80 % diagnosed on first urine, 15 % on second, and rest on the third.

A-58. (**a**) **More sensitive for high-grade lesions**

The sensitivity of urine cytology for high-grade lesions is 79 % (specificity is >95 %) and the sensitivity of urine cytology for low-grade lesions is 30 % (specificity is 80 %). Washings of ureter and pelvis have lower sensitivity and prone to have false positivity due to marked cellularity

A-59. (**e**) **All of the above**

Urolithiasis, chemotherapy, polyomavirus infection, and seminal vesicle cells all are causes of false-positive diagnosis in urine cytology due to their ability to cause nuclear enlargement, hyperchromasia, and atypia that can be misdiagnosed as carcinoma in urine cytology.

Instrumentation and calculi may induce a reactive process with active appearing proliferating epithelial cells that vary in cell size and exhibit nuclear hyperchromasia. The dislodged cells often occur in clusters and sheets unlike the single cells spontaneously shed from tumors. When exfoliated these cells can mimic low-grade tumors and they would not be misinterpreted as high-grade carcinomas. Clinical information may be critical for proper evaluation. Intravesical bacillus Calmette-Guerin (BCG) is utilized widely in the treatment of superficial bladder carcinoma. It induces a chronic inflammatory response, sometimes with granuloma formation. Urothelial cells show marked degenerative changes and are mixed with inflammatory cells and histiocytes. It may be difficult to distinguish degenerating malignant cells from degenerating benign epithelial cells or monocytes. Chemotherapeutic drugs, and particularly mitomycin C and thiotepa, can induce similar effects. Cyclophosphamide is known to cause severe atypia of urothelium mimicking carcinoma and in fact may be a carcinogen for the bladder. Human polyomavirus reactivation – this virus causes smudgy nuclear degeneration with or without hyperchromasia that may mimic carcinoma cells for the inexperienced. Ileal loop – in post-cystectomy patients, ileal urine specimens are typically very cellular with abundant degenerated cells. This background may mask the presence of a few isolated malignant cells.

A-60. **(e) Umbrella cells are more common in voided urine.**

The umbrella cells are a common component of the urine sediment regardless of the type of sample or collection technique. They are the largest of the urothelial cells and may have single, double, or multiple nuclei. Their abundant cytoplasm is usually eosinophilic, finely granular, and sometimes vacuolated, with a cell membrane that is sharply demarcated and often slightly rolled. Nuclei may vary in size but they are spherical or slightly ovoid with finely textured chromatin and a well-defined nuclear membrane. Large multinucleated umbrella cells are particularly common in washings and brushing specimens. The mechanism of formation of these giant cells is not clear but appears to be an artifact.

A-61. **(d) A positive UroVysion FISH result indicates the presence of a urothelial neoplasm.**

A positive UroVysion FISH result indicates the presence of a urothelial neoplasm. This statement is not true. UroVysion test is a multi-target, multicolor fluorescence in situ hybridization (FISH) assay that searches for abnormalities in chromosomes 3 (polysomy),7 (polysomy), 17 (polysomy), and 9 (deletion of 9p21). The sensitivity of the test is 84 % and the specificity is 92 %. Therefore, it has false positivity and a positive UroVysion FISH result may NOT indicate the presence of a urothelial neoplasm. However, in the presence of highly atypical suspicious cells, the sensitivity and the specificity is very high and most likely indicative of urothelial carcinoma. The test is FDA approved. The start-up costs are very high, since a quality immunofluorescence microscope with 4 filters connected to a computer with a digital camera is required in addition to dark-field space and technical personnel licensed for complex procedures.

UroVysion FISH test is basically a cytogenetics test that searches for abnormalities in chromosomes 3 (polysomy), 7 (polysomy), 9 (deletion of 9p21), and 17 (polysomy). According to the protocol, at least 25 nuclei must be recordable before a specimen can be considered informative.

Reading List

Bardales RH. Practical urologic cytopathology. New York: Oxford University Press; 2002.

Bibbo M, Kern WH. Chapter 15. Urinary tract. In: Bibbo M, Wilbur DC, editors. Comprehensive cytopathology. 3rd ed. Philadelphia: Saunders Elsevier; 2008. p. 409–38.

DeMay RM. Chapter 5. Urine. In: DeMay RM, editor. The art & science of cytopathology. 2nd ed. Chicago: ASCP Press; 2012. p. 436–89.

Khalbuss WE, Monaco SE, Pantanowitz L. Chapter 11. Urine. In: The ASCP quick compendium of cytopathology. 2013; p. 184–211.

Layfield LJ, Elsheikh TM, Fili A, Nayar R, Shidham V. Papanicolaou Society of Cytopathology Review of the state of the art and recommendations of the Papanicolaou Society of Cytopathology for urinary cytology procedures and reporting: the Papanicolaou Society of Cytopathology Practice Guidelines Task Force. Diagn Cytopathol. 2004;30(1):24–30.

Melamed M. Chapter 22. The lower urinary tract in the absence of cancer. In: Koss LG, Melamed MR, editors. Koss' diagnostic cytology and its histopathologic bases. 5th ed. Philadelphia: Lippincott Williams & Wilkins; 2006a. p. 568–642.

Melamed M. Chapter 23. Tumors of the urinary tract in urine and brushings. In: Koss LG, Melamed MR, editors. Koss' diagnostic cytology and its histopathologic bases. 5th ed. Philadelphia: Lippincott Williams & Wilkins; 2006b. p. 777–846.

Quiroga-Garza G, Nassar D, Khalbuss WE, Monaco SE, Pantanowitz L. Vegetable cell contaminants in urinary bladder diversion cytology specimens. Acta Cytol. 2012;56(3):271–6.

Renshaw AA. Chapter 3. Urine & bladder washings. In: Cibas ES, Ducatman BS, editors. Cytology diagnostic principles & clinical correlates. 3rd ed. Philadelphia: Saunders Elsevier; 2009. p. 105–28.

Soft Tissue and Bone Fine-Needle Aspiration

12

Ehab A. ElGabry and Walid E. Khalbuss

Contents

12.1 **Image-Based Questions 1–42** 671

12.2 **Text-Based Questions 43–90** 701

12.3 **Answers and Discussion of Image-Based Questions 1–42** 706

12.4 **Answers and Discussion of Text-Based Questions 43–90** 712

Reading List 716

Table 12.1 Major cytomorphological pattern categories of soft tissue lesions

Myxoid
Spindle cell
Round cell
Pleomorphic
Polygonal/epithelioid

Table 12.2 Chromosomal translocations in sarcomas

Tumor type	Associated translocation
Alveolar rhabdomyosarcoma	t(2;13)(q35;q14)
	t(1;13)(p36;q14)
Alveolar soft part sarcoma	t(X;17)(p11.2;q25)
Angiomatoid fibrous histiocytoma	t(12;16)(q13;p11)
Clear cell sarcoma	t(12;22)(q13;q12)
Congenital fibrosarcoma/congenital mesoblastic nephroma	t(12;15)(p13;q25)
Dermatofibrosarcoma protuberant	t(17;22)(q22;q13)
Desmoplastic small round cell tumor	t(11;22)(p13;q12)
Endometrial stromal sarcoma	t(7;17)(p15;q21)
Ewing sarcoma/peripheral primitive neuroectodermal tumor	t(11;22)(q24;q12)
	t(21;22)(q22;q12)
	t(7;22)(p22;q12)
	t(17;22)(q12;q12)
	t(2;22)(q33;q12)
	t(16;21)(p11;q22)
Inflammatory myofibroblastic tumor	t(1;2)(q22;p23)
	t(2;19)(p23;p13)
	t(2;17)(p23;q23)
Low-grade fibromyxoid sarcoma	t(7;16)((q33;p11)
Myxoid chondrosarcoma	t(9;22)(q22;q12)
	t(9;15)(q22;q21)
	t(9;17)q22;q11)
Myxoid liposarcoma	t(12;16)(q13;p11)
	t(12;22)(q13;q12)
Synovial sarcoma	t(X;18)(p11;q11)

E.A. ElGabry, MD (✉)
Department of Pathology, University of Pittsburgh Medical Center (UPMC)-Shadyside, 5150 Centre Avenue; POB2, Suite 201, Pittsburgh, PA 15232, USA
e-mail: drgabry2013@gmail.com

W.E. Khalbuss, MD, PhD, FIAC
Department of Pathology, GE Clarient Diagnostic Services, 31 Columbia, Aliso Viejo, California, 92656, USA
e-mail: Walid.khalbuss@ge.com

W.E. Khalbuss, Q.K. Li (eds.), *Diagnostic Cytopathology Board Review and Self-Assessment*,
DOI 10.1007/978-1-4939-1477-7_12, © Springer Science+Business Media New York 2015

Table 12.3 Differential diagnosis of soft tissue round blue cell tumors

Ewing sarcoma/PNET
Rhabdomyosarcoma
Poorly differentiated synovial sarcoma
Desmoplastic sarcoma
Neuroblastoma
Malignant lymphoma

Table 12.4 Common benign soft tissue lesions with spindle morphology

Neural origin: schwannoma, neurofibroma
Adipocytic: spindle cell lipoma and fibrolipoma
Muscle origin: leiomyoma and fibromatosis
Miscellaneous: granulomas and nodular fasciitis

Table 12.5 Common malignant soft tissue lesions with spindle morphology

Fibrosarcoma
Leiomyosarcoma
Synovial sarcoma
Malignant peripheral nerve sheath tumors (MPNST)
Kaposi sarcoma
Low-grade fibromyxoid sarcoma
Gastrointestinal stromal tumor (GIST)
Malignant fibrous histiocytoma (MFH)
Malignant spindle cell melanoma
Malignant spindle cell carcinoma

Table 12.6 Common benign lesions with myxoid morphology

Ganglion cysts
Nodular Fasciitis
Myxoma
Spindle cell lipoma
Myxoid neurofibroma

Table 12.7 Common malignant lesions with myxoid morphology

Myxoid liposarcoma
Myxoid chondrosarcoma
Myxofibrosarcoma
Chordoma
Low-grade fibromyxoid sarcoma
Mucinous metastatic carcinoma

Table 12.8 Common soft tissue tumors with epithelioid cells predominance

Benign
Rhabdomyoma
Granular cell tumor (frequently benign)
Malignant
Epithelioid sarcoma
Epithelioid variant of leiomyosarcoma
Epithelioid variant of angiosarcoma
Malignant peripheral nerve sheath tumor
Malignant extrarenal rhabdoid tumor (ERT)
Pleomorphic rhabdomyosarcoma (PR)
Clear cell sarcoma
Alveolar soft part sarcoma
Metastatic tumors (melanoma, carcinoma, mesothelioma)
Indeterminate malignant potential
Epithelioid hemangioendothelioma

Table 12.9 Common soft tissue lesions with pleomorphic morphology

Myxofibrosarcoma
Liposarcoma
Rhabdomyosarcoma
Osteosarcoma

Table 12.10 Immunostain panels for metastatic carcinoma of unknown origin (female)

CK7; CK20
Mammaglobin; ER
TTF1
CEA
CA19-9
S100; synaptophysin
WT-1

Table 12.11 Immunostain panels for metastatic carcinoma of unknown origin (male)

CK7; CK20
TTF1
PSA
CEA; CA19-9
S100; synaptophysin

12.1 Image-Based Questions 1–42

Figs. 12.1, 12.2, and 12.3

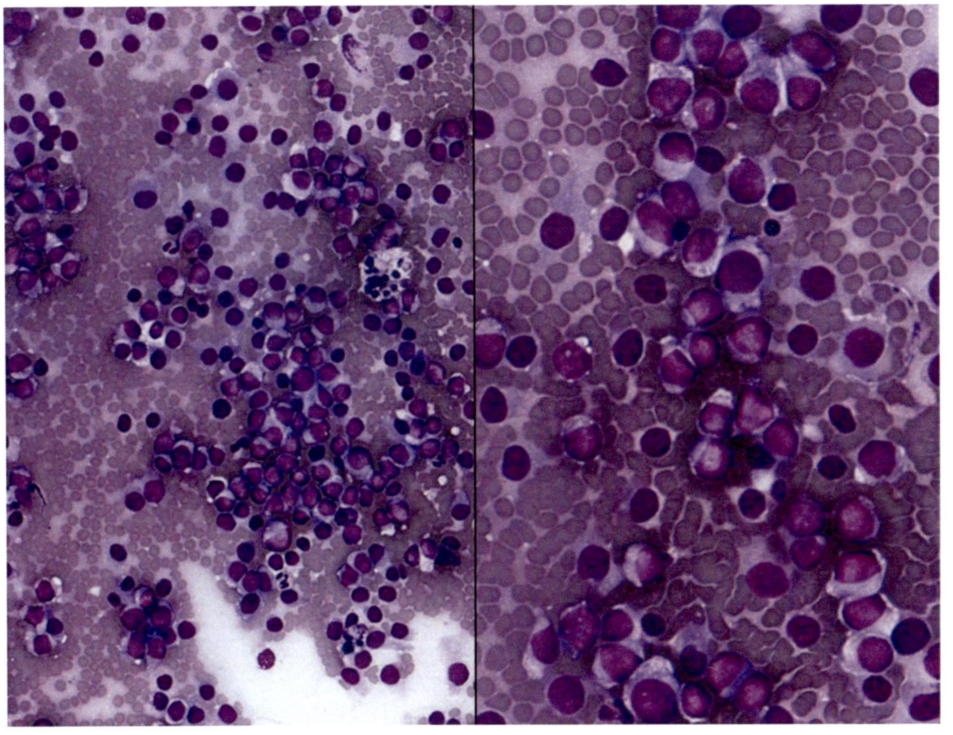

Q-1. A 15-year-old female presented with progressive pain in the left thigh for a period of 2 months. Physical examination revealed local tenderness and swelling over the proximal and mid-thirds of the left thigh. A biopsy of the mass was done. Immunohistochemistry studies were negative for pan-CK, chromogranin, and CD45. Immunostains for synaptophysin, CD99, and PAS-D are positive. FNA of the mass is shown in the images provided. What is the most likely diagnosis?
(a) Non-Hodgkin lymphoma
(b) Carcinoma
(c) Small cell carcinoma
(d) Ewing sarcoma
(e) Rhabdomyosarcoma

Q-2. What is the most likely translocation?
(a) t(x;17)(p11.2;q25)
(b) t(11;22) with EWSR1-FLI1 fusion
(c) t(12;22)(q13;q12)
(d) t(12;16)(q13;p11)
(e) None of the above

Q-3. Which of the following is true regarding this lesion?
(a) *Electron microscopy is needed for diagnosis.*
(b) There is a high rate of lymph node metastases.
(c) Most common skeletal sites include the skull.
(d) Response to preoperative chemotherapy is a major independent prognostic factor.
(e) They are extremely common in patients older than 30.

Figs. 12.4 and 12.5

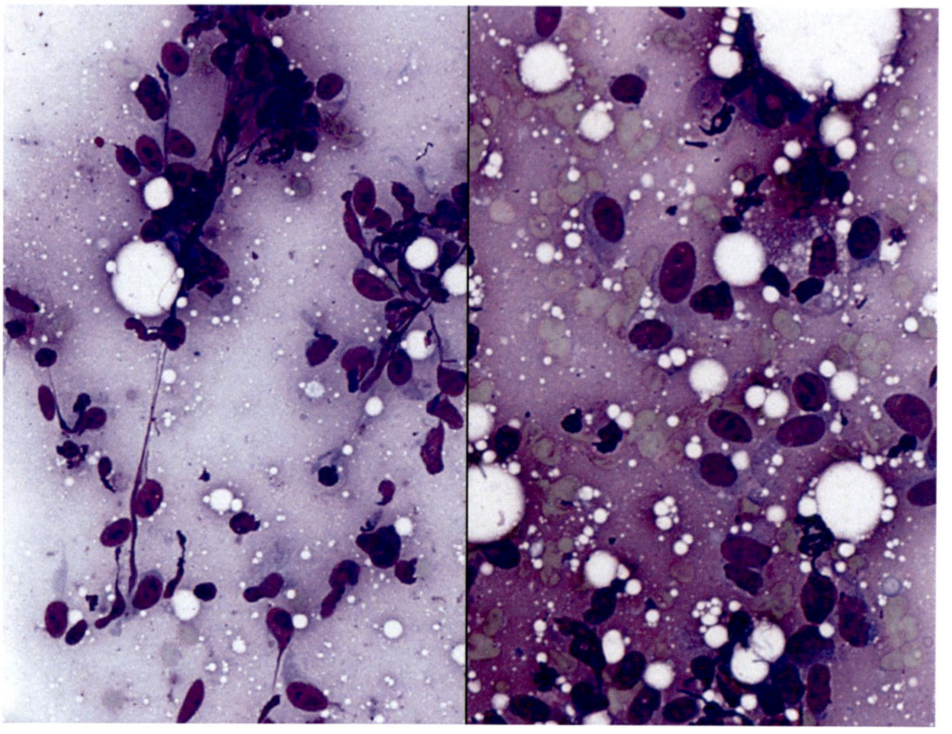

Q-4. A 78-year-old woman was diagnosed with a poorly differentiated ductal carcinoma of the right breast for which she underwent conservative surgery. In addition, she received tamoxifen treatment and postoperative radiation. During a routine follow-up 8 years later, she presented with 1.5 cm area of purple skin lesion at the upper inner quadrant of the right breast associated with peau d'orange. FNA of the mass was performed and shown in the image provided. What is the most likely diagnosis?

(a) Hemangioma
(b) Epithelioid variant of angiosarcoma
(c) Recurrent breast cancer
(d) Melanoma
(e) Spindle cell variant of angiosarcoma

Q-5. Which of the following statement/s regarding this lesion is/are false?

(a) Immunostains would stain positive for CD31.
(b) This lesion is always negative for cytokeratin stains.
(c) This lesion usually stain negative for FLI-1.
(d) A and B.
(e) B and C.

Fig. 12.6

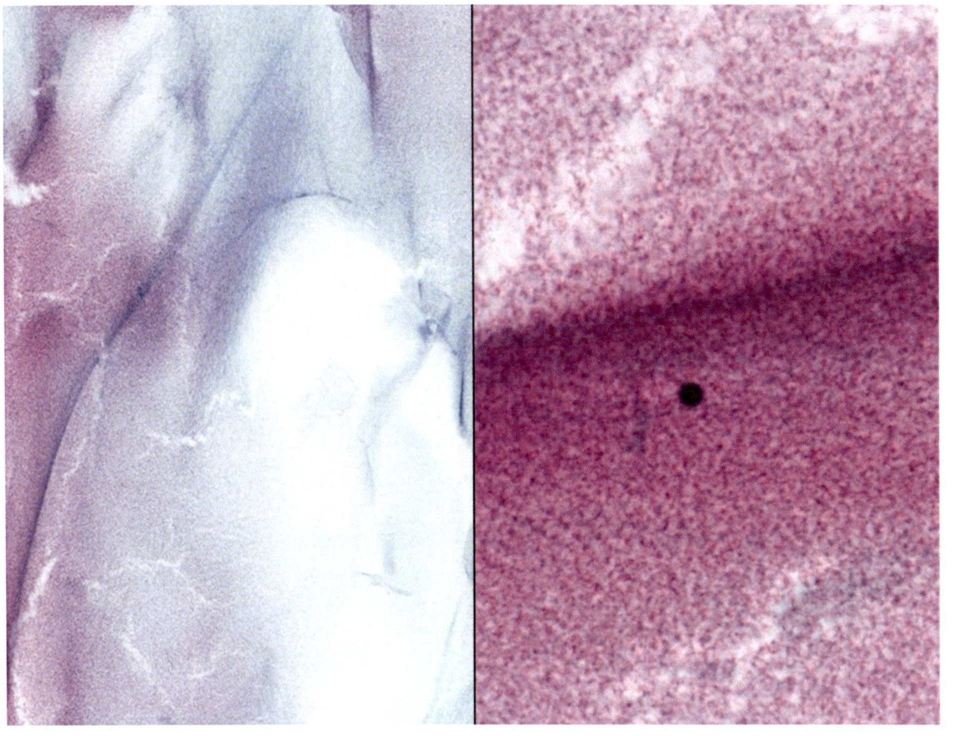

Q-6. A 55-year-old Caucasian man with right groin hernia underwent inguinal hernioplasty. Three days later, the patient presented with a right groin fluctuating mass beneath the surgical wound. No fever or redness seen. FNA of the mass revealed clear yellow fluid that is paucicellular, containing only few degenerated histiocytes and occasional lymphocytes. What is the most likely diagnosis?

(a) Ganglion cyst
(b) Hematoma
(c) Seroma
(d) Myxoma
(e) Abscess

Figs. 12.7 and 12.8

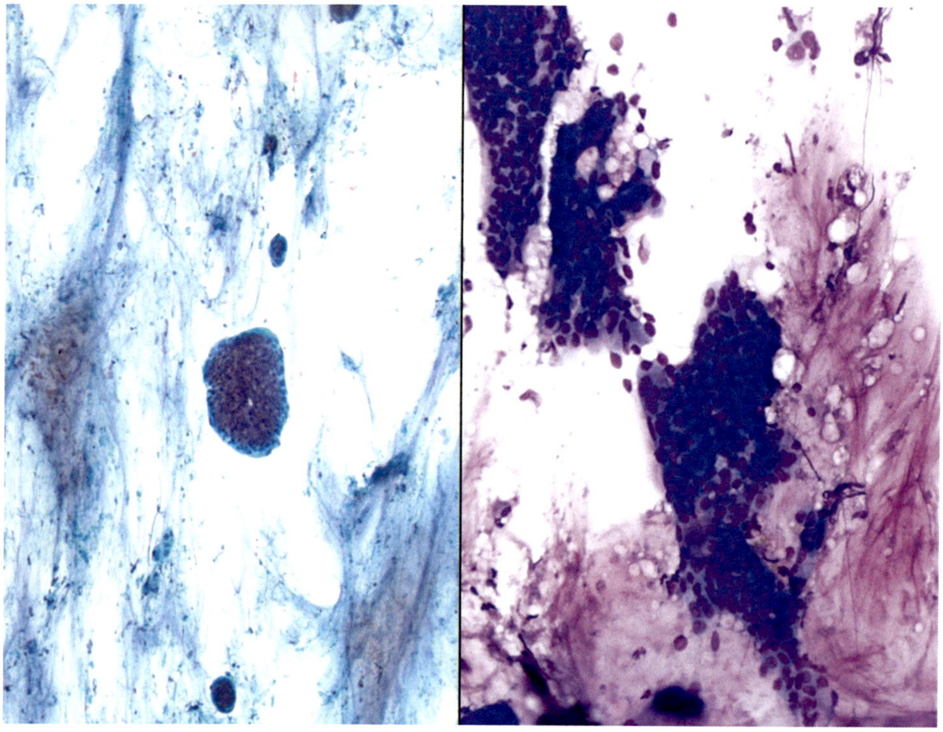

Q-7. A 73-year-old smoker women presents with a neck soft tissue mass. The patient has a past medical history of colonic carcinoma. Fine-needle aspiration of the mass is demonstrated in the provided images. What is the most likely diagnosis?
(a) Lymphoma
(b) Myxoma
(c) Cellular myxoma
(d) Metastatic mucinous carcinoma
(e) Chordoma

Q-8. Immunostains were done, and the immune profile of the lesion is CK20+, CK7−, CEA+, and CDx2+. Based on the immune profile, what is the most likely diagnosis?
(a) Breast
(b) Colon
(c) Lung
(d) Pancreas
(e) Kidney

Figs. 12.9 and 12.10

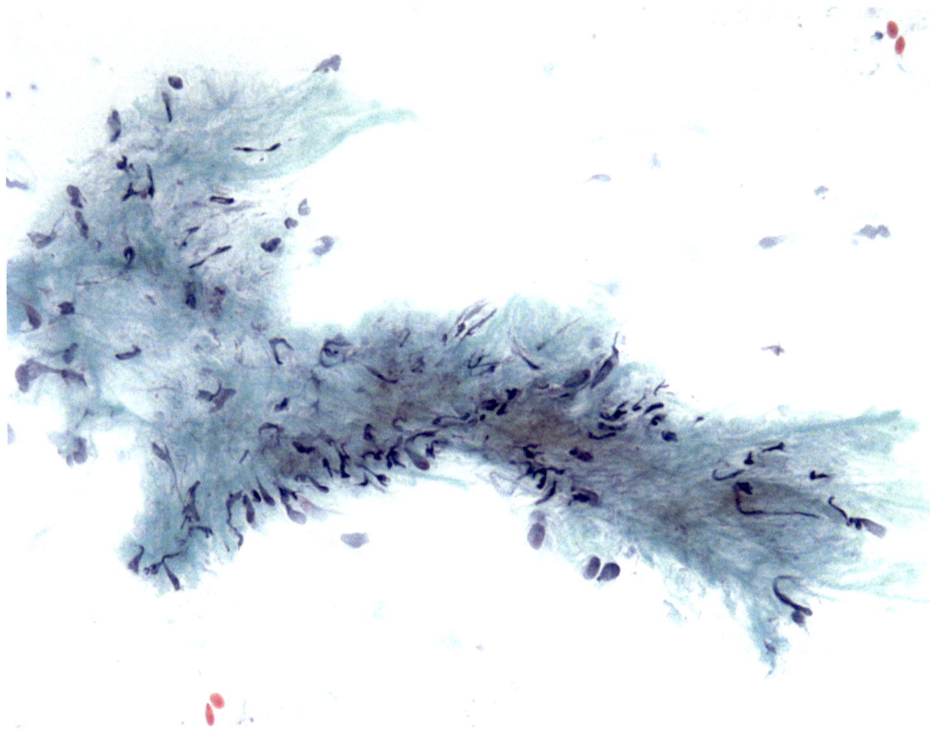

Q-9. 40-year-old man presented with a rapidly growing 4 cm lesion on his forearm. FNA of the mass revealed zonation effect with hypocellular and hypercellular areas and spindle cell predominance with some chronic inflammatory cells. Histologic sections displayed storiform pattern with numerous mitoses. What is the most likely diagnosis?
(a) Schwannoma
(b) Fibromatosis
(c) Nodular fasciitis
(d) Neurofibroma
(e) Leiomyoma

Q-10. Which of the following statements is false regarding this lesion?
(a) *It is a slowly growing mass.*
(b) It is a rapidly growing mass.
(c) Most frequently affect the forearm.
(d) Spontaneous regression may happen.
(e) Peak incidence in the fourth decade of life.

Figs. 12.11, 12.12, and 12.13

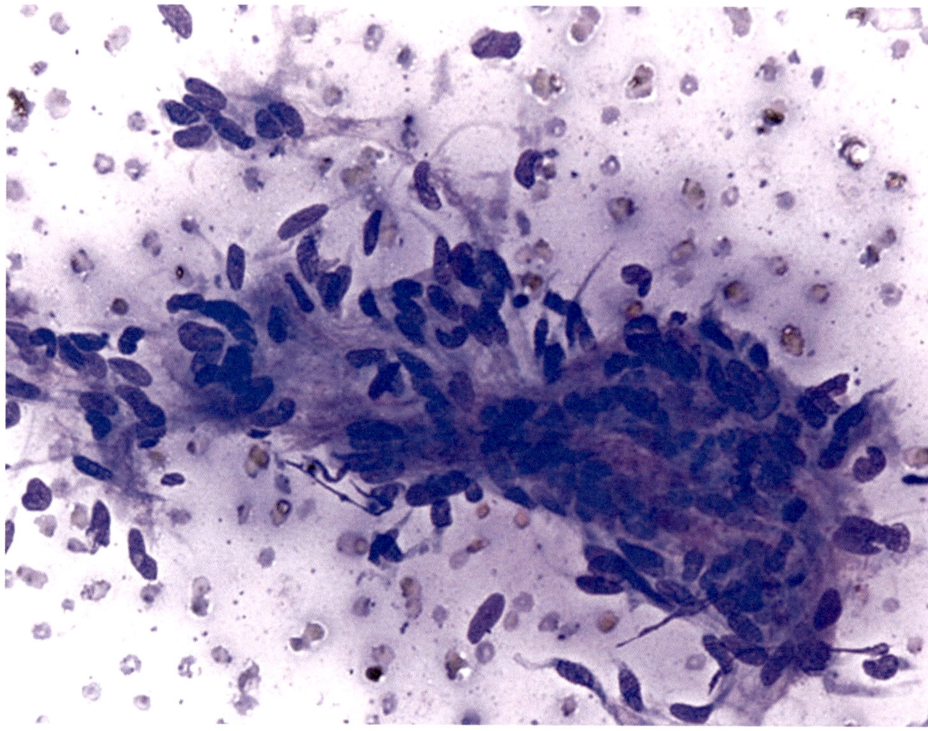

Q-11. A 24-year-old HIV-positive male who has not been compliant with his highly active antiretroviral therapy has reported a new onset of purple lesions on both legs. FNA aspirates of the lesions were done, and the smears are shown in the provided images. What is the most likely diagnosis?
(a) Granuloma
(b) Spindle cell melanoma
(c) Nodular fasciitis
(d) Angiosarcoma
(e) Kaposi sarcoma

Q-12. Which of the following descriptions is not consistent with cytologic smears of Kaposi sarcoma?
(a) Loosely cohesive clusters of bland spindle cells with large oval nuclei.
(b) May resemble granulomas.
(c) Numerous plasmacytoid lymphocytes are frequently seen.
(d) Romanowsky stain may show metachromatic stroma.
(e) Neoplastic cells may show nuclear streak artifacts.

Q-13. Which of the following immunostaining profiles would be most consistent with the diagnosis?
(a) CD31+
(b) CD34+
(c) HHV8+
(d) All of the above
(e) A and C only

Figs. 12.14 and 12.15

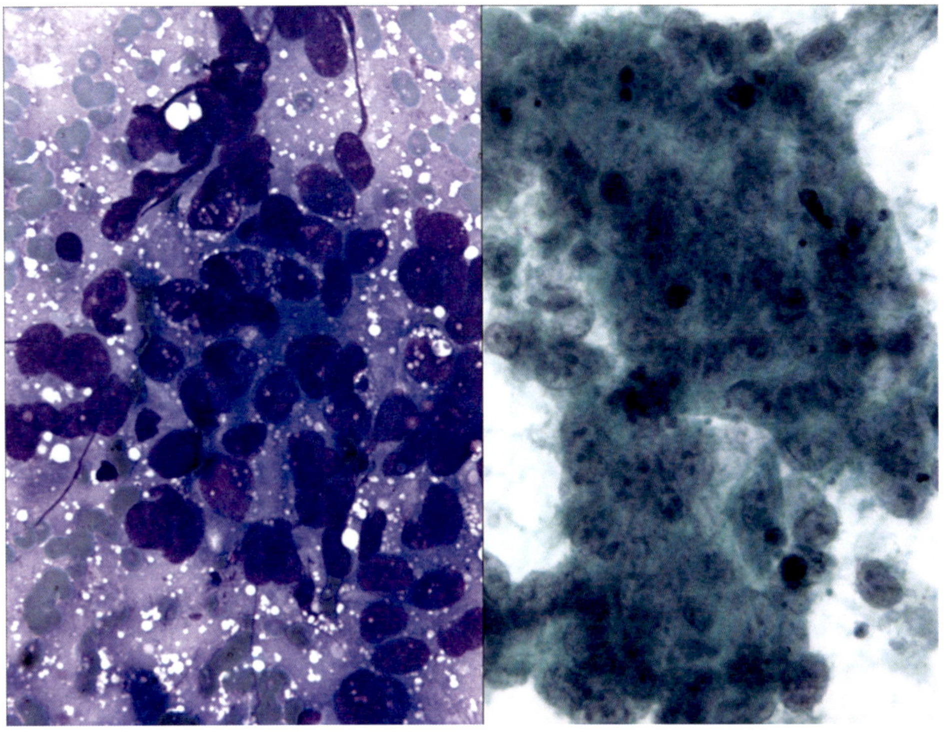

Q-14. A 24-year-old man presents with a painful, tender, popliteal mass measuring 2×2 cm. FNA of the mass is done and shown in the provided images. What is the most likely diagnosis?

(a) Synovial sarcoma
(b) Bursitis
(c) Synovitis
(d) Spindle cell carcinoma
(e) Hematoma

Q-15. Ancillary testing (immunostains and FISH) of this lesion may show:

(a) CD99 positive
(b) The presence of the t(x;18)(p11;q11) translocation by FISH
(c) Positive immunostaining for cytokeratin and EMA
(d) Positive immunostaining for Bcl2
(e) All of the above

Fig. 12.16

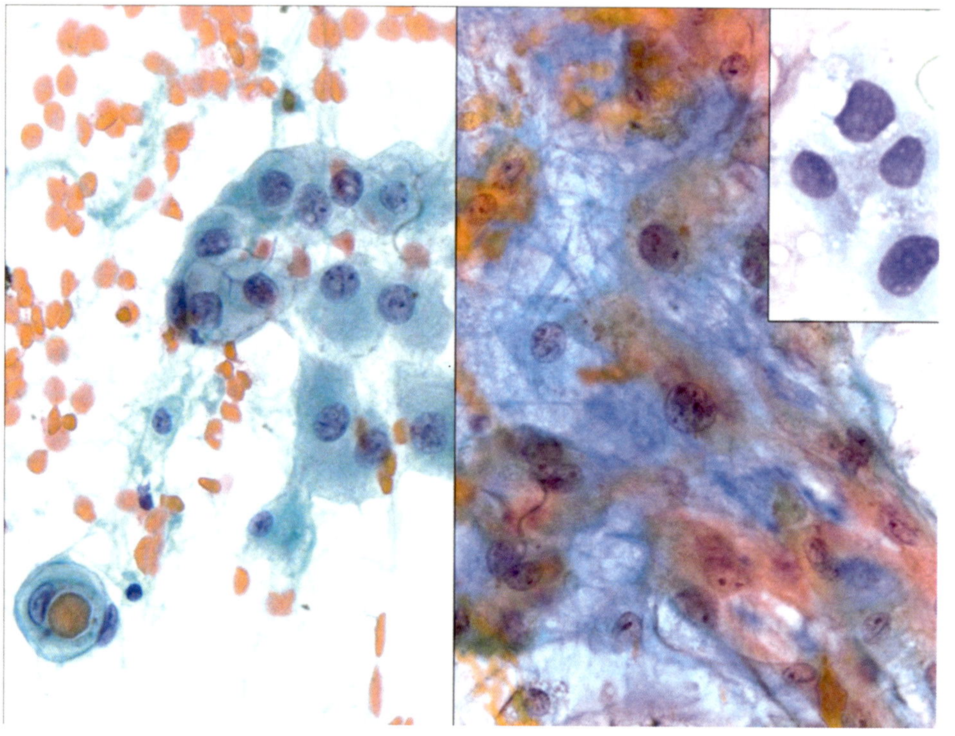

Q-16. A 75-year-old man who presented with progressive lower back pain for 9 months was found to have a sacrococcygeal mass on physical exam. FNA of the mass revealed large cells with multivacuolated cytoplasm in an abundant myxoid matrix. Using immunostains of the lesion showed: S100 +, EMA +, cytokeratin +, and CEA −. The most likely diagnosis is:
(a) Myxoma
(b) Myxofibrosarcoma
(c) Parachordoma
(a) Chordoma
(b) Metastatic mucinous adenocarcinoma

Fig. 12.17

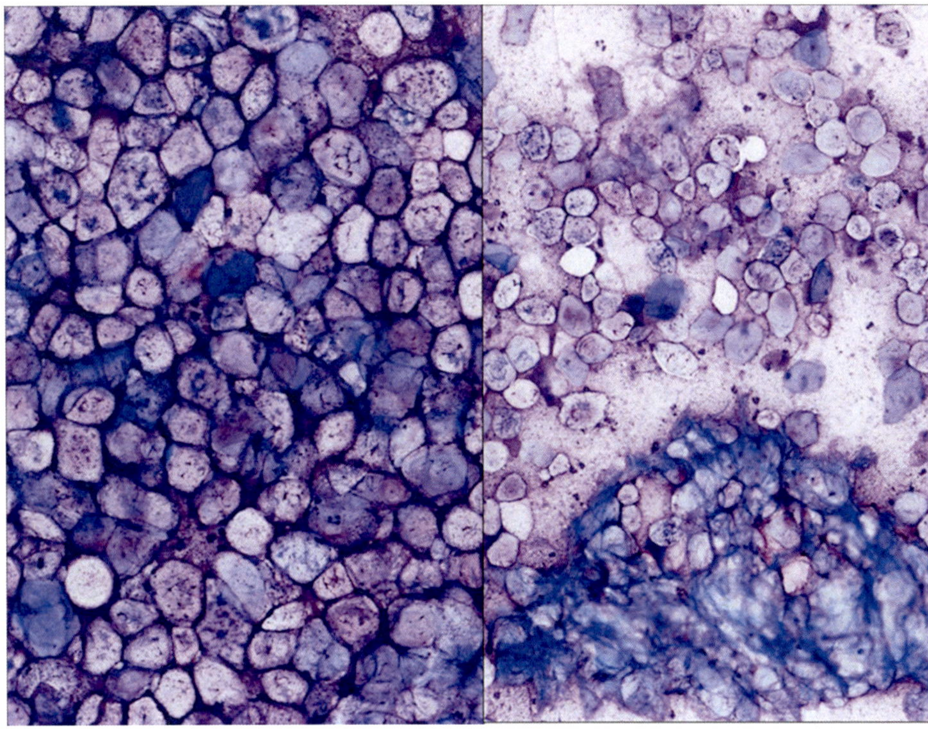

Q-17. A 25-year-old man had a painless 1 cm bump on his face. FNA aspirate of the mass is shown in the following images. What is your diagnosis?

(a) Epidermal inclusion cyst
(b) Fat necrosis
(c) Herpes simplex infection
(d) Human papilloma virus

Fig. 12.18

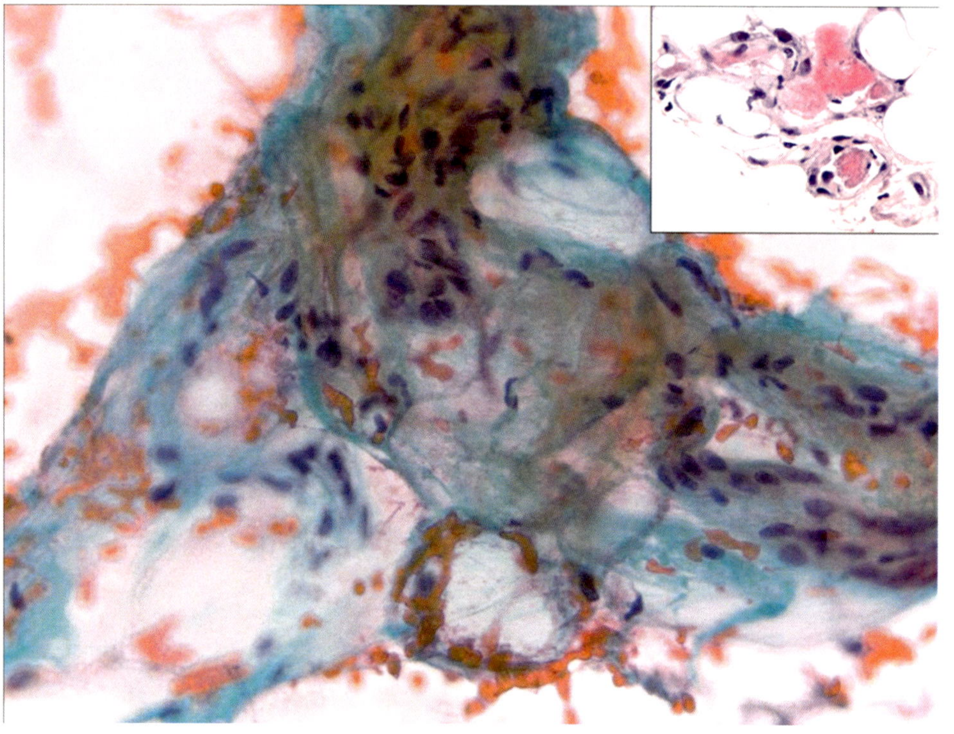

Q-18. A 14-year-old female developed 2 cm painful subcutaneous nodules on the forearm. FNA of the nodule is shown in these images. What is your diagnosis?

(a) Liposarcoma
(b) Lipoma
(c) Hibernoma
(d) Hemangioma
(e) Angiolipoma

Fig. 12.19

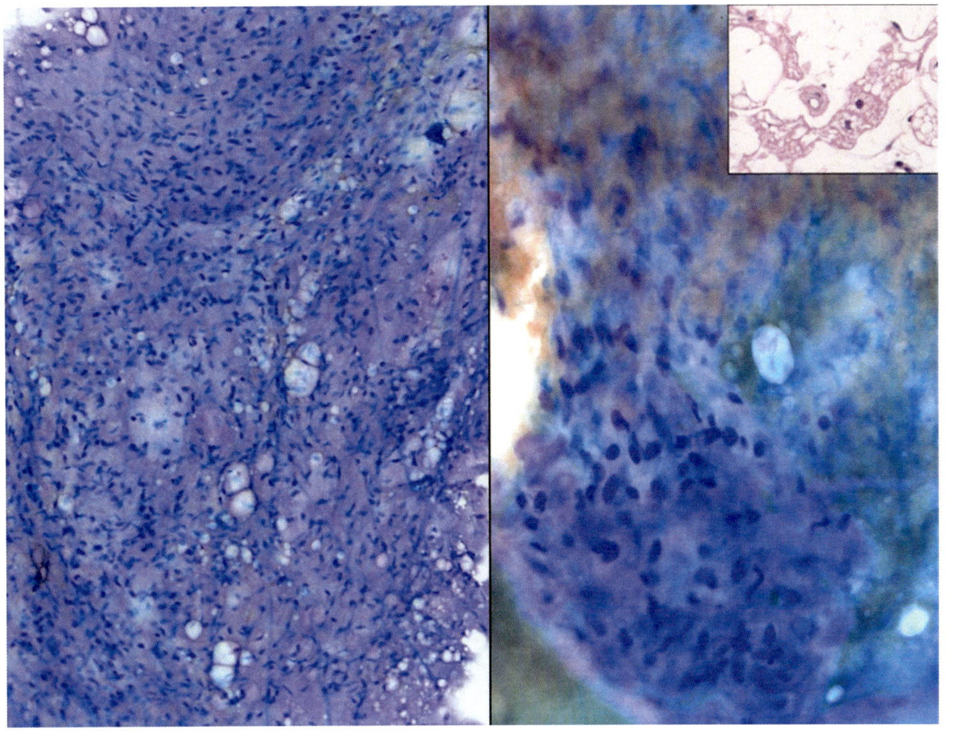

Q-19. A 26-year-old man developed a 2.7 cm soft mobile mass in the left shoulder area. FNA aspirate of the mass is displayed. What is your diagnosis?
(a) Liposarcoma
(b) Lipoma
(c) Hibernoma
(d) Hemangioma
(e) Angiolipoma

Figs. 12.20 and 12.21

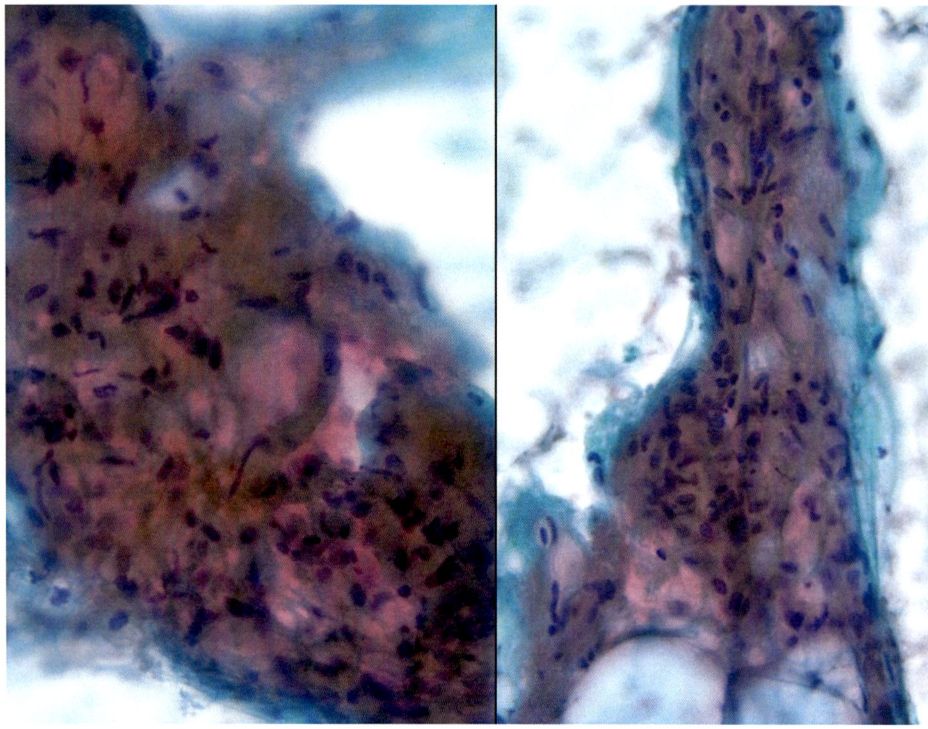

Q-20. A 50-year-old male developed a radiological abnormal mass in the gluteal area. The cellular features of the FNA aspirate of the mass is shown in these images. The most likely diagnosis is:
(a) Atypical lipomatous tumor
(b) Lipoma
(c) Pleomorphic liposarcoma
(d) Myxoid liposarcoma
(e) Angiosarcoma

Q-21. FISH studies for the mass will most likely show:
(a) Amplification of the murine double minute 2 (MDM2) oncogene
(b) t(2;13)(q35;q14)
(c) No amplification of the murine double minute 2 (MDM2) oncogene
(d) A and B only
(e) None of the above

Fig. 12.22

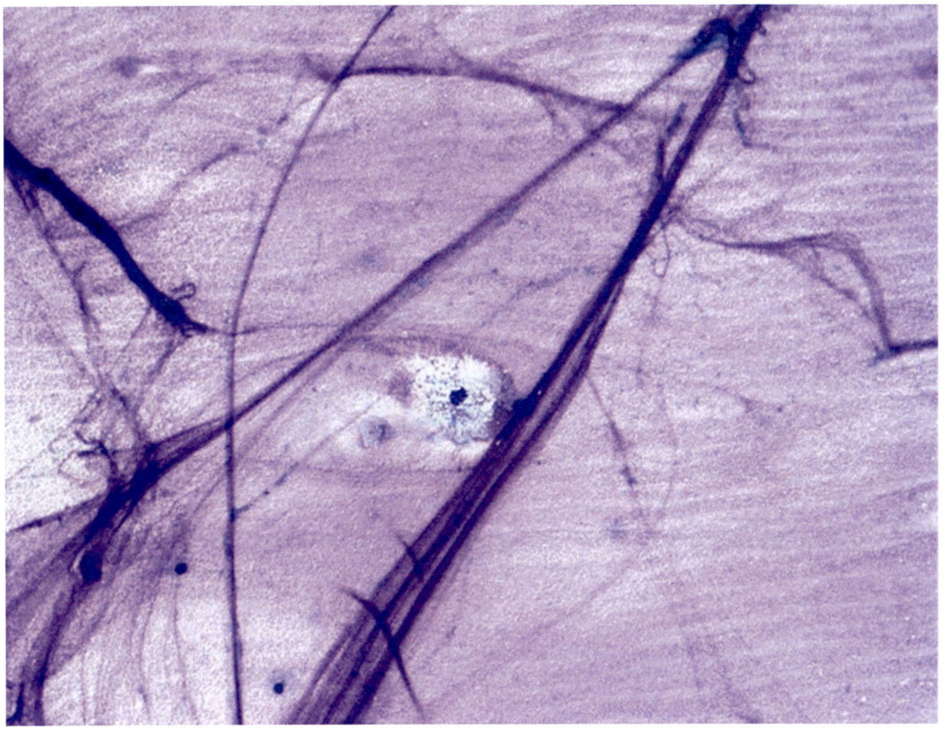

Q-22. The FNA aspirate shown is from a painless, slowly growing, and well-circumscribed tumor in the thigh of a 45-year-old man. The aspirate showed a clear gel-like material. What is your diagnosis?

(a) Ganglion cyst
(b) Seroma
(c) *Myxoma*
(d) Myxoid liposarcoma
(e) Chordoma

Fig. 12.23

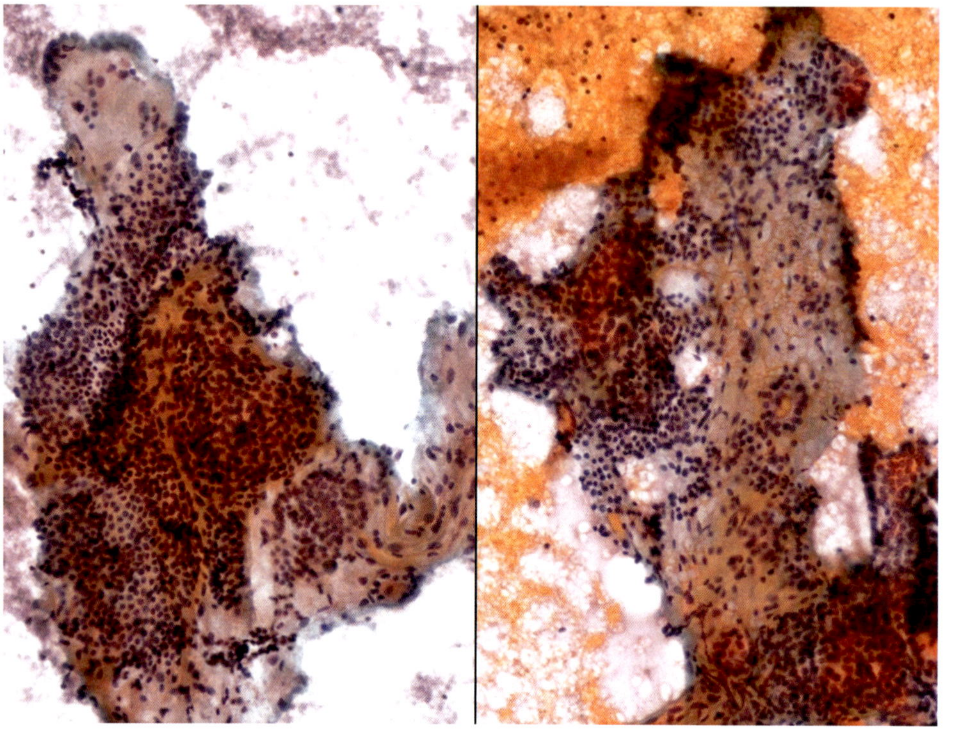

Q-23. The FNA aspirate displayed is from a deep-seated soft tissue thigh mass. The patient has a history of Gardner's syndrome. What is your diagnosis?
(a) Gastrointestinal stromal tumor (GIST)
(b) Nodular fasciitis
(c) Cellular myxoma
(d) Fibromatosis
(e) Schwannoma

Figs. 12.24 and 12.25

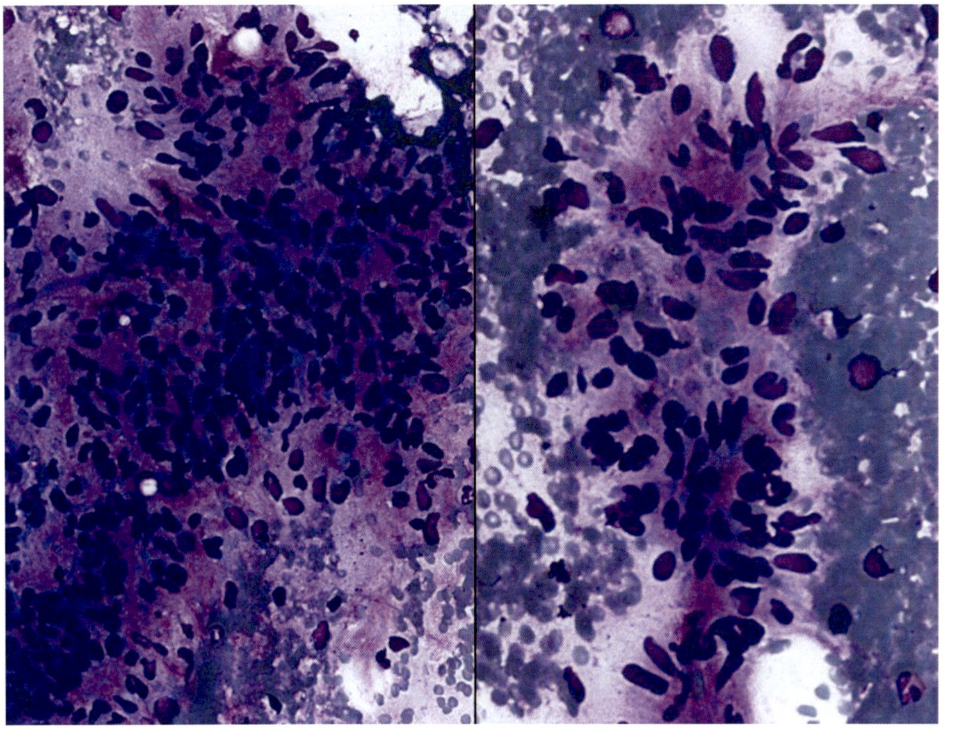

Q-24. A 45-year-old man with history of neurofibromatosis presented with a deep mass of the neck. FNA aspirate of the mass is highly cellular (see images). What is the most likely diagnosis?
(a) *Malignant peripheral nerve sheath tumor (MPNST)*
(b) Schwannoma
(c) Neurofibroma
(d) Nodular fasciitis
(e) Fibromatosis

Q-25. The tumor would most likely stain positive for:
(a) EMA
(b) Solitary fibrous tumor
(c) *S100*
(d) CD45
(e) Desmin

Fig. 12.26

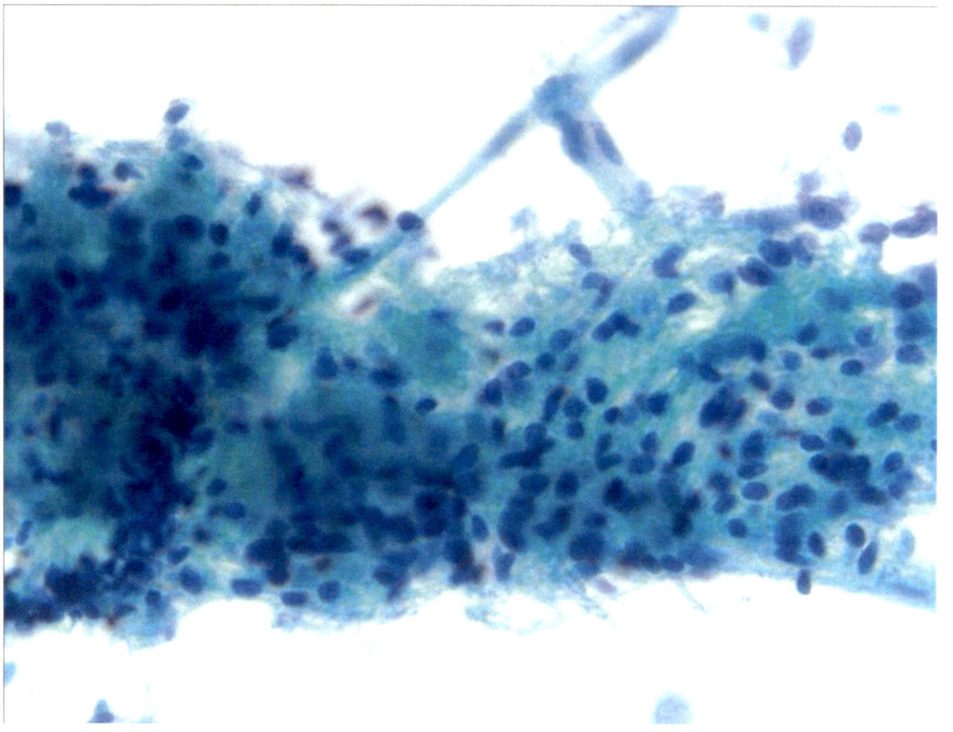

Q-26. The following image is from a FNA of a mass of the arm of a 35-year-old man. The cellular features are most consistent with the diagnosis of:

(a) Atypical lipomatous tumor
(b) Solitary fibrous tumor
(c) Rhabdomyoma
(d) Lymphoma
(e) Metastatic carcinoma of unknown origin

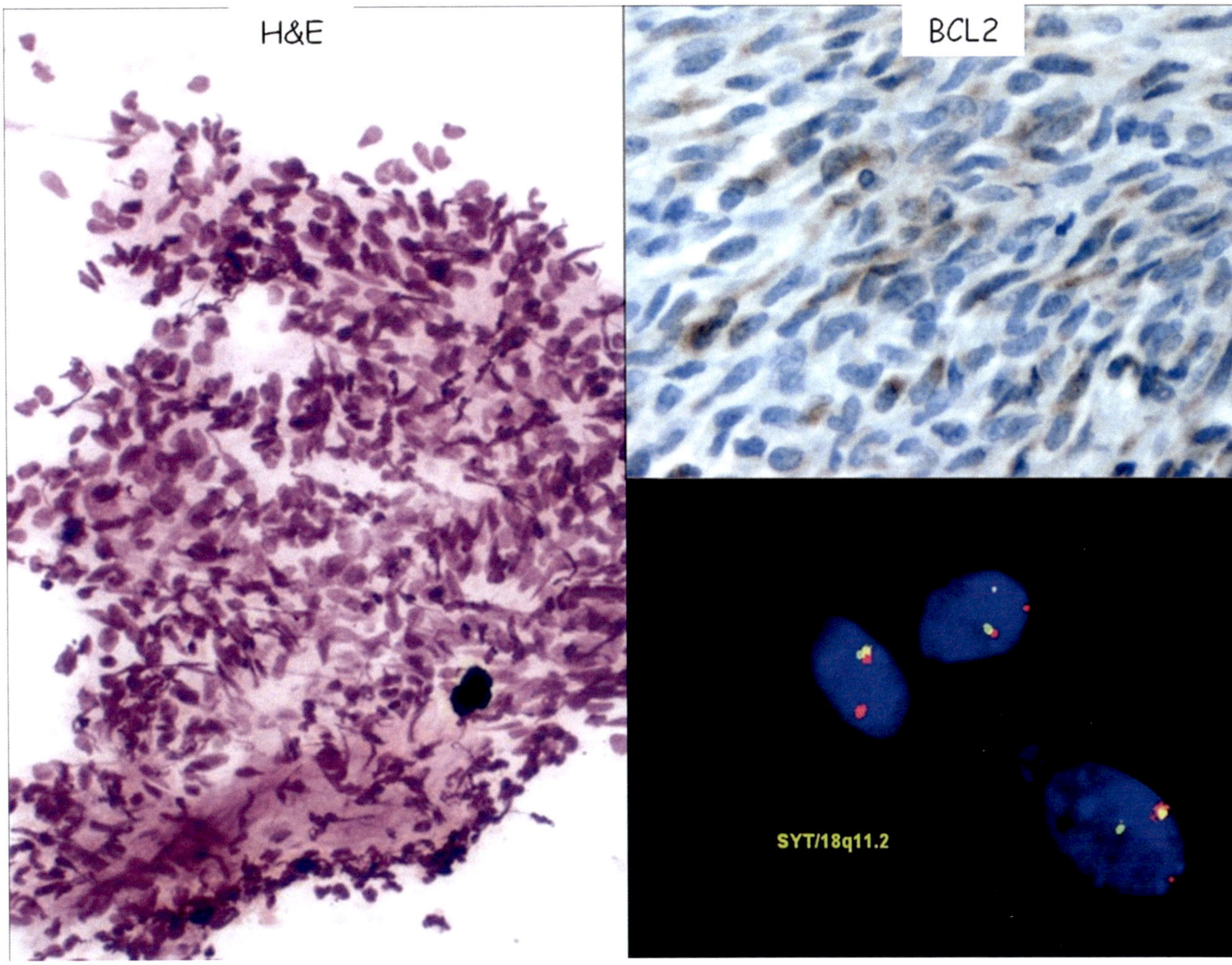

Fig. 12.27

Q-27. The tumor may stain positive for:

(a) CD34
(b) CD99
(c) S100
(d) *All of the above*
(e) A and C only

Figs. 12.28 and 12.29

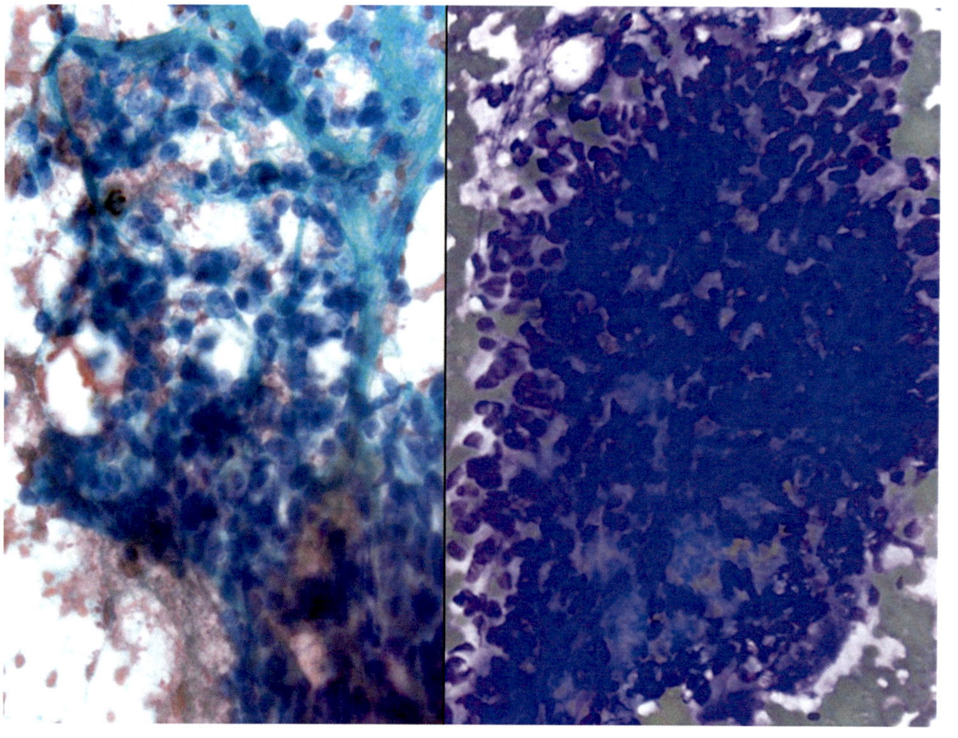

Q-28. The following two figures represent FNA aspirate and ancillary testing of a forearm mass from a 29-year-old male. What is the most likely diagnosis?
(a) Liposarcoma
(b) Synovial sarcoma
(c) Nodular fasciitis
(d) Rhabdomyosarcoma
(e) Rhabdomyoma

Q-29. The tumor may stain positive for:
(a) CK
(b) EMA
(c) BCL2
(d) None of the above
(e) All of the above

Fig. 12.30

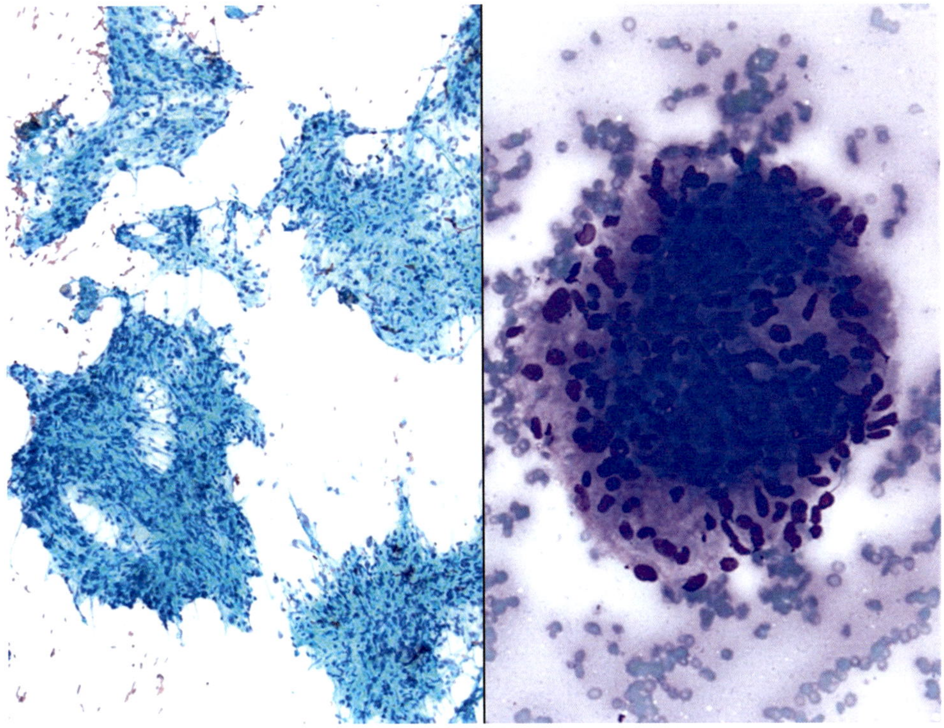

Q-30. The FNA aspirate of an ill-defined large thigh mass from a 33-year-old male is shown. What is the most likely diagnosis?
(a) Liposarcoma
(b) Ewing/PNET
(c) Leiomyosarcoma
(d) Rhabdomyosarcoma
(e) Leiomyoma

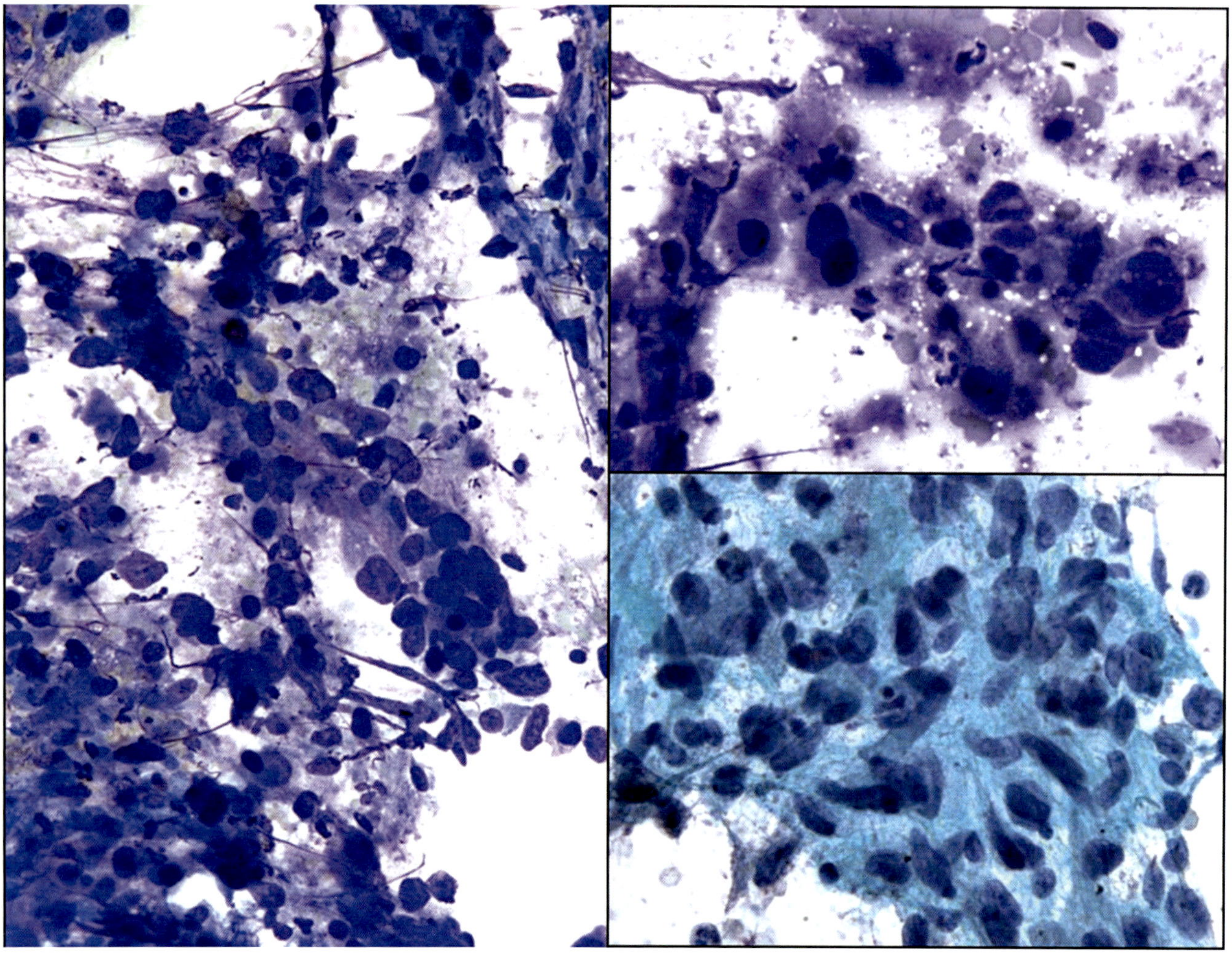

Fig. 12.31

Q-31. The FNA aspirate of a large femur mass from a 39-year-old male is displayed in these images. What is the most likely diagnosis?

(a) *Osteosarcoma*
(b) Ewing/PNET
(c) Metastatic adenocarcinoma
(d) Rhabdomyosarcoma
(e) Plasmacytoma

Fig. 12.32

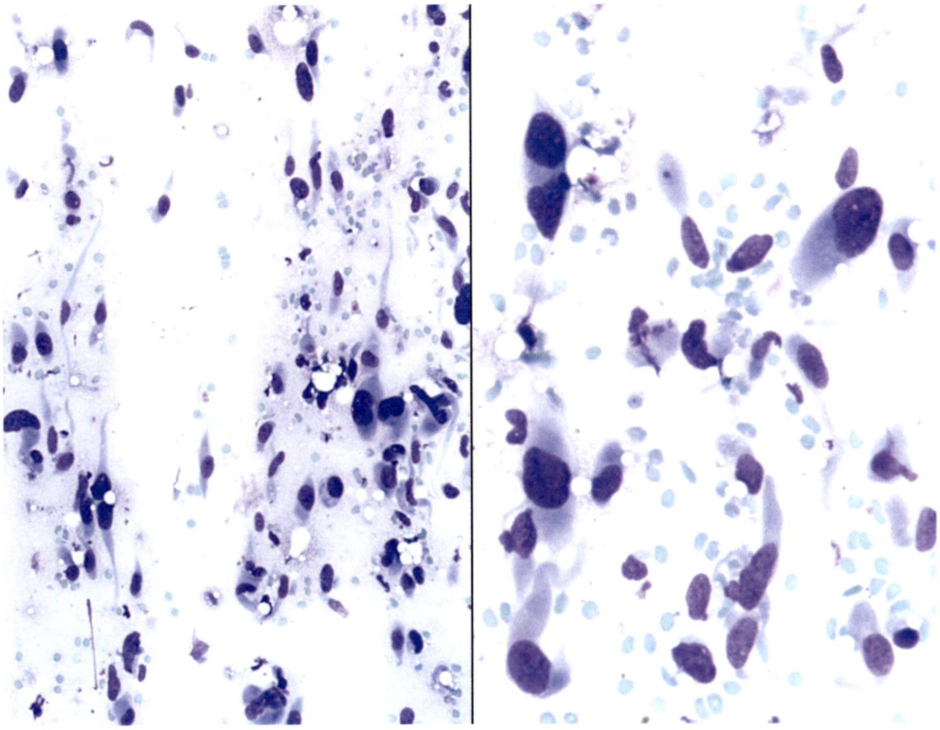

Q-32. All the following statements are true regarding the lesion shown in the image except:
(a) Retroperitoneal tumors in women may stain positive for estrogen.
(b) It is a malignant tumor of skeletal muscle origin.
(c) It may be associated with EBV infection in immunocompromised patients.
(d) It may stain positive for desmin.
(e) It may stain positive for caldesmon.

Fig. 12.33

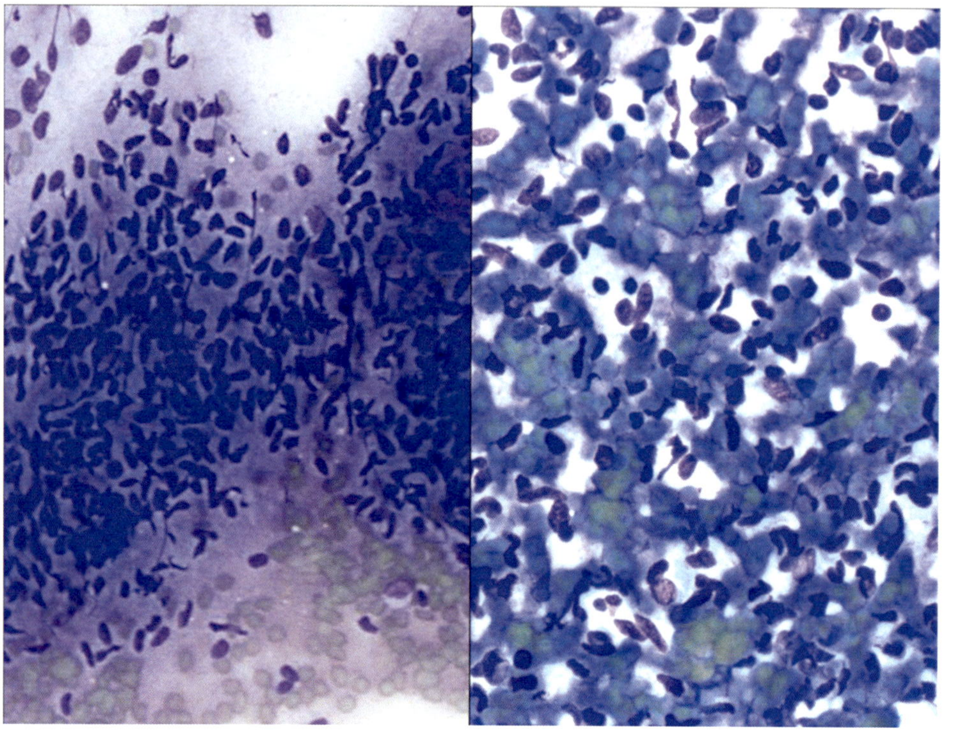

Q-33. Which of the following is a true statement about the lesion shown in the image?
(a) It comprises approximately 20 % of all soft tissue tumors:
(b) Have a very high tendency to affect children.
(c) Most frequently present as a deep-seated lesion.
(d) Most cases are malignant.
(e) Most cases show benign outcome.

Fig. 12.34

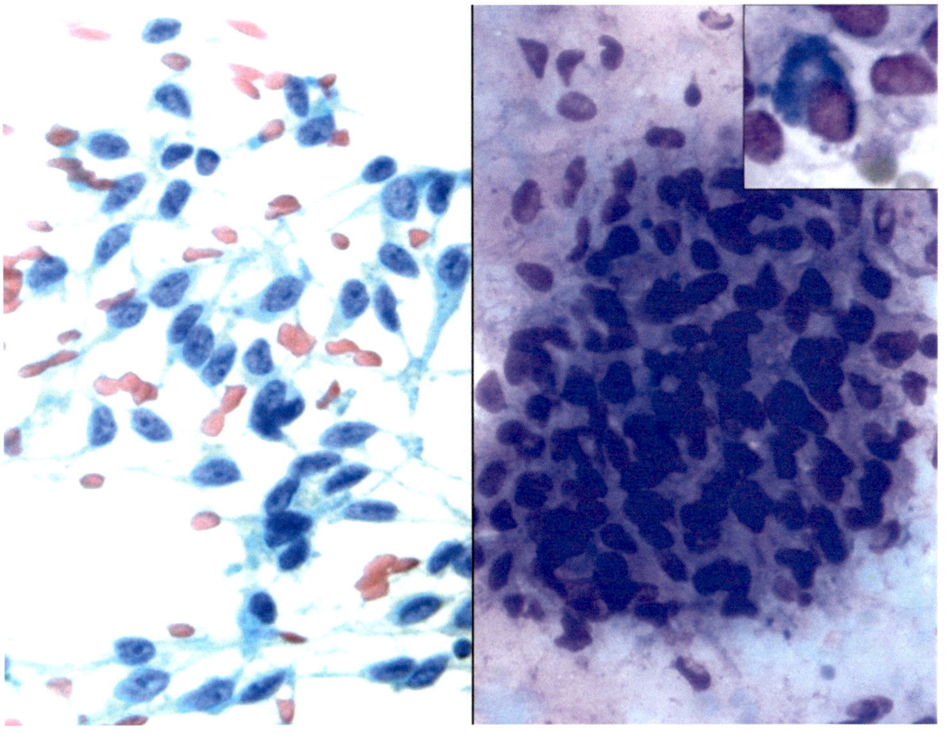

Q-34. The image provided shows a FNA of a face lesion. The lesion is positive for HMB45. What is the most likely diagnosis?
(a) Spindle cell melanoma
(b) MPNST
(c) Synovial sarcoma
(d) Malignant fibrohistiocytoma
(e) Fibrosarcoma

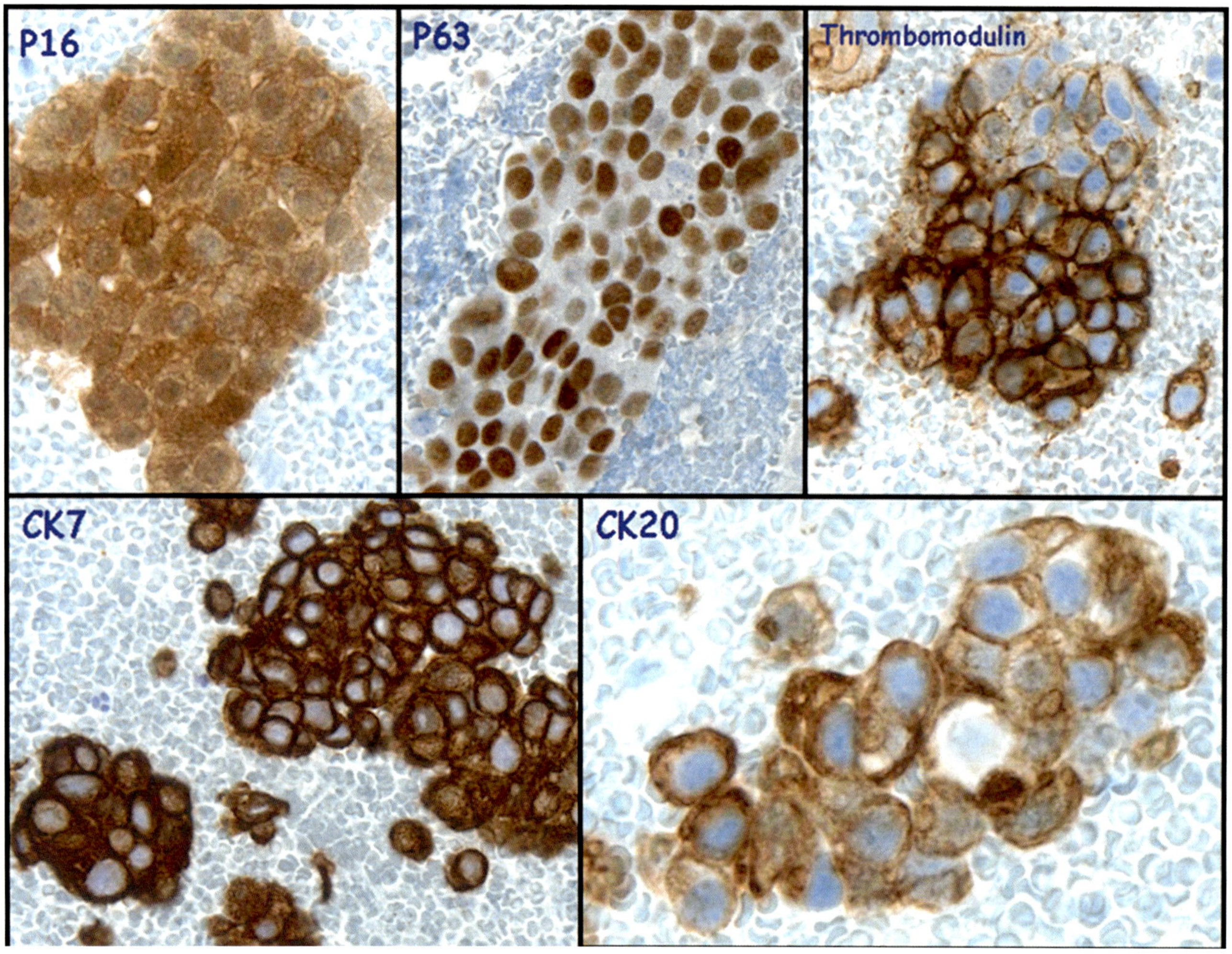

Fig. 12.35

Q-35. A 68-year-old man with no history of malignancy presented with a sacral lytic lesion. Immunostains were done and are shown in the image provided. Based on the immunohistochemistry profile, what is the most likely diagnosis?
(a) Metastatic breast carcinoma
(b) Metastatic colon carcinoma
(c) Metastatic urothelial carcinoma
(d) Synovial sarcoma
(e) Epithelioid variant of angiosarcoma

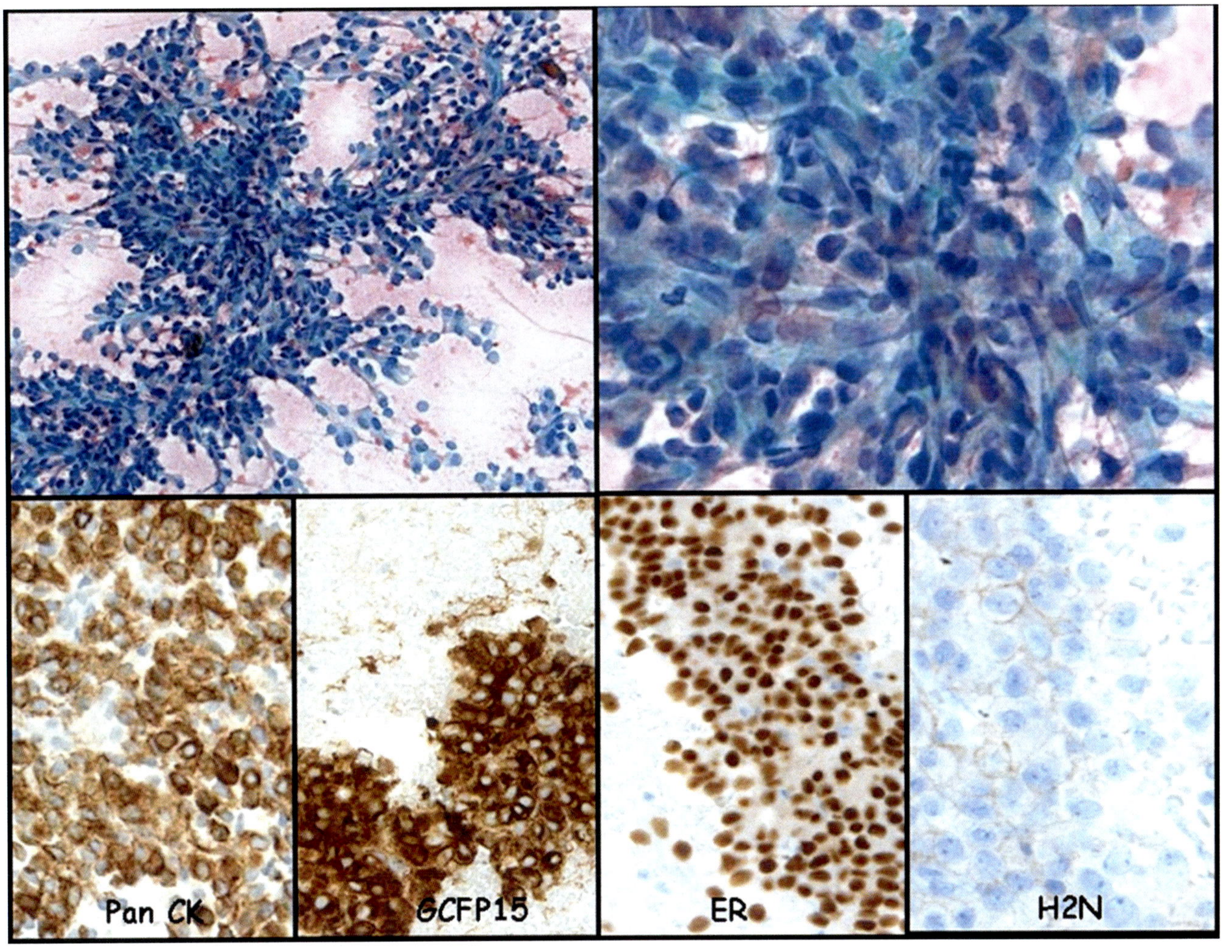

Fig. 12.36

Q-36. A 65-year-old woman had an arm lesion. FNA was done and is shown with immunohistochemistry staining. Based on the images provided, what is the most likely diagnosis?

(a) Metastatic breast ductal carcinoma
(b) Metastatic colon carcinoma
(c) Metastatic lung carcinoma
(d) Metastatic renal cell carcinoma
(e) Epithelioid variant of angiosarcoma

Fig. 12.37

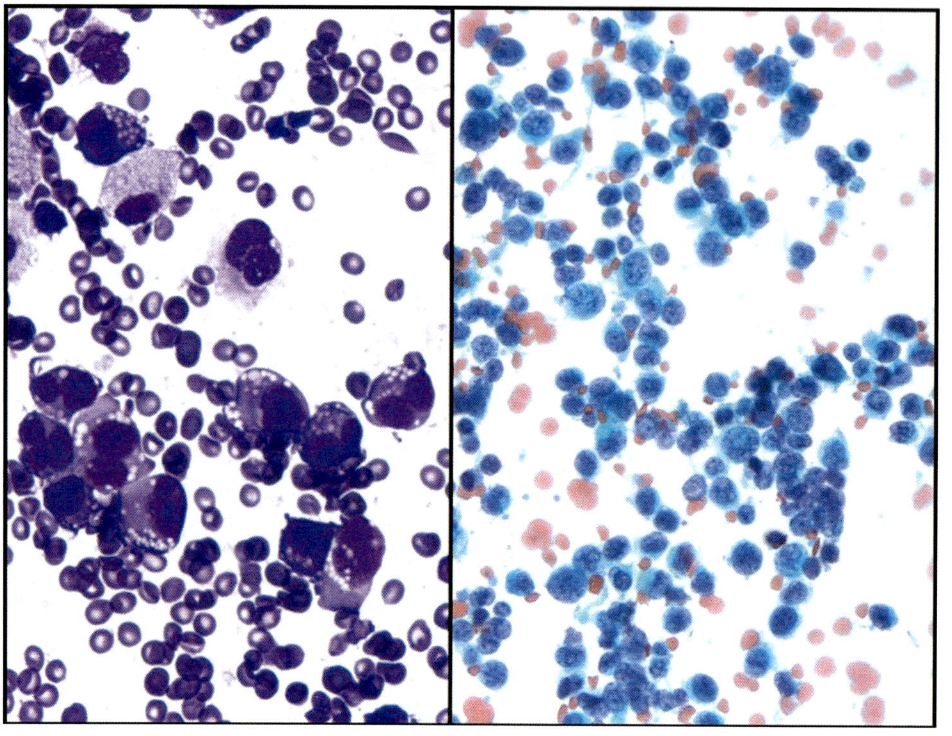

Q-37. A 12-year-old boy presented with a forearm lesion. FNA was done and is shown. FISH studies of the lesion showed t(2;13)(q35;q14). What is the diagnosis based on the images provided and the FISH result?

(a) Chordoma
(b) Alveolar rhabdomyosarcoma
(c) Leiomyosarcoma
(d) Pleomorphic rhabdomyosarcoma
(e) None of the above

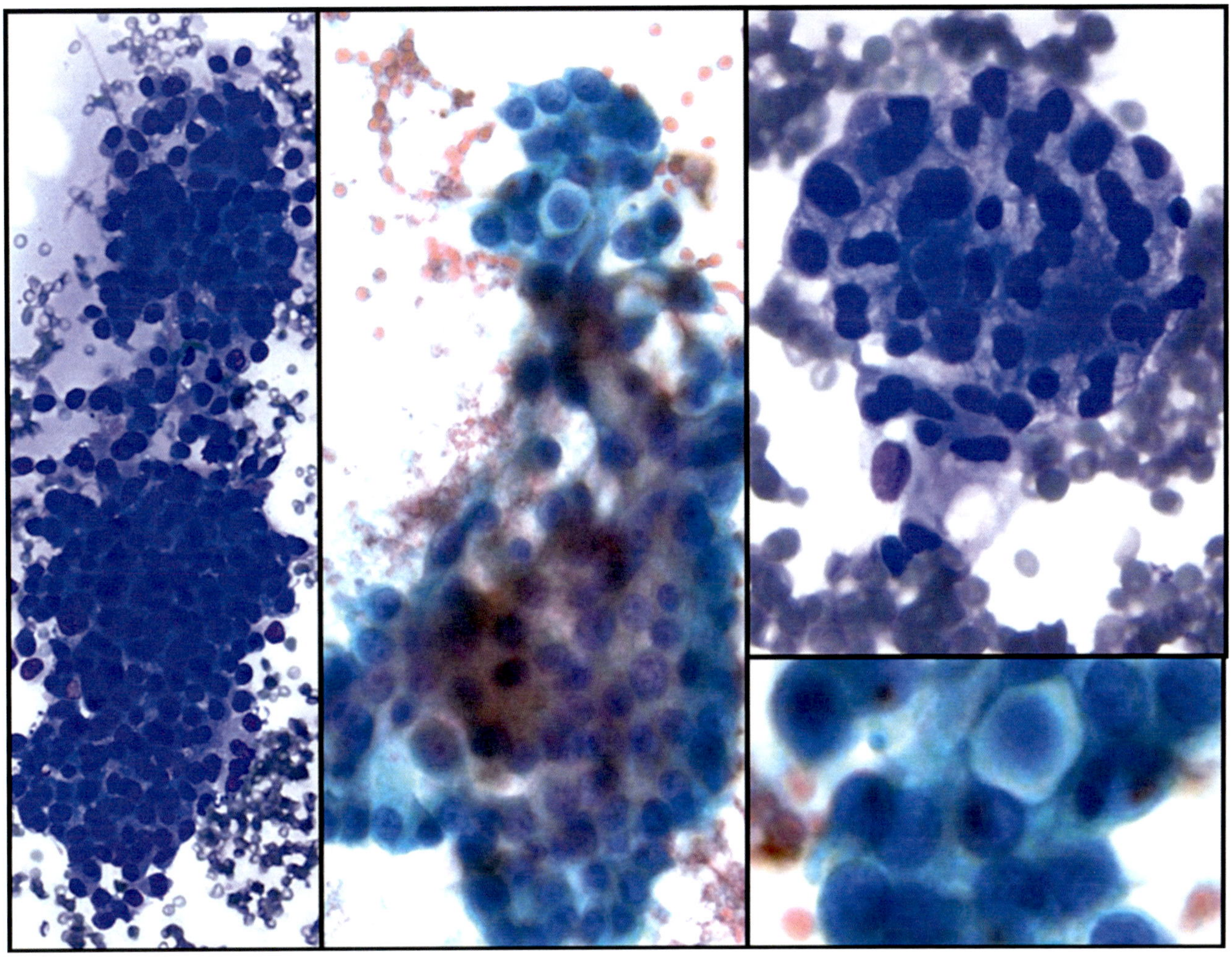

Fig. 12.38

Q-38. A 75-year-old male with no history of malignancy presented with a lytic lesion in the spine. FNA was done and is shown. What is the most likely diagnosis?

(a) Metastatic prostate adenocarcinoma
(b) Metastatic colon carcinoma
(c) Metastatic lung carcinoma
(d) Metastatic urothelial carcinoma
(e) None of the above

Figs. 12.39 and 12.40

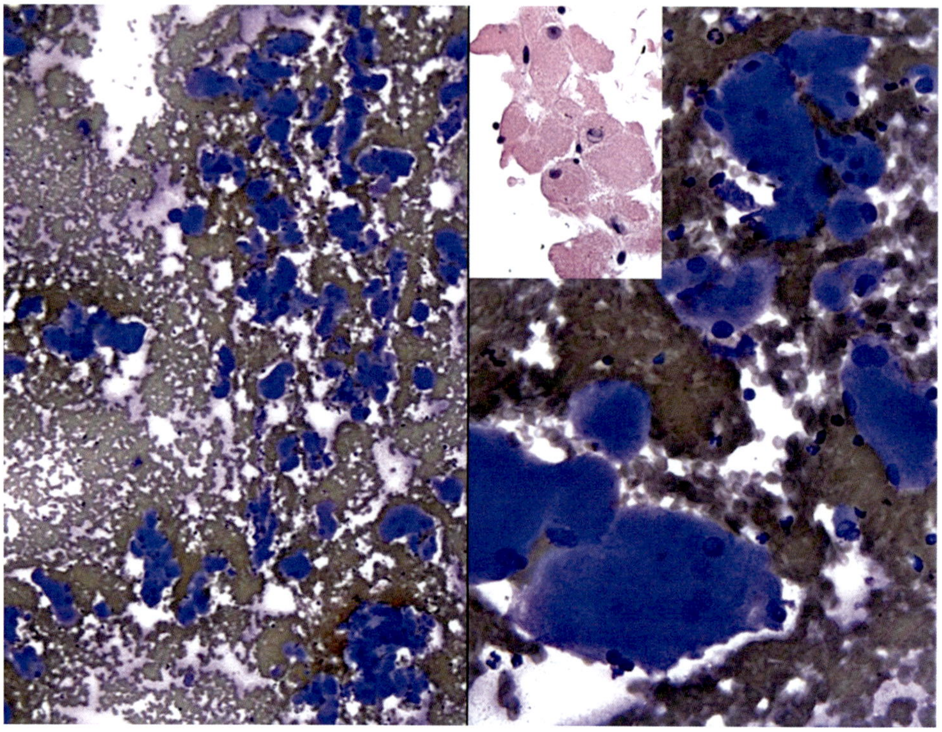

Q-39. A 65-year-old woman presented with a mass in the oral cavity. FNA was done and is shown. What is the most likely diagnosis?
(a) Rhabdomyoma
(b) Chordoma
(c) Granuloma
(d) Granular cell tumor
(e) None of the above

Q-40. The lesion shown in the image would most likely stain positive for:
(a) Desmin
(b) Myogenin
(c) EMA
(d) A and B
(e) None of the above

Fig. 12.41

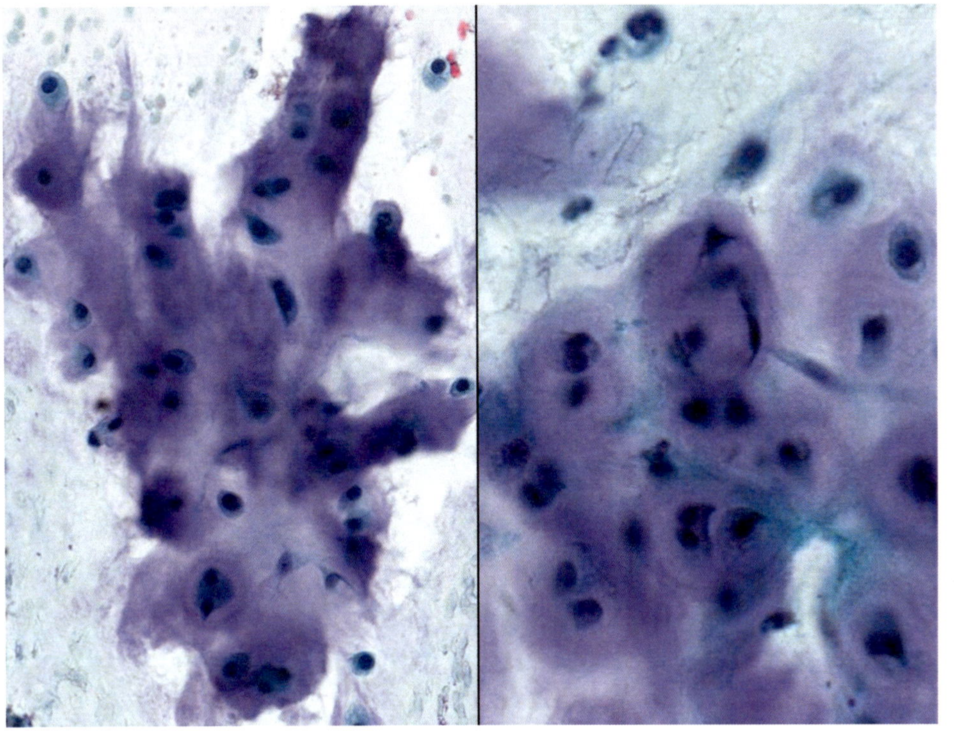

Q-41. A 48-year-old man presents with a lytic bone lesion in the pelvis. FNA specimen of the lesion is shown in these images. What is the most likely diagnosis?
(a) Osteosarcoma
(b) Low-grade chondrosarcoma
(c) Dedifferentiated chondrosarcoma
(d) High-grade chondrosarcoma
(e) None of the above

Fig. 12.42

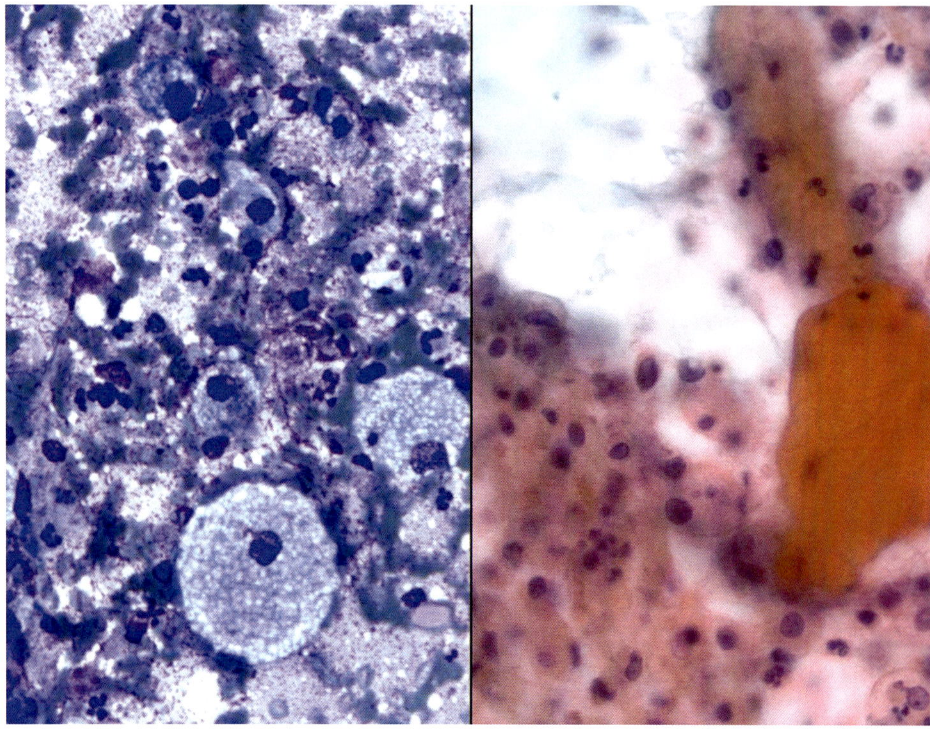

Q-42. A **7**-year-old girl presented to the emergency department with a palpable lump in the left leg. The patient has a recent history of a blunt trauma to the leg. What is the most likely diagnosis?

(a) Osteosarcoma
(b) Liposarcoma
(c) Lipoma
(d) Fat necrosis
(e) None of the above

12.2 Text-Based Questions 43–90

Q-43. Advantages of FNA of soft tissue and bone lesions include all of the following except:
(a) Simple and inexpensive procedure.
(b) On-site evaluation of sample adequacy.
(c) Limited experience needed to aspirate and interpret samples.
(d) Minimal morbidity.
(e) Ancillary studies may be done on cell blocks.

Q-44. The most useful role of FNA in the initial diagnosis of bone and soft tissue lesions is to:
(a) Render definitive diagnosis of the lesions
(b) Provide additional tissue for immunohistochemistry studies
(c) Provide additional tissue for molecular studies
(d) Render preliminary diagnosis and triage lesions according to tissue origin (sarcoma vs. lymphoma vs. carcinoma)
(e) Sample fibrous lesions

Q-45. Fine-needle aspiration of fibrotic or necrotic lesions may most likely cause:
(a) False-negative diagnoses
(b) False-positive diagnoses
(c) Accurate diagnoses
(d) Adequate sample
(e) Contamination of tissue planes

Q-46. Following a systemic pattern recognition diagnostic approach to soft tissue lesions can:
(a) Enhance the diagnostic yield of the less experienced cytopathologist
(b) Confuse the less experienced cytopathologist
(c) Increase the cost of the procedure
(d) Obviate the need for immunohistochemistry
(e) Obviate the need for cytogenetic studies

Q-47. The most common soft tissue neoplasm that occurs in adults is:
(a) Liposarcoma
(b) Lipoma
(c) Adult rhabdomyoma
(d) Schwannoma
(e) Solitary fibrous tumor

Q-48. Which of the following is NOT true regarding lipoma?
(a) Adipocytes have bland nuclei without atypia.
(b) Adipocytes are frequently destructed during specimen processing.
(c) Smears rarely show single adipocytes.
(d) Adipocytes are generally large, univacuolated, and uniform in size and shape.
(e) Lipoma has distinctive histological features different from subcutaneous adipose tissue.

Q-49. Which of the following is true regarding hibernoma?
(a) It is a malignant lipomatous tumor.
(b) It rarely contains capillaries.
(c) Myxoid stroma is usually a very prominent feature.
(d) Characteristic hibernoma cells are multivacuolated with granular cytoplasm.
(e) Characteristic hibernoma cells are univacuolated with clear cytoplasm.

Q-50. The most common soft tissue sarcoma of adults is:
(a) Liposarcoma
(b) Chondrosarcoma
(c) Osteosarcoma
(d) Ewing sarcoma
(e) Angiosarcoma

Q-51. Which is of the following is a false statement regarding liposarcoma?
(a) Well-differentiated liposarcoma frequently presents as a deep-seated retroperitoneal tumor.
(b) The identification of lipoblasts is very specific for the diagnosis of liposarcoma.
(c) FNA specimens of liposarcoma usually contain large tissue fragments.
(d) Lipoblasts are multivacuolated cells with atypical scalloped nuclei.
(e) Pleomorphic liposarcoma is a rare variant of liposarcoma.

Q-52. Branching blood vessels with "chicken wire" appearance is characteristic of:
(a) Well-differentiated liposarcoma
(b) Atypical lipomatous tumor
(c) Pleomorphic liposarcoma
(d) Dedifferentiated liposarcoma
(e) Myxoid liposarcoma

Q-53. The detection of t(12;16)(q13;p11) reciprocal translocation indicates:
(a) Myxoid liposarcoma
(b) Pleomorphic liposarcoma
(c) Round cell liposarcoma
(d) A and C
(e) None of the above

Q-54. Which is true about ganglion cyst?
(a) Frequently occurs on the planter surface of the foot.
(b) Show abundant granular myxoid material and histiocytes.
(c) Mostly affects older patients above 70 years old.
(d) Unlike synovial cysts, they communicate with joint spaces.
(e) Usually are of large sizes (>5 cm).

Q-55. Which is true regarding intramuscular myxoma?
(a) It frequently presents with mitosis and necrosis.
(b) Microscopic examination shows abundant myxoid background with plenty of atypical cells and lymphocytes.
(c) Radiation therapy is the treatment of choice.
(d) It is a benign lesion.
(e) Surgery is rarely effective.

Q-56. Tumors with positive EWSR1 gene rearrangements include?
(a) Ewing sarcoma/PNET
(b) Clear cell sarcoma
(c) Angiomatoid fibrous histiocytoma
(d) All of the above
(e) A and B only

Q-57. Which is of the following statements is false regarding lipoblasts?
(a) They have scalloped nuclei.
(b) They have spindle-shaped nuclei.
(c) May be confused with multivacuolated macrophages.
(d) Cytoplasmic lipid droplets compress the nuclei.
(e) They may aid in the diagnosis of liposarcoma.

Q-58. Carney's complex may include all of the following except:
(a) Cushing syndrome
(b) Lentiginosis
(c) Gastrointestinal stromal tumor
(d) Heart myxoma
(e) Cutaneous myxoma

Q-59. Regarding dedifferentiated liposarcomas, which of the following is false?
(a) Dedifferentiated liposarcomas have worse prognosis than other types of pleomorphic sarcomas.
(b) Dedifferentiated liposarcomas have better prognosis than other types of pleomorphic sarcomas.
(c) They can demonstrate an abrupt transition from well-differentiated liposarcoma to a non-lipogenic sarcoma.
(d) Clinically they usually present as a large painless mass.

Q-60. Which of the following is NOT true about myxofibrosarcoma?
(a) Most frequently presents in superficial location.
(b) Most frequently presents in a deep-seated location.
(c) It was previously called "malignant fibrous histiocytoma (MFH)."
(d) More common in the elderly group.
(e) It can arise in the retroperitoneum.

Q-61. Which of the following sarcomas have a relatively higher potential for lymph node metastasis?
(a) Myxofibrosarcoma
(d) Clear cell sarcoma
(c) Rhabdomyosarcoma
(d) Synovial sarcoma
(e) All of the above

Q-62. Which of the following statements is false regarding myxofibrosarcoma?
(a) FNA may show pseudolipoblasts.
(b) Its subtypes include: myxoid, pleomorphic, giant cell, and inflammatory type.
(c) Myxoid subtype has worse prognosis than pleomorphic subtype.
(d) Histological sections may show the classic herring bone growth pattern.
(e) Cytologically, it has a wide range of atypia.

Q-63. Which of the following is true about chordoma?
(a) It is a benign mesenchymal neoplasm.
(b) Physaliphorous cells are key diagnostic feature.
(c) Females are affected twice as often as males.
(d) Most frequently present in the lower extremity.
(e) Peak incidence in the second decade of life.

Q-64. Which of the following statements best describes physaliphorous cells?
(a) Bland spindle-shaped cells
(b) Large cells with bubbly cytoplasm
(c) Small cells with finely granular cytoplasm
(d) Large cells with scalloped nuclei
(e) Spindle with cigar-shaped nuclei

Q-65. Which of the following is false regarding myxoid chondrosarcoma?
(a) They may occur in bone.
(b) They may occur in soft tissue.
(c) They often stain positive for cytokeratin.
(d) They share some chordoma features.
(e) Extraskeletal myxoid chondrosarcoma affect more men than women.

Q-66. Benign soft tissue lesions with spindle cell morphology include all of the following except?
(a) Nodular fasciitis
(b) Schwannoma
(c) Granulomatous inflammation
(d) Fibromatosis
(e) Gastrointestinal stromal tumors (GIST)

Q-67. Which is a false statement regarding desmoid tumors?
(a) May be associated with familial adenomatosis polyposis (FAP).
(b) Stain positively for beta-catenin.
(c) FNA displays low to moderate cellularity.
(d) Often display high mitotic activity and cellular atypia.
(e) Typically show uniform bland spindled cells with elongated nuclei.

Q-68. Which of the following statements correctly describes schwannoma features?
(a) Antoni A area is hypocellular with myxomatous changes.
(b) Antoni B area is hypercellular and demonstrates numerous Verocay bodies.
(c) Verocay bodies consist of a stacked arrangement of two palisading rows of nuclei separated by an acellular zone.
(d) Verocay bodies are spindle-shaped cells with intranuclear inclusions.
(e) Schwannoma cells have rounded nuclei with prominent nucleoli.

Q-69. Microscopic examination of neurofibroma lesions may reveal:
(a) Schwann cells
(b) Physaliphorous cells
(c) Fibroblasts
(d) All of the above
(e) A and C only

Q-70. All of the following statements about malignant peripheral nerve sheath tumor (MPNST) are correct except:
(a) Associated with neurofibromatosis (NF) in 90 % of cases.
(b) Associated with neurofibromatosis (NF) in 50 % of cases.
(c) It is a deeply seated tumor.
(d) It has the propensity to recur locally and frequently metastasize.
(e) In comparison to other neurogenic tumors, it displays higher degree of cytological atypia.

Q-71. Which of the following cytomorphological features are associated with malignant peripheral nerve sheath tumor (MPNST)?
(a) Spindle cells
(b) Palisading features
(c) Wavy nuclei with tapered ends
(d) All of the above
(e) A and C only

Q-72. Which of the following statements best describe FNA of hemangiomas?
(a) FNA may reveal vascular coils containing bland spindle cells.
(b) FNA is frequently nondiagnostic.
(c) FAN is frequently diagnostic.
(d) A and C.
(e) A and B.

Q-73. Etiological factors for angiosarcoma may include:
(a) History of previous radiation treatment
(b) Maffucci syndrome
(c) Coagulopathies
(d) All of the above
(e) A and C only

Q-74. Which of the following is false regarding synovial sarcoma?
(a) The monophasic variant shows predominantly round cell pattern.
(b) The biphasic variant display spindle and epithelial components.
(c) FISH testing may indicate the presence of the t(x;18)(p11;q11) translocation.
(d) It is generally more frequent in males haphazardly arranged in clusters of cells.
(e) It can stain positive for CD99.

Q-75. Which of the following descriptions is consistent with osteosarcoma?
(a) Mostly affects children under the age of 5
(b) Most frequently affects epiphysis of long bones
(c) Can be associated with Paget's disease

(d) Often stains positive for EMA
(e) No reported associations with previous radiation exposure

Q-76. Which is a false statement about fibrosarcoma?
(a) Five-year survival rate less than 50 %
(b) Five-year survival rate more than 90 %
(c) It is a rare tumor.
(d) Infantile type has a better prognosis.
(e) Most cases of infantile fibrosarcoma contain the chromosomal translocation t(12;15)(p13;q26) with NTRK3-ETV6 fusion.

Q-77. Which is a true statement/s regarding spindle cell melanoma?
(a) It usually stains positive for S100.
(b) It usually stains positive for HMB45.
(c) FNA is usually hypercellular with many dissociated cells and rare clustering.
(d) All of the above.
(e) A and C only.

Q-78. Which is a false statement regarding rhabdomyosarcoma?
(a) It is has an embryonal, alveolar, and pleomorphic subtypes.
(b) It always stains negative for synaptophysin and chromogranin.
(c) In alveolar rhabdomyosarcoma (RMS), FISH may detect the FKHR breakpoint.
(d) PCR can be used in alveolar RMS to identify FKHR-PAX3/PAX7 fusion transcripts.
(e) It can occasionally stain positive for CD99.

Q-79. All of the following statements regarding Ewing sarcoma are correct except:
(a) Ewing sarcoma is more common in bones than in soft tissues.
(b) It predominantly affect children and young adults.
(c) On rare occasions, it may stain positive for cytokeratins.
(d) Most commonly they have t(11;22) tanslocation with EWSR1-FLI1 fusion.
(e) It usually stains negative for glycogen.

Q-80. Which of the following statements correctly describe Homer Wright rosettes?
(a) In contrast to Flexner-Wintersteiner rosettes, they do not have empty lumens.
(b) The fibrillary lumen material may stain positive for S100.
(c) They are associated with neuroblastoma, medulloblastoma, and primitive neuroectodermal tumors (PNETs).
(d) All of the above.
(e) B and C only.

Q-81. Which of the following statement/s are true regarding neuroblastoma?
(a) Most frequently occur before the age of 5 years.
(b) Metastasis may be the first presentation of the disease.
(c) N-myc amplification denotes better prognosis.
(d) All of the above.
(e) A and B only.

Q-82. Which of the following immunohistochemistry profiles support the diagnosis of desmoplastic small round cell tumor (DSRCT)?
(a) EMA positive
(b) Dot-like and paranuclear positivity for desmin
(c) CD56 positive
(d) S100, synaptophysin, and chromogranin positive
(e) All of the above

Q-83. Which of the following does not correctly describe paraganglioma?
(a) It is synonymous with chemodectoma.
(b) It can be benign or malignant.
(c) They are hypovascular tumors.
(d) The tumor cells tumor are positive for NSE, chromogranin, and synaptophysin.
(e) The cytoplasm of the tumor cells is moderately abundant and may contain eosinophilic granules.

Q-84. All of the following statements are correct regarding clear cell sarcoma except:
(a) It is also called malignant melanoma of the soft parts.
(b) It is usually negative for S100, HMB45, MITF, and melan A.
(c) FISH can demonstrate their characteristic t(12;22)(q13;q12) translocation.
(d) Tumor cells may show multinucleation.
(e) They can be confused for metastatic melanoma.

Q-85. Which immunohistochemistry profile would support the diagnosis of synovial sarcoma when differentiating it from other spindle cell malignancies?
(a) CK +, EMA +, S100 +, HMB-45 –, desmin –, CD99 +, CD117 –, H-caldesmon –
(b) CK –, EMA –, S100 –, HMB-45+, desmin –, CD99 –, CD117 –, H-caldesmon –
(c) CK +, EMA +, S100 +, HMB-45 +, desmin +, CD99 –, CD117 –, H-caldesmon –
(d) CK–, EMA –, S100 +, HMB-45 –, desmin +, CD99 +, CD117 +, H-caldesmon +
(e) None of the above

Q-86. All the following statements regarding alveolar soft part sarcoma are correct except:
(a) It is a rare tumor affecting mainly children and young adults.
(b) The characteristic rod-shaped or rhomboid crystals seen in histology are frequently seen in cytology specimens.
(c) FNA aspirate frequently display hemorrhagic or granular backgrounds and naked nuclei.
(d) It may stain positive for PAS (diastase resistant).
(e) None of the above.

Q-87. When differentiating round cell malignancy, which of the following is correct?
(a) Small cell carcinoma: CK+, synaptophysin+, CD56 +, CD45 –, PLAP –, CD99–, desmin –
(b) Lymphoma: CK–, CD56 –, CD45+, PLAP –, CD99–, CD117–, desmin –
(c) Rhabdomyosarcoma: CK +, CD56 +, CD45 –, CD99 +, CD117–, desmin +, myogenin –
(d) All of the above
(e) A and B only

Q-88. Which is false regarding giant cell of the bone?
(a) It is a high-grade malignancy that accounts for 12 % of all bone tumors.
(b) Although locally aggressive with very rare metastases.
(c) Diagnosis require the presence of both ovoid mononuclear and osteoclast-like giant cells with similar nuclear features.
(d) The knee is a common site.
(e) It usually affects young adults (20–40 years).

Q-89. Bacillary angiomatosis is usually associated with:
(a) Herpes simplex
(b) *Mycobacteria*
(c) *Cryptococcus neoformans*
(d) *Bartonella henselae*
(e) *Histoplasma capsulatum*

Q-90. All the following statements regarding pigmented villonodular synovitis of the tendon sheath are correct except:
(a) Intranuclear inclusions can be seen.
(b) It is synonymous with diffuse-type giant cell tumor of the tendon sheath.
(c) FNA aspirates reveal mononuclear histiocytes admixed with multinucleate osteoclast-like giant cells.
(d) Tumor cells may contain hemosiderin crystals.
(e) FNA aspirates show clusters of epithelioid spindle cells in a hemorrhagic background.

12.3 Answers and Discussion of Image-Based Questions 1–42

A-1. **(d) Ewing Sarcoma**
Ewing sarcoma (ES) mainly affects children and young adults. It rarely occurs after the age of 30. It is one of the "small round blue cell" tumor families. For practical purposes, ES and PNET can be considered as one entity where ES is more undifferentiated while PNET displays some neural differentiation. The figure provided shows a hypercellular FNA aspirate (DQ stain) with single and clusters of small blue round cells depicting two populations larger, paler cells and smaller, darker, lymphocyte-like cells. In general, the cells show scant cytoplasm, hyperchromatic nuclei with no noticeable nucleoli. Other features that may be seen in ES include: rosette formation and necrotic background. Clinical history, chromosomal studies, and immunohistochemistry play a critical role in the differential of blue cell tumors. Electron microscopy is rarely used now for these tumors. This case was negative for CD45, essentially ruling out lymphoma and negative muscle markers. In addition, it was positive for synaptophysin, CD99, and PAS-D thus supporting Ewing sarcoma diagnosis. However, CD99 can also be positive with other tumors, and hence it is not specific for the diagnosis. The best confirmatory testing for this entity is FISH testing.

A-2. **(b) t(11;22) with EWSR1-FL1 fusion**
Ewing sarcoma is associated with several translocations involving the EWSR1 and ETS family of genes; however, t(11;22) with EWSR1-FLI1 fusion is the most common translocation (90 % of cases). For the other choices provided, translocation t(12;22)(q13;q12) is seen in clear cell sarcoma, while t(12;16)(q13;p11) is seen in myxoid liposarcoma, and t(x;17)(p11.2;q25) denotes alveolar soft part sarcoma.

A-3. **(d) Response to preoperative chemotherapy is a major independent prognostic factor.**
The tumor stage at time of diagnosis is the main prognostic factor. In addition, response to preoperative chemotherapy is a major independent prognostic factor. Higher degree of histological tumor necrosis denotes better response. Grading tumor necrosis can be assessed as follows: grade I, tumor necrosis of less than 50 %; grade II, tumor necrosis of 51–90 %; grade III, 91–99 % tumor necrosis; and grade IV, absence of viable tumor cells.

A-4. **(b) Epithelioid variant of angiosarcoma**
Radiation-induced angiosarcomas are aggressive tumors that may develop after many years in women with history of radiation therapy of the breast. The two common variants include spindle and epithelioid cell angiosarcoma. On cytologic examination, the spindle cell variant would display an oval- or spindle-shaped hyperchromatic, pleomorphic nuclei with prominent nucleoli of variable sizes and fine-to-coarse chromatin. Multinucleation is rare. On the other hand, the epithelioid variant can present with numerous multinucleated cells with irregular pleomorphic nuclei showing coarse chromatin and large or multiple nucleoli. On DQ stain, cytoplasmic microvacuoles can be detected. The FNA aspirate morphology displayed is most consistent with the epithelioid variant of angiosarcoma. In practice, a panel of immunostains to further differentiate carcinoma vs. melanoma vs. sarcoma is needed.

A-5. **(b) This lesion is always negative for cytokeratin stains.**
In general, angiosarcomas express the various vascular antigens, including von Willebrand factor, CD31, CD34 (nonspecific, can be negative), VEGFR-3 (variable staining), and FLI-1 (nuclear staining). Since cytokeratin can be expressed in about one third of soft tissue angiosarcomas, particularly the epithelioid subtype, it has a minimal value in discriminating between angiosarcoma and carcinoma.

A-6. **(c) Seroma**
The main point of this question is to realize that clinical history and findings of physical exam can provide invaluable clues for diagnosis of hypocellular myxoid lesions as well as all other soft tissue lesions. Seroma is an accumulation of fluid in a tissue that usually occurs after any surgery and is a frequent complication after mastectomy. FNA aspirate should yield a clear yellow fluid. Cytologically, it presents with degenerated histiocytes and few lymphocytes in a hypocellular edematous background that should not be confused for a myxoma. Infected seromas will have clinical signs of infection (redness, hotness, and fever), and the aspirate will contain many polymorphonuclear leukocytes.

A-7. **(d) Metastatic mucinous carcinoma**
Metastatic mucinous carcinomas should always be ruled out in myxoid soft tissue lesions with epithelioid cell morphology. It is usually seen in older patients. FNA shows abundant mucinous material with floating epithelioid cells. The cells can be arranged singly or in small or large clusters. Signet ring cell morphology may be observed in some cells, and the tumor cells may show variable nuclear atypia.

A-8. (**b**) **Colon**
Clinical history of malignancy and immunohistochemistry panels can be very helpful in detecting primary sites of the cancer. For example, metastases of breast origin may be ER+, PR+, GCDFP +, and mammaglobin+, whereas adenocarcinomas from the lung will be CK7+, CK20+, TTF-1+, and surfactant protein A+. An example of immunostaining profile is CK20+, CK7-, CEA+, and CDx2+ is indicative of colon origin.

A-9. (**c**) **Nodular fasciitis**
The clinical presentation and the cytologic features description are most consistent of nodular fasciitis. The classic picture manifests as a rapidly enlarging mass in young adult that may regress spontaneously with the forearm being the most common location. FNA my show mixed cytomorphological patterns with zonation: hypocellular and hypercellular areas and mixed cellularity with spindle cells predominance. Such cells have a small amount of pale cytoplasm and relatively uniform oval-to-elongated nuclei with finely granular chromatin and usually inconspicuous nucleoli.

A-10. (**a**) **It is a slowly growing mass.**
Nodular fasciitis is a reactive appearing proliferation of fibroblasts and myofibroblasts in a myxoid background with culture-like appearance and vascular proliferation. Rapid growth is one of the key clinical clues to the diagnosis. It usually affects young adults with the flexor forearm, chest, and back being common sites. It generally arises from superficial fascia; however, it can occasionally be intramuscular or intravascular. In soft tissue lesions, correlation with the clinical presentation is essential for making the correct diagnosis.

A-11. (**e**) **Kaposi sarcoma**
KS presents mainly with mucocutaneous lesions that evolve from early patch to plaque lesions and may grow into larger tumor nodules. It is associated with human herpesvirus type 8 (KSHV/HHV8). Cytomorphology aspirates of KS shows single and scattered tissue fragments composed of loosely cohesive clusters of spindle cells. The spindle cells are bland with moderate cytoplasm forming tapering tails that blend with adjacent cells. The nuclei are large, oval with smooth contour, evenly dispersed chromatin, and inconspicuous nucleoli.

A-12. (**c**) **Numerous plasmacytoid lymphocytes are frequently seen.**
Cytomorphology aspirates of KS typically show loose cohesive clusters of bland spindle cells. They may resemble granulomas. Using Romanowsky stain, the background stroma may appear metachromatic. Neoplastic cells may show nuclear streak artifact. Plasmacytoid lymphocytes are not one of the typical features seen.

A-13. (**d**) **All of the above**
Kaposi sarcoma generally stains positive for CD31, CD34 (D2-40), and HHV8 (LNA-1).

A-14. (**a**) **Synovial sarcoma** mostly affects males (15 and 40 years). Because of its slowly growing nature, it is often misdiagnosed for benign lesions (bursitis or synovitis). The image shown displays feature consistent with monomorphic synovial sarcoma. It shows monotonous population of spindle cells arranged in sheets. The cells have scant granular cytoplasm, elongated hyperchromatic nuclei with irregular nuclear borders, multiple conspicuous nucleoli, and coarse chromatin. The clinical history and the cytology are most consistent with synovial sarcoma (monophasic variant).

A-15. (**e**) **All of the above**
In general, synovial sarcoma is positive for CD99, EMA, and CK (particularly the epithelioid component) and bcl2 (particularly spindle component). In addition, the presence of t(x;18)(p11;q11) translocation can be detected by FISH.

A-16. (**d**) **Chordoma**
Both the clinical presentation and the cytomorphological features support the diagnosis of chordoma. Chordoma is a slow-growing painful, low-grade malignant mesenchymal neoplasm that commonly arises in bone sites. The sacrum and coccyx are affected frequently. The classic FNA morphology of chordoma will show abundant myxoid matrix, the characteristic physaliphorous cells with their large bubbly cytoplasm, and small mononuclear cells with granular cytoplasm. Physaliphorous cells may sometimes mimic lipoblasts. Immunostains of chordoma will show positivity for S100, EMA, and cytokeratin (CK).

A-17. (**a**) **Epidermal inclusion cyst**
The images show anucleated squamous cells and keratin, without inflammation. The clinical presentation

and the cytomorphological features are consistent with epidermal inclusion cyst.

A-18. (e) **Angiolipoma**
Angiolipomas usually present as painful, multiple, subcutaneous nodule most commonly on the forearm or the chest. They usually affect young adults and are rare in children or elderly patients. They consist of mature adipocytes, thin-walled vessels, and characteristic fibrin thrombi within blood vessels.

A-19. (c) **Hibernia**
Hibernoma is a rare brown fat benign lipomatous tumor that affects adults. FNAs tend to be cellular and composed of delicate capillaries and mature adipocytes. Hibernoma cells are large, rounded, finely multivacuolated cells with granular cytoplasm. Caution must be taken since the tumor may occasionally show large lipoblast-like cells that may lead to the misdiagnosis of liposarcoma.

A-20. (a) **Atypical lipomatous tumor**
Atypical lipomatous tumor and well-differentiated liposarcoma are essentially synonymous. FNA specimens show variably sized, univacuolated adipocytes intermixed with blood and extracellular fat. Lipoblasts with their characteristic indented scalloped nuclei are a key finding to make this diagnosis.

A-21. (a) **Amplification of the murine double minute 2 (MDM2) oncogene**
FISH study for well-differentiated liposarcoma will reflect amplification of (MDM2) oncogene. t(2;13)(q35;q14) indicate alveolar rhabdomyosarcoma.

A-22. (c) **Myxoma**
Myxoma is a benign, painless tumor that affects adults (30–70 years).

The specimen is hypocellular with a myxoid background, rare scattered histiocytes, and bland epithelioid mesenchymal cells. The cells can be single or in small clusters admixed with foamy histiocytes. Mitoses, atypia, and necrosis are usually absent. In conjunction with clinical history, the findings seen in the provided images are most consistent with myxoma.

A-23. (d) **Fibromatosis**
Desmoid tumors are deep soft tissue tumors occurring mostly on the trunk or proximal limbs. They may be associated with Gardner's syndrome. FNA shows a population of short, bland, bipolar spindle cells with mild atypia in a collagenized or myxoid stroma. The cells display uniform distribution within the stromal matrix with no special pattern. They have elongated nuclei, fine granular chromatin, and small nucleoli. In addition, numerous naked nuclei may also be seen. The differential diagnosis includes smooth muscle tumors, GIST, and cellular myxoma.

A-24. (a) **Malignant peripheral nerve sheath tumor (MPNST)**
Malignant peripheral nerve sheath tumor (MPNST) is a deep-seated tumor. In 50 % of cases, it is associated with neurofibromatosis (NF). In comparison to other neurogenic tumors, it is relatively hypercellular with more cytological atypia. The cytomorphological features of MPNST consist of spindle cells with wavy tapered end nuclei and may have palisading features. Cells have notable cytological atypia with course and hyperchromatic chromatin.

A-25. (c) **S100**
Compared to schwannoma and neurofibroma which usually show S100 diffuse and strong positivity, malignant peripheral nerve sheath tumor (MPNST) will likely show weaker and focal staining with S100. MPNST would most likely have a negative reaction for all other listed answer choices.

A-26. (b) **Solitary fibrous tumor**
Solitary fibrous tumor (SFT) is a fibroblastic mesenchymal tumor that may be located superficially or in deep soft tissues. This uncommon tumor affects adults and occasionally children. SFT can be seen in various locations such as the extremities, head and neck, thoracic wall, pleura, retroperitoneum, and mediastinum. Most cases are benign. Only a few are malignant tumors. These tumors have a prominent hemangiopericytic branching vascular pattern. Myxoid or cystic change can be seen. FNA shows predominance of spindle cells or in some cases a mixture of spindle and round cells. Single cells and naked nuclei may be present in variable numbers. When large tissue fragments are present, they often contain numerous capillaries. Tumor cells are round, medium sized with scant cytoplasm and display mild cytological atypia. Some cells may appear plasmacytoid due to the peripheral location of their nuclei. Benign solitary fibrous tumors cannot be differentiated from malignant ones on cytological grounds alone, because malignant tumors often lack atypia. In some cases of malignant SFT, one may find hyper-

cellular aspirates with notable atypia, increased mitoses, and necrosis.

A-27. (**d**) **All of the above**
Typically, solitary fibrous tumors are positive for CD34 and CD99 and may possibly stain positive for EMA, BCL2, SMA, and S100.

A-28. (**d**) **Synovial sarcoma**
The first step in the diagnostic approach to soft tissue masses is to categorize the lesion to one of the main patterns: lipomatous, round cell, spindle cell, epithelioid/polygonal, or myxoid. This tumor belongs to the spindle cell group, where it shows a monotonous population of short spindle cells with scant granular cytoplasm, elongated hyperchromatic nuclei, irregular nuclear borders, multiple conspicuous nucleoli, and coarse chromatin. These features are consistent with synovial sarcoma (monophasic variant), however, and as with all soft tissue tumors, ancillary studies (IHC and genetic) along with clinical/radiological correlation are required.

A-29. (**e**) **All of the above**
Synovial sarcoma are usually positive for cytokeratin and EMA (90 % positivity in the epithelial component), bcl2 (in the spindle cell component), calponin, and CD99. In addition, FISH study should be done to further confirm the presence of the t(x;18)(p11;q11) translocation.

A-30. (**c**) **Leiomyosarcoma**
As previously stated, the first step in the diagnostic approach to soft tissue tumors is to triage the lesion to one of the main patterns. This case displays predominantly spindle morphology, making leiomyosarcoma and leiomyoma the main diagnostic differentials. The cytomorphology presented in this case is predominantly spindled. Cells show cigar-shaped nuclei, irregular coarse chromatin, and nonvisible nucleoli. The chromatin features and the degree of atypia favor a diagnosis of leiomyosarcoma than leiomyoma. Leiomyosarcoma may sometimes present in fascicle arrangement or display nuclei palisading. Ancillary studies with clinical/radiological correlation are required for further diagnostic confirmation.

A-31. (**c**) **Osteosarcoma**
Osteosarcomas are high-grade malignant tumors of the bone in which the neoplastic cells produce osteoid. They can be categorized as bone/osteoid predominant (osteoblastic), chondroid predominant (chondroblastic), minimal bone or cartilage matrix with high-grade spindle cell morphology (fibroblastic), or having other unusual histological forms. The cytology specimens are cellular in a hemorrhagic background. The cells may be single and present in clusters. They display marked variation in size and shape, hyperchromasia, irregular nuclear membranes, prominent nucleoli, and atypical mitoses. The presence of osteoid matrix (best seen in DQ stain) can be very helpful in the diagnosis. Correlation with radiographic findings is crucial for the proper diagnosis. Occasionally, osteosarcoma may show multinucleated neoplastic cells or plasmacytoid cells. The cytomorphological features does not support other answer choices: Ewing/PNET is part of the round small blue cell differential which is not consistent with the image provided. The absence of plasma cells rules out plasmacytoma, no signet/columnar cells with visible cytoplasmic vacuolations rule out adenocarcinoma, and rhabdomyosarcoma belongs to the round cell differential.

A-32. (**b**) **It is a malignant tumor of skeletal muscle origin.**
The image shown is of myxoid leiomyosarcoma. The tumor is of smooth muscle origin and can be associated with EBV infection in patients with AIDS or transplant. The cytomorphology presented in this case shows spindle. Cells show cigar-shaped nuclei, irregular coarse chromatin, and nonvisible nucleoli in a myxoid background. In general, they stain positive for alpha-smooth muscle actin, desmin, calponin, and caldesmon. In addition, retroperitoneal LMS affecting women may stain positive for ER receptors.

A-33. (**e**) **Most cases are benign.**
The image shows solitary fibrous tumor (SFT) which is a rare tumor affecting mostly adults and may be located superficially or in deep soft tissues. FNA shows a predominance of spindle cells with few round cells. Tumor cells have scant cytoplasm and display mild cytological atypia. Most cases are benign. Because malignant tumors often lack atypia, benign SFT cannot be differentiated from malignant ones on the basis of cytologic assessment.

A-34. (**a**) **Spindle cell melanoma**
The image shows spindle cells arranged in both isolated pattern and clusters. They have a well-demarcated abundant cytoplasm with some cells showing plasmacytoid morphology. The inset shows a cell with a dark/blue-black pigment. The morphology and the positive staining for HMB45 make the diagnosis of spindle cell melanoma more likely than other question choices.

Spindle cell melanoma is a morphologic variant of melanoma with an incidence of 3–14 %. The differential diagnosis include: MFH, fibrosarcoma, MPNST, clear cell sarcoma, synovial sarcoma, and pleomorphic carcinoma. The tumor stains positive for S100, HMB45, and melan A. HMB45 is more specific than S100 for melanoma diagnosis.

A-35. (c) **Metastatic urothelial carcinoma**
Although clinical history is most useful in the diagnosis of metastatic malignancy, the workup for patients who first present with metastasis can be challenging. Immunohistochemistry can be very helpful in delineating the origin of the tumor. The immunohistochemistry profile may show CK7+, CK20+, and P63, and thrombomodulin+is consistent with metastatic urothelial carcinoma.

A-36. (a) **Metastatic breast ductal carcinoma**
The distinction between metastatic carcinoma vs. sarcoma is important since the treatment would be different. The FNA specimen image shows cluster of large polygonal cells with large nuclei and visible macronucleoli. Some isolated cells can all be seen in the background. The immunohistochemistry profile shows the tumor to be positive for pan-CK, GFCP15, ER, and weak positivity for HER2-N. The immunoprofile and the FNA morphology are most consistent with metastatic breast ductal carcinoma.

A-37. (b) **Alveolar rhabdomyosarcoma**
The FNA aspirate is highly cellular and shows single cells and some cells in loose groups. The cells are large, polygonal with abundant sharply demarcated cytoplasm that contains vacuoles. The nucleoli are round, hyperchromatic with prominent nucleoli. Some of the cells have eccentric nuclei (plasmacytoid/rhabdoid morphology). Binucleated and multinucleation are also seen. The morphology and the FISH studies results of positive t(2;13)(q35;q14) indicate alveolar rhabdomyosarcoma.

A-38. (b) **Metastatic urothelial carcinoma**
In general, clinical history and ancillary studies are indispensable tools when making diagnostic decisions about the origin of metastatic malignancies. However, the cytomorphology of the lesions can also offer valuable clues. The FNA specimen shows a loosely cohesive cluster of pleomorphic large cells with abundant cytoplasm and relatively distinct cell borders. Nuclei are large and hyperchromatic with irregularly distributed granular chromatin and prominent nucleoli. Eosinophilic intracytoplasmic inclusion (Melamed-Wolinska bodies) is seen. Although they have no specific diagnostic value, their presence supports a urothelial origin. In practice, a definite cytologic diagnosis should not be rendered on cell morphology alone. Ancillary studies must be ordered (refer to Question 83 for the immunoprofile of urothelial tumors); however, the cytological features described are mostly suggestive of metastatic urothelial carcinoma.

A-39. (a) **Rhabdomyoma**
Rhabdomyoma is a rare benign skeletal muscle tumor. Extracardiac rhabdomyoma occurs most frequently in the oral cavity, larynx, and pharynx. In this case, the FNA smear is showing large cells with abundant granular cytoplasm. The nuclei are round, and some cells show multinucleation. The features and the clinical history are most consistent with rhabdomyoma.

A-40. (d) **A and B**
The typical rhabdomyoma immunohistochemical profile would reveal the cells to be positive for desmin and myoglobin. In addition to PAS+, diastase sensitive detects glycogen. The tumor is negative for keratin, EMA, CD68, and S100 may show weak positivity on occasions.

A-41. (b) **Low-grade chondrosarcoma**
Chondrosarcomas are malignant tumors that can arise in the bone or in the soft tissue. They produce chondroid matrix. The most frequent sites are the pelvis, or the diaphysis or metaphysis of long bones. The tumor grading from I to III affect both treatment and prognosis. Chondrosarcomas are classified as classic (conventional), dedifferentiated, mesenchymal myxoid, and clear cell. The FNA image shows a classic chondrosarcomas, with lower-grade features: cells in lacunae in a cartilaginous matrix with rounded and centrally placed nuclei with some cells showing prominent nucleoli. Some cells show binucleation. The cells have well-defined borders with pale cytoplasm and a bright magenta cartilaginous matrix. These features are more consistent with low-grade conventional chondrosarcoma. Higher grades will show crowding and higher cellularity. In dedifferentiated chondrosarcoma, both classic low-grade elements and undifferentiated sarcomatoid elements will be seen. The transition from one zone to the other can be abrupt or gradual. A sampling error may yield only the cells of poorly differentiated sarcoma and lead to misdiagnosis.

A-42. (**d**) **Fat necrosis**

Fat necrosis of the subcutaneous tissue usually affects women and young children. It generally follows minor trauma such as fall or blunt injury and usually appears on the shins, thighs, arms, breasts, and buttocks. Clinically, it may present as a lump, skin discoloration, or a painful region. In the absence of history of injury, the clinical picture may be confused for a neoplastic disorder. The FNA specimen show lipid-laden macrophages (lipophages) with abundant vacuolated cytoplasm. In addition, degenerating histiocytes with opaque pyknotic nuclei are seen. The clinical history and the cytomorphology are most consistent with fat necrosis.

12.4 Answers and Discussion of Text-Based Questions 43–90

A-43. **(c) Limited experience needed to aspirate and interpret samples**
One of the major challenges of interpretation of soft tissue FNA biopsies is the lack of expertise among most cytopathologists in this field. The vast diverse patterns of soft tissue lesions and the relative low volume of cases seen by the pathologist in their daily practice contribute to the steep learning curve of this subspecialty. The remainder of the answer choices is considered advantages to FNA of soft tissue lesions.

A-44. **(d) Triage lesions according to tissue origin (sarcoma vs. lymphoma vs. carcinoma)**
Since providing a definitive diagnosis of soft tissue lesions using FNA is frequently not feasible nor recommended, the most useful role for FNA in clinical practice is to help with the initial triaging of the lesions into benign/inflammatory vs. malignant, in addition to providing tissue of origin (sarcoma vs. lymphoma vs. carcinoma) if malignant.

A-45. **(a) False-negative diagnoses**
Tumors with marked necrosis or fibrotic areas may most likely cause false-negative diagnoses mostly attributed to sampling errors.

A-46. **(a) Enhance the diagnostic yield of the less experienced cytopathologist**
As discussed previously, the paucity of exposure to soft tissue FNA specimens pose a real challenge to the practicing cytopathologist. Following systemic pattern recognition, diagnostic approaches may help patching the lack of expertise and enhance the diagnostic yield of the less experienced cytologist.

A-47. **(b) Lipoma**
Lipoma is the most common soft tissue neoplasm that occurs in adults.

A-48. **(e) Lipoma has distinctive histologic features different from subcutaneous adipose tissue.**
The cytomorphology of lipoma will show large univacuolated, uniform adipoctyes with bland nuclei. No distinctive morphologic features will help in the differentiating lipoma from the subcutaneous adipose tissue. Accordingly, the clinical presentation and the aspiration of a mass by the cytopathologist are key in making the diagnosis of lipoma.

A-49. **(d) Characteristic hibernoma cells are multivacuolated with granular cytoplasm.**
Hibernoma is an uncommon benign lipomatous tumor. It frequently yields cellular FNA aspirates of mature adipocytes with numerous capillaries and characteristic multivacuolated cells with granular cytoplasm (hibernoma cells).

A-50. **(a) Liposarcoma**
The most common soft tissue sarcoma in adults is liposarcoma.

A-51. **(b) The identification of lipoblasts is very specific for the diagnosis of liposarcoma.**
Lipoblasts are multivacuolated cells with atypical scalloped nuclei. This key finding is extremely helpful in diagnosing liposarcoma; however, it is not entirely specific for the diagnosis of liposarcoma. In fact, some benign lipomatous lesions (as fat necrosis) may show lipoblast-like cells.

A-52. **(e) Myxoid liposarcoma**
Myxoid liposarcoma present with abundant myxoid background. Tissue fragments contain extensive capillaries and mesenchymal cells. They may show lipoblasts. The mesenchymal cells can have scant cytoplasm or a cytoplasm with long fibrillary processes. They display pleomorphic nuclei with oval or plump morphology. In addition, branching blood vessels with "chicken wire" appearance is characteristic of this tumor.

A-53. **(d) A and C**
Cytogenetic studies demonstrate myxoid liposarcoma and round cell liposarcoma to have identical reciprocal chromosomal translocation t(12;16)(q13;p11). This fact indicates that the two tumors constitute a single entity, with pure myxoid lesions depicting the lowest grade of the range and pure round cell liposarcomatous lesions representing the highest grade of the range.

A-54. **(b) Show abundant granular myxoid material and histiocytes**
Ganglion cysts are small (usually <2 cm) masses frequently located on the dorsal surface of the wrist. They usually affect younger patients, and they do not communicate with joint spaces. Microscopically, FNA aspirates will reveal histiocytes in an abundant myxoid background. Histiocytes may form small groups or present as single cells. The typical histiocytic immunohistochemical profile should stain positive for CD68 and negative for cytokeratin.

A-55. **(d) It is a benign lesion.**
Intramuscular myxoma is a benign tumor "myxo is greek for mucous" that usually present as painless, slowly growing gelatinous mass which frequently involve the thigh muscles. FNA aspirates are generally hypocellular, hypovascular, with bland uniform shaped cells (spindle, round to oval, or satellite) floating in an abundant myxoid background. The cells display bland morphology with no atypia, mitosis, or necrosis. Please note that a cellular variant exists and represents an intermediate group between intramuscular myxoma and low-grade myxofibrosarcoma. Surgery is the treatment of choice.

A-56. **(d) All of the above**
The differential diagnosis of the family of tumors with positive EWSR1 gene rearrangements include: Ewing sarcoma, desmoplastic small round cell tumor, clear cell sarcoma, extraskeletal myxoid chondrosarcoma, angiomatoid fibrous histiocytoma, liposarcoma (subsets), and myoepithelial tumor of soft tissue. Accurate diagnosis of the mentioned tumors is essential for proper prognostic triaging and subsequent treatment strategies; accordingly, cytogenetic evaluation of this group of tumors is indicated.

A-57. **(b) They have spindle-shaped nuclei.**
Classically, lipoblasts are multivacuolated cells, with intracytoplasmic lipid droplets compressing the nucleus leading to its characteristic scalloped "resembling the shell of scallop fish" shaped borders. Mimickers of lipoblasts include multivacuolated macrophages that contain lipid and/or mucin droplets. Although the presence of lipoblasts can help enormously in the diagnosis of liposarcoma, their identification is not entirely specific for the diagnosis.

A-58. **(c) Gastrointestinal stromal tumor**
There are two distinct entities: Carney's triad (gastrointestinal stromal tumor + pulmonary chondroma + adrenal paraganglioma) and Carney's complex (heart and skin myxomas, skin hyperpigmentation "lentiginosis," and endocrine over activity). The point of this question is to raise the awareness to this distinction.

A-59. **(a) Dedifferentiated liposarcomas have worse prognosis than other types of pleomorphic sarcomas.**
Dedifferentiated liposarcoma have distinct zones of well-differentiated liposarcoma and non-lipogenic sarcoma that presents clinically as a large painless mass. The transition from one zone to the other can be abrupt or gradual. In general, it has a better prognosis than other pleomorphic sarcomas.

A-60. **(b) Most frequently presents in a deep-seated location.**
Approximately two thirds of myxofibrosarcoma present as superficial lesions mainly confined to the deep dermis and subcutaneous fat of the limbs. This clinical information can be useful in differentiating myxofibrosarcoma from other myxoid soft tissue lesions with higher predilection to present as deeply seated lesions.

A-61. **(e) All of the above**
In general, sarcomas rarely if ever metastasize to lymph nodes. However, few sarcomas have a relatively higher potential to do so. This limited group of sarcomas include: myxofibrosarcoma, clear cell sarcoma, rhabdomyosarcoma, and synovial sarcoma.

A-62. **(c) Myxoid subtype has worse prognosis than pleomorphic subtype.**
Myxofibrosarcoma have many subtypes including: myxoid, pleomorphic, giant cell, and inflammatory type. The myxoid and pleomorphic types are the most prevalent with the myxoid type having a better prognosis.

A-63. **(b) Physaliphorous cells are key diagnostic feature.**
Chordoma is a rare slowly growing, low-grade malignant neoplasm arising from the notochord. Men are affected twice as often as women with a peak incidence in the fifth and sixth decades of life. The tumor has a tendency to affect the axial skeleton with the sacrococcygeal and the base of the skull being the most frequent sites involved. Microscopically, the most characteristic feature is physaliphorous cells floating in an abundant myxoid matrix.

A-64. **(b) Large cells with bubbly cytoplasm**
The word physaliphorous is derived from the Greek word for bubble (physallis). These cells are large with multivacuolated cytoplasm that gives the characteristic bubbly appearance. Although there is some resemblance to lipoblasts, physaliphorous nuclei are not scalloped.

A-65. **(c) They often stain positive for cytokeratins.**
Myxoid chondrosarcoma may affect the bone or soft tissue. Using DQ stain, FNA specimens show abundant extracellular myxoid matrix with hyaline cartilage occasionally seen. In general, the degree of cellularity is in direct portion to the tumor grade

(the higher the grade, the higher the cellularity). The tumor may resemble some chordoma features. Myxoid chondrosarcoma rarely stain positive for cytokeratin or EMA.

A-66. (e) **Gastrointestinal stromal tumors (GIST)**
Advancements in molecular diagnostics have altered our understanding of GIST biology.

In the past, the majority of GIST tumors were thought to be benign. Currently, all GIST tumors are believed to have malignant potential.

A-67. (d) **Often display high mitotic activity and cellular atypia**
Desmoid tumors may arise as a part of Gardner's syndrome, familial adenomatosis polyposis (FAP), or sporadically. FNA specimens display uniform bland spindled cells with oblong nuclei. Classically, the tumor show minimal atypia with no-to-rare mitosis.

A-68. (c) **Verocay bodies consist of a stacked arrangement of two palisading rows of nuclei separated by an acellular zone.**
Schwannoma is a benign tumor derived from schwann cells. Classically, it presents with biphasic morphology with a hypercellular zone (Antoni A) and myxoid hypocellular zone (Antoni B): Verocay bodies consist of stacked arrangement of two palisading rows of nuclei separated by an acellular zone that most likely represent fibrillary process. Verocay bodies are most often seen in the cellular zone (Antoni A).

A-69. (e) **A and C only**
Microscopic examination of neurofibroma may reveal schwann cells and fibroblasts. Physaliphorous cells are characteristic of chordoma.

A-70. (a) **Associated with neurofibromatosis in 90 % of cases.**
Malignant peripheral nerve sheath tumor (MPNST) is a deep-seated tumor. In 50 % of cases, it is associated with neurofibromatosis (NF). In comparison to other neurogenic tumors, it is relatively hypercellular with more cytological atypia. It has a high predilection for local recurrence and frequent distant metastases.

A-71. (d) **All of the above**
The cytomorphological features of MPNST include spindle or epithelioid cells with wavy nuclei, coarse hyperchromatic chromatin, and possible palisading. In addition, mitotic figures and necrosis may be seen.

A-72. (e) **A and B**
Hemangiomas are common benign vascular neoplasms with no predilection to specific body site or patient age. In most cases, FNAs tend to show blood only aspirates rendering them nondiagnostic. Occasionally, it may show compact dense vascular coils containing bland, elongated spindle cells in a bloody background. Classically, the cells would display scant/moderate cytoplasm, bland nuclei with occasional nuclear grooves, and small nucleoli.

A-73. (d) **All of the above**
Angiosarcomas are vascular sarcomas with endothelial cell features and two common morphologies: spindle and epithelioid cell angiosarcoma. They may be associated with coagulopathies, Maffucci syndrome, and postradiation for other malignancies. Maffucci syndrome is a sporadic disease that had been reported to present with multiple enchondromas, hemangiomas, and lymphangiomas.

A-74. (a) **The monophasic variant shows predominantly round cell pattern.**
A monophasic variant of synovial sarcoma most commonly presents with spindle cell pattern although a monophasic epithelioid pattern can also exist. Otherwise, all the other answer choices are correct.

A-75. (c) **Can be associated with Paget's disease**
Osteosarcomas are high-grade malignant tumors of the bone that rarely affects children under 5 years of age. These tumors most frequently affect the metaphysic of long bones. Osteosarcomas may be primary or secondary (e.g., status post radiation treatment or in association with Paget's disease). Osteosarcoma secondary to Paget's disease usually affect patients above the age of 40. The tumors should stain negative for EMA.

A-76. (c) **Five-year survival rate more than 90 %**
Fibrosarcoma is a rare tumor. It has two types: adult and infantile. The 5-year survival rate is poor (<50 %). The infantile type frequently contains the chromosomal translocation t(12;15)(p13;q26) with NTRK3-ETV6 fusion and generally has a better prognosis.

A-77. (d) **All of the above**
Spindle cell melanoma is a variant that may mimic other spindle cell sarcomas. It usually stains positive for HMB45, melan A, and S-100 and tyrosinase and MITF. FNA aspirates are generally cellular with many single cells.

A-78. (b) **It always stains negative for synaptophysin and chromogranin.**
Rhabdomyosarcoma (RMS) is a malignant tumor with muscle differentiation that has the following subtypes: embryonal, alveolar, and pleomorphic subtypes. In alveolar RMS, FISH may detect the FKHR breakpoint, and PCR helps to identify FKHR-PAX3/PAX7 fusion transcripts. It is of note that the tumor may occasionally stain positive for synaptophysin, chromogranin, and CD99.

A-79. (e) **It usually stains negative for glycogen.**
Ewing sarcoma/PNET affects bones more than soft tissues and occurs predominantly in patients aged (5–25 years). Immunoprofile of the tumor frequently reveals positivity for PAS (glycogen) and CD99. Rare positivity for cytokeratins is reported. They have t(11;22) tanslocation with EWSR1-FLI1 fusion (90 %).

A-80. (d) **All of the above**
Homer Wright pseudorosettes are formed by cells with nuclei arranged around a central area of fibrillary neuropil material that usually stains positive for S100. Flexner-Wintersteiner rosettes are true rosette (empty lumen) and are characteristic of retinoblastoma. Homer Wright rosettes can be associated with neuroblastoma, medulloblastoma, and PNETs.

A-81. (e) **A and B only**
Neuroblastoma is a malignant small round cell tumor mostly seen before the age of 5 years (90 % of cases). Unfortunately, the first presentation of the disease may be nodal or bone metastasis. N-myc amplification usually implies worse prognosis.

A-82. (e) **All of the above**
Desmoplastic small round cell tumor (DSRCT) is a rare neoplasm with a poor prognosis that usually affects males. In general, the immunoprofile would show positivity for EMA, desmin, S100, CD56, NSE, chromogranin, and synaptophysin. Characteristically it shows a dot-like and paranuclear staining with desmin. Tumor cells can also be positive for CD99 and WT1.

A-83. (c) **They are hypovasuclar tumors.**
Paraganglioma is currently the most accepted term used to describe these lesions that were previously called chemodectoma, carotid body tumor, or glomus. Paragangliomas are tumors of neural crest origin that can be benign or malignant. They are very vascular tumors, and they stain positive for NSE, chromogranin, and synaptophysin. Tumor cells have abundant cytoplasm that frequently contain eosinophilic granules.

A-84. (b) **It is usually negative for S100, HMB45, MITF, and melan A.**
Clear cell sarcoma, also called malignant melanoma of the soft parts, is a rare sarcoma mainly affecting young adults (30–40 years). Tumor is usually positive for S100, HMB45, MITF, and melan A; thus, it can be confused for a metastatic melanoma. FISH can play an important role in the diagnosis since it can be the characteristic t(12;22)(q13;q12) translocation. FNA specimens may show tumor cells that are round, oval, or polygonal. The cells may display multinucleation. The cytoplasm of tumor cells is moderately abundant and may show vacuolization. In addition, individual cells may contain melanin pigment. Oval or round eccentric nuclei with occasional intranuclear inclusion are often seen and may display multiple nucleoli. Vacuolated, lacy, or tigroid backgrounds can exist.

A-85. (a) **A. CK+, EMA+, S100 +, HMB45 –, desmin –, CD99 +, CD117 –, H-caldesmon –**
The differential of spindle cell malignancy would focus on triaging the tumor to spindle cell melanoma, spindle cell carcinoma, or spindle cell sarcoma. Immunohistochemistry can offer great help in this process. The key is to be aware that although cytokeratin is mainly used to rule out carcinoma, focal CK expression can be seen in sarcomas such as synovial sarcoma, Ewing sarcoma, and epithelioid sarcoma. In addition, synovial sarcoma may also show positivity for EMA. It is of note that S100 is more sensitive for melanoma, while HMB45 is more specific, accordingly both should be ordered when ruling out melanoma. Synovial sarcoma may be positive or negative for S100; however, HMB45 positivity should raise the suspicious of melanoma.

A-86. (b) **The characteristic rod-shaped or rhomboid crystals seen in histology are frequently seen in cytology specimens.**
Alveolar part sarcoma is a very rare soft tissue tumor affecting mostly older children and young adults. Although it is a slowly growing tumor, it is reported to have early metastases to the lungs, bones, and brain. FNA aspirate frequently display large, polygonal tumor cells with abundant, fragile, granular cytoplasm, and centrally located nuclei with prominent nucleoli. Hemorrhagic or granular backgrounds with naked nuclei are commonly seen. Unlike histology

specimens, the characteristic rod-shaped or rhomboid crystals are not usually seen in cytology specimens. The tumor may stain positive for PAS.

A-87. **(e) A and B only**
Differential diagnosis of round cell malignancy may include: lymphoma, small cell carcinoma, seminoma, Ewing/PNET, desmoplastic small round cell tumor (DSRCT), and rhabdomyosarcoma. In addition to clinical correlation, IHC can be very helpful. In general, CK is positive in most carcinomas. In addition to synaptophysin and chromogranin, small cell carcinoma can stain positive for cd56 and NSE. Except for anaplastic large cell lymphoma and immunoblastic lymphoma, CD45 is otherwise a reliable lymphoma marker. However, if lymphoma is suspected, fresh tissue should be always submitted for flow cytometry. PLAP is a useful marker for seminoma. Rhabdomyosarcoma mostly stain positive for desmin and myogenin.

A-88. **(a) It is a high-grade malignancy that accounts for 12 % of all bone tumors.**
Giant cell tumor (GCT) of the bone is a low-grade malignancy accounting for approximately or 4 % of all primary bone tumors. It generally affects young adults (20–40 years) with the knee being the most frequent. Although locally aggressive, they rarely metastasize. Specific diagnosis requires the presence of a combination of ovoid mononuclear and osteoclast-like giant cells with similar nuclei.

A-89 **(a) *Bartonella henselae* infection**
Bartonella henselae infection (cat scratch disease) causes bacillary angiomatosis with a vascular proliferation associated with a neutrophilic infiltrate.

A-90. **(e) FNA aspirates show clusters of epithelioid spindle cells in a hemorrhagic background.**
Pigmented villonodular synovitis represents the diffuse type of giant cell tumor of the tendon sheath. FNA aspirates reveal mononuclear histiocytes admixed with multinucleate osteoclast-like giant cells. Both the histiocytes and the giant cells share the same nuclear features. Tumor cells may contain brown golden hemosiderin crystals. Intranuclear inclusions may be seen.

Reading List

Czerniak B, Tuziak T. Chapter 35. Soft tissue lesions. In: Koss LG, Melamed MR, editors. Koss' diagnostic cytology and its histopathologic bases. 5th ed. Philadelphia: Lippincott Williams & Wilkins; 2006. p. 1302–39.

Czerniak B, Tuziak T, Kram A, Ayal A. Chapter 36. Bone tumors. In: Koss LG, Melamed MR, editors. Koss' diagnostic cytology and its histopathologic bases. 5th ed. Philadelphia: Lippincott Williams & Wilkins; 2006. p. 1340–74.

Khalbuss WE, Monaco SE, Pantanowitz L. Chapter 19. Soft tissue and bone. In: Quick compendium of cytopathology. The ASCP; 2013. p. 412–47.

Khalbuss WE, Parwani AV. Cytopathology of soft tissue & bone lesions. New York: Springer; 2011. p. 1–244.

Khalbuss WE, Teot LA, Monaco SE. Diagnostic accuracy and limitations of fine needle aspiration cytology of bone and soft tissue lesions: a review of 1,114 cases with cytological-histologic correlation. Cancer Cytopathol. 2010;118:24–32.

Layfield LJ, Bedrossian CW, Crim JR, Palombini L. Musculoskeletal cytohistology. Cambridge: Cambridge University Press; 2012.

Qian X. Chapter 16. Soft tissue. In: Cibas ES, Ducatman BS, editors. Cytology diagnostic principles & clinical correlates. 3rd ed. Philadelphia: Saunders Elsevier; 2009. p. 451–522.

Yoshino N, Kojima T, Asami S, et al. Diagnostic significance and clinical applications of chimeric genes in Ewing's sarcoma. Biol Pharm Bull. 2003;26:585–8.

Application of Molecular Diagnostics to Cytopathology

13

Momin T. Siddiqui

Contents

13.1 **Questions 1–20** 720

13.2 **Answers and Discussion of Questions 1–20** 724

Reading List 734

Table 13.1 Introduction: Molecular testing and cytology

Diagnostic molecular testing is now being increasingly applied to cytopathologic specimens such as urines, fine-needle aspirations, and bronchial and bile duct brushings, to name a few. Molecular tests using a cytopathologic specimen combine the application of molecular biology techniques, cytomorphology, and principles of the molecular mechanisms of disease for diagnosis and treatment of various diseases. As this process continues, the importance of a combined cytomorphological and molecular approach that maintains the diagnostic cytopathologist at the core of the clinical decision-making process is of great value to the patients and cannot be emphasized enough
Molecular biology commonly refers to nucleic acid (RNA, DNA) techniques, even though proteins are technically "molecular" level moieties. Although immunoperoxidase staining technology is the indicator for a set of underlying molecular interactions, immunoperoxidase technology is not considered molecular biology. However, many of the targets of the immunohistochemical procedures are proteins derived from aberrant genes including tumor suppressor genes, cell cycle regulators, oncogenes, and tumor-specific cytokine genes. The techniques that are commonly used clinically include polymerase chain reaction, Southern blot analysis, in situ hybridization, in situ PCR, sequencing, and microarray technologies and are now more frequently being employed in the clinical laboratory for diagnostic purposes. Cytopathologic specimens are generally of a smaller size, which may limit the number of target nucleic acids/proteins present, for molecular analysis. The molecular techniques most commonly utilized in cytopathologic preparations include in situ hybridization and polymerase chain reaction methods featuring DNA or RNA amplification
Many molecular genetic techniques, new probes and markers, and emerging targets are investigated or under investigations for their potential clinical value in identifying and characterizing malignancies encountered in cytopathologic specimens. In recent years, there has been greater integration of molecular diagnostics into the practice of cytopathology and has already been shown to be essential to better patient care and management. The patient is hence the primary beneficiary of this evolution in the evolving practice of cytopathology in gynecologic, exfoliative, and fine-needle aspiration specimens

M.T. Siddiqui, MD (✉)
Department of Pathology and Laboratory Medicine,
Emory University Hospital, 1364 Clifton Road NE,
Atlanta, GA 30322, USA
e-mail: mtsiddi@emory.edu

W.E. Khalbuss, Q.K. Li (eds.), *Diagnostic Cytopathology Board Review and Self-Assessment*,
DOI 10.1007/978-1-4939-1477-7_13,

Table 13.2 Utility of polymerase chain reaction (PCR) technology in cytopathologic specimens

PCR is now most often used in the cytology laboratory for identifying infectious organisms, detecting gene mutations in solid tumors, and detecting occult lymphoma by B- and T-cell clonal gene rearrangement assays
1. PCR in detection and diagnosis of infectious diseases
This methodology has been particularly successful in diagnosing viral infections in cytopathologic specimens. For human papillomavirus detection, PCR-based methods have been used to detect the "high-risk" types of HPV infection in cervicovaginal cytopathologic samples. In addition, liquid-based gynecologic cytopathologic samples can also be used for PCR detection of herpes virus infection. In *Chlamydia trachomatis* and *Neisseria gonorrhoeae* detection, PCR methods are also available for use with liquid-based gynecology cytopathologic samples. Finally, rapid DNA probe tests that use the technique of nucleic acid hybridization for identifying infectious organisms (mycobacteria) isolated from culture of cytopathologic samples, such as body cavity fluids or pulmonary samples, are also now commercially available
2. PCR and lymphoproliferative diseases
PCR-based techniques using DNA from fine-needle aspirates and other cytopathologic specimens can help in the identification of B- and T-cell clonality in malignant lymphomas and may complement and in some cases may even outperform conventional classic morphologic assessment. Detecting specific chromosomal translocations also can be useful in diagnosing lymphomas. A high percentage of follicular lymphomas have the t(14;18) translocation (BCL2), which can be detected by a PCR-based assay. A second translocation that can be detected is the t(11;14) associated with mantle cell lymphoma. Leukemia is another example of a disease for which molecular assays are helpful at diagnosis, staging, or in measuring minimal residual disease. Diagnosis of recurrence in fluid specimens or a fine-needle aspirate can rely on the B and T clonality assay or on tests for one of the many characteristic translocations (e.g., BCR-ABL)
3. PCR and solid tumors
Application of PCR-based assays for oncogene mutations or amplifications or tumor suppressor gene deletions or mutations as well as other genetic abnormalities is useful in diagnosing solid tumor malignancies and is now being done on fine-needle aspirates. A variety of molecular assays for oncogene activation such as *RAS*, *BRAF*, *KIT*, *EGFR*, tumor suppressor gene expression loss (p53), DNA instability (microsatellite analyses), and other abnormalities have demonstrated clinical utility in cytopathologic specimens. Oncogene mutation assays may prove more sensitive and specific for the presence of certain malignancies than conventional cytology for fine-needle aspiration specimens and fluid samples. Identifying gene mutations by PCR and sequencing methods in a variety of cytopathologic samples has shown promise in increasing the sensitivity of cytopathologic diagnoses and in detecting cancerous and precancerous lesions prior to the evidence of recognizable morphologic changes. PCR can be used to detect a variety of tumor-specific genetic abnormalities, such as unique translocations in sarcoma, *KIT* gene mutation in gastrointestinal stromal tumor, or *BRAF* mutation in papillary thyroid carcinoma

Table 13.3 Testing for telomerase activity and microsatellite instability

These are additional PCR-based assays, which may include gene sequencing, used to complement cytopathologic diagnoses. A PCR procedure can identify telomerase, an enzyme which is often detected in rapidly proliferating cells, in a variety of cytopathologic samples as an indicator of malignancy or precancerous lesions. A modified PCR method to identify telomerase activity, the telomere repeat amplification protocol (TRAP), has been applied to a variety of cytologic samples including cervical-vaginal, effusion, fine-needle aspirates, and, to the largest extent, urinary cytology. Detection of telomerase levels has added a new dimension to conventional cytology in increasing the sensitivity and specificity for the detection of recurrent urothelial malignancy
PCR-based testing does have limitations and mostly are confined to the amount and quality of DNA required for the assay to provide optimal results. Generally, needle washes in ethanol or methanol fixatives are best. Cells stored in tissue culture mediums (such as RPMI) or even buffered saline also are satisfactory, as are the majority of the proprietary fixatives used for monolayer preparations. However, formalin alters the DNA and is not recommended

Table 13.4 Fluorescent in situ hybridization testing (FISH) on cytopathologic specimens

This technique allows microscopic visualization of a labeled nucleic acid probe with either a fluorescent label (FISH) or chromogenic color reaction (brightfield ISH). FISH tests allow for the detection of numerical and structural abnormalities of chromosomes and have been applied to cytopathologic samples obtained from body cavity fluids, exfoliative cytology specimens, and fine-needle aspirates. FISH testing lends itself particularly well to use in cytologic preparations because the cells are already disaggregated and in a single layer, hence yielding highly sensitive results. A variety of preparations can be used such as air-dried smears, ethanol, methanol, and Carnoy's fixed preparations. Each year our knowledge of the number of chromosomal translocations associated with specific solid tumors increases. Some of these translocations can assist in making difficult morphologic diagnoses
Two examples are the t(11;22) translocation of Ewing sarcoma or the t(X;18) translocation in synovial sarcoma. These translocations can be detected by reverse transcriptase-PCR or by FISH testing

Table 13.5 Applications of in situ hybridization technique for detection of infectious diseases

The in situ hybridization technique has been successfully applied to cytologic samples, particularly for diagnosing viral infections
It has been applied for detecting HPV DNA in cervicovaginal cytology specimens

Table 13.6 Applications of situ hybridization technique in lymphoproliferative diseases

FISH can be used to detect tumor-specific chromosomal abnormalities in B-cell lymphomas that are difficult to differentiate based on cytomorphology alone. The FISH technique has proved to be particularly useful for detecting BCR-ABL or cryptic 12;21 gene translocation in leukemias and for detecting MYC, BCL2, or CCND1 (BCL1) translocation in lymphomas
Cytologic smears and aspirates may actually be a better sample type than tissue biopsies for performing chromosomal translocation analysis by FISH

Table 13.7 Applications of in situ hybridization technique in solid tumors

FISH testing can be used for detecting gains or losses in chromosomes. Chromosomal aneusomies that have been detected by FISH testing have also correlated well with tumor grade, stage, detection of recurrence, and the ability to detect micrometastasis. Detection of bladder cancer in urothelial cytology specimens, using a multiprobe assay such as the Abbott/Vysis UroVysion test, is a prime example of utilizing this testing modality. This assay shows improved sensitivity over cytology for detecting urothelial carcinoma in urinary cytology specimens such as bladder washings or renal pelvic washings. The same multiprobe FISH assay has also shown promise in detecting malignant bile duct strictures using routine biliary cytology samples. Finally, multiprobe FISH has shown clinical utility in identifying early genetic changes of lung carcinoma in pulmonary cytology
The FISH method has also been developed to perform tumor prognosis assays such as *N-MYC* amplification in neuroblastoma and HER2/*neu* (ERBB2) oncogene copy number as a prognostic or predictive indicator in breast cancers

13.1 Questions 1–20

Q-1. Conventional karyotypic analysis and FISH can reveal specific chromosomal abnormalities characteristic of commonly encountered renal tumors on fine-needle aspirations. Which of the following statement is NOT true?
- (a) Conventional clear cell RCC is strongly associated with deletions on chromosome 3p.
- (b) The papillary subtype of RCC is typically associated with trisomy/tetrasomy 7, trisomy 17, and the loss of the Y chromosome.
- (c) Trisomies of chromosomes 3, 12, 16, and 20 can be present in papillary subtype of RCC, and their presence has been associated with increased propensity for local invasion and metastasis.
- (d) Xp11.2 translocation RCC is not recognized as a distinct entity in the 2004 World Health Organization classification of renal tumors.
- (e) Oncocytoma can show loss of chromosome 1 and/or 14 and 1 sex chromosome, most often the Y chromosome and rearrangement of 11q13, with t(9;11) and t(5;11).

Q-2. Which of the following statements is correct regarding FISH analysis of fine-needle aspirates from a lymph node?
- (a) Demonstration of the t(11;14)(q13;q32) translocation by FISH between *IGH* and *CCND1* will support the diagnosis of mantle cell lymphoma rather than SLL/CLL.
- (b) Translocation of the *BCL2* gene, a hallmark of follicular lymphoma, occurs in 100 % of diffuse large B-cell lymphomas (DLBCLs).
- (c) *MYC* gene rearrangement can be observed in up to 50 % of diffuse large B-cell lymphomas (DLBCLs).
- (d) Diffuse large B-cell lymphomas (DLBCLs) may have abnormalities of the 3q27 region involving the BCL6 gene in up to 1 % of cases.
- (e) Chromosomal translocations associated with extranodal marginal zone lymphoma of mucosa-associated lymphoid tissue (MALT lymphoma) only include t(11;18)(q21;q21).

Q-3. Which of the following is not an indication for FISH testing in urine samples?
- (a) Atypical urinary cytology
- (b) Follow-up evaluation after intravesical BCG treatment
- (c) Upper urinary tract cytology with numerous umbrella cells
- (D) Surveillance urinary cytology, after transurethral resection
- (e) Hematuria in patients with an increased risk of UC

Q-4. Which of the following statements regarding cytologic evaluation of tuberculous lymphadenitis is false?
- (a) PCR has been found to be very sensitive and specific in fine-needle aspiration of TB LAP with maximum sensitivity in cases of necrosis with or without granulomas.
- (b) PCR is the most rapid method of identifying M. tuberculosis to the species level in cytologic samples of tuberculous lymphadenitis.
- (c) A confident diagnosis of TB can be rendered on cytology when a combination of epithelioid cell granulomas and caseous necrosis with or without multinucleated giant cell is seen.
- (d) Cytomorphology cannot be supplemented with AFB smear and culture wherever required and PCR should be kept as a reserve method for equivocal cases.
- (e) All the above statements are true.

Q-5. Which of the following statements regarding FISH UroVysion assay on urine samples is false?
- (a) Presence of equal to or >4 morphologically abnormal cells (large nuclear size, irregular shape, and patchy 4,6-diamidino-2-phenylindole staining) of 25 analyzed cells that demonstrate either polysomy of equal to or >2 chromosomes 3, 7, and 17 in the same cell.
- (b) Homozygous deletion of 9p21 in 12 of 25 cells.
- (c) If there is only tetrasomy, then there should be at least ten abnormal cells to qualify the FISH result as positive.
- (d) FISH test is based primarily on aneuploidy or polysomy for equal to or >2 chromosomes and, thus, is optimized toward diagnosing patients with high-grade UC.
- (e) Polysomy is the most infrequent chromosomal abnormality and usually is identified in high-grade UC.

Q-6. Which of the following statements is correct regarding cerebrospinal fluid evaluation for herpes simplex encephalitis?
- (a) Visual detection of herpes virus in CSF samples is the gold standard for diagnosis.
- (b) PCR-based testing for herpes virus in CSF samples is the gold standard for diagnosis.

(c) False-negative PCR results have not been observed during the early course of herpes virus infection.
(d) PCR testing for herpes virus has very high sensitivity but a low specificity.
(e) PCR testing of CSF samples should be performed 10 days after the onset of symptoms for optimal results.

Q-7. Metastatic squamous cell carcinoma from head and neck primaries to neck lymph nodes is frequently diagnosed by fine-needle aspiration. Which statement is false?
(a) Fine-needle aspiration cytology can easily ascertain the primary site of metastatic disease on morphology alone.
(b) Squamous cell carcinoma associated with low-risk HPV subtypes is not noted in these aspirates.
(c) In situ hybridization testing can easily be performed to detect HPV-induced primary oropharyngeal squamous cell carcinoma.
(d) Immunohistochemical analysis utilizing p16 is very useful to detect metastatic disease arising from an oropharyngeal primary tumor.
(e) Testing algorithms for detecting HPV 16 in these cytologic specimens include molecular, in situ hybridization (ISH), and immunohistochemical (IHC) studies.

Q-8. Ewing's sarcoma/primitive neuroectodermal tumor (ES/PNET) of the kidney can be diagnosed by fine-needle aspiration samples. Which of the following statement is incorrect?
(a) The molecular marker of ES/PNET is the EWS/FLI1 gene fusion, which may be detected from standard cytogenetic studies showing the chromosomal translocation t(11;22)(q24;q12) or by fluorescence in situ hybridization (FISH) or RT-PCR.
(b) DNA sequencing of the PCR fragments can confirm the type I transcript in most cases, as this is the most prevalent translocation, joining exon 7 of EWS and exon 6 of FLI-1 (type I) and is reportedly found in 65–75 % of patients.
(c) The applicability of RT-PCR on FNA of ES/PNET has made it possible to render an accurate diagnosis on aspiration material, thereby obviating the need for an open biopsy or core biopsy.
(d) ES/PNET can also show intense cytoplasmic MIC-2 immunoreactivity and can be distinguished by the use of other IHC markers and molecular expression of SYT/SSX translocation.
(e) PNET/ES tumors have been reported to be positive for MIC-2 in 84–100 % of cases.

Q-9. Which of the following statements regarding breast cancer hormone receptor status evaluation on cell blocks from fine-needle aspiration samples is correct?
(a) The routine method for detecting ER and PR expression is FISH, whereas HER2 overexpression can be detected by IHC and/or FISH.
(b) The IHC analysis of ER, PR, and HER2 expression has been standardized for formalin-fixed, paraffin-embedded tissue sections.
(c) IHC and FISH methods, which are approved by the US Food and Drug Administration (FDA) for the assessment of breast carcinoma, require tissue samples to be fixed in 50 % neutral-buffered formalin.
(d) The guidelines also require validation of HER2 testing by documenting 100 % concordance rates between IHC HER2 positive and IHC HER2 negative with FISH amplified and non-amplified cases, respectively.
(e) All the above statements are correct.

Q-10. Papillary thyroid carcinoma can metastasize to the neck lymph nodes. These lymph nodes can be evaluated by fine-needle aspiration. The following statements regarding these aspirates are all true except:
(a) Measurements of thyroglobulin (Tg) levels in the rinse of the aspiration biopsy needle have been proposed for detection of neck lymph node metastasis from PTC in patients after total thyroidectomy and radioiodine ablation.
(b) The cases with Tg levels ≥10 ng/ml usually correlate with a diagnosis of PTC on follow-up.
(c) Following total thyroidectomy for thyroid cancer, serum Tg should be undetectable, and any detectable serum Tg indicates neoplastic thyroid foci.
(d) Tg is undetectable in 20 % of patients with isolated lymph node metastases during thyroid hormone treatment and in 5 % after thyroid hormone withdrawal.
(e) All the above statements are false.

Q-11. Pleural micrometastasis from a lung primary can be detected with a high degree of sensitivity and specificity using which of the following technique?
(a) RT-PCR detection of vascular endothelial growth factor (VEGF) mRNA alone.
(b) Immunohistochemical positivity of cytokeratin 7.
(c) RT-PCR detection of endostatin mRNA alone.
(d) Calretinin-negative pleural fluids.
(e) RT-PCR detection of both VEGF mRNA and endostatin mRNA.

Q-12. Which of the following statement regarding dual-translocation or double-hit lymphomas (DTL) is False?

(a) The morphologic and immunophenotypic spectrum of most of these neoplasms overlaps with Burkitt's lymphoma (BL) and diffuse large B-cell lymphoma (DLBCL).
(b) B-cell lymphomas with concurrent *IGH/BCL2* and *MYC* rearrangements are termed dual-translocation or double-hit lymphomas (DTL).
(c) Large cells with centroblastic nuclear features and dark-blue (basophilic) cytoplasm, followed by the presence of apoptotic bodies and marked nuclear pleomorphism in cytologic samples are commonly noted.
(d) FISH analysis for *IGH/BCL2* and *MYC* translocations is not helpful in diagnosing this entity.
(e) These tumors have a highly aggressive behavior and a poor prognosis.

Q-13. The utilization of targeted therapy for non-small cell lung cancers involves molecular testing for mutations in EGFR and KRAS. Which of the following statement is true?

(a) EGFR is a transmembrane receptor protein with an extracellular binding domain and a nuclear tyrosine kinase domain.
(b) Cancer cells with EGFR mutations not only possess a growth advantage over those with wild-type EGFR but also show decreased sensitivity to the anti-EGFR tyrosine kinase inhibitors (TKIs).
(c) KRAS mutation may be a predictor for resistance to TKIs therapy in patients with NSCLC and a prognostic marker, although it is still controversial whether KRAS can predict resistance to TKIs.
(d) EGFR mutations are uncommon in lung adenocarcinoma.
(e) EGFR and KRAS mutations do not vary in different ethnicities.

Q-14. All of the following statements regarding molecular testing on lung cancer cytology samples are true except:

(a) The highest and lowest mutation rates of EGFR have been observed in adenocarcinoma and squamous carcinoma, respectively.
(b) KRAS mutations in exon 1 (codons 21 and 13) are predominant.
(c) EGFR and KRAS mutations are also found to be mutually exclusive.
(d) Samples with sparse cellularity (<500 tumor cells) have a higher PCR failure rate to detect gene mutations.
(e) It has been noted that no significant difference in the mutation rates between samples obtained by cytology versus histology occur.

Q-15. All statements regarding cryopreservation of patient FNA specimens for future nucleic acid-based molecular testing are true except:

(a) To maximize RNA integrity (high-quality RNA), devitalization time (Td) should be kept to 6 h or less.
(b) Post-aspiration processing time (Tp) should be kept to 1 h or less.
(c) The amount of time samples are frozen (tested up to 27 weeks) does not seem to affect the quality of the RNA recovered.
(d) Presence of cellular necrosis associated with the sample appears to decrease the overall quality of RNA recovered.
(e) In cryopreservation, potential benefit of preserving viability is not maintained.

Q-16. Which of the following stains are would be most useful in evaluating atypical cells identified in breast fine-needle aspiration samples?

(a) Cytokeratin 5/6
(b) P63
(c) Cytokeratin 5/6 and p63
(d) P53
(e) Calponin

Q-17. The following statements regarding somatic genetic alterations in papillary thyroid carcinoma (PTC) are correct except:

(a) The most frequent BRAF genetic alteration is a point mutation involving the substitution of thymine, 1799th nucleotide at 15th BRAF exon with adenine (T1799A).
(b) BRAF mutation involving V600E is highly specific for PTC among other primary thyroid neoplasms.
(c) Combination of cytology and BRAF testing positively identifies 80.0 % of PTCs preoperatively
(d) The BRAF V600E point mutation has not been reported in any follicular carcinoma, adenoma, or benign thyroid nodule.
(e) All the above statements are false.

Q-18. Sputum cytology can be helpful in diagnosing lung cancers. The following statements are all correct except:

(a) Identification of *HYAL2* and *FHIT* tumor suppressor genes can help detect abnormal cells in 55 % cytologically negative sputum from lung cancer patients, suggesting that testing for genetic aberrations in sputum samples could be more sensitive than cytology in identifying cancer cells.

(b) Magnetic cell sorting (MACS) is a process of immunomagnetic cell selection based on the recognition of cell-specific antibodies coupled to magnetic beads. MACS has been used in sputum samples to improve diagnosis of lung cancer.

(c) MACS enrichment for bronchial epithelial cells can average 36-fold over the original sputum in one step, yielding at least 2.3×10^5 cells with >40 % purity per sample.

(d) Utilizing MACS with anti-CD14 and anti-CD16 antibody beads does not deplete macrophages and neutrophils.

(e) Detection of *FHIT* aberrations in enriched sputum produces higher sensitivity compared with unprocessed sputum, leading to greater accuracy in genetic diagnosis of lung cancer in sputum samples.

Q-19. The following statements regarding utility of fine-needle aspiration in diagnosing metastatic malignant melanomas are all true except:

(a) *BRAF* V600E mutation in metastatic melanomas from fine-needle aspirates can be identified.

(b) In aspirates with *BRAF* V600E mutation, the patients developed metastatic disease in a shorter time period compared to those without this mutation.

(c) Metastatic melanomas identified on fine-needle aspirates with *BRAF* V600E mutations tend to acquire metastatic potential at lower Clark's invasion level and lower thickness.

(d) *BRAF* V600E mutation is identified in 100 % of fine-needle aspirates from metastatic melanomas.

(e) Assessing for the *BRAF* V600E mutation in fine-needle aspirates of metastatic melanomas can add to prognostic information.

Q-20. Pathway Tissue of Origin Test has been used in cytologic samples and may identify the primary sites of metastatic disease. Which of the following statements is not true?

(a) The Pathwork Tissue of Origin Test (Pathwork Diagnostics, Redwood City, CA) is a microarray-based gene expression test.

(b) The test can be performed on cytologic samples that have been stored from 5 to 15 years.

(c) Expression levels of 2,000 genes to classify tumors by similarity scores (SS) into 15 sites of origin are utilized in this test.

(d) The analyzed specimen needs to be non-necrotic, with abundant tumor content (>60 %) and few inflammatory cells.

(e) Pathwork Diagnostics does not report scores >5 and <20 because concordance with the tissue of origin in specimens with those scores is poor, and thus scores within this range should not be used for clinical management.

13.2 Answers and Discussion of Questions 1–20

A-1. (d) **Xp11.2 translocation RCC is recognized as a distinct entity in the 2004 World Health Organization classification of renal tumors.**
Cytologically, the most prominent feature on Diff-Quik-stained slides in an aspirate is the presence of numerous follicular structures with epithelial cells (one to more layers) surrounding a dense, hyalinized central core. This microscopic finding can be recapitulated in the cell block. On Papanicolaou-stained slides, the cells surrounding hyalinized globules and bands are even more evident. In addition, true papillary structures are also found. Hence, to differentiate it morphologically from a papillary renal cell carcinoma, karyotypic analysis and FISH testing are very important.

Conventional cytogenetics and FISH have revealed characteristic chromosomal abnormalities in a variety of renal tumors. For instance, the conventional, clear cell RCC is strongly associated with deletions on chromosome 3p, which harbors tumor suppressor gene loci including the Von Hippel-Lindau (VHL) gene. Loss of 3p can occur through simple interstitial or terminal deletions, loss of chromosome 3, and unbalanced translocations. The papillary subtype of RCC is typically associated with trisomy/tetrasomy 7, trisomy 17, and the loss of the Y chromosome. The presence of only these abnormalities has been associated with lack of metastatic potential. Additional trisomies of chromosomes 3, 12, 16, and 20 can be present, and their presence has been associated with increased propensity for local invasion and metastasis. In contrast to papillary RCCs, chromophobe RCCs are associated with low chromosome number because of specific loss of the second copy of chromosomes 1, 2, 6, 10, 13, 17, and 21. In this regard, the detection of multiple monosomies by FISH analysis can be helpful in accurately classifying oncocytic neoplasms on FNA, especially in cases where the distinction of chromophobe RCCs from oncocytomas is difficult because of overlapping cytomorphological features and/or equivocal results on immunohistochemistry. From a cytogenetic standpoint, oncocytoma can be classified into three groups: those with loss of chromosome 1 and/or 14 and 1 sex chromosome, most often the Y chromosome; those with rearrangement of 11q13, with t(9;11) and t(5;11) among the most frequent translocations observed; and those with heterogeneous abnormalities, including both numerical and structural aberrations. Finally, the Xp11.2 translocation RCC is recognized as a distinct entity in the 2004 World Health Organization classification of renal tumors. The most common translocations are t(X;1)(p11.2;q21) and t(X;17)(p11.2;q25) resulting in fusions of the *TFE3* gene on Xp11.2 with *PRCC* in 1q21 and *ASPL* in 17q25, respectively.

A-2. (a) **Demonstration of the t(11;14)(q13;q32) translocation by FISH between *IGH* and *CCND1* will support the diagnosis of mantle cell lymphoma rather than SLL/CLL.**
In SLL/CLL cases with a CD23-negative flow cytometry profile, the differential diagnosis includes mantle cell lymphoma and SLL/CLL. Demonstration of the t(11;14)(q13;q32) translocation by FISH between *IGH* and *CCND1* will support the diagnosis of mantle cell lymphoma rather than SLL/CLL.

FISH analysis has become very important in demonstrating the characteristic gene translocations for some malignant lymphomas. The most specific translocations can be helpful for ruling in or out a specific diagnosis. The following are some of the commonly noted findings on FISH analysis in malignant lymphomas.

Burkitt's lymphomas can have *MYC* translocations at band 8q24 to the IGH (14q32) locus or, less commonly, to the IGL (22q11) or IGL (2p12) light-chain loci. Follicular lymphomas genetically are characterized by the translocation t(14;18)(q32;q21) and *BCL2* gene rearrangement. The t(11;14)(q13;q32) between *IGH* and the cyclin D1 (*CCND1*) gene is present in almost all cases of mantle cell lymphoma and is considered the primary genetic event. Diffuse large B-cell lymphomas (DLBCLs) may have abnormalities of the 3q27 region involving the BCL6 gene in up to 30 % of cases. Translocation of the *BCL2* gene, a hallmark of follicular lymphoma, occurs in 20–30 % of DLBCL, and an *MYC* gene rearrangement can be observed in up to 10 % of DLBCL. Chromosomal translocations associated with extranodal marginal zone lymphoma of mucosa-associated lymphoid tissue (MALT lymphoma) include t(11;18)(q21;q21), t(1;14)(p22;q32), t(11;18)(q32;q21), and t(3;14)(p14.1;q32) and result in the production of a chimeric protein (apoptosis inhibitor 2 [API2]-MALT1) or in the transcriptional deregulation of the genes *BCL10*, *MALT1*, and forkhead box p1 (*FOXP1*), respectively. In SLL/CLL cases with a CD23-negative flow cytometry profile, the differential diagnosis includes mantle cell lymphoma and SLL/CLL. Demonstration of the t(11;14)(q13;q32) translocation by FISH between *IGH* and *CCND1* will support the diagnosis of mantle cell lymphoma rather than SLL/CLL, because this translocation is present in almost all mantle cell lymphomas. The use of interphase FISH for the detection of t(11;14)(q13;q32) translocation in the diagnosis of mantle cell lymphoma on FNA specimens has been documented in the literature.

A-3. (c) **Upper urinary tract cytology with numerous umbrella cells.**

Although upper urinary tract cytology usually comprises of atypical urothelial cells and may require additional FISH analysis for detection of urothelial carcinoma. The sample when it presents with only umbrella cells is not ideal for submission for FISH testing since these are indicative of a mature urothelial lining.

Urinary bladder cancer is the sixth most frequent cancer to be found in developed countries. These patients can have a long-term survival, especially in low-grade urothelial carcinoma, and hence need lifelong monitoring. The cost per patient with bladder cancer from diagnosis to death is highest of all cancers. The majority (70 %) of bladder cancers are non-muscle invasive (stage pTa,pT1 and carcinoma in situ). Among these, 70 % are low-grade noninvasive (pTa) tumors that often recur but almost never progress to life-threatening disease. Combined cystoscopy and cytology are the gold standard for diagnosis and follow-up of urothelial carcinoma (UC). The high specificity for the diagnosis of high-grade UC is an undisputed strength of urinary cytology. Urinary cytology is very useful in detecting non-visible carcinoma in situ at cystoscopy. However, urinary cytology performs weakly in low-grade UC due to an overlap of cytological features with benign urothelial cells. In addition, there is a commonly used but poorly defined category of atypical cytology that has questionable significance. Development and progression of cancer are driven by genetic aberrations such as mutations and chromosome and gene copy number abnormalities. Fluorescence in situ hybridization (FISH) is a robust technique for the detection of chromosome copy number gains (polysomies), gains or amplifications and deletions of DNA loci, and translocations in urinary cancers. The multiprobe FISH UroVysion assay (Abbott Molecular Inc., Des Plaines, Ill., USA) for the enumeration of chromosomes 3, 7, and 17 and the locus-specific identifier for the region at 9p21 was developed to overcome the diagnostic limitations of urinary cytology. The 4 probes were selected since increased copy numbers (polysomies) of the chromosomes 3, 7, and 17 had been found to be particularly frequent in bladder cancer. Deletion of 9p21, the site of the tumor suppressor gene *P16*, is also common and occurs early in the development of both papillary and flat urothelial neoplasia. Subsequent progression is associated with chromosomal instability leading to aneuploidy with multiple chromosomal aberrations. UroVysion FISH has a sensitivity of 90–100 % for the detection of invasive bladder cancer (pT1–4) and a specificity of greater than 95 %. In the clinically far less relevant category of low-grade noninvasive bladder cancer, utilizing FISH increases the sensitivity of cytology from 25 to 60–75 %.

A-4. (d) **Cytomorphology can be easily supplemented with AFB smear and culture wherever required, and PCR should be kept as a reserve method for equivocal cases**, especially in developing nations where tuberculous lymphadenitis is rampant and can be easily diagnosed on aspirate samples morphologically exhibiting a combination of epithelioid cell granulomas and caseous necrosis with or without multinucleated giant cells. A supplementary AFB smear can also be cost effectively performed to confirm the cytologic impression. PCR techniques can also be easily performed to identify M. tuberculosis to the species level in cytologic samples of tuberculous lymphadenitis and has been found to be very sensitive and specific; however, especially in a developing nation where cost-effective techniques are more user friendly, its role is best limited to equivocal cases.

A-5. (e) **Polysomy is the most frequent chromosomal abnormality and usually is identified in high-grade UC.**

The other statements are all true regarding evaluation of the sample submitted for FISH testing.

The FDA has approved use of the multiprobe FISH test for the detection of recurrent UC and the evaluation of hematuria. A positive FISH result is defined as the presence of equal to or >4 morphologically abnormal cells (large nuclear size, irregular shape, and patchy 4,6-diamidino-2-phenylindole staining) of 25 analyzed cells that demonstrate either polysomy of equal to or >2 chromosomes 3, 7, and 17 in the same cell or homozygous deletion of 9p21 in 12 of 25 cells. Polysomy is the most frequent chromosomal abnormality and usually is identified in high-grade UC. Homozygous deletion of 9p21 refers to the absence of both gold signals that are used to hybridize to the 9p21 gene; as a sole manifestation of malignancy, this finding is far less frequent than polysomy. In addition to these, it is also recommend that if there is only tetrasomy, then there should be at least ten abnormal cells to qualify the FISH result as positive. The acceptance of the FISH assay as an adjunct to cytology generally is favorable and has been reported that FISH had higher sensitivity for all grades and stages of UC than conventional cytology alone in detecting UC. It should be noted, however, that the FISH test is based primarily on aneuploidy or polysomy for equal to or >2 chromosomes and, thus, is optimized toward diagnosing patients with high-grade UC.

A-6. (b) **PCR-based testing for herpes virus in CSF samples is the gold standard for diagnosis.**
Herpes simplex virus (HSV) is the most frequently identified cause of acute infectious encephalitis worldwide. Herpes simplex encephalitis (HSE) presents with a wide range of symptoms making clinical diagnosis difficult. In adults, it is associated with HSV type 1 infection, which results in focal necrotizing encephalitis. The diagnosis of HSE relies on the detection of viral DNA in cerebrospinal fluid (CSF) samples by a highly sensitive (95–100 %) and specific (94–100 %) polymerase chain reaction (PCR) test. Hence molecular tests, such as PCR-based testing, are the "gold standard" for diagnosis. False-negative PCR results have been observed during the early course of HSE and after more than 10 days of disease evolution. Before the use of antiviral drugs, the case-fatality ratio (CFR) was about 70 % versus 50 % with vidarabine and 14–20 % with acyclovir (ACV) treatment, and most surviving patients had severe sequelae. Hence, ACV should be administered as early as possible and even before the laboratory confirmation of the diagnosis is available, as any delay may result in permanent cognitive or physical impairment of the patient. The usual course of treatment is to give 10 mg/kg t.i.d. of ACV for 2 or 3 weeks. However, the marketing recommendations of ACV stipulate a 10-day treatment course in the case of HSE but also state that the duration of ACV "should be adapted to the condition of the patient and response to treatment." Despite early treatment, some patients may still experience a poor outcome. Hence PCR-based testing of CSF samples is very important for reducing morbidity and mortality in these patients.

A-7. (a) **Fine-needle aspiration cytology can easily ascertain the primary site of metastatic disease on morphology alone.**
Squamous cell carcinoma (SCC) represents the most common malignancy of the head and neck, with 25,000–30,000 cases reported in the USA, annually. A subset of these patients present with cervical lymph node metastasis as the initial presentation, with a further subset of patients presenting without a clinically apparent primary site. Fine-needle aspiration cytology is the mainstay in diagnosing this metastatic SCC. In patients with cervical lymph node metastasis of SCC, there are no consistent and reliable cytologic features that indicate tumor origin. Immunohistochemical markers may aid in delineating the epithelial nature of the process but fail to aid in distinguishing the primary site. In this scenario, imaging studies and endoscopic nonselective biopsies may be performed in an attempt to identify the primary site. When the primary site still remains unknown, the patient may undergo wide field, rather than localized radiation with a definite increase in morbidity. Studies have indicated that in these cases of metastatic oropharyngeal SCC in cervical lymph nodes (diagnosed by fine-needle aspiration), human papillomavirus (HPV), specifically type 16, plays a significant role in the biology of these tumors. Recent literature reports now also indicate that certain high-risk HPV subtypes such as HPV 16 are noted within a subset of oropharyngeal SCC with distinct clinical characteristics. Patients with HPV-positive SCC tend to lack the lifestyle risk factors (betel nut chewing, smoking) and be of slightly younger age. Testing algorithms for HPV 16 include molecular, in situ hybridization (ISH) and immunohistochemical (IHC) studies. Although molecular testing offers specificity, the lack of access, significant cost, and turnaround time affects its clinical utility. Alternatively, surrogate markers using ISH and IHC stains offer benefits in terms of ease of use/interpretation, access, cost, and turnaround time. p16 is a cyclin-dependent kinase inhibitor that functions to slow progression through the cell cycle. HPV oncoproteins lead to inactivation of the retinoblastoma (Rb) gene, a tumor suppressor gene. Rb inactivation leads to an upregulation of various cell cycle-associated proteins, including p16. p16 expression can be detected by immunohistochemistry and is useful for detecting metastatic oropharyngeal SCC in neck lymph nodes.

A-8. (d) **ES/PNET can also show intense cytoplasmic MIC-2 immunoreactivity and can be distinguished by the use of other IHC markers and molecular expression of SYT/SSX translocation.**
This is incorrect since this is noted in synovial sarcoma.

Ewing's sarcoma/primitive neuroectodermal tumor (ES/PNET) of the kidney affects young adults with a rapid clinical progression and significant mortality owing to late diagnosis, early metastasis, and advanced stage at presentation. The diagnosis is based on the cytomorphological features (round cell morphology with rosette formation), immunohistochemistry (MIC2 and neural markers expression), and molecular pathology (EWS translocation). The differential diagnosis of small round cell tumors localized to the kidney is broad and, besides ES/PNET, includes blastemal Wilms' tumor (WT), small-cell neuroendocrine carcinoma, lymphoma, neuroblastoma (NB), desmoplastic small round cell tumor (DSRCT), and synovial sarcoma (SS). It is important to correctly classify these tumors for appropriate treatment. ES/PNET of the kidneys tends to be a high-stage, aggressive neoplasm that requires more extensive therapy as compared to other tumors. A primary PNET of the kidney can be diagnosed by fine-needle aspiration (FNA) and immunohistochemistry (IHC) and subsequently confirmed by reverse transcriptase-polymerase chain reaction (RT-PCR). The clinical classic triad of symptoms, including hematuria, pain, and palpable mass, occurs in most patients with renal ES/PNET. Radiologic finding is nonspecific and shows evidence of a large heterogeneous tumor and is useful only for staging of the disease process and not for diagnosis per se. The diagnosis of ES/PNET is based on the pathologic findings. The cytologic finding of a poorly differentiated, highly cellular small round cell tumor forming rosettes and pseudorosettes is an indication of ES/PNET; however, the diagnosis needs confirmation using IHC and/or molecular pathologic examination. Small round blue cell tumors do pose diagnostic problems in FNA because the cytomorphological differentiating features are subtle. This differential diagnosis is further complicated by the relatively rare occurrence of most of these entities in the kidney. The role of FNA in the diagnosis of these small round cell lesions has gained much importance during the past decade. ES/PNET is frequently misdiagnosed as blastema-predominant WT, both being monotonous round cell tumors. ES/PNET on cytology reveals variably cohesive clusters of small round cells with irregular nuclei and the typical "Ewingoid" or pale nuclear chromatin and direct perivascular arrangement. Apoptotic cells, mitosis, and necrosis are easily identified. The intracytoplasmic glycogen also produces a "tigroid background" in the MGG-stained smear. The features favoring the diagnosis of WT are the presence of a discrete population of monomorphic round cells with a high nuclear/cytoplasmic (N/C) ratio with opened-up chromatin and inconspicuous nucleoli comprising the blastemal component along with evidence of epithelial and mesenchymal differentiation. However, in up to one-third of cases, the aspirate is blastema-predominant and requires immunohistochemistry which may be performed on the cell block or smears of FNA. In WT, positivity for vimentin, low-molecular weight cytokeratin, epithelial membrane antigen, and WT-1 is noted. Metastatic renal NBs are also similar morphologically to renal ES/PNET. However, 90 % of NB occurs by age of 5 years, and features facilitating this diagnosis include round cell population with coarse chromatin and frequent rosette formation with or without ganglionic differentiation in a fibrillary background. Again, differentiating features are not always present and IHC is very useful to differentiate it from ES/PNET because NBs are consistently positive for NSE and chromogranin and negative for MIC2 and FLI-1. Further RT-PCR for tyrosine hydroxylase and dopa decarboxylase is useful to confirm a diagnosis of neuroblastoma. PNET/ES tumors have been reported to be positive for MIC-2 in 84–100 % of cases. MIC-2 analysis is very helpful in the diagnosis of ES/PNET tumors in FNA biopsy material since it provides a strong positive confirmatory marker for this tumor. However, MIC2 expression is not pathognomonic for ES/PNET. There have been reports of positive staining of some of the other small blue cell malignancies including WT, T-cell lymphoblastic lymphomas, SS, and rhabdomyosarcoma. ES/PNET typically show diffuse and membranous positivity as was seen in the index case in contrast to the other tumors where the staining is focal and weak and predominantly cytoplasmic. Diffuse cytoplasmic staining for MIC-2 in PNET has also been reported in one study. SS show intense cytoplasmic MIC-2 immunoreactivity and can be distinguished by the use of other IHC markers and molecular expression of SYT/SSX translocation. Negative reaction with other generalized markers like LCA, cytokeratin, and connective tissue antigens tends to exclude most other small round cell tumors. Hence, it is necessary to use MIC-2 among a panel of IHC markers and correlate results with clinical features and cytologic findings.

Although immunohistochemistry is an invaluable adjunct which is routinely performed in every diagnostic laboratory, the specificity of molecular markers in the diagnosis of small blue round cell tumors makes their demonstration an attractive alternative option. The value of RT-PCR as an ancillary technique in the FNA diagnosis of small round cell tumors has been recently highlighted. The molecular marker of PNET is the EWS/FLI1 gene fusion, which may be detected from standard cytogenetic studies showing the chromosomal translocation t (11;22)(q24;q12) or by fluorescence in situ hybridization (FISH) or RT-PCR. The variable lengths of the PCR fragments require verification of the specificity of the PCR product to exclude false-positive results owing to nonspecific amplification. This is usually achieved either by DNA sequencing or by hybridization of PCR fragments with specific probes. DNA sequencing of the PCR fragments can confirm the type I transcript in most cases, as this is the most prevalent translocation, joining exon 7 of EWS and exon 6 of FLI-1 (type I) and is reportedly found in 65–75 % of patients. Further, the outcome of tumors with a EWS-FLI-1 type I fusion transcript is better outcome when compared the type II fusion transcript. The use of fine-needle aspirate for molecular analysis has obvious advantages as it provides fresh tumor cells. The problems associated with stored histological paraffin blocks in RT-PCR interpretation like false-positive due to cross contamination and false-negative results due to poor processing of specimens are circumvented. The applicability of RT-PCR on FNA has made it possible to render an accurate diagnosis on aspiration material, thereby obviating the need for an open biopsy or core biopsy.

A-9. (**b**) **The IHC analysis of ER, PR, and HER2 expression has been standardized for formalin-fixed, paraffin-embedded tissue sections.**

The prognostic and therapeutic implications of estrogen receptor (ER), progesterone receptor (PR), and human epidermal growth factor 2 (HER2) status in breast carcinomas are well established. Up to 75 % of primary breast carcinomas express ER, and about 50 % of these tumors coexpress PR. Only a minority of breast carcinomas have no ER or PR expression (20 %), and an even smaller percentage of primary breast carcinomas express PR but not ER (<10 %). HER2 overexpression is present in 20–30 % of breast carcinomas and should be evaluated by immunohistochemistry (IHC) and/or fluorescence in situ hybridization (FISH) according to The American Society of Clinical Oncology and College of American Pathologists (ASCO/CAP) guidelines for all primary breast carcinomas. The routine method for detecting ER and PR expression is IHC, whereas HER2 overexpression can be detected by IHC and/or FISH. The IHC analysis of ER, PR, and HER2 expression has been standardized for formalin-fixed, paraffin-embedded tissue sections. Therefore, accurate detection of these prognostic markers is essential, and consistent results can be achieved by compliance with the ASCO/CAP national guidelines. The guidelines also require validation of HER2 testing by documenting 95 % concordance rates between IHC HER2 positive and IHC HER2 negative with FISH amplified and non-amplified cases, respectively. The detection of these markers on FNA samples has been studied extensively on direct smears, cytospin slides, LB preparations, and CB sections with variable success rates. Cell blocks from aspirates of breast carcinoma should also be processed with a formalin fixative as recommended by the above guidelines; however, if formalin-free fixatives are used in cytology, validation of ER, PR, and HER2 IHC results is very essential before these hormone receptor status results can be used for therapeutic purposes. IHC and FISH methods, which are approved by the US Food and Drug Administration (FDA) for the assessment of breast carcinoma, require tissue samples to be fixed in 10 % neutral-buffered formalin. The use of an ideal fixative for FNA material and the development of optimal processing conditions to preserve antigenicity of tumor cells are however still very essential for the accurate determination of marker status on cell-block preparations and continue to be a subject of ongoing research. Following the current well-established guidelines is crucial; however, all new techniques, including alternative fixatives which may be used in the future, should be validated before they are used for or either diagnostic prognostic purposes.

A-10. (**e**) **All the above statements are false.**

Explanation: Lymph node metastases are common in patients with papillary thyroid carcinoma (PTC), with an incidence as high as 50 %. Many patients have clinically negative nodes on preoperative evaluation and are later found to have central lymph node metastases. Clinical examination may detect lymph node involvement in 15–30 % of patients. However, occult metastases may be observed in up to 90 % of patients. Although the prognosis of PTC is usually favorable, approximately 5–20 % of these patients develop local or regional recurrences after the initial surgery. Different tools have been proposed to identify metastatic lymph nodes at the onset or during the follow-up of thyroid cancer. Among these, whole body scanning with radioiodine, measurement of basal and stimulated serum thyroglobulin (Tg) levels and high-resolution ultrasound, and fine-needle aspiration FNA and FNA-Tg levels have all been studied. Measurements of Tg in the rinse of the aspiration biopsy needle have been proposed for detection of neck lymph node metastasis from PTC in patients after total thyroidectomy and radioiodine ablation.

Tg is a glycoprotein produced only by thyroid follicular cells and is produced by almost all differentiated thyroid cancer tissues. Following total thyroidectomy for thyroid cancer, serum Tg should be undetectable, and any detectable serum Tg indicates neoplastic thyroid foci. The highest sensitivity is attained following thyroid hormone withdrawal or stimulation with recombinant human thyroid-stimulating hormone. Tg is undetectable in 20 % of patients with isolated lymph node metastases during thyroid hormone treatment and in 5 % after thyroid hormone withdrawal. The measurement of Tg levels does not localize neoplastic foci. Ultrasound and US-guided fine-needle aspiration cytology are the most useful techniques for diagnosing nodal metastases. Confirmation of malignancy in lymph nodes with a suspicious sonographic appearance can be achieved by FNA. False-negative FNA results are unavoidable and occur in 6–8 % of cases. These false negatives could be due to the absence of tumor cells in the FNA specimen, cystic changes in metastatic lymph nodes, or partial or focal involvement of the lymph node. Several studies have reported that FNA-Tg identifies PTC metastases of the neck lymph nodes with higher sensitivity and specificity than FNA alone. FNA-Tg level assay is inexpensive and easy to perform on FNA samples reliable even in very small lesions and has a high diagnostic accuracy. Particularly important are the results in the category of atypical/suspicious for PTC recurrence. The cases with Tg levels ≥10 ng/ml usually correlate with a diagnosis of PTC on follow-up.

A-11. (e) **RT-PCR detection of both VEGF mRNA and endostatin mRNA.**

Explanation: To distinguishing metastatic malignant cells from reactive mesothelial cells in body cavity fluid can be very challenging when there are relatively few metastatic cells. Immunocytochemistry can greatly aid in such diagnostic dilemmas, but currently available immunohistochemical markers have varying sensitivity and specificity for mesothelial cells or metastatic carcinomas. False-negative results of cytological examination of body cavity fluids can thus be a serious problem. Recently, RT-PCR techniques have been evaluated for the detection of cancer cells in pleural effusion of patients with lung cancer. Diagnosis of pleural effusions of patients with lung cancer by means of detecting tumor marker mRNA in occult lung cancer cells has also been reported. Vascular endothelial growth factor (VEGF) is an angiogenic growth factor which plays a role in the formation of pleural effusions from patients with lung cancer and has proved to be a useful marker in detecting malignancies. Although many known angiogenesis inducing factors, including VEGF and tumor necrosis factor alpha, are present in the pleural fluid. Anti-angiogenic factors, such as endostatin in pleural effusions, have also been found to be useful in detecting metastatic disease in pleural fluids. Endostatin is an angiogenesis inhibitor that is an endogenously produced proteolytic fragment of type XVIII collagen. Both angiogenic factors and angiogenesis inhibitors are likely contributors to the formation of effusion in the pleural space. When combinations of VEGF mRNA and endostatin mRNA are evaluated together, they can yield a sensitivity of 95.7 % and accuracy of 93.8 % for detecting pleural micrometastases. Earlier diagnosis of malignant pleural effusions thus may be established by detecting VEGF mRNA and endostatin mRNA by RT-PCR when used in a combination.

A-12. (d) **FISH analysis for IGH/BCL2 and MYC translocations is not helpful in diagnosing this entity. This is incorrect since these translocations can be detected by FISH analysis.**

B-cell lymphomas exhibiting both *IGH*/*BCL2* and *MYC* rearrangements are termed dual-translocation or double-hit lymphomas (DTL). They are characterized by complex karyotypes accompanied by a highly aggressive behavior, followed by a poor prognosis. The morphologic and immunophenotypic spectrum of DTL overlaps with Burkitt's lymphoma (BL) and diffuse large B-cell lymphoma (DLBCL). They are currently categorized as B-cell lymphoma, unclassifiable, with features intermediate between DLBCL and BL (U-DLBCL/BL). The most common cytomorphologic features that are noted on cytologic examination of DTL are a predominance of large cells with centroblastic nuclear features and dark-blue (basophilic) cytoplasm, followed by presence of apoptotic bodies and marked nuclear pleomorphism. The prevalence of dual translocation in B-cell lymphoma may be difficult to detect for two main reasons. First, the diagnosis may be difficult, because only recently have a few series provided detailed clinical and histopathologic descriptions of this entity and the features required for a diagnosis based on criteria defined by the World Health Organization (WHO) classification. Second, well-documented dual translocation is also reported sometimes in morphologically typical DLBCL and even in follicular lymphomas. In these samples that lack any morphologic trigger for testing, investigation of *MYC* and *BCL2* translocation usually has been initiated only because of unusual clinical behavior.

Although DTL is unusual, cases will eventually be encountered by a cytopathologist who routinely diagnoses lymphoma samples, and the clinical opportunity for a more aggressive treatment will be missed unless appropriate investigations are initiated. Preceding or concurrent surgical pathology specimens may reveal features of conventional DLBCL or even follicular lymphomas, and cytology samples, such as fluids like cerebrospinal fluid, may provide the only material for diagnosis. Hence, a cytomorphologic picture of large cells with deeply basophilic cytoplasm, cytoplasmic vacuoles, and frequent segmented nuclei, particularly in fine-needle aspiration smears and especially in patients with clinically aggressive and/or unusual clinical features, should trigger FISH analysis for *IGH*/*BCL2* and *MYC* translocations to identify DTL.

A-13. (**c**) **KRAS mutation may be a predictor for resistance to TKIs therapy in patients with NSCLC and a prognostic marker, although it is still controversial whether KRAS can predict resistance to TKIs.**

Targeted therapy in lung cancer is currently used on patients with non-small cell lung cancers (NSCLC) and mutations in epidermal growth factor receptor (EGFR). EGFR is a transmembrane receptor protein with an extracellular binding domain and a cytoplasmic tyrosine kinase domain. Ligand binding with transforming growth factor α (TGF-α) and epidermal growth factor (EGF) results in autophosphorylation of key tyrosine residues in the receptor cytoplasmic domain and further activation of downstream signaling events that trigger antiapoptosis, cell proliferation, angiogenesis, tumor invasion, and metastasis. Malignant cells with EGFR mutations possess a growth advantage over those with wild-type EGFR but also show increased sensitivity to the anti-EGFR tyrosine kinase inhibitors (TKIs). TKIs (gefitinib and erlotinib) that can block ligand binding have produced favorable treatment responses in patients who have advanced NSCLC with mutated EGFR. In addition, the presence of EGFR mutations can be used as a prognostic factor. EGFR mutations are most common in lung adenocarcinoma. The mutation frequencies vary among ethnic groups and are seen more commonly in Asians (20–40 %) than among Caucasians (5–20 %). Mutations in EGFR exons 18–21 occur in the majority, and these are usually deletions in exon 19 and point mutations in exon 21. Another marker frequently tested in patients with NSCLC is Kristen-Rous sarcoma virus (KRAS) gene. KRAS mutation may also be a predictor for resistance to TKIs therapy in patients with NSCLC and a prognostic marker. Although it is still controversial whether KRAS can predict resistance to TKIs. A major challenge in evaluating TKI treatment efficacy in patients with advanced NSCLC is the complexity of EGFR and KRAS mutations, which vary by ethnicity, sex, and smoking history. Resistance to TKI therapy is also associated with new mutations. Therefore, assessment of EGFR and KRAS status in patients with NSCLC is crucial to determine the benefits of targeted therapies using TKI. With the increased use of endobronchial ultrasound-guided (EBUS) biopsy for staging and diagnosis of lung cancer, EBUS FNA cytology specimens may be the only tissue source for diagnosis and molecular testing. If routine cytology specimens could be used more often, then more invasive procedures performed to obtain sufficient tumor tissue for molecular testing can be reduced or avoided.

A-14. (**d**) Samples with sparse cellularity (<500 tumor cells) have a higher PCR failure rate to detect gene mutations. This statement is false since the data indicates that only samples with sparse cellularity (<300 tumor cells) have a higher PCR failure rate to detect these gene mutations. This can happen when only a few passes from a fine-needle aspiration with relatively limited material are collected and may result in suboptimal material for molecular testing.

Clinical validity of using cytology specimens for molecular testing has been studied using cytology specimens, mainly smears and cell-block material, in lung cancer patients for molecular testing to detect epidermal growth factor receptor (EGFR) and Kristen-Rous sarcoma virus (KRAS) gene mutations. An overall high efficiency using cytology specimens for molecular testing to detect EGFR or KRAS mutation in lung cancer patients has also been observed. The use of routinely processed cytology specimens (including EBUS, CT, and US-guided fine-needle aspirations) for molecular testing has also been validated in a recent study. It has also been shown that the two major cytology preparations, smears and cell block, are equally good for molecular testing. The data indicates that only samples with sparse cellularity (<300 tumor cells) have a higher PCR failure rate to detect these gene mutations. This can happen when only a few passes from a fine-needle aspiration with relatively limited material are collected and may result in suboptimal material for molecular testing. It has been noted that no significant difference in the mutation rates between samples obtained by cytology versus histology occur. Good correlations between cytology classifications and the frequencies of EGFR and KRAS mutations have also been identified in cytology samples. The highest and lowest mutation rates of EGFR have been observed in adenocarcinoma and squamous carcinoma, respectively. EGFR exons 19 and 21 are most frequently detected in cytology samples, accounting for 65 % of mutations in the tested EGFR exons. KRAS mutations in exon 1 (codons 21 and 13) are predominant. In addition, EGFR and KRAS mutations are also found to be mutually exclusive. In summary, clinical utilization of routine cytology specimens, including EBUS, CT/US fine-needle aspirations are a reliable source for molecular testing to detect EGFR or KRAS mutations in lung cancer patients.

A-15. (**e**) In cryopreservation, potential benefit of preserving viability is not maintained. This is a false statement, since with cryopreservation, there is not only preservation of morphology and nucleic acids, but there is the potential additional benefit of preserving viability as well. Banking of cryopreserved cytology specimens could be an important cost-effective asset in the development of molecular diagnostics using cytologic specimens.

Frozen-tissue banks are now recognized as crucial resources for the future growth of clinical molecular test development. The feasibility of prospectively banking cytology specimens has been evaluated on a limited basis. The major utility of developing such a resource would be the preservation of diseased cell types that would not be available for research or clinical testing by other means. Certain conditions and cell types, such as metastatic disease and premalignant tumors, may only ever be sampled via aspiration cytology. Translational research and molecular test development in these areas would be greatly facilitated if there were protocols set in place for banking fine-needle aspiration (FNA) specimens. One recent study has tested whether cryopreservation of patient FNA specimens could serve as a suitable method for banking diagnostic material for future nucleic acid-based molecular testing. It primarily focused on the quality of RNA that could be recovered from such specimens because RNA is the nucleic acid most susceptible to degradation. To maximize the number of molecular testing applications using RNA, a high level of RNA integrity is most desirable. DNA integrity was not evaluated here, but in general, it is much more resistant to degradation than RNA. The findings of this study can be summarized as follows. To maximize RNA integrity (high-quality RNA), devitalization time (Td) should be kept to 6 h or less and post-aspiration processing time (Tp) to 1 h or less. For the majority of clinically obtained FNA samples, this can be done easily. Conversely, the amount of time samples are frozen (tested up to 27 weeks) does not seem to affect the quality of the RNA recovered. Third, the presence of cellular necrosis associated with the sample appears to decrease the overall quality of RNA recovered. In further support of this interpretation, it was observed that all samples with >30 % necrosis had associated RNA degradation. Finally, the evaluation of the morphological characteristics of cryopreserved FNAs showed that while there were some occasional artifactual changes in morphology, the ability to identify diseased versus non diseased cell types can be maintained. This is important because it permits the use of purification processes that depend on visual identification of cells, such as laser-capture microdissection. In conclusion, with cryopreservation, there is not only preservation of morphology and nucleic acids, but there is the potential additional benefit of preserving viability as well. Banking of cryopreserved cytology specimens could be an important cost-effective asset in this development of molecular diagnostics.

A-16. (**c**) **Cytokeratin 5/6 and p63.**
These two stains when used in combination are very helpful in identifying myoepithelial cells within atypical epithelial groups of cells in breast aspirates. The presence of myoepithelial cells in breast aspirates is generally indicative of a benign lesion rather than a malignant tumor.

The National Cancer Institute (NCI) has a recommended classification for breast fine-needle aspirations. There are five categories identified in this classification: benign, atypical, suspicious, malignant, or unsatisfactory. In proliferative breast lesions with or without atypia, the recommended category is atypical. About 30–45 % of breast fine-needle aspiration cytology specimens are diagnosed as atypical and later are found to be malignant or atypical ductal lesions on histologic follow-up. In addition, studies have also shown a variable rate of sensitivity (82.5–98.2 %), specificity (77.4–100 %), and accuracy (79–97 %) of breast fine-needle aspiration cytology for diagnosing tumors. The limited ability of breast fine-needle aspirates to distinguish proliferative breast lesions such as atypical ductal hyperplasia (ADH), ductal carcinoma in situ (DCIS), and low-grade invasive carcinoma, coupled with the lack of uniformity in the reporting of breast fine-needle aspirations, have contributed to the emergence of core needle biopsy of breast lesions as a preferred diagnostic modality. Immunohistochemical staining may be helpful in further classifying these breast aspiration cases with atypical findings. Cytokeratin (CK) 5/6, a specific high-molecular weight cytokeratin, is present in myoepithelial cells of benign breast parenchyma. Benign ductal epithelial hyperplasia originates from committed stem cells that are CK5/6-positive cells, whereas malignant proliferations lack CK5/6 immunohistochemical expression. Therefore, assessing CK5/6 expression by immunohistochemistry might minimize the false-negative and false-positive diagnoses. Another marker for myoepithelial cells is p63, which is a nuclear stain. This may also help in assessing atypical breast lesions. Hence, CK 5/6 and p63 immunohistochemical staining can be a useful diagnostic adjunct to differentiate benign from malignant epithelial proliferations in breast fine-needle aspiration specimens.

A-17. (e) **All the above statements are false.**
Explanation: Papillary thyroid carcinoma (PTC) is the most common malignancy of the thyroid gland (80 % of all thyroid cancers). Recent research has shown that over 80 % of PTC have a somatic genetic alteration, which include BRAF gene mutations, RET gene mutations, RET/PTC rearrangements, and RAS mutations. These mutations also appear to be mutually exclusive. BRAF gene mutations have been reported in 50–80 % of PTC, the most prevalent genetic alteration encountered in PTC. The most frequent BRAF genetic alteration is a point mutation involving the substitution of thymine, 1799th nucleotide at 15th BRAF exon with adenine (T1799A). The latter refers to coding changes in codon 600 and causes the production of glutamate instead of valine (V600E). This oncogenic mutation results in the activation of the mitogen-activated protein kinase signaling pathway and the malignant transformation of follicular cells. Although it has been reported in tumors of other organs, BRAF mutation involving V600E is highly specific for PTC among other primary thyroid neoplasms. The BRAF V600E point mutation has not been reported in any follicular carcinoma, adenoma, or benign thyroid nodule. In addition, the presence of BRAF mutation has also been associated with aggressive tumor characteristics, such as extra-thyroidal extension, lymph node involvement, resistance to radioactive iodide, and tumor recurrence. Therefore, the detection of BRAF V600E mutation, using fine-needle aspiration (FNA) biopsy material, would not only assist preoperative diagnosis of PTC but also provide prognostic implications to guide subsequent patient management. Approximately 60–70 % of thyroid nodules which undergo fine needle aspiration are classified as benign, whereas 4–10 % of nodules are malignant. The remaining 20–30 % present equivocal findings, which are not diagnostic of either a benign nodule or malignancy. The new Bethesda system for the classification of thyroid FNA, cases that are classified as "atypia of undetermined significance" or "suspicious," have a risk of malignancy of 10–15 % and 60–70 %, respectively. The current guidelines recommend repeat FNA for patients with a diagnosis of "atypia of undetermined significance" and lobectomy with or without intraoperative consultation for those with a "suspicious" diagnosis. However, intraoperative analysis of frozen sections does not always provide a definitive diagnosis. As a result, there may be significant management ramifications, ranging from delaying any necessary surgery to avoiding more definitive initial surgical treatment. BRAF V600E point mutation thus may be very helpful in identification of PTC preoperatively. In a recent study, 84 and 17 % of positive and equivocal (both indeterminate and suspicious) cases were found to have mutated BRAF, respectively. In addition, the combination of cytology and molecular analysis positively identified 80.0 % of PTCs preoperatively, which is a 26 % increase in the number of correctly identified PTC when compared with cytologic diagnosis alone.

A-18. (d) **Utilizing MACS with anti-CD14 and anti-CD16 antibody beads does not deplete macrophages and neutrophils.**
This statement is not true since MACS does lead to enrichment of bronchial epithelial cells in sputum cytology samples.

Sputum cytology specimens comprise of exfoliated epithelial cells from the bronchial tree and have been considered diagnostic material for diagnosing lung cancers. Morphologic analysis of sputum by cytology has been used for the early diagnosis of lung cancer, particularly squamous cell carcinoma and small-cell carcinoma. However, the sensitivity for it is very low, because sputum cytology depends mainly on both the skills of the person collecting the specimen as well as the cytopathologist interpreting the cytology sample. Bronchial epithelial cells may be limited in number in sputum samples; hence, cytocentrifuge slides are needed to have enough bronchial epithelial cells to be analyzed, making sputum cytology very labor-intensive and time-consuming. Instead of observing morphologic characterization by cytology, molecular genetic study of sputum could identify the cells containing tumor-related genetic aberrations, which occur in microscopically normal-appearing epithelium and are specific signs of the progression of tumorigenesis. A study has found that the combined assessment of deletions of both *HYAL2* and *FHIT* tumor suppressor genes could detect abnormal cells not only in all the cytologically positive sputum but also in 55 % cytologically negative sputum from lung cancer patients, suggesting that testing for genetic aberrations in sputum samples could be more sensitive than cytology in identifying cancer cells. Therefore, molecular genetic studies might overcome the limitation of sputum cytology and detect genetically abnormal cells that may not be detected on cytologic examination, providing a potential diagnostic tool for early-stage lung cancer. The use of sputum for molecular genetic analyses can be limited by its cellular heterogeneity, which includes about 1 % bronchial epithelial cells. The large excess of macrophages and neutrophils that account for >95 % sputum cell population can obscure detection and quantitation of neoplastic changes occurring in the bronchial epithelial cells. Therefore, enrichment of bronchial epithelial cells before the actual detection procedure can improve the efficiency and accuracy of genetic and cytologic diagnosis of lung cancer in sputum samples. Magnetic cell sorting (MACS) is a process of immunomagnetic cell selection based on the recognition of cell-specific antibodies coupled to magnetic beads. MACS has been developed to specifically separate rare circulating tumor cells from whole blood for predicting recurrence in patients with solid cancers. Concentrated and purified bronchial epithelial cells from sputum thus may improve diagnosis of lung cancer in sputum samples. A study has been done utilizing MACS with anti-CD14 and anti-CD16 antibody beads to specifically deplete macrophage and neutrophils and enrich bronchial epithelial cells from sputum of stage I NSCLC patients, cancer-free heavy smokers, and healthy nonsmokers. The enriched sputum was analyzed by using fluorescence in situ hybridization (FISH) for the detection of genetic deletion of *FHIT*. This study demonstrates that the MACS enrichment for bronchial epithelial cells could average 36-fold over the original sputum in one step, yielding at least 2.3×10^5 cells with >40 % purity per sample. Furthermore, the enrichment for respiratory epithelial cells could increase the diagnostic value of sputum and efficiency of genetic and cytology analysis of lung cancer. MACS is a simple and fast enrichment strategy, because it simultaneously depletes macrophages and neutrophils, while enriching exfoliated bronchial cells in a single process, decreasing the time consumption to less than 1 h. Finally, the MACS strategy is a relatively inexpensive and high-throughput enrichment procedure that could easily be available and accessible in many clinical settings. This study demonstrated that the detection of *FHIT* aberrations in the enriched sputum produced higher sensitivity compared with unprocessed sputum, implying that the enrichment could improve the accuracy of genetic diagnosis of lung cancer in sputum samples. The MACS does not alter the structure, function, or activity status of enriched cells, which, therefore, could also have the potential to be used for analysis of other forms of biomarkers in the early detection of lung cancer.

A-19. **(d) *BRAF* V600E mutation is identified in 100 % of fine-needle aspirates from metastatic melanomas.**

This statement is not true since only 38.6 % of the metastatic melanoma cases in a recent study were able to identify this mutation on aspirate samples.

Metastatic malignant melanoma is incurable in the majority of patients with current therapeutic options. Several agents targeted at different points in signaling pathways of cell proliferation and melanoma progression have been tested with very limited success. One of the most important phenomenon in the development of melanoma is the activation of the RAS-RAF-mitogen-activated protein kinase (MAPK) pathway. RAS-regulated kinases, encoded by *BRAF*, mediate cell growth and malignant transformation. Sorafenib is the first oral multi-kinase inhibitor to be developed that targets and inhibits Raf kinases (RAF-1, wild-type BRAF, and BRAF V600E) and has demonstrated antitumor effects in metastatic renal cell carcinoma. If the response to RAF kinase inhibition is dependent on the presence of an activated BRAF protein, it will be necessary to evaluate cases of malignant melanoma for the presence or absence of *BRAF* mutations. In a recent study, *BRAF* V600E mutation in fine-needle aspirates from metastatic melanomas was evaluated. The results showed that 38.6 % of metastatic melanomas possess this type of somatic mutation. The presence of *BRAF* V600E mutation did not correlate to any of the cytological cell types. In addition, the melanoma cases with a *BRAF* V600E mutation had a tendency for a shorter time for developing metastatic disease compared to those cases without mutation. Moreover, comparison of histologic corresponding primary tumors revealed that melanomas with *BRAF* V600E tended to acquire metastatic potential at lower Clark's invasion level and lower thickness. This may indicate that assessing the *BRAF* V600E mutation in melanomas can add prognostic information to the traditional markers such as tumor thickness and invasion level. Mutated tumors may thus have a more aggressive clinical course because such melanomas metastasize at an earlier stage.

A-20. **(b) The test can be performed on cytologic samples that have been stored from 5 to 15 years.**
A recent study utilized samples which were stored from <1 to 7 years. This time frame has been currently found to be true.

Tumors with an unknown primary represent 4–5 % of all new cancers in the United States and the primary site of the tumor cannot be identified, even after an extensive clinical workup. This workup is costly and includes imaging tests, laboratory tests, and immunohistochemical (IHC) stains for specific tumor sites. Identifying the tissue of origin in patients with these unknown primary tumors is essential for determining the best therapeutic approach since it has been shown that patients who receive a primary tumor diagnosis have longer survival rates when compared with those who don't. Cell blocks prepared from cytologic body fluid specimens such as pleural, peritoneal, or pericardial fluids are often the first pathologic specimen received for clinical evaluation. These cell blocks are often used to provide a diagnosis of malignancy and to identify the primary site. The challenges associated with identifying a tissue of origin have led to the emergence of molecular-based assays for this purpose. The main molecular approaches used are gene expression microarrays and polymerase chain reaction (PCR) assays, which are the bases of several commercially available assays. The Pathwork Tissue of Origin Test (Pathwork Diagnostics, Redwood City, CA) is a microarray-based gene expression test that uses the expression levels of 2,000 genes to classify tumors by similarity scores (SS) into 15 sites of origin. Because the median survival time for patients with malignant effusions is <6 months, the ability to use cell blocks from body fluids with molecular tests that aid in identifying the primary tumor site of metastatic carcinoma can be valuable in selecting appropriate therapy. A recent study evaluated the use of cell blocks from body fluids as a specimen type for the Pathwork Tissue of Origin Test. Seventeen body fluid specimens of known origin were processed with the Tissue of Origin Test, and the accurate tissue of origin was predicted in 94.1 % of cases that met specimen entry criteria. This study found that in order to obtain an accurate result with cytologic specimens on the Pathwork test, it is important for the analyzed specimen to be non-necrotic, with abundant tumor content (>60 %) and few inflammatory cells or mesothelial cells. This highlights the importance of correctly qualifying the percentage of tumor cells in a given specimen before performing gene expression analysis with microarrays. Although in this study all SS values were reported, in clinical practice, Pathwork Diagnostics does not report scores >5 and <20 because concordance with the tissue of origin in specimens with those scores is poor and thus scores within this range should not be used for clinical management. However, values <5 have been reported to be useful for ruling out possible sites of origin. The results of the current study indicate that cell blocks from cytology specimens yield RNA of acceptable quantity and quality with which to perform a microarray assay such as the Tissue of Origin Test. The samples were stored from <1 to 7 years, indicating that sample age does not adversely affect the results of this assay.

Reading List

Clark DP. Molecular diagnostics on thyroid fine-needle aspirations: the pathway to value creation. Cancer Cytopathol. 2010;118(1):14–6.

Khalbuss WE, Monaco SE, Pantanowitz L. Chapter 7: Cytology techniques & ancillary studies in non-gynecological cytopathology. In: The ASCP quick compendium (QC) of cytopathology. Chicago: ASCP Press; 2013. p. 84–111.

Krishnamurthy S. Applications of molecular techniques to fine-needle aspiration biopsy. Cancer. 2007;111(2):106–22.

Rimm DL. New technologies and the future of cytopathology. ASC Bulletin. 2004;41(6):104–7.

Salto-Tellez M, Koay ESC. Molecular diagnostic cytopathology: definitions, scope and clinical utility. Cytopathology. 2004;15:252–5.

ERRATUM TO

Lung Cytopathology (Bronchial and Aspiration Cytology)

Qing Kay Li and Walid E. Khalbuss

W.E. Khalbuss, Q.K. Li (eds.), *Diagnostic Cytopathology Board Review and Self-Assessment*, DOI 10.1007/978-1-4939-1477-7_1, © Springer Science+Business Media New York 2015

DOI 10.1007/978-1-4939-1477-7_14

The below figures were missed in chapter 1. Please find the new figures.

The online version of the original chapter can be found at http://dx.doi.org/10.1007/978-1-4939-1477-7_1

Q.K. Li, MD, PhD (✉)
Department of Pathology, The Johns Hopkins University School of Medicine, The Johns Hopkins Bayview Medical Center, 4940 Eastern Avenue, AA Building, Room 154B, Baltimore, MD 21224-2780, USA
e-mail: qli23@jhmi.edu

W.E. Khalbuss, MD, PhD, FIAC
Department of Pathology, GE Clarient Diagnostic Services, 31 Columbia, Aliso Viejo, California, 92656, USA
e-mail: Walid.khalbuss@ge.com

W.E. Khalbuss, Q.K. Li (eds.), *Diagnostic Cytopathology Board Review and Self-Assessment*, DOI 10.1007/978-1-4939-1477-7_14, © Springer Science+Business Media New York 2015

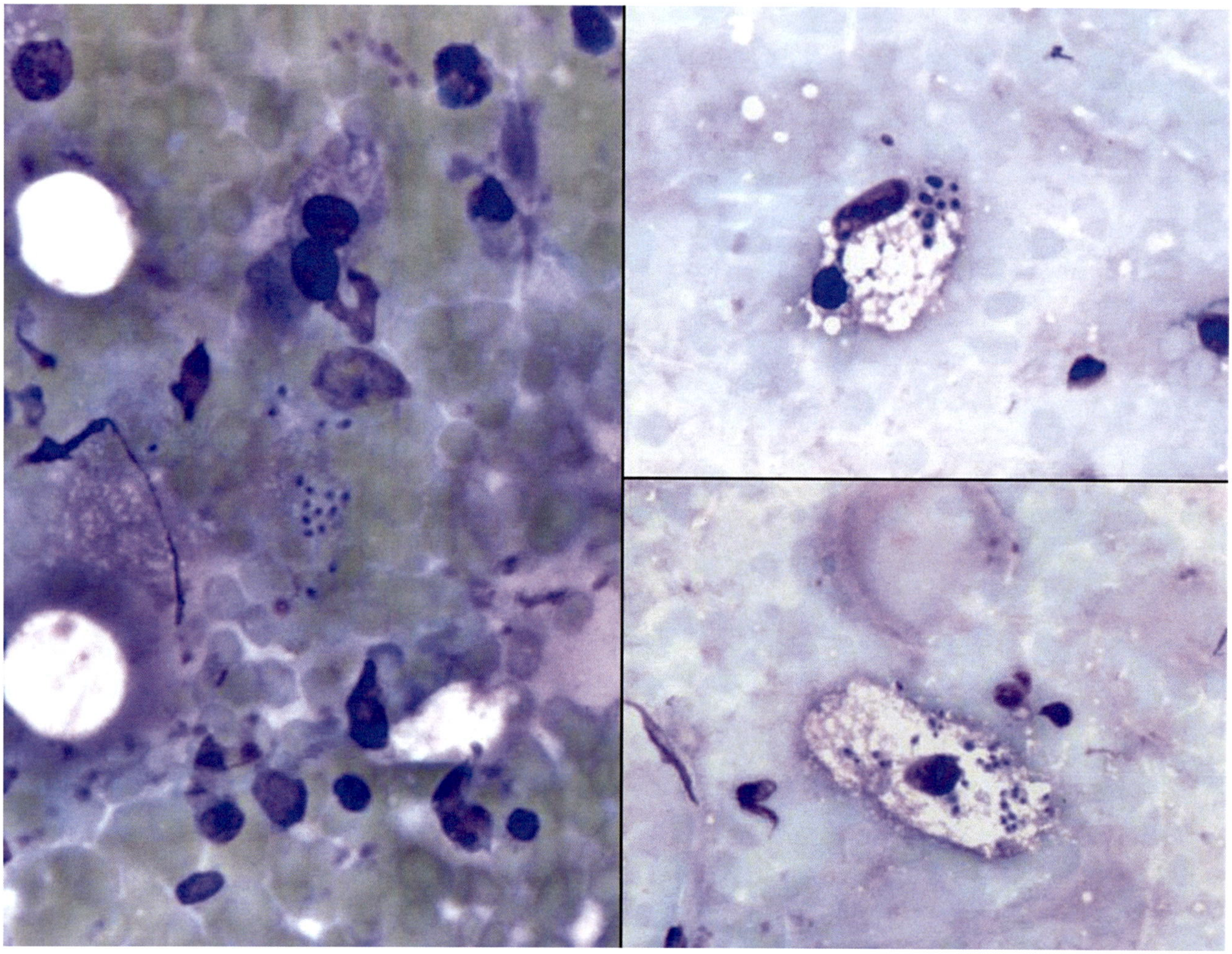

Fig. 1.9

Fig. 1.10

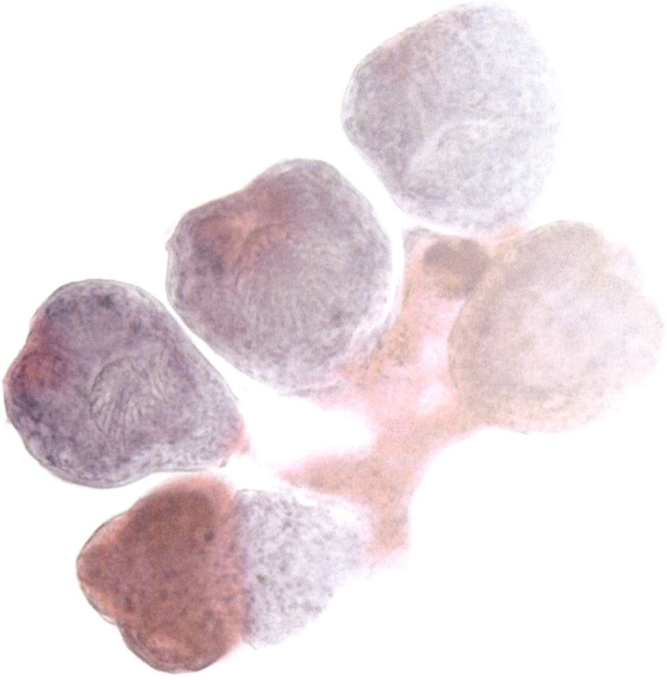

Fig. 1.11

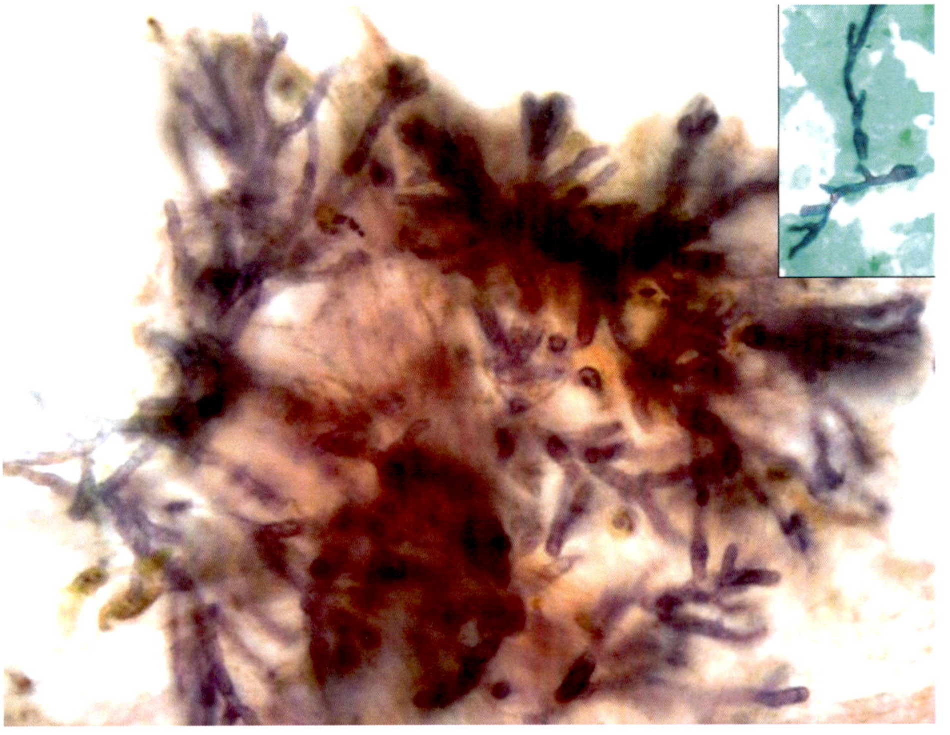

Fig. 1.12

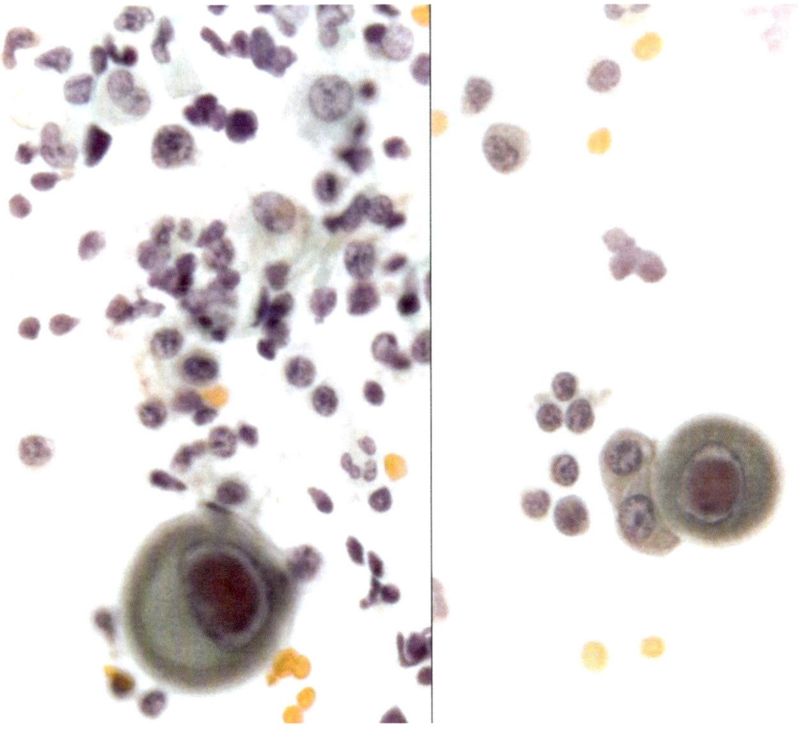

Fig. 1.13

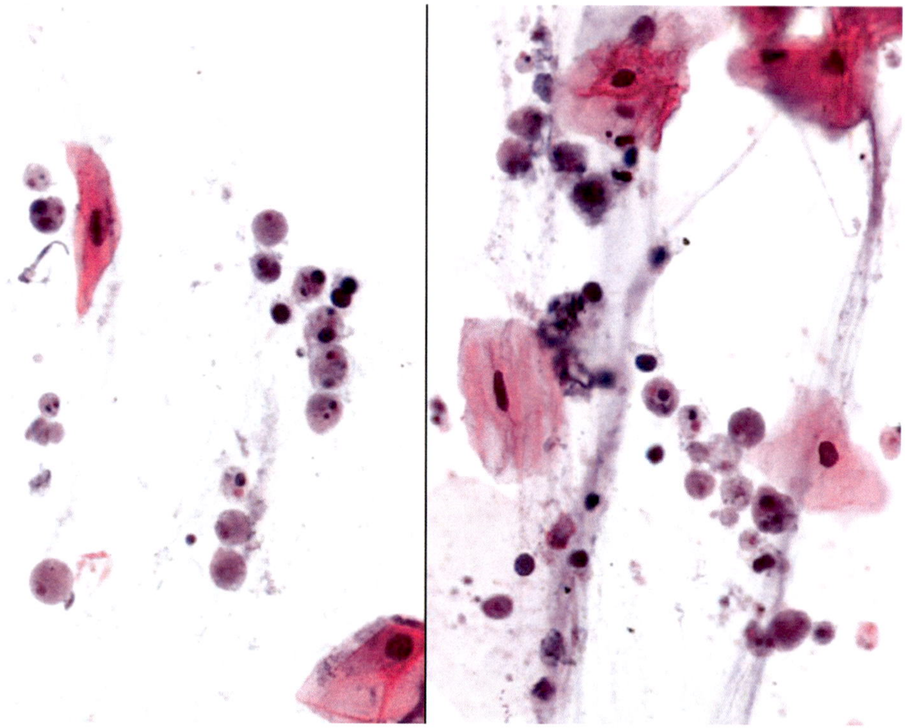

Fig. 1.14

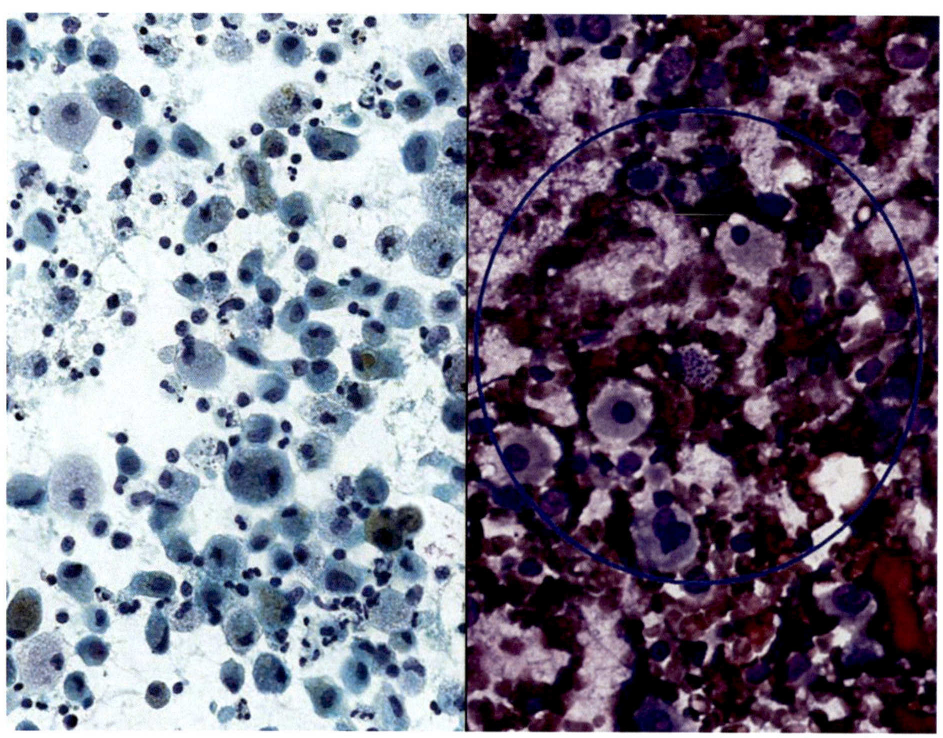

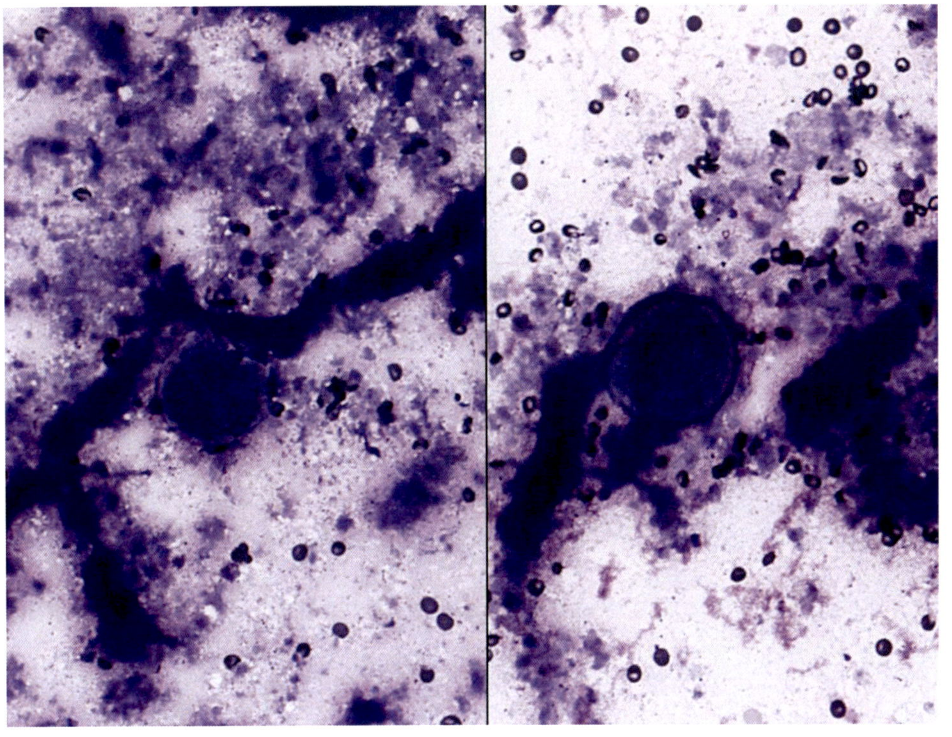

Fig. 1.15

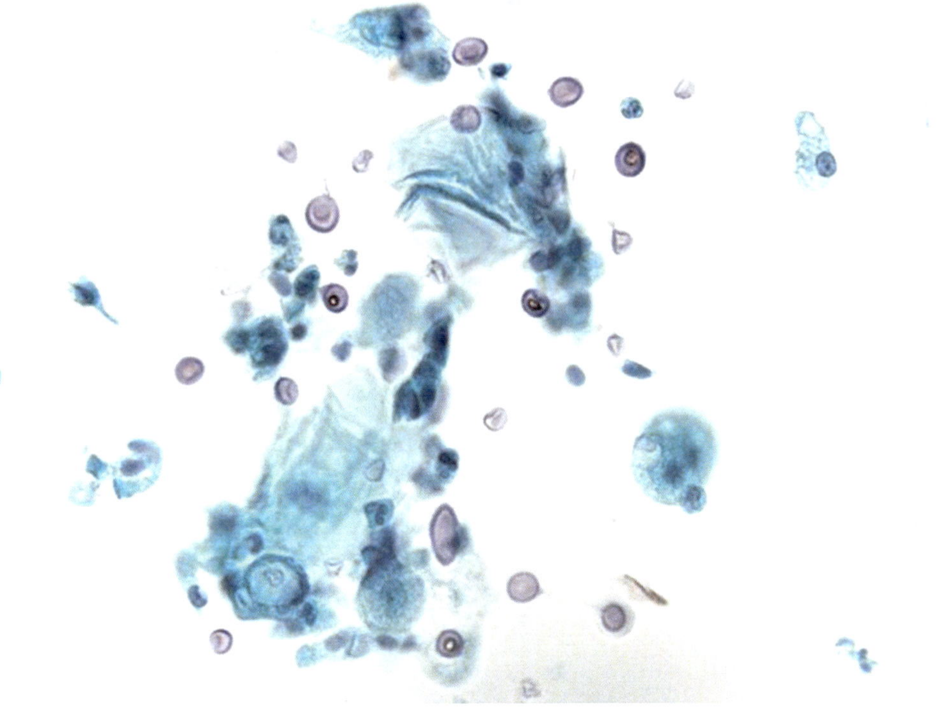

Fig. 1.16

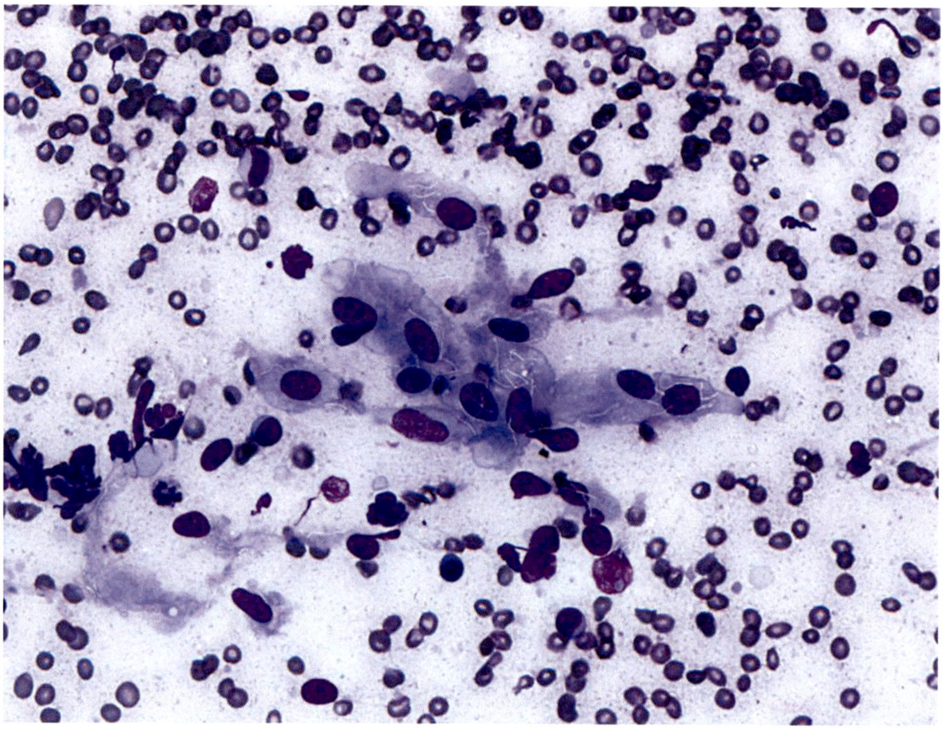

Fig. 1.17

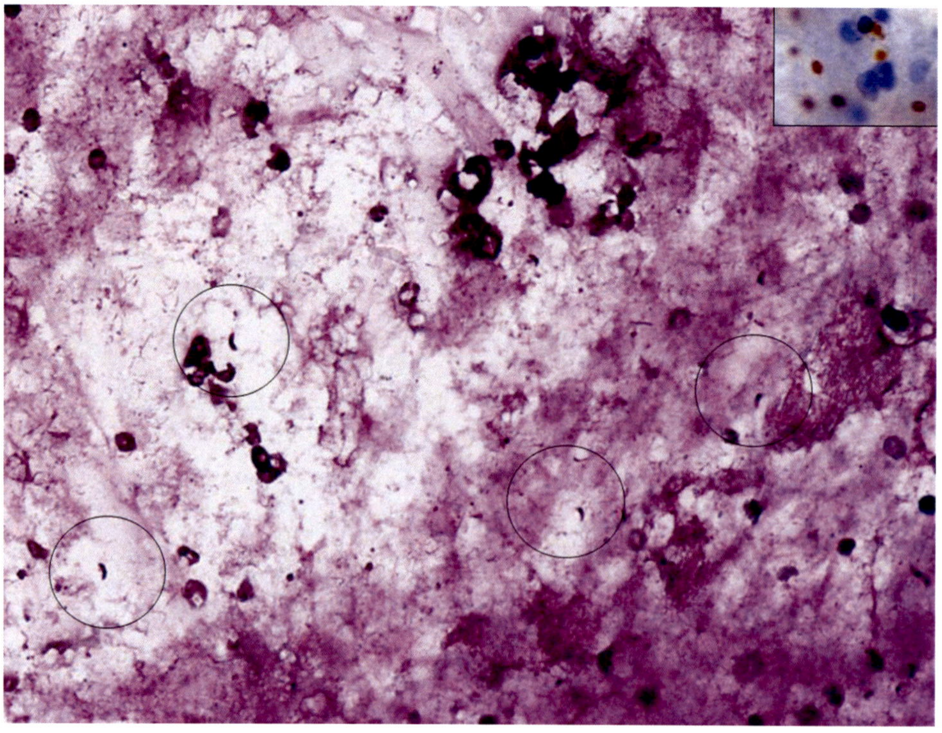

Fig. 1.18

Fig. 1.19

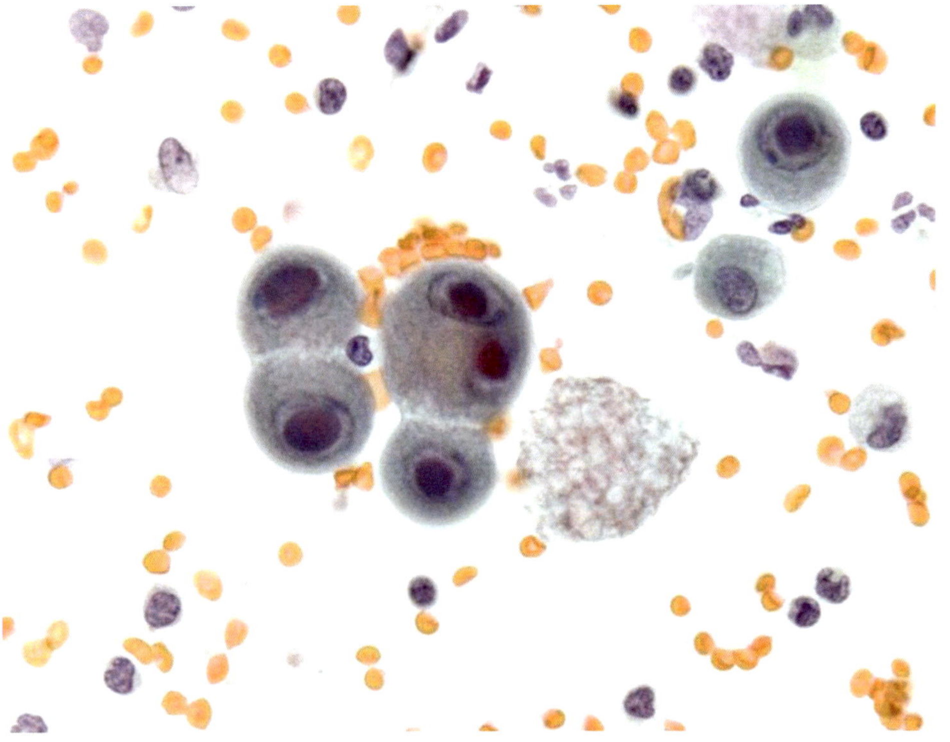

Fig. 1.20

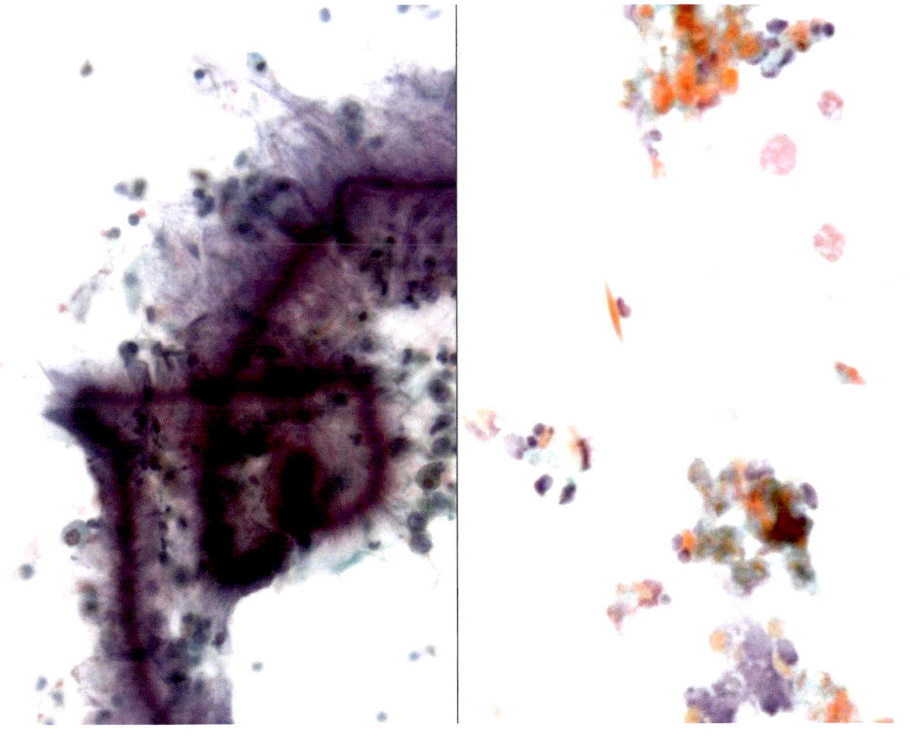

Index

A

Abundant granular cytoplasm, 604, 616–617
Abundant granular myxoid, 704, 714
Acellular matrix material, 403
Acinic cell carcinoma (ACC), 472
  abundant vacuolated cytoplasm, 397, 407
  bland small cells, 397, 400, 407, 408
  cellular with neoplastic acinar cells, 357, 403
  glandular structures and single cells, 493, 517
  naked nuclei and cytoplasmic debris, 378, 405
  pancreaticoblastoma, 515, 520
  salivary gland neoplasms, 357, 403
Actinomysis, 432, 459
Acute bacterial meningitis, 206, 230
Acute cystitis, 627, 661
Acute meningitis, 220, 237
Acute myeloid leukemia (AML), 223, 237
Acute suppurative lymphadenitis, 321, 345
Adenocarcinoma(s)
  adenoma/adenocarcinoma, 404, 553, 566
  biopsy specimen, bone lesion with metastatic, 86, 109
  brushing cytology, 558, 570
  cell block preparation, 26, 27, 28, 97
  colonic, 552, 565
  with cytoplasmic mucin, 25, 97
  Diff-Quik stain, 29, 52, 54, 97–98, 101–102
  duct, 514, 519
  dyscohesive individual cells, 554, 566
  esophagus-gastric junction, 557, 567
  FNA, 559, 571–572
  granular, 480, 516
  hepatoid type, 511, 518
  hyperchromatic cells, 544, 545, 564
  jaundice patient, 543, 563
  with lepidic growth pattern, 87, 111, 117
  with micropapillary and/lepidic growth pattern, 90, 118
  moderately differentiated, 474, 484, 488, 508, 516–518
  with mucinous features, 38, 99
  mucinous noncystic (*see* Mucinous noncystic adenocarcinoma)
  papanicolaou preparation, 40, 41, 47, 53, 71, 99, 100, 101, 105
  poorly differentiated, 42, 88, 99, 113–114, 487, 509, 517, 518
  prominent nucleoli, 558, 570
  undifferentiated, 492, 517
  well-differentiated, 24, 97, 491, 507, 514, 517, 518, 519
Adenoid cystic carcinoma
  basaloid cells and matrix globules, 402, 410
  basaloid neoplasm, 404
  perineural invasion, 402, 409
  pleomorphic adenoma, 408
  submandibular gland, 362, 403
  three-dimensions, 362, 403
  Warthin tumor and mucoepidermoid carcinoma, 401, 409
Adenomatoid nodules, 255, 258, 293
Adenosquamous carcinoma, 481, 516
Adrenal cortical adenoma, 592, 609
Adrenal cortical carcinoma, 593, 603, 610, 614
Adrenal FNAs
  components, 576
  neoplastic conditions, 576–577
ALCL. *See* Anaplastic large cell lymphoma (ALCL)
ALK-positive large B-cell lymphoma, 342, 353
Alveolar macrophages
  abundant, 86, 109
  and amorphous/foamy material, 93
  and curschmann spirals, 86, 108
  degenerated, 51, 101
Alveolar proteinosis
  amorphous material, 93
  coarsely granular eosinophilic to cyanophilic debris, 92
  idiopathic disease, 88, 114
Alveolar rhabdomyosarcoma, 698, 712
Alveolar soft part sarcoma, 707, 717–718
AML. *See* Angiomyolipoma (AML)
Anaplastic carcinoma
  keratins, 279, 300
  neutrophilic cannibalism, 278, 299
  pleomorphic cells, 279, 300
  sarcomas, 279, 300
  tumor cells, 278, 299
  UC, 278, 299
  visceral metastases, 279, 300
Anaplastic large cell lymphoma (ALCL)
  FNA, axillary neoplasm, 327, 345
  lymphoglandular bodies, 338, 349
  T-cell lymphomas, 338, 348–349
Anaplastic lymphomakinase (ALK)
  EML4-ALK, 86, 90, 108, 117
  non-small cell lung carcinoma, 90, 117
Ancillary testing, 679, 709
Angiolipomas, 682, 710
Angiomyolipoma (AML), 452, 464, 584, 607
Angiosarcoma, 705, 716
Aseptic meningitis, 206, 231
Aspergillosis
  allergic bronchopulmonary, 14, 94
  calcium oxalate crystals, 14, 94
  characterization, 87, 99, 111
  conidial forms, 14, 94
  immunocytochemistry, 14, 94
  invasive pulmonary, 14, 94
Asthma, 23, 96–97
Astrocytoma, 220, 236

W.E. Khalbuss, Q.K. Li (eds.), *Diagnostic Cytopathology Board Review and Self-Assessment*,
DOI 10.1007/978-1-4939-1477-7, © Springer Science+Business Media New York 2015

Atypia of undetermined significance/follicular lesion of undetermined significance (AUS/FLUS)
Atypical lipomatous tumor, 684, 710

B
Bacillary angiomatosis, 707, 718
Bacillus Calmette-Guerin (BCG) therapy, 657, 668
Barrett mucosa
  dysplasia, 559, 572
  glandular cells, 559, 571
  high-grade dysplasia, adenocarcinoma, 559, 572
Bartonella henselae infection, 707, 718
B-cell lymphoma
  c-Myc immunohistochemical stain, 340, 351
  CNS tumor, 217, 235
  EBV, 217, 235
  metastatic carcinoma, 208, 231
  predominant of CD20+ cells, 657, 667
BCG therapy. *See* Bacillus Calmette-Guerin (BCG) therapy
Beckwith–Wiedmann Syndrome, 515, 520
Benign bile duct epithelial cells, 446, 452, 461, 463, 464
Benign biliary epithelium
  columnar epithelial cells, 510, 518
  honey comb pattern, 505, 518
Benign glandular cells
  bland basal nuclei, 557, 567
  colon brushing, 549, 563
Benign renal cyst, 581, 606–607
Benign renal tubular cells, 579, 606
BerEP4, 88, 114
Bile duct brushing cytology
  adenocarcinomas, 527, 560
  Barrett esophagus, 526, 560
  benign-appearing gastric mucosa, 531, 561
  biliary stricture and the placement, 558, 570
  gastric mucosa, reactive changes, 532, 561
  HIV-positive patient, heart burn and weight loss, 528, 560
  HSV infection, 528, 560
  hyperchromatic nuclei, 557, 568
  squamous cell carcinomas, 529, 530, 560–561
  vegetable cells, 537, 562
Bile duct hamartoma, 424, 458
Biliary tree brushing
  adenocarcinoma, 543, 563
  HCC, 548, 564–565
  lymphoma, 547, 564
  melanoma, 546, 564
Bipolar nuclei, 177, 194
BL. *See* Burkitt's-like lymphoma (BL)
Bladder
  detection, 721
  FISH, 727
  gall, 473
  thyroid transcription factor 1 (TTF1), 195
  urinary cancer, 727
Bladder malignancy subtyping, 619
Bladder neoplasms, 658, 669
Bland nuclei, 604, 616–617
Bone
  acute leukemia, 201, 230
  Burkitt lymphoma, 186
  Ewing's sarcoma, 179
  giant cell tumor, 346
  Hürthle cell carcinoma, 264, 295
  LE cells, 196
  lesion with metastatic lung adenocarcinoma, 86, 109
  malignancy, 207, 231
  megakaryocytic cells, 216, 235
  metastatic giant cell tumor, 492
  RCC, 457
  visceral metastases, 278, 300
Bone fine-needle aspiration (FNA)
  alveolar rhabdomyosarcoma, 698, 712
  angiolipomas, 682, 710
  atypical lipomatous tumor, 684, 710
  chordoma, 680, 709
  epidermal inclusion cyst, 681, 709–710
  epithelioid variant of angiosarcoma, 674, 708
  ES, 673, 708
  fibromatosis, 686, 710
  hibernoma, 683, 710
  Kaposi sarcoma, 678, 679, 709
  leiomyosarcoma, 691, 711
  low-grade chondrosarcoma, 701, 712
  metastatic mucinous carcinoma, 676, 708
  metastatic urothelial carcinoma, 699, 712
  MPNST, 687, 710
  nodular fasciitis, 677, 709
  osteosarcomas, 692, 711
  rhabdomyoma, 700, 712
  seroma, 675, 708
  SFT, 688, 710–711
  spindle cell melanoma, 695, 711–712
  synovial sarcoma, 690, 711
Branchial cleft cysts
  intrathyroidal, 285, 301
  papillary carcinoma, 247, 290
  squamous cells, 247, 290
Breast carcinoma, GIST, 538, 562
Bronchial epithelial cells
  reactive (*see* Reactive bronchial cells)
  without cilia, 88, 113
Bronchial reserve cells, 77, 105–106
Bronchioalveolar macrophages
  adenocarcinomas and signet ring cell carcinomas, 57, 70, 102, 104
  cytoplasmic pigments/vacuoles, 57, 70, 102, 104
  degenerated, 62, 103
  and goblet cells, 103
Bronchoalveolar carcinoma, 87, 111, 174, 189
Bronchoalveolar lavage (BAL), 88, 113
Bronchoscopic washing, 87, 112
Bubbly cytoplasm, 704, 715
Burkitt's-like lymphoma (BL), 172, 176, 186–187, 193, 454, 468
  c-Myc immunohistochemical stain, 340, 351
  cytoplasmic vacuoles, 326, 345
  EBV, 338, 348
  endemic and sporadic, 341, 353
  immunocompromised patients, 336, 347

C
Calretinin, 88, 114
CAM 5.2, 515, 520
Candida albicans, 657, 668
Carcinoembryonic antigen (CEA), 88, 114
Carcinoid
  acini and pseudorosette structures, 4, 92
  cellular arrangement and tumor cell morphology, 89, 116
  exophytic endobronchial lesion, 8, 92
  LCNEC, 89, 116
  nuclear molding and crowding, 558, 571

plasmacytoid and occasional pleomorphic cells, 556, 566
salt-and-pepper stippled chromatin, 8, 92
tumor-like nuclei with markedly atypia and enlargement, 89, 116
CD15, 88, 114
CD10 negativity, lymphoglandular bodies, 330, 346
Cellular degeneration, 657, 668
Cellular pleomorphic adenoma, 404
Cellular with neoplastic acinar cells, 403
Cerebral infarction, 224, 238
Cerebrospinal fluid (CSF)
adenocarcinoma, 227, 228, 239
blood contamination, 207, 212, 231, 234
brain hemorrhage/bleeding, 212, 234
brain tissue, 215, 235
carcinoma, 208, 211, 231–233
CNS tumor, 217, 235
corpora amylacea, 217, 235
cytokeratin, 220, 236
cytomorphology, 200
ependyma, 211, 233
flow cytometry, 225, 238
germinal matrix, 211, 224, 233, 238
leptomeningeal, 217, 235
leukemia (*see* Leukemia)
lumbar puncture, 212, 234
lymphocytes, 209, 232
lymphoid cells, 210, 233
malignancy, 207, 231
melanoma, 219, 236
meningeal malignancy, 211, 212, 233, 234
metastatic melanoma, 205, 230
multiple myeloma, 203, 210, 230, 232
myeloid blasts, 225, 238
neutrophils, 206, 207, 212, 231, 234
Ommaya reservoir, 210, 232
optimal cells, 212, 234
PCR-based testing, 728
red blood cells, 206, 212, 231, 234
viral DNA, 728
Charcot–Leyden crystal, 90, 96, 118, 178, 196
Chemotherapy, independent prognostic factor, 673, 708
Chicken wire, 703, 714
Cholangiocarcinoma
bile and sinusoidal capillary, 452, 463
CEA, CK7 and CD15, 464
cirrhotic liver, 455, 468
clear cytoplasm, atypical cells, 454, 467
dispersed tumor cells, 454, 467
endoscopic ultrasound-guided FNA (EUS-FNA), 429, 459
HepPar1, 453, 465
numerous naked nuclei, 452, 463
pseudointranuclear inclusions, 454, 467
risk factors, cirrhosis, 452, 464
spindle cells, 453, 465–466
Chondrocytes, 213, 235
Chordoma, 680, 709
Chromosome 9 alteration, urothelial carcinoma, 657, 667
Chromosome X translocations, 604, 614–615
Chronic sialadenitis, 404
Cirrhosis, 175, 190, 452, 464
Classical Hodgkin lymphoma (CHL), 323, 345
Clear cell renal cell carcinomas (RCCs), 580, 585, 604, 606–608, 616
Clear cell sarcoma, 706, 717
CLL/SLL
del 13q14.3, 340, 352
mature B-lineage lymphocytes, 339, 350
17p deletion, 337, 348
prominent nucleoli, 324, 345
Clumped chromatin, 86, 109
CMV. *See* Cytomegalovirus (CMV)
C-Myc immunohistochemical stain
B-cell lymphomas, 340, 351
Burkitt lymphoma, 340, 351
lymphoid neoplasms, 340, 351
Coccidioidomycosis, 18, 95
Collagen balls, 124, 179
Colloid nodules
cystic degeneration, 254, 293
MNG, 253, 292
oncocytic (Hurthle) cells, 254, 293
watery colloid, 253, 292
Colon, 676, 709
adenocarcinoma, 451, 462
characteristics, 89, 115
metastatic carcinoma, 31, 33, 98
picket fence appearance, 89, 115
Corpora amylacea, 646, 664
Cryptococcosis
Cryptococcus gattii, 19, 95–96
infection of *Cryptococcus neoformans,* 7, 19, 50, 92, 95–96, 101
Cryptococcus neoformans
differential diagnosis, 210, 232
fungal meningitis, 210, 232
immunocompromised patient, 320, 344–345
mucin stain, 222, 225, 237, 238
mucopolysaccharide, 211, 233
PAS stain, 221, 237
CSF. *See* Cerebrospinal fluid (CSF)
CT-guided transthoracic needle biopsy, 177, 195–196
Cyclophosphamide therapy, 658, 668
Cyst contents, CEA levels, 515, 520
Cystic RCCs. *See* Cystic renal cell carcinomas (RCCs)
Cystic renal cell carcinomas (RCCs), 583, 603, 607, 614
Cystoscopic surveillance protocols, 657, 667
Cytokeratin, 674, 705, 708, 715–716
Cytokeratin 7, 515, 520
Cytology. *See also* Cerebrospinal fluid (CSF)
basal cell adenoma/adenocarcinoma, 403
bile duct brushing (*see* Bile duct brushing cytology)
bronchial and aspiration (*see* Lung cytopathology)
Burkitt lymphoma diagnosis, 346
follicular lymphoma, 348
liver FNAs (*see* Liver FNAs)
lymphocytic proliferation, 351
and molecular testing (*see* Molecular testing and cytopathology)
mucinous neoplasms IPMN, 519
Rosai-Dorfman disease, 348
salivary duct carcinoma, 410
serous fluid (*see* Serous fluid cytopathology)
Cytomegalovirus (CMV), 657, 667
cytomegaly, 15, 94
description, 94
and HSV, 15, 94
immunocytochemistry/in situ hybridization, 15, 94
infection, 559, 560, 572
and PCP, 22, 96
pneumonia, 15, 94
pulmonary macrophages, endothelial cells and fibroblasts, 15, 94
Cytomorphological features, MPNST, 705, 716
Cytoplasmic debris, 405, 407

D
Decoy cells, 657, 667
Dedifferentiated liposarcomas, 704, 715
Dermatopathic lymphadenopathy, 338, 349
Desmoplastic small round cell tumor (DSRCT), 706, 717
Diff-Quik stain, 606, 609, 611, 614, 616
Diffuse large B cell lymphoma (DLBCL), 428, 458, 468, 588, 608–609
  B-cell lymphoma, 342, 353
  hyperchromatic nuclei and irregular nuclear membrane, 559, 569–570
  stomach bleeding, 536, 562
  three-dimensional clusters, atypical cells, 559, 569
DLBCL. *See* Diffuse large B cell lymphoma (DLBCL)
DSRCT. *See* Desmoplastic small round cell tumor (DSRCT)
Duct adenocarcinoma, 515, 519–520
Duct epithelium, 404
Duodenal contaminant, 483, 516
Dysgerminoma, 157, 184

E
Echinococcosis, 13, 93–95
Endobronchial ultrasound-guided transbronchial needle aspiration (EBUS-TBNA), 86, 108
  clinical utilization, 733
  FNA cytology specimens, 732
  staging and diagnosis, 731
Endocrine tumor, 437, 460
Endometrial cells, 653, 665
Endoscopic US-guided FNA, 514–515, 519
Entamoeba gingivalis infection, 16, 94–95
Ependymal cells
  and choroid plexus, 211, 233
  CSF, 214, 235
  leptomeningeal cells, 210, 232
  malignancy, 207, 231
  neutrophils, 207, 231
Ependymoma, 220, 236
Epidermal growth factor receptor (EGFR)
  adenocarcinoma with micropapillary and lepidic growth pattern, 90, 118
  and *KRAS*, 86, 90, 108, 109, 117
  mutation and overexpression, 90, 117
  tyrosine kinase, 90, 117, 119
Epidermal inclusion cyst, 681, 709–710
Epithelial cells, 404
Epithelioid angiosarcoma (EAS) and EHE, 88, 113
Epithelioid spindle cells, 707, 718
Epithelioid variant of angiosarcoma, 674, 708
Epstein–Barr virus (EBV), 218, 236
  neutrophilic infiltrate, 340, 351
  PTLD, 338, 349
ES. *See* Ewing sarcoma (ES)
EUS-FNA biopsy, submucosal lesions, 557–558, 569
Ewing sarcoma (ES), 673, 706, 708, 717
Ewing's sarcoma/primitive neuroectodermal tumor (ES/PNET)
  clinical progression, 728–729
  FISH, 730
  FNA role, 729
  IHC and RT-PCR, 729
  immunohistochemistry, 729
  metastatic renal NBs, 729
  MIC2 and neural markers expression, 729
  SYT/SSX translocation, 729
EWSR1 gene rearrangements, 704, 715
Extramedullary hematopoiesis, 445, 461

F
Fat necrosis, 702, 713
Fibrolamellar hepatocellular carcinoma, 442, 461
Fibromatosis, 686, 710
Fibrosarcoma, 706, 716
Fine granular (salt-and-pepper) chromatin pattern, 175, 191–192
Fine needle aspiration (FNA). *See also* Bone fine-needle aspiration (FNA)
  adenosquamous carcinoma, 316, 344
  advantages, 703, 714
  ALK positivity, 327, 345
  "atypia of undetermined significance", 734
  axillary neoplasm, 327, 345
  biliary tree brushing, 540
  biliary tree stent placement, 541
  biopsy material, 734
  Castleman disease, 318, 344
  CD138, 340, 352
  cell block/smear, 729
  chromophobe RCCs, 726
  CLL/SLL, 324, 345
  cytology of the liver, 300, 304 (*See also* Liver FNAs)
  desmin, 340, 352
  diagnostic problems, 729
  differentiated squamous cell carcinoma, 559
  EBUS-TBNA, 86, 108
  esophagus-gastric junction, 557
  false-negative, 731
  fibrotic/necrotic lesions, 703, 714
  FNA-Tg, 730, 731
  GIST, 557
  hemangiomas, 705, 716
  HHV-8, 317, 344
  liver (*see* Fine needle aspiration (FNA))
  lung (*see* Fine needle aspiration (FNA))
  lymph node, 339, 350
  lymphoma, 569, 571
  MALT lymphoma, 114, 558, 569
  mandibular lesion, 326, 345
  medium-sized lymphoid cells, 325, 345
  myogenin, 340, 352
  myogenin, desmin, CD138 and SMA, 340, 352
  nucleic acid-based molecular testing, 724
  pancreas (*see* Pancreatic FNA)
  percutaneous, 90, 118 (*see also* Percutaneous FNA)
  poorly differentiated adenocarcinoma, 88, 113
  renal and adrenal lesions (*see* Renal and adrenal lesions, differential diagnosis)
  retroperitoneal lymphadenopathy, 559
  RT-PCR, 730
  sarcoma, 312, 343
  sarcoma *vs.* lymphoma *vs.* carcinoma, 703, 714
  seminomas/dysgerminoma, 184
  sessile submucosal mass, 557
  SLE lymphadenopathy, 341, 353
  SMA, 340, 352
  thyroid (*see* Thyroid FNA)
  transbronchial (*see* Transbronchial FNA biopsy)
Flat carcinoma in situ (CIS), 658, 668–669
Flbrotic or necrotic lesions, 703, 714
Flow cytometry, 88, 114
  acute leukemia, 230

CD138-positive cells, 341, 352
immunophenotyping, 114
leptomeningeal metastasis, 234
lymphocytosis (lymphocytic effusion), 180
plasmacytoma, 340–341, 352
Fluorescence in situ hybridization (FISH)
ALK-FISH assay, 108
cytopathologic specimens, 720
IGH and CCND1, 726–727
IGH/BCL2, 731–732
lymph node, 722
oncocytic neoplasms, 726
and RT-PCR, 730
studies, 684
urothelial carcinoma, 727
UroVysion assay, 722
Focal nodular hyperplasia, 448, 462
Follicular lymphoma
axillary node, CD10 and Bcl-6, 340, 351–352
B-cell markers, 337, 348
Follicular neoplasms (FNs)
adenoma, 262, 295
colloids, 261, 294
hyperplastic nodules, 259, 294
microfollicles, 261, 262, 294, 295
MNG, 259, 294
papillary carcinoma, 259, 262, 294, 295
Follicular variant of PTC (FVPC), 273, 298

G

Ganglion cysts, 704, 714
Gastric mucosa
benign gastric ulcer, 533, 561
reactive changes, 532, 561
Gastrointestinal stromal tumor (GIST), 416, 456, 704, 705, 715, 716
Gastrointestinal (GI) tract lesions, cytology
adenocarcinoma, 534, 561
adenoma, 539, 562–563
benign components and conditions, 524
biliary tree adenocarcinoma, chemo-and radiation therapy, 542, 563
bipolar nuclei, 194
coarse chromatin and large prominent nucleoli, 557, 567–568
contaminants, 514, 519
leiomyosarcoma, 557, 568
malignant conditions, 525
MALT lymphomas, 558, 569
naked nuclei, 194
neutral mucin, 191
reactive glandular cells, 540, 541, 563
signet ring cell carcinoma, stomach, 535, 561–562
spindle-shaped/epithelioid tumor cells, 557, 568
synaptophysin, chromogranin and CD56, 557, 567
GCT. *See* Giant cell tumor (GCT)
Germinoma, 220, 236
Giant cell tumor (GCT), 707, 718
GIST. *See* Gastrointestinal stromal tumor (GIST)
GI tract and bile duct brushing cytology, differential diagnosis
colon adenomas, adenocarcinomas, 565–566
cytomegalovirus (CMV) infection, 560
cytomorphology, tumor cells, 562
leiomyosarcoma, 568
reactive atypia, adenocarcinomas, 561
spindle cell lesion, FNA cytology, 562
Glioblastoma multiforme, 218, 236
Glomeruli, 578, 604, 606, 615
Goblet cell
bronchial washing and BAL specimen, 63, 103
bronchioalveolar macrophages, 103
hyperplasia (*see* Goblet cell hyperplasia)
Goblet cell hyperplasia
adenocarcinomas and signet ring cell carcinomas, 64, 103–104
mucinfilled cytoplasm and "signet ring" appearance, 36, 98–99
reactive bronchial epithelium, 48, 100
Granular adenocarcinoma, 480, 516
Granulomatous inflammation, 658, 668
Diff-Quik preparation, 55, 102
sarcoidosis and malignant lesions, 55, 102
Granulomatous reactions, 405
Graves disease
flame cells, 251, 291–292
follicular cells, 251, 291
IgG antibodies, 251, 292

H

Hairy cell leukemia, 341, 352, 353
Hamazaki-Wesenberg bodies, 336, 347
Hashimoto thyroiditis (HT), 260, 294
HCC. *See* Hepatocellular carcinoma (HCC)
Health Care Financing Administration (HCFA), 91, 119
Hemangioma, 422, 457
Hepatoblastoma, 440, 460–461
Hepatocellular carcinoma (HCC), 90, 97, 110, 115, 118, 242
abdominal pain, jaundice and liver masses, 421, 457, 548, 564–565
bile and sinusoidal capillary, 452, 463
biliary brush specimen, 559
chromatin, 415, 456
and CMV, 344
dense cytoplasm and distinct cell border, 455, 468
diagnosis, 450, 462
DLBCL, 458
fatty change, 452, 463
fibrolamellar, 442, 461, 466
focal nodular hyperplasia, 462
HepPar1, 453, 465
intermediate-sized tumor cells, 453, 466
intranuclear inclusions, 176, 192
metastic melanoma, 460, 511
panel (HepPar1, CD10, CAM5.2 and CK8/18), 452, 464
pleural effusion, 144, 182
poorly differentiated, 447, 461–462
preserved reticulin scaffold pattern, 453, 454, 464, 466
sinusoidal capillaries, 454, 467
well-differentiated, 426, 453, 458, 465
Hep Par 1 (hepatocyte Paraffin 1) antibody, 453, 465
Herpes simplex virus (HSV), 10, 93, 94, 96, 658, 668
bile duct brushing cytology, 528, 560
Cowdry A bodies, 555, 566
multinucleation, 557, 568
Herpes virus infection, 658, 668
Hibernia, 683, 710
Hibernoma cells, 703, 714
High-grade malignancy, 707, 718
Histiocytes, 704, 714
Histoplasmosis, 12, 17, 93, 95
HMB45, 89, 115
HMGI(Y) gene on chromosome 6p21, 89, 116

Hodgkin lymphoma, 149, 183
mixed cellularity, 337, 348
nodular lymphocyte-predominant, 337, 348
sinus histiocytosis, FNA, 341, 353
Homer Wright rosettes, 706, 717
Honey comb pattern, 404
HSV. *See* Herpes simplex virus (HSV)
Hürthle cell neoplasms
benign thyroid lesions, 289, 304
eosinophilic cytoplasms, 260, 294
HT, 260, 294
lymphocytic thyroiditis, 263, 295
metastatic carcinoma, 264, 295
microfollicles, 263, 295
nuclei, 263, 295
psammoma bodies, 289, 304
radioiodine scan, 265, 296
renal cell carcinoma, 260, 294
Hyaline matrix globules, 403
Hyaluronic acid–alcian blue, 176, 194
Hydatid disease, 13, 93–95
Hyperchromatic nucleoli and clumped chromatin, 86, 109, 407
Hypovasuclar tumors, 706, 717

I
IHC markers S100, 89, 115
Immune markers, 88, 114
Immunocytochemistry, 93, 94
ASCO/CAP guidelines, 730
cytospin slides, 205, 230
FN, 262, 295
formalin-free fixatives, 730
HER2 overexpression, 730
Hürthle cell, 264, 295
Hürthle cell neoplasm, 262, 295
lobular carcinoma, 204, 230
markers, 731
molecular expression and markers (*see* Ewing's sarcoma/primitive neuroectodermal tumor (ES/PNET))
prognostic and therapeutic implications, 730
RT-PCR, 729
stains, 728, 736
"Immunocyt" test, 657, 667
Immunoglobulin G (IgG), 251, 292
Immunostaining, 676, 678
panels, metastatic carcinoma
female, 672
male, 672
Inflammatory myofibroblastic tumor (IMT), 90, 116–117
In-situ hybridization
cystoscopy, 727
HPV-induced detection, 723
infectious diseases detection, 721
in lymphoproliferative diseases, 721
in solid tumors, 721
Intracranial hemorrhage, 224, 237
Intraductal papillary mucinous cyst (IPMN), 514, 519
Intramuscular myxoma, 704, 715
Intranuclear inclusions, 176, 192, 658, 668
Intrathecal, 201, 210, 230, 232
Irregular nuclear membrane
adenocarcinoma, 97
and hyperchromasia, 87, 110
nuclei, 99, 100

K
Kaposi sarcoma (KS), 317, 344, 678, 708, 709
Karetin debris and biopsy, 68, 104
Kikuchi lymphadenitis
extensive neutrophilic infiltrate, 339, 350
occasional lymphocytes, 337, 347
Kristen-Rous sarcoma virus (KRAS)
cytology samples, 733
and EGFR, 732
in lung cancer patients, 733
mutation, 724
NSCLC, 732
TKIs therapy, 732
KS. *See* Kaposi sarcoma (KS)

L
LE cells. *See* Lupus erythematosus (LE) cells
Leiomyosarcoma, 691, 711
Leishmaniasis, 320, 337, 348
Lepra bacilli, 336, 347
Leptomeningeal metastasis, 210, 212, 232, 234
acute bacterial meningitis, 206, 230
CSF, 210, 232
lobular carcinoma, 204, 230
lung cancer, 206
lymphoma, 208, 217, 231, 235
Leukemia
CNS, 211, 233
CSF, 201, 230
false-positive diagnosis, 211, 233
intrathecal chemotherapy effect, 201, 230
Lymphoblastic and Burkitt lymphoma, 211, 233
Liesegang rings, 582, 607
Lipoblasts, 703, 704, 714, 715
Lipoma, 703, 714
Liposarcoma, 703, 714
Liver cytology, differential diagnosis. *See* Liver FNAs
Liver FNAs
actinomysis, 432, 459
benign bile duct epithelial cells, 446, 452, 461, 463, 464
benign components, 412
benign hepatocytes, 452, 463
bile duct hamartoma, 424, 458
breast cancer, DLBCL, 428, 458
cholangiocarcinoma (*see* Cholangiocarcinoma)
colon adenocarcinoma, 451, 453, 462, 466
endocrine tumor, 437, 460
extramedullary hematopoiesis, 445, 461
fibrolamellar HCC, 442, 461
focal nodular hyperplasia, 448, 462
HCC (*see* Hepatocellular carcinoma (HCC))
hemangioma, 422, 457
hepatic AML, 452, 464
hepatoblastoma, 440, 460–461
hyperchromatic and prominent nucleoli, 454, 467
lymphoma, 453, 465
metastatic adenocarcinoma, 423, 430, 436, 457, 459, 460
metastatic carcinoid, 427, 433, 458, 459
metastatic cell carcinoma, 414, 449, 456, 462
metastatic endocrine tumor, 459–460
metastatic leiomyosarcoma, 443, 461
metastatic melanoma, 420, 438, 457, 460
metastatic RCC, 419, 457
metastatic urothelial cell carcinoma, 418, 456–457
mucinous adenocarcinomas, ovary, 431, 459

naked nuclei, 425, 453, 458, 466
neoplastic lesions, 413
normal liver cells, 435, 439, 444, 460, 461
oral contraceptives, 452, 462
paranuclear blue bodies, cytoplasm, 453, 466
poorly differentiated adenocarcinoma, 416, 456
S100, HMB45 and melanin A, 417, 456
well-differentiated HCC, 426, 458
Wilm's tumor, 441, 461
Low-grade B cell lymphoma, 589, 609
Low-grade chondrosarcoma, 701, 712
Lumbar puncture, 208, 210, 212, 231, 232, 234
Lung cytopathology
abundant alveolar macrophages, 86, 109
adenocarcinomas (*see* Adenocarcinoma(s))
ALK gene, 86, 108
ALK gene rearrangement, *EML4-ALK*, 90, 117
alveolar macrophages, 86, 108
alveolar proteinosis, 88, 114
architectural patterns, 88, 113
aspergillosis, 14, 87, 94, 111
asthma, 23, 96–97
atypical and typical carcinoid, 89, 116
benign component, 2
benign mesothelial cells, 86, 109–110
BerEP4, 88, 114
bilateral lung infiltrations, 87, 112
bone lesion with metastatic lung adenocarcinoma, 86, 109
bronchial reserve cells, 77, 105–106
bronchioalveolar macrophages, 57, 70, 102, 104
bronchoalveolar carcinoma, 87, 111
bronchoalveolar lavage, 88, 113
bronchoscopic washing, 87, 112
calretinin, 88, 114
carcinoid (*see* Carcinoid)
CD15, 88, 114
CEA, 88, 114
Charcot-Leyden crystal, 90, 118
CK20 and CDX2, 89, 115
clusters of bronchial epithelial cells without cilia, 88, 113
clusters of ciliated bronchial epithelium (creola bodies), 86, 108–109
CMV, 15, 22, 94, 96
coccidioidomycosis, 18, 95
colon, 89, 115
color and volume of specimen, 91, 119
cough, fever and weight loss, 7
cryptococcosis (*see* Cryptococcosis)
curschmann spirals, 86, 108
degenerated alveolar macrophages, 51, 101
EBUS-TBNA, 86, 108
echinococcosis (hydatid disease), 13, 93–94
EGFR and *KRAS* mutations, 86, 109
EHE and EAS, 88, 113
Entamoeba gingivalis infection, 16, 94–95
flow cytometry, 88, 114
goblet cell, 63, 103
goblet cell hyperplasia (*see* Goblet cell hyperplasia)
granulomatous inflammation, 55, 102
HCFA, 91, 119
hilar lymph node, 89, 115
histoplasmosis, 12, 17, 93, 95
HIV-positive patient, 5, 6
HMB45, 89, 115
HMGI(Y) gene on chromosome 6p21, 89, 116
HSV infection, 10, 93
hyperchromatic nucleoli and clumped chromatin, 86, 109
IHC markers S100, 89, 115
immune markers, 88, 114
immunostains of cytokeratin, 87, 111–112
IMT, 90, 116–117
intercellular windows, 90, 117–118
irregular nuclear membrane and hyperchromasia, 87, 110
karetin debris and biopsy, 68, 104
KRAS mutations, 91, 119
KRAS protein and EGFR tyrosine kinase, 90, 117
lower mitotic rate and absence of necrosis, 89, 116
make cell block and perform silver stain, 89, 114
Melanin A, 89, 115
metastatic breast carcinoma, 89, 115
metastatic carcinoma, breast, 30, 33, 98
metastatic carcinoma, colon, 31, 34, 98
metastatic melanoma, 89, 115
metastatic synovial sarcoma, 56, 102
microbiology culture and core biopsy, 88, 114
micropapillary/lepidic growth, 90, 118
mitosis and necrosis, 87, 112
monomorphous population of lymphocytes, 87, 111
Mucormycosis (zygomycosis), 9, 92–93
mutation and overexpression, *EGFR* gene, 90, 117
necrotic debris, 86, 110
neoplastic lesions, 3
neutrophils, 90, 116
non-diagnostic specimen, 67, 104
nuclear grooves, 87, 111
nuclei with marked variation in size and shape, 87, 112
p53, 88, 114
pancoast tumor, 89, 115–116
PCP (*see Pneumocystis jiroveci (carinii)* pneumonia (PCP))
percutaneous FNA, 90, 118
prominent nucleoli, 88, 89, 112–113, 115
pulmonary hamartoma, 89, 116
reactive bronchial cells (*see* Reactive bronchial cells)
reactive squamous cells, 66, 104
renal cell carcinoma, 87, 110
sarcoidosis, 88, 114
shared cell borders, 86, 110
signet ring-like cells, 88, 113
significant variation of nuclear size and shape, 90, 118
small cell carcinoma (*see* Small cell carcinoma)
squamous cell carcinoma (*see* Squamous cell carcinoma)
squamous cells with reactive atypia, 65, 104
strongyloidiasis, 6, 92
TB, 20, 96
toxoplasmosis, 21, 96
transbronchial fine-needle aspiration biopsy, 86, 109
TTF, 88, 114
WT1, 88, 114
Lung, metastatic carcinoma
CNS, 202, 230
fatal cancer, 202, 230
leukemia/lymphoma, 208, 231
lobular carcinoma, 204, 230
Lung/squamous cell carcinoma, 223, 237
Lupus erythematosus (LE) cells, 125, 178, 179, 196
Lymph node cytopathology
acid-fast stain, 331, 343
Auramine O, 336, 347
CD103+, CD25+, CD23–, 341, 353
CD138, plasma cells, 313, 343
cohesive proliferation, 332, 346
cyclin D1, 331, 343

Lymph node cytopathology (*cont.*)
  denatured DNA and immunoglobulin, 341, 353
  histiocytic lymphoma, 338, 349
  leishmanial infection, 337, 348
  malignant effusion, 336, 347
  Melan-A, 311, 343
  metastatic renal cell carcinoma, 334, 346
  mixed inflammatory response, 318, 344
  molecular testing, 336, 347
  monospot test, 339, 350
  morphology, malignant cells, 339, 351
  multinucleated giant cells, 315, 343–344
  nasopharyngeal carcinoma and seminoma, 338, 349
  rituxan (rituximab) chemotherapy, 336, 347
  sarcoidosis, 339, 350
  tall columnar cells, 339, 350
  triple therapy, 341, 352
  WT-1 and calretinin, 314, 343
Lymph node metastasis, 704, 715
Lymphocytes
  chronic/subacute/viral meningitis, 210, 232
  metastatic adenocarcinoma, 210, 232
  monomorphous population, 87, 111
  T-cell lymphoma, 210, 232
Lymphocytic thyroiditis
  follicular cells, 249, 291
  Hurthle cells, 250, 291
  noniatrogenic hypothyroidism, 249, 291
  PTC, 249, 291
Lymphocytosis (lymphocytic effusion), 133, 177, 180, 194
Lymphoepithelial island, 405
Lymphoglandular bodies, 403, 404
Lymphoma, 501, 517, 603, 614

M

MA. *See* Metanephric adenoma (MA)
Magnetic cell sorting (MACS)
  anti-CD14 and anti-CD16 antibody, 735
  bronchial epithelial cells, 734
  HYAL2 and *FHIT* genes, 735
  sputum cytology specimens, 734
Malakoplakia, 658, 668
Malignant lymphoma, 628, 661
Malignant peripheral nerve sheath tumor (MPNST), 687, 705, 710, 716
Malignant tumor, skeletal muscle origin, 693, 711
MALT lymphomas
  chronic autoimmune conditions, 337, 348
  GI, 558, 569
  lymphoglandular bodies, 558, 569
Mantle cell lymphoma
  Bcl-1, 329, 346
  infectious mononucleosis, 339, 351
  marginal zone/MALT lymphoma, 339, 351
MDM2 oncogene. *See* Murine double minute 2 (MDM2) oncogene
Medullary carcinoma
  amyloid, 275, 298
  cytoplasmic granules, 277, 299
  differential diagnosis, 276, 299
  dyscohesive cells, 275, 298
  metachromatic cytoplasmic granules, 276, 299
  oncocytic tumors, 276, 299
  serum calcitonin levels, 275, 298
  thyroglobulin, 275, 298
Medullary thyroid carcinoma (MTC), 275, 288, 298, 302
Medulloblastoma
  astrocytoma, 225, 238
  CNS tumors, 217, 235
  small cell carcinoma, 218, 236
Megakaryocytes, 216, 235
Melamed-Wolinska bodies, 642, 658, 663–664, 668
Melanin, 89, 115, 220, 236
Meningitis
  aseptic, 206, 231
  Cryptococcus neoformans, 210, 221, 232, 237
  cytological examination, CSF, 206, 230–231
  lymphocytes, 221, 237
  mucin stain, 226, 238
  sarcoidosis, 224, 238
  tuberculosis, 211, 233
Merkel cell tumor, 403
Metanephric adenoma (MA), 590, 609
Metaplastic squamous cells, 406
Metastasis
  adenocarcinoma, 202, 230
  B-cell lymphoma, 208, 231
  cystic lesions, 247, 290
  Hürthle cell carcinoma, 264, 295
  leptomeningeal, 204, 212, 230, 234
  liver FNAs (*see* Liver FNAs)
  lobular carcinoma, 204, 230
  and lung mass, 37, 99
  medullary carcinoma, 276, 299
  medulloblastoma, 220, 236
  melanoma, 205, 228, 230, 239
  neck lymph node, 730
  PTC, 271, 297
  renal cell carcinoma, 281, 300
  SCC, 728
  squamous cell carcinoma, 282, 301
Metastatic adenocarcinoma, 204, 230, 436, 460
  BerEP4, Napsin A, TTF1, Calretinin, WT1 and P53, 174, 188
  lung, 423, 452, 457, 465
Metastatic basal cell carcinoma, 404
Metastatic basaloid squamous cell carcinoma, 404
Metastatic breast carcinoma, 89, 115
Metastatic breast ductal carcinoma, 697, 712
Metastatic carcinoid, 427, 433, 458, 459
Metastatic carcinoma
  of breast, 30, 33, 98
  of colon, 31, 34, 98
  to liver, 300
  to lung (*see* Lung, metastatic carcinoma)
Metastatic colonic adenocarcinoma, 635, 662
Metastatic endocrine tumor, 459–460
Metastatic endometrial adenocarcinoma, 656, 666
Metastatic endometrial carcinoma, 597, 611
Metastatic HCC. *See* Metastatic hepatocellular carcinoma (HCC)
Metastatic hepatocellular carcinoma (HCC), 598, 611
Metastatic leiomyosarcoma, 443, 461
Metastatic lung small cell carcinoma, 645, 664
Metastatic melanoma, 89, 115, 420, 457, 594, 610
  BRAF testing, 339, 350
  Melan-A, 319, 344
  pleomorphic plasmacytoid cells, 335, 346
  prostate carcinoma, 332, 346
Metastatic mucinous adenocarcinoma, 309, 343, 600, 611
Metastatic mucinous adenocarcinoma of the ovary, 431, 459
Metastatic mucinous carcinoma, 676, 708
Metastatic papillary thyroid carcinoma, 308, 343
Metastatic prostate adenocarcinoma, 430, 459

Metastatic prostate carcinoma, 602, 612
Metastatic renal cell carcinoma, 500, 517
Metastatic small cell carcinoma, 414, 456, 498, 517, 595, 610
Metastatic squamous cell carcinoma, 449, 462, 599, 611
Metastatic synovial sarcoma, 56, 102
Metastatic urothelial cell carcinoma, 418, 456–457, 596, 610, 696, 699, 712
Mikulicz disease, 405
Mitoses, 404
Mitosis and necrosis, 87, 112
MNG. *See* Multinodular goiter (MNG)
Molecular testing and cytopathology
  BRAF V600E mutation, 724–725, 734–735
  cryopreservation, 724, 733
  cytokeratin 5/6 and p63, 724, 733–734
  cytologic samples, 725, 735
  cytomorphology, 722, 727
  description, 719
  ES/PNET, 723, 728–730
  false-negative FNA, 731
  FISH, 720
  FNA cytology, 723, 728
  IGH and CCND1, 722, 726–727
  IGH/BCL2 and MYC translocations, 724, 731–732
  IHC analysis, 723, 730
  in situ hybridization technique (*see* In-situ hybridization)
  KRAS mutation, 724, 732
  lymph node metastases, 730
  MACS, 724–725, 734–735
  PCR-based testing, 722–723, 728
  PCR technology, 720
  polysomy, 722, 727–728
  RT-PCR detection, 723, 731
  telomerase activity and microsatellite instability, 720
  upper urinary tract cytology, 722, 727
  Xp11.2 translocation, 722, 726
Mollaret meningitis, 224, 226, 238
Monomorphous population of cells, 604, 615
Monotonous rounded nuclei, 404
MPNST. *See* Malignant peripheral nerve sheath tumor (MPNST)
Mucicarmine, 175, 191
Mucinous cystic neoplasm (MCN), 475, 494, 516, 517
Mucinous metaplasia, 405
Mucinous noncystic adenocarcinoma
  adenoma, 497, 503, 517, 518
  endocrine tumor, 504, 518
  polyhedral cells, 485, 516
  signet ring cells, 477, 516
  three-dimensional pattern, 476, 516
Mucoepidermoid carcinomas, 407, 408
Mucormycosis (zygomycosis), 9, 92–93
Multinodular goiter (MNG), 253, 292
Multiple myeloma, 203, 210, 230
Murine double minute 2 (MDM2) oncogene, 684, 710
Mycobacterium avium, 336, 347
Mycosis fungoides
  CD4+/CD8–/CD34–, 328, 345–346
  lymphoproliferative disorder, 328, 345
  nuclear contour irregularities, 328, 345
  variable chromatin patterns, 328, 345
Myelolipomas
  adrenal gland, 322, 345
  HMB45 negative, 322, 345
Myoepithelial carcinoma, 405, 407
Myoepithelial cells, 404, 406
Myoepithelioma, 407
Myxofibrosarcoma, 704, 715
Myxoid chondrosarcoma, 705, 715–716
Myxoid cytoplasm, 235
Myxoid, hyalinized stroma, 472
Myxoid leiomyosarcoma, 693, 711
Myxoid liposarcoma, 703, 714
Myxoid matrix
  carcinoma expleomorphic adenoma, 407
  pleomorphic adenoma with tyrosine crystalloids, 407
Myxoma, 685, 710

N
Naked nuclei, metastatic breast carcinoma, 176, 194
Necrosis, 657, 667
Necrotic debris, 86, 93, 104, 106, 107, 110, 406
Necrotizing granulomatous inflammation, 657, 668
Neoplasms (uncommon), kidney and adrenal gland myelolipomas, 345
Neoplastic cells, 404
NETs. *See* Neuroendocrine tumors (NETs)
Neuroblastoma, 706, 717
Neuroendocrine tumors (NETs), 175, 190, 191, 403
Neurofibroma lesions, 705, 716
Neurosyphilis, 210, 232
Neutrophils, 90, 116
Nodular fasciitis, 677, 709
Nontyrosine crystalloids, 404
Normal adrenal cortical cells, 591, 609
Normal liver cells, 435, 439, 444, 460, 461
Normal pancreatic tissue, 478, 516
Nuclear enlargement and variation, 603, 613
Nuclear grooves, 87, 111, 175, 190, 454, 466
Numerous naked nuclei, 603, 613
Numerous plasmacytoid lymphocytes, 678, 709

O
Oncocytic carcinoma, 407
Oncocytic mucoepidermoid carcinoma, 406
Oncocytomas, 408, 586, 604, 605, 608, 615, 617
Osteosarcoma, 692, 711

P
P53, 88, 110, 114
Paget's disease, 705, 716
Pancoast tumor, 89, 115–116
Pancreatic cystic lesions, 473
Pancreatic endocrine neoplasm (PEN), 472
Pancreatic FNA
  ACC and PEN, 472
  adenocarcinoma, 472
  aspirate, 495, 517
  CEA, 489, 517
  cell arrangement, 514, 519
  cystic lesions, 473
  differentiated adenocarcinoma, 474, 516
  drinking coffee, 514, 519
  duct epithelium, 486, 516
  duodenal contaminant, 483, 516
  endocrine tumor, 490, 514, 517, 519
  focal mucinous lining, 515, 520
  gastric contaminant, 479, 516
  indications, contraindication and accuracy, 471
  MCN, 475, 516

Pancreatic FNA (*cont.*)
- metastatic neoplasms, 473
- moderately differentiated adenocarcinoma, 482, 484, 516
- mucinous cystadenocarcinoma, 490, 517
- noncystic adenocarcinoma, 476, 516
- normal pancreatic tissue, 478, 516
- ovarian stroma, 514, 519
- pseudopapillary tumor, 502, 518
- S100 and HMB45, 499, 517
- small cell carcinoma, 513, 518
- stomach, 514, 519

Pancreaticoblastoma, 515, 520
Pancreatic pseudocyst, 514, 519
Papillary RCCs, 604, 615
Papillary thyroid carcinoma (PTC), 343, 350
- basophilic structures, 286, 302
- benign thyroid lesions, 267, 268, 296, 297
- BRAF gene mutations, 734
- cervical lymphadenopathy, 266, 296
- collagen balls, 179
- colloids, 267, 296
- columnar cell variant, 274, 298
- cyst lining, 514
- cysts, 270, 297
- cytoplasmic inclusion, 272, 298
- Diff-Quick stain, 268, 297
- diffuse sclerosing, 274, 298
- FN, 272, 297
- FVPC, 273, 298
- immunoreaction, 271, 297
- intraductal mucinous tumor, 474–476, 483
- intranuclear inclusion, 268, 297
- malignancy, 266, 296
- metastatic adenocarcinoma of the lung, 457, 459
- MNG, 272, 298
- mucosal folds, 108
- neoplastic cells, 266, 286, 296, 301
- nonneoplastic thyroglossal cyst, 270, 297
- nucleoli, 266, 296
- psammoma bodies, 183, 186, 267, 296
- PTC (*see* Papillary thyroid carcinoma (PTC))
- RCCs, 726
- recurrence, 731
- red blood cells, 272, 298
- renal cell carcinoma, 140, 181–182, 726
- somatic genetic alterations, 724
- tall-cell variant, 274, 298
- ThinPrep smears, 269, 297
- thyroid carcinoma, 110, 181, 192
- thyroidectomy and radioiodine ablation, 730–731
- total thyroidectomy, 272, 297
- urothelial neoplasia, 727

Parathyroid adenoma
- cytoplasm, 284, 301
- focal nuclear pleomorphism, 284, 301
- hypercalcemia, 284, 301
- nuclei, 287, 302
- thyroglobulin, 284, 301
- vascular structures, 287, 302

Patent urachus, 658, 669
PCP. *see Pneumocystis jiroveci (carinii)* pneumonia (PCP)
Pediatric nodal marginal zone lymphoma, 342, 353
PEL. *See* Primary effusion lymphoma (PEL)
Percutaneous FNA, 90, 118
Peripheral T-cell lymphoma NOS, 342, 354
Peutz–Jeghers Syndrome, 515, 520
Pheochromocytoma, 601, 612
Physaliphorous cells, 704, 715
Plasma cell leukemia and cells, 341–342, 353
Plasmacytoid, 406
Plasmacytoid myoepithelial cells, 407
Pleomorphic adenoma
- amylase crystalloids, 398, 408
- characteristics, 398, 407
- chondromyxoid matrix, 372, 404
- diagnostic pattern, 370, 404
- epithelial cells, 365, 404
- extracellular material, 399, 408
- fibrillary matrix, 370, 404
- mucoepidermoid carcinomas, 398, 408
- myoepithelial cells, 365, 404
- plasmacytoid, 385, 406
- with tyrosine crystalloids, 393, 407
- tyrosine rich crystals, 401, 409
- Warthin tumors, 398, 399, 407, 408

Pleomorphic appearance, 98, 102, 113, 115, 116
Pleomorphic features
- and abundant cytoplasm, 209, 232
- astrocytoma, 219, 236
- carcinoid tumor, 566
- giant tumor cells, 517
- glioblastoma multiforme, 218, 236
- HCC, 457, 462, 564–565
- hepatoblastoma, 460
- Hodgkin cells, 562
- Hürthle cell neoplasm, 263, 295
- lobular carcinoma, 204, 230
- metastatic prostate adenocarcinoma, 459
- MTC, 275, 288, 298, 302
- nuclear, 731
- plasmacytoid, 568
- plasmacytoid cells, 335, 346
- sinusoidal capillaries, 467
- three-dimensional group, 518
- tumor cells, 463
- Wilm's tumor, 461

Pleomorphic sarcomas, 704, 715
Pneumocystis jiroveci (carinii) pneumonia (PCP)
- aspergillosis, 87, 111
- cell block and perform silver stain, 89, 114
- and CMV, 22, 96
- coccidioidomycosis, 18, 95
- cytological features, 5, 92
- histoplasmosis, 12, 93
- immunocompromised patients, 11, 93
- toxoplasmosis, 21, 96

Pneumothorax, 174, 175, 189–190
Polymerase chain reaction (PCR), 93, 94, 96
- in cytopathologic specimens, 720
- failure rate, 731
- HSC, 728
- RT-PCR, 729, 731

Polyomavirus immunostain (SV40), 625, 660
Polyomavirus infection, 630, 657, 661, 667
Post-transplant lymphoproliferative disorders (PTLD), EBV, 338, 349
Precursor T-cell lymphoblastic lymphoma, 338, 349
Primary adenosquamous carcinoma, 515, 520
Primary cutaneous ALCL, 336, 347
Primary effusion lymphoma (PEL), 148, 175, 183, 192
Prominent nucleoli, 175, 176, 190, 193, 407, 453, 465
Psammoma bodies, 176, 193, 403
Pseudointranuclear inclusions, 454, 467

Pseudomyxoma peritonei, 169, 186
Pulmonary adenocarcinoma, 340, 352
Pulmonary hamartoma, 89, 116
Pyknotic nuclei, 176, 193, 454, 467–468

R

RCC. *See* Renal cell carcinoma (RCC)
Reactive biliary epithelium, 506, 518
Reactive bronchial cells
  and *Candida,* 39, 99
  epithelial cells, 35, 43, 44, 45, 46, 69, 76, 98, 100, 104, 105
  and mucin vacuole, 75, 105
Reactive glandular cells
  abdominal pain and enlarged liver, 540, 563
  biliary tree stent placement, 541, 563
  coarse chromatin and irregular nuclear membrane, 559, 572
  cytological features, 550, 565
  dispersed large polygonal cells, 559, 572
  hyperchromatic nuclei, 559, 572
  multinucleation and prominent small nucleoli, 551, 565
  radiation-and chemotherapy-induced, 557, 567
Reactive lymphadenopathy, 317, 344
Reactive lymphoid hyperplasia, 336, 347
Reactive mesothelial cells
  breast cancer, radiation and chemotherapy, 153, 184
  bronchoalveolar carcinoma, 174, 189
  cell block preparation, 156, 184
  hepatitis C and liver nodules, 150, 183
  lung mass and pleural effusion, 138, 181
  "signet ring" cells, 175, 190
  "Window" between atypical cells, 174, 188
Reactive urothelial cells, 621, 636, 640, 660, 662, 663
Reed–Sternberg cells, EBV stains LMP-1, 323, 345
Renal and adrenal lesions, differential diagnosis
  adrenal cortical adenoma, 592, 609
  adrenal cortical carcinoma, 593, 610
  AML, 584, 607
  benign renal cyst, 581, 606–607
  benign renal tubular cells, 579, 606
  clear cell RCC, 580, 585, 606–608
  cystic renal cell carcinoma (RCC), 583, 607
  DLBCL, 588, 608–609
  glomerulus, 578, 606
  liesegang rings, 582, 607
  low-grade B cell lymphoma, 589, 609
  MA, 590, 609
  metastatic endometrial carcinoma, 597, 611
  metastatic HCCs, 598, 611
  metastatic melanoma, 594, 610
  metastatic mucinous adenocarcinoma, 600, 611
  metastatic prostate carcinoma, 602, 612
  metastatic small cell carcinoma, 595, 610
  metastatic squamous cell carcinoma, 599, 611
  metastatic urothelial cell carcinoma, 596, 610
  neoplastic conditions, 576–577
  normal adrenal cortical cells, 591, 609
  oncocytoma, 586, 608
  pheochromocytoma, 601, 612
  urothelial cell carcinomas, 587, 608
Renal cell carcinoma (RCC), 87, 110, 419, 457
  breast and lung cancers, 281, 301
  epithelial fragments vascularization, 281, 300
  esophagus, 281, 300–301
  FN, 281, 300
  plasmacytoma, 281, 300
Renal transplantation, 174, 189
Rhabdomyoma, 700, 712
Rhabdomyosarcoma (RMS), 129, 180, 407, 706, 717
Rheumatoid pleuritis, 166, 177, 185, 196
RMS. *See* Rhabdomyosarcoma (RMS)
Rosai-Dorfman disease, 337, 348
Round cell
  diagnosis, 729
  ependymal cells, 214, 235
  FNA, 337
  glioblastoma multiforme, 218, 236
  lesions, 729
  morphology, 729
  nuclei, 518
  rosettes and pseudorosettes, 729

S

Salivary duct, 405
Salivary gland fine-needle aspiration
  acinic cell carcinoma (*see* Acinic cell carcinoma (ACC))
  acute sialadenitis, 369, 404
  adenocarcinoma, 359, 386, 403, 406
  adenoid cystic carcinoma (*see* Adenoid cystic carcinoma)
  basal cell adenoma/adenocarcinoma, 359, 386, 403, 406
  basaloid neoplasm, 374, 404–405
  benign acini, 366, 404
  benign duct epithelium, 367, 404
  benign intra-parotid lymph node, 373, 404
  canalicular adenoma, 401, 409
  carcinoma expleomorphic adenoma, 392, 407
  caused by ischemic changes, 401, 409
  chronic sialadenitis, 371, 404
  common salivary gland tumor, 402, 410
  cryptococcal sialadenitis, 390, 406
  epithelial myoepithelial carcinoma, 363, 403
  granulomatous sialadenitis, 381
  hemangioma, 401, 409
  hyaline globules, 401, 409
  intercalated duct, 401, 409
  low grade mucoepidermoid carcinoma, 375, 405
  lymphoepithelial cyst, 401, 409
  lymphoepithelial sialadenitis, 382, 405–406
  metastatic melanoma, 388, 406
  metastatic renal cell carcinoma, 394, 407
  metastatic rhabdomyosarcoma, 396, 407
  metastatic spindle cell melanoma, 377, 405
  minor salivary glands, 401, 409
  mucoepidermoid carcinoma, 360, 387, 403, 406
  neuroendocrine carcinoma, 358, 403
  oncocytoma, 395, 407
  palate, 401, 409
  pleomorphic adenoma (*see* Pleomorphic adenoma)
  polymorphous low grade adenocarcinoma, 364, 376, 404
  salivary duct carcinoma, 361, 402, 403, 410
  sarcomatous changes, 380, 405
  schwannoma, 384, 406
  sebaceous differentiation, 368, 404
  sialadenitis, 401, 409
  squamous cell carcinoma, 402, 410
  Warthin tumor (*see* Warthin tumor)
Sarcoidosis, 88, 102, 114
Sarcoma
  chromosomal translocations, 671
  vs. lymphoma *vs.* carcinoma, 703, 714
Scattered tumor cells, 603, 613

Schwannoma, 405, 705, 716
Seroma, groin hernia, 675, 708
Serous fluid cytopathology
  benign components, 122
  Burkitt lymphoma, 172, 186–187
  calretinin, TTF and BerEP4, 154, 184
  CD56, 142, 177, 182, 194–195
  cell block preparation, 175, 192
  collagen ball, 124, 179
  endometriosis, 161, 185
  eosinophilic pleural effusion (EPF), 187
  Ewing's sarcoma, 127, 179
  Hodgkin lymphoma, 149, 183
  hyperchromatic nucleoli and clumped chromatin, 174, 188–189
  immunostains of synaptophysin, chromogranin, CD56 and CD45, 177, 195
  lupus erythematosus (LE) cells, 125, 179
  lymphocytosis (lymphocytic effusion), 133, 180
  lymphomatous effusion, 130, 180
  malignant conditions, 123
  mesothelial cell hyperplasia, 132, 180
  mesothelioma, 128, 135, 174, 175, 179, 181, 188, 191
  metastatic adenocarcinoma of lung, 141, 163, 182, 185
  metastatic breast lobular carcinoma, 126, 179
  metastatic colonic adenocarcinoma, 145, 182
  metastatic dysgerminoma, 157, 184
  metastatic hepatocellular carcinoma, 144, 182
  metastatic melanoma, 134, 136, 165, 180–181, 185
  metastatic mucinous adenocarcinomas, 146, 155, 182–184
  metastatic papillary renal cell carcinoma, 140, 181–182
  metastatic serous carcinoma, 152, 171, 183, 186
  metastatic signet ring cell carcinoma, 139, 181
  metastatic squamous cell carcinoma, 131, 137, 147, 151, 168, 180, 181, 183, 186
  monomorphous population of lymphocytes, 174, 189
  mucinous adenocarcinomas, 146, 182–183
  NSE, synaptophysin, S100 and GFAP, 143, 182
  primary effusion lymphoma (PEL), 148, 183
  pseudomyxoma peritonei, 169, 186
  reactive mesothelial cells, 138, 150, 153, 156, 158–160, 162, 164, 167, 170, 181, 183–186
  rhabdomyosarcoma, 129, 180
  rheumatoid pleuritis, 166, 185
  shared cell borders, 174, 188
SFT. *See* Solitary fibrous tumor (SFT)
Sheets and dispersed polygonal cells, 603, 613
Signet ring cell carcinoma
  GI EUS-FNA, 558, 570
  large prominent nucleoli, 559, 571
Signet ring cells, 139, 175, 181, 190
Signet ring-like cells, 88, 101–104, 113
Small cell carcinoma
  abundant cytoplasm, 175, 191
  cell block preparation, 49, 101
  Diff-Quik preparation, 32, 98
  lung, 177, 195
  papanicolaou preparation, 37, 99
  perihilar lymph node, 338, 349–350
  plasmacytoid morphology, 319, 344
  scant cytoplasm and high N:C ratio, 85, 107
  transthoracic FNA, 90, 118
Small pyknotic nuclei, 605, 617
Soft tissue, 116, 200, 242
  caldesmon, 343
  cytomorphological pattern categories, 671
  diagnostic approach, 703, 714
  differential diagnosis, 672
  epithelioid cells predominance, 672
  FNA biopsies, 703, 714
  myxoid morphology, 672
  neoplasm, adults, 703, 714
  pleomorphic morphology, 672
  reactive changes, mesenchymal cells, 343
  spindle morphology, 672
Solid pseudopapillary neoplasm (SPN), 472
Solid pseudopapillary tumor, 514, 519
Solitary fibrous tumor (SFT), 688, 689, 694, 710–711
Spinal tap. *See* Lumbar puncture
Spindle cell(s), 92, 109, 113, 114, 116, 117
  angiomyolipoma, 568
  calcitonin, 288, 302
  cholangiocarcinoma, 453, 465–466
  FNA cytology, 562
  GIST, 456, 562
  hemangioma, 457
  HHV-8, 344
  leiomyosarcoma, 461, 568
  melanoma, 276, 299, 695, 706, 711–712, 716
  metastatic, 405
  morphology, 705, 716
  MTC, 277, 299
  neoplastic cells, 275, 298
  neuroendocrine cell features, 568
  poorly differentiated adenocarcinoma, 175, 191
  reactive lymphadenopathy, 344
  S100, HMB45 and melanin A, 176, 193–194
  tissue culture medium, 254, 293
Spindle-shaped nuclei, 704, 715
Splenic marginal zone lymphoma, 341, 352, 353
Squamous cell carcinoma, 658, 669
  bile duct brushing cytology, 529, 530, 560–561
  bronchi, 87, 110
  Diff-Quik stain, 59–61, 102–103
  large prominent nucleoli, 559, 571
  papanicolaou stain, 78, 80, 81, 83, 106, 107
  poorly differentiated, 58, 72, 73, 74, 82, 102, 105–107
  sputum specimen, 84, 107
  well-differentiated, 65, 104
Squamous cells, reactive atypia, 65, 104
Squamous intraepithelial lesion, low grade (CIN-1), 634, 662
Squamous metaplasia, 405
S100, stain positive, 687, 710
Stains negative
  glycogen, 706, 717
  synaptophysin and chromogranin, 706, 717
Strongyloidiasis, 6, 92
Synaptophysin
  aspirate, 496, 517
  eccentric nuclei, 512, 518
  and keratin, 515, 520
  and trypsin, 515, 520
Synaptophysin and chromogranin, 706, 717
Synovial sarcoma, 405, 679, 690, 705, 706, 709, 711, 716, 717
Systemic lupus erythematosus (SLE) lymphadenopathy, 341, 353

T

T-cell lymphoblastic lymphoma, 340, 351
Thick-walled blood vessels, 603, 613–614
Three-dimensional clusters of cells, 604, 616–617

Thyroid FNA
adenomatoid nodules, 255, 258, 293
anaplastic carcinoma, 278, 279, 289, 299–300, 303
AUS/FLUS, 257, 293
B-cell lymphoma, 289, 303
benign thyroid nodule, 245, 290
branchial cleft cysts, 247, 285, 290, 301
calcitonin, 288, 302
colloid nodules, 253, 254, 292–293
cysts, 246, 290
differential diagnosis, 243, 244
follicular cells, 246, 290
follicular neoplasm (*see* Follicular neoplasms (FNs))
Graves disease, 251, 291–292
Hürthle cell neoplasms, 260, 289, 294, 304
hyperthyroidism, 252, 292
insular carcinoma/PDC, 289, 303
large cell lymphoma, 280, 300
lymphocytic thyroiditis, 249, 250, 291
malignancy risk, 242
melanoma, 283, 301
metastatics, malignancy, 244
MTC, 275–277, 298, 299
necrosis, 289, 303
neutrophilic cannibalism, 289, 303
nodules, 241–243
parathyroid adenoma, 284, 301
pleomorphic cells, 289, 303
PTC (*see* Papillary thyroid carcinoma (PTC))
radioactive iodine, 252, 292
renal cell carcinoma, 281, 300–301
squamous cell carcinoma, 282, 301
subacute thyroiditis, 248, 291
T4 and TSH levels, 256, 293
trabecular tumor, 244
UC, 289, 303
visceral metastases, 289, 304
Toxoplasma meningoencephalitis, 221, 237
Toxoplasmosis, 21, 96
Transbronchial FNA biopsy, 86, 109, 112
Transbronchial needle aspiration (TBNA), 108
Transcription factor E3 *(TFE3)* gene, 604, 614–615
T(12;16)(q13;p11) reciprocal translocation, 703, 714
Tuberculosis (TB), 20, 96
Tuberculosis meningitis, 211, 233
Tumor necrosis, 654, 665–666
Tumors, elderly male patients, 603, 614
T(11;22) with EWSR1-FL1 fusion, 673, 708
Tyrosinase rystalloids, 408

U

Ultrasound-guided thoracentesis, 177, 196
Undifferentiated carcinoma (UC), 289, 303
Unsatisfactory, obscuring lubricants, 637, 662–663
Urine cytopathology. *See also* Urine specimen
bladder malignancy subtyping, 619
malignancy criteria, urothelial carcinomas, 620
testing, 619
Urine specimen
acute cystitis, 627, 661
benign, negative for malignant, 624, 660
bladder neoplasms, 658, 669
Candida albicans, 657, 668
columnar cells and urothelial cells, basal, 647, 664
corpora amylacea, 646, 664
cystitis glandularis/cystitis cystica, 651, 665
cytology images, 642, 643, 663–664
endometrial cells, 653, 665
Enterobius vermicularis, 648, 664–665
false-positive diagnosis, 658, 669
high grade urothelial carcinoma, 631, 638, 661–663
immediate cytopreparation, 657, 667–668
low grade, 622, 629, 660, 661
Melamed-Wolinska bodies, 642, 663–664
melanoma, 652, 665
metastatic colonic adenocarcinoma, 635, 662
metastatic endometrial adenocarcinoma, 655, 666
metastatic lung small cell carcinoma, 645, 664
midstream clean-catch urine, 658, 669
polyomavirus immunostain (SV40), 625, 660
polyomavirus infection, 630, 639, 661, 663
reactive urothelial cells, 621, 636, 640, 649, 660, 662, 663, 665
repeat sampling, 633, 644, 662, 664
sensitivity, 658, 669
squamous intraepithelial lesion, low grade (CIN-1), 634, 662
suspicious, malignant lymphoma, 628, 661
tumor necrosis, 654, 665–666
umbrella cells, 570, 658
unsatisfactory, non-urothelial elements, 650, 665
unsatisfactory, obscuring lubricants, 637, 662–663
urolithiasis, 641, 663
urothelial carcinoma, 623, 632, 660, 662
urothelial carcinoma in situ (CIS), 626, 660–661
UroVysion FISH Testing, 570, 659
Urolithiasis, 641, 663
Urothelial carcinoma
cell carcinoma, 418, 456–457
cytological features, 727
cytomorphologic features, high grade, 638, 663
FISH, 657, 667
FISH analysis, 727
high-grade, small cell features, 631, 661–662
high grade, squamous differentiation, 623, 655, 660, 666
high-grade tumors, 632, 662
low grade, 622, 629, 660, 661
low-grade carcinoma, 727
malignancy criteria, 620
necrosis, 657, 667
neoplasia, 727
perinuclear haloes, 657, 667
Urothelial carcinoma in situ (CIS), 626, 660–661
Urothelial cell carcinoma, 587, 604, 608, 615
Urothelial cells, cytomegalovirus (CMV), 657, 667
UroVysion FISH Testing, 570, 659

V

Ventriculoperitoneal shunts, 224, 238
Viral lymphadenopathy, 318, 344
V-Ki-ras2 Kirsten rat sarcoma viral oncogene homolog *(KRAS)*
and *EGFR,* 86, 90, 108, 117
non-smokers, 91, 119
protein on activity of EGFR tyrosine kinase, 90, 117
Voided urine, 657, 667
Von Hippel–Lindau Syndrome, 515, 520

W
Warthin–Finkeldey cells, 341, 353
Warthin tumor, 402, 410
 diagnostic, 389, 406
 lymphocytes, 356, 402, 403, 409–410
 oncocytes, 356, 403
 salivary duct system, 401, 409
 squamous etaplasia, 379, 405
 squamous metaplasia, 391, 406–407
Well-differentiated hepatocellular carcinoma (HCC), 426, 453, 458, 465
Wilm's tumor, 441, 461

X
Xp11.2 translocation
 conventional cytogenetics and FISH, 726
 immunohistochemistry, 726
 papanicolaou-stained slides, 726

FSC
www.fsc.org
MIX
Papier | Fördert
gute Waldnutzung
FSC® C083411

Kolibri 360 GmbH
Ferdinand-Jühlke-Straße 7
99095 Erfurt, Deutschland
produktsicherheit@kolibri360.de